*Goldfrank's*

# CLINICAL MANUAL OF TOXICOLOGIC EMERGENCIES

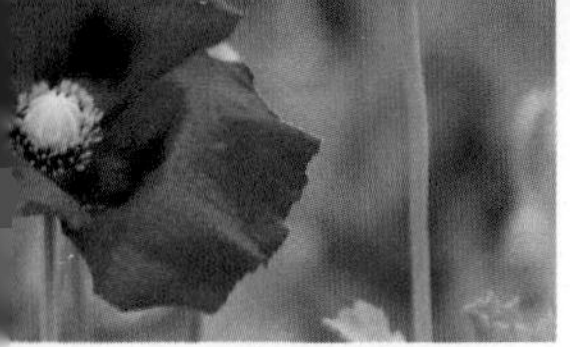

# EDITORS


**Robert S. Hoffman, MD, FAACT, FRCP Edin, FEAPCCT**
Professor of Emergency Medicine and Medicine
New York University Grossman School of Medicine
Ronald O. Perelman Department of Emergency Medicine, NYU Grossman School of Medicine
Emergency Physician
Bellevue Hospital Center and NYU Langone Health
New York, New York

**Sophie Gosselin, MD, CSPQ, FRCPC, FACMT, FAACT**
Emergency Physician and Medical Toxicologist
Consultant, Centre antipoison du Québec, Québec, Canada
Chief of Department of Emergency Medicine, Centre intégré de santé et services Sociaux de la Montérégie-Centre, Hôpital Charles Lemoyne, Greenfield Park, Québec, Canada.
Professor, Department of Family Medicine and Emergency Medicine, Faculté de Médecine et des Sciences de la Santé, Université de Sherbrooke, Sherbrooke, Québec, Canada

**Lewis S. Nelson, MD, MBA, FAACT, FACEP, FACMT, FASAM**
Professor and Chair, Department of Emergency Medicine
Professor of Pharmacology, Physiology, and Neuroscience
Rutgers New Jersey Medical School
Director, Division of Medical Toxicology and Addiction Medicine
Chief of Service, Emergency Department, University Hospital of Newark
Senior Consultant, New Jersey Poison Information & Education System
Newark, New Jersey

**Mary Ann Howland, PharmD, DABAT, FAACT**
Professor of Pharmacy
St. John's University College of Pharmacy and Health Sciences
Adjunct Professor of Emergency Medicine
New York University Grossman School of Medicine
Ronald O. Perelman Department of Emergency Medicine, NYU Grossman School of Medicine
Bellevue Hospital Center and NYU Langone Health
Senior Consultant in Residence
New York City Poison Control Center
New York, New York

**Neal A. Lewin, MD, FACEP, FACMT, FACP**
Druckenmiller Professor of Emergency Medicine and Professor of Medicine
New York University Grossman School of Medicine
Ronald O. Perelman Department of Emergency Medicine, NYU Grossman School of Medicine
Director, Didactic Education
Emergency Medicine Residency
Attending Physician, Emergency Medicine and Internal Medicine
Bellevue Hospital Center and NYU Langone Health
New York, New York

**Silas W. Smith, MD, FACEP, FACMT**
JoAnn G. and Kenneth Wellner Associate Professor of Emergency Medicine
Chief, Division of Quality, Safety, and Practice Innovation
Affiliate Faculty, Institute for Innovations in Medical Education
Emergency Physician
Ronald O. Perelman Department of Emergency Medicine, NYU Grossman School of Medicine
Bellevue Hospital Center and NYU Langone Health
New York, New York

**Lewis R. Goldfrank, MD, FAAEM, FAACT, FACEP, FACMT, FACP**
Professor of Emergency Medicine
New York University Grossman School of Medicine
Emergency Physician
Ronald O. Perelman Department of Emergency Medicine, NYU Grossman School of Medicine
Bellevue Hospital Center and NYU Langone Health
Medical Director, New York City Poison Control Center
New York, New York

*Goldfrank's*

# CLINICAL MANUAL OF TOXICOLOGIC EMERGENCIES

Second Edition

**Robert S. Hoffman, MD, FAACT, FRCP Edin, FEAPCCT**

**Sophie Gosselin MD, CSPQ, FRCPC, FACMT, FAACT**

**Lewis S. Nelson, MD, MBA, FAACT, FACEP, FACMT, FASAM**

**Mary Ann Howland, PharmD, DABAT, FAACT**

**Neal A. Lewin, MD, FACEP, FACMT, FACP**

**Silas W. Smith, MD, FACEP, FACMT**

**Lewis R. Goldfrank, MD, FAAEM, FAACT, FACEP, FACMT, FACP**

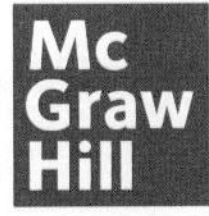


New York Chicago San Francisco Athens London Madrid Mexico City
Milan New Delhi Singapore Sydney Toronto

**Goldfrank's Clinical Manual of Toxicologic Emergencies, Second Edition**



1 2 3 4 5 6 7 8 9 LWI 28 27 26 25 24 23

ISBN 978-1-260-47499-2
MHID 1-260-47499-2

## NOTICE

Medicine is an ever-changing science. As new research and clinical experience broaden our knowledge, changes in treatment and drug therapy are required. The authors and the publisher of this work have checked with sources believed to be reliable in their efforts to provide information that is complete and generally in accord with the standards accepted at the time of publication. However, in view of the possibility of human error or changes in medical sciences, neither the authors nor the publisher nor any other party who has been involved in the preparation or publication of this work warrants that the information contained herein is in every respect accurate or complete, and they disclaim all responsibility for any errors or omissions or for the results obtained from use of the information contained in this work. Readers are encouraged to confirm the information contained herein with other sources. For example and in particular, readers are advised to check the product information sheet included in the package of each drug they plan to administer to be certain that the information contained in this work is accurate and that changes have not been made in the recommended dose or in the contraindications for administration. This recommendation is of particular importance in connection with new or infrequently used drugs.

This book was set in Kepler by KnowledgeWorks Global Ltd.
The editors were Kay Conerly, Jennifer Bernstein, and Sylvia Choi.
The production supervisor was Catherine Saggese.
Project management was provided by Revathi Viswanathan of KnowledgeWorks Global Ltd.
The designer was Mary McKeon.

This book is printed on acid-free paper.

**Library of Congress Cataloging-in-Publication Data**

Names: Hoffman, Robert S. (Robert Steven), 1959- author. | Nelson, Lewis S. 1963- Goldfrank's toxicologic emergencies.
Title: Goldfrank's Clinical manual of toxicologic emergencies / Robert S. Hoffman, Sophie Gosselin, Lewis S. Nelson, Neal A. Lewin, Mary Ann Howland, Silas W. Smith, Lewis R. Goldfrank.
Other titles: Manual of toxicologic emergencies
Description: Second edition. | New York : McGraw Hill, [2023] | Preceded by: Goldfrank's manual of toxicologic emergencies / Robert S. Hoffman ... [et al.]. c2007. | Summary: "The condensed, clinically focused companion to the world-renowned Goldfrank's Toxicologic Emergencies. The Manual portable and ideal for students, nurses, pharmacists, and physicians in the clinical practice setting. It focuses on assessment and management for immediate care of poisoned patients. Many tables and figures throughout facilitate quick referencing of critical information"—Provided by publisher.
Identifiers: LCCN 2023007491 (print) | LCCN 2023007492 (ebook) | ISBN 9781260474992 (paperback ; alk. paper) | ISBN 1260474992 (paperback ; alk. paper) | ISBN 9781260475005 (ebook)
Subjects: MESH: Emergencies | Poisoning | Poisons | Handbook
Classification: LCC RA1224.5 (print) | LCC RA1224.5 (ebook) | NLM QV 607 | DDC 615.9/08—dc23/eng/20230429
LC record available at https://lccn.loc.gov/2023007491
LC ebook record available at https://lccn.loc.gov/2023007492

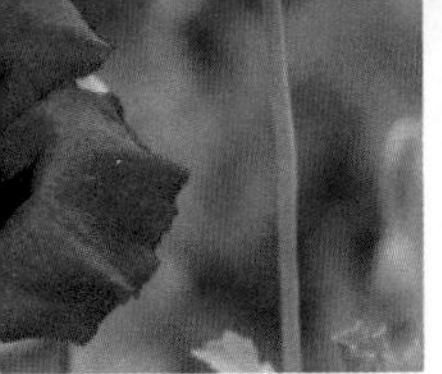

# DEDICATION

To the staffs of our hospitals, emergency departments, intensive care units, and outpatient sites, who have worked with remarkable courage, concern, compassion, and understanding in treating the patients discussed in this text and many thousands more like them.

To the Emergency Medical Services personnel who have worked so faithfully and courageously to protect our patients' health and who have assisted us in understanding what happens in the home and the field.

To the Poison Center staff, who have quietly and conscientiously integrated their skills with ours to serve these patients and prevent many patients from ever requiring a hospital visit.

To all the faculty, fellows, residents, nurses, nurse practitioners, physician assistants, and medical and pharmacy students who have studied toxicology with us, whose inquisitiveness has helped us continually strive to understand complex and evolving problems and develop methods to teach them to others. (Editors)

To my wife Ali; my children Casey and Jesse; my parents; and my friends, family, and colleagues for their never-ending patience and forgiveness for the time I have spent away from them; to the many close colleagues and committee members who have helped me understand the fundamentals of evidence-based medicine and challenged me to be clear, precise, and definitive when making treatment recommendations. (R.S.H.)

To my husband Daniel, my friends and family for understanding "me-time" spent on this book; to colleagues and students for continually asking interesting questions to help find better ways to care for our patients. (S.G.)

To my wife Laura for her unwavering support; to my children Daniel, Adina, and Benjamin for their fresh perspective, youthful insight, and appreciation of my passion; to my parents Myrna of blessed memory and Dr. Irwin Nelson for the foundation they provided; and to my family, friends, and colleagues who keep me focused on what is important in life. (L.N.)

To my husband Bob; to my children Robert, Marcy and her husband Doug, and my grandchildren Joey and Kenzie; to the loving memory of my father and mother; and to family, friends, colleagues, and students for all their help and continuing inspiration. (M.A.H.)

To my wife Gail Miller; my sons Jesse Miller Lewin, MD, and Justin Miller Lewin, MD, and my daughters-in-law Alana Amarosa Lewin, MD, and Alice Tang, MD; my granddaughter Isabelle Rose Lewin; my grandsons Charles Andrew Lewin and Parker Tang Lewin, and in memory of my parents. To all my patients, students, residents, fellows, and colleagues who constantly stimulate my being a perpetual student. (N.L.)

To my wife Helen, for her resolute support, understanding, and patience; to my children Addison and Alston, for their boundless enthusiasm, inquisitiveness, and spirit; and to my parents. (S.W.S.)

To my children Rebecca and Ryan, Jennifer, Andrew and Joan, Michelle (deceased) and James; to my grandchildren Benjamin, Adam, Sarah, Kay, Samantha, Herbert, Jonah, Susie, and Sasha, who have kept me acutely aware of the ready availability of possible poisons; and to my wife, partner, and best friend Susan (deceased) whose support was essential to help me in the development of the first ten editions and whose contributions continue to inspire me and will be found throughout the text. (L.G.)

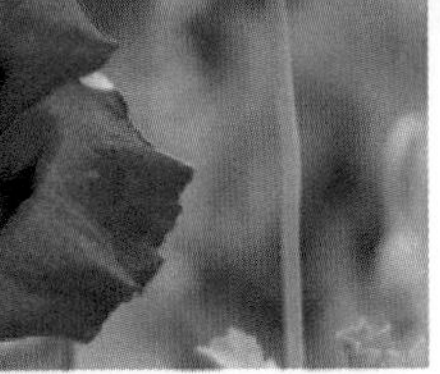

# CONTENTS

## M. OCCUPATIONAL AND ENVIRONMENTAL TOXINS

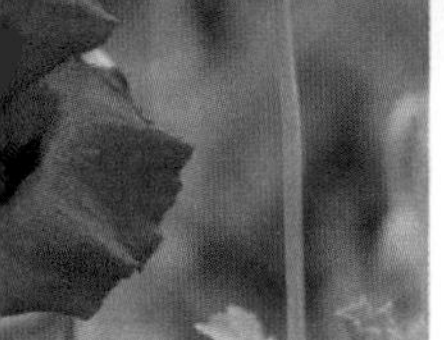

# CONTRIBUTORS
## to GOLDFRANK'S TOXICOLOGIC EMERGENCIES, 11TH EDITION from which this Manual is derived


**Theodore C. Bania, MD, MS**
Assistant Professor of Emergency Medicine
Director of Research and Toxicology
Mt. Sinai West and Mt. Sinai St. Luke's Hospitals
Department of Emergency Medicine
Associate Dean for Human Subject Research
Associate Director Program for the Protection of Human Subjects
Icahn School of Medicine at Mount Sinai
New York, New York
*Antidotes in Brief: A23, Lipid Emulsion*

**Fermin Barrueto Jr., MD, MBA, FACEP**
Volunteer Associate Professor of Emergency Medicine
University of Maryland School of Medicine
Baltimore, Maryland
Senior Vice President
Chief Medical Officer
University of Maryland Upper Chesapeake Health
Bel Air, Maryland
*Chapter 86, Sodium Monofluoroacetate and Fluoroacetamide*

**James David Barry, MD**
Clinical Professor of Emergency Medicine
University of California, Irvine School of Medicine
Irvine, California
Associate Director, Emergency Department
Long Beach VA Medical Center
Long Beach, California
*Chapter 28, Antimalarials*

**Michael C. Beuhler, MD**
Professor of Emergency Medicine
Carolinas HealthCare System
Medical Director, Carolinas Poison Center
Charlotte, North Carolina
*Chapter 85, Phosphorus*

**Steven B. Bird, MD**
Professor of Emergency Medicine
University of Massachusetts Medical School
UMass Memorial Medical Center
Worcester, Massachusetts
*Chapter 63, Chromium*

**Eike Blohm, MD**
Assistant Professor of Surgery
Division of Emergency Medicine
Toxicology Consultant Northern New England Poison Center
University of Vermont Larner College of Medicine
University of Vermont Medical Center
Burlington, Vermont
*Chapter 89, Marine Envenomations*

**Keith J. Boesen, PharmD, FAZPA**
Instructor, University of Arizona College of Pharmacy
Director, Arizona Poison and Drug Information Center
Tucson, Arizona
*Special Considerations: SC9, Exotic Nonnative Snake Envenomations*

**Kelly A. Green Boesen, PharmD**
Clinical Pharmacist
Tucson, Arizona
*Special Considerations: SC9, Exotic Nonnative Snake Envenomations*

**George M. Bosse, MD**
Professor of Emergency Medicine
University of Louisville School of Medicine
Medical Director, Kentucky Poison Center
Louisville, Kentucky
*Chapter 20, Antidiabetics and Hypoglycemics/Antiglycemics*

**Nicole C. Bouchard, MD, FACMT, FRCPC**
Assistant Clinical Professor of Emergency Medicine
Donald and Barbara Zucker School of Medicine at Hofstra/Northwell
Emergency Physician
Lenox Health in Greenwich Village, Northwell Health
New York, New York
*Chapter 26, Thyroid and Antithyroid Medications*

**Jeffrey R. Brubacher, MD, MSc, FRCPC**
Associate Professor of Emergency Medicine
University of British Columbia
Emergency Physician
Vancouver General Hospital
Vancouver, British Columbia, Canada
*Chapter 32, β-Adrenergic Antagonists*

**D. Eric Brush, MD, MHCM**
Clinical Associate Professor of Emergency Medicine
University of Massachusetts Medical School
Division of Toxicology
Director of Clinical Operations
UMass Memorial Medical Center
Worcester, Massachusetts
*Chapter 89, Marine Envenomations*

**Michele M. Burns, MD, MPH**
Assistant Professor of Pediatrics and Emergency Medicine
Harvard Medical School
Director, Medical Toxicology Fellowship
Medical Director, Regional Center for Poison Control and Prevention
Attending Physician, Pediatric Emergency Medicine
Boston Children's Hospital
Boston, Massachusetts
*Chapter 71, Silver*

**Diane P. Calello, MD**
Associate Professor of Emergency Medicine
Rutgers New Jersey Medical School
Executive and Medical Director
New Jersey Poison Information and Education System
Newark, New Jersey
*Chapter 66, Lead*
*Chapter 70, Selenium*

**Jennifer L. Carey, MD**
Assistant Professor of Emergency Medicine
Division of Medical Toxicology
University of Massachusetts Medical School
UMass Memorial Medical Center
Worcester, Massachusetts
*Chapter 52, Hallucinogens*

**Gar Ming Chan, MD, FACEM**
Emergency Medicine Specialist
Calvary Health Care, Lenah Valley
Tasmania, Australia
*Chapter 64, Cobalt*

**Yiu-Cheung Chan, MD, MBBS, FRCS (Ed), FHKCEM, FHKAM**
Consultant, Accident and Emergency Department,
United Christian Hospital
Hong Kong Poison Information Centre
Hong Kong SAR, China
*Chapter 87, Strychnine*

**Nathan P. Charlton, MD**
Associate Professor of Emergency Medicine
Program Director, Medical Toxicology
University of Virginia School of Medicine
Charlottesville, Virginia
*Chapter 93, Smoke Inhalation*

**Betty C. Chen, MD**
Assistant Professor of Emergency Medicine
University of Washington School of Medicine
Harborview Medical Center
Toxicology Consultant, Washington Poison Center
Seattle, Washington
*Chapter 31, Antithrombotics*
*Antidotes in Brief: A17, Prothrombin Complex Concentrates and Direct Oral Anticoagulant Antidotes*

**Jason Chu, MD**
Associate Professor of Emergency Medicine
Icahn School of Medicine at Mount Sinai
Emergency Physician and Medical Toxicologist
Mt. Sinai West and Mt. Sinai St. Luke's Hospitals
New York, New York
*Chapter 25, Antimigraine Medications*

**Richard F. Clark, MD**
Professor of Emergency Medicine
Director, Division of Medical Toxicology
University of California, San Diego
San Diego, California
*Antidotes in Brief: A37, Antivenom: Spider*
*Antidotes in Brief: A38, Antivenom: Scorpion*

**John A. Curtis, MD**
Emergency Physician
Cheshire Medical Center-Dartmouth Hitchcock Keene
Keene, New Hampshire
*Chapter 69, Nickel*

**Michael A. Darracq, MD, MPH**
Associate Professor of Clinical Emergency Medicine
University of California, San Francisco (UCSF)-Fresno
Medical Education Program
Department of Emergency Medicine
Division of Medical Toxicology
Fresno, California
*Antidotes in Brief: A37, Antivenom: Spider*
*Antidotes in Brief: A38, Antivenom: Scorpion*

**Andrew H. Dawson, MBBS, FRACP, FRCP, FCCP**
Clinical Professor of Medicine, University of Sydney
Clinical Director, NSW Poisons Information Centre
Director, Clinical Toxicology
Royal Prince Alfred Hospital
Sydney, Australia
*Chapter 80, Barium*

**Francis Jerome DeRoos, MD**
Associate Professor of Emergency Medicine
Perelman School of Medicine at the University of Pennsylvania
Hospital of the University of Pennsylvania
Philadelphia, Pennsylvania
*Chapter 34, Miscellaneous Antihypertensives and Pharmacologically Related Agents*

**Suzanne Doyon, MD, MPH, ACEP, FACMT, FASAM**
Assistant Professor of Emergency Medicine
Medical Director, Connecticut Poison Control Center
University of Connecticut School of Medicine
Farmington, Connecticut
*Chapter 21, Antiepileptics*

**Michael Eddleston, BM, ScD**
Professor of Clinical Toxicology
University of Edinburgh
Consultant Clinical Toxicologist
Royal Infirmary of Edinburgh and National Poisons Information Service, Edinburgh
Edinburgh, United Kingdom
*Chapter 83, Insecticides: Organic Phosphorus Compounds and Carbamates*

**Brenna M. Farmer, MD**
Assistant Professor of Clinical Medicine
Weill Cornell Medical College of Cornell University
Emergency Physician
Assistant Program Director of Emergency Medicine
New York-Presbyterian Hospital
Director of Patient Safety
Weill Cornell Emergency Department
New York, New York
*Chapter 53, γ-Hydroxybutyric Acid (γ-Hydroxybutyrate)*
*Chapter 57, Aluminum*

**Brandy Ferguson, MD**
Assistant Professor of Emergency Medicine
New York University School of Medicine
Emergency Physician
Ronald O. Perelman Department of Emergency Medicine
Bellevue Hospital Center and NYU Langone Health
New York, New York
*Chapter 101, Hazardous Materials Incident Response*

**Denise Fernández, MD**
Assistant Professor of Emergency Medicine
Albert Einstein College of Medicine
Medical Toxicologist
Emergency Physician
Jacobi Medical Center/North Central Bronx Hospital
Bronx, New York
*Chapter 55, Nicotine*

**Laura J. Fil, DO, MS**
Adjunct Professor
Department of Primary Care
Touro College of Osteopathic Medicine
Middletown, New York
Emergency Physician
Department of Emergency Medicine
Vassar Brothers Medical Center
Poughkeepsie, New York
*Chapter 12, Food Poisoning*

**Lindsay M. Fox, MD**
Assistant Professor of Emergency Medicine
Rutgers New Jersey Medical School
University Hospital
Toxicology Consultant, New Jersey Poison Information and Education System
Newark, New Jersey
*Chapter 16, Plant- and Animal-Derived Dietary Supplements*

**Jessica A. Fulton, DO**
Emergency Physician
Grandview Hospital
Sellersville, Pennsylvania
*Chapter 76, Caustics*

**Howard L. Geyer, MD, PhD**
Assistant Professor of Neurology
Director, Division of Movement Disorders
Montefiore Medical Center
Albert Einstein College of Medicine
Bronx, New York
*Chapter 11, Botulism*
*Antidotes in Brief: A6, Botulinum Antitoxin*

**Marc Ghannoum, MD, MSc**
Associate Professor of Medicine
University of Montreal
Nephrology and Internal Medicine
Verdun Hospital
Montreal, Québec, Canada
*Chapter 4, Principles and Techniques Applied to Enhance Elimination*

**Beth Y. Ginsburg, MD**
Assistant Professor of Emergency Medicine
Icahn School of Medicine at Mount Sinai
New York, New York
Emergency Physician
Elmhurst Hospital Center
Elmhurst, New York
*Chapter 17, Vitamins*

**Jeffrey A. Gold, MD**
Professor of Medicine
Chief, Division of Pulmonary and Critical Care (Interim)
Associate Director, Adult Cystic Fibrosis Center
Oregon Health and Science University
Portland, Oregon
*Chapter 50, Alcohol Withdrawal*

**David S. Goldfarb, MD, FASN**
Professor of Medicine and Physiology
New York University School of Medicine
Clinical Chief, Nephrology Division
NYU Langone Health
Chief, Nephrology Section
New York Harbor VA Healthcare System
Consultant, New York City Poison Control Center
New York, New York
*Chapter 4, Principles and Techniques Applied to Enhance Elimination*

**Lewis R. Goldfrank, MD, FAAEM, FAACT, FACEP, FACMT, FACP**
Professor of Emergency Medicine
New York University Grossman School of Medicine
Emergency Physician
Ronald O. Perelman Department of Emergency Medicine, NYU Grossman School of Medicine
Bellevue Hospital Center and NYU Langone Health
Medical Director, New York City Poison Control Center
New York, New York
*Chapter 1, Initial Evaluation of the Patient: Vital Signs and Toxic Syndromes*
*Chapter 2, Principles of Managing the Acutely Poisoned or Overdosed Patient*
*Chapter 90, Mushrooms*
*Chapter 91, Plants*

**Sophie Gosselin, MD, CSPQ, FRCPC, FACMT, FAACT**
Emergency Physician and Medical Toxicologist
Consultant, Centre antipoison du Québec, Québec, Canada
Chief of Department of Emergency Medicine, Centre intégré de santé et services Sociaux de la Montérégie-Centre, Hôpital Charles Lemoyne, Greenfield Park, Québec, Canada.
Professor, Department of Family Medicine and Emergency Medicine, Faculté de Médecine et des Sciences de la Santé, Université de Sherbrooke, Sherbrooke, Québec, Canada
*Chapter 22, Antihistamines and Decongestants*
*Antidotes in Brief: A23, Lipid Emulsion*

**Howard A. Greller, MD, FACEP, FACMT**
Department of Clinical Medicine, Affiliated Medical Professor
City University of New York School of Medicine
Director of Research and Medical Toxicology
SBH Health System Department of Emergency Medicine
St. Barnabas Hospital
Bronx, New York
*Chapter 43, Lithium*

**Hallam Melville Gugelmann, MD, MPH**
Assistant Clinical Professor
Division of Clinical Pharmacology and Medical Toxicology, Department of Medicine, University of California, San Francisco
Emergency Physician, CPMC St. Luke's Hospital Emergency Department
Assistant Medical Director, California Poison Control System-San Francisco Division
San Francisco, California
*Chapter 34, Miscellaneous Antihypertensives and Pharmacologically Related Agents*

**David D. Gummin, MD, FAACT, FACEP, FACMT**
Professor of Emergency Medicine, Pediatrics, Pharmacology and Toxicology
Section Chief, Medical Toxicology
Medical College of Wisconsin
Medical Director, Wisconsin Poison Center
Milwaukee, Wisconsin
*Chapter 78, Hydrocarbons*

**Caitlin J. Guo, MD, MBA**
Assistant Professor of Anesthesiology, Perioperative Care and Pain Medicine
New York University School of Medicine
Attending Physician
Bellevue Hospital Center and NYU Langone Health
New York, New York
*Chapter 38, Inhalational Anesthetics*
*Chapter 39, Neuromuscular Blockers*
*Antidotes in Brief: A24, Dantrolene Sodium*

**Amit K. Gupta, MD**
Assistant Professor of Emergency Medicine
Seton Hall Medical School
Assistant Residency Director, Department of Emergency Medicine
Hackensack University Medical Center
Hackensack, New Jersey
*Chapter 51, Disulfiram and Disulfiramlike Reactions*

**Jason B. Hack, MD**
Professor of Emergency Medicine
Program Director, Division of Medical Toxicology
The Warren Alpert Medical School of Brown University
Rhode Island Hospital
Providence, Rhode Island
*Chapter 35, Cardioactive Steroids*

**In-Hei Hahn, MD, FACEP, FACMT**
Expedition Medical Officer
Research Associate
Division of Paleontology
American Museum of Natural History
New York, New York
*Chapter 88, Arthropods*

**Stephen A. Harding, MD**
Assistant Professor of Emergency Medicine
Henry J. N. Taub Department of Emergency Medicine
Baylor College of Medicine
Houston, Texas
*Chapter 57, Aluminum*

**Rachel Haroz, MD**
Assistant Professor of Emergency Medicine
Cooper University Health Care
Camden, New Jersey
*Chapter 53, $\gamma$-Hydroxybutyric Acid ($\gamma$-Hydroxybutyrate)*

**Ashley Haynes, MD, FACEP**
Assistant Professor of Emergency Medicine
Division of Toxicology
University of Texas Southwestern Medical School
Attending Physician
Parkland Hospital
Clements University Hospital
Children's Medical Center
Dallas, Texas
*Chapter 74, Antiseptics, Disinfectants, and Sterilants*
*Antidotes in Brief: A5, Sodium Bicarbonate*

**Robert G. Hendrickson, MD, FACMT, FAACT**
Professor of Emergency Medicine
Program Director, Fellowship in Medical Toxicology
Associate Medical Director, Oregon Poison Center
Oregon Health and Science University
Portland, Oregon
*Chapter 6, Acetaminophen*
*Antidotes in Brief: A3, N-Acetylcysteine*

**Fred M. Henretig, MD, FAAP, FACMT**
Professor Emeritus of Pediatrics
Perelman School of Medicine, University of Pennsylvania
Senior Toxicologist, The Poison Control Center at the Children's Hospital of Philadelphia
Philadelphia, Pennsylvania
*Chapter 66, Lead*

**Christina H. Hernon, MD**
Lecturer in Emergency Medicine
Harvard Medical School
Department of Emergency Medicine
Division of Medical Toxicology
Cambridge Health Alliance
Cambridge, Massachusetts
*Chapter 29, Antituberculous Medications*

**Elizabeth Quaal Hines, MD**
Clinical Assistant Professor of Pediatrics
Division of Pediatric Emergency Medicine
University of Maryland School of Medicine
Toxicology Consultant, Maryland Poison Center
Baltimore, Maryland
*Chapter 67, Manganese*

**Lotte C. G. Hoegberg, MS (Pharm), PhD, FEAPCCT**
Pharmacist, Medical Toxicologist
The Danish Poisons Information Centre
Department of Anesthesia and Intensive Care
Copenhagen University Hospital Bispebjerg
Copenhagen, Denmark
*Chapter 3, Techniques Used to Prevent Gastrointestinal Absorption*

**Robert J. Hoffman, MD, MS, FACMT, FACEP**
Medical Director, Qatar Poison Center
Sidra Medicine
Doha, Qatar
*Chapter 36, Methylxanthines and Selective α-Adrenergic Agonists*

**Robert S. Hoffman, MD, FAACT, FRCP Edin, FEAPCCT**
Professor of Emergency Medicine and Medicine
New York University Grossman School of Medicine
Ronald O. Perelman Department of Emergency Medicine, NYU Grossman School of Medicine
Emergency Physician
Bellevue Hospital Center and NYU Langone Health
New York, New York
*Chapter 1, Initial Evaluation of the Patient: Vital Signs and Toxic Syndromes*
*Chapter 2, Principles of Managing the Acutely Poisoned or Overdosed Patient*
*Chapter 48, Cocaine*
*Chapter 61, Cadmium*
*Chapter 72, Thallium*
*Antidotes in Brief: A26, Benzodiazepines*
*Antidotes in Brief: A27, Thiamine Hydrochloride*
*Antidotes in Brief: A31, Prussian Blue*

**Michael G. Holland, MD, FEAPCCT, FAACT, FACMT, FACOEM, FACEP**
Clinical Professor of Emergency Medicine
SUNY Upstate Medical University
Syracuse, New York
Medical Toxicologist, Upstate New York Poison Center
Syracuse, New York
Director of Occupational Medicine, Glens Falls Hospital Center for Occupational Health
Glens Falls, New York
Senior Medical Toxicologist, Center for Toxicology and Environmental Health
North Little Rock, Arkansas
*Chapter 84, Insecticides: Organic Chlorines, Pyrethrins/Pyrethroids and Insect Repellents*

**Christopher P. Holstege, MD**
Professor of Emergency Medicine and Pediatrics
Chief, Division of Medical Toxicology
University of Virginia School of Medicine
Medical Director, Blue Ridge Poison Center
University of Virginia Health System
Charlottesville, Virginia
*Chapter 96, Cyanide and Hydrogen Sulfide*

**William J. Holubek, MD, MPH, CPE, FACEP, FACMT**
Vice President of Medical Affairs
WellStar Atlanta Medical Center
Atlanta, Georgia
*Chapter 8, Nonsteroidal Antiinflammatory Drugs*

**Fiona Garlich Horner, MD**
Clinical Assistant Professor of Emergency Medicine
Keck School of Medicine of the University of Southern California
Los Angeles, California
*Antidotes in Brief: A26, Benzodiazepines*

**Mary Ann Howland, PharmD, DABAT, FAACT**
Professor of Pharmacy
St. John's University College of Pharmacy and Health Sciences
Adjunct Professor of Emergency Medicine
New York University Grossman School of Medicine
Ronald O. Perelman Department of Emergency Medicine, NYU Grossman School of Medicine
Bellevue Hospital Center and NYU Langone Health
Senior Consultant in Residence
New York City Poison Control Center
New York, New York
*Chapter 1, Initial Evaluation of the Patient: Vital Signs and Toxic Syndromes*
*Chapter 2, Principles of Managing the Acutely Poisoned or Overdosed Patient*
*Antidotes in Brief: A1, Activated Charcoal*
*Antidotes in Brief: A2, Whole-Bowel Irrigation and Other Intestinal Evacuants*
*Antidotes in Brief: A3, N-Acetylcysteine*
*Antidotes in Brief: A4, Opioid Antagonists*
*Antidotes in Brief: A7, Deferoxamine*
*Antidotes in Brief: A9, Octreotide*
*Antidotes in Brief: A10, L-Carnitine*
*Antidotes in Brief: A11, Physostigmine Salicylate*
*Antidotes in Brief: A12, Folates: Leucovorin (Folinic Acid) and Folic Acid*
*Antidotes in Brief: A15, Pyridoxine*
*Antidotes in Brief: A18, Vitamin* $K_1$
*Antidotes in Brief: A19, Protamine*
*Antidotes in Brief: A20, Glucagon*
*Antidotes in Brief: A22, Digoxin-Specific Antibody Fragments*
*Antidotes in Brief: A25, Flumazenil*
*Antidotes in Brief: A26, Benzodiazepines*
*Antidotes in Brief: A28, Dimercaprol (British Anti-Lewisite or BAL)*
*Antidotes in Brief: A29, Succimer (2,3-dimercaptosuccinic acid) and DMPS (2,3-dimercapto-1-propanesulfonic acid)*
*Antidotes in Brief: A30, Edetate Calcium Disodium* ($CaNa_2EDTA$)
*Antidotes in Brief: A32, Calcium*
*Antidotes in Brief: A33, Fomepizole*
*Antidotes in Brief: A34, Ethanol*
*Antidotes in Brief: A35, Atropine*
*Antidotes in Brief: A36, Pralidoxime*
*Antidotes in Brief: A41, Hydroxocobalamin*
*Antidotes in Brief: A42, Nitrites (Amyl and Sodium) and Sodium Thiosulfate*
*Antidotes in Brief: A43, Methylene Blue*

**Nicholas B. Hurst, MD, MS, FAAEM**
Assistant Professor of Emergency Medicine
Medical Toxicology Consultant
Arizona Poison and Drug Information Center
University of Arizona College of Medicine-Tucson
Tucson, Arizona
*Special Considerations: SC9, Exotic Nonnative Snake Envenomations*

**David H. Jang, MD, MSc, FACMT**
Assistant Professor of Emergency Medicine
Divisions of Medical Toxicology and Critical Care Medicine (ResCCU)
Perelman School of Medicine, University of Pennsylvania
Philadelphia, Pennsylvania
*Chapter 33, Calcium Channel Blockers*
*Chapter 46, Amphetamines*

**David N. Juurlink, MD, PhD, FRCPC, FAACT, FACMT**
Professor of Medicine, Pediatrics and Health Policy, Management and Evaluation
Director, Division of Clinical Pharmacology and Toxicology
University of Toronto
Senior Scientist, Institute for Clinical Evaluative Sciences
Medical Toxicologist, Ontario Poison Centre
Toronto, Ontario, Canada
*Chapter 40, Antipsychotics*

**Bradley J. Kaufman, MD, MPH, FACEP, FAEMS**
Associate Professor of Emergency Medicine
Donald and Barbara Zucker School of Medicine at Hofstra/Northwell
Hempstead, New York
Emergency Physician
Long Island Jewish Medical Center
New Hyde Park, New York
First Deputy Medical Director
Fire Department of the City of New York
New York, New York
*Chapter 101, Hazardous Materials Incident Response*

**Brian S. Kaufman, MD**
Professor of Medicine, Anesthesiology, Neurology and Neurosurgery
New York University School of Medicine
NYU Langone Health
New York, New York
*Chapter 38, Inhalational Anesthetics*

**William Kerns II, MD, FACEP, FACMT**
Professor of Emergency Medicine and Medical Toxicology
Division of Medical Toxicology
Department of Emergency Medicine
Carolinas Medical Center
Charlotte, North Carolina
*Antidotes in Brief: A21, High-Dose Insulin*

**Hong K. Kim, MD, MPH**
Assistant Professor of Emergency Medicine
University of Maryland School of Medicine
Baltimore, Maryland
*Chapter 75, Camphor and Moth Repellents*

**Mark A. Kirk, MD**
Associate Professor of Emergency Medicine
University of Virginia
Charlottesville, Virginia
Director, Chemical Defense
Countering Weapons of Mass Destruction
Department of Homeland Security
Washington, District of Columbia
*Chapter 93, Smoke Inhalation*
*Chapter 96, Cyanide and Hydrogen Sulfide*

**Cathy A. Kondas, MD, MBS**
Assistant Professor of Psychiatry
New York University School of Medicine
Attending Psychiatrist
Director, Women's Mental Health Fellowship
Associate Director, Consultation-Liaison Psychiatry
Bellevue Hospital Center
New York, New York
*Special Considerations: SC3, Patient Violence*

**Andrea Martinez Kondracke, MD**
Assistant Professor of Psychiatry and Internal Medicine
New York University School of Medicine
Division Chief, Department of Medical Psychiatry and Consultation Liaison Psychiatry
Bellevue Hospital Center
New York, New York
*Special Considerations: SC3, Patient Violence*

**Jeffrey T. Lai, MD**
Assistant Professor of Emergency Medicine
Department of Emergency Medicine
University of Massachusetts Medical School
UMass Memorial Medical Center
Worcester, Massachusetts
*Chapter 29, Antituberculous Medications*

**Melisa W. Lai-Becker, MD, FACEP, FAAEM**
Instructor in Emergency Medicine
Harvard Medical School
Chief, CHA Everett Hospital Emergency Department
Director, CHA Division of Medical Toxicology
Cambridge Health Alliance
Boston, Massachusetts
*Chapter 71, Silver*

**Jeff M. Lapoint, DO**
Director, Division of Medical Toxicology
Department of Emergency Medicine
Southern California Permanente Group
San Diego, California
*Chapter 47, Cannabinoids*

**David C. Lee, MD**
Professor of Emergency Medicine
Donald and Barbara Zucker School of Medicine at Hofstra/Northwell
Hempstead, New York
Chair, Department of Emergency Medicine
WellSpan York Hospital
York, Pennsylvania
*Chapter 45, Sedative-Hypnotics*

**Joshua D. Lee, MD**
Associate Professor of Population Health
New York University School of Medicine
New York, New York
*Special Considerations: SC5, Prevention, Treatment, and Harm Reduction Approaches to Opioid Overdoses*

**Justin M. Lewin, MD**
Assistant Professor of Psychiatry
New York University School of Medicine
Comprehensive Psychiatric Emergency Program
Consultation-Liaison Psychiatry
Bellevue Hospital Center
New York, New York
*Special Considerations: SC3, Patient Violence*

**Neal A. Lewin, MD, FACEP, FACMT, FACP**
Druckenmiller Professor of Emergency Medicine and Professor of Medicine
New York University Grossman School of Medicine
Ronald O. Perelman Department of Emergency Medicine, NYU Grossman School of Medicine
Director, Didactic Education
Emergency Medicine Residency
Attending Physician, Emergency Medicine and Internal Medicine
Bellevue Hospital Center and NYU Langone Health
New York, New York
*Chapter 1, Initial Evaluation of the Patient: Vital Signs and Toxic Syndromes*
*Chapter 2, Principles of Managing the Acutely Poisoned or Overdosed Patient*

**Erica L. Liebelt, MD, FACMT**
Clinical Professor of Pediatrics and Emergency Medicine
University of Washington School of Medicine
Medical/Executive Director
Washington Poison Center
Seattle, Washington
*Chapter 41, Cyclic Antidepressants*

**Zhanna Livshits, MD**
Assistant Professor of Medicine
Weill Cornell Medical College of Cornell University
Emergency Physician and Medical Toxicologist
New York Presbyterian Weill Cornell Medical Center
New York, New York
*Chapter 62, Cesium*

**Heather Long, MD**
Associate Professor of Emergency Medicine
Director, Medical Toxicology
Albany Medical Center
Albany, New York
*Chapter 54, Inhalants*

**Scott Lucyk, MD, FRCPC**
Clinical Assistant Professor of Emergency Medicine
Medical Toxicologist
Associate Medical Director, Poison and Drug Information Service (PADIS)
Program Director, Clinical Pharmacology and Toxicology
Alberta Health Services
Calgary, Alberta, Canada
*Special Considerations: SC1, Decontamination Principles: Prevention of Dermal, Ophthalmic and Inhalational Absorption*

**Daniel M. Lugassy, MD**
Assistant Professor of Emergency Medicine
Medical Director, New York Simulation Center for the Health Sciences (NYSIM)
New York University School of Medicine
Division of Medical Toxicology
Ronald O. Perelman Department of Emergency Medicine
Emergency Physician, Bellevue Hospital Center and NYU Langone Health
Toxicology Consultant
New York City Poison Control Center
New York, New York
*Chapter 10, Salicylates*

**Nima Majlesi, DO**
Assistant Professor of Emergency Medicine
Donald and Barbara Zucker School of Medicine at Hofstra/Northwell
Director of Medical Toxicology
Staten Island University Hospital
Staten Island, New York
*Chapter 73, Zinc*

**Alex F. Manini, MD, MS, FACMT, FAACT**
Professor of Emergency Medicine
Division of Medical Toxicology
Icahn School of Medicine at Mount Sinai
Elmhurst Hospital Center
New York, New York
*Chapter 44, Monoamine Oxidase Inhibitors*

**Jeanna M. Marraffa, PharmD, DABAT, FAACT**
Associate Professor of Emergency Medicine
Clinical Toxicologist
Assistant Clinical Director, Upstate New York Poison Center
Upstate Medical University
Syracuse, New York
*Chapter 13, Dieting Xenobiotics and Regimens*

**Maryann Mazer-Amirshahi, PharmD, MD, MPH**
Associate Professor of Emergency Medicine
Georgetown University School of Medicine
Emergency Physician,
Department of Emergency Medicine
MedStar Washington Hospital Center
Washington, District of Columbia
*Chapter 30, Antidysrhythmics*

**Nathanael J. McKeown, DO, FACMT**
Assistant Professor of Emergency Medicine
Oregon Health & Science University
Medical Toxicologist
Oregon Poison Center
Chief, Emergency Medicine Service
VA Portland Health Care System
Portland, Oregon
*Chapter 6, Acetaminophen*

**Maria Mercurio-Zappala, RPh, MS**
Assistant Professor of Emergency Medicine
New York University School of Medicine
Ronald O. Perelman Department of Emergency Medicine
Associate Director
New York City Poison Control Center
New York, New York
*Chapter 72, Thallium*

**Stephen W. Munday, MD, MPH, MS**
Chair, Department of Occupational Medicine and Chief Medical Toxicologist
Sharp Rees-Stealy Medical Group
San Diego, California
*Chapter 59, Arsenic*

**Mark J. Neavyn, MD**
Assistant Professor of Emergency Medicine
Program Director, Fellowship in Medical Toxicology
University of Massachusetts Medical School
UMass Memorial Medical Center
Worcester, Massachusetts
*Chapter 52, Hallucinogens*

**Lewis S. Nelson, MD, MBA, FAACT, FACEP, FACMT, FASAM**
Professor and Chair, Department of Emergency Medicine
Professor of Pharmacology, Physiology, and Neuroscience
Rutgers New Jersey Medical School
Director, Division of Medical Toxicology and Addiction Medicine
Chief of Service, Emergency Department, University Hospital of Newark
Senior Consultant, New Jersey Poison Information & Education System
Newark, New Jersey
*Chapter 1, Initial Evaluation of the Patient: Vital Signs and Toxic Syndromes*
*Chapter 2, Principles of Managing the Acutely Poisoned or Overdosed Patient*
*Chapter 9, Opioids*
*Chapter 30, Antidysrhythmics*
*Chapter 50, Alcohol Withdrawal*
*Chapter 65, Copper*
*Chapter 91, Plants*
*Chapter 94, Simple Asphyxiants and Pulmonary Irritants*
*Antidotes in Brief: A4, Opioid Antagonists*
*Antidotes in Brief: A26, Benzodiazepines*
*Special Considerations: SC2, Transdermal Toxicology*

**Vincent Nguyen, MD**
Assistant Professor of Emergency Medicine
Medical Toxicologist
Albert Einstein College of Medicine
Jacobi Medical Center/North Central Bronx Medical Center
The Bronx, New York
*Antidotes in Brief: A8, Dextrose (D-Glucose)*

**Sean Patrick Nordt, MD, PharmD, DABAT, FAACT, FAAEM, FACMT**
Associate Dean, Academic Affairs
Gavin Herbert Endowed Professor of Pharmacy
Chief Medical Officer
Chapman University School of Pharmacy
Crean College of Health and Behavioral Sciences
Chapman University
Adjunct Associate Professor of Emergency Medicine
Department of Emergency Medicine
University of California, Irvine
Irvine, California
*Chapter 19, Pharmaceutical Additives*

**Ruben E. Olmedo, MD**
Associate Clinical Professor of Emergency Medicine
Icahn School of Medicine at Mount Sinai
Director, Division of Toxicology
Mount Sinai Hospital
New York, New York
*Chapter 56, Phencyclidine and Ketamine*

**Dean Olsen, DO**
Assistant Professor of Emergency Medicine and Toxicology
NYIT College of Osteopathic Medicine
Old Westbury, New York
Director, Residency in Emergency Medicine
Nassau University Medical Center
East Meadow, New York
*Chapter 9, Opioids*

**Robert B. Palmer, PhD, DABAT, FAACT**
Assistant Clinical Professor of Emergency Medicine (Medical Toxicology)
University of Colorado School of Medicine
Attending Toxicologist
Medical Toxicology Fellowship Program
Rocky Mountain Poison and Drug Center
Denver, Colorado
*Special Considerations: SC10, Assessment of Ethanol-Induced Impairment*

**Jeanmarie Perrone, MD, FACMT**
Professor of Emergency Medicine
Director of Medical Toxicology
Perelman School of Medicine, University of Pennsylvania
Philadelphia, Pennsylvania
*Chapter 18, Iron*

**Anthony F. Pizon, MD**
Associate Professor of Emergency Medicine
University of Pittsburgh School of Medicine
Chief, Division of Medical Toxicology
University of Pittsburgh Medical Center
Pittsburgh, Pennsylvania
*Chapter 92, Native (US) Venomous Snakes and Lizards"*
*Antidotes in Brief: A39, Antivenom for North American Venomous Snakes (Crotaline and Elapid)*

**Dennis P. Price, MD**
Assistant Professor of Emergency Medicine
New York University School of Medicine
Emergency Physician
Ronald O. Perelman Department of Emergency Medicine
Bellevue Hospital Center and NYU Langone Health
New York, New York
*Chapter 97, Methemoglobin Inducers*

**Jane M. Prosser, MD**
Medical Toxicologist
Emergency Physician
Department of Emergency Medicine
Kaiser Permanente Northern California
Kaiser Permanente
Vallejo, California
*Special Considerations: SC4, Internal Concealment of Xenobiotics*

**Rama B. Rao, MD, FACMT**
Associate Professor of Medicine
Weill Cornell Medical College of Cornell University
Chief, Division of Medical Toxicology
Emergency Physician
New York-Presbyterian Hospital
New York, New York
*Chapter 60, Bismuth*
*Special Considerations: SC6, Intrathecal Administration of Xenobiotics*
*Special Considerations: SC11, Organ Procurement from Poisoned Patients*

**Joseph G. Rella, MD**
Assistant Professor of Medicine
Weill Cornell Medical College of Cornell University
Emergency Physician
New York-Presbyterian Hospital
New York, New York
*Chapter 100, Radiation*
*Antidotes in Brief: A44, Potassium Iodide*
*Antidotes in Brief: A45, Pentetic Acid or Pentetate (Zinc or Calcium) Trisodium (DTPA)*

**Daniel J. Repplinger, MD**
Assistant Clinical Professor of Emergency Medicine
University of California, San Francisco
Zuckerberg San Francisco General Hospital
San Francisco, California
*Chapter 88, Arthropods*

**Morgan A. A. Riggan, MD, FRCPC**
Assistant Professor of Emergency Medicine
Western University
Emergency Physician
London Health Sciences Centre
London, Ontario, Canada
Medical Toxicologist
Poison and Drug Information Service (PADIS)
Alberta Health Services
Calgary, Alberta, Canada
*Chapter 78, Hydrocarbons*

**Darren M. Roberts, MBBS, PhD, FRACP**
Conjoint Associate Professor
University of New South Wales
Consultant Physician and Clinical Toxicologist
St. Vincent's Hospital and New South Wales Poisons Information Centre
Sydney, Australia
*Chapter 82, Herbicides*

**Anne-Michelle Ruha, MD**
Professor of Internal Medicine and Emergency Medicine
Departments of Internal Medicine and Emergency Medicine
University of Arizona College of Medicine—Phoenix
Department of Medical Toxicology
Banner—University Medical Center Phoenix
Phoenix, Arizona
*Chapter 92, Native (US) Venomous Snakes and Lizards*
*Antidotes in Brief: A39, Antivenom for North American Venomous Snakes (Crotaline and Elapid)*

**Cynthia D. Santos, MD**
Assistant Professor of Emergency Medicine
Emergency Physician
University Hospital of Newark
Rutgers New Jersey Medical School
Toxicology Consultant
New Jersey Poison Information and Education System
Newark, New Jersey
*Chapter 7, Colchicine, Podophyllin, and the Vinca Alkaloids*

**Daniel Schatz, MD**
Addiction Medicine Fellow
Department of Medicine
New York University School of Medicine
Bellevue Hospital Center
New York, New York
*Special Considerations: SC5, Prevention, Treatment, and Harm Reduction Approaches to Opioid Overdoses*

**Capt. Joshua G. Schier, MD, MPH, USPHS**
Lead, Environmental Toxicology Team
Centers for Disease Control and Prevention
Assistant Professor of Emergency Medicine
Emory University School of Medicine
Associate Director, Emory/CDC Medical Toxicology Fellowship
Consultant, Georgia Poison Center
Atlanta, Georgia
*Chapter 7, Colchicine, Podophyllin, and the Vinca Alkaloids*
*Special Considerations: SC8, Diethylene Glycol*

**David T. Schwartz, MD**
Associate Professor of Emergency Medicine
New York University School of Medicine
Emergency Physician
Ronald O. Perelman Department of Emergency Medicine
Bellevue Hospital Center and NYU Langone Health
New York, New York
*Chapter 5, Principles of Diagnostic Imaging*

**Shahin Shadnia, MD, PhD, FACMT**
Professor of Clinical Toxicology
Head of Clinical Toxicology Department
School of Medicine
Shahid Beheshti University of Medical Sciences
Chairman of Loghman Hakim Hospital Poison Center
Tehran, Iran
*Chapter 81, Fumigants*

**Lauren Kornreich Shawn, MD**
Assistant Professor of Emergency Medicine
Icahn School of Medicine at Mount Sinai
Mount Sinai St. Luke's, Mount Sinai West
New York, New York
*Chapter 15, Essential Oils*

**Farshad Mazda Shirazi, MSc, MD, PhD, FACEP, FACMT**
Associate Professor of Emergency Medicine, Pharmacology and Pharmacy Practice and Science
University of Arizona College of Medicine—Tucson
Program Director, Medical Toxicology
Medical Director, Arizona Poison and Drug Information Center
Tucson, Arizona
*Special Considerations: SC9, Exotic Nonnative Snake Envenomations*

**Silas W. Smith, MD, FACEP, FACMT**
JoAnn G. and Kenneth Wellner Associate Professor of Emergency Medicine
Chief, Division of Quality, Safety, and Practice Innovation
Affiliate Faculty, Institute for Innovations in Medical Education
Emergency Physician
Ronald O. Perelman Department of Emergency Medicine, NYU Grossman School of Medicine
Bellevue Hospital Center and NYU Langone Health
New York, New York
*Chapter 1, Initial Evaluation of the Patient: Vital Signs and Toxic Syndromes*
*Chapter 2, Principles of Managing the Acutely Poisoned or Overdosed Patient*
*Antidotes in Brief: A1, Activated Charcoal*
*Antidotes in Brief: A2, Whole-Bowel Irrigation and Other Intestinal Evacuants*
*Antidotes in Brief: A6, Botulinum Antitoxin*
*Antidotes in Brief: A9, Octreotide*
*Antidotes in Brief: A12, Folates: Leucovorin (Folinic Acid) and Folic Acid*
*Antidotes in Brief: A13, Glucarpidase (Carboxypeptidase $G_2$)*
*Antidotes in Brief: A14, Uridine Triacetate*
*Antidotes in Brief: A16, Magnesium*
*Antidotes in Brief: A20, Glucagon*
*Antidotes in Brief: A22, Digoxin-Specific Antibody Fragments*
*Antidotes in Brief: A32, Calcium*

**Craig G. Smollin, MD, FACMT**
Associate Professor of Emergency Medicine
Program Director, Medical Toxicology
University of California, San Francisco
Medical Director, California Poison Control System–San Francisco Division
San Francisco, California
*Chapter 48, Cocaine*

**Sari Soghoian, MD, MA**
Associate Professor of Emergency Medicine
New York University School of Medicine
New York, New York
Clinical Coordinator, Korle Bu Teaching Hospital
Department of Emergency Medicine
Accra, Ghana
*Chapter 55, Nicotine*
*Chapter 67, Manganese*

**Kambiz Soltaninejad, PharmD, PhD**
Associate Professor of Toxicology
Department of Forensic Toxicology
Legal Medicine Research Center
Legal Medicine Organization
Tehran, Iran
*Chapter 81, Fumigants*

**Meghan B. Spyres, MD**
Assistant Professor of Clinical Emergency Medicine
Division of Medical Toxicology
University of Southern California, Keck School of Medicine
Los Angeles, California
*Chapter 46, Amphetamines*

**Samuel J. Stellpflug, MD, FAACT, FACMT, FACEP, FAAEM**
Associate Professor of Emergency Medicine
University of Minnesota Medical School
Minneapolis, Minnesota
Director, Clinical Toxicology
Regions Hospital
Saint Paul, Minnesota
*Antidotes in Brief: A21, High-Dose Insulin*

**Christine M. Stork, BS, PharmD, DABAT, FAACT**
Professor of Emergency Medicine
Clinical Director, Upstate NY Poison Center
Upstate Medical University
Syracuse, New York
*Chapter 27, Antibacterials, Antifungals, and Antivirals*
*Chapter 42, Serotonin Reuptake Inhibitors and Atypical Antidepressants*

**Mark K. Su, MD, MPH**
Associate Professor of Emergency Medicine
New York University School of Medicine
Emergency Physician
Ronald O. Perelman Department of Emergency Medicine
Bellevue Hospital Center and NYU Langone Health
Director, New York City Poison Control Center
New York, New York
*Chapter 31, Antithrombotics*
*Chapter 77, Hydrofluoric Acid and Fluorides*
*Antidotes in Brief: A17, Prothrombin Complex Concentrates and Direct Oral Anticoagulant Antidotes*

**Jeffrey R. Suchard, MD**
Professor of Clinical Emergency Medicine and Pharmacology
University of California, Irvine School of Medicine
Irvine, California
*Chapter 98, Chemical Weapons*
*Chapter 99, Biological Weapons*

**Payal Sud, MD, FACEP**
Assistant Professor of Emergency Medicine
Donald and Barbara Zucker School of Medicine at Hofstra/Northwell
Hempstead, New York
Director of Performance Improvement
Department of Emergency Medicine
Long Island Jewish Medical Center
Assistant Program Director
Medical Toxicology Fellowship
Northwell Health
New Hyde Park, New York
*Chapter 45, Sedative-Hypnotics*

**Young-Jin Sue, MD**
Clinical Associate Professor of Pediatrics
Albert Einstein College of Medicine
Attending Physician, Pediatric Emergency Services
The Children's Hospital at Montefiore
Bronx, New York
*Chapter 68, Mercury*

**Kenneth M. Sutin, MS, MD, FCCP, FCCM**
Professor of Anesthesiology
New York University School of Medicine
Attending Physician, Department of Anesthesiology
Bellevue Hospital Center
New York, New York
*Chapter 39, Neuromuscular Blockers*
*Antidotes in Brief: A24, Dantrolene Sodium*

**Matthew D. Sztajnkrycer, MD, PhD**
Professor of Emergency Medicine
Mayo Clinic College of Medicine and Science
Staff Toxicologist
Minnesota Poison Control System
Rochester, Minnesota
*Chapter 37, Local Anesthetics*

**Asim F. Tarabar, MD, MS**
Assistant Professor of Emergency Medicine
Yale University School of Medicine
Director, Medical Toxicology
Yale New Haven Hospital
New Haven, Connecticut
*Chapter 58, Antimony*

**Stephen R. Thom, MD, PhD**
Professor of Emergency Medicine
Director of Research
University of Maryland School of Medicine
Baltimore, Maryland
*Antidotes in Brief: A40, Hyperbaric Oxygen*

**Christian Tomaszewski, MD, MS, MBA, FACMT, FACEP**
Professor of Clinical Emergency Medicine
University of California, San Diego Health
Chief Medical Officer, El Centro Regional Medical Center
San Diego, California
*Chapter 95, Carbon Monoxide*

**Stephen J. Traub, MD**
Associate Professor of Emergency Medicine
Mayo Clinic College of Medicine and Science
Chairman, Department of Emergency Medicine
Mayo Clinic Arizona
Phoenix, Arizona
*Chapter 61, Cadmium*

**Michael G. Tunik, MD**
Associate Professor of Emergency Medicine and Pediatrics
New York University School of Medicine
Director of Research, Division of Pediatric Emergency Medicine
Emergency Physician
Ronald O. Perelman Department of Emergency Medicine
Bellevue Hospital Center and NYU Langone Health
New York, New York
*Chapter 12, Food Poisoning*

**Matthew Valento, MD**
Assistant Professor of Emergency Medicine
Site Director for Medical Toxicology
University of Washington School of Medicine
Attending Physician
Harborview Medical Center
Seattle, Washington
*Chapter 41, Cyclic Antidepressants*

**Susi U. Vassallo, MD**
Professor of Emergency Medicine
New York University School of Medicine
Emergency Physician
Ronald O. Perelman Department of Emergency Medicine
Bellevue Hospital Center and NYU Langone Health
New York, New York
*Chapter 14, Athletic Performance Enhancers*

**Larissa I. Velez, MD, FACEP**
Professor of Emergency Medicine
University of Texas Southwestern Medical School
Vice Chair of Education
Program Director of Emergency Medicine
Department of Emergency Medicine
University of Texas Southwestern Medical Center
Staff Toxicologist, North Texas Poison Center
Dallas, Texas
*Antidotes in Brief: A8, Dextrose (D-Glucose)*

**Lisa E. Vivero, PharmD**
Drug Information Specialist
Irvine, California
*Chapter 19, Pharmaceutical Additives*

**Richard Y. Wang, DO**
Senior Medical Officer
National Center for Environmental Health
Centers for Disease Control and Prevention
Atlanta, Georgia
*Chapter 23, Chemotherapeutics*
*Chapter 24, Methotrexate, 5-Flourouracil, and Capecitabine*
*Special Considerations: SC7, Extravasation of Xenobiotics*

**Paul M. Wax, MD**
Clinical Professor of Emergency Medicine
University of Texas Southwestern Medical School
Dallas, Texas
Executive Director
American College of Medical Toxicology
Phoenix, Arizona
*Chapter 74, Antiseptics, Disinfectants, and Sterilants*
*Antidotes in Brief: A5, Sodium Bicarbonate*

**Sage W. Wiener, MD**
Assistant Professor of Emergency Medicine
SUNY Downstate Medical Center College of Medicine
Director of Medical Toxicology
SUNY Downstate Medical Center/Kings County Hospital
Brooklyn, New York
*Chapter 79, Toxic Alcohols*

**Rachel S. Wightman, MD**
Assistant Professor of Emergency Medicine
Division of Medical Toxicology
The Warren Alpert Medical School of Brown University
Rhode Island Hospital
Providence, Rhode Island
*Chapter 76, Caustics*

**Luke Yip, MD**
Consultant and Attending Staff Medical Toxicologist
Denver Health
Rocky Mountain Poison and Drug Center
Department of Medicine
Section of Medical Toxicology
Denver, Colorado
Senior Medical Toxicologist
Centers for Disease Control and Prevention
Office of Noncommunicable Diseases, Injury, and Environmental Health
National Center for Environmental Health/Agency for Toxic Substances and Disease Registry
Atlanta, Georgia
*Chapter 49, Ethanol*

**Erin A. Zerbo, MD**
Assistant Professor of Psychiatry
Associate Director, Medical Student Education in Psychiatry
Rutgers New Jersey Medical School
Newark, New Jersey
*Special Considerations: SC3, Patient Violence*

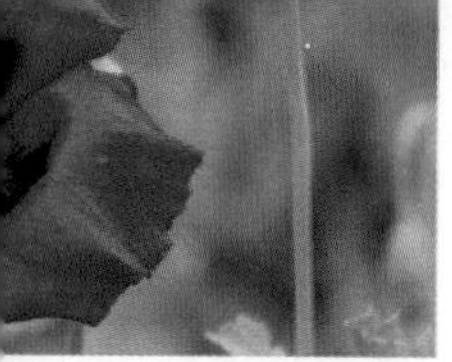

# PREFACE

*Goldfrank's Clinical Manual of Toxicologic Emergencies* is a distillation of the essential clinical information provided in the 11th edition of *Goldfrank's Toxicologic Emergencies.* Designed to stimulate interest in the management of exposed and poisoned patients, this manual is for students and bedside practitioners, including pharmacists, nurses, advanced practice providers, and physicians. It specifically focuses on those healthcare professionals who need the essential information for their daily care of poisoned patients.

Ever since the first edition of the Manual was published in 2007 as a companion to the 8th edition of the main textbook, the editors have received many requests for updates. Although our work on the main textbook is relentless, we decided that the time was right to revise this companion book. Although many of the fundamentals of pharmacology and toxicology remain sound, our approach to patients with toxicologic emergencies continues to evolve based on scientific advances and the ever-changing epidemiological landscape of available xenobiotics.

Unlike the previous edition of this Manual, we included only the clinical chapters from the main textbook. While this decision may require novice readers to refer to the main textbook for core knowledge, it allowed us to preserve the rigor of the clinical chapters while also including critical images and tables from the main textbook, in order to provide a focused approach designed for bedside application. This Manual also serves as a learning tool for others who may prefer a more portable resource. Thus, while the chapters follow the same overall organization as the 11th edition of *Goldfrank's Toxicologic Emergencies*, the chapter numbers differ. In the main textbook, chapters are followed by "Antidotes in Depth," which provide extensive information for more than 40 therapeutic interventions. Here, each "Antidote in Brief" describes essential clinical toxicological interventions.

While this handbook is designed to stand alone, it is truly a companion work to the main textbook, which provides extensive background information and references, and to the Study Guide, which offers self-assessment questions and directed learning.

We hope that this updated edition meets your educational needs and allows you to improve the care of your patients. As always, we encourage your comments and thoughtful feedback. We will do our best to incorporate your suggestions into future editions.

**The Editors**

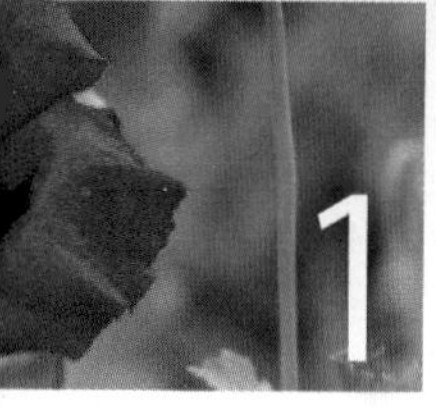

# 1 INITIAL EVALUATION OF THE PATIENT: VITAL SIGNS AND TOXIC SYNDROMES

For more than 200 years, health care providers have attempted to standardize their approach to the assessment of patients. At the New York Hospital in 1865, pulse rate, respiratory rate, and temperature were incorporated into the bedside chart and called "vital signs." It was not until the early part of the 20th century that blood pressure determination also became routine. Additional components of the present standard emergency assessment, such as oxygen saturation by pulse oximetry, capillary blood glucose, and pain severity, are sometimes considered vital signs. Although they are essential components of the clinical evaluation and are important considerations throughout this text, they are not discussed in this chapter but can be found in other relevant sections.

In the practice of medical toxicology, vital signs play an important role beyond assessing and monitoring the overall status of a patient, because they frequently provide valuable physiologic clues to the toxicologic etiology and severity of an illness. Table 1–1 presents the normal vital signs for various age groups. Published normal values likely have little relevance for an acutely ill or anxious patient in the emergency setting, yet that is precisely the environment in which abnormal vital signs must be identified and addressed. Descriptions of vital signs as "normal" or "stable" are too nonspecific to be meaningful and therefore should never be accepted as defining normalcy in an individual patient. Only a complete assessment of a patient can determine whether or not a particular vital sign is truly clinically normal in the particular clinical setting. **No patient should be considered too agitated, too young, or too gravely ill for the practitioner to obtain a complete set of vital signs; indeed, these patients urgently need a thorough evaluation.**

The vital signs must be recorded as accurately as possible on arrival and repeated periodically as clinically indicated to identify trends. Meticulous attention to both the initial and repeated determinations of vital signs is of extreme importance in identifying a pattern of changes suggesting a particular xenobiotic or group of xenobiotics. The value of serial monitoring of the vital signs is demonstrated by the patient who presents with anticholinergic toxicity and receives the antidote, physostigmine. In this situation, it is important to recognize when tachycardia becomes bradycardia (eg, anticholinergic syndrome followed by cholinergic syndrome due to physostigmine excess).

The assessment starts by analyzing diverse information, including vital signs, history, and physical examination. Mofenson and Greensher coined the term toxidromes from the words *toxic syndromes* to describe the groups of signs and symptoms that consistently result from particular toxins. These syndromes are usually best described by a combination of the vital signs and clinically apparent end-organ manifestations. Table 1–2 describes the most typical toxidromes. This table includes only vital signs that are thought to be characteristically abnormal or pathognomonic and directly related to the toxicologic effect of the xenobiotic. A detailed analysis of each sign, symptom, and toxic syndrome can be found in the pertinent chapters throughout the text. In this chapter, the most typical toxic syndromes are considered to enable the appropriate assessment and differential diagnosis of a poisoned patient. In considering a toxic syndrome, the reader should always remember that the actual clinical manifestations of a poisoning are far more variable than the syndromes described in Table 1–2, especially when coingestants are ingested.

**TABLE 1–1 Normal Vital Signs by Age[a]**

| *Age* | *Systolic BP (mm Hg)* | *Diastolic BP (mm Hg)* | *Pulse (beats/min)* | *Respirations (breaths/min)* |
|---|---|---|---|---|
| Adult | 120 | 80 | 50–90 | 16–24 |
| 16 years | ≤120 | <80 | 80 | 16–30 |
| 12 years | 119 | 76 | 85 | 16–30 |
| 10 years | 115 | 74 | 90 | 16–30 |
| 6 years | 107 | 69 | 100 | 20–30 |
| 4 years | 104 | 65 | 110 | 20–30 |
| 4 months | 90 | 50 | 145 | 30–35 |
| 2 months | 85 | 50 | 145 | 30–35 |
| Newborn | 65 | 50 | 145 | 35–40 |

[a]The normal rectal temperature is defined as 95.0°F to 100.4°F (35°–38°C) for all ages. For children 1 year of age or younger, these values are the mean values for the 50th percentile. For older children, these values represent the 90th percentile at a specific age for the 50th percentile of weight in that age group.

These respiration values were determined in the emergency department and may be environment and situation dependent.

BP = blood pressure.

## BLOOD PRESSURE

Xenobiotics cause hypotension by four major mechanisms: decreased peripheral vascular resistance, decreased myocardial contractility, dysrhythmias, and depletion of intravascular volume (Table 1–3). Hypertension from xenobiotics is caused by CNS sympathetic overactivity, increased myocardial contractility, increased peripheral vascular resistance, or a combination thereof.

**TABLE 1–2 Toxic Syndromes**

| Group | Vital Signs BP | P | R | T | Mental Status | Pupil Size | Peristalsis | Diaphoresis | Other |
|---|---|---|---|---|---|---|---|---|---|
| Anticholinergics | –/↑ | ↑ | ± | ↑ | Delirium | ↑ | ↓ | ↓ | Dry mucous membranes, flush, urinary retention |
| Cholinergics | ± | ± | ± | – | Normal to depressed | ± | ↑ | ↑ | Salivation, lacrimation, urination, diarrhea, bronchorrhea, fasciculations, paralysis |
| Ethanol or sedative–hypnotics | ↓ | ↓ | ↓ | –/↓ | Depressed, agitated | ± | ↓ | – | Hyporeflexia, ataxia |
| Opioids | ↓ | ↓ | ↓ | ↓ | Depressed | ↓ | ↓ | – | Hyporeflexia |
| Serotonin toxicity | ↑ | ↑ | –/↑ | ↑ | Normal to agitated delirium | –/↑ | ↑ | ↑ | Clonus, tremor, seizures |
| Sympathomimetics | ↑ | ↑ | ↑ | ↑ | Agitated | ↑ | –/↑ | ↑ | Tremor, seizures, diaphoresis |
| Withdrawal from ethanol or sedative–hypnotics | ↑ | ↑ | ↑ | ↑ | Agitated, disoriented, hallucinations | ↑ | ↑ | ↑ | Tremor, seizures, diaphoresis |
| Withdrawal from opioids | ↑ | ↑ | – | – | Normal, anxious | ↑ | ↑ | ↑ | Vomiting, rhinorrhea, piloerection, diarrhea, yawning |

↑ = increases; ↓ = decreases; ± = variable; – = change unlikely; BP = blood pressure; P = pulse; R = respirations; T = temperature.

## PULSE RATE

Extremely useful clinical information can be obtained by evaluating the pulse rate (Table 1–4). The normal heart rate for adults was defined by consensus studies suggesting that 95% of the population has bradycardia and tachycardia thresholds of 50 beats/min and 90 beats/min, making absolute definitions unrealistic, particularly in the ED. Because pulse rate is the net result of a balance between sympathetic (adrenergic) and parasympathetic (muscarinic and nicotinic) tone, many xenobiotics that exert therapeutic or toxic effects or cause pain syndromes, hyperthermia, or volume depletion also affect the pulse rate. The inability to differentiate easily between sympathomimetic and anticholinergic xenobiotic effects by vital signs alone illustrates the principle that no single vital sign abnormality can definitively establish a toxicologic diagnosis.

**TABLE 1–3 Common Xenobiotics That Affect the Blood Pressure**

| Hypotension | Hypertension |
|---|---|
| $\alpha_1$-Adrenergic antagonists | $\alpha_1$-Adrenergic agonists |
| $\alpha_2$-Adrenergic agonists (central) | $\alpha_2$-Adrenergic agonists (central) (early) |
| β-Adrenergic antagonists | $\alpha_2$-Adrenergic antagonists |
| $\beta_2$-Adrenergic agonists | Ergot alkaloids |
| Angiotensin-converting enzyme inhibitors | Ethanol and sedative–hypnotic withdrawal |
| Angiotensin receptor blockers | Lead (chronic) |
| Antidysrhythmics | Monoamine oxidase inhibitors (overdose early and drug–food interaction) |
| Calcium channel blockers | Nicotine (early) |
| Cyanide | Phencyclidine |
| Cyclic antidepressants | Sympathomimetics |
| Ethanol and other alcohols | |
| Iron | |
| Methylxanthines | |
| Nitrates and nitrites | |
| Nitroprusside | |
| Opioids | |
| Phenothiazines | |
| Phosphodiesterase-5 inhibitors | |
| Sedative–hypnotics | |

## RESPIRATORY RATE

Although respirations are typically assessed initially for rate alone, careful observation of the depth and pattern is essential (Table 1–5). Hyperventilation means an increase in minute ventilation above normal and it may result from tachypnea, hyperpnea, or both. When hyperventilation results solely or predominantly from hyperpnea, clinicians may miss this important finding entirely, instead erroneously describing such a hyperventilating patient as normally ventilating or even hypoventilating if bradypnea is also present. Similarly hypoventilation means a decreased minute ventilation and can result from bradypnea or hypopnea or both.

## TEMPERATURE

Temperature evaluation and control are critical, yet our ability to recognize abnormal temperatures by clinical examination is limited. The risks of inaccuracy are substantial when an oral temperature is taken in a tachypneic patient, an axillary temperature or a temporal artery temperature is taken in any patient (especially those found outdoors), or a tympanic temperature is taken in a patient with cerumen impaction.

**TABLE 1–4 Common Xenobiotics That Affect the Pulse Rate**

| Bradycardia | Tachycardia |
|---|---|
| $\alpha_2$-Adrenergic agonists (central) | $\alpha_1$-Adrenergic antagonists |
| β-Adrenergic antagonists | Anticholinergics |
| Baclofen | Antipsychotics |
| Calcium channel blockers (nondihydropyridine) | β-Adrenergic agonists |
| Carbamates | Cyclic antidepressants |
| Cardioactive steroids | Disulfiram–ethanol interaction |
| Ciguatoxin | Ethanol and sedative–hypnotic withdrawal |
| Ergot alkaloids | Iron |
| γ-Hydroxybutyric acid | Methylxanthines |
| Opioids | Phencyclidine |
| Organic phosphorus compounds | Sympathomimetics |
| Synthetic cannabinoids | Thyroid hormone |
| | Thiamine deficiency |
| | Yohimbine |

**TABLE 1–5 Common Xenobiotics That Affect Respiration**

| *Bradypnea* | *Tachypnea* |
|---|---|
| $\alpha_2$-Adrenergic agonists (central) | Cyanide |
| Botulinum toxin | Dinitrophenol and congeners |
| Carbamates | Epinephrine |
| Elapidae venom | Ethylene glycol |
| Ethanol and other alcohols | Hydrogen sulfide |
| γ-Hydroxybutyric acid | Methanol |
| Magnesium | Methemoglobin producers |
| Neuromuscular blockers | Methylxanthines |
| Opioids | Nicotine (early) |
| Organic phosphorus compounds | Pulmonary irritants |
| Sedative–hypnotics | Salicylates |
| Tetanospasmin | Sympathomimetics |
| Tetrodotoxin | |

**TABLE 1–6 Common Xenobiotics That Affect Temperature[a]**

| *Hyperthermia* | *Hypothermia* |
|---|---|
| Anticholinergics | $\alpha_2$-Adrenergic agonists (central) |
| Chlorophenoxy herbicides | Anesthetics (general and intravenous) |
| Dinitrophenol and congeners | Cannabinoids |
| Malignant hyperthermia[a] | Carbon monoxide |
| Monoamine oxidase inhibitors | Ethanol |
| Neuroleptic malignant syndrome[a] | γ-Hydroxybutyric acid |
| Phencyclidine | Hypoglycemics |
| Salicylates | Opioids |
| Sedative–hypnotic or ethanol withdrawal | Sedative–hypnotics (particularly barbiturates) |
| Serotonin toxicity[a] | Thiamine deficiency |
| Sympathomimetics | |
| Thyroid hormone | |

[a]Xenobiotic-related syndromes.

Obtaining **rectal temperatures** ($T_r$) using a nonglass probe is essential for safe and accurate temperature determinations in agitated individuals and is considered the standard method of temperature determination in this textbook.

Hypothermia ($T_r$ <95.0°F; <35°C) and hyperthermia ($T_r$ >100.4°F; >38°C) are common manifestations of toxicity. Severe or significant hypothermia and hyperthermia, unless immediately recognized and managed appropriately, may result in grave complications and inappropriate or inadequate resuscitative efforts. Life-threatening hyperthermia (T >106°F; >41.1°C) from any cause may lead to extensive rhabdomyolysis, myoglobinuric kidney failure, and direct liver and brain injury and must therefore be identified and corrected immediately. Hypothermia is probably less of an immediate threat to life than hyperthermia, but it requires rapid appreciation, accurate diagnosis, and skilled management because it may suggest energy failure. Table 1–6 is a representative list of xenobiotics that affect body temperature.

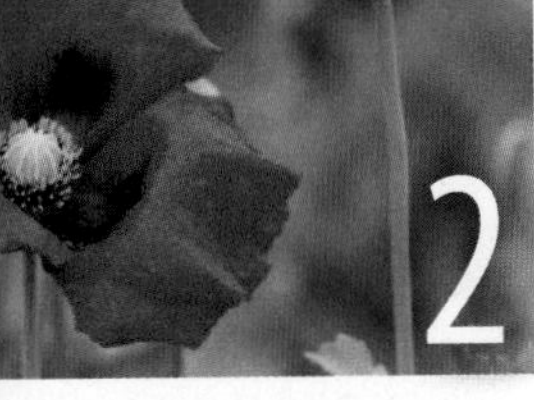

# 2 PRINCIPLES OF MANAGING THE ACUTELY POISONED OR OVERDOSED PATIENT

## OVERVIEW

For more than 5 decades, medical toxicologists and poison information specialists have used a clinical approach to poisoned or overdosed patients that emphasizes treating the patient rather than treating the poison. Too often in the past, patients were initially ignored while attention was focused on the ingredients listed on the containers of the product(s) to which they presumably were exposed. However, astute clinicians must always be prepared to administer a specific antidote immediately in instances when nothing else will save a patient, such as with cyanide poisoning. Moreover, after resuscitative antidotes are given, all poisoned or overdosed patients benefit from an organized, rapid clinical management plan also known as a toxicological risk assessment.

With the widespread availability of accurate rapid bedside testing for capillary blood glucose, pulse oximetry for oxygen saturation, and end-tidal $CO_2$ monitors, clinicians can safely provide rational, individualized approaches to determine the need for, and in some instances more precise amounts of, dextrose, thiamine, naloxone, and oxygen. Likewise, appreciation of the potential for significant adverse effects associated with all types of gastrointestinal (GI) decontamination interventions and recognition of the absence of clear evidence-based support of efficacy have led to abandoning of syrup of ipecac-induced emesis, an almost complete elimination of orogastric lavage, and a significant reduction in the routine use of activated charcoal. The value of whole-bowel irrigation (WBI) with polyethylene glycol electrolyte solution (PEG-ELS) appears to be much more specific and limited than originally thought, and some of the limitations and (uncommon) adverse effects of activated charcoal are now more widely recognized (Chap. 3). However, as with many issues in clinical medicine, properly selected procedures performed in properly selected patients can lead to an acceptable risk-benefit profile. Routine exclusion of GI decontamination procedures is not optimal and can lead to suboptimal care manifested as increased toxic effects and prolonged use of health care resources. Similarly, interventions to eliminate absorbed xenobiotics from the body are now much more narrowly defined or, in some cases, have been abandoned. Multiple-dose activated charcoal (MDAC) is useful for select but not all xenobiotics. Ion trapping in the urine is only beneficial, achievable, and relatively safe when the urine can be maximally alkalinized in a limited number of cases (Antidotes in Brief: A5). Finally, the roles of hemodialysis, hemoperfusion, and other extracorporeal techniques are now much more specifically defined (Chap. 4). Thus, this chapter represents our current efforts to formulate a logical and effective approach to managing a patient with probable or actual toxic exposure.

The management of most patients with toxicologic clinical syndromes cannot be based on specific antidotal therapies but rather relies on the application of directed supportive or pharmacologic care. Table 2–1 provides a recommended stock list of antidotes and therapeutics for the treatment of poisoned or overdosed patients. Consensus antidote stocking guidelines exist as well.

## MANAGING ACUTELY POISONED OR OVERDOSED PATIENTS

Rarely, if ever, are all of the circumstances involving a poisoned patient known. The history may be incomplete, unreliable, or unobtainable; multiple xenobiotics may be involved; and even when a xenobiotic etiology is identified, it may not be easy to determine whether the problem is an overdose, an allergic or idiosyncratic reaction, or a drug–drug interaction. The patient's presenting signs and symptoms may force an intervention at a time when there is almost no information available about the etiology of the patient's condition (Table 2–2).

### Initial Management of Patients with a Suspected Exposure

The clinical approach to the patient potentially exposed to a xenobiotic begins with the recognition and treatment of life-threatening conditions, including airway compromise, breathing difficulties, and circulatory problems such as hemodynamic instability and serious dysrhythmias. After the "ABCs" (airway, breathing, and circulation) are addressed, the patient's level of consciousness should be assessed because it helps determine the techniques to be used for further management of the exposure.

### Management of Patients with Altered Mental Status

Figure 2–1 provides an approach to these patients. Within the first 5 minutes of managing a patient with an altered mental status (AMS), five therapeutic interventions should be administered if indicated and not contraindicated:

1. Supplemental oxygen to treat xenobiotic-induced hypoxia
2. Hypertonic dextrose: 0.5 to 1.0 g/kg of $D_{50}W$ for an adult or a more dilute dextrose solution ($D_{10}W$ or $D_{25}W$) for a child; the dextrose is administered as an IV bolus as specific or empiric therapy for documented or suspected hypoglycemia when rapid confirmation is unavailable (Antidotes in Brief: A8)
3. Thiamine (100 mg IV for an adult; usually unnecessary for a child) to prevent Wernicke encephalopathy in patients at risk (Antidotes in Brief: A27)
4. Naloxone (0.04 mg IV with upward titration) for an adult or child with opioid-induced respiratory compromise (Antidotes in Brief: A4)
5. Rectal temperature and initiation of appropriate cooling or warming measures if hyperthermia or hypothermia are present

**TABLE 2–1 Antidotes and Therapeutics for the Treatment of Poisonings and Overdoses[a]**

| Therapeutics[b] | Indications | Therapeutics[b] | Indications |
|---|---|---|---|
| Acetylcysteine (p. 66) | Acetaminophen and other causes of hepatotoxicity | Fomepizole (p. 548) | Ethylene glycol, methanol, diethylene glycol |
| Activated charcoal (p. 22) | Adsorbent xenobiotics in the GI tract | Glucagon (p. 301) | β-Adrenergic antagonists, CCBs |
| Antivenom (*Centruroides* spp) (p. 615) | Scorpion envenomation | Glucarpidase (p. 220) | Methotrexate |
| Antivenom (*Crotalinae*) (p. 658) | Crotaline snake envenomations | Hydroxocobalamin (p. 691) | Cyanide |
| Antivenom (*Micrurus fulvius*) (p. 658) | Coral snake envenomations | Idarucizumab (p. 285) | Dabigatran |
| Antivenom (*Latrodectus mactans*) (p. 613) | Black widow spider envenomations | Insulin (p. 331) | β-Adrenergic antagonists, CCBs, hyperglycemia |
| Antivenom (*Synanceja* spp) (p. 624) | Stonefish envenomation | Iodide (SSKI) (p. 724) | Radioactive iodine ($I^{131}$) |
| Atropine (p. 586) | Bradydysrhythmias, cholinesterase inhibitors (organic phosphorus compounds, physostigmine) muscarinic mushrooms (*Clitocybe*, *Inocybe*) ingestions | Lipid emulsion (p. 331) | Local anesthetics |
| Benzodiazepines (p. 401) | Seizures, agitation, stimulants, ethanol and sedative–hypnotic withdrawal, cocaine, chloroquine, organic phosphorus compounds | Magnesium sulfate injection (p. 271) | Cardioactive steroids, hydrofluoric acid, hypomagnesemia, ethanol withdrawal, torsade de pointes |
| Botulinum antitoxin (Heptavalent) (p. 114) | Botulism | Methylene blue (1% solution) (p. 701) | Methemoglobinemia, ifosfamide, vasoplegic syndrome, shock |
| Calcium chloride, calcium gluconate (p. 532) | Fluoride, hydrofluoric acid, ethylene glycol, CCBs, hypermagnesemia, β-adrenergic antagonists, hyperkalemia | Naloxone (p. 90) | Opioids, clonidine |
| L-Carnitine (p. 195) | Valproic acid: hyperammonemia | Norepinephrine | Hypotension |
| Cyanide kit (nitrites, p. 693; sodium thiosulfate, p. 693) | Cyanide | Octreotide (p. 184) | Insulin secretagogue–induced hypoglycemia |
| Cyproheptadine (p. 364) | Serotonin toxicity | Oxygen (Hyperbaric) (p. 683) | Carbon monoxide, cyanide, hydrogen sulfide |
| Dantrolene (p. 346) | Malignant hyperthermia | D-Penicillamine (p. 473) | Copper |
| Deferoxamine (p. 166) | Iron, aluminum | Phenobarbital (p. 418) | Seizures, agitation, stimulants, ethanol and sedative–hypnotic withdrawal |
| Dextrose in water (50% adults; 20% pediatrics; 10% neonates) (p. 181) | Hypoglycemia | Phentolamine (p. 399) | Vasoconstriction: cocaine, MAOI interactions, epinephrine, and ergot alkaloids |
| Digoxin-specific antibody fragments (p. 319) | Cardioactive steroids | Physostigmine (p. 206) | Anticholinergics |
| Dimercaprol (British anti-Lewisite [BAL]) (p. 457) | Arsenic, mercury, gold, lead | Polyethylene glycol electrolyte lavage solution (p. 25) | Decontamination |
| Diphenhydramine (p. 351) | Dystonic reactions, allergic reactions | Pralidoxime (p. 588) | Acetylcholinesterase inhibitors (organic phosphorus compounds and carbamates) |
| DTPA (p. 726) (calcium trisodium pentetate) | Radioactive isotopes; americium, curium, plutonium | Protamine (p. 291) | Heparin anticoagulation |
| Edetate calcium disodium (calcium disodium versenate, $CaNa_2EDTA$) (p. 488) | Lead, other selected metals | Prussian blue (p. 508) | Thallium, cesium |
| Ethanol (p. 550) | Ethylene glycol, methanol, diethylene glycol | Pyridoxine (vitamin $B_6$) (p. 262) | Isoniazid, ethylene glycol, gyromitrin-containing mushrooms |
| Flumazenil (p. 381) | Benzodiazepines | Sodium bicarbonate (p. 104) | Ethylene glycol, methanol, salicylates, cyclic antidepressants, methotrexate, phenobarbital, quinidine, chlorpropamide, class I antidysrhythmics, chlorophenoxy herbicides, sodium channel blockers |
| Folinic acid (p. 217) | Methotrexate, methanol | Starch (p. 516) | Iodine |
| | | Succimer (p. 485) | Lead, mercury, arsenic |
| | | Thiamine (vitamin $B_1$) (p. 412) | Thiamine deficiency, ethylene glycol, chronic ethanol consumption ("alcoholism") |
| | | Uridine triacetate (p. 223) | Fluorouracil, capecitabine |
| | | Vitamin $K_1$ (p. 289) | Warfarin or rodenticide anticoagulants |

[a]Each emergency department should have the vast majority of these antidotes immediately available; some of these antidotes may be stored in the pharmacy, and others may be available from the Centers for Disease Control and Prevention, but the precise mechanism for locating each one must be known by each staff member.

[b]A detailed analysis of each of these antidotes is found in the text in the Antidotes in Brief section on the page cited to the right of each antidote or therapeutic listed.

CCB = calcium channel blocker; DTPA = diethylenetriaminepentaacetic acid; EDTA = ethylenediamine tetraacetic acid; GI = gastrointestinal; MAOI = monoamine oxidase inhibitor; SSKI = saturated solution of potassium iodide.

**TABLE 2–2 Clinical and Laboratory Findings in Poisoning and Overdose**

| | |
|---|---|
| Agitation | Anticholinergics,[a] hypoglycemia, phencyclidine, sympathomimetics,[b] synthetic cannabinoid receptor agonists, withdrawal from ethanol and sedative–hypnotics |
| Alopecia | Alkylating agents, radiation, selenium, thallium |
| Ataxia | Benzodiazepines, carbamazepine, carbon monoxide, ethanol, hypoglycemia, lithium, mercury, nitrous oxide, phenytoin |
| Blindness or decreased visual acuity | Caustics (direct), cisplatin, cocaine, ethambutol, lead, mercury, methanol, quinine, thallium |
| Blue skin | Amiodarone, FD&C #1 dye, methemoglobinemia, silver |
| Constipation | Anticholinergics,[a] botulism, lead, opioids, thallium (severe) |
| Deafness, tinnitus | Aminoglycosides, carbon disolfide, cisplatin, loop diuretics, macrolides, metals, quinine, quinolones, salicylates |
| Diaphoresis | Amphetamines, cholinergics,[c] hypoglycemia, opioid withdrawal, salicylates, serotonin toxicity, sympathomimetics,[b] withdrawal from ethanol and sedative–hypnotics |
| Diarrhea | Arsenic and other metals, boric acid (blue-green), botanical irritants, cathartics, cholinergics,[c] colchicine, iron, lithium, opioid withdrawal, radiation |
| Dysesthesias, paresthesias | Acrylamide, arsenic, ciguatera, cocaine, colchicine, thallium |
| Gum discoloration | Arsenic, bismuth, hypervitaminosis A, lead, mercury |
| Hallucinations | Anticholinergics,[a] dopamine agonists, ergot alkaloids, ethanol, ethanol and sedative–hypnotic withdrawal, LSD, phencyclidine, sympathomimetics,[b] tryptamines |
| Headache | Carbon monoxide, hypoglycemia, MAOI–food interaction (hypertensive crisis), serotonin toxicity |
| Metabolic acidosis (elevated anion gap) | Methanol, uremia, ketoacidosis (diabetic, starvation, alcoholic), paraldehyde, metformin, iron, isoniazid, lactic acidosis, cyanide, protease inhibitors, ethylene glycol, salicylates, toluene |
| Miosis | Cholinergics,[c] clonidine, opioids, phencyclidine, phenothiazines |
| Mydriasis | Anticholinergics,[a] botulism, opioid withdrawal, sympathomimetics[b] |
| Nystagmus | Barbiturates, carbamazepine, carbon monoxide, dextromethorphan, ethanol, lithium, MAOIs, phencyclidine, phenytoin, quinine, synthetic cannabinoid receptor agonists |
| Purpura | Anticoagulant rodenticides, corticosteroids, heparin, pit viper venom, quinine, salicylates, anticoagulants, levamisole |
| Radiopaque ingestions | Arsenic, halogenated hydrocarbons, iodinated compounds metals (eg, iron, lead), potassium compounds |
| Red skin | Anticholinergics,[a] boric acid, disulfiram, hydroxocobalamin, scombroid, vancomycin |
| Rhabdomyolysis | Carbon monoxide, doxylamine, HMG-CoA reductase inhibitors, sympathomimetics,[b] *Tricholoma equestre mushrooms* |
| Salivation | Arsenic, caustics, cholinergics,[c] clozapine, ketamine, mercury, phencyclidine, strychnine |
| Seizures | Bupropion, camphor, carbon monoxide, cyclic antidepressants, *Gyromitra* mushrooms, hypoglycemia, isoniazid, methylxanthines, ethanol and sedative–hypnotic withdrawal |
| Tremor | Antipsychotics, arsenic, carbon monoxide, cholinergics,[c] ethanol, lithium, mercury, methyl bromide, sympathomimetics,[b] thyroid hormones |
| Weakness | Botulism, diuretics, magnesium, paralytic shellfish, steroids, toluene |
| Yellow skin | APAP (late), pyrrolizidine alkaloids, β carotene, amatoxin mushrooms, dinitrophenol |

[a]Anticholinergics, including antihistamines, atropine, cyclic antidepressants, and scopolamine.

[b]Sympathomimetics, including adrenergic agonists, amphetamines, cocaine, and ephedrine.

[c]Cholinergics, including muscarinic mushrooms; organic phosphorus compounds and carbamates, including select Alzheimer disease drugs and physostigmine; and pilocarpine and other direct-acting xenobiotics.

APAP = acetaminophen; HMG-CoA = 3-hydroxy-3-methyl-glutaryl-CoA; LSD = lysergic acid diethylamide; MAOI = monoamine oxidase inhibitor.

## Further Evaluation of All Patients with Suspected Xenobiotic Exposures

Vital signs should be obtained serially and a full physical examination should be performed. Toxicologic etiologies of abnormal vital signs and physical findings are summarized in Tables 1–1 to 1–6. Toxic syndromes, sometimes called "toxidromes," are summarized in Table 1–2.

Typically, in the management of patients with toxicologic emergencies, there is both a necessity and an opportunity to obtain various diagnostic studies and ancillary tests interspersed with stabilizing the patient's condition, obtaining the history, and performing the physical examination. For most patients with unintentional exposures or intended self-harm the routine use of laboratory testing is of limited value. Specifically, urine and serum drug screens add little if anything to clinical management and are often misleading or misinterpreted. Rather targeted laboratory testing is preferred as guided by the history and physical examination.

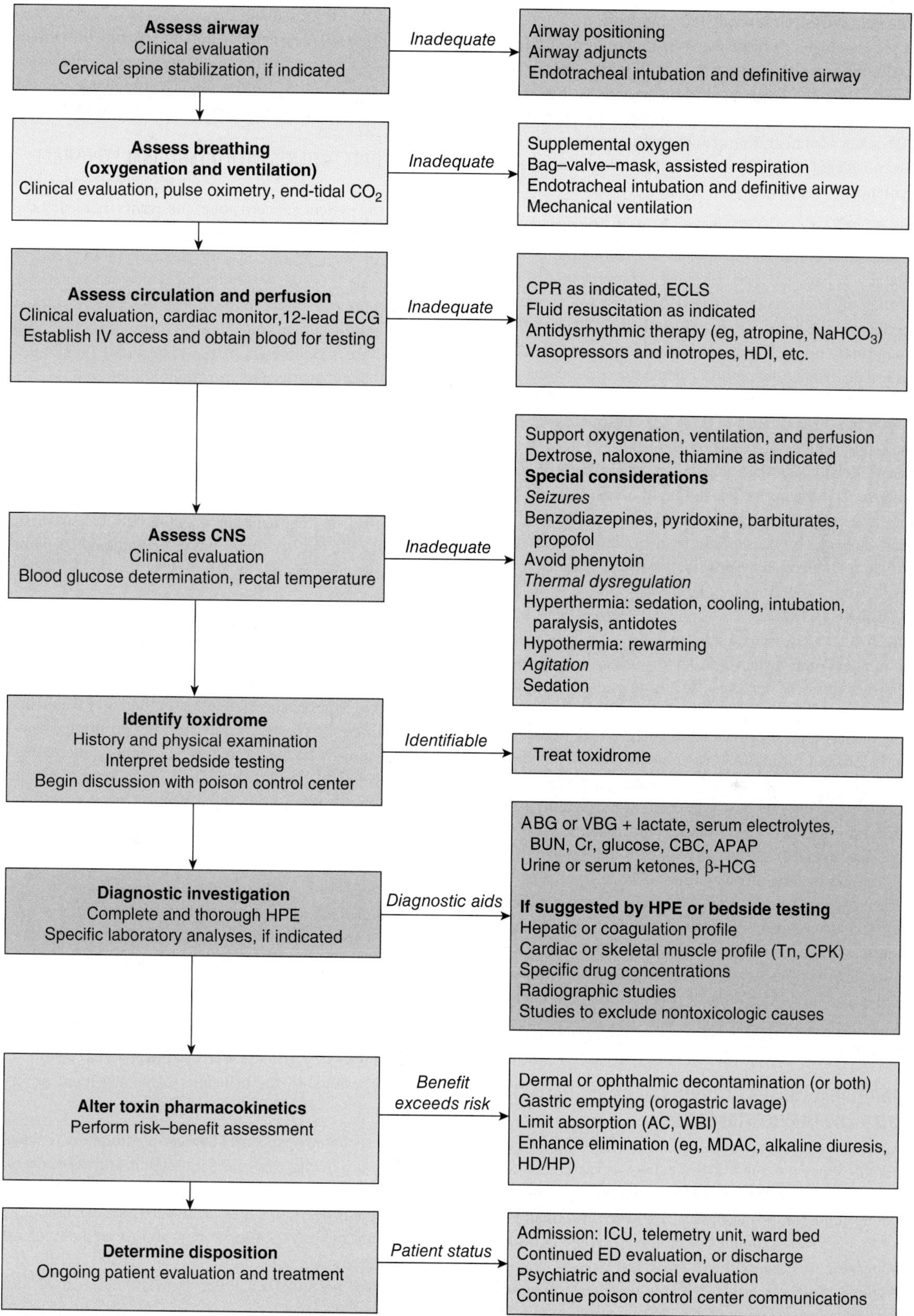


**FIGURE 2–1.** This algorithm is a basic guide to the management of poisoned patients. A more detailed description of the steps in management may be found in the accompanying text. This algorithm is only a guide to actual management, which must, of course, consider the patient's clinical status. ABG = arterial blood gas; AC = activated charcoal; APAP = acetaminophen; β-HCG = β-human chorionic gonadotropin; CBC = complete blood count; CNS = central nervous system; CPK = creatine phosphokinase; CPR = cardiopulmonary resuscitation; Cr, creatinine; ECG = electrocardiograph; ECLS = extracorporeal life support; HD = hemodialysis; HDI = high-dose insulin; HP = hemoperfusion; HPE = history and physical examination; ICU = intensive care unit; MDAC = multiple-dose activated charcoal; Tn = troponin; VBG = venous blood gas; WBI = whole-bowel irrigation.

### The Role of Gastrointestinal Decontamination

A series of highly individualized treatment decisions regarding limiting the exposure to the xenobiotic follow the initial stabilization and assessment of the patient. As noted previously and as discussed in detail in Chap. 3, evacuation of the GI tract or administration of activated charcoal can no longer be considered standard or routine toxicologic care for most patients.

### Eliminating Absorbed Xenobiotics from the Body

Discussions of the indications for and techniques of manipulating urinary pH (ion trapping), diuresis, hemodialysis, hemoperfusion, continuous renal replacement therapy, and exchange transfusion are found in Chap. 4. Alkalinization of the urinary pH with sodium bicarbonate is used to enhance salicylate elimination (other xenobiotics are discussed in Chap. 4), and sodium bicarbonate also prevents toxicity from methotrexate (Antidotes in Brief: A5). If extracorporeal elimination is contemplated, hemodialysis is used for patients who overdose with salicylates, methanol, ethylene glycol, lithium, valproic acid, and other xenobiotics that are either dialyzable or cause fluid and electrolyte abnormalities. Plasmapheresis and exchange transfusion are used to eliminate xenobiotics with large molecular weights that are not dialyzable.

## AVOIDING PITFALLS

The history alone is not a reliable indicator of which patients require naloxone, hypertonic dextrose, thiamine, and oxygen. Instead, the need for these therapies should be evaluated and performed if indicated (unless specifically contraindicated) only after a clinical assessment for all patients with AMS. Attributing an AMS to alcohol because of an odor on a patient's breath is potentially misleading. Small amounts of alcohol or alcoholic beverage congeners generally produce the same breath odor as do intoxicating amounts. Conversely, even when an extremely high blood ethanol concentration is confirmed by laboratory analysis, it is dangerous to ignore other possible causes of an AMS. Because some individuals with an alcohol use disorder are alert with ethanol concentrations in excess of 500 mg/dL, a concentration that would result in coma and possibly apnea and death in a nontolerant person, finding a high ethanol concentration does not eliminate the need for further search into the cause of a depressed level of consciousness.

## ADDITIONAL CONSIDERATIONS IN MANAGING PATIENTS WITH A NORMAL MENTAL STATUS

As in the case of patients with AMS, vital signs must be obtained and recorded. If the patient is alert, talking, and in no respiratory distress, all that remains to document are the respiratory rate and rhythm. Because the patient is alert, additional history should be obtained, keeping in mind that information regarding the number and types of xenobiotics ingested, time elapsed, prior vomiting, and other critical information may be unreliable. Speaking to a friend or relative of the patient may provide an opportunity to learn useful and reliable information regarding the exposure, the patient's frame of mind, a history of previous exposures, and the type of support that is available if the patient is discharged from the ED. At times, it is essential to initially separate the patient from any relatives or friends to obtain greater cooperation from the patient and avoid violating confidentiality and because the interpersonal anxiety may interfere with therapy.

## APPROACHING PATIENTS WITH INTENTIONAL EXPOSURES

Initial efforts at establishing rapport with the patient by indicating to the patient concern about the events that led to the ingestion and the availability of help after the xenobiotic is removed (if such procedures are planned) often facilitate management. If GI decontamination is deemed beneficial, the reason for and nature of the procedure should be clearly explained to the patient together with reassurance that after the procedure is completed, there will be ample time to discuss his or her concerns and provide additional care.

## SPECIAL CONSIDERATIONS FOR MANAGING PREGNANT PATIENTS

In general, a successful outcome for both the mother and fetus depends on optimum management of the mother. Proven effective treatment for a potentially serious toxic exposure to the mother should never be withheld based on theoretical concerns regarding the fetus.

### Physiologic Factors

A pregnant woman's total blood volume and cardiac output are elevated through the second trimester and into the later stages of the third trimester. This means that signs of hypoperfusion and hypotension manifest later than they would in a woman who is not pregnant, and when they do, uterine blood flow may already be compromised. Maintaining the patient in the left-lateral decubitus position helps prevent supine hypotension resulting from impairment of systemic venous return by compression of the inferior vena cava.

### Use of Antidotes

Limited data are available on the use of antidotes in pregnancy. In general, antidotes should not be used if the indications for use are equivocal. On the other hand, antidotes should not be withheld if they have the potential to reduce potential maternal morbidity and mortality as the health of the fetus is directly linked to that of the mother.

## MANAGEMENT OF PATIENTS WITH CUTANEOUS EXPOSURE

In all of these cases, the principles of management are as follows:

1. Avoid secondary exposures by wearing protective (rubber or plastic) gowns, gloves, eye protection, and shoe covers. Cases of serious secondary poisoning have occurred in emergency personnel after prolonged skin contact with xenobiotics such as organic phosphorus compounds on the victim's skin or clothing.
2. Remove the patient's clothing, place it in plastic bags, and then seal the bags.
3. Wash the patient with soap and copious amounts of water twice regardless of how much time has elapsed since the exposure.

4. Make no attempt to neutralize an acid with a base or a base with an acid. Further tissue damage may result from the heat generated by the exothermic reaction.
5. Avoid using any greases or creams because they will only keep the xenobiotic in close contact with the skin and ultimately make removal more difficult.

Special Considerations: SC1 discusses the principles of preventing dermal absorption.

## MANAGEMENT OF PATIENTS WITH OPHTHALMIC EXPOSURES

The eyes should be irrigated with the eyelids fully retracted for no less than 20 minutes. To facilitate irrigation, an anesthetic should be used, and the eyelids should be kept open with an eyelid retractor. An adequate irrigation stream is obtained by running 1 L of 0.9% sodium chloride through regular IV tubing held a few inches from the eye or by using an irrigating lens. Checking the eyelid fornices with pH paper strips is important to ensure adequate irrigation; the pH should normally be 6.5 to 7.6 if accurately tested, although when using paper test strips, the measurement will often be near 8.0. SC1 describes the management of toxic ophthalmic exposures in more detail.

## IDENTIFYING PATIENTS WITH NONTOXIC EXPOSURES

The following general guidelines for determining that an exposure is either nontoxic or minimally toxic will assist clinical decision making:

1. Identification of the product and its ingredients is possible.
2. None of the United States Consumer Product Safety Commission's "signal words" (CAUTION, WARNING, or DANGER) appear on the product label.
3. The route of exposure is known.
4. A reliable approximation of the maximum exposure quantity is able to be made.
5. Based on the available medical literature and clinical experience, the potential effects related to the exposure are expected to be benign or at worst self-limited and not likely to require the patient to access health care.
6. The patient is asymptomatic or has developed the maximal expected self-limited toxicity.
7. Adequate time has occurred to assess the potential for the development of toxicity.

For any patient in whom there is a question about the nature of the exposure, it is not appropriate to consider that exposure nontoxic. All such patients, and all patients for whom the health care provider is unsure of the risks associated with a given exposure, should be referred either to the regional poison control center or health care facility for further evaluation.

## DISPOSITION OF PATIENTS

The poison control center must determine the need for direct medical care in a hospital or whether the patient has had a nontoxic exposure (discussed earlier) and can be managed at home. In the ED, many patients are discharged after their evaluation and treatment and after psychiatric and social services evaluations are obtained as needed. Among clinically ill poisoned patients, the decision is generally simplified based on the relative abilities of the various units within the medical facility. Critical care units expend the highest level of resources to assure both intensive monitoring and the provision of timely care and are necessary for patients who are currently ill or currently stable but likely to decompensate. See Table 2–3 for a description of patients best suited

**TABLE 2–3 Define the Indications for Intensive Care Unit Admission**

| *Patient Characteristics* | *Xenobiotic Characteristics* | *Capabilities of the Inpatient or Observation Unit* |
|---|---|---|
| Does the patient have any signs of serious end-organ toxicity?<br>Are the end-organ effects progressing?<br>Are laboratory data suggestive of serious toxicity?<br>Is the patient a high risk for complications requiring ICU intervention?<br>  Seizures<br>  Unresponsive to verbal stimuli<br>  Level of consciousness impaired to the point of potential airway compromise<br>  $PCO_2$ >45 mm Hg<br>  Systolic blood pressure <80 mm Hg (in an adult)<br>  Cardiac dysrhythmias (ventricular dysrhythmias, high-grade conduction abnormalities)<br>  Abnormal ECG complexes and intervals (QRS duration ≥0.10 seconds; QT interval prolongation)<br>  Refractory or recurrent hypoglycemia<br>Is the patient at high risk for complications such as aspiration pneumonitis, anoxic brain injury, rhabdomyolysis, or compartment syndrome?<br>Does the patient have preexisting medical conditions that could predispose to complications?<br>  Alcohol or drug dependence<br>  Liver disease<br>  Acute kidney injury or chronic kidney disease<br>  Heart disease<br>  Pregnancy: Is the xenobiotic or the antidote teratogenic?<br>Is the patient suicidal? | Are there known serious sequelae (eg, cyclic antidepressants, CCBs)?<br>Can the patient deteriorate rapidly from its toxic effects?<br>Is the onset of toxicity likely to be delayed (eg, modified-release preparation, slowed GI motility, or delayed toxic effects)?<br>Does the xenobiotic have effects that will require cardiac monitoring?<br>Is the amount ingested a potentially serious or potentially lethal dose?<br>Are xenobiotic concentrations rising?<br>Is the required or planned therapy unconventional (eg, large doses of atropine for treating overdoses of organic phosphorus compounds; or high dose insulin for CCB overdose)?<br>Does the therapy have potentially serious adverse effects?<br>Is there insufficient literature to describe the potential human toxic effects?<br>Are potentially serious coingestants likely (must take into account the reliability of the history)? | Does the admitting health care team appreciate the potential seriousness of a toxicologic emergency?<br>Is the nursing staff:<br>  Familiar with this toxicologic emergency?<br>  Familiar with the potential for serious complications?<br>Is the staffing adequate to monitor the patient?<br>  What is the ratio of nurses to patients?<br>  Are time-consuming nursing activities required and realistic?<br>Can a safe environment be provided for a suicidal patient?<br>  Can a patient have suicide precautions and monitoring with a medical floor bed?<br>  Can a one-to-one observer be present in the room with the patient?<br>  Can the patient be restrained or sedated? |

CCB = calcium channel blocker; ECG = electrocardiogram; GI = gastrointestinal; ICU = intensive care unit.

for admission to a critical care unit. Determining the optimal disposition for a poisoned patient requires an evaluation of the nature of the exposure, the patient, and the capabilities of the community and the institution. Most often such decisions are made conservatively and cautiously, given the unpredictable nature of human poisoning.

## ENSURING AN OPTIMAL OUTCOME

The best way to ensure an optimal outcome for the patient with a suspected toxic exposure is to apply the principles of basic and advanced life support in conjunction with a planned and stepwise approach toxicologic risk assessment. Always bear in mind that a toxicologic etiology or co-etiology for any abnormal conditions necessitates modifying whatever standard approach is typically brought to the bedside of a severely ill patient. Involvement of the expertise of a poison control center, a medical toxicologist, or a clinical toxicologist can help direct both diagnosis and management strategies to improve the efficiency of the patient's care and the outcome. The thoughtful combination of stabilization, general management principles, and both empiric and specific treatment when indicated will result in successful outcomes in the majority of patients with actual or suspected exposures.

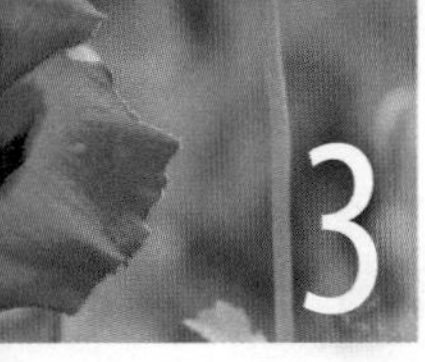

# 3 TECHNIQUES USED TO PREVENT GASTROINTESTINAL ABSORPTION

Gastrointestinal (GI) decontamination is a highly controversial issue in medical toxicology. It can play an essential role in the initial phase of management of orally poisoned patients and frequently is the only treatment available other than routine supportive care. Unfortunately, as is true in most areas of medical toxicology, rigorous studies that demonstrate the effects of GI decontamination on clinically meaningful endpoints are difficult to perform and few of such studies are published. The heterogeneity of poisoned patients demands that very large, randomized studies be performed because patients who present to an emergency department (ED) typically have both unreliable or imprecise ingestions histories and low-risk or multiple xenobiotics exposures (Chap. 2). These factors, as well as other significant sources of bias, are often hidden in the inclusion and exclusion criteria of even the best available studies. Numerous determinants contribute to the difficulties in designing and completing studies that provide sound evidence for or against a particular therapeutic option. As might be suspected, no available study provides adequate guidance for the management of a patient who has definitely ingested an unknown xenobiotic at an unknown time. Fortunately, in most cases, there is some component of the history or clinical presentation that offers insight into the nature of the ingested xenobiotic (Chap. 1). It is our recommendation that decontamination should rarely be omitted unless a minimally toxic exposure has occurred.

The reported trends in the use of GI decontamination demonstrate a continued decline in the United States (US). The frequency of activated charcoal (AC) use declined from 4.6% of all exposures in 2006 to 1.97% in 2015, and a similar decline was observed in the frequency of orogastric lavage (4.2% in 2006 to 0.08% in 2015) and whole-bowel irrigation (WBI) (0.11% in 2006 to 0.08% in 2015). The decline in the use of GI decontamination likely results from an epidemiologic shift in developed countries away from overdoses of more difficult to treat or more lethal xenobiotics, such as salicylates, theophylline, barbiturates, and cyclic antidepressants, toward benzodiazepines, prescription opioids, serotonergic reuptake inhibitors, and acetaminophen (APAP), with a natural resultant decrease in morbidity and mortality or the availability of an excellent antidote. Although true for developed countries, studies in developing countries indicate a different pattern of poisonings, with patients ingesting xenobiotics such as organic phosphorus compounds and other pesticides and herbicides with a more lethal toxicologic profile.

Similarly, the use of orogastric lavage is continually declining. The frequency of orogastric lavage varies from lowest frequency (percent of lavage compared with total decontaminations modalities using AC, orogastric lavage, and WBI) in North America (0.08%, US) and Scandinavia (7.9%–9%; Denmark and Norway), in Mediterranean countries and Russia (30%–33%; Spain, Palestine, and Russia), to the highest frequency in Asia and South American countries, India (34%–50%), Nepal (43%), and Bolivia (96%). As noted earlier, the frequency tends to correlate with the type of xenobiotic ingested, with the highest frequency of lavage in regions where insecticides such as organic phosphorus compounds and carbamates are more commonly ingested. Additionally, the use of decontamination seems to correlate inversely with availability of costly antidotes and ICUs.

This chapter does not discuss details with regard to the risk assessment and general principles of managing acutely poisoned or overdosed patients; these issues are discussed in Chap. 2. Rather, the focus is on when to do GI decontamination and what exactly to do. Detailed discussions of AC and WBI are found in the corresponding Antidotes in Brief sections, Activated Charcoal (Antidotes in Brief: A1) and Whole-Bowel Irrigation and Other Intestinal Evacuants (Antidotes in Brief: A2). In addition, when the ingested xenobiotic is known, readers should also refer to the decontamination sections found in Chapters 6–100 and Special Considerations SC1, which offer insight into xenobiotic-specific issues that may alter decontamination strategies.

The efficacy of techniques used to prevent absorption of xenobiotics from the GI tract depends on one simple concept: **At the time of the intervention, there must be enough xenobiotic in the GI tract to alter the patient's outcome if absorbed.**

## TIME

Ingestion is the most common route of exposure in poisoning in the US and many other countries. After ingestion, rates of absorption of pharmaceuticals are based on pharmacokinetic studies that are typically performed on fasting healthy human volunteers given a minimal number of pills with a small amount of liquid. In contrast, most overdose patients take large numbers of pills with some liquid or food. Gastric emptying time is prolonged by the presence of food or other solids compared with liquids.

Case reports and clinical practice demonstrate that poisoned patients still have xenobiotics in their stomachs as residuals or pharmacobezoars, from hours up to several days after ingestion and even on autopsy. In a prospective study of 85 poisoned patients, markedly prolonged gastric emptying half-lives and gastric hypomotility were demonstrated using gastric scintigraphy. Similarly, using upper GI endoscopy in 167 adult patients presenting to an ED after an oral drug overdose, residual gastric contents were found in 60% of the patients presenting more than 1 hour after ingestion. In fact, many patients had significant material remaining in the stomach many hours later.

Although the ability of xenobiotics to be removed by orogastric lavage is variable and unknown, the ability of AC to prevent absorption by adsorption of the xenobiotic is

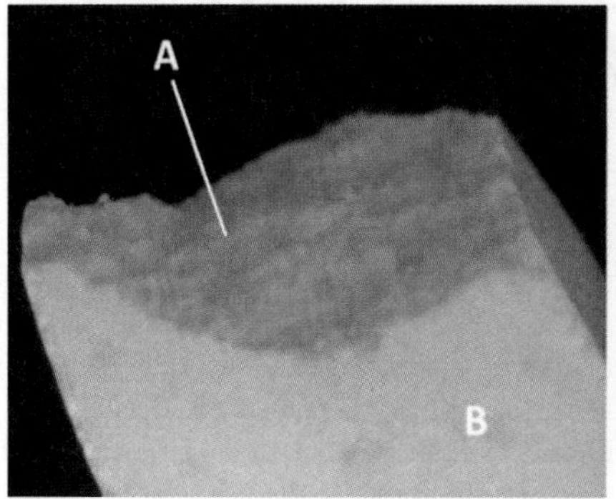


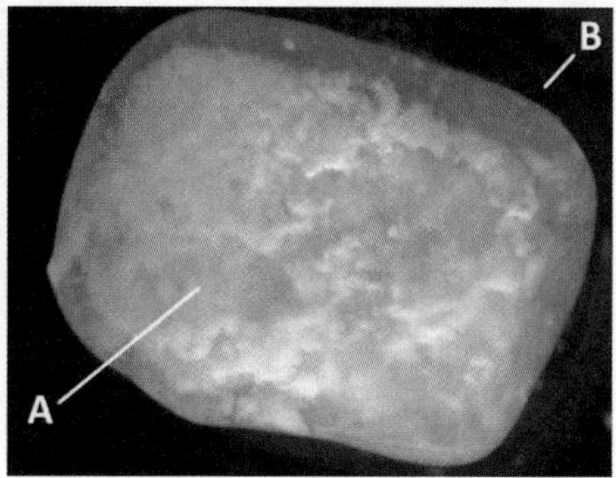


**FIGURE 3–1.** Acetaminophen 500-mg extended-release tablet microscopy. The tablet cut was in halves and showed as the dry tablet at the left and after incubation in 1 L of simulated gastric fluid for 4 hours at 37°C. **A,** Tablet core. **B,** Hydrogel polymer coating material (*left*) forming the swelled gel-layer (*right*) surface of the tablet. (*Used with permission from Lotte C. G. Hoegberg as supervisor, mentor and collaborator with Refsgaard F, Petersen SH. In Vitro Investigation of Potential Pharmacobezoar Formation and Their Dissolution of Extended Release Tablets [master's thesis]. Copenhagen: Section of Toxicology, Department of Pharmacy, School of Pharmaceutical Sciences, Faculty of Health Sciences, University of Copenhagen; 2016.*)

likely beneficial far later than the 1 hour that is commonly promoted in many clinical scenarios rather than a blanket one-size-fits-all dogma. Additional factors to consider are the changes in drug delivery systems that are more commonly available in recent years. They include hydrophilic matrix systems, in which the polymeric coating swells in contact with an aqueous medium to form a gel layer on the surface of the tablet (Fig. 3–1), which tends to cause tablet adherence in aqueous acidic media (Fig. 3–2). This adherence is recognized in growing reports of pharmacobezoars, in which the active xenobiotic is ultimately released by dissolution, diffusion, or erosion. The release of xenobiotic(s) retained within the pharmacobezoar is slower compared with the release from individual tablets because the surface-to-volume ratio is lower, thereby reducing the rate of dissolution. The time to appearance of symptoms in the patient is expected to be both delayed and prolonged and the maximum serum concentration possibly lower, but as long as the xenobiotic(s) remains in the pharmacobezoar, continuous release will occur. There are no specific rules that adequately predict when pharmacobezoars form or in which patients they form, and after they have formed, pharmacobezoars are difficult to identify. Evidence of continuing absorption should raise suspicion for pharmacobezoar formation.

## OROGASTRIC LAVAGE

The principal theory governing orogastric lavage for gastric emptying is very simple: if a portion of a xenobiotic with substantial toxic potential is removed before absorption, toxicity should be either prevented or diminished. The relevant amount of xenobiotic that needs to be removed to obtain a beneficial treatment effect varies depending on the xenobiotic, the amount ingested, the overall health of the patient, and the shape of the dose–response curve for the individual xenobiotic. The xenobiotic size also has to be retrievable through the lumen of the tube used for the procedure. Even though the benefit of orogastric lavage is debated, many publications demonstrate that there is a continued frequent or routine use of orogastric lavage around the world. Unfortunately, most reports fail to quantify the amount of xenobiotic removed.

Several clinical trials attempted to define the role of gastric emptying in poisoned patients. Although all of these studies were limited because of the inclusion of a large number of low-risk patients, numerous restrictive exclusion criteria, and methodologic biases, they clearly demonstrated that many patients can be successfully managed without orogastric lavage. No new clear evidence to support the clinical effectiveness of orogastric lavage is available, and studies and reports describe a modest, varied, and unreliable effect.

The ability to visualize fragments before determination of the need for GI decontamination has revitalized interest in selected use of orogastric lavage, and studies and case reports evaluate the amount of xenobiotic in the stomach before the initiation of orogastric lavage. Gastric tablet fragments that are identified by endoscopy confirm gastric presence of the ingested xenobiotic and a potential benefit from orogastric lavage. Additionally, direct visualization allows observation of the effectiveness of orogastric lavage. Similarly, approaches have been taken using abdominal computed tomography and transabdominal ultrasonography with limited results.

The clinical parameters listed in Table 3–1 help to identify individuals for whom orogastric lavage is usually not indicated based on a risk-to-benefit analysis. In contrast, for a small subset of patients (Table 3–1), gastric emptying is still recommended. Time is an important consideration because for orogastric lavage to be beneficial, a consequential amount of xenobiotic must still be present in the stomach. Demographic studies have found that very few poisoned patients arrive at the ED within 1 to 2 hours of ingestion. In most studies, the average time from ingestion to presentation is approximately 3 to 4 hours, with significant variations. This delay diminishes the likelihood of recovering a large percentage of the xenobiotic from the stomach to reduce a grave or possible lethal amount to a survivable amount except in those who have taken a massive amount. As discussed earlier, there is growing evidence to support the delayed persistence

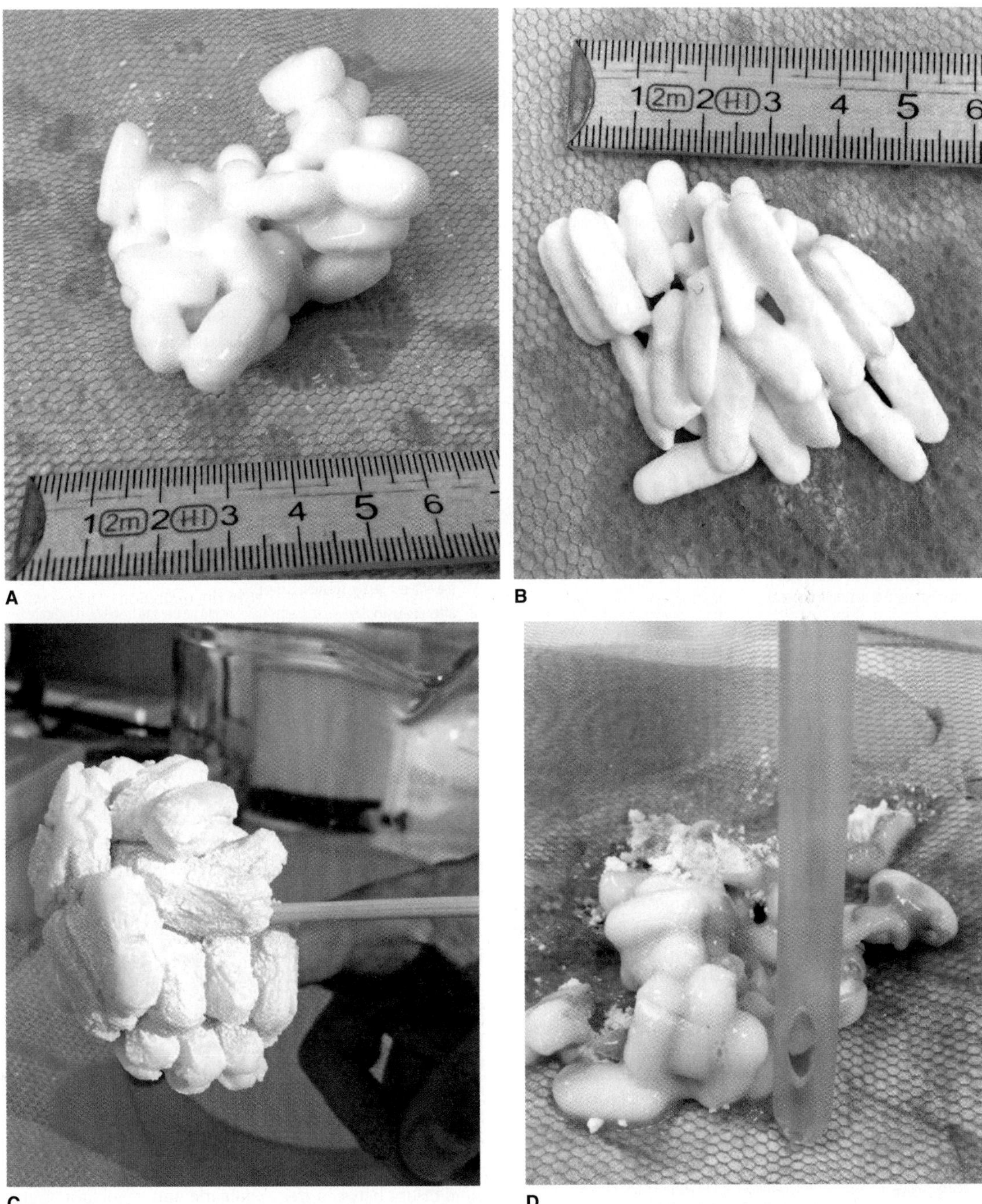


**FIGURE 3–2.** Pharmacobezoar formation of four different extended-release formulations. A total of 30 tablets were incubated in 1 L of simulated gastric fluid (Ph.Eur., omitting pepsin) for up to 48 hours at 37°C. **A,** Acetaminophen extended release, 500 mg, 4 hours. **B,** Acetaminophen combined immediate and extended release, 665 mg, 4 hours. **C,** Verapamil extended release, 240 mg, 48 hours. **D,** Quetiapine extended release, 50 mg, 4 hours, and orogastric tube size 30 Fr. (*Used with permission from Lotte C. G. Hoegberg as supervisor, mentor and collaborator with Refsgaard F, Petersen SH. In Vitro Investigation of Potential Pharmacobezoar Formation and Their Dissolution of Extended Release Tablets [master's thesis]. Copenhagen: Section of Toxicology, Department of Pharmacy, School of Pharmaceutical Sciences, Faculty of Health Sciences, University of Copenhagen; 2016.*)

of significant amounts of drug in the stomach of selected overdose patients, thereby invalidating any concept of a hard stop occurring 60 minutes post ingestion.

Assessment of whether or not orogastric lavage is appropriate for a patient must include an evaluation for potential contraindications and an evaluation of airway protection. (Table 3–2). In some cases, orogastric lavage delays AC administration further, and it is reasonable to eliminate orogastric lavage and only administer AC in cases when the benefits of orogastric lavage are estimated to be minimal

**TABLE 3–1 Risk Assessment: When to Consider Orogastric Lavage**

| *Orogastric Lavage Is Usually Not Indicated*[a] | *Orogastric Lavage Is Indicated*[b] |
|---|---|
| The xenobiotic has limited toxicity at almost any dose.<br>Although the xenobiotic ingested is potentially toxic, the dose ingested is likely less than that expected to produce significant illness.<br>The ingested xenobiotic is well adsorbed by AC, and the amount ingested is not expected to exceed the adsorptive capacity of AC.<br>Significant spontaneous emesis has already occurred.<br>The patient presents many hours postingestion and has minimal signs or symptoms of poisoning.<br>The ingested xenobiotic has a highly efficient antidote (eg, APAP and *N*-acetylcysteine).<br>The procedure cannot be accomplished appropriately or safely (wrong tube size, lack of provider skill, anticipated extant esophageal or gastric injury, etc.) | The ingested xenobiotic is known to produce life-threatening toxicity *or* the patient has obvious signs or symptoms of life-threatening toxicity and<br>• There is reason to believe that, given the time of ingestion, a significant amount of the ingested xenobiotic is still present in the stomach *or*<br>• The ingested xenobiotic is not adsorbed by AC or AC is unavailable *or*<br>• Although the ingested xenobiotic is adsorbed by AC, the amount ingested exceeds the AC–xenobiotic ratio of 10:1 even when using a dose of AC that is twice the standard dose recommended *and*<br>• The patient has not had spontaneous emesis *or*<br>• No highly effective specific antidote exists or alternative therapies (eg, hemodialysis) pose a significant risk to the patient. |

[a]Patients who fulfill some of these criteria can be decontaminated safely with activated charcoal alone or in many cases require no decontamination at all.
[b]Patients who fulfill these criteria should undergo orogastric lavage *if* there are no contraindications or other compelling time-dependent interventions. For individuals who meet some of these criteria but who are judged not to be candidates for orogastric lavage, single- or multiple-dose activated charcoal or whole-bowel irrigation (or both) should be used.

AC = activated charcoal; APAP = acetaminophen.

to initiate the fastest decontamination procedure. The procedure should always be performed by trained health care professionals and in health care settings. When deciding whether to actually perform orogastric lavage for a poisoned patient, these indications, contraindications, and potential adverse effects must be considered. Table 3–3 summarizes our recommended technique of orogastric lavage.

**TABLE 3–2 Orogastric Lavage: Indications and Contraindications**

| *Indications* | *Contraindications* |
|---|---|
| The patient meets some of the criteria for orogastric lavage (Table 3–1).<br>The benefits of orogastric lavage outweigh the risks. | The patient does not meet any of the criteria for orogastric lavage (Table 3–1).<br>The patient has lost or will likely lose his or her airway protective reflexes without being intubated. (After intubation, orogastric lavage can be performed if otherwise indicated.)<br>Ingestion of a xenobiotic with a high aspiration potential (eg, a hydrocarbon) in the absence of endotracheal intubation.<br>Ingestion of an alkaline caustic.<br>Ingestion of a foreign body (eg, a drug packet).<br>The patient is at risk of hemorrhage or gastrointestinal perforation because of underlying pathology, recent surgery, or another medical condition that could be further compromised by the use of orogastric lavage.<br>Ingestion of a xenobiotic in a form known to be too large to fit into the lumen of the lavage tube (eg, many modified-release preparations). |

**TABLE 3–3 Technique for Performing Orogastric Lavage**

**Select the correct tube size**

Adults and adolescents: 36–40 Fr
Children: 22–28 Fr

**Procedure**

1. If there is potential for airway compromise, endotracheal intubation should precede orogastric lavage.
2. The patient should be kept in the left lateral decubitus position if possible. Because the pylorus points upward in this orientation, this positioning theoretically helps prevent the xenobiotic from advancing through the pylorus during the procedure.
3. Before insertion, the proper length of tubing to be passed should be measured and marked on the tube. The length should allow the most proximal tube opening to be passed beyond the lower esophageal sphincter.
4. After the tube is inserted, it is essential to confirm that the distal end of the tube is in the stomach by withdrawal of material; injecting air; or if unable to clinically confirm placement, use radiographic confirmation.
5. Any material present in the stomach should be withdrawn.
6. In adults, 250-mL aliquots of a room temperature 0.9% saline lavage solution is instilled via a funnel or lavage syringe. In children, aliquots should be 10–15 mL/kg to a maximum of 250 mL.
7. Orogastric lavage should continue for at least several liters in an adult and for at least 0.5 to 1.0 L in a child or until a colorless particulate matter returns and the effluent lavage solution is clear.
8. After orogastric lavage, the same tube should be used to instill AC if indicated.
9. The tube should be withdrawn/removed.

## ACTIVATED CHARCOAL

Activated charcoal is an effective method for reducing the absorption of many xenobiotics. For certain xenobiotics, it also enhances elimination through interruption of either the enterohepatic or enteroenteric cycle. Its superb adsorptive properties theoretically make it the most useful management strategy for undifferentiated patients with acute oral overdoses.

### Mechanism

The entire effect of AC takes place in the GI tract. Oral AC is not absorbed through the wall of the GI tract but rather passes straight through the gut unchanged. To be adsorbed to AC, the xenobiotic must be dissolved in the GI liquid phase and be in physical contact with the AC. The possible sites of adsorption are demonstrated in Fig. 3–3. The surface (internal and external) of AC is specifically manufactured to chemically adsorb certain xenobiotics. Activated charcoal forms an equilibrium between free xenobiotic and xenobiotic that is adsorbed to it through relatively weak intermolecular forces.

$$\text{Free xenobiotic} + \text{AC} \Leftrightarrow \text{Xenobiotic–AC complex}$$

Desorption of the adsorbed xenobiotic occurs slowly over time and is best studied for acid toxins as they move from the acidic environment of the stomach through the alkaline small bowel. But if sufficient AC is present, the equilibrium remains shifted toward the xenobiotic–AC complex.

### Efficacy

However, as is true for the other methods of GI decontamination, there is a lack of sound evidence of its benefits as defined by clinically meaningful endpoints. Thus, evaluations

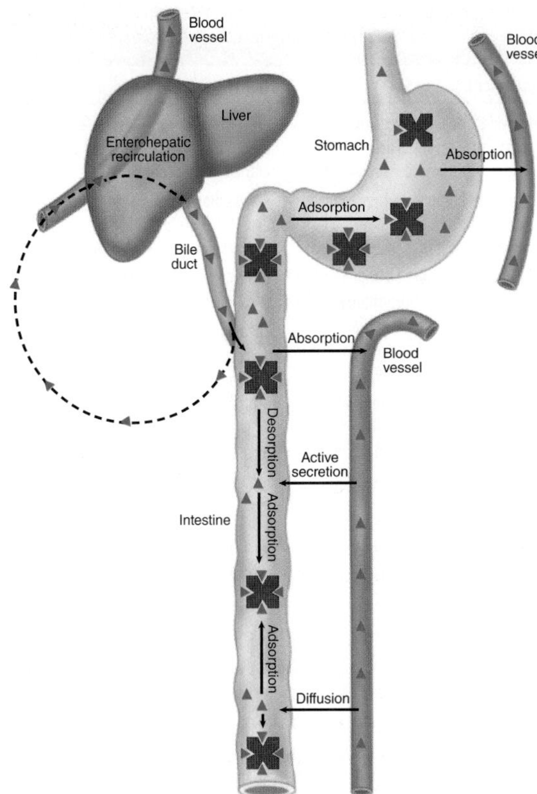


**FIGURE 3–3.** Mechanism of xenobiotic (▼) removal by AC in the luminal space of the gastrointestinal tract. The position of systemic xenobiotic absorption depends on the physical chemical characteristics of the xenobiotic and takes place from stomach, intestine, or both. Xenobiotic reentry into the luminal space can take place by enterohepatic recirculation and enteroenteric recirculation by active secretion and passive diffusion. Excess and continued supply of activated charcoal facilitates adsorption of recycled xenobiotic and favors continued active and passive diffusion of xenobiotic to the luminal space and adsorption of xenobiotic.

of the efficacy of AC are often performed by comparisons of pharmacokinetic parameters, such as area under the blood xenobiotic concentration–time curve (AUC), maximum blood concentration of the xenobiotic (Cmax), time to maximum blood concentration (Tmax), and elimination half-life ($t_{½}$). More novel approaches include population pharmacokinetics. In contrast, several randomized controlled trials fail to show a benefit of AC over either emesis or no therapy at all. Most suffer from inclusion of a large number of low-risk patients and selection biases from extensive exclusion criteria.

Theoretically, early administration of AC to a patient presenting with a significant oral overdose of a potentially toxic xenobiotic would lower systemic exposure to that xenobiotic and thus be of benefit to the patient. The precise definition of "early" is yet to be defined; however, a range of reports show significant beneficial effects even if dosing is delayed up to 4 hours after the xenobiotic ingestion. It should be clear that the commonly promulgated limitation of a 1-hour time frame should serve as a guideline rather than an absolute endpoint. It is only logical that if an intervention is effective at 59 minutes, it will also be beneficial at 61 minutes. Because after massive life-threatening ingestions, the absorption of xenobiotics is prolonged, **there is no exact time limit for AC use.** It is therefore recommended to administer AC to *prevent absorption* in poisoned patients even when they present late to medical care if there is a potential for clinically significant ongoing absorption. Additional benefits on enhanced elimination are discussed later.

## Prehospital Use

Prehospital use of AC has not gained wide acceptance because of unfounded concerns that it would not be administered properly by the untrained lay public and that many children would refuse to drink the charcoal slurry. In fact, an 18-month consecutive case series demonstrated that AC could be administered successfully in the home when given by the lay public. Home use of AC significantly reduced the time to AC administration after xenobiotic ingestion from a mean of 73 ± 18.1 minutes for ED treatment to a mean of 38 ± 18.3 minutes for home treatment. Additionally, prehospital AC did not markedly delay transport or arrival of overdose patients into the ED and was generally safe in 441 cases collected retrospectively in which prehospital AC was given. Complications included emesis in 6.6% of the patients, as well as hypotension, hypoxia, and declining mental status, but authors attributed these events to the xenobiotic ingested rather than the AC itself.

Many authorities recommend that AC should neither be a standard nor be administered at home and that administration should only be carried out by health professionals. However, we recommend that prehospital AC be used in rural and remote areas if the transport time to health care facilities exceeds the time frame of possible beneficial effect of AC, and its administration is expected to reduce the risk of appearance of life-threatening symptoms, but only after consultation with a knowledgeable health care professional.

## Dosing

The optimal dose of oral AC has never been fully established. Information concerning the maximum adsorptive capacity of AC for the particular xenobiotic ingested permits a theoretical calculation of an adequate dose, assuming that the amount of xenobiotic ingested is known. However, clinicians must remain cognizant of the risk of approaching or exceeding the adsorptive capacity of the standard dose of approximately 1 g/kg of body weight of AC. While more AC will theoretically improve this binding ratio, 1 g/kg of AC is about as much as most people can tolerate in a single dose based on the amount of water required to suspend AC for ingestion.

The idea that a fixed ratio of AC to xenobiotic is appropriate for all xenobiotics is clearly inappropriate. It is possible, however, to develop a logical approach to dosing based on available data. The effect of the ratio of AC to xenobiotic is such that theoretically increasing the ratio enhances the completeness of adsorption corresponding to a higher percentage of adsorption and total amount of adsorbed xenobiotic (Fig. 3–4). Thus the optimal AC dose is theoretically the minimum dose that completely adsorbs the ingested

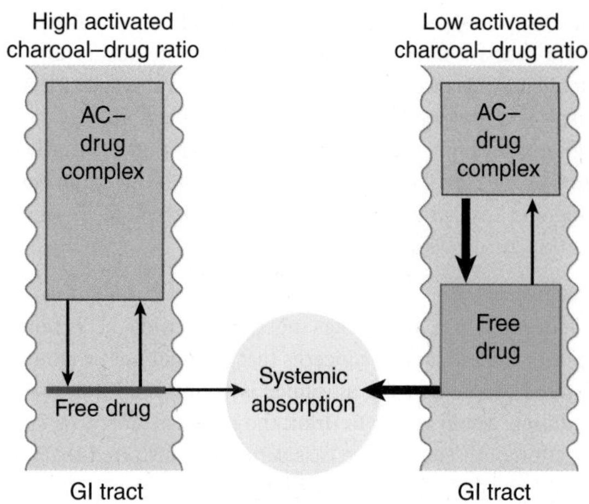


**FIGURE 3–4.** The effect of high and low ratios of AC to xenobiotic in the gastrointestinal (GI) tract. The reduced systemic absorption achieved when the AC–xenobiotic ratio is high (*left*) is compared with the increased systemic absorption at a low activated charcoal–xenobiotic ratio (*right*).

xenobiotic and, if relevant, that maximizes enhanced elimination. The results of in vitro studies show that the ideal AC–xenobiotic ratio varies widely, but a common recommendation is to deliver an AC–xenobiotic ratio of 10:1, or 50 to 100 g of AC to adult patients (0.5 to 1.0 g/kg of body weight in children), whichever is greater. From a theoretical perspective, this amount will adsorb 5 to 10 g of a xenobiotic, which should be adequate for most poisonings. These recommendations are generally based more on AC tolerance than on efficacy. When calculation of a 10:1 ratio exceeds these recommendations and the ingestion is potentially severely toxic, either orogastric lavage should be performed expeditiously before dosing of AC or multiple-dose AC (MDAC) therapy should be administered.

### Methods to Increase the Palatability of Activated Charcoal

Activated charcoal has a pronounced gritty texture, and it immediately sticks in the throat because it adheres to the mucosal surfaces and begins to cake. In addition, the black appearance and insipid taste of AC make it less attractive. There have been numerous attempts at making AC more appealing. The general recommendation, however, remains that AC should be mixed with water or other carbonated beverages to mask the texture.

### Effect on Oral Therapeutics

The nonspecific nature and high adsorptive capacity of AC raise concerns about the simultaneous use of orally administered therapeutics. It would be expected that therapeutics administered shortly before or simultaneously with AC would be extensively adsorbed, greatly reducing therapeutic efficacy. Caution is advised to prevent both underdosing and overdosing of needed therapeutics.

### Contraindications and Complications

Few clinically significant adverse effects are associated with the use of AC for poisoned patients. Adverse GI effects are most commonly described, but the frequency varies, and it might be difficult to differentiate from adverse effects resulting from the ingested xenobiotic. Pulmonary aspiration of gastric contents containing AC and inadvertent direct instillation of AC into the lungs from a misplaced nasogastric tube are rare but severe events that might lead to airway obstruction, bronchospasm, hypoxemia, aspiration, permanent lung injury, and even death. Although relatively few reports of clinically significant emesis and pulmonary aspiration resulting from the administration of AC exist, the severity of these complications is clear. Consequently, it is important to evaluate whether AC therapy is likely to be beneficial based on the indications and contraindications listed in Table 3–4. This is especially true in small children, in whom the risks of nasogastric tube use often outweigh the benefits of AC.

**TABLE 3–4 Single-Dose Activated Charcoal Therapy: Indications and Contraindications**

| *Indications* | *Contraindications* |
|---|---|
| The patient does not meet criteria for orogastric lavage (Table 3–1) or orogastric lavage is likely to be harmful. | Activated charcoal is known not to adsorb a clinically meaningful amount of the ingested xenobiotic. |
| The patient has ingested a potentially toxic amount of a xenobiotic that is well adsorbed by AC. | Airway protective reflexes are absent or expected to be lost, and the patient is not intubated. |
| The ingestion occurred within a time frame amenable to adsorption by AC or clinical factors are present that suggest that not all of the xenobiotic has already been systemically absorbed. | Gastrointestinal perforation is likely, as in cases of caustic ingestions. |
| Patients who have potentially life-threatening toxicity regardless of the time since ingestion as long as no absolute contraindications exist. | Therapy will likely increase the risk and severity of aspiration, such as in the presence of hydrocarbons with a high aspiration potential. |
| | Endoscopy will be an essential diagnostic modality (caustics). |

## MULTIPLE-DOSE ACTIVATED CHARCOAL

Multiple-dose AC is defined as at least two sequential doses of AC, but in many cases, the actual number of doses administered is substantially greater. This technique serves two purposes: (1) to prevent ongoing absorption of a xenobiotic that persists in the GI tract (such as modified-release preparation) and (2) to enhance elimination in the postabsorptive phase by either disrupting enterohepatic recirculation or enteroenteric recirculation ("gut dialysis").

Volunteer studies demonstrate that MDAC increases the elimination of a large number of xenobiotics. Unfortunately, many of the most life-threatening ingestions have never been studied for MDAC administration. A large trial of all ingestions that compared SDAC, MDAC, and no therapy failed to show any clinical benefit of either AC regimen. However, another randomized controlled study was unique in that the design only included patients who ingested life-threatening doses of yellow oleander seeds. In this study, the use of MDAC significantly reduced the likelihood of death and secondary outcomes included life-threatening cardiac dysrhythmias, dose of atropine used, need for anti-digoxin Fab fragments, need for cardiac pacing, admission to the ICU, and length of stay. It is uncertain whether these

**TABLE 3–5 Multiple-Dose Activated Charcoal Therapy: Indications and Contraindications**

| *Indications* | *Contraindications* |
|---|---|
| Ingestion of a life-threatening amount of *Amanita* spp., amiodarone, amitriptyline, carbamazepine, colchicine, dextropropoxyphene, digitoxin, digoxin, disopyramide, dosulepin, duloxetine, diquat, *Gymnopilus penetrans*, lamotrigine, nadolol, phenobarbital, phenylbutazone, phenytoin, piroxicam, quetiapine, quinine, sotalol, theophylline, valproic acid, verapamil, or vinorelbine. | Any contraindication to single-dose activated charcoal. |
| Ingestion of a life-threatening amount of a xenobiotic that undergoes enterohepatic or enteroenteric recirculation and that is adsorbed to activated charcoal. | The presence of an ileus or other causes of diminished peristalsis. |
| Ingestion of a significant amount of any slowly released xenobiotic or of a xenobiotic known to form concretions or bezoars. | |

results can be extended to other clinical situations. Based on the available data we recommend MDAC for the indications listed in Table 3–5. The technique is summarized in Table 3–6.

### Contraindications and Complications

Table 3–5 summarizes the contraindications for MDAC therapy. Similar to single-dose AC, MDAC can produce emesis, with subsequent pulmonary aspiration of gastric contents containing AC. Sorbitol seems to increase the risk of emesis. It is intuitive that these risks are greater with MDAC than with single-dose therapy, but the risk is still estimated to be very low (less than 1% in one study). Readers are referred to Antidotes in Brief: A1 for a more detailed discussion of single-dose AC and MDAC therapy.

**TABLE 3–6 Technique of Administering Multiple-Dose Activated Charcoal Therapy**

Initial dose orally or via orogastric or nasogastric tube:

Adults and children: 1 g/kg of body weight or a 10:1 ratio of activated charcoal to xenobiotic, whichever is greater. After massive ingestions, 2 g/kg of body weight is reasonable if such a large dose can be tolerated.

Repeat doses orally or via orogastric or nasogastric tube:

Adults and children: 0.5 g/kg of body weight every 4–6 h for 12–24 h in accordance with the dose and dosage form of xenobiotic ingested (larger doses or shorter dosing intervals are reasonable in high-risk cases).

**Procedure**

1. Add eight parts of water to the selected amount of powdered form. All formulations, including prepacked slurries, should be shaken well for at least 1 min to form a transiently stable suspension before the patient drinks or has it instilled via orogastric or nasogastric tube.
2. A cathartic can be added to AC *for the first dose only* when indicated. Cathartics should not be administered routinely and never be repeated with subsequent doses of activated charcoal.
3. If the patient vomits the dose of activated charcoal, it should be repeated. Smaller, more frequent doses or continuous nasogastric administration is better tolerated. Administration of an antiemetic is recommended.
4. If a nasogastric or orogastric tube is used for MDAC administration, time should be allowed for the last dose to pass through the stomach before the tube is removed. Suctioning the tube itself before removal will theoretically lessen the risk of subsequent activated charcoal aspiration.

MDAC = multiple-dose activated charcoal.

## WHOLE-BOWEL IRRIGATION

Whole-bowel irrigation represents a method of purging the GI tract in an attempt to expeditiously achieve gut clearance and prevent further absorption of xenobiotics. This is achieved through the oral or nasogastric administration of large amounts of an osmotically balanced polyethylene glycol electrolyte lavage solution (PEG-ELS). The current evidence for the clinical efficacy of WBI is divergent, depending on the xenobiotic and its formulation. Volunteer studies often offer extreme variability in results, and significant variations are noted when individual subjects are simultaneously given three different modified-release xenobiotics. Case reports and series demonstrate the overall safety of WBI as well as some beneficial effects on secondary endpoints, but the benefits remain generally theoretical. When experimental, theoretical, and anecdotal human experience is considered, the use of WBI with PEG-ELS is reasonable for patients with potentially toxic ingestions of modified release pharmaceuticals and substantial amounts of metals. Other indications include the ingestion of large amounts of a xenobiotic with a slow absorptive phase in which morbidity is expected to be high, the ingested xenobiotic is not adsorbed by AC, and other methods of GI decontamination are unlikely to be either safe or beneficial. The removal of packets of xenobiotics from body packers can be considered a unique indication for WBI (Special Considerations: SC4). Table 3–7 summarizes the indications and contraindications for WBI.

## CATHARTICS

At present, there is no indication for the routine use of cathartics as a method of either limiting absorption or enhancing elimination. It is reasonable to administer a single dose as an adjunct to AC therapy when there are no contraindications and constipation or an increased GI transit time is expected. Multiple-dose cathartics should never be used, and magnesium- and phosphate-containing cathartics should be avoided in patients with kidney disease (Antidotes in Brief: A2).

**TABLE 3–7 Whole-Bowel Irrigation: Indications and Contraindications**

| *Indications* | *Contraindications* |
|---|---|
| Potentially toxic ingestions of sustained-release and modified release drugs. | Airway protective reflexes are absent or expected to become so in a patient who is not intubated. |
| Ingestion of a toxic amount of a xenobiotic that is not adsorbed to AC when other methods of GI decontamination are not possible or not efficacious. | The GI tract is not intact. There are signs of ileus, obstruction, significant GI hemorrhage, or hemodynamic instability that might compromise GI motility. |
| Removal of illicit drug packets from body packers. | Persistent vomiting. |
| | Signs of leakage from cocaine packets (indication for surgical removal). |

GI = gastrointestinal.

Adapted from Shargel L, Yu A: *Applied Biopharmaceutics and Pharmacokinetics*, 3rd ed. Norwalk, CT: Appleton & Lange; 1993.

## SURGERY AND ENDOSCOPY

Surgery and endoscopy are occasionally indicated for decontamination of poisoned patients. As might be expected, no controlled studies have been conducted, and potential indications are based largely on case reports and case series. The most robust data comes from patients who intentionally use their gastrointestinal tracts to smuggle drugs and is discussed in depth in Special Considerations: SC4. Over the years, case reports presented mixed results for the endoscopic removal of drug packets, pharmacobezoars, or foreign material from the stomach. At present, this method is not routinely recommended for the removal of drug packets because of the concern regarding packet rupture. The procedure is reasonable for removal of a compact pharmacobezoar containing a xenobiotic causing severe and continued poisoning. Occasionally bezoars that cannot be effectively treated with AC or by orogastric lavage can be fragmented and retrieved endoscopically. Under exceptional circumstances, there is certainly a precedent for attempting this procedure in a highly controlled setting such as an ICU or operating room.

## OTHER ADJUNCTIVE METHODS USED FOR GASTROINTESTINAL DECONTAMINATION

Pharmaceuticals that either speed up GI passage or slow down gastric emptying were administered in an attempt to minimize the absorption of a xenobiotic. In all cases, the results were negligible, and the potential risks of administering additional pharmacologically active xenobiotics to an already poisoned patient seem to outweigh any benefit. Interventions that reduce the absorption of xenobiotics from the GI tract other than AC were also studied, including sodium polystyrene sulfonate for lithium or thallium overdose. Human studies showed minimal decreased absorption and increased clearance of lithium when sodium polystyrene sulfonate was administered, and it is therefore not routinely recommended. Similarly, case reports describe the use of the lipid-lowering resins cholestyramine and colestipol to interrupt the enterohepatic circulation of digoxin, digitoxin, and chlordane to increase elimination. With the increased use of AC and availability of digoxin-specific Fab fragments, indications for lipid-lowering resins for cardioactive steroid ingestions seem obsolete except in countries where digoxin-specific Fab fragments are not available.

## POST–BARIATRIC SURGERY PATIENTS

Patients who have undergone bariatric surgery represent a subgroup of patients who need special caution before GI decontamination procedures can be initiated. Bariatric surgery procedures differ, but they all alter the gastric anatomy and reduce the gastric volume significantly. Unfortunately, no studies have investigated the optimal GI decontamination procedure in this subgroup of patients, and until studies are available, caution is required. Limited data are available, and a single report demonstrated that orogastric lavage was impossible because of resistance in the midesophagus. A retrospective poison control center study in 19 cases reported very poor results from orogastric lavage in four post bariatric surgery patients, with minor gastric bleeding caused by the procedure in one of these patients.

We recommend against orogastric lavage in a patient who has undergone bariatric surgery because the placement of a gastric tube possesses a risk of perforation and other injuries. Also, the reduced gastric volume makes it impossible for the patient to hold more than an estimated volume of 100 mL of fluid at the time. Dosing of AC is possible but should be divided into smaller portions using a maximum volume of 100 mL. WBI is reasonable after ingestion of large amounts of slow-release formulations.

## GENERAL GUIDANCE

The trends in GI decontamination have dramatically shifted toward less intervention over the years with no apparent worsening of outcome. These trends highlight the benign nature, in the developed world, of many exposures and the benefits of good supportive care in the typical patient for whom the interventions of GI decontamination represent more risk than benefit. In contrast, in clear cases of life-threatening ingestion, most poison control centers and toxicologists recommend some intervention. This distinction serves as a reminder that the existing studies and consensus statements cannot be applied to all cases and that a lack of data produces significant uncertainty in choices for GI decontamination in either atypical or severely poisoned patients.

It is essential to note that only one study, the oleander comparison of SDAC vs MDAC mentioned above, has ever demonstrated a survival advantage for any form of GI decontamination of poisoned patients. Its unique design, involving a cohort of patients with life-threatening toxicity, forces a reassessment of all previous and subsequent literature and confirms that the principles of decontamination are sound. It also suggests that the failure of most studies to demonstrate a benefit results not from a failure of the techniques used but from applying decontamination techniques to subsets of patients who were likely to have good outcomes regardless of intervention. By consulting experts within clinical and medical toxicology, treating clinicians will be assisted in the risk assessment and evaluation of poisoned patients, and guidelines for specific management can be provided, thereby initially obtaining correct and goal-directed treatment.

Special Considerations

# SC1 DECONTAMINATION PRINCIPLES: PREVENTION OF DERMAL, OPHTHALMIC AND INHALATIONAL ABSORPTION

## DECONTAMINATION PRINCIPLES: PREVENTION OF DERMAL, OPHTHALMIC, AND INHALATIONAL ABSORPTION

The benefits of decontamination by removal or neutralization of a xenobiotic are severalfold and include (1) prevention of further absorption and toxicity in exposed patients, (2) prevention of secondary contamination of other staff or equipment, and (3) prevention of contamination of the health care facility and other patients. Because of the risk of injury to the provider, the use of appropriate personal protective equipment (PPE) is paramount before initiation of patient decontamination. This Special Consideration focuses on situations that require health care facility–based dermal, ophthalmic, and pulmonary decontamination. Mass casualty events, the incident command system, and prehospital decontamination are covered in detail elsewhere (Chap. 101).

## HAZARDOUS MATERIALS (HAZMAT)

Decontamination should be initiated by first responders. However, up to 80% of patients from a scene of xenobiotic release self-present to a hospital without undergoing any prior decontamination. After the Tokyo sarin gas subway attacks in 1995, many patients presented directly to a hospital as their first site of health care contact. Hospital-based decontamination attempts were not universal, with a limited number of patients receiving a change of clothes or shower, which resulted in approximately 23% of staff experiencing symptoms consistent with secondary contamination. Thus hospital personnel must have the appropriate knowledge and follow an organized approach to decontamination to ensure their personal safety and the safety of other health care providers and patients. Close cooperation between the emergency department (ED) and prehospital providers, including HAZMAT teams responding to the initial site of exposure, helps to identify the xenobiotic involved and helps to guide decontamination efforts.

In addition, patients from industrial incidents often present with traumatic injuries or multiorgan dysfunction that requires appropriate basic and advanced life support measures. Evaluation and support of patient airway, breathing, and circulation should ideally be done concomitantly with decontamination efforts, as long as health care providers are protected using appropriate PPE.

## DECONTAMINATION

### Dermal Exposures

Patients exposed to liquids, aerosols, or solids require dermal decontamination. Patients who have undergone appropriate prehospital decontamination and those exposed to gases and vapors without gross contamination of clothes do not pose a risk of secondary contamination to health care workers. These patients should proceed directly to the treatment area without further ED dermal decontamination and assist in their own decontamination efforts if possible. Methods of dermal decontamination include physical removal (clothing removal, removal of visible solid particles), adsorption (Fuller earth, activated charcoal, flour), dilution (flushing), or acts to neutralize the xenobiotic.

### Physical Removal

The most important step is to remove contaminated clothing, which removes from 75% to 90% of the contaminants. Clothing should be cut off rather than pulled off because pulling off clothing will worsen contaminant exposure to the patient and health care staff. Clothing and personal belongings should be double bagged in sealed plastic bags with the patient's information written on it. Dermal decontamination may also include physical removal of the xenobiotic with forceps or gentle removal with brushing or use of a towel or straight edge on the skin. Abrasive cleansers are not recommended as they increase systemic absorption. Flushing the skin with copious amounts of water effectively removes most materials.

A method of dry decontamination using activated charcoal, flour, or Fuller earth is suggested to adsorb certain nerve agents and sulfur mustard, after which the adsorbed compound is gently brushed or wiped off with a towel. The US military utilizes a carbon-based adsorbent–polystyrene polymeric–ion exchange resin for local, dermal decontamination. Although dry decontamination is effective for localized exposures, it is unlikely to be useful in the hospital setting and therefore is not recommended because a lack of familiarity will delay more effective decontamination.

### Dilution and Neutralization

Water only, soap and water, and 0.5% hypochlorite solutions are used to decontaminate skin after hazardous material exposures. The solution must be readily available, nonirritating, rapid acting, and not produce toxic end products or enhance absorption. Regardless of the solution used, the most important factor is that it must be done as soon as possible to minimize local and systemic toxicity. Flushing contaminated skin with high volumes of low-pressure water will aid in physical removal and significant dilution of the xenobiotic. A military study showed that even an oil-based xenobiotic was removed from 90% of subjects within 30 seconds and 100% of subjects at 90 seconds using a water only decontamination method. Overall, showering with tepid water and liquid soap (mild, nonabrasive soap such as hand dishwashing soap) is the most effective, easiest, and most readily available method for removing hazardous materials from patients' hair and skin. Gentle scrubbing downward from head to toe with care taken to avoid contaminating unexposed areas is recommended. If there is significant contamination of the hair it is reasonable to decontaminate the hair first with the head down to prevent secondary contamination of the back and chest which are now exposed. Recommendations for duration of water-based decontamination range from 3 to 30 minutes. It is reasonable to wash exposed areas with tepid water and liquid soap for 5 to 15 minutes, with an additional 10 to 15 minutes for contaminated open wounds. Although some data support the use of specialty solutions, these are not generally available, will delays attempting to obtain them will likely increase patient injury, and therefore are not recommended at this time.

In certain instances, use of water may actually worsen toxicity. Exceptions to the water-first approach are solid alkali metals, including sodium, potassium, and lithium, because water causes these metals to form their corresponding bases (sodium, potassium, or lithium hydroxide) and liberate a substantial amount of heat. In addition, alkyl metals such as alkyl of aluminum, zinc, magnesium, or lithium cause similar reactions. Radioactive compounds (cesium and rubidium) also react on contact with water. Specific dusts (pure magnesium, white phosphorus, sulfur, strontium, titanium, uranium, yttrium, zinc, and zirconium) spontaneously ignite on contact with air. If these compounds are suspected on patient skin or clothing, residual metal should be removed with forceps and stored in mineral oil. Since identification is often delayed and because the time to removal is paramount, unless these exceptions are clearly known or extremely highly suspected, exposed patients should be immediately washed with copious amounts of soap and water.

### Ophthalmic Exposures

Acids and alkalis are the most commonly implicated xenobiotics in ophthalmic chemical exposures. The severity of ophthalmic burns is determined by several factors, including solution concentration, pH, duration of exposure, extent of surface damaged, and degree of intraophthalmic penetration. Liquids are most commonly implicated in ophthalmic exposures, but gases can dissolve on the surface of the eye and be absorbed. Solids or powders also lead to ophthalmic injury if not removed promptly.

### Decontamination

Contact lenses should be carefully removed to prevent any additional injury to the eye and allow adequate irrigation. The single most important intervention after ophthalmic chemical injuries is immediate and copious irrigation because concentrated solutions penetrate the eye within seconds to minutes. Overly complicated ocular decontamination protocols lead to uncertainty and delays in initiating treatment. Copious irrigation of the eye should be started promptly because time to irrigation is the most important factor. Any solution with a pH between 5 and 9 and temperature between 10° and 42°C is adequate for initial irrigation.

To adequately irrigate the eye and surrounding structures, the eye should be held open and continuously flushed. Topical anesthetic should be applied before initiation to limit pain, irritation and reflex blepharospasm. Solution can either be poured slowly into the eyes by gently pulling apart the patient's eyelids and tilting the head to the side or by using specially designed lenses that are placed beneath the eyelids to be in direct contact with the surface of the eye to enable direct flushing. The patient should be instructed to roll the eyeball to remove any particles retained beneath the eyelids. The eyelids should be gently everted to assess for the presence of particulate debris that should be removed using a moist cotton tip. Irrigation should be continued for cycles of 10 to 15 minutes followed by pH rechecks. Ocular pH should be checked using litmus paper with a goal to continue irrigation until the pH is 7.5 to 8. Copious flushing normalizes the pH at the ophthalmic surface; however, the pH is not always reflective of the deeper structures of the globe, because xenobiotics will penetrate deeper into the eye. Ophthalmic burns from strong or concentrated acids or alkalis require irrigation for at least 2 to 3 hours and immediate ophthalmologic consultation. Further treatments including cycloplegics, mydriatics, steroids, and topical antibiotics are beyond the scope of this chapter and should be discussed with an ophthalmologist.

### Inhalational Exposures

Removal of xenobiotics from the pulmonary tree is performed using bronchoalveolar lavage. It is rarely indicated when the xenobiotic is not able to rapidly diffuse from the pulmonary system and is expected to continually damage the lungs if left in place, such as the carbonaceous material that accumulates after smoke inhalation.

## SPECIFIC DECONTAMINATION EXAMPLES

### Caustics

A review of controlled clinical studies concluded that water was the best decontaminating solution for dermal caustic exposures and that time to decontamination was the most important factor in limiting morbidity and improving outcomes. Other solutions were investigated for the purpose of "active rinsing." They are postulated to not only provide the irrigation benefits of water but also act to neutralize the offending xenobiotic. A review of an emergency rinsing solution suggested it was a safe and effective method for improving healing time, healing sequelae, and pain management for chemical burns involving the skin and eyes of humans. However, lack of treatment randomization, observer blinding, uncertain initial time to decontamination between the groups, and significant conflicts of interest limit the applicability of the studies. Further research and increased availability of amphoteric, emergency rinsing solutions are required before this can be recommended as a first-line therapy in preference to rapid and widely available water rinsing.

### Hydrofluoric Acid

Hydrofluoric acid is a weak acid (pKa = 3.2) that can cause severe burns and life-threatening electrolyte abnormalities. Standard decontamination includes immediate and prolonged water rinsing of exposed areas followed closely by administration of calcium gluconate by one of several routes (Chap. 77). Dermal or ophthalmic exposures to hydrofluoric acid to the skin or eyes should be flushed with plain water or 0.9% saline for at least 20 minutes. Once again, because rigorous studies with amphoteric salts provide unimpressive results, this method cannot be recommended over water for the treatment of hydrofluoric acid exposures.

### Phenol

Concentrated phenol solutions cause severe chemical burns. After exposure to concentrated solutions, skin will turn white initially followed by yellow-brown discoloration. Because toxicity is often significant, adequate dermal decontamination is essential. In experimental models, low molecular weight (300-400 D) polyethylene glycol (PEG) and isopropyl alcohol (IPA) washes were more effective than the other treatments at reducing morphologic changes, including papillary dermal edema, pyknotic basal cells, and collagen necrosis. However, in another experimental model, PEG formulated with industrial methylated spirits did not outperform water at limiting systemic phenol absorption. Given the inconclusive findings, decontamination using inexpensive, readily available tepid water should be performed. Further studies on the safety and efficacy of using IPA and PEG–IMS are required before their use should be routinely applied to patients with phenol burns presenting to hospital.

### Unknown Xenobiotics

Patients often present to health care facilities after exposure to an unknown xenobiotic. In these cases, patients should have clothing removed and affected areas washed with tepid water and liquid soap for 5 to 15 minutes, with an additional 10 to 15 minutes for contaminated open wounds. Ophthalmic exposures should have immediate water irrigation for cycles of 10 to 15 minutes followed by pH rechecks with goal pH of 7.5 to 8.

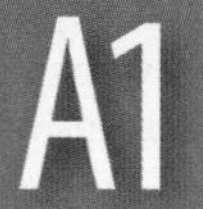


# ACTIVATED CHARCOAL

## INTRODUCTION

Activated charcoal (AC) is used to prevent absorption or enhance elimination of a potentially toxic xenobiotic. A detailed discussion of the merits of AC as a decontamination strategy is presented in Chap. 3.

## HISTORY

Charcoal, a fine, black, odorless powder, has been recognized for more than two centuries as an effective adsorbent of many substances. Bertrand attributed his survival in 1811 from separate mercuric chloride and arsenic trioxide ingestions to their antecedent admixture with charcoal. In 1830, Touéry demonstrated the powerful adsorbent qualities of charcoal by ingesting several lethal doses of strychnine mixed with charcoal in front of colleagues, suffering no ill effects. Holt first used charcoal to "save" a patient from mercury bichloride poisoning in 1834. However, it was not until the 1940s that Andersen began to systematically investigate the adsorbency of charcoal and demonstrated that charcoal is an excellent, broad-spectrum gastrointestinal (GI) adsorbent.

## PHARMACOLOGY

### Chemistry and Preparation

Activated charcoal is produced by pyrolysis of various carbonaceous materials followed by treatment at high temperatures (600°–900°C) with a variety of oxidizing (activating) agents to increase adsorptive capacity through formation of an internal maze of pores. Typical AC surface areas average 800 to 1,200 $m^2/g$.

### Mechanism of Action

The actual adsorption of a xenobiotic by AC relies on hydrogen bonding, ion–ion, dipole, and van der Waals forces, suggesting that most xenobiotics are best adsorbed by AC in their dissolved, nonionized form.

### Pharmacokinetics

Activated charcoal is pharmacologically inert and not absorbed. Its GI transit time is influenced by many factors mainly relating to the ingested xenobiotic (type and quantity), the patient (fasting, hydration status, perfusion), and other treatments (associated cathartics or evacuants).

### Pharmacodynamics

The adsorption rate to AC depends on external surface area, and the adsorptive capacity depends on the far larger internal surface area. When the AC surface area is large, the adsorptive capacity is increased, but affinity is decreased because van der Waals forces and hydrophobic forces diminish. Weak bases are best adsorbed to AC at basic pHs, and weak acids are best adsorbed to AC at acidic pHs. Activated charcoal decreases the systemic absorption of most xenobiotics. Notable xenobiotics not amenable to AC are small and often charged molecules such as the alcohols, acids, alkalis, iron, lead, lithium, magnesium, potassium, and sodium salts. Although the binding of AC to cyanide is less than 4%, because the usual toxic dose of cyanide is small, 50 g of AC would theoretically bind more than 10 lethal doses of potassium cyanide.

The efficacy of AC is directly related to the quantity administered. A 10:1 AC-to-xenobiotic ratio is the dose typically recommended based on experimental data. A meta-analysis of 64 controlled volunteer studies demonstrated that the percentage of reduction in xenobiotic exposure provided by AC followed a sigmoidal dose–response curve. Activated charcoal to xenobiotic ratios of 1:1, 5:1, 10:1, 20:1, 25:1, and 50:1 reduced xenobiotic exposures by 9.0%, 30.2%, 44.6%, 58.9%, 62.9%, and 73.0%, respectively. In vitro studies demonstrate that adsorption begins within about 1 minute of AC administration but does not achieve equilibrium for 10 to 25 minutes.

The clinical efficacy of AC to prevent absorption is inversely related to the time elapsed after ingestion and depends largely on the rate of absorption of the xenobiotic. According to the same meta-analysis of volunteer studies mentioned above, the median reductions of xenobiotic exposure when AC was administered at 0 to 5 minutes, 30 minutes, 60 minutes, 120 minutes, 180 minutes, 240 minutes, and 360 minutes after ingestion were 88.4%, 48.5%, 38.4%, 24.4%, 13.6%, 27.4%, and 11%, respectively. After systemic absorption or parenteral administration, AC can enhance elimination of select xenobiotics through enterohepatic and enteroenteric recirculation.

Desorption (xenobiotic dissociation from AC) can occur, especially for weak acids, as the AC–xenobiotic complex transits the stomach and intestine and as the pH changes from acidic to basic. Desorption can lead to ongoing systemic xenobiotic absorption over days. The clinical effects of desorption can be minimized by providing sufficient AC to overcome the decreased affinity of the xenobiotic secondary to pH change, such as by using multiple-dose AC (MDAC).

### Concomitant Administration of Activated Charcoal with Cathartics or Evacuants

Cathartics are often used with AC; however, evidence suggests that AC alone is comparably effective to AC plus a single dose of cathartic (sorbitol or magnesium citrate). If a cathartic is used, it should be used only once. Repeated doses of any cathartic are associated with salt and water depletion, hypotension, and severe or fatal fluid and electrolyte derangements. Whole-bowel irrigation (WBI) with PEG electrolyte lavage solution can significantly decrease the in vitro and in vivo adsorptive capacity of AC. Activated charcoal and WBI interactions are further discussed in Antidotes in Brief: A2.

## ROLE OF ACTIVATED CHARCOAL IN GASTROINTESTINAL DECONTAMINATION

### Single-Dose Activated Charcoal (SDAC)

When evaluating SDAC alone, a meta-analysis of 64 controlled volunteer studies found significant reductions in ingested xenobiotic amounts when SDAC was provided in appropriate quantity (eg, a 10:1 AC: xenobiotic ratio) and within 240 minutes of exposure. Research subsequent to this meta-analysis continued to confirm a pharmacokinetic advantage of SDAC in volunteer studies. For some new pharmaceuticals such as rivaroxaban and apixaban a benefit was demonstrated as late as 6 to 8 hours post ingestion, likely because these xenobiotics undergo extensive enterohepatic recirculation. In a pharmacokinetic and pharmacodynamic evaluation of escitalopram overdosed patients, SDAC reduced the absorbed fraction by 31% and reduced the risk of QT interval prolongation by approximately 35% for escitalopram doses above 200 mg. In patients with venlafaxine overdoses, SDAC significantly decreased the odds of having a seizure compared with no decontamination. In patients presenting with quetiapine overdoses, SDAC administration within 2 hours reduced the probability of intubation by 7% for a 2 g ingestion and by 17% for a 10 g ingestion.

### Multiple-Dose Activated Charcoal (MDAC)

Multiple-dose AC functions both to prevent the absorption of xenobiotics that are slowly absorbed from the GI tract and to enhance the elimination of suitable xenobiotics via enterohepatic recirculation. Multiple-dose AC decreases xenobiotic absorption when large amounts of xenobiotics are ingested and dissolution is delayed (eg, masses, bezoars), when xenobiotic formulations exhibit a delayed or prolonged release phase (eg, enteric coated, extended release), when GI motility is impaired because of coingestants, or when reabsorption can be prevented (eg, enterohepatic circulation of active xenobiotic, active metabolites, or conjugated xenobiotic hydrolyzed by gut bacteria to active xenobiotic).

The ability of MDAC to enhance elimination is demonstrated in multiple volunteer studies. Successful MDAC requires the a large amount of the xenobiotic to be in the blood compartment (low volume of distribution), have limited protein binding, and have prolonged endogenous clearance. In experimental studies, xenobiotics with the longest intrinsic plasma half-lives seemed to demonstrate the largest percent reduction in plasma half-life when MDAC was used. Clinical benefit has been demonstrated for a few xenobiotics with significant toxicity such as salicylates, phenobarbital, theophylline, and phenytoin. The most compelling evidence of MDAC's benefits in the overdose setting comes from a randomized study in patients with severe cardiac toxicity caused by yellow oleander seeds. When compared to a single dose of AC, MDAC was associated with fewer deaths and fewer life-threatening dysrhythmias and a reduced need for antidote.

Ultimately, the decision to administer SDAC or MDAC should involve a patient-tailored, risk-to-benefit analysis. Potential adverse effects are weighed against the particular ingested xenobiotic, its quantity, and formulation; dose–response curve of the xenobiotic; the impact of SDAC or MDAC on this curve; the time since ingestion; coingestants; gastric motility and contents; available antidotes, therapies, and medical support; the severity of presentation; anticipated sequelae; patient cooperativity; and other patient-specific factors and comorbidities.

## ADVERSE EFFECTS AND SAFETY ISSUES

Contraindications to AC include presumed GI perforation or obstruction or the need for endoscopic visualization (eg, in caustic ingestions). To prevent aspiration pneumonitis from oral AC administration, an airway assessment must occur, and potential airway compromise should be excluded. With decreased bowel function, repeat doses of AC should be withheld or delayed until the stomach can be decompressed to decrease the risk of subsequent vomiting and aspiration.

Although the use of AC is relatively safe, emesis, which typically occurs after rapid administration; constipation; and diarrhea are frequently reported after AC administration. Serious adverse effects of AC include pulmonary aspiration of AC with or without gastric contents, leading to airway obstruction (potentially of rapid onset), acute respiratory distress syndrome, bronchiolitis obliterans, and death; peritonitis from spillage of enteric contents, including AC, into the peritoneum after GI perforation; and intestinal obstruction and pseudo-obstruction, especially after repeated AC doses in the presence of either dehydration or prior bowel adhesions. Complications observed with SDAC increase with MDAC.

## PREGNANCY AND LACTATION

The safety of AC in pregnancy is undetermined. The benefit of preventing absorption with AC should outweigh the risk of administration to the pregnant patient. Single-dose AC and MDAC have been safely administered to pregnant patients as part of poisoning management. The lack of absorption of AC would not predispose it to breast milk excretion, although definitive safety in lactation has not been established.

## DOSING AND ADMINISTRATION

The optimal SDAC dose is unknown. However, most authorities recommend a minimum oral AC dose of 1 g/kg of body weight or a 10:1 ratio of AC to xenobiotic, up to an amount that can be tolerated by the patient and safely administered, which usually represents 50 to 100 g in adults. Activated charcoal that is not premixed is best administered as a slurry in a 1:8 ratio of AC to suitable liquid, such as water or carbonated beverage to mask the granular texture of AC.

### Prehospital Administration

Prehospital AC administration by emergency medical personnel expedites the administration after overdose. However, the implementation costs and potential adverse effects have to be weighed against the small number of patients who would actually benefit. A prospective poison control center case series demonstrated successful home AC administration. A review of AC in the home suggested variable success depending on the parent and child. One additional retrospective review determined that prehospital paramedic-administered AC did not increase EMS encounter duration. A retrospective review of poisoned children concluded that those who were preannounced to an emergency department by the poison control center received AC earlier (59 minutes) than patients without a referral (71 minutes).

### Hospital Administration

Offering AC in an opaque, decorated, covered cup and a straw facilitates administration in children. The black color and gritty nature of AC have led to the development of many formulations to improve palatability and patient acceptance. Most additives do not decrease the adsorptive capacity; however, improvements in palatability and acceptance have been minimal or nonexistent with all of these formulations. Most patients prefer either cola-flavored drink or chocolate milk or other additives.

### Multiple-Dose Activated Charcoal Administration

An initial AC loading dose should be administered to adults and children in an attempt to achieve an AC-to-xenobiotic ratio of 10:1 or 1 g/kg of body weight (if the xenobiotic exposure amount is unknown). After the initial AC loading dose of 1 g/kg, subsequent doses of 0.5 g/kg (~25–50 g in adults) every 4 hours for up to 12 to 24 hours can be administered based on the clinical condition of the patient.

## FORMULATION AND ACQUISITION

Activated charcoal is supplied in bottles or tubes as a ready-to-use aqueous suspension in multiple-dose formulations (eg, suspensions of 15 g, 25 g, and 50 g of AC in 72 mL, 120 mL, and 240 mL at a fixed concentration of 208 mg/mL AC). Although the aqueous suspension is preferred, some AC suspensions are also premixed with sorbitol (eg, 25 and 50 g AC with 48 or 96 g of sorbitol to yield 208 mg/mL of AC and 400 mg/mL of sorbitol). When not premixed, it is recommended to create a slurry of AC in a 1:8 ratio of AC to suitable liquid (eg, water). We recommend against the routine use of AC that is premixed with sorbitol as part of an MDAC regimen.

Antidotes in Brief

# A2 WHOLE-BOWEL IRRIGATION AND OTHER INTESTINAL EVACUANTS

## INTRODUCTION

One approach to altering the pharmacokinetics of a xenobiotic is to administer a gastrointestinal (GI) evacuant. Selected patients benefit from minimizing systemic exposure by decreasing GI transit time and increasing rectal evacuation. The most effective process of evacuating the GI tract in poisoned patients is referred to as whole-bowel irrigation (WBI). Whole-bowel irrigation is typically accomplished using polyethylene glycol with a balanced electrolyte lavage solution (PEG-ELS). Unless stated otherwise, WBI will mean WBI with PEG-ELS. A detailed discussion of the merits of WBI in the context of various decontamination strategies is provided in Chap. 3.

## HISTORY

In 1625 while endeavoring to recover from a febrile illness, Johann Glauber drank from a well from which he later isolated *sal mirabile,* now known as sodium sulfate, $Na_2SO_4$. Subsequent discoveries of naturally occurring purgatives included Epsom salts (magnesium sulfate) and sodium phosphate. Polyethylene glycol was initially introduced in 1957 as a nonabsorbable marker for the study of human fat, carbohydrate, and protein absorption. In 1973, Hewitt and colleagues reported on WBI in clinical practice using their method of "whole-gut irrigation" with a solution of sodium chloride, potassium chloride, and sodium bicarbonate in distilled water to prepare the large bowel for surgery. In 1976, WBI was used therapeutically in a patient who ingested 300 lead air-gun pellets and who had no effective effluent to oral magnesium sulfate purgation.

## PHARMACOLOGY

### Nomenclature

Laxatives promote a soft-formed or semifluid stool within 6 hours to 3 days. Cathartics promote a rapid, watery evacuation within 1 to 3 hours. The term *purgative* relates the force associated with bowel evacuation. Promotility xenobiotics stimulate GI motor function via the enteric nervous system through a variety of acetylcholine, dopamine, guanylate cyclase-C, motilin, opioid, and serotonin receptor and intestinal chloride channel interactions.

Laxatives are further classified into categories of bulk-forming, softener or emollient, lubricant, stimulant or irritant, saline, hyperosmotic, and evacuant. Bulk-forming laxatives include high-fiber products such as methylcellulose, polycarbophil, and psyllium; softeners or emollients include docusate calcium. Mineral oil is the sole lubricant. These cathartics are not used therapeutically in medical toxicology because their onset of action is delayed. Stimulant or irritant laxatives include anthraquinones (sennosides, aloe, and casanthranol), diphenylmethane (bisacodyl), and castor oil. Saline (meaning salt) cathartics, which include magnesium citrate, magnesium hydroxide, magnesium sulfate, sodium phosphate, and sodium sulfate, are used infrequently. Hyperosmotic xenobiotics, generally nonabsorbable sugars and alcohols, including sorbitol and lactulose, are occasionally used in poisoned patients. The most common process of evacuating the intestinal tract in poisoned patients is WBI with PEG-ELS.

### Chemistry and Preparation

The addition reaction of ethylene oxide to an ethylene glycol equivalent polymerizes ethylene oxide into PEG. The number after PEG represents its average molecular weight (MW). Polyethylene glycol 3350 used in pharmaceutical, personal care, and food applications is water soluble. Polyethylene glycol 3350 without electrolytes is sold for nonprescription use for short-term treatment of constipation. Whole-bowel irrigation used in poison management is typically accomplished using PEG 3350 added to a balanced electrolyte lavage solution (PEG-ELS), which contains an isotonic mixture of sodium sulfate, sodium bicarbonate, sodium chloride, and potassium chloride.

### Mechanisms of Action

The effects of saline cathartics are largely attributed to their relatively nonabsorbable ions that establish an osmotic gradient and draw water into the gut. The increased water leads to increased intestinal pressure and a subsequent increase in intestinal motility. A lack of endogenous hydrolytic enzymes allows sorbitol, lactulose, and sodium sulfate to reach the colon unchanged. Colonic bacteria metabolize sorbitol into acetic and short-chain fatty acids and lactulose into lactic acid and small amounts of formic and acetic acids. This results in a slight acidification of colonic contents, an increase in osmotic pressure that draws water into the lumen, and stimulation of colonic propulsive motility. Long-chain PEGs (eg, MW ~3,350 Da) are nonabsorbable, isosmotic, indigestible molecules that remain in the colon together with the water diluent, resulting in WBI primarily by the mechanical effect of large-volume lavage. The balanced electrolyte solution significantly reduces the risk of electrolyte and metabolic abnormalities and helps preclude fluid shifts across the GI mucosa. Promotility xenobiotics such as metoclopramide and erythromycin stimulate gut motor function. Metoclopramide mediates 5-hydroxy tryptamine ($5HT_4$) receptor agonist and dopamine ($D_2$) receptor antagonist activity, which both result in increased acetylcholine release and GI motility. Erythromycin stimulates gut motor function via direct stimulation of GI motilin receptors.

### Pharmacokinetics

Absorption of magnesium, phosphate, and other electrolytes contained in hypertonic products is well described. In one prospective, nonrandomized study, 9 of 14 patients developed elevated magnesium concentrations (2.2–5.0 mEq/L) after multiple doses of magnesium-containing cathartics were administered. During the 24 hours after administration of oral sodium phosphate solution in seven healthy volunteers, serum phosphorus reached a mean peak concentration of 7.6 mg/dL (range, 3.6–12.4 mg/dL), and ionized calcium reached a mean nadir concentration of 4.6 mg/dL (range, 4.4–5.2 mg/dL). Sorbitol and PEG are not absorbed.

### Pharmacodynamics

In one systematic review, the mean transit times after administration of sorbitol, magnesium citrate, magnesium sulfate, and sodium sulfate were 0.9 to 8.5 hours, 3 to 14 hours, 9.3 hours, and 4.2 to 15.4 hours, respectively. Sorbitol produced stools in the shortest amount of time, which also was associated with the highest incidence of nausea, vomiting, generated gas, and flatus. In comparison, patients ingesting PEG-ELS (1.2–1.8 L/h until the rectal effluent was clear) completed their colonic preparation goals within 1.5 to 3 hours after averaging a total of 5.5 L per patient (range, 3–8 L).

## ROLE OF GASTROINTESTINAL EVACUATION IN POISONING MANAGEMENT

Cathartics should not be used in the routine management of overdosed patients. When comparing the efficacy of a single dose of activated charcoal (AC) alone with that of AC plus a single dose of cathartic, studies suggest the combination to be equal to, slightly better than, or even slightly worse than AC alone. In human volunteer studies, 3 to 5 hours of WBI with PEG-ELS was more effective than AC with sorbitol for enteric-coated acetylsalicylic acid (ASA) when administered 4 hours after ingestion, decreased peak lithium concentrations and lithium area under the plasma drug concentration versus time curve (AUC) compared with volunteers; decreased the bioavailability of two sustained-release medications; and propelled radiopaque markers through the gut more efficiently than control participants. However, multiple studies highlight the limited utility of WBI to assist in the prevention of absorption of relatively rapidly absorbed xenobiotics. Reports suggest successful WBI use in the management of overdoses of iron, sustained-release theophylline, sustained-release verapamil, modified-release fenfluramine, zinc sulfate, lead, arsenic trioxide, arsenic-containing herbicide, mercuric oxide powder, strontium, potassium chloride capsules, clonidine and fentanyl transdermal patches, and in body packers. Whole-bowel irrigation for 5 hours after ingestion of 10 fluorescent coffee beans by each of seven volunteers removed an average of only four beans (range, 1–8). Similar failures are reported with jequirity beans (*Abrus precatorius*), iron, and button batteries.

Whole-bowel irrigation is recommended for evacuation of highly toxic xenobiotics with a slow absorption phase and not adsorbed to AC (eg, iron, lead, lithium, potassium). When AC is expected to be of benefit, it is recommended that it be administered prior to WBI to achieve its greatest effect.

### Internal Drug Concealment

The approach to patients with internal concealment and enteral transport of illicit substances (eg, cocaine, heroin, amphetamines, and hashish) is comprehensively reviewed in Special Considerations: SC4.

## ADVERSE EFFECTS AND SAFETY ISSUES

Potential adverse effects associated with various cathartics and promotility xenobiotics include salt and water depletion, hypernatremia, hypermagnesemia, hyperphosphatemia, hypokalemia, and metabolic (contraction) alkalosis, absorption of magnesium or other absorbable electrolytes, activation of the renin–angiotensin–aldosterone system, phosphate-induced nephropathy, and colonic fermentation of digestible sugars. Frail elderly patients, children, and those with decreased kidney function are most susceptible to adverse effects. Multiple-dose AC regimens containing 70% sorbitol used to enhance elimination cause severe cathartic-related adverse effects (salt and water depletion). The potential for sorbitol-related adverse events from the unintentional use of repetitive AC dosing was emphasized by a survey revealing that 16% of hospitals surveyed only stocked AC premixed with sorbitol. Thus, if sorbitol is administered with AC, it should for a single dose only.

Contraindications to WBI include prior, current, or anticipated diarrhea; salt and water depletion; significant GI anatomical or functional compromise such as colitis, hemorrhage, ileus, obstruction, perforation, or toxic megacolon; an unprotected or compromised airway; and hemodynamic instability. Adverse effects resulting from the use of WBI include vomiting, particularly after rapid administration, abdominal bloating, fullness, cramping, flatulence, and pruritus ani. Typically, patients need to remain near a commode for at least 4 to 6 hours and as long as 24 hours to complete WBI therapy. Slow or low-volume administration of WBI results in sodium absorption and should be avoided.

Unintentional administration of WBI by other than the enteral route has occurred. A 4-year-old child inadvertently received 390 mL of WBI intravenously with no obvious adverse result. In contrast, several reports demonstrate acute respiratory distress syndrome (ARDS) after WBI inadvertently enters the trachea.

## XENOBIOTIC, ACTIVATED CHARCOAL, AND WHOLE-BOWEL IRRIGATION INTERACTIONS

Theoretically, WBI might worsen drug toxicity by facilitating drug dissolution because of the addition of the large volume of WBI, increasing drug solubility (lower molecular weight PEGs are used as pharmaceutical excipients and solvents), or through compromise of the adsorbent benefits of coadministered AC. In a simulated gastric fluid model containing 5 g of acetaminophen (APAP) and 0.5 L of WBI, APAP concentrations were increased at all time points and the AUC 315 mg-min/L was increased to 6233 mg-min/L compared to 0.9% sodium chloride control. In a prospective, randomized, crossover study of 10 volunteers administered 75 mg/kg of a bilayer, delayed-release APAP preparation, WBI initiated 30 minutes after ingestion resulted in a statistically insignificant decrease in the APAP AUC.

Several in vitro studies with cocaine, chlorpromazine, fluoxetine, salicylate, and theophylline demonstrate that the addition of WBI to AC significantly decreases the adsorptive capacity of AC. The most likely explanation is competition with the AC surface for solute adsorption. In a controlled study evaluating the effect of WBI added to AC, effects were variable depending on the study drug. A case report documents a rapid increase in carbamazepine concentrations temporally related to the initiation of WBI. A similar rapidly increasing drug concentration occurred after the initiation of WBI in a patient with a reported 10 g phenytoin overdose. Caution is advised when giving WBI to patients who have ingested large amounts of drug that might exceed solubility or who received large amounts of charcoal previously.

## PREGNANCY AND LACTATION

Commercial preparations of WBI are pregnancy category C. Whole-bowel irrigation with large volumes of fluid was used successfully in pregnant women at 26 and 38 weeks of gestation. The lack of absorption of WBI would not predispose it to excretion in breast milk, although definitive safety in lactation is not established.

## DOSING AND ADMINISTRATION

The recommended dose of WBI is 0.5 L/h or 25 mL/kg/h for small children and 1.5 to 2.0 L/h or 20 to 30 mL/min for adolescents and adults. Whole-bowel irrigation solution is administered orally or through a nasogastric tube for 4 to 6 hours or until the rectal effluent becomes clear. If the xenobiotic being removed is radiopaque, a diagnostic imaging technique demonstrating the absence of the xenobiotic is a reasonable clinical endpoint (Special Considerations: SC4). An antiemetic such as metoclopramide or a 5-$HT_3$ serotonin antagonist is recommended for the treatment of nausea or vomiting.

## FORMULATION AND ACQUISITION

The original WBI solution was GoLYTELY. This solution contained PEG with electrolytes and sodium sulfate as an added laxative. Colyte is similar to GoLYTELY. NuLYTELY is a PEG formulation with 52% less total salt than GoLYTELY and no added sodium sulfate. These changes decreased the salty taste and the risk of fluid- or electrolyte-related complications. Available WBI products (eg, GoLYTELY, Colyte, NuLYTELY, TriLyte) differ slightly in their composition. All contain PEG 3350 with varying amounts of sodium chloride, potassium chloride, sodium sulfate, and sodium bicarbonate, which upon reconstitution yield the following concentrations: sodium, 65 to 125 mEq/L; potassium, 5 to 10 mEq/L; chloride, 35 to 53 mEq/L; bicarbonate, 17 to 20 mEq/L; and sulfate, 0 to 80 mEq/L.

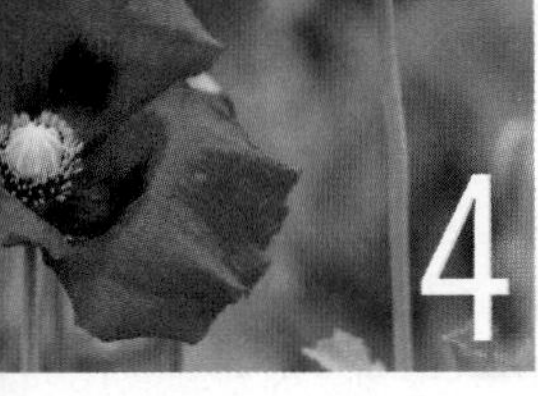

# 4 PRINCIPLES AND TECHNIQUES APPLIED TO ENHANCE ELIMINATION

Enhancing the elimination of a xenobiotic from a poisoned patient is a logical step after initial stabilization of the airway, breathing, and circulation; supportive measures; and techniques to inhibit absorption. Table 4–1 lists methods that might be used to enhance elimination. In this chapter, hemodialysis, hemoperfusion, and hemofiltration are considered *extracorporeal treatments* (ECTRs) because xenobiotic removal occurs in a blood circuit outside the body.

## EPIDEMIOLOGY

Although undoubtedly an underestimate of true use, enhanced elimination techniques were performed relatively infrequently in the cohorts of millions of patients reported by the American Association of Poison Control Centers (AAPCC) National Poison Data System (NPDS). Alkalinization of the urine was reportedly used 11,651 times, multiple-dose activated charcoal (MDAC) 1,104 times, hemodialysis 2,663 times, and hemoperfusion 49 times.

Lithium and ethylene glycol were the most common xenobiotics for which hemodialysis was used between 1985 and 2014 (Fig. 4–1).

Very few prospective, randomized, controlled clinical trials have been conducted to determine which groups of patients actually benefit from enhanced elimination of various xenobiotics and which modalities are most efficacious. For most poisonings, it is unlikely that such studies will ever be performed, given the relative scarcity of appropriate cases of sufficient severity and because of the many variables that would hinder controlled comparisons. Thus, limited evidence deemed of high quality exists. Fortunately, in the absence of robust evidence, consensus-based recommendations have now been published and are being developed to guide clinical decisions. The American Academy of Clinical Toxicology (AACT) and the European Association of Poisons Centres and Clinical Toxicologists (EAPCCT) published joint position papers on urine alkalinization and MDAC. The Extracorporeal Treatments in Poisoning (EXTRIP) work group has published several recommendations regarding the indications for dialysis and other ECTRs for overdose (see also http://extrip-workgroup.org).

**TABLE 4–1 Potential Methods of Enhancing Elimination of Xenobiotics**

| *Occurring Inside the Body* | *Occurring Outside the Body (Extracorporeal)* |
|---|---|
| Cerebrospinal fluid replacement | Exchange transfusion |
| Forced diuresis | Hemodialysis |
| Manipulation of urine pH | Hemofiltration and hemodiafiltration |
| Metal chelators | Hemoperfusion (charcoal, resin) |
| Multiple-dose activated charcoal | Liver support devices |
| Peritoneal dialysis | Plasmapheresis |
| Resins (Prussian blue, sodium polystyrene sulfonate, cholestyramine, colestipol) | |

## GENERAL INDICATIONS FOR ENHANCED ELIMINATION

Enhanced elimination is generally indicated for several types of patients, with the preexisting condition that the responsible xenobiotic is removable.

- *Patients who fail to respond adequately to comprehensive supportive care.*
- *Patients in whom the normal route of elimination of the xenobiotic is impaired.*
- *Patients in whom the amount of xenobiotic absorbed or its high concentration in serum indicates that serious morbidity or mortality is likely.*
- *Patients with concurrent disease or in an age group (very young or old) associated with increased risk of morbidity or mortality from the overdose.*
- *Patients with concomitant electrolyte disorders that could be corrected with hemodialysis.*

Ideally, these techniques are applied to poisonings for which studies suggest an improvement.

The need for extracorporeal elimination is less clear for patients who are poisoned with xenobiotics that are known to be removed by an ECTR but that cause limited morbidity if supportive care is provided. Relatively high rates of endogenous clearance would also make extracorporeal elimination redundant. Also, ECTR should be avoided if other more effective and less invasive modalities are available.

## CHARACTERISTICS OF XENOBIOTICS APPROPRIATE FOR EXTRACORPOREAL THERAPY

The appropriateness of any modality for increasing the elimination of a given xenobiotic depends on various properties of the molecules in question. Effective removal by the ECTR and other methods listed in Table 4–1 is limited by a number of factors, including a large volume of distribution (Vd), molecular, and compartmental factors. The Vd relates to the concentration of the xenobiotic in the blood or serum as a proportion of the total body burden. The Vd can be envisioned as the apparent volume in which a known total dose of drug is distributed before metabolism and excretion occur:

$$\text{Vd (L/kg)} \times \text{Patient weight (kg)} = \text{Dose (mg)/Concentration (mg/L)}$$

The larger the Vd, the less the xenobiotic is present in the blood compartment for elimination. A xenobiotic with a Vd below 1 L/kg is usually considered amenable to extracorporeal elimination. Additionally, a low percentage of protein binding and a small molecular weight are required for effective hemodialysis. Of note, kinetic parameters after an overdose often differ from those after therapeutic or experimental doses. The most important is saturation of protein binding, which happens for some xenobiotics at higher concentrations. Hemoperfusion and plasmapheresis can overcome some limitations of protein binding and molecular

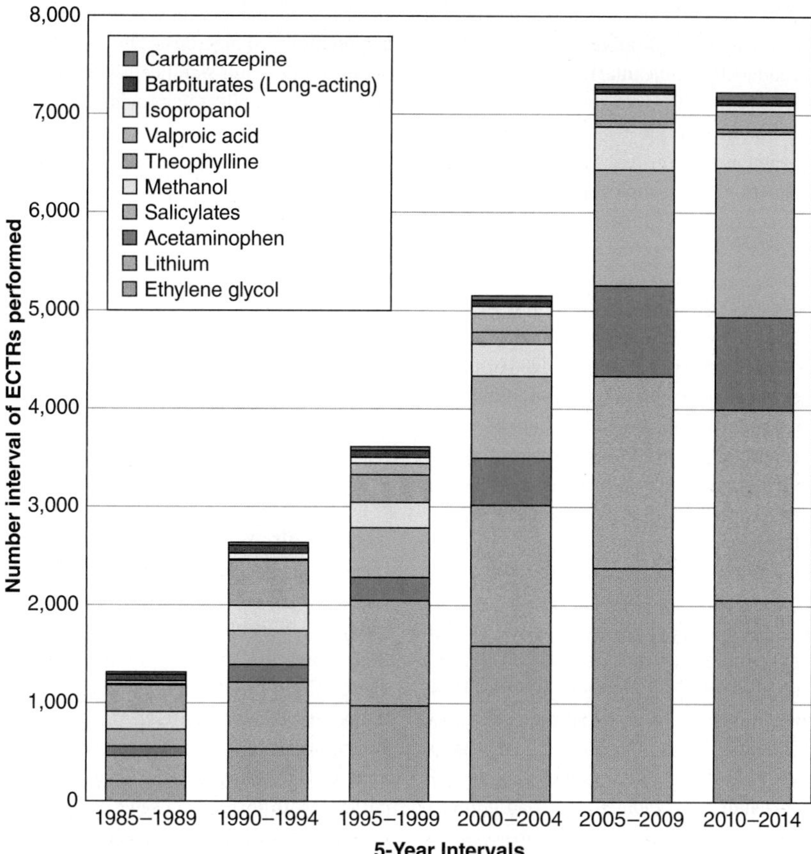


**FIGURE 4–1.** Xenobiotics that were most commonly reported by the AAPCC as treated with extracorporeal therapies per 5-year intervals. ECTR = extracorporeal treatment.

weight. Finally, any technique of enhanced elimination, a generally accepted principle, is worthwhile only if a large portion of total body drug burden can be eliminated or if total body clearance of the xenobiotic is increased by a factor of at least 2. This substantial increase is easier to achieve when the xenobiotic has a low endogenous clearance.

## TECHNIQUES TO ENHANCE REMOVAL OF XENOBIOTICS

Although the efficacy of, or need for, removal of many xenobiotics remains controversial, consensus regarding the indications for these procedures has developed. This consensus has led to consistent application of several techniques of enhanced elimination for some toxic exposures that occur relatively more frequently.

### Multiple-Dose Activated Charcoal: "Gastrointestinal Dialysis"

Oral administration of multiple doses of activated charcoal increases elimination of some xenobiotics present in the blood. This modality is discussed in more detail in Antidotes in Brief: A1 and will not be discussed here.

### Resins

Resins are sometimes used in poisoning management. They can reduce the bioavailability of ingested drugs and act as decontaminants, similarly to activated charcoal. In addition, however, they can promote elimination of certain xenobiotics by enhancing their back-diffusion from plasma to gut (gastrointestinal dialysis) and interrupt enterohepatic recirculation.

The most commonly used resins are sodium polystyrene sulfonate (Kayexalate), cholestyramine, and Prussian blue. Sodium polystyrene sulfonate is an ion exchanger that is used regularly for hyperkalemia in patients with chronic kidney disease. Limited data now exist on its potential use in lithium poisoning, although treatment results in hypokalemia. Prussian blue is also an ion exchanger used for treatment of poisoning by cesium or thallium (Antidotes in Brief: A31). Cholestyramine, a bile acid sequestrant, binds several xenobiotics, including digoxin, ibuprofen, and mycophenolate mofetil, although its application in poisoning is doubtful (Chap. 35).

### Forced Diuresis

Forced diuresis by volume expansion with isotonic sodium-containing solutions, such as 0.9% sodium chloride and lactated Ringer (LR) solution with or without the addition of a diuretic, increases renal clearance of some molecules. This therapy would theoretically be most useful for xenobiotics such as lithium for which the glomerular filtration rate (GFR) is an important determinant of excretion. In people with normal extracellular fluid (ECF) volume, the increase in GFR and increase in xenobiotic renal elimination expected with plasma volume expansion is variable and unpredictable and not likely to be clinically significant. However, in patients who have contraction of the ECF volume, repletion of ECF volume with 0.9% sodium chloride will increase GFR and suppress proximal tubular sodium reabsorption. The result is an increase in excretion of low-molecular-weight xenobiotics such as lithium. After the ECF volume is restored, the continued infusion of 0.9% sodium chloride will not enhance elimination of lithium to any major extent.

The major risk of excessive volume repletion is ECF volume overload, manifested by pulmonary and cerebral edema. This complication is particularly likely in patients with baseline chronic kidney disease or congestive heart failure. In general, because of these risks and the limited benefit, forced diuresis is not recommended routinely. However, forced diuresis is used to treat xenobioitic-induced hypercalcemia, which can result from excessive ingestion of calcium supplements or vitamin D.

### Manipulations of Urinary pH

Many xenobiotics are weak acids or bases that are ionized in aqueous solution to an extent that depends on the pKa of the xenobiotic and the pH of the solution. Knowing these variables, the Henderson-Hasselbalch equation can be used to determine the relative proportions of the acids, bases, and buffer pairs. Whereas cell membranes are relatively impermeable to ionized or polar molecules (eg, an unprotonated salicylate anion), nonionized, nonpolar forms (eg, the protonated, noncharged salicylic acid) cross more easily. As xenobiotics pass through the kidney, they may be filtered, secreted, and reabsorbed. If the urinary pH is manipulated to favor the formation of the ionized form in the tubular lumen, the xenobiotic is trapped in the tubular fluid and is not passively reabsorbed into the bloodstream. This is referred to as ion trapping. To make manipulation of urinary pH worthwhile, the renal excretion of the xenobiotic must be a major route of elimination.

Alkalinization of the urine to enhance elimination of weak acids has a role for salicylates, phenobarbital, chlorpropamide, formate, diflunisal, fluoride, methotrexate, and the herbicide 2,4-dichlorophenoxyacetic acid (2,4-D). Alkalinization is achieved by the intravenous administration of sodium bicarbonate (1–2 mEq/kg rapid initial infusion with additional dosing) to increase urinary pH to 7 to 8. This degree of alkalinization will be difficult, if not impossible, if metabolic acidosis and acidemia are present. As for the case of 0.9% sodium chloride or LR, there is a risk of ECF volume overload with sodium bicarbonate administration. Hypernatremia may also occur, especially if sodium bicarbonate is given as a hypertonic solution. Bicarbonaturia is also associated with urinary potassium losses, so the patient's serum potassium concentration should be monitored frequently and the appropriate dose of potassium administered as long as GFR is not impaired. A further complication of alkalemia is a decrease of ionized calcium.

Acidification of the urine by systemic administration of HCl or $NH_4Cl$ to enhance elimination of weak bases, such as phencyclidine or the amphetamines, is not useful and is potentially dangerous. The technique was abandoned because it does not significantly enhance removal of xenobiotics and is complicated by acidemia.

### Peritoneal Dialysis

Peritoneal dialysis (PD) is a technique in which a solution is introduced into the abdomen via a catheter so that the patient's peritoneum can act as a membrane across which water, solutes, and xenobiotics are exchanged with the blood. Although PD is a relatively simple method to enhance xenobiotic elimination, it is too slow to be clinically useful. Consequently, PD is not the ECTR of choice unless other more efficient techniques are unavailable. Besides exchange transfusion, it may be the only practical option in small children when experience with extracorporeal techniques in younger age groups is lacking or until a child can be transported to an appropriate center where hemodialysis can be performed.

### Hemodialysis

During conventional hemodialysis, blood and countercurrent dialysate are separated by a semipermeable membrane (*dialyzer*). Xenobiotics then diffuse across the membrane from blood into the dialysate down the concentration gradients (Fig. 4–2). Blood is pumped through one lumen of a temporary dialysis catheter, passed through the machine, and returned to the venous circulation through the second lumen. The utility of hemodialysis for the treatment of patients with toxicity caused by lithium, toxic alcohols, salicylates, or theophylline is unquestionable and is not dealt with here; each of these xenobiotics is described in detail in separate chapters that also review their toxicity and indications for extracorporeal therapies. This section describes the hemodialysis procedure and its application in general.

Prompt consultation with a nephrologist is always indicated in the case of poisoning with a xenobiotic that might benefit from extracorporeal removal. To perform hemodialysis, a nephrologist must be available in addition to a nurse. The dialysis machine requires preparation, and a vascular access catheter must be inserted. A delay, ranging from 1 to several hours before hemodialysis can be instituted should be anticipated, particularly during hours when the hospital dialysis unit, if there is one, is closed.

Vascular access is obtained via a double-lumen catheter that is made of silicon, polyethylene, polyurethane, or polytetrafluoroethylene (Teflon). The hollow-fiber dialyzer, almost universally used today, is composed of thousands of blood-filled capillary tubes held together in a bundle and bathed in the machine-generated dialysate. Hemodialysis efficacy for poisonings with low-molecular-weight xenobiotics improves with the use of larger membranes with larger clearances. "High-flux," synthetic dialyzers have larger pores and increased surface area that allow greater clearance of larger molecules.

To limit the risk of hemodynamic instability during hemodialysis, the blood lines and artificial kidney (the dialysis membrane) should be primed with an appropriate volume of fluid at the onset of the procedure. Computerized machines allow fine control of ultrafiltration rates to limit volume

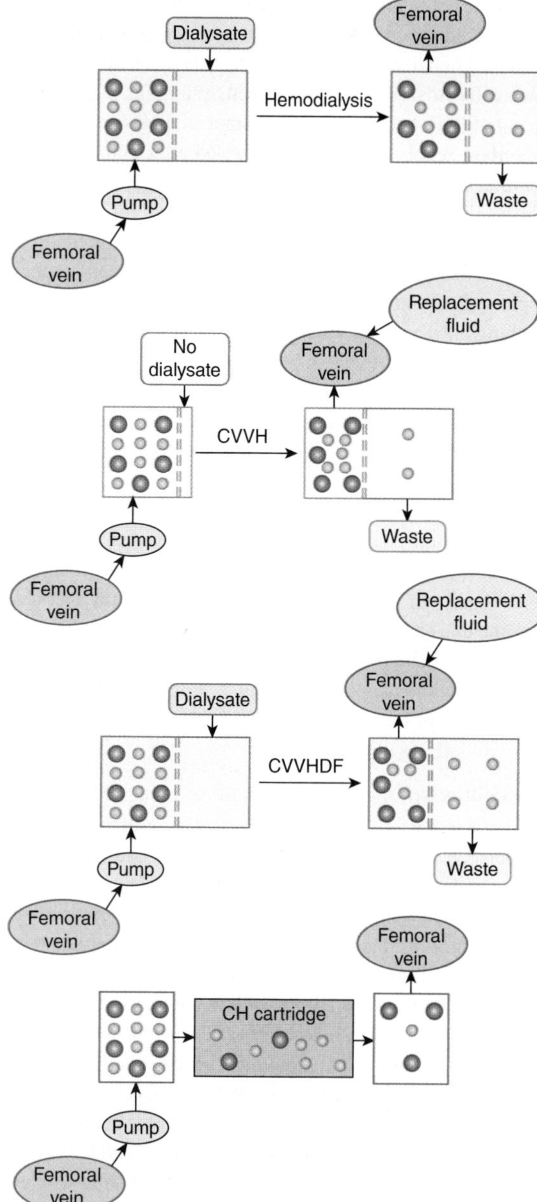


**FIGURE 4–2.** Comparative schematic layouts of hemodialysis (HD), continuous venovenous hemofiltration (CVVHDF), continuous venovenous hemofiltration with dialysis (CVVHD), and hemoperfusion (HP). *Red circles* are high-molecular-weight (MW) xenobiotics, such as methotrexate, whose high MW makes them too large to be removed by HD. *Yellow circles* are low MW diffusible solutes such as urea or methanol. In dialysis, solute moves across a semipermeable membrane (*dashed lines*) from a solution in which it is present in a high concentration (blood) to one in which it is at a low concentration (dialysate). In CVVH and CVVHDF, plasma moves across a similar membrane in response to hydrostatic pressures; replacement fluid must be provided. The latter also uses a dialysate to augment clearance. The availability of blood pumps has made arteriovenous modalities nearly obsolete. Charcoal hemoperfusion (CH) requires movement of blood through a sorbent-containing cartridge and does not include dialysis or hemofiltration.

losses; in the past, imprecise calculations and manipulations led to frequent episodes of hypotension. Hypotension still occurs in some in critically ill patients but can often be corrected with 0.9% sodium chloride, colloid, vasopressors, or inotropes. Full anticoagulation with heparin is usually required to avoid clotting of the circuit. In poisoned patients, hemodialysis is usually performed for 4 to 8 hours but needs to be prolonged in some cases if there is a large poison body burden, as is sometimes necessary for toxic alcohols.

**TABLE 4–2 Characteristics of Xenobiotics That Allow Clearance by Hemodialysis, Hemoperfusion, and Hemofiltration**

| *For All Three Techniques* | *For Hemodialysis* | *For Hemoperfusion* | *For Hemofiltration* |
|---|---|---|---|
| Low Vd (<1 L/kg) | MW <5,000 Da | MW <50,000 Da | MW <40,000 Da |
| Single-compartment first-order kinetics | Low protein binding | Adsorption by activated charcoal | Low protein binding |
| Low endogenous clearance (<4 mL/min/kg) | | | |

MW = molecular weight; Vd = volume of distribution.

Table 4–2 lists the characteristics of xenobiotics that make them amenable to hemodialysis. These requirements greatly reduce the number of xenobiotics that can be expected to be cleared by dialysis. During hemodialysis, clearance of a xenobiotic ($Cl_x$) can be calculated by:

$$Cl_x = Q_p \times ER$$

where $Q_p$ is the plasma flow rate and ER is the extraction ratio.

$$Q_p = Q_b \times (1 - Hct)$$

where $Q_b$ is blood flow rate and Hct is hematocrit. The ER is a measure of the percentage of xenobiotic passing through the artificial kidney or charcoal hemoperfusion cartridge. This can be calculated as:

$$ER = \frac{C_{in} - C_{out}}{C_{in}} \times 100$$

where $C_{in}$ is the concentration of the xenobiotic in blood entering the system and $C_{out}$ is the concentration in blood leaving the system.

Thus:

$$Cl_x = [Q_p (C_{in} - C_{out})]/C_{in}$$

With the current routine use of high flux membranes, hemodialysis appears, in some cases, to be as efficient as hemoperfusion to remove certain xenobiotics. In addition to removing xenobiotics, hemodialysis can correct acid–base and electrolyte abnormalities such as metabolic acidosis or alkalosis, hyperkalemia, and ECF volume overload. Consequently, hemodialysis is preferred, if not essential, for poisonings characterized by these disorders, especially when clearance rates resulting from hemoperfusion and hemodialysis are relatively similar.

An important unwanted effect of hemodialysis is the removal of therapeutic drugs and antidotes. Doses of these xenobiotics need to be increased during dialysis or administered immediately afterward. Examples include ethanol, fomepizole, *N*-acetylcysteine, many antibiotics, and water-soluble vitamins.

### Hemoperfusion

During hemoperfusion, blood is pumped via a catheter through a cartridge containing a very large surface area of sorbent, either activated charcoal or a resin, on to which the xenobiotic can be directly adsorbed (Fig. 4–2). The activated charcoal sorbent is coated with a very thin layer of polymer membrane such as cellulose acetate to prevent direct contact between blood and sorbent, improve biocompatibility, and help prevent activated charcoal embolization. Other adsorptive resins were used for hemoperfusion in the past, such as the synthetic Amberlite XAD-2 and XAD-4 and anion exchange resins such as Dow 1X-2. None of these resins is currently approved or available for use in the United States, but they remain available in other countries.

The adsorptive capacity of the cartridge is reduced with use because of deposition of cellular debris and blood proteins and saturation of active sites by the xenobiotic in question. Hemoperfusion is typically performed for 4 to 6 hours at flow rates that usually cannot exceed 250 mL/min because of the risk of hemolysis.

The characteristics of xenobiotics that make them amenable to hemoperfusion (Table 4–2) differ slightly from those for hemodialysis in that hemoperfusion is not as limited by plasma protein binding. Unfortunately, when xenobiotics are poorly adsorbed by activated charcoal, hemoperfusion becomes useless. Hemodialysis and hemoperfusion are sometimes combined to optimize clearance, with greater removal rates than with either procedure alone, although it is unclear if this marginal benefit outweighs the cost and added complication rates of this combination.

A practical problem limiting the use of charcoal hemoperfusion is the availability of the cartridges. The cartridges are expensive (~$600 compared with the maximal cost for a high-flux dialysis membrane of less than $40), especially if cartridges are replaced regularly. Some have expiration dates, limiting their shelf life. Complications of hemoperfusion are more common than with hemodialysis: thrombocytopenia, leukopenia, and hypocalcemia. Finally, hemoperfusion cannot correct acid–base or electrolyte abnormalities and cannot provide ultrafiltration if volume overload occurs.

Although hemoperfusion has historically been considered the preferred method to enhance the elimination of carbamazepine, phenobarbital, phenytoin, and theophylline (Table 4–3), older comparisons of hemodialysis and hemoperfusion clearance rates are now obsolete. The most frequent indication for charcoal hemoperfusion in the past was theophylline toxicity, and theophylline is rarely used today. As in the case of hemodialysis, doses of drugs used therapeutically will need to be increased if they are removed by hemoperfusion.

### Liver Support Devices

A newer concept for poisonings is that of liver support devices or liver dialysis. Several techniques have been developed; the following three are the most common. (1) Single-pass albumin dialysis (SPAD) is similar to hemodialysis but has albumin added to the dialysate in counter-directional flow, which is then discarded after passing through a filter. (2) The Molecular Adsorbents Recirculation System (MARS) is identical to SPAD, but the albumin-enhanced dialysate (with the adsorbed xenobiotics) is itself recycled after going through another dialysis circuit and through both resin and activated charcoal cartridges. (3) The Prometheus system is a device that combines albumin adsorption with high-flux hemodialysis after selective filtration of the albumin fraction through a polysulfone filter. In all of these techniques, the dialysate bathing the fibers contains human serum albumin that binds the xenobiotic of interest. A steep concentration gradient from blood to dialysate is established so that even highly protein-bound xenobiotics can be removed from the plasma. The membrane is impermeable to albumin, which remains in the dialysate.

These extracorporeal devices are all able to remove protein-bound xenobiotics, but their use in poisoning remains limited to rare case reports. These devices are mostly used in patients with hepatic encephalopathy and liver failure and as a bridge to hepatic transplantation. Whether these relatively expensive (in excess of $10,000 per treatment), complicated, and nonspecific procedures would offer benefit in a handful of instances in which protein binding limits removal of xenobiotics is not known.

### Hemofiltration

Hemofiltration is the movement of plasma across a semipermeable membrane in response to an active hydrostatic pressure by convection. In pure hemofiltration, there is no dialysate solution on the other side of the dialysis membrane (Fig. 4–2). Molecules are transported across the membrane with plasma water, a mechanism known as *convective transport* or *bulk flow*. The ECF volume status of the patient determines whether replacement of all or some of the filtered plasma is indicated. Compared with hemodialysis (diffusion), hemofiltration favors the elimination of larger xenobiotics (eg, myoglobin, molecular weight = 17,000 Da) but is slightly less effective for the removal of smaller molecules. Because most xenobiotics of interest in toxicology are smaller than 1,000 Da, it is unclear if hemofiltration has any advantage over pure hemodialysis. Solute clearance can be significantly enhanced by combining both diffusion and convection, a technique known as *hemodiafiltration*. Table 4–2 summarizes the properties of xenobiotics that make them amenable to hemofiltration.

### Continuous Techniques

Continuous techniques are referred to collectively as modalities of *continuous renal replacement therapy* (CRRT). The blood flow and effluent flow are lower than those administered during intermittent techniques, so the achievable xenobiotic clearance is lower. However, what they lack in removal rates is compensated by longer administration (they can be performed without interruption for several days).

For all of these procedures, the patient usually must be fully anticoagulated. Continuous techniques include

**TABLE 4–3 Properties of Xenobiotics Grouped by Benefit of Extracorporeal Techniques for Elimination**

| *Xenobiotic* | *MW (Da)* | *Water Soluble* | *Vd (L/Kg)* | *Protein Binding (%)* | *Endogenous Clearance (mL/min/kg)* | *Comments* |
|---|---|---|---|---|---|---|
| ***Clinically Beneficial*** | | | | | | |
| Bromide | 35 | Yes | 0.7 | 0 | 0.1 | Falsely elevated chloride measurement |
| Caffeine | 194 | Yes | 0.6 | 36 | 1.3 | Hyperglycemia, hypokalemia, metabolic acidosis |
| Ethylene glycol | 62 | Yes | 0.6 | 0 | 2.0 | Oxaluria, kidney failure |
| Diethylene glycol | 106 | Yes | 0.5 | 0 | NA | Kidney failure |
| Isopropanol | 60 | Yes | 0.6 | 0 | 1.2 | No acidosis, ketosis and ketonuria |
| Lithium | 7 | Yes | 0.8 | 0 | 0.4 | Low anion gap, low CL in kidney failure |
| Metformin | 129 | Yes | 3–5 | 0 | 8 | Very low CL in kidney failure |
| Methanol | 32 | Yes | 0.6 | 0 | 0.7 | Risk of CNS hemorrhage |
| Propylene glycol | 76 | Yes | 0.6 | 0 | 1.7 | Lactic acidosis |
| Salicylate | 138 | Yes | 0.2 | 50 (saturable) | 0.9 | CL and protein binding ↓, with ↑ dose; HD also corrects electrolytes and acid–base disturbance |
| Theophylline | 180 | Yes | 0.5 | 56 | 0.7 | HP and HD can also be combined |
| Valproic acid | 144 | Yes | 0.2 | 90 (saturable) | 0.1 | ↑ Concentrations associated with ↓ % protein binding, HD also clears ammonia when elevated |
| ***Possibly Clinically Beneficial*** | | | | | | |
| Acetaminophen | 151 | Yes | 0.9 | 30 | 2.0 | For coma and mitochondrial injury |
| Amatoxins | 373–990 | Yes | 0.3 | 0 | 2.7–6.2 | Possibly effective if performed within the first 24 h of exposure |
| Aminoglycosides | >500 | Yes | 0.3 | 1.5 | <10 | CL ↓ with kidney failure |
| Atenolol | 255 | Yes | 1.0 | 2.5 | <5 | Useful if CL ↓ caused by kidney failure |
| Carbamazepine | 236 | No | 1.4 | 74 | 1.3 | CL ↑ in patients on long-term therapy |
| Disopyramide | 340 | No | 0.6 | 1.2 | 1.6 | Protein binding ↓ as concentration ↑ |
| Fluoride | 19 | Yes | 0.3 | 50 | 2.5 | Hypocalcemia may be improved by HD |
| Methotrexate | 454 | Yes | 0.6 | 50 | 1.5 | Urine alkalinization is indicated, good antidote |
| Paraquat | 186 | Yes | 1.0 | 6 | 24.0 | Tight tissue binding precludes efficacy unless initiated early |
| Phenobarbital | 232 | No | 0.5 | 24 | 0.1 | Only for prolonged coma |
| Phenytoin | 252 | No | 0.6 | 90 | 0.3 | CL ↓ as dose ↑; HD efficient |

CL = clearance; CNS = central nervous system; HD = hemodialysis; HF = hemofiltration; HP = hemoperfusion; MW = molecular weight; NA = not available; Vd = volume of distribution.

*continuous venovenous hemofiltration* (CVVH), *continuous venovenous hemodialysis* (CVVHD), and *continuous venovenous hemodiafiltration* (CVVHDF) (Fig. 4–2).

There are several possible advantages of continuous modalities; the major benefits are a slower fluid removal rate and solute flux, which are pertinent for acutely ill patients who are hemodynamically unstable, fluid overloaded, and oliguric. Another practical advantage of CRRT is that the procedure is usually done in ICUs by ICU nurses, and when available in such units, it might not require dialysis personnel. In clinical toxicology, CRRT is sometimes used after hemodialysis or hemoperfusion to further remove a xenobiotic, especially those that distribute slowly from tissue-binding sites or from the intracellular compartment. However, because the rate of removal with CRRT is considerably inferior to that achieved by intermittent hemodialysis or hemoperfusion, it is not ideal for severely poisoned patients.

For these reasons, intermittent hemodialysis is preferable over CRRT for removal of xenobiotics. Continuous modalities are best suited for hemodynamically unstable patients who require net ultrafiltration, although this situation is infrequent unless oliguric acute kidney injury is present.

### Plasmapheresis and Exchange Transfusion

Plasmapheresis and exchange transfusion are intended to eliminate xenobiotics that are either extremely large (>100,000 Da, typified by immunoglobulins) or extensively protein bound. The xenobiotic to be eliminated should also have limited endogenous metabolism to make pheresis or exchange worthwhile. Plasmapheresis is particularly expensive, and both pheresis and exchange transfusion expose the patient to the risks of infection with plasma- or bloodborne diseases. Replacement of the removed plasma during plasmapheresis can be accomplished with fresh-frozen plasma, albumin, or combinations of both. Exchange transfusion may be an appropriate technique in the management of small infants or neonates in whom hemodialysis or hemoperfusion is often technically difficult or impossible, such as in the neonatal population.

## OTHER TECHNIQUES TO ENHANCE ELIMINATION

Further discussions of some of the techniques to enhance elimination that are not discussed here may be found in Special Considerations: SC6 (cerebrospinal fluid drainage and replacement), Antidotes in Brief: A22 (toxin-specific antibodies), and Chap. 66 (chelation). All of these techniques have limited and very specific indications. A summarized approach to the use of ECTRs is shown in Fig. 4–3.

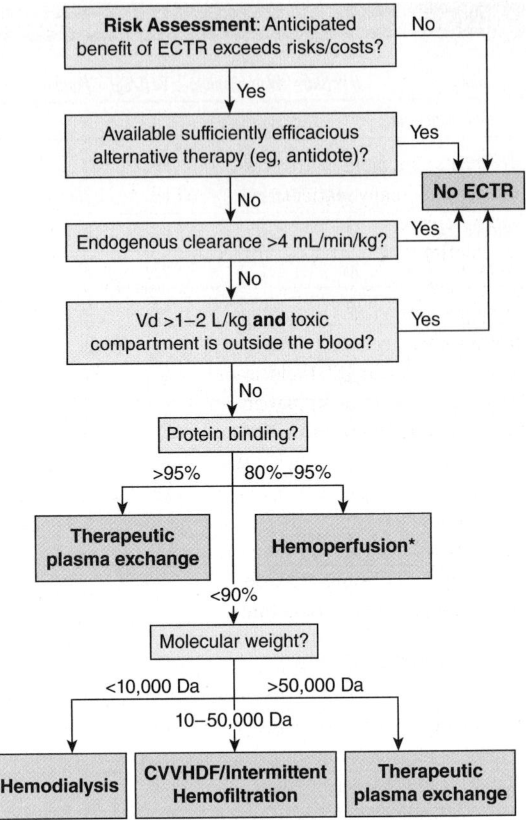


**FIGURE 4–3.** Clinical approach to consideration of using an extracorporeal treatment (ECTR) in a poisoning situation. This assessment requires analysis of the patient's condition, the specific xenobiotic, alternative treatments, molecular and toxicokinetic characteristics, and available modalities. *If the xenobiotic is adsorbed to activated charcoal, hemoperfusion is preferred; if not, then evaluate based on molecular weight.

## TOXICOLOGY OF HEMODIALYSIS

Patients with chronic kidney failure are repeatedly exposed to nearly 600 L of water each week during the course of their hemodialysis treatments that is derived from municipal reservoirs. Problems with dialysate generation therefore have the potential to be lethal to this population by exposing them to significant quantities of toxins. There are two potential sources of dialysate contamination: the municipal reservoirs and water treatment plants and the dialysis unit. Water contamination should be especially suspected when multiple dialysis patients experience similar symptoms nearly simultaneously.

Contamination of dialysate from the municipal water supply may occur as a result of xenobiotic runoff into reservoirs or as a result of inadvertent or intentional addition of a chemical by the municipality. Chlorine and chloramine are frequently added to municipal water supplies to control bacterial populations. However, chlorine may combine with nitrogenous compounds and form chloramine, which causes nausea, vomiting, methemoglobinemia, and hemolytic anemia. Chloramine has been blamed for decreased bone marrow sensitivity to erythropoietin.

Water from the municipal supply may be treated in a variety of ways. It first enters the dialysis unit and is treated with a water softener to remove calcium and magnesium. It is then run through an activated charcoal bed to adsorb chloramine, which could be lethal if left in place. Most commonly, water for dialysate is then generated by reverse osmosis, a process that requires that water, in response to applied hydrostatic pressure (and against the osmotic gradient), cross a membrane that is relatively impermeable to solutes, leaving them behind. Current requirements are that water be highly purified but not sterile, because bacteria cannot cross from the dialysate into the blood. However, small quantities of endotoxin (molecular weight, 5–15,000 Da) can cross, particularly in situations that include the use of high-flux membranes.

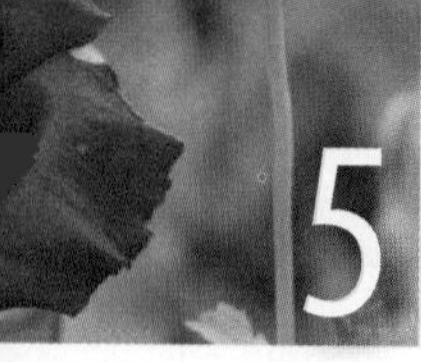

# 5 PRINCIPLES OF DIAGNOSTIC IMAGING

Diagnostic imaging plays a significant role in the management of many patients with toxicologic emergencies. Radiography can confirm a diagnosis (eg, by visualizing the xenobiotic), assist in therapeutic interventions such as monitoring gastrointestinal (GI) decontamination, and detect complications of the xenobiotic exposure (Table 5–1).

Conventional radiography is readily available in the emergency department (ED) and is the imaging modality most frequently used in acute patient management. Other imaging modalities are used in certain toxicologic emergencies, including computed tomography (CT); enteric and intravascular contrast studies; ultrasonography; transesophageal echocardiography (TEE); magnetic resonance imaging (MRI) and magnetic resonance angiography (MRA); and nuclear scintigraphy, including positron emission tomography (PET) and single-photon emission tomography (SPECT).

## VISUALIZING THE XENOBIOTIC

A number of xenobiotics are radiopaque and can potentially be detected by conventional radiography. Radiography is most useful when a substance that is known to be radiopaque is ingested or injected. If the toxic material itself is available for examination, it can be radiographed outside of the body to detect its radiopacity or any radiopaque contents (Fig. 75–1).

## RADIOPACITY

The radiopacity of a xenobiotic is determined by several factors. First, the intrinsic radiopacity of a substance depends on its physical density (g/cm$^3$) and the atomic numbers of its constituent atoms. Biologic tissues are composed mostly of carbon, hydrogen, and oxygen and have an average atomic number of approximately 6. Substances that are more radiopaque than soft tissues include bone, which contains calcium (atomic number 20), radiocontrast agents containing iodine (atomic number 53) and barium (atomic number 56), iron (atomic number 26), and lead (atomic number 82). Some xenobiotics have constituent atoms of high atomic number, such as chlorine (atomic number 17), that contribute to their radiopacity.

The thickness of an object also affects its radiopacity. Finally, the radiographic appearance of the surrounding area also affects the detectability of an object. A moderately radiopaque tablet is easily seen against a uniform background, but in a patient, overlying bone or bowel gas often obscures the tablet.

## ULTRASONOGRAPHY

Compared with conventional radiography, ultrasonography theoretically is a useful tool for detecting ingested xenobiotics because it depends on echogenicity rather than radiopacity for visualization. Reliably finding pills scattered throughout the GI tract, which often contains air and feces that block the ultrasound beam, is a formidable task. In a well-controlled trial comparing participants who ingested 50 enteric-coated placebo tablets with control participants, ultrasonography of the stomach had a sensitivity of only 62.5% at the time of ingestion and 20.8% after 1 hour and a specificity of 58.3% and 79%, respectively. Ultrasonography, therefore, has limited clinical practicality and is therefore not routinely recommended.

## INGESTION OF AN UNKNOWN XENOBIOTIC

The number of potentially ingested xenobiotics that are radiopaque is limited. In addition, the radiographic appearance of an ingested xenobiotic is not sufficiently distinctive to determine its identity (Fig. 5–1). However, when ingestion of a radiopaque xenobiotic such as ferrous sulfate tablets or another metal with a high atomic number is suspected, abdominal radiographs are helpful.

A short list of the more consistently radiopaque xenobiotics is summarized in the mnemonic CHIPES—chloral hydrate, "heavy metals," iron, phenothiazines, and enteric-coated and sustained-release preparations. The CHIPES mnemonic has several limitations. It does not include all of the pills that are radiopaque in vitro such as acetazolamide and busulfan. Most radiopaque medications are only moderately radiopaque, and when ingested, they dissolve rapidly, becoming difficult or impossible to detect. Pill formulations of fillers, binders, and coatings vary among manufacturers, and even a specific product can change depending on the date of manufacture. Furthermore, the insoluble matrix of some sustained-release preparations is radiopaque when seen on a radiograph.

## EXPOSURE TO A KNOWN XENOBIOTIC

When a xenobiotic that is known to be radiopaque is involved in an exposure, radiography plays an important role in patient care. Radiography can confirm the diagnosis of a radiopaque xenobiotic exposure, quantify the approximate amount of xenobiotic involved, and monitor its removal from the body.

### Iron Tablet Ingestion

Adult-strength ferrous sulfate tablets are readily detected radiographically because they are highly radiopaque and disintegrate slowly when ingested (Fig. 5–2). Some iron preparations are not radiographically detectable. Liquid, chewable, or encapsulated ("Spansule") iron preparations rapidly fragment and disperse after ingestion (Chap. 18). Even when intact, these preparations are less radiopaque than ferrous sulfate tablets.

### Metals

Metals, such as arsenic, cesium, lead, manganese, mercury, potassium, and thallium, are often detected radiographically. An example of metal exposure is leaded ceramic glaze (Fig. 5–3).

**TABLE 5–1** Examples of Xenobiotics with Diagnostic Imaging Findings

| *Xenobiotic* | *Imaging Study*[a] | *Findings* |
|---|---|---|
| Amiodarone | Chest | Phospholipidosis (interstitial and alveolar filling), pulmonary fibrosis |
| Asbestos | Chest | Interstitial fibrosis (asbestosis), calcified pleural plaques, mesothelioma |
| Beryllium | Chest | Acute: airspace filling; chronic: hilar adenopathy |
| Body packers and body stuffers | Abdominal<br>Enteric contrast or abdominal CT<br>Ultrasonography | Ingested packets, ileus, bowel obstruction<br>Retained packets, bowel obstruction or perforation<br>Ingested packets |
| Carbon monoxide | Head CT, MRI<br>SPECT, PET | Bilateral basal ganglion lucencies, white matter demyelinization<br>Cerebral dysfunction |
| Caustic ingestion | Enteric contrast<br>CT | Esophageal perforation or stricture |
| Chemotherapeutics (busulfan, bleomycin) | Chest | Interstitial pneumonitis |
| Cholinergics | Chest | Diffuse airspace filling (bronchorrhea) |
| Cocaine | Chest, abdominal<br>Noncontrast, head CT, MRI, TEE<br>SPECT, PET | Diffuse airspace filling, pneumomediastinum, pneumothorax, aortic dissection, perforation<br>SAH, intracerebral hemorrhage, infarction<br>Cerebral dysfunction, dopamine receptor downregulation |
| Corticosteroids | Skeletal | Avascular necrosis (femoral head), osteoporosis |
| Ethanol | Chest<br>Head CT, MRI<br>SPECT, PET | Dilated cardiomyopathy, aspiration pneumonitis, rib fractures<br>Cortical atrophy, cerebellar atrophy, SDH (head trauma)<br>Cerebellar and cortical dysfunction |
| Fluorosis | Skeletal | Osteosclerosis, osteophytosis, ligament calcification |
| Hydrocarbons (low viscosity) | Chest | Aspiration pneumonitis |
| Inhaled allergens | Chest | Hypersensitivity pneumonitis |
| Injection drug use | Chest, skeletal, cranial CT | Septic emboli, pneumothorax, osteomyelitis (axial skeleton), AIDS-related infections |
| Iron | Abdominal | Radiopaque tablets |
| Irritant gases | Chest | Diffuse airspace filling thorax |
| Lead | Skeletal<br>Abdominal | Metaphyseal bands in children (proximal tibia, distal radius), bullets (dissolution near joints)<br>Ingested leaded paint chips or other leaded compounds |
| Manganese | MRI brain | Basal ganglia and midbrain hyperintensity |
| Mercury (elemental) | Abdominal, skeletal, or chest | Ingested, injected, or embolic deposits |
| Metals (Pb, Hg, Tl, As) | Abdominal | Ingested xenobiotic |
| Nitrofurantoin | Chest | Hypersensitivity pneumonitis |
| Opioids | Chest<br>Abdominal | ARDS<br>Ileus |
| Phenytoin | Chest, CT | Hilar lymphadenopathy, pseudolymphoma |
| Procainamide, isoniazid, hydralazine | Chest<br>Echocardiogram | Pleural and pericardial effusions (xenobiotic-induced lupus syndrome)<br>Pericardial effusion |
| Salicylates | Chest | ARDS |
| Silica, coal dust | Chest | Interstitial fibrosis, hilar adenopathy (egg-shell calcification) |
| Thorium dioxide | Abdominal | Hepatic and splenic deposition |

[a]Conventional radiography unless otherwise stated.

AIDS = acquired immune deficiency syndrome; ARDS = acute respiratory distress syndrome; CT = computed tomography; MRI = magnetic resonance imaging; PET = positron emission tomography; SAH = subarachnoid hemorrhage; SDH = subdural hematoma; SPECT = single-photon emission tomography; TEE = transesophageal echocardiography.

***Mercury.*** Unintentional ingestion of elemental mercury previously occurred when a glass thermometer or a long intestinal tube with a mercury-containing balloon broke. Liquid elemental mercury can be injected subcutaneously or intravenously. Radiographic studies assist in débridement by detecting mercury that remains after the initial excision (Fig. 5–4). Elemental mercury that is injected intravenously produces a dramatic radiographic picture of pulmonary embolization.

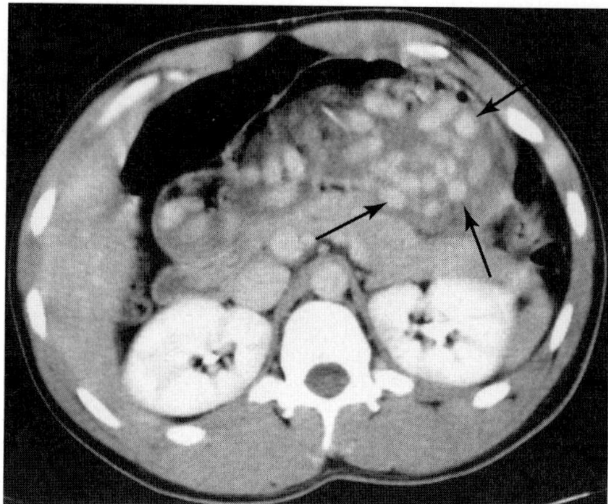

**FIGURE 5–1.** Ingestion of an unknown substance. A 46-year-old man presented to the emergency department with a depressed level of consciousness. Because he also complained of abdominal pain and mild diffuse abdominal tenderness, a computed tomography (CT) scan of the abdomen was obtained. The CT scan revealed innumerable tablet-shaped densities within the stomach (*arrows*). The CT finding was suspicious for an overdose of an unknown xenobiotic. Orogastric lavage was attempted, and the patient vomited a large amount of whole navy beans. Computed tomography is able to detect small, nearly isodense structures such as these that cannot be seen using conventional radiography. *(Used with permission from Dr. Earl J. Reisdorff, MD, Michigan State University, Lansing, MI.)*

***Lead.*** Ingested lead is detected only by abdominal radiography, such as in a child with lead poisoning who has ingested paint chips (Fig. 66–7). Radiography can confirm the source of lead poisoning by revealing metallic material in the joint or CSF (Fig. 5–5).

### Xenobiotics in Containers

In some circumstances, ingested xenobiotics are seen even though they are of similar radiopacity to surrounding soft tissues. If a xenobiotic is ingested in a container, the container itself will be visible (Special Considerations: SC4).

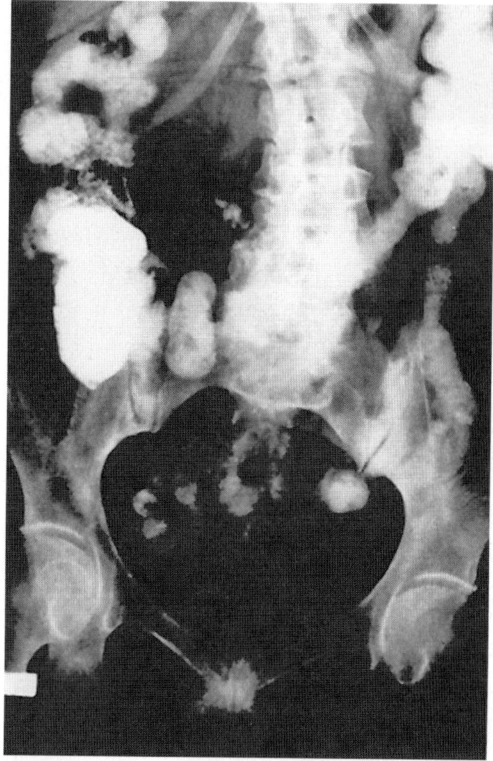

**FIGURE 5–3.** An abdominal radiograph of a patient who intentionally ingested ceramic glaze containing 40% lead. *(Used with permission from the Fellowship in Medical Toxicology, NYU School of Medicine, New York City Poison Control Center.)*

***Body Packers.*** "Body packers" are individuals who smuggle large quantities of illicit drugs across international borders in securely sealed packets. The uniformly shaped, oblong packets are seen on abdominal radiographs either because there is a thin layer of air or metallic foil within the container wall or because the packets are outlined by

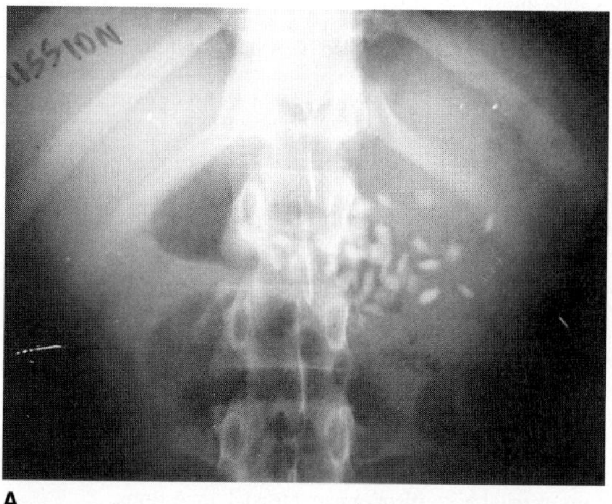

A

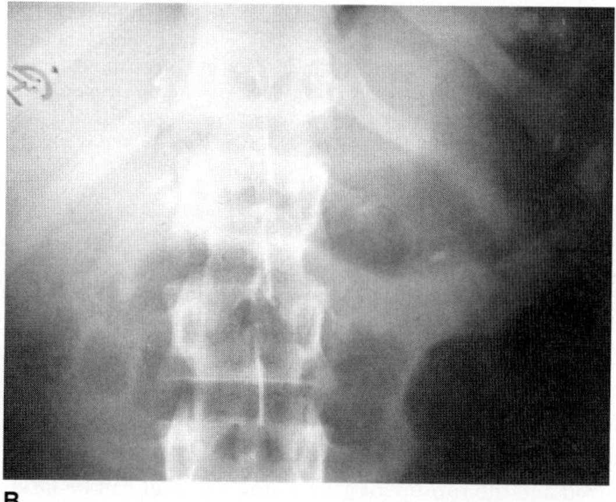

B

**FIGURE 5–2.** Iron tablet overdose. (**A**) Identification of the large amount of radiopaque tablets confirms the diagnosis in a patient with a suspected iron overdose and permits rough quantification of the amount ingested. (**B**) After emesis and whole-bowel irrigation, a second radiograph revealed some remaining tablets and indicated the need for further intestinal decontamination. *(Used with permission from the Fellowship in Medical Toxicology, NYU School of Medicine, New York City Poison Control Center.)*

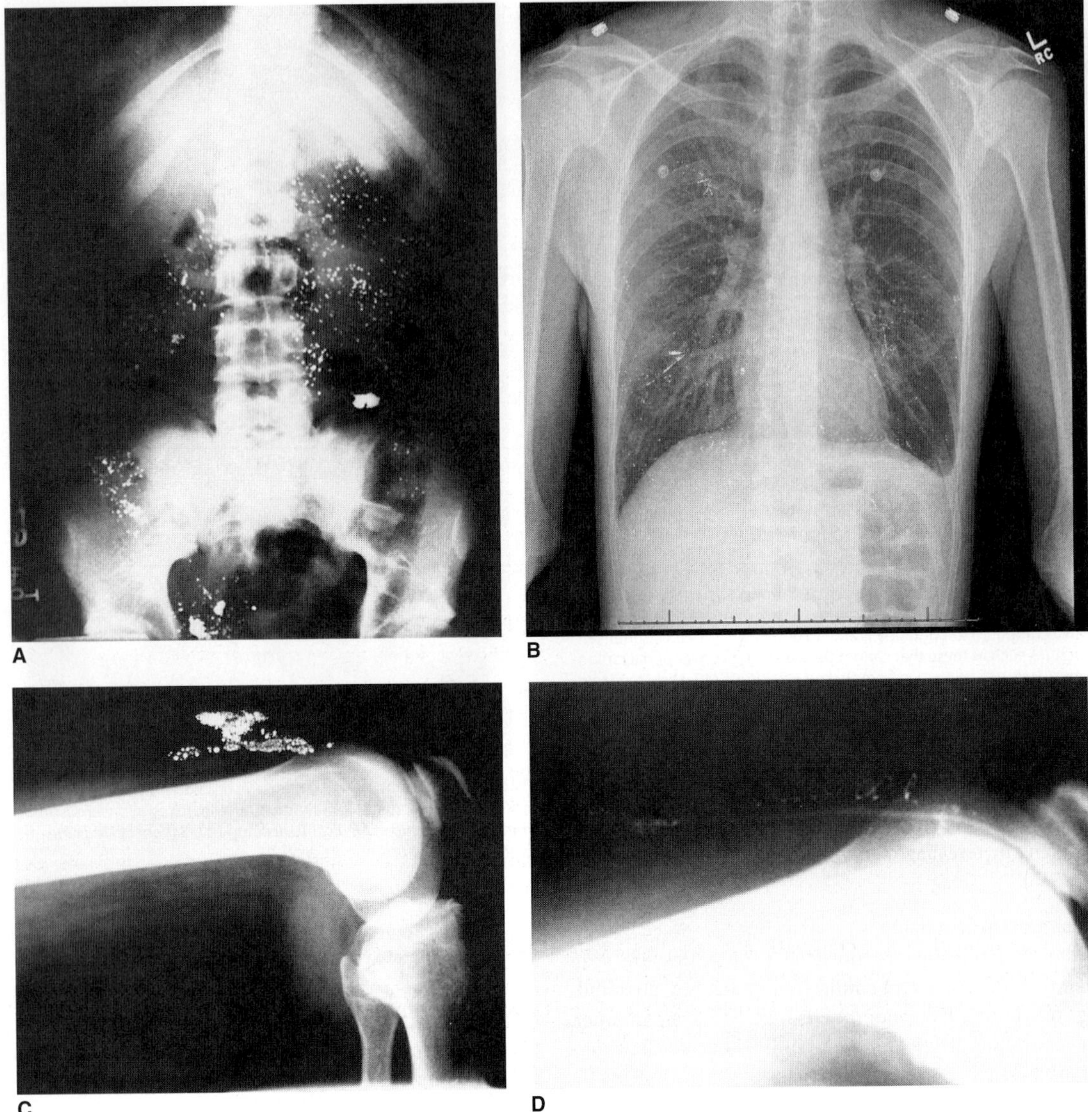

**FIGURE 5–4.** Elemental mercury exposures. (**A**) Unintentional rupture of a Cantor intestinal tube distributed mercury throughout the bowel. (**B**) Chest radiograph following intravenous mercury injection. (**C**) Subcutaneous injection of elemental mercury is readily detected radiographically. Because mercury is systemically absorbed from subcutaneous tissues, it must be removed by surgical excision. (**D**) A radiograph after surgical débridement reveals nearly complete removal of the mercury deposit. Surgical staples and a radiopaque drain are visible. *(Image A used with permission from Dr. Alexander Baxter, Department of Radiology, New York; image B reproduced with permission Allen B, Desai B, Beattie LK. A rare cause of chest pain: disseminated elemental mercury microthromboembolism, 2016;5(1), 11-18; and images C and D used with permission from the Fellowship in Medical Toxicology, NYU School of Medicine, New York City Poison Control Center.)*

bowel gas (Fig. 5–6). The sensitivity of abdominal radiography for such packets is high, in the range of 85% to 90%. The major role of radiography is as a rapid screening test to confirm the diagnosis in individuals suspected of smuggling drugs, such as persons being held by airport customs agents. However, because packets are occasionally not visualized and the rupture of even a single packet can be fatal, abdominal radiography should not be relied on to exclude the diagnosis of body packing. Ultrasonography is used to rapidly detect packets, although it also should not be relied on to exclude such a life-threatening ingestion. Computed tomography without oral contrast is more sensitive than radiography and ultrasonography.

***Body Stuffers.*** A "body stuffer" is an individual who, in an attempt to avoid imminent arrest, hurriedly ingests contraband in insecure packaging. The risk of leakage from such haphazardly constructed containers is high. Unfortunately, radiographic studies cannot reliably confirm or exclude such ingestions.

## Halogenated Hydrocarbons

Some halogenated hydrocarbons are visualized radiographically. Radiopacity is proportionate to the number of chlorine

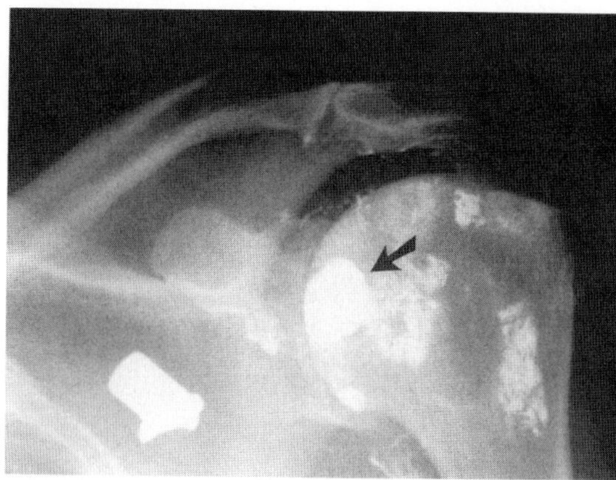

**FIGURE 5–5.** A "lead arthrogram" discovered many years after a bullet wound to the shoulder. At the time of the initial injury, the bullet was embedded in the articular surface of the humeral head (*arrow*). The portion of the bullet that protruded into the joint space was surgically removed, leaving a portion of the bullet exposed to the synovial space. A second bullet was embedded in the muscles of the scapula. Eight years after the injury, the patient presented with weakness and anemia. Extensive lead deposition throughout the synovium is seen. The blood lead concentration was 91 mcg/dL. *(Used with permission from the Fellowship in Medical Toxicology, NYU School of Medicine, New York City Poison Control Center.)*

atoms. Both carbon tetrachloride ($CCl_4$) and chloroform ($CHCl_3$) are radiopaque. Because these liquids are immiscible in water, a triple layer is seen within the stomach on an upright abdominal radiograph—an uppermost air bubble, a middle radiopaque chlorinated hydrocarbon layer, and a lower gastric fluid layer.

### Moth Repellants

Some types of moth repellants (mothballs) can be visualized by radiography. If the patient is known to have ingested a moth repellant but the nature of the moth repellant is unknown, the difference in radiopacity helps determine the type. Radiographs of the moth repellant outside of the patient can distinguish these two types (Fig. 75–1).

### Radiolucent Xenobiotics

A radiolucent xenobiotic is often visible because it is less radiopaque than surrounding soft tissues. Hydrocarbons such as gasoline are relatively radiolucent when embedded in soft tissues. The radiographic appearance resembles subcutaneous gas as seen in a necrotizing soft tissue infection (Fig. 5–7).

## EXTRAVASATION OF INTRAVENOUS CONTRAST MATERIAL

Extravasation of intravenous (IV) radiographic contrast material is a common occurrence. In most cases, the volume extravasated is small, and there are no clinical sequelae. Rarely, a patient has an extravasation large enough to cause cutaneous necrosis and ulceration. The incidence of sizable extravasations has increased because of the use of rapid-bolus automated power injectors for CT studies. Fortunately, nonionic low-osmolality contrast solutions are currently nearly always used for these studies. The treatment of contrast extravasation has not been studied in a large series of human participants and is therefore controversial. The affected extremity should be elevated to promote drainage, and the intermittent application of ice packs is recommended to lower the incidence of ulceration.

## VISUALIZING THE EFFECTS OF A XENOBIOTIC ON THE BODY

The lungs, central nervous system (CNS), GI tract, and skeleton are the organ systems that are most amenable to diagnostic imaging. Disorders of the lungs and skeletal system are seen by plain radiography. For abdominal pathology, contrast studies and CT are more useful, although plain radiographs can diagnose intestinal obstruction, perforation, and radiopaque foreign bodies. Imaging of the CNS uses CT, MRI, and nuclear scintigraphy (PET and SPECT).

### Skeletal Changes Caused by Xenobiotics

A number of xenobiotics affect bone mineralization. Toxicologic effects on bone result in either increased or decreased density (Table 5–2). With lead poisoning, the metaphyseal regions of rapidly growing long bones develop transverse bands of increased density along the growth plate (Fig. 5–8). Lead lines are caused by the toxic effect of lead on bone growth and do not represent deposition of lead in bone. Lead impedes resorption of calcified cartilage in the zone of provisional calcification adjacent to the growth plate. Fluoride poisoning also causes a diffuse increase in bone mineralization (Fig. 5–9).

Skeletal disorders associated with focal diminished bone density (or mixed rarefaction and sclerosis) include osteonecrosis, osteomyelitis, and osteolysis. Osteonecrosis, also known as avascular necrosis, most often affects the femoral head, humeral head, and proximal tibia. Radiographically, focal skeletal lucencies and sclerosis are seen, ultimately with loss of bone volume and collapse (Fig. 5–10A). Osteomyelitis is a serious complication of injection drug use. It usually affects the axial skeleton, especially the vertebral bodies, as well as the sternomanubrial and sternoclavicular joints (Figs. 5–10B and C). Spinal epidural abscesses causing spinal cord compression accompany vertebral osteomyelitis. Radiographic findings are negative early in the disease course before skeletal changes are visible, and the diagnosis is confirmed by MRI or CT (Fig. 5–10D).

### Pulmonary and Other Thoracic Problems

Chest radiographic findings suggest certain diseases, although the diagnosis ultimately depends on a thorough clinical history. Many pulmonary disorders are radiographically detectable because they result in fluid accumulation within the normally air-filled lung. Fluid accumulates within the alveolar spaces or interstitial tissues of the lung, producing the two major radiographic patterns of pulmonary disease, airspace filling and interstitial lung disease (Table 5–3). Most xenobiotics are widely distributed throughout the lungs and produce diffuse rather than focal radiographic abnormalities.

***Diffuse Airspace Filling.*** Overdose with various xenobiotics, including salicylates, opioids, and paraquat, causes acute respiratory distress syndrome (ARDS) with or without diffuse alveolar damage and characterized by leaky capillaries

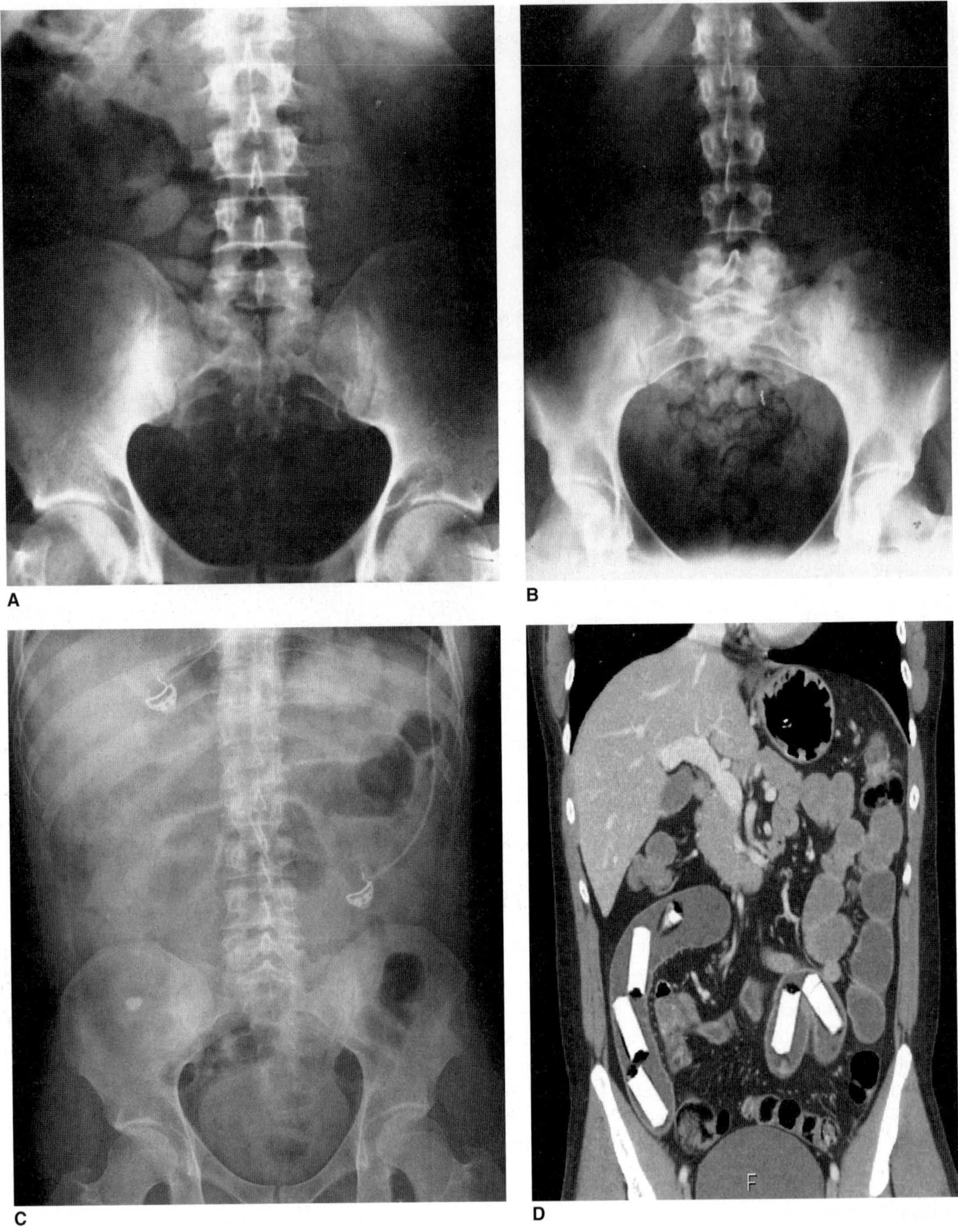


**FIGURE 5–6.** Three "body packers" showing the various appearances of drug packets. Drug smuggling is accomplished by packing the gastrointestinal tract with large numbers of manufactured, well-sealed containers. (**A**) Multiple oblong packages of uniform size and shape are seen throughout the bowel. (**B**) The packets are visible in this patient because they are surrounded by a thin layer of air within the wall of the packet. (**C** and **D**) Small bowel obstruction caused by drug packets in a man who developed abdominal pain and vomiting 1 day after arriving on a plane flight from Colombia. Computed tomography confirmed bowel obstruction, and the patient underwent laparotomy and removal of 15 packets through an enterotomy. *(Images A and B used with permission from Dr. Emil J. Balthazar, Department of Radiology, Bellevue Hospital Center. Images C and D used with permission from the Fellowship in Medical Toxicology, New York University School of Medicine, New York City Poison Center.)*

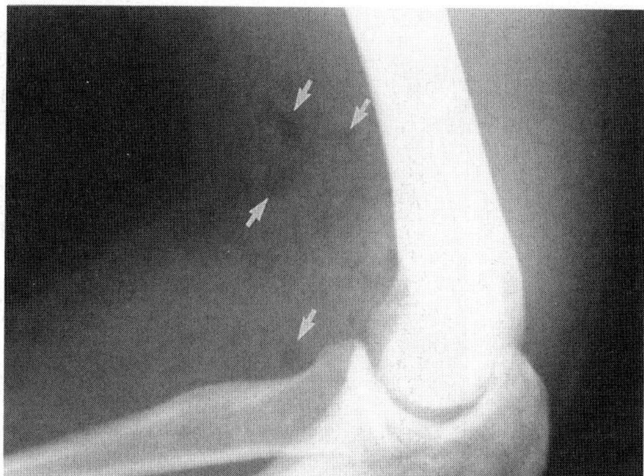

**FIGURE 5–7.** Subcutaneous injection of gasoline into the antecubital fossa. The radiolucent hydrocarbon mimics gas in the soft tissues that is seen with a necrotizing soft tissue infection such as necrotizing fasciitis or gas gangrene (*arrows*). *(Used with permission from the Fellowship in Medical Toxicology, NYU School of Medicine, New York City Poison Control Center.)*

(Fig. 5–11). There are, of course, many other causes of ARDS, including sepsis, anaphylaxis, and major trauma.

*Focal Airspace Filling.* Focal infiltrates are usually caused by bacterial pneumonia, although aspiration of gastric contents also causes localized airspace disease. Aspiration occurs during sedative–hypnotic or alcohol intoxication or during a seizure. During ingestion, low-viscosity hydrocarbons often enter the lungs while they are being swallowed. There is a typical delay in the development of radiographic abnormalities, and the chest radiograph abnormalities appear over the first 6 hours after the ingestion. During aspiration, the most dependent portions of the lung are affected. When the patient is upright at the time of aspiration, the lower lung segments are involved. When the patient is supine, the posterior segments of the upper and lower lobes are affected.

**TABLE 5–2 Xenobiotic Causes of Skeletal Abnormalities**

| *Increased Bone Density* | *Diminished Bone Density (Either Diffuse Osteoporosis or Focal Lesions)* |
|---|---|
| *Metaphyseal bands (children)*<br>Lead, bismuth, phosphorus: chondrosclerosis caused by toxic effect on bone growth | Corticosteroids:<br>Osteoporosis: diffuse<br>Osteonecrosis: focal avascular necrosis of the femoral head; loss of volume with both increased and decreased bone density<br>Also occurs in alcoholism, bismuth arthropathy, Caisson disease (dysbarism), trauma |
| *Diffuse increased bone density*<br>Fluorosis: osteosclerosis (hyperostosis deformans), osteophytosis, ligament calcification; usually involves the axial skeleton (vertebrae and pelvis) and can cause compression of the spinal cord and nerve roots<br>Hypervitaminosis A (pediatric): cortical hyperostosis and subperiosteal new bone formation; diaphyses of long bones have an undulating appearance<br>Hypervitaminosis D (pediatric): generalized osteosclerosis, cortical thickening, and metaphyseal bands | Hypervitaminosis D (adult): focal or generalized osteoporosis<br>Injection drug use: osteomyelitis (focal lytic lesions) caused by septic emboli; usually affects vertebral bodies and sternomanubrial joint<br>Vinyl chloride monomer: acroosteolysis (distal phalanges) |

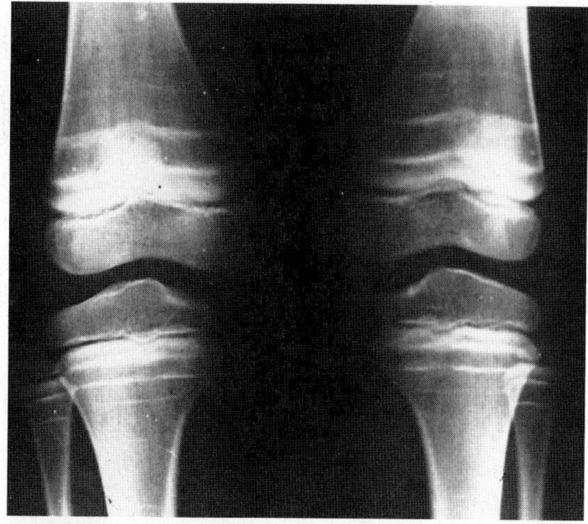

A

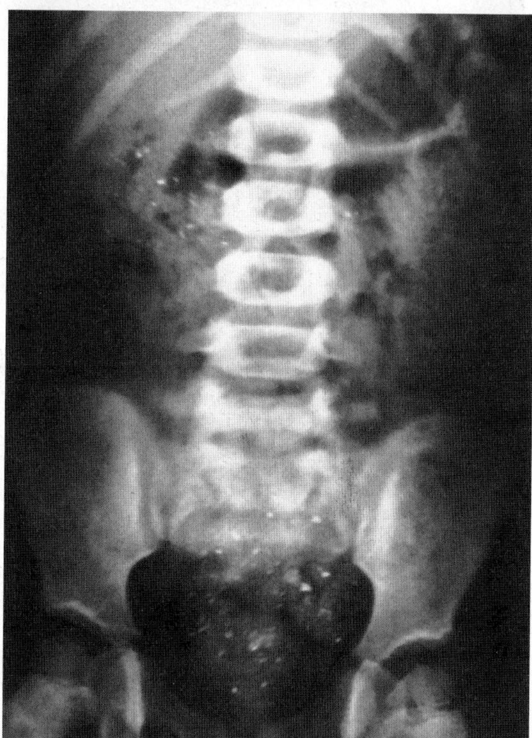

B

**FIGURE 5–8.** (**A**) A radiograph of the knees of a child with lead poisoning. The metaphyseal regions of the distal femur and proximal tibia have developed transverse bands representing bone growth abnormalities caused by lead toxicity. The multiplicity of lines implies repeated exposures to lead. (**B**) The abdominal radiograph of the child shows many radiopaque flakes of ingested leaded paint chips. Lead poisoning also caused abnormally increased cortical mineralization of the vertebral bodies, which gives them a boxlike appearance. *(Used with permission from Dr. Alexander Baxter, Department of Radiology, New York.)*

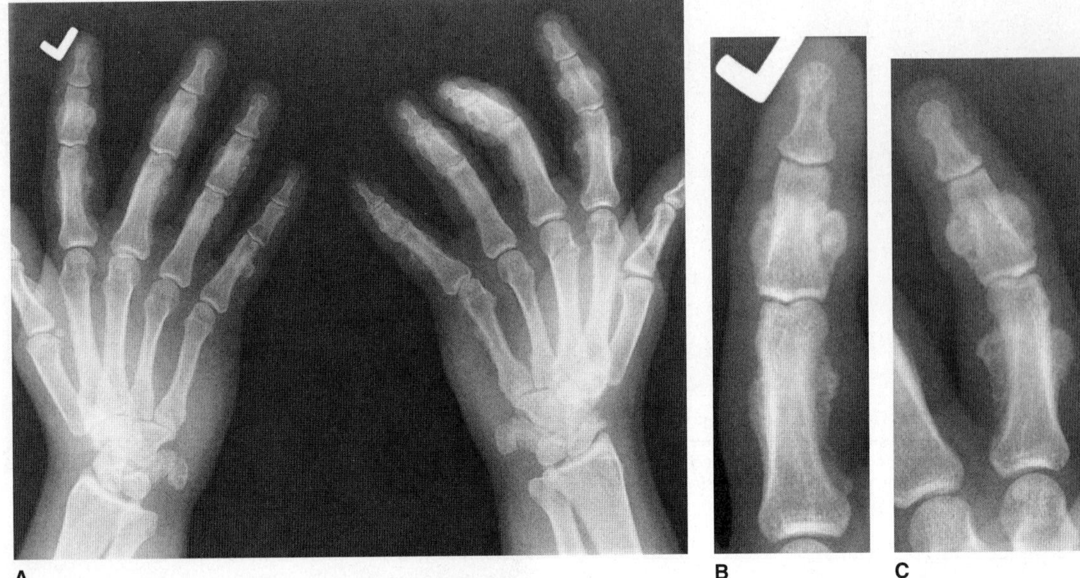


**FIGURE 5–9.** Skeletal fluorosis. A 28-year-old man developed progressive muscle and joint pain over 3 to 4 weeks particularly involving his hands with thickening of his fingers. The results of an evaluation for inflammatory rheumatologic disorders were negative. Radiographs of his hands showed exuberant periosteal new bone formation known as "periostitis deformans," which is characteristic of skeletal fluorosis. Further questioning revealed that the patient had been "huffing" the propellant of "Dust Off"; 225 cans were found at his residence. The propellant is difluoroethane (Freon 152a). The hydrocarbon is dehalogenated in the liver, and chronic exposure results in fluoride toxicity. *(Used with permission from Dr. Eric Lavonas, Rocky Mountain Poison and Drug Center, Denver Health and Hospital Authority, Denver, CO, and Dr. Shawn M. Varney, Department of Emergency Medicine, San Antonio Military Medical Center, TX.)*

***Multifocal Airspace Filling.*** Multifocal airspace filling occurs with septic pulmonary emboli, which is a complication of injection drug use and right-sided bacterial endocarditis. The foci of pulmonary infection often undergo necrosis and cavitation.

***Interstitial Lung Diseases.*** Toxicologic causes of interstitial lung disease include hypersensitivity pneumonitis, use of medications with direct pulmonary toxicity, and inhalation or injection of inorganic particulates. On the chest radiograph, acute and subacute disorders cause a fine reticular or reticulonodular pattern. Chronic interstitial disorders cause a coarse reticular "honeycomb" pattern.

***Hypersensitivity Pneumonitis.*** Hypersensitivity pneumonitis is a delayed-type hypersensitivity reaction to an inhaled or ingested allergen. Inhaled organic allergens such as those in moldy hay (farmer's lung) and bird droppings (pigeon breeder's lung) cause hypersensitivity pneumonitis in sensitized individuals. The chest radiograph findings are normal or show fine interstitial or alveolar infiltrates. Chronic hypersensitivity pneumonitis causes progressive dyspnea, and the radiograph shows interstitial fibrosis.

***Particulates.*** Inhaled inorganic particulates, such as asbestos, silica, and coal dust, cause pneumoconiosis. This is a chronic interstitial lung disease characterized by interstitial fibrosis and loss of lung volume. Intravenous injection of illicit xenobiotics that have particulate contaminants, such as talc, causes a chronic interstitial lung disease known as talcosis.

***Pleural Disorders.*** Asbestos-related calcified pleural plaques develop many years after asbestos exposure (Fig. 5–12). These lesions do not cause clinical symptoms and have only a minor association with malignancy and interstitial lung disease. Asbestos-related pleural plaques should not be called *asbestosis* because that term refers specifically to the interstitial lung disease caused by asbestos. Pleural plaques must be distinguished from mesotheliomas, which are not calcified, enlarge at a rapid rate, and erode into nearby structures such as the ribs.

Pneumothorax and pneumomediastinum are associated with illicit drug use. These complications are related to the route of administration rather than to the particular drug. Barotrauma associated with the Valsalva maneuver or intense inhalation with breath holding during the smoking of "crack" cocaine or marijuana results in pneumomediastinum (Fig. 5–13A).

***Lymphadenopathy.*** Phenytoin causes drug-induced lymphoid hyperplasia with hilar lymphadenopathy. Chronic beryllium exposure results in hilar lymphadenopathy that mimics sarcoidosis, with granulomatous changes in the lung parenchyma. Silicosis is associated with "eggshell" calcification of hilar lymph nodes.

***Cardiovascular Abnormalities.*** Dilated cardiomyopathy occurs in chronic alcoholism and exposure to cardiotoxic medications such as doxorubicin. Enlargement of the cardiac silhouette is also caused by a pericardial effusion, which accompanies drug-induced lupus. Aortic dissection is associated with use of cocaine and amphetamines. The chest radiograph shows an enlarged or indistinct aortic knob and an enlarged ascending or descending aorta (Figs. 5–13B to D).

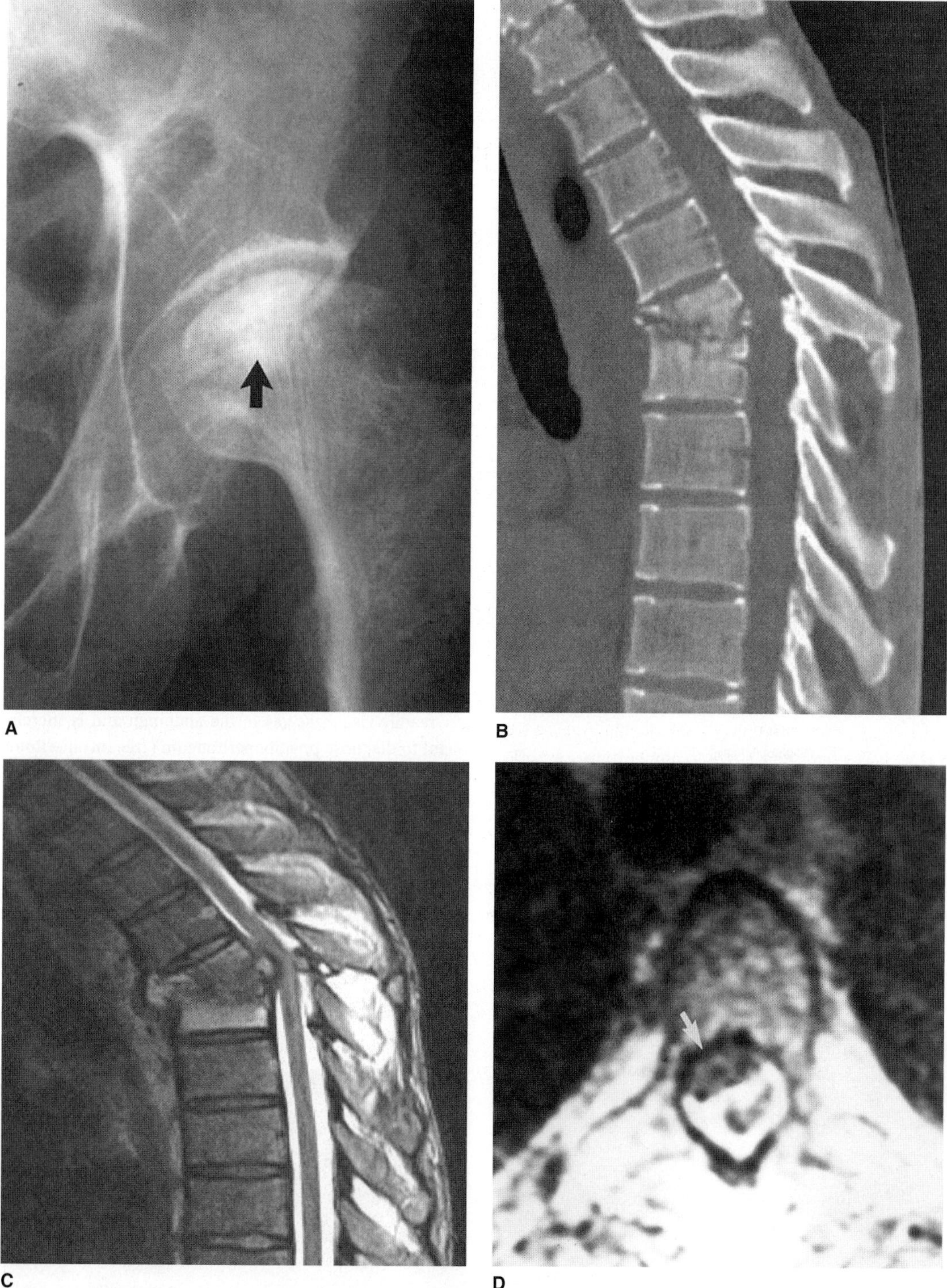


**FIGURE 5–10.** Focal loss of bone density and collapse: (**A**) Avascular necrosis causing collapse of the femoral head in a patient with long-standing steroid-dependent asthma (*arrow*). (**B** and **C**) Vertebral osteomyelitis in an injection drug user who presented with posterior thoracic pain for 2 weeks and then lower extremity weakness. As seen on computed tomography (CT), the infection begins in the intervertebral disk and then spreads to the adjacent vertebral bodies. Magnetic resonance image shows extension into the spinal canal causing spinal cord compression. (**D**) An injection drug user with thoracic back pain, leg weakness, and low-grade fever. Radiographic and CT findings of the spine were negative. Magnetic resonance image showing an epidural abscess (*arrow*) compressing the spinal cord. The cerebrospinal fluid in the compressed thecal sac is bright on this T2-weighted image. *(Reproduced with permission from Schwartz DT, Reisdorff EJ: Emergency Radiology. New York, NY: McGraw-Hill; 2000.)*

**TABLE 5–3 Chest Radiographic Findings in Toxicologic Emergencies**

| *Radiographic Finding* | *Responsible Xenobiotic* | *Disease Processes* |
|---|---|---|
| Diffuse airspace filling | Opioids | ARDS |
| | Paraquat | |
| | Salicylates | |
| | Irritant gases: $NO_2$ (silo filler's disease), phosgene ($COCl_2$), $Cl_2$, $H_2S$ | |
| | Organic phosphorus compounds, carbamates | Cholinergic stimulation (bronchorrhea) |
| | Alcoholic cardiomyopathy, cocaine, doxorubicin, cobalt | Congestive heart failure |
| Focal airspace filling | Low-viscosity hydrocarbons | Aspiration pneumonitis |
| | Gastric contents aspiration: CNS depressants, alcohol, seizures | |
| Multifocal airspace filling | Injection drug use | Septic emboli |
| Interstitial patterns | Inhaled organic allergens: farmer's lung, pigeon-breeder's lung | Hypersensitivity pneumonitis |
| Fine or coarse reticular or reticulonodular pattern | Nitrofurantoin, penicillamine | |
| Patchy airspace filling seen in some cases | Chemotherapeutics: bleomycin, busulfan, carmustine, cyclophosphamide, methotrexate | Cytotoxic lung damage |
| | Amiodarone | Phospholipidosis |
| | Talcosis (illicit drug contaminant) | Injected particulates |
| | Pneumoconiosis: asbestosis, beryllIosis (chronic), coal dust, silicosis | Inhaled inorganic particulates |

ARDS = acute respiratory distress syndrome; CNS = central nervous system.

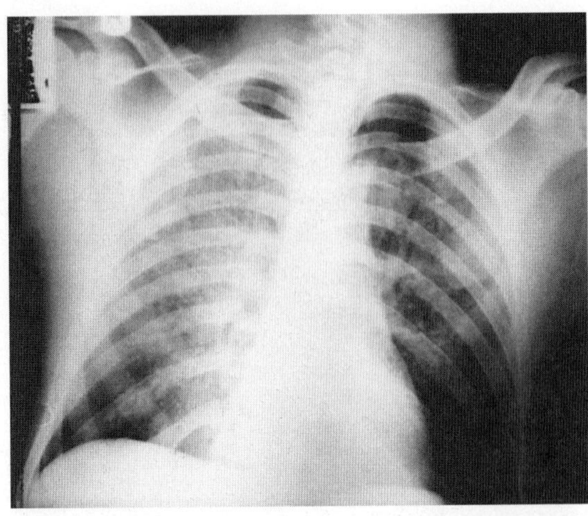

**FIGURE 5–11.** Diffuse airspace filling. The chest radiograph of a patient who had recently injected heroin intravenously and presented with respiratory distress and acute respiratory distress syndrome. The heart size is normal.

## Abdominal Problems

Abdominal imaging modalities include conventional radiography, CT, GI contrast studies, and angiography. Conventional radiography is limited in its ability to detect most intraabdominal pathology because most pathologic processes involve soft tissue structures that are not well seen. Plain radiography readily visualizes gas in the abdomen and is therefore useful to diagnose pneumoperitoneum (free intraperitoneal air) and bowel distension caused by mechanical obstruction or diminished gut motility (adynamic ileus). Other abnormal gas collections, such as intramural gas associated with intestinal infarction, are seen infrequently (Table 5–4).

***Pneumoperitoneum.*** Gastrointestinal perforation is diagnosed by the visualization of free intraperitoneal air under the diaphragm on an upright chest radiograph (Fig. 5–14). Esophageal and gastric perforations occur after the ingestion of

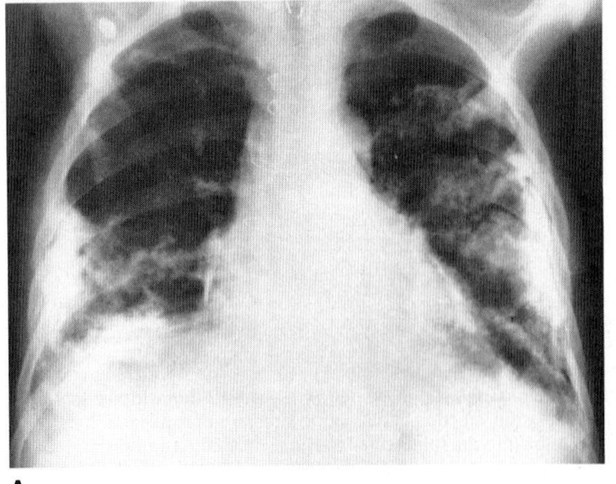

A

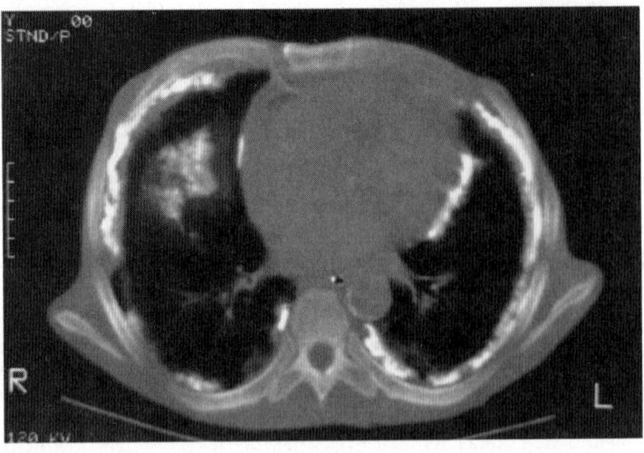


B

**FIGURE 5–12.** (**A**) Calcified plaques typical of asbestos exposure are seen on the pleural surfaces of the lungs, diaphragm, and heart. The patient was asymptomatic; this was an incidental radiographic finding. (**B**) The computed tomography (CT) scan demonstrates that the opacities seen on the chest radiograph do not involve the lung itself. A lower thoracic image shows calcified pleural plaques (the diaphragmatic plaque is seen on the *right*). The CT scan confirms that there is no interstitial lung disease ("asbestosis"). *(Used with permission from the Fellowship in Medical Toxicology, NYU School of Medicine, New York City Poison Control Center.)*

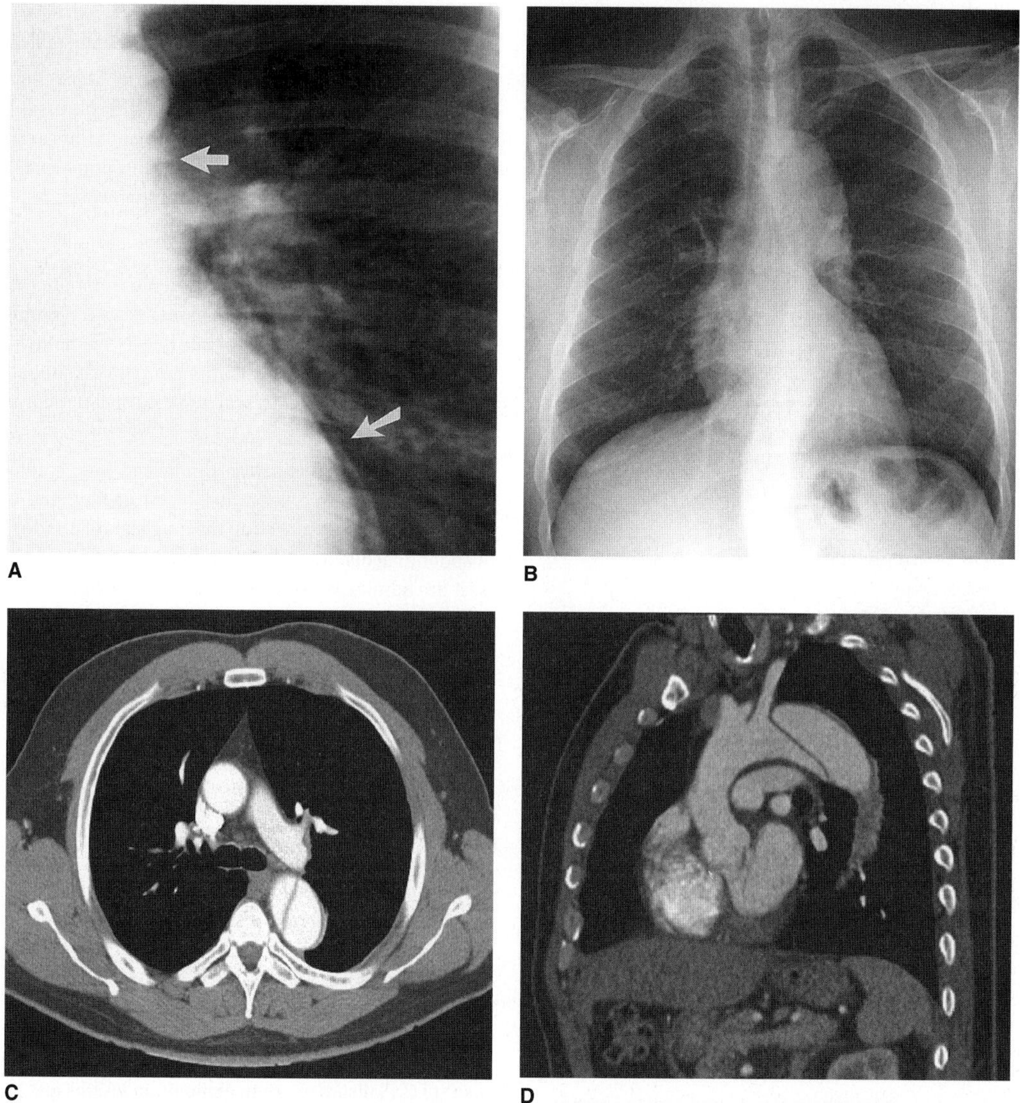


**FIGURE 5–13.** Two patients with chest pain after cocaine use. (**A**) Pneumomediastinum after forceful inhalation while smoking "crack" cocaine. A fine white line representing the pleura elevated from the mediastinal structures is seen (*arrows*). The patient's chest pain resolved during a 24-hour period of observation. (**B** to **D**) Thoracic aortic dissection after cocaine use. The patient presented with chest pain radiating to the back. He had a history of hypertension and was noncompliant with medications. Chest radiography shows an enlarged aorta caused by aortic wall weakening secondary to his long-standing hypertension. Computed tomography angiography shows the intraluminal dissection flap originating at the left subclavian artery and extending into the descending aorta. *(Used with permission from the Fellowship in Medical Toxicology, NYU School of Medicine, New York City Poison Control Center.)*

caustics such as iron, alkali, or acid; after forceful emesis; or as a complication of orogastric lavage. Esophageal perforation causes pneumomediastinum and mediastinitis.

***Obstruction and Ileus.*** Mechanical bowel obstruction is caused by large intraluminal foreign bodies such as a body packer's packets or a medication bezoar. Adynamic ileus results from the use of opioids, anticholinergics, and tricyclic antidepressants. Because adynamic ileus occurs in many diseases, the radiographic finding of an ileus is not helpful diagnostically. When the distinction between obstruction and adynamic ileus cannot be made based on the abdominal radiographs, abdominal CT can clarify the diagnosis.

***Mesenteric Ischemia.*** In most patients with intestinal ischemia, plain abdominal radiographs show only a nonspecific or adynamic ileus pattern. In a small proportion of patients with ischemic bowel (5%), intramural gas is seen. Rarely, gas is also seen in the hepatic portal venous system. Computed tomography is better able to detect signs of mesenteric ischemia, particularly bowel wall thickening. Intestinal ischemia and infarction infrequently are caused by the use of cocaine; other sympathomimetics; and the ergot alkaloids, all of which induce mesenteric vasoconstriction.

***Gastrointestinal Hemorrhage and Hepatotoxicity.*** Radiography is not usually helpful in the diagnosis of such common abdominal

**TABLE 5–4 Plain Abdominal Radiography in Toxicologic Emergencies**

| *Radiographic Finding* | *Xenobiotic* |
|---|---|
| Pneumoperitoneum (hollow viscus perforation) | Caustics: iron, alkali, acids<br>Cocaine<br>GI decontamination (ipecac, lavage tube) |
| Mechanical obstruction (intraluminal foreign body)<br>Intestinal, Gastric outlet, Esophageal } Upper GI series | Foreign-body ingestion<br>Body packer<br>Enteric-coated pills<br>Bezoar |
| Ileus (diminished gut motility) | Antimuscarinics<br>Cyclic antidepressants<br>Mesenteric ischemia caused by cocaine, oral contraceptives, cardioactive steroids<br>Hypokalemia<br>Hypomagnesemia<br>Opioids |
| Intramural gas (intestinal infarction)<br>Bowel wall thickening<br>Hepatic portal venous gas ($H_2O_2$)<br>(CT is more sensitive) | Calcium channel blockers<br>Cocaine<br>Ergot alkaloids<br>Oral contraceptives |
| Foreign-body ingestion | Bismuth subsalicylate<br>Body packers and stuffers<br>Calcium carbonate<br>Enteric-coated and sustained-release tablets<br>Iron pills<br>Metals (As, Cs, Hg, K, Pb, Tl)<br>Pica (calcareous clay) |
| Nephrocalcinosis | Calcium<br>Vitamin D |

CT = computed tomography; GI = gastrointestinal.

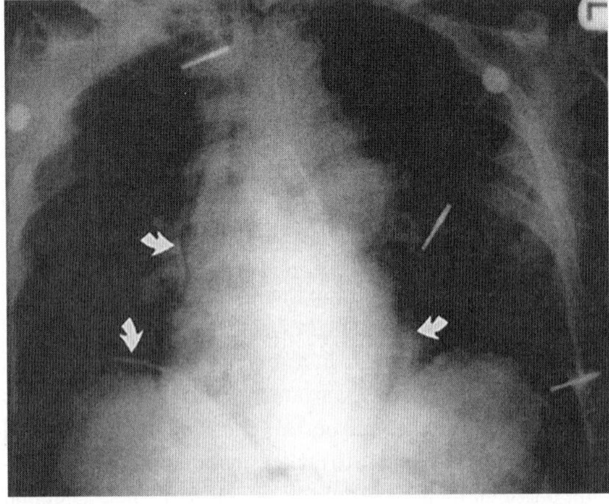

**FIGURE 5–14.** Gastrointestinal perforation after gastric lavage with a large-bore orogastric tube. The upright chest radiograph shows air under the right hemidiaphragm and pneumomediastinum (*arrows*). An esophagram with water-soluble contrast did not demonstrate the perforation. Laparotomy revealed perforation of the anterior wall of the stomach. *(Used with permission from the Fellowship in Medical Toxicology, NYU School of Medicine, New York City Poison Control Center.)*

complications as GI hemorrhage and hepatotoxicity unless the bleeding is due to ingestion of ferrous sulfate tablets.

***Contrast Esophagram and Upper Gastrointestinal Series.*** Ingestion of a caustic causes severe damage to the mucosal lining of the esophagus. This can be demonstrated by a contrast esophagram. However, in the acute setting, upper endoscopy should be performed rather than an esophagram because it provides more information about the extent of injury and prognosis. In addition, administration of barium will coat the mucosa, making endoscopy difficult. Computed tomography is a noninvasive means to assess degree of esophageal injury and estimate the risk of later developing an esophageal stricture. For later evaluation, a contrast esophagram identifies mucosal defects, scarring, and stricture formation (Fig. 5–15).

***Abdominal Computed Tomography.*** Computed tomography provides great anatomic definition of intraabdominal organs and plays an important role in the diagnosis of a wide variety of abdominal disorders. In most cases, both oral and IV contrast are administered. Oral contrast delineates the intestinal lumen. Intravenous contrast is needed to reliably detect lesions in hepatic and splenic parenchyma, the kidneys, and the bowel wall. Hepatic portal venous gas is well visualized after ingestion of high-concentration hydrogen peroxide (Fig. 5–16). Ingested foreign bodies, such as a body packer's packets, are detected on noncontrast CT (Fig. 5–6D) and Special Considerations: SC4.

***Vascular Lesions.*** Angiography detects such complications of injection drug use as venous thrombosis and arterial laceration causing pseudoaneurysm formation. Intravenous injection of amphetamine, cocaine, or ergotamine causes necrotizing angiitis that is associated with microaneurysms, segmental stenosis, and arterial thrombosis (Fig. 5–17).

## Neurologic Problems

Diagnostic imaging studies have revolutionized the management of CNS disorders. Both acute brain lesions and chronic degenerative changes are detected (Table 5–5).

***Imaging Modalities.*** Computed tomography can directly visualize brain tissue and many intracranial lesions. Computed tomography is the imaging study of choice in the emergency setting because it readily detects acute intracranial hemorrhage as well as parenchymal lesions that are causing mass effect. Computed tomography is fast, is widely available on an emergency basis, and can accommodate critical patient support and monitoring devices. Infusion of IV contrast further delineates intracerebral mass lesions such as tumors and abscesses.

*Magnetic resonance imaging* (MRI) has largely supplanted CT in nonemergency neurodiagnosis. It offers better anatomic discrimination of brain tissues and areas of cerebral edema and demyelinization. However, MRI is no better than CT in detecting acute blood collections or mass lesions. In the emergency setting, the disadvantages of MRI outweigh its strengths. Magnetic resonance imaging is often readily available on an emergency basis, but image acquisition time is long, and critical care supportive and

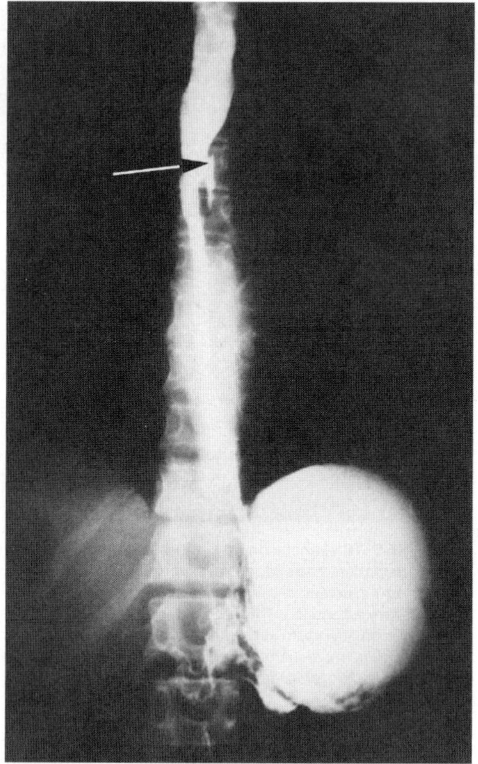
A

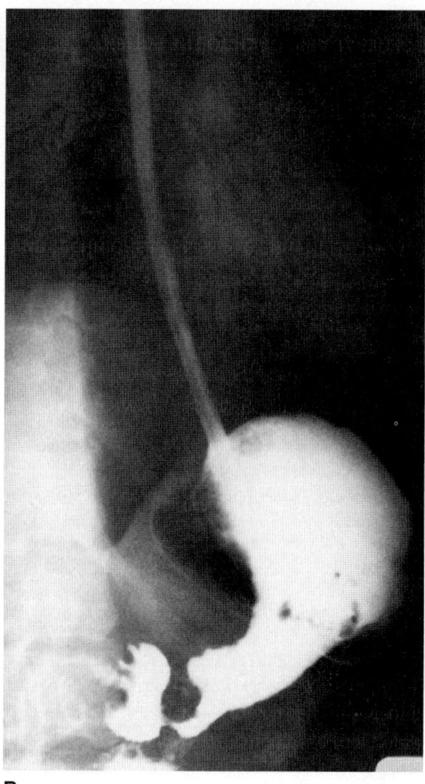
B

**FIGURE 5–15.** (**A**) A barium swallow performed several days after ingestion of liquid lye shows intramural dissection and extravasation of barium with early stricture formation. (**B**) At 3 weeks after ingestion, there are an absence of peristalsis, diffuse narrowing of the esophagus, and reduction in size of the fundus and antrum of the stomach as a result of scarring. *(Used with permission from Dr. Alexander Baxter, Department of Radiology, New York.)*

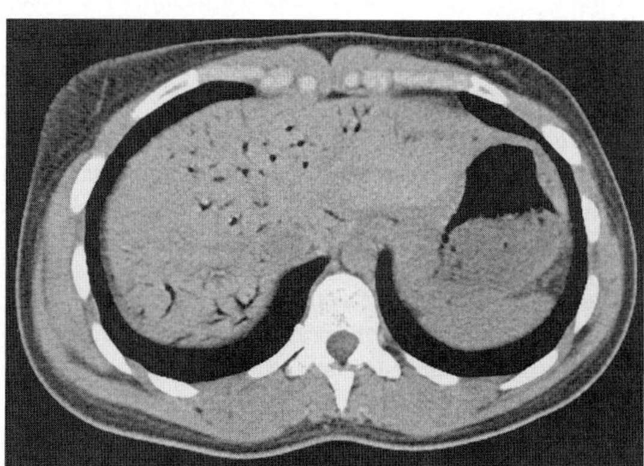

**FIGURE 5–16.** Abdominal computed tomography showing extensive hepatic portal venous gas in a woman who inadvertently ingested a small quantity of commercial concentration (35%) hydrogen peroxide. She also had gastric and esophageal erosions on endoscopy and was treated successfully with antacids and hyperbaric oxygen. *(Used with permission from Dr. Alexander Baxter, Department of Radiology, New York.)*

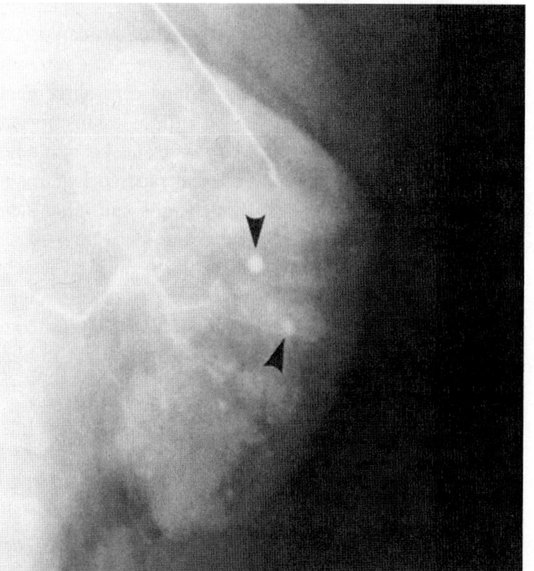

**FIGURE 5–17.** A selective renal angiogram in an injection methamphetamine user demonstrating multiple small and large aneurysms (arrowheads). *(Used with permission from Dr. Alexander Baxter, Department of Radiology, New York.)*

**TABLE 5–5 Cranial Computed Tomography (Noncontrast) in Toxicologic Emergencies**

| *Computed Tomography Finding* | *Brain Lesion* | *Xenobiotic Etiology* |
|---|---|---|
| Hemorrhage | Intraparenchymal hemorrhage<br>Subarachnoid hemorrhage | Sympathomimetics: cocaine ("crack"), amphetamine, phenylpropanolamine, phencyclidine, ephedrine, pseudoephedrine<br>Mycotic aneurysm rupture (IDU) |
| | Subdural hematoma | Trauma secondary to ethanol, sedative–hypnotics, seizures<br>Anticoagulants, NSAIDs, ASA |
| Brain lucencies | Basal ganglia focal necrosis (also subcortical white matter lucencies) | Carbon monoxide, cyanide, hydrogen sulfide, manganese, toxic alcohols |
| | Stroke: vasoconstriction | Sympathomimetics: cocaine ("crack"), amphetamine, phenylpropanolamine, phencyclidine; ephedrine, pseudoephedrine; ergotamine |
| | Mass lesion: tumor, abscess | Septic emboli, AIDS-related CNS toxoplasmosis or lymphoma |
| Loss of brain tissue | Atrophy: cerebral, cerebellar | Alcoholism, toluene |

CNS = central nervous system; IDU = injection drug use; NSAIDs = nonsteroidal antiinflammatory drugs; ASA = aspirin.

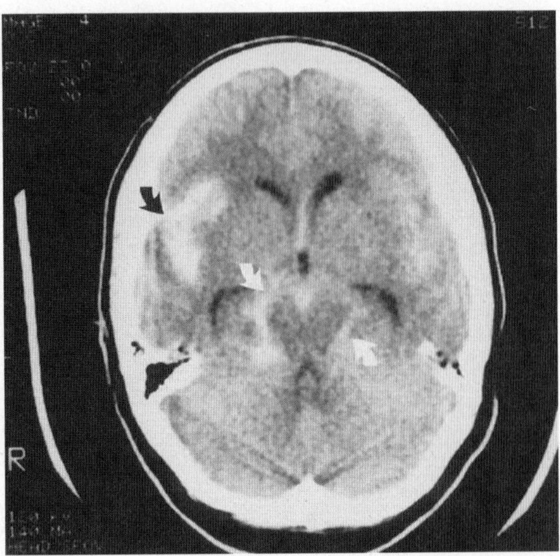


**FIGURE 5–18.** Subarachnoid hemorrhage after intravenous cocaine use. The patient had sudden severe headache followed by a generalized seizure. Extensive hemorrhage is seen surrounding the midbrain (*white arrows*) and in the right Sylvian fissure (*black arrow*). Angiography revealed an aneurysm at the origin of the right middle cerebral artery. *(Used with permission from The Fellowship in Medical Toxicology, New York University School of Medicine, New York City Poison Center.)*

monitoring devices are often incompatible with magnetic resonance scanning machines.

*Nuclear scintigraphy* that uses CT technology (SPECT and PET) is being used as a tool to elucidate functional characteristics of the CNS. Examples include both immediate and long-term effects of various xenobiotics on regional brain metabolism, blood flow, and neurotransmitter function.

***Emergency Cranial Computed Tomography Scanning.*** An emergency noncontrast CT scan is obtained to detect acute intracranial hemorrhage and focal brain lesions causing cerebral edema and mass effect. Patients with these lesions present with focal neurologic deficits, seizures, headache, or altered mental status. Toxicologic causes of intraparenchymal and subarachnoid hemorrhage include cocaine and other sympathomimetics (Fig. 5–18). Cocaine-induced vasospasm causes ischemic infarction, although this is not well seen by CT until 6 to 24 or more hours after onset of the neurologic deficit (Fig. 5–19). Drug-induced CNS depression, most commonly ethanol intoxication, predisposes the patient to head trauma, which may result in a subdural hematoma or cerebral contusion.

***Xenobiotic-Mediated Neurodegenerative Disorders.*** A number of xenobiotics directly damage brain tissue, producing morphologic changes that may be detectable using CT and especially MRI. Such changes include generalized atrophy, focal areas of neuronal loss, demyelinization, and cerebral edema. Imaging abnormalities help establish a diagnosis or predict prognosis in a patient with neurologic dysfunction after a xenobiotic exposure. In some cases, the imaging abnormality will suggest a toxicologic diagnosis in a patient with a neurologic disorder in whom a xenobiotic exposure was not suspected clinically.

***Atrophy.*** With long-term ethanol use, there is a widespread loss of neurons and resultant atrophy. In some individuals with alcoholism, the loss of brain tissue is especially prominent in the cerebellum.

***Focal Lesions.*** Carbon monoxide poisoning produces focal degenerative lesions in the brain. In about half of patients with severe neurologic dysfunction after carbon monoxide poisoning, CT scans show bilateral symmetric lucencies in the basal ganglia, particularly the globus pallidus (Fig. 5–20). The basal ganglia are especially sensitive to hypoxic damage because of their limited blood supply and high metabolic requirements. Basal ganglion lucencies, white matter lesions, and atrophy are caused by other xenobiotics such as methanol, ethylene glycol, cyanide, hydrogen sulfide, inorganic and organic mercury, manganese, heroin, barbiturates, chemotherapeutics, solvents such as toluene, and podophyllin.

**Posterior Reversible Encephalopathy Syndrome.** A wide range of medical conditions and medications cause symmetrical cortical and subcortical white matter changes that are reversible when the condition or xenobiotic is removed. This was formerly termed *reversible leukoencephalopathy syndrome*, but because the changes are not limited to the white matter and often involve the occipital lobes, it is now more commonly known as *posterior reversible encephalopathy syndrome*. However, this term too has been questioned because the changes are often more diffuse. The clinical manifestations include

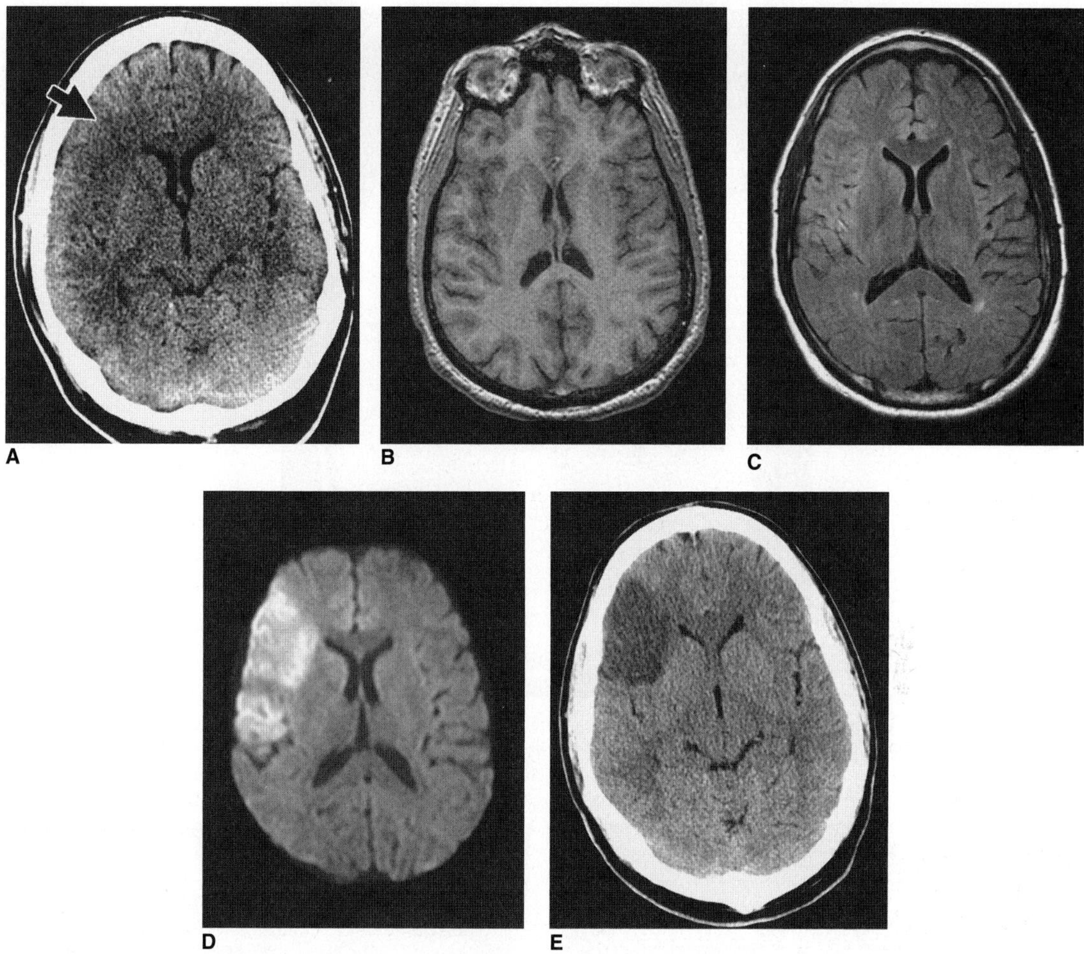

**FIGURE 5–19.** Acute stroke confirmed by diffusion-weighted magnetic resonance image (MRI). A 39-year-old man presented with left facial weakness that began 3 hours earlier after smoking crack cocaine. He also complained of left arm "tingling" but had normal examination findings. An emergency noncontrast computed tomography (CT) scan was obtained that was interpreted as normal (**A**), although in retrospect, there was subtle loss of the normal gray–white differentiation (*arrow*). Magnetic resonance imaging was obtained to confirm that the facial palsy was a stroke and not a peripheral seventh cranial nerve palsy. Standard MRI sequences (T1-weighted, T2-weighted, and fluid-attenuated inversion recovery) were normal in this early ischemic lesion (**B** and **C**). Diffusion-weighted imaging is able to show such early ischemic change—cytotoxic (intracellular) edema (**D**). The patient's facial paresis improved but did not entirely resolve. A repeat CT scan 2 days later showed an evolving (subacute) infarction with vasogenic edema (**E**). Infarction was presumably caused by vasospasm because no carotid artery lesion or cardiac source of embolism was found. *(Reproduced with permission from Schwartz DT: Emergency Radiology: Case Studies. New York, NY: McGraw-Hill; 2008.)*

headache, visual disturbance, altered mental status, and seizures (Fig. 5–21). These reversible cerebral disorders are distinct from irreversible white matter disease termed *toxic leukoencephalopathy*. This is associated with various cancer chemotherapeutics, carbon monoxide, toluene, methanol, and heroin inhalation on aluminum foil ("chasing the dragon").

***Nuclear Scintigraphy.*** Whereas both CT and MRI display cerebral anatomy, nuclear medicine studies provide functional information about the brain. Nuclear scintigraphy uses radioactive isotopes that are bound to carrier molecules (ligands). The choice of ligand depends on the biologic function being studied. Brain cells take up the radiolabeled ligand in proportion to their physiologic activity or the regional blood flow. The radioactive emission from the isotope is detected by a scintigraphic camera, which produces an image showing the quantity and distribution of tracer. Better anatomic detail is provided by using CT techniques to generate cross-sectional images. There are two such technologies: SPECT and PET. These imaging modalities are used in the research and clinical settings to study the neurologic effects of particular xenobiotics and the mechanisms of xenobiotic-induced neurologic dysfunction.

Both PET and SPECT are used to study the effects of various xenobiotics on cerebral function. In patients with severe neurologic dysfunction after carbon monoxide poisoning, SPECT regional blood flow measurements show diffuse hypometabolism in the frontal cortex. In patients who chronically use cocaine, SPECT blood flow scintigraphy demonstrates focal cortical perfusion defects. The extent of these perfusion deficits correlates with the frequency of drug use.

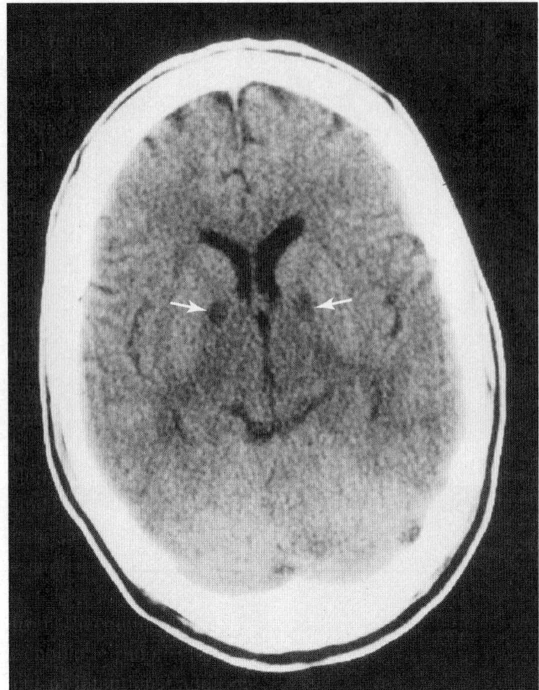

**FIGURE 5–20.** A head computed tomography scan of a patient with mental status changes after carbon monoxide poisoning. The scan shows characteristic bilateral symmetrical lucencies of the globus pallidus (*arrows*). *(Used with permission from Dr. Paul Blackburn, Maricopa Medical Center, Arizona.)*

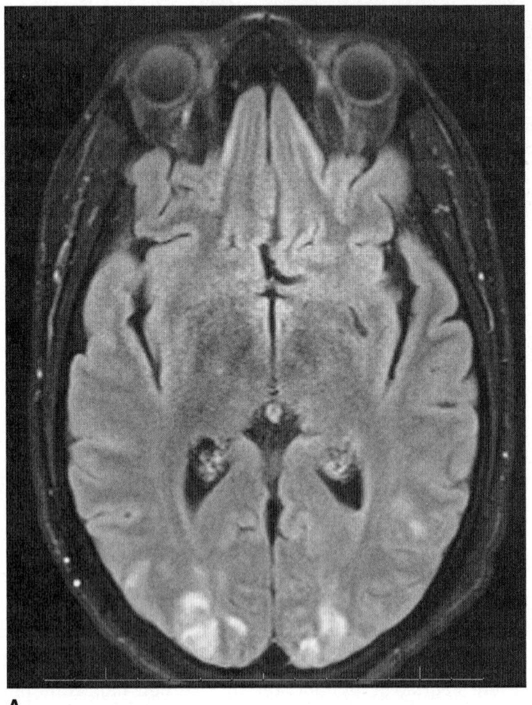

**A**

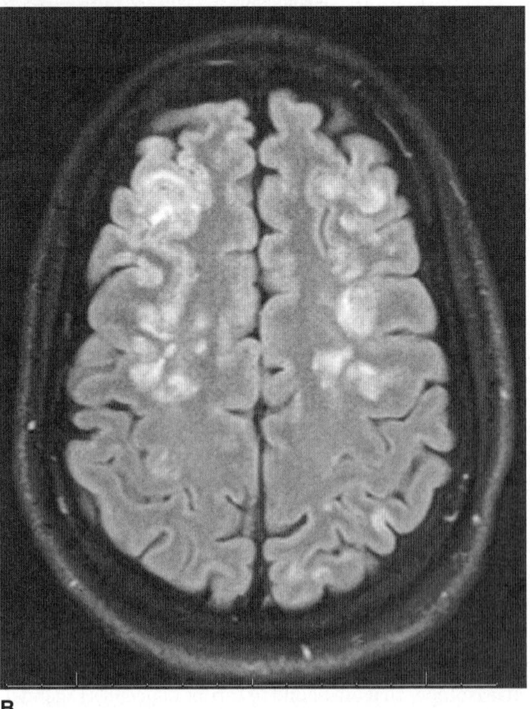

**B**

**FIGURE 5–21.** Posterior reversible encephalopathy syndrome (PRES) caused by cyclosporine. A 29-year-old man with severe aplastic anemia was treated with stem cell transplantation and cyclosporine to prevent subsequent graft-versus-host disease. The next day, he developed headache followed by a generalized tonic-clonic seizure with a prolonged postictal period. The head computed tomography scan was normal, and magnetic resonance imaging (MRI) revealed symmetric areas of fluid-attenuated inversion recovery hyperintensity involving the cortex and subcortical white matter of the occipital, frontal, and parietal lobes (**A** and **B**). Cyclosporine was stopped. The next day, he returned to his normal mental status. Follow-up MRI 1 week later revealed near-complete resolution (**C** and **D**). *(Used with permission from Dr. Alexander Baxter, Department of Radiology, New York University School of Medicine.)*

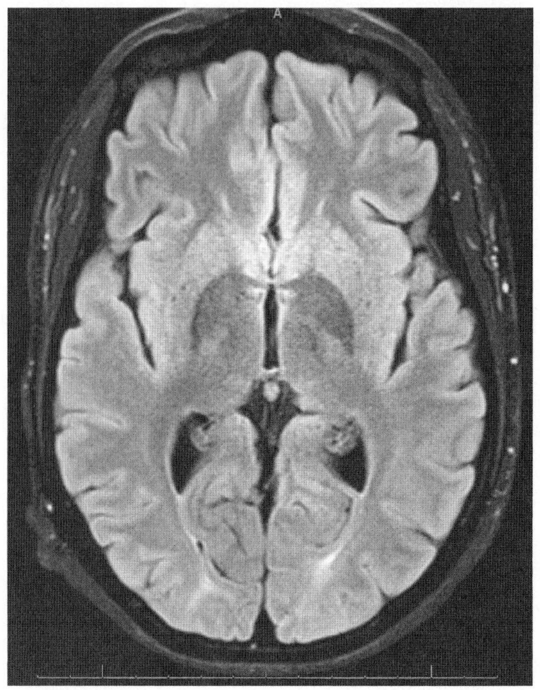


C

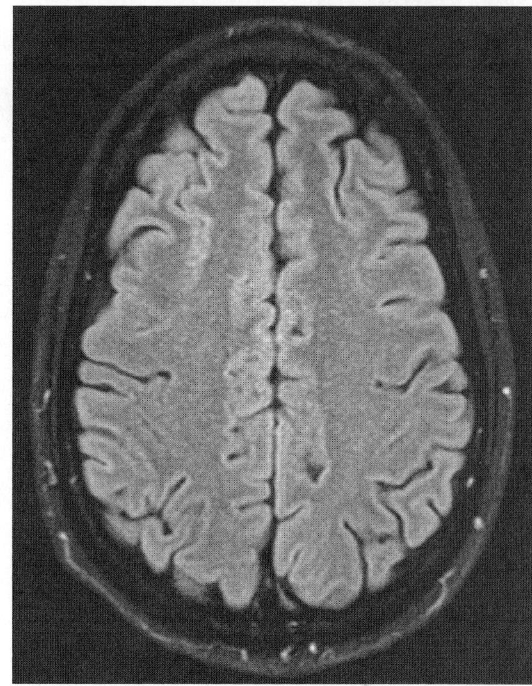

D

**FIGURE 5–21.** *(Continued)*

Focal perfusion defects probably represent local vasculitis or small areas of infarction.

There are many advances in the use of these imaging modalities, and initial applications are being applied to patient care. These imaging modalities are capable of demonstrating abnormalities in many patients with xenobiotic exposures, although other patients with significant cerebral dysfunction have normal study findings.

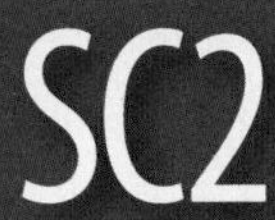



# SC2 TRANSDERMAL TOXICOLOGY

## HISTORY AND CURRENT USE

Applying a xenobiotic to the skin to treat a systemic medical condition is not new. Ointments and other salves have been applied topically for thousands of years for the treatment of local and systemic diseases. Over recent decades, an increasing number of medications have been formulated in transdermal delivery systems, or patches. Certain medications, such as testosterone, can be administered as a spray or gel. Further, xenobiotics are absorbed transdermally, as occurs with nicotine following direct exposure to moist tobacco leaf in patients with "green tobacco sickness" or following direct contact with organic phosphorus pesticide spraying.

The skin is the largest organ system in the body. There are several benefits of transdermal delivery of xenobiotics. This route provides a noninvasive means to administer xenobiotics. Patches can be left in place for long periods of time, which improves compliance and results in steady plasma concentrations that reduce side effects. Avoidance of first-pass metabolism permits delivery of poorly orally bioavailable xenobiotics. However, because absorption through the skin following simple application is passive, there is a large degree of variability among both patients and xenobiotics.

## TRANSDERMAL ADMINISTRATION PHARMACOLOGY

### Passive Administration

In order to reach the systemic circulation, a xenobiotic applied to the stratum corneum (horny layer) must initially pass through about a dozen layers of keratinized epidermal cells and then into the dermis. The keratinaceous horny layer is impervious to water because of the presence of ceramides, fatty acids, and other lipids. A xenobiotic must be sufficiently lipid soluble to partition into the stratum corneum and sufficiently water soluble to partition out from the stratum corneum into underlying tissue. This ability is described by the octanol–water partition coefficient and varies widely among xenobiotics.

Molecules with intermediate partition coefficients have adequate lipid solubility to permit diffusion through stratum corneum while still having sufficient water solubility to allow partitioning into the lower layers of the epidermis. Permeation enhancers improve absorption by solubilizing the xenobiotic or altering the characteristics of the stratum corneum, effectively increasing the lipid solubility of the xenobiotic. An alternative means of enhancing lipophilicity is the addition of organic functional groups to create a prodrug that is cleaved once absorbed. Even with these advances, only a few medications have the essential molecular requirements to be systemically delivered by the transdermal route. The upper limit of the molecular weight of an acceptable xenobiotic is 500 Da, and the xenobiotic must be sufficiently potent to exert the desired effect at concentrations that can reliably be obtained.

The ability to cross the dermis is related to the concentration gradient provided by the transdermal patch. To allow sufficient delivery, a large amount of medication is contained in the apparatus to maintain the concentration gradient over time. For example, the 50-μg/hr fentanyl patch (which delivers 1.2 mg daily) contains 8.4 mg (8,400 μg) of fentanyl in the patch. Upon completion of the 3-day use of a fentanyl patch, the amount of fentanyl remaining in a patch ranged from 28% to 85%.

Applying xenobiotics to broken skin or tissue lacking a stratum corneum, such as the mucosa, results in a substantial increase in absorption. Other properties of the skin that account for pharmacokinetic variability include hydration status and temperature. Absorption also varies based on the site of application on the body and on both the thickness of the stratum corneum and the blood flow.

### Active Administration

Because passive administration is highly limited, active methods involving physical or mechanical methods of enhancing delivery are generally superior. The delivery of xenobiotics of differing lipophilicity and molecular weight including proteins, peptides, vaccines, and oligonucleotides is improved by active energy-requiring techniques such as electroporation, iontophoresis, and ultrasonography (Tables SC2–1 and SC2–2).

### Patch Technology

In most current patches, the xenobiotic to be delivered is incorporated into the adhesive layer to reduce the delay to absorption. Multiple layers of adhesive are often separated by membranes that regulates release. To allow a longer duration of xenobiotic delivery, a reservoir is often added. This compartment contains the medication in solution or suspension, and a rate-regulating membrane ensures that the release follows zero-order kinetics to avoid fluctuations in concentration. Increasing the surface area of contact by enlarging the patch proportionally increases the amount of xenobiotic

**TABLE SC2–1 Examples of Xenobiotics Available in Patch Formulations**

| | |
|---|---|
| Buprenorphine | Nicotine |
| Camphor | Nitroglycerin |
| Clonidine | Norelgestromin/ethinyl estradiol |
| Donepezil | Oxybutynin |
| Dextroamphetamine | Rivastigmine |
| Estradiol | Rotigotine |
| Estradiol/levonorgestrel | Scopolamine |
| Fentanyl | Selegiline |
| Granisetron | Testosterone |
| Methylphenidate | Wintergreen oil |
| Lidocaine | |

| TABLE SC2–2 Description of Active Transdermal Drug Delivery Systems |
|---|
| *Electroporation:* uses high-voltage microsecond duration electrical pulses to create transient pores within the skin (for larger molecules such as peptides). |
| *Iontophoresis:* uses electrodes to pass a small current through a xenobiotic (pilocarpine for sweat testing for cystic fibrosis and for lidocaine). |
| *Microneedle-based devices:* approximately 10–100 µm in length, and are generally arranged in arrays on patch devices. Each microneedle is coated in the xenobiotic to be delivered, and the small size avoids the production of pain. |
| *Needleless injection:* compressed air is used to force xenobiotics across the skin surface, and may deliver local anesthetics prior to intravenous line placement. |
| *Ultrasound:* low-frequency ultrasound to promote transcutaneous delivery, also called sonophoresis. |

delivered. The membrane itself is not altered. Removal of the rate-regulating membrane, however, results in rapid absorption of toxic quantities of xenobiotic. Incorporating the xenobiotic into a fabric mesh (matrix patch) eliminates the reservoir and reduces the risk for unintentional toxicity and abuse. These matrix patches can be safely cut to change the dosage delivered without risking spillage.

### Pharmacokinetics

The initial detection of xenobiotic in the serum following transdermal application is delayed compared to other routes of administration. The delay is dependent on the properties of the xenobiotic, the skin, and the environment. For example, fentanyl concentrations will not be detected in the serum for at least 1 to 2 hours after placement of a patch, and the peak therapeutic concentration is typically achieved after 24 h. It is exactly for this reason that the fentanyl patch is not indicated for the treatment of acute pain.

The pharmacokinetics of serial patches is based on removal of the patch after the specified time period and application of a new patch at a different location. This allows a new subcutaneous depot to form while the existing depot from the initial patch is absorbed. If applied to the same location, the dose in the adhesive that is designed for more rapid absorption will combine with the existing depot and alter the clinical pharmacokinetics possibly leading to an overdose. Washing the skin or removing the patch will not result in a rapid fall in serum concentrations or a reduction in clinical effect. Rather, the concentration and clinical effects will resolve over several hours because of the persistence of the dermal depot, which is not removed by cleansing.

## ADVERSE EFFECTS

There is substantial risk of variation in absorption as a result of changes in ambient conditions. For example, when patches are exposed to heat (endogenous or exogenous such as fever or a heating pad) patients absorb drug at a rate greater than expected due to vasodilation. Certain patches, such as those with a metal backing, will frequently become exceedingly hot during exposure to magnetic resonance imaging studies and result in burns. Because transdermal systems require that large amounts of xenobiotic be present within the transdermal patch itself, to maximize the transcutaneous gradient, much of the xenobiotic typically remains in the patch at the prescribed time of removal raising issues of safe disposal. This is especially true for unsupervised exposure in children and as an abuse potential among others if the leftover content in the patch is chewed, ingested, brewed, or otherwise retrieved. Because many prescribers are unfamiliar with the dosing and initiation of therapy with transdermal products, those xenobiotics with consequential adverse effects in overdose, such as fentanyl, are commonly linked to poor outcomes even with intended therapeutic use.

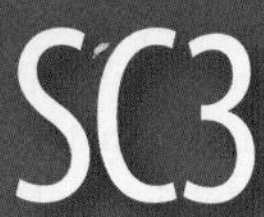



# SC3 PATIENT VIOLENCE

The aggressive and/or violent patient presents unique challenges. Aggressive individuals are difficult to treat, and they tend to elicit strong negative reactions in hospital personnel. Violence directed against healthcare workers is commonplace within the healthcare setting and is particularly prominent in the inpatient psychiatry ward and emergency department settings. Workplace violence occurs so frequently that there is a perception among healthcare workers that being subjected to violence from patients or families is an expected part of their job. Workplace violence is classified into 4 broad categories that are dependent on the relationship of the perpetrator to the workplace. In type I, there is no association between the perpetrator and the workplace and the event is usually of criminal intent (theft, assault). In type II, the most common type in the hospital setting, the perpetrator is a patient, visitor, family member or customer with or without an acute health condition exhibiting the violent behavior. In general, these acts of violence occur while workers are performing basic work functions such as an intoxicated patient who punches a nurse while obtaining vital signs. In type III, the perpetrator is a current or former employee and perpetrates a violent act against another employee. In type IV, the perpetrator has a personal relationship with a specific employee but not with the institution.

The section below addresses the differential diagnosis of violent behavior, predictions of violence, the pharmacotherapy for the treatment of aggressive and/or agitated behavior, and the use of seclusion and physical restraint. It also provides an overview of potential risk factors for violent behavior.

## Differential Diagnosis

There are many causes of violent behavior; some are social, medical, or biological in nature. The most common characteristic of the violent patient is alteration in mental status. Factors such as metabolic derangements, exposure to xenobiotics (both licit and illicit), withdrawal syndromes, seizures, head trauma, stroke, infectious diseases, psychosis, cognitive impairment, and personality disorder all predispose a patient to aggression and violence. Additionally, patients with severe pain, delirium, or extreme anxiety often respond to the efforts of emergency personnel with resistance, hostility, or overt aggression. Once confused, the patient often misinterprets health care efforts in a paranoid manner and becomes violent under circumstances that would not normally be sufficient to provoke a violent outburst in that individual.

## Prediction of Violence

Although there is a high expectation that violence is predictable, there are no reliable predictors of violence. Prior history of violence is postulated as a risk factor for future violence. Predicting violent behavior based on medical diagnosis is unfruitful and leads to bias or discrimination. Studies of emergency department violence show the following risk factors for violence: the presence of guns, area of gang activity, low socioeconomic status, and interacting with patients who were recently given bad news.

## Substance Use and Violence

The association between substance use and violence is well established. Alcohol is found in the offender, the victim, or both in as many as two-thirds of homicides and serious assaults. Substance use is seldom the sole cause, but interacts with other physiologic, cognitive, psychological, situational, and cultural factors including any underlying mental illness. A tripartite model for substance-related violence is described:

1. systemic violence related to the sale and distribution of drugs,
2. economic compulsive violence associated with profit-oriented criminal activity to maintain the expenses of an individual's substance use disorder, and
3. psychopharmacologic violence resulting from the direct effects of using the particular xenobiotic.

Toxicity can cause disinhibition, impulsivity, perceptual disturbance, paranoia, irritability, misinterpretation, affective instability, and/or confusion. Withdrawal syndromes also promote aggressive behavior for a multitude of reasons, including physical discomfort, anticipatory anxiety, stigmatization, irritability as a direct result of withdrawal, and withdrawal-related delirium.

## Mental Illness and Violence

Several studies show an association between mental illness and increased risk for violence. Although persons with psychotic disorders are not generally aggressive, hallucinations lead to aggression when patients explicitly follow the instructions of a violent command hallucination. Paranoid ideation that leads an individual to believe that she or he is at imminent risk of bodily harm is an example of thoughts that lead psychotic patients to be aggressive. In patients with schizophrenia, having a co-occurring substance use disorder more than triples the rate of violence. In addition to substance abuse and severe mental illnesses, researchers have consistently found a greater prevalence of personality disorders among individuals who become violent in an inpatient setting as compared to nonviolent inpatients. Antisocial personality disorder is the condition most strongly associated with both substance use and aggression.

## Alternative Etiologies

Delirium from any underlying condition is a cause of aggression. Patients are often confused, frightened, or frankly psychotic as a result of impaired perception. A risk of violence is also associated with stable cognitive dysfunction such as traumatic brain injury and dementia. These patients are often unable to engage in a rational manner, and verbal de-escalation attempts are often unsuccessful or even futile.

### Assessment of the Violent Patient

The comprehensive evaluation of the violent patient includes a complete physical examination with the intent of revealing the underlying cause of the violent behavior as well as ensuring the discovery of secondary patient injuries. Recommended assessment includes vital signs including a core temperature, rapid blood chemistries (glucose, electrolytes), a complete blood count, liver function tests, kidney function tests, thyroid function tests, and urinalysis. The need for lumbar puncture and/or neuroimaging is best guided by clinical history and physical examination.

### Treatment

There are 3 main approaches to controlling aggressive behavior in order of escalation: First and foremost, there is verbal de-escalation. When this has failed, medical anxiolysis and sedation will be the next approach. Finally, under the most extreme circumstances where there is significant risk for harming self or others, the use of physical restraints is indicated to permit pharmacologic intervention.

### Verbal De-escalation

Because of several high-profile deaths involving restraints, there is a continued focus on advancing techniques and training in de-escalation. These techniques use both verbal and nonverbal communication, and include designating a single individual to talk to a patient, building rapport, listening and understanding in a calm and compassionate manner, using a calm voice, making eye contact, and focusing on the person and not the behavior while avoiding multiple stimuli. Many hospitals have behavioral response teams. The purpose of these teams is to respond, assess, protect, and treat the patient with behavioral disturbances. The teams are generally multidisciplinary in nature and consist of mental health, medical, and security professionals.

### Psychopharmacologic Interventions

The goal of acute pharmacologic intervention for agitated or violent behavior is to target the suspected cause of the agitation while regaining behavioral control and ensuring safety. For example, the patient in alcohol withdrawal presenting with agitation would benefit from a benzodiazepine, whereas an antipsychotic could be detrimental and lead to unnecessary side effects (Chap. 50). Haloperidol is safely used in the treatment of agitation and aggression in patients with psychoses and delirium or acute ethanol intoxication to avoid the additional sedating effects of benzodiazepines. It can be administered orally, intravenously, or intramuscularly. Dosing intervals range from 30 minutes to 2 hours, with a usual regimen of haloperidol 2.5 mg to 5 mg; most patients respond after 1 to 3 doses. During a behavioral crisis, most psychiatrists would switch to a second-generation antipsychotic such as olanzapine or add a mood stabilizer such as valproic acid rather than continue to titrate haloperidol because of escalating risks of side effects as haloperidol dose is increased (such as extrapyramidal symptoms and QT interval prolongation). Droperidol is an older antipsychotic that is rarely used as an antipsychotic in the United States but widely used elsewhere. Evidence overall supports its use as a first-line treatment option for acute agitation. Although midazolam is proven to induce adequate sedation more rapidly than droperidol, 15 versus 30 minutes, respectively, midazolam also has a significantly higher rate of needing additional medication for sedation, when compared to droperidol, but this allows interval reassessment. Droperidol is often given intramuscularly at doses 5 to 10 mg every 3 to 4 hours as needed (Chap. 40). Various benzodiazepines are quite effective for sedation; their use has been examined in patients with psychoses, stimulant toxicity, sedative–hypnotic and alcohol withdrawal, and postoperative agitation. The advantages and disadvantages are described in detail in Antidotes in Brief A26: Benzodiazepines. A 2016 review compared the use of benzodiazepines, antipsychotics, and combined therapy in the treatment of agitated patients in the emergency department. This review concluded that more patients remained sedated with combination therapy compared to benzodiazepines alone. Additionally, antipsychotic monotherapy and combinations both required fewer repeated administrations for sedation than benzodiazepines alone. Benzodiazepine monotherapy was also associated with a higher incidence of adverse events than the antipsychotics alone or combinations. We recommend the use of antipsychotic monotherapy in the presumed psychiatric agitation in those primarily calm enough to be cared for by a psychiatrist with limited likelihood of a consequential toxicologic problem, whereas diazepam or midazolam should be used in treating undifferentiated episodes of toxicity and agitation. When appropriate regimens of monotherapy fail, a combination of benzodiazepines and antipsychotics is reasonable. There is no role for the combination of an antihistamine with a benzodiazepine and an antipsychotic.

There are multiple indications for the use of ketamine within the field of medicine, including a potential treatment for major depressive disorders, as well as use in the emergency department as sedation for procedures and for intubation. Ketamine is an antagonist of the glutamate *N*-methyl-D-aspartate (NMDA) receptor that is a dissociative anesthetic, which provides both analgesia and amnesia. The few studies on the prehospital administration of ketamine to treat agitation reported intubation rates between 39% and 63%. This is in comparison to ketamine use in other more controlled settings. Given the conflicting and limited data on its safety in treating agitation, ketamine is not recommended as a first-line therapy to treat agitation in the emergency department setting, and physicians should use caution when using ketamine given concerns for significant adverse events, which means evaluation for airway compromise and resuscitative preparedness.

If a patient is agitated in the context of alcohol intoxication, we recommend antipsychotics and we suggest that benzodiazepines should be avoided because of the potential to cause additive respiratory depression. Antipsychotics, particularly low-potency antipsychotics (such as chlorpromazine), lower the seizure threshold in animals, so their use for patients with cocaine/amphetamine toxicity or alcohol/sedative–hypnotic withdrawal is not recommended. In contrast, benzodiazepines have a unique role in the treatment of agitation secondary to cocaine toxicity (Chap. 48 and Antidotes in Brief: A26).

### Physical Restraint

Isolation and mechanical restraints are also used in the treatment of violent behavior. Isolation or seclusion can help to diminish environmental stimuli and thereby reduce hyperreactivity. However, because seclusion is defined by a condition of very limited interactive and environmental cues, it is not indicated for patients with unstable medical conditions, delirium, dementia, self-injurious behavior such as cutting or head banging, or those who are experiencing extrapyramidal reactions as a consequence of antipsychotics such as an acute dystonic reaction. Mechanical restraint is used to prevent patient and staff injury. All facilities should have clear, written policy guidelines for restraint that address monitoring, reassessment, documentation, and provisions for patient comfort.

See Tables SC3–1 and SC3–2 for violence warning signs and the S.A.F.E.S.T. approach, which is an approach to the violent patient.

| TABLE SC3–1 Violence Warning Signs |
|---|
| Agitated movements |
| Body posturing, rapid/shallow breathing |
| Clenched fists |
| Loud vocalizations |
| Pacing |
| Staring |
| Striking at inanimate objects |
| Threatening statements |

| TABLE SC3–2 | S.A.F.E.S.T. Approach |
|---|---|
| Spacing | Maintain a safe distance<br>Allow both patient and you to have equal access to the door (but you should be closest)<br>Do not touch the patient |
| Appearance | Maintain empathetic and professional detachment<br>Use one primary person to build rapport<br>Have security available as a show of strength |
| Focus | Watch the patient's hands<br>Look for potential weapons<br>Watch for escalating agitation |
| Exchange | Attempt to de-escalate by use of calm/continuous talking<br>Avoid punitive or judgmental statements<br>Use good listening skills<br>Elicit patient cooperation by targeting the current problem |
| Stabilization | By the least restrictive and most appropriate approach(s) possible:<br>Physical restraints<br>Sedation (benzodiazepines)<br>Antipsychotics |
| Treatment | Treat underlying cause<br>May need to treat involuntarily |

Data from FitzGerald D: S.A.F.E.S.T. Approach. *Tactical Intervention Guided Emergency Response (TIGER)* Textbook; 2003.

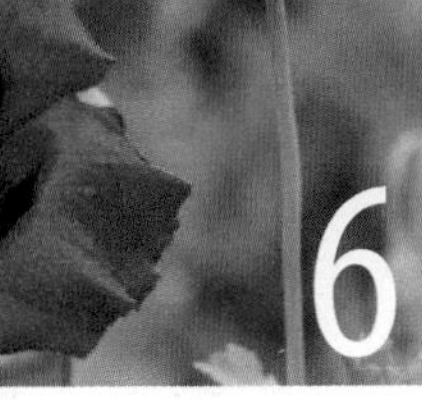

A. Analgesics and Antiinflammatory Medications

# 6 ACETAMINOPHEN

## HISTORY AND EPIDEMIOLOGY

By the late 1800s, both phenacetin and acetanilide were used as analgesics and antipyretics, but their acceptance was limited by significant side effects, including methemoglobinemia. *N*-Acetyl-*p*-aminophenol is abbreviated as APAP (*N*-**a**cetyl-***p***-**a**mino**p**henol) and is referred to as acetaminophen in the United States (US), Canada, Japan, and several other countries and as paracetamol in most other areas of the globe. Acetaminophen has since proved to be a remarkably safe medication at appropriate dosages, which has led to its popularity. Unfortunately, APAP toxicity is the leading cause of fulminant hepatic failure in most developed nations.

Acetaminophen is available in myriad single-medication dose formulations and delivery systems and in a variety of combinations with opioids, other analgesics, sedatives, decongestants, expectorants, and antihistamines. The diversity and wide availability of APAP products dictate that the potential for APAP toxicity be evaluated not only after identified ingestions but also after exposure to unknown or multiple xenobiotics in settings of intentional overdose, abuse, and therapeutic misadventures.

## PHARMACOLOGY

Acetaminophen is an analgesic and antipyretic with weak peripheral antiinflammatory and antiplatelet properties. Analgesic activity is reported at a serum [APAP] of 10 μg/mL (66 μmol/L) and antipyretic activity at 4 to 18 μg/mL (26.5-119 μmol/L). Acetaminophen has a unique mechanism of action among the analgesic antipyretics. Most of the nonsteroidal antiinflammatory drugs (NSAIDs) occupy the cyclooxygenase (COX) binding site on the enzyme prostaglandin $H_2$ synthase ($PGH_2$) and prevent arachidonic acid from physically entering the site and being converted to prostaglandin $H_2$. Acetaminophen also inhibits prostaglandin $H_2$ production but does so indirectly by reducing a heme on the peroxidase (POX) portion of the $PGH_2$, and indirectly inhibiting COX activation. In this way, APAP function is highly dependent on cellular location and intracellular conditions. Acetaminophen strongly inhibits prostaglandin synthesis where concentrations of POX and arachidonic acid ("peroxide tone") are low, such as in the brain. In conditions of high peroxide tone, such as inflammatory cells and platelets, prostaglandin synthesis is less affected by APAP. This dissociation explains the strong central antipyretic and analgesic effect of APAP but weak peripheral antiinflammatory and antiplatelet effects.

## PHARMACOKINETICS

Immediate-release APAP is rapidly absorbed with a time to peak [APAP] of approximately 30 minutes for liquid formulations and 45 minutes for tablets. Extended-release APAP has a time to peak of 1 to 2 hours but is almost entirely absorbed by 4 hours. The time to peak is delayed by food and coingestion of opioids or antimuscarinics. The oral bioavailability is 60% to 98%, and the volume of distribution (Vd) is approximately 1 L/kg. Peak [APAP] after recommended doses typically ranges from 8 to 20 μg/mL (53-132 μmol/L). Acetaminophen is available in the intravenous (IV) form and as a prodrug (eg, propacetamol). In adults, peak [APAP] after a 1 g infusion is approximately 30 μg/mL (198 μmol/L) and after a 2 g infusion is approximately 75 μg/mL (496 μmol/L). Acetaminophen has total protein binding of 10% to 30% that does not change in overdose. Acetaminophen metabolism is detailed in Figure 6–1. The elimination half-life of APAP is approximately 2 to 3 hours after a nontoxic dose but is prolonged in patients who develop hepatotoxicity.

## TOXICOKINETICS

After most oral overdoses, the majority of APAP absorption occurs within 2 hours, and peak plasma concentrations generally occur within 4 hours. Later peaks, double or multiple peaks are documented with large ingestions (> 50 g) or xenobiotics that decrease gastrointestinal mobility. The amount of NAPQI formed is increased out of proportion to the APAP dose and accounts for up to 20% to 50% of metabolism in patients with hepatotoxicity. The toxicokinetics of IV APAP are largely unknown.

## PATHOPHYSIOLOGY

After therapeutic APAP dosing, GSH (glutathione) supply and turnover far exceed that required to detoxify NAPQI. With ample GSH supply, NAPQI is largely bound by GSH, and no toxicity occurs. After overdose, the rate and quantity of NAPQI formation excedes supply and turnover of GSH, resulting in the release of NAPQI within the cell. In animal experiments, hepatotoxicity becomes evident only when hepatic [GSH] decreases to 30% of baseline.

When NAPQI formation overwhelms the supply of thiol-containing compounds, it covalently binds proteins throughout the cell, inducing a series of events that result in cell death. Ultimately, the mitochondrial permeability transition (MPT) pores open, causing mitochondrial membrane permeability, decreased mitochondrial respiration, and decreased adenosine triphosphate (ATP) synthesis. Furthermore, MPT opening leads to release of intermembrane proteins and ultimately leads to DNA fragmentation and cellular necrosis. The final pathway of hepatic cell death is predominantly cellular necrosis. Apoptosis occurs early in APAP toxicity or after activation of the immune system in response to cellular necrosis but is not likely the major mechanism of cellular toxicity.

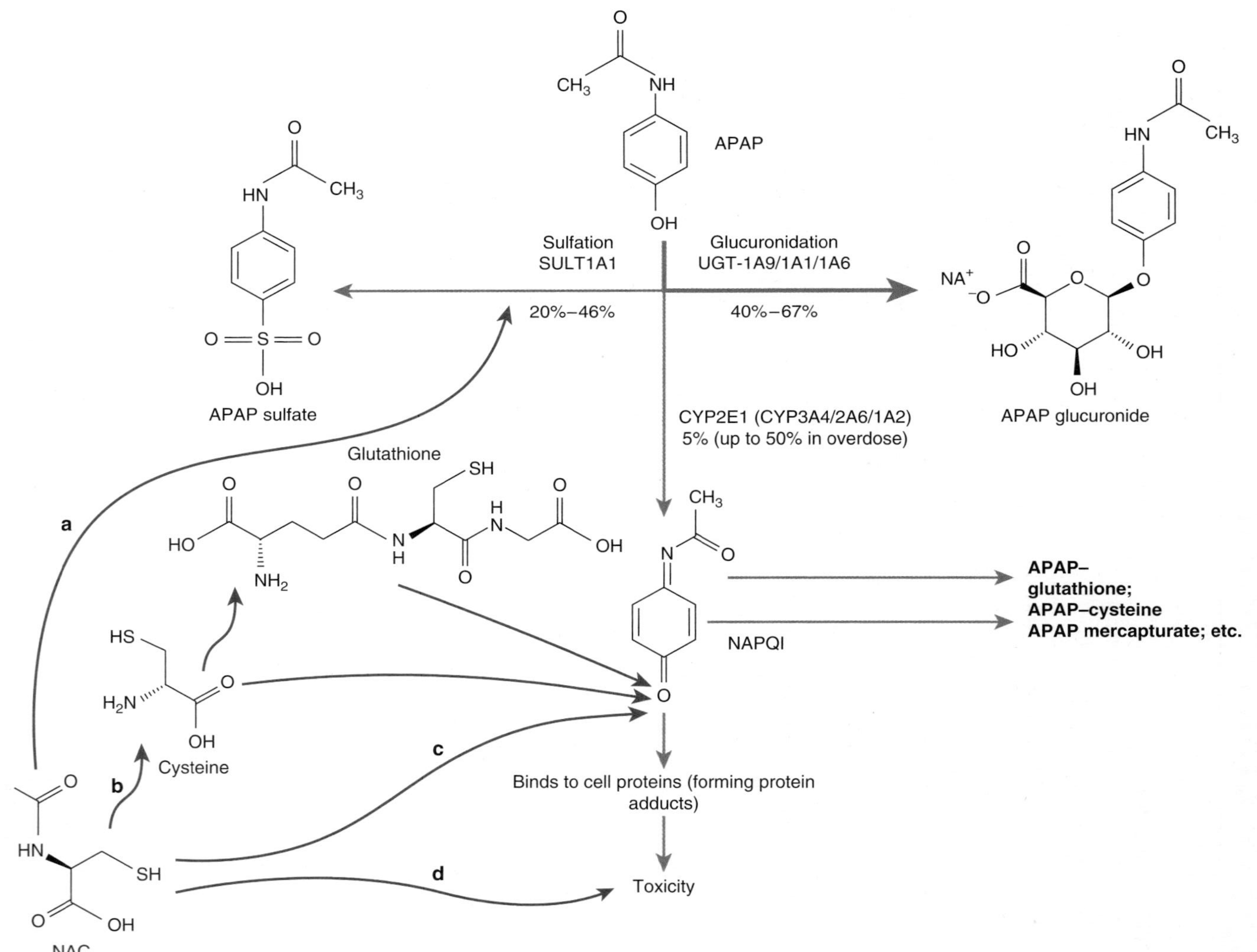


**FIGURE 6–1.** Important routes of acetaminophen (APAP) metabolism in humans and mechanisms of *N*-acetylcysteine (NAC) hepatoprotection. (a) *N*-Acetylcysteine augments sulfation; (b) NAC is a glutathione (GSH) precursor; (c) NAC is a GSH substitute; and (d) NAC improves multiorgan function during hepatic failure and possibly limits the extent of hepatocyte injury. APAP = *N*-acetyl-*p*-aminophenol; NAPQI = *N*-acetyl-*p*-benzoquinoneimine.

Macrophages, neutrophils, and inflammatory cells infiltrate after necrosis, followed by a cascade of inflammatory cytokines that contribute to further hepatocellular destruction.

Hepatotoxicity initially and most profoundly occurs in hepatic zone III (centrilobular) because this zone is the area with the largest concentration of oxidative metabolism (CYP2E1). In more severe hepatotoxicity, necrosis extends into zones II and I, destroying the entire hepatic parenchyma. Kidney injury after acute overdose is typically acute tubular necrosis that is most likely caused by local production of NAPQI. Direct injury to organs other than the liver and kidney is rarely reported. The mechanism of early central nervous system (CNS) depression after APAP ingestion is undefined, but theoretical mechanisms include serotonin and opioid effects as well as APAP-induced CNS GSH depletion. Early after massive APAP ingestion, metabolic acidosis and elevated lactate result from alterations in mitochondrial respiratory function. Rare cases of metabolic acidosis with 5-oxoprolinemia and 5-oxoprolinuria are reported and this may be indicative of genetic polymorphisms of GSH synthetase and 5-oxoprolinase.

## CLINICAL MANIFESTATIONS

The clinical course of acute APAP toxicity is typically divided into four stages. During stage I, hepatic injury has not yet occurred, and even patients who ultimately develop severe hepatotoxicity are often asymptomatic. Clinical findings, when present, are nonspecific and include nausea, vomiting, malaise, pallor, and diaphoresis. Laboratory indices of hepatic function are normal. Stage II represents the onset of hepatic injury, which occurs in fewer than 5% of those who overdose, largely because of lower toxic dose. The aspartate aminotransferase (AST) is the most sensitive widely available measure to detect the onset of hepatotoxicity, and AST abnormalities always precede evidence of actual hepatic dysfunction. The AST elevation most commonly begins within 24 hours after ingestion and is nearly universal by 36 hours. In the most severely poisoned patients, AST may increase as early as 12 hours after ingestion. The alanine aminotransferase (ALT) concentration elevates shortly after the AST, but they peak at similar concentrations, and AST decreases earlier than the ALT. Of note, both [AST] and [ALT] are markers of hepatotoxicity, but because [AST] rises and decreases earlier than [ALT], we recommend using AST for detecting early hepatotoxicity and for determining hepatic recovery. In all other cases, AST and ALT are interchangeable and are described generically as aminotransferases in this chapter.

Stage III, defined as the time of maximal hepatotoxicity, most commonly occurs between 72 and 96 hours after ingestion. The clinical manifestations of stage III include fulminant hepatic failure with encephalopathy and coma and, rarely, hemorrhage. Concentrations of AST and ALT above 10,000 IU/L are common, even in patients without other evidence of hepatic failure. Much more important than the degree of [aminotransferase] elevation, abnormalities of PT and INR, glucose, lactate, creatinine, and pH are essential determinants of prognosis and treatment. Kidney function abnormalities are rare (< 1%) overall, but they occur in as many as 25% of patients with significant hepatotoxicity and in 50% to 80% of those with hepatic failure. After acute ingestions, elevations of [creatinine] typically occur between 2 and 5 days after ingestion, peak on days 5 to 7 (range, 3–16 days), and normalize over 1 month. Fatalities from fulminant hepatic failure generally occur between 3 and 5 days after an acute overdose.

Stage IV is recovery. Survivors have complete hepatic regeneration, and no cases of chronic hepatic dysfunction are reported. The rate of recovery varies; in most cases, [AST], pH, PT, and INR, and [lactate] are normal by 7 days in survivors of acute overdoses. Alanine aminotransferase concentration ([ALT]) remains elevated longer than [AST], and [creatinine] may be elevated for more than 1 month. The recovery time is much longer in severely poisoned patients, and hepatic histologic abnormalities potentially persist for months.

## DIAGNOSTIC TESTING

### Assessing the Risk of Toxicity

***Principles Guiding the Diagnostic Approach.*** Most patients with APAP exposures do not develop toxicity, and the overall mortality rate after acute APAP ingestion is less than 0.5%. However, APAP is now the leading cause of acute liver failure (ALF) in the US and much of the developed world. When evaluating risk, it is useful to separate different categories of APAP exposure as discussed below.

***Risk Determination After Acute Overdose.*** Acute overdose usually is defined as a single ingestion, although many patients actually overdose incrementally over a brief period of time. For purposes of this discussion, an *acute overdose* is somewhat arbitrarily defined as one in which the entire ingestion occurs within a single 4-hour period. Doses of at least 12 g (~150 mg/kg) in an adult or 200 to 350 mg/kg in a child are necessary to cause hepatotoxicity in most patients. The dose history should be used in the assessment of risk only if there is reliable corroboration or direct validation. Suicidal patients who deny ingesting APAP have a measurable concentration in 1.4% to 8.4% of cases and 0.2% to 2.2% require treatment. Therefore, when the history suggests possible risk, the patient should be further assessed with measurement of a serum [APAP].

Interpretation of [APAP] after acute exposures is based on the Rumack-Matthew nomogram (Fig. 6–2). The nomogram is designed and validated using a single value obtained at or greater than 4 hours after ingestion to allow for complete APAP absorption. Although patients who develop hepatotoxicity typically have APAP half-lives greater than 4 hours, plotting multiple points on the nomogram or using an APAP half-life to determine risk is not adequately studied and has significant limitations. It is important to realize that the line was based on [aminotransferase] elevation rather than on hepatic failure or death, and it was chosen to be very sensitive, with little regard to specificity. Without antidotal therapy, only 60% of those with an initial APAP above the original (200) line will develop hepatotoxicity as defined by [aminotransferases] above 1,000 IU/L. The line used in the US runs parallel to the original line but was arbitrarily lowered by 25% to add even greater sensitivity. The lower line is often referred to as the *treatment line* or *150 line*. The treatment line

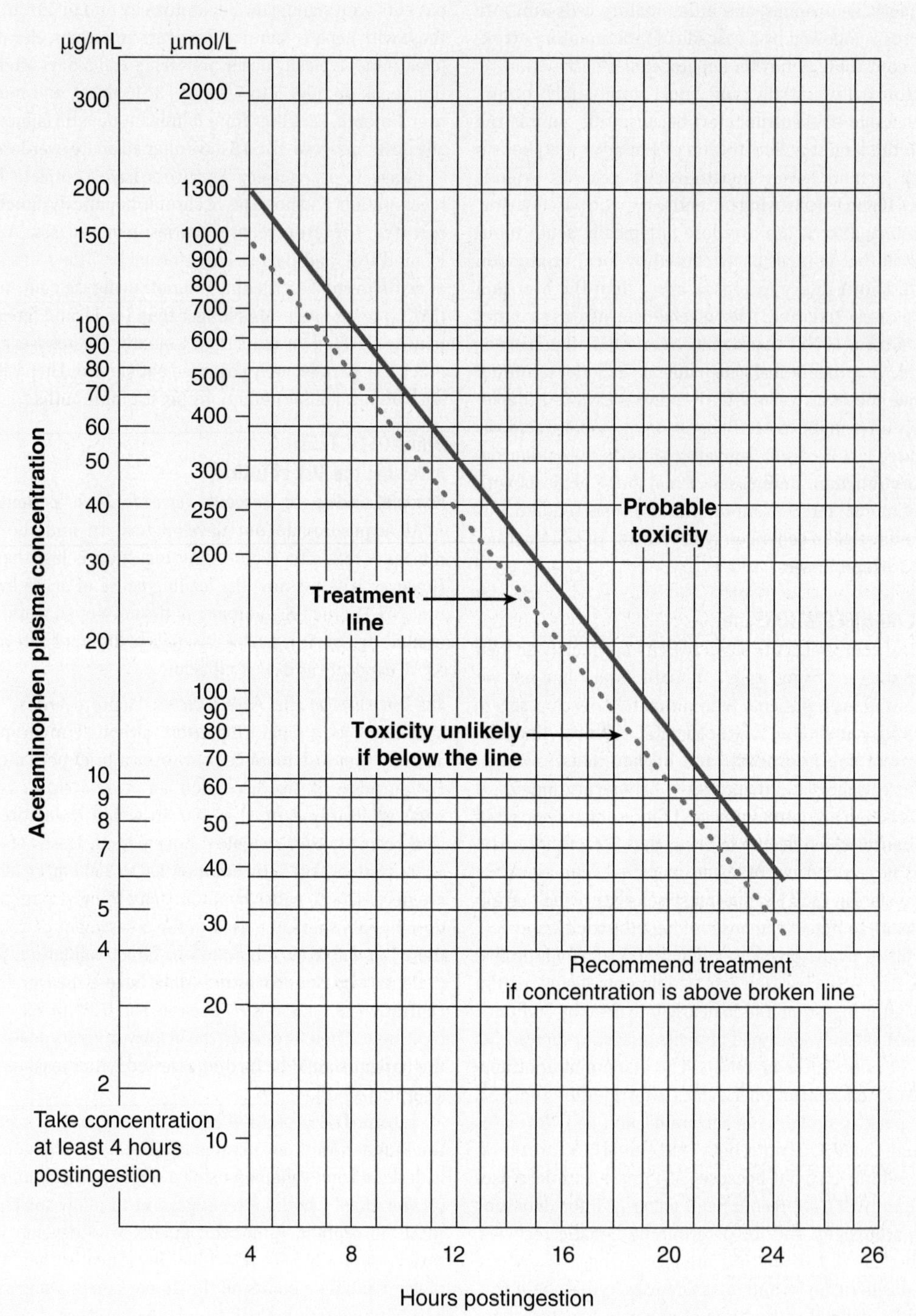


**FIGURE 6–2.** Rumack-Matthew nomogram (reconstructed) for determining the risk of acetaminophen (APAP)-induced hepatotoxicity after a single acute ingestion. Serum [APAP] above the treatment line on the nomogram indicates the need for *N*-acetylcysteine therapy. *(Reproduced with permission from Tintinalli JE Stapczynski S, Ma OJ, et al. Tintinalli's Emergency Medicine: A Comprehensive Study Guide, 8th ed. New York, NY: McGraw-Hill Education; 2016.)*

is one of the most sensitive screening tools used in medicine. The incidence of nomogram failures using this line in the US is only 1% to 3%. The United Kingdom uses a single nomogram line starting at 100 µg/mL at 4 hours ("100 line") for all acute APAP ingestions.

Based on these observations and more than 25 years of use, the 150 line is adequate in nearly all cases and is reliable when rigorously followed. When using the APAP nomogram, it is essential to precisely define the time window during which APAP ingestion occurred and, if the time is unknown, to use the *earliest possible time* as the time of ingestion. Using this approach, patients with an [APAP] below the treatment line, even if only slightly so, do not require further evaluation or treatment for acute APAP overdose.

The goal should be to determine an [APAP] at the earliest point at which it will be meaningful in decision making. Therefore, measurement of an [APAP] 4 hours after ingestion or as soon as possible thereafter is used to confirm the patient's risk of toxicity and thus the need to initiate NAC. Although it is optimal to start NAC therapy as soon as possible after confirmation of risk, NAC is nearly 100% effective if started before 8 hours after ingestion. This allows clinicians some leeway to wait for the laboratory results before starting therapy in patients in whom the history of ingestion suggests that the 4-hour [APAP] will fall below the treatment line. However, it should be noted that delaying NAC therapy longer than 8 hours after ingestion increases the patient's risk. If there is any concern about the availability of an [APAP] before this time, then treatment with NAC should be initiated. In such cases, the [APAP] still should be determined as soon as possible. When the results become available, they should be interpreted according to the treatment line on the APAP nomogram and NAC either continued or discontinued on the basis of this result. In the unusual circumstance in which no determination of an [APAP] can ever be obtained, evidence of possible risk by history alone is sufficient to initiate and complete a course of NAC therapy. Measurement of the [APAP] between 2 and 4 hours after ingestion is only helpful to exclude ingestion of APAP. If an [APAP] is undetectable in this time frame, significant APAP overdose is likely excluded. Concentrations obtained prior to 2 hours after ingestion should never be acted upon because of their imprecision as predictors of toxicity and the lack of benefit of early treatment

### Determination of Risk When the Acetaminophen Nomogram Is Not Applicable

***Risk Determination When Time of Ingestion Is Unknown.*** The *earliest possible time* of ingestion ("worst-case scenario") is used for risk-determination purposes. If this time window cannot be established or is so broad that it encompasses a span of more than 24 hours, then the following approach is suggested. Determine both the [APAP] and [AST]. If the [AST] is elevated, regardless of the [APAP], treat the patient with NAC. If the time of ingestion is completely unknown and the [APAP] is detectable, it is prudent to assume that the patient is at risk and to initiate treatment with NAC. If the [APAP] is undetectable and the [AST] is within the normal range for the local laboratory, there is little evidence that subsequent consequential hepatic injury is possible and NAC is unnecessary.

***Risk Assessment After Extended-Release Acetaminophen.*** Following ingestion of extended-release formulations, a small number of patients have an initial [APAP] below the treatment line but then have a subsequent [APAP] above the treatment line ("nomogram crossing"). While it is unclear whether nomogram crossing is correlated with outcome, it is common practice to obtain serial [APAP] every 2 hours until a clear downward trend is obtained. Any [APAP] above the nomogram treatment line is an indication to begin antidotal therapy.

***Intravenous Acetaminophen.*** Experience with patients with IV APAP overdose is limited. Hepatotoxicity and liver failure are described after single erroneous supratherapeutic doses of 75 to 150 mg/kg. Cases of hepatotoxicity with liver failure are reported after repeated therapeutic dosing (59–77 mg/kg/day) in severely catabolic patients over 3 to 5 days. There is no evidence for the use of the nomogram in patients with IV overdose. Given the limited data and that iatrogenic errors are usually quantifiable, it seems reasonable to treat patients given more than 60 mg/kg of IV APAP in a single dose and to treat until the [APAP] is undetectable. Finally, it is also reasonable to treat patients receiving multiple therapeutic doses of IV APAP with NAC if there is evidence of hepatotoxicity or if there is evidence of APAP accumulation (eg, the [APAP] is above therapeutic concentrations that are expected for the last dose).

***Risk Determination After Repeated Supratherapeutic Ingestions (or Chronic Overdose).*** No well-established guidelines are available for determining risk after chronic exposure to APAP. The chronic ingestion of "maximal therapeutic" doses (3–4 g/day) in normal adults without special comorbidities is safe. Although therapeutic dosing appears to be safe, repeated supratherapeutic ingestions (RSTIs) may lead to toxicity. The risk of hepatotoxicity is likely proportional to both the total amount of APAP ingested and the duration of the exposure; however, exact cutoffs for safe dosing are difficult to determine and are likely subject to factors related to the individual.

Conceptually, the groups that are at "high risk" for hepatotoxicity after RSTI of APAP have potentially increased activity of CYP2E1 and therefore proportionally increased NAPQI formation or have decreased GSH stores and turnover rate. Many reported cases of APAP toxicity from RSTI involve patients who have a factor or factors that influence their GSH supply or turnover, NAPQI production, or both, including infants with febrile illness who received excessive dosing, chronic heavy ethanol users, catabolic postsurgical patients, and patients chronically taking CYP-inducing medications. Catabolic states enhance CYP2E1 activity and shunt hepatic metabolism to gluconeogenesis, leading to decreased glucose precursors for glucuronidation and subsequent increased production of NAPQI.

To determine the need for NAC, evaluate the patient's risk based on dosing history and other risk factors and then use limited laboratory testing that consists of an [APAP] and [AST], with additional testing as indicated by these results and other clinical features. The objective is to identify the two conditions that warrant NAC therapy: remaining APAP yet to be metabolized and potentially serious hepatic injury.

In asymptomatic patients, a reasonable approach is to perform laboratory evaluation for adults who have ingested more than 200 mg/kg/day (or 10 g/day, whichever is less) in a 24-hour period or more than 150 mg/kg/day (or 6 g/day, whichever is less) in a 48-hour period. In children younger than 6 years of age, laboratory evaluation is reasonable if the reported ingestion is more than 100 mg/kg/day during a

72-hour period or longer. After a patient is determined to be at risk, the [APAP] and [AST] should be determined.

Using the strategy described here, patients with an elevated [AST] are considered at risk, regardless of their [APAP]. An [APAP] is useful in patients with a normal [AST] as a tool to determine only whether sufficient APAP remains to lead to subsequent NAPQI formation and delayed hepatotoxicity. In many cases, the [AST] is normal, and the [APAP] is undetectable, obviating the need for NAC. If the [AST] is normal, then the patient is considered at risk if the [APAP] is 10 μg/mL (66 μmol/L) or above. Patients who are identified as at risk, with either an elevated [AST] *or* an elevated [APAP], should be treated with NAC.

Patients who develop a highly elevated [AST] after chronic APAP overdose should be treated with NAC and further evaluated with laboratory tests to assess hepatotoxicity and prognosis. Initial elevations of INR or [creatinine] are markers of poor prognosis in RSTI of APAP.

### Risk Determination After Acetaminophen Exposure in Children

Serious hepatotoxicity or death after acute APAP overdose is extremely rare in children. Predominant theories for resistance to toxicity include a relative hepatoprotection in children because of increased sulfation capacity or differences in the characteristics of childhood poisonings, including smaller ingested doses, overestimation of liquid doses, and unique formulations (pediatric elixirs contain propylene glycol, which inhibits CYP2E1). The use of the nomogram and other stratification tools described above are applicable for pediatric patients.

### Risk Determination After Acetaminophen Exposure in Pregnancy

The initial risk of toxicity in a pregnant woman is similar to that of a nonpregnant patient. No alteration of the treatment line is necessary. In fact, there are no reported cases of fetal or maternal toxicity in women with an [APAP] below the treatment line or in those treated with NAC within 10 hours of an acute ingestion. Pregnant women who develop APAP toxicity in the first trimester have an increased risk of spontaneous abortion, fetal demise is described in the second trimester, and those who develop APAP toxicity after about 20 weeks of gestation have a potential risk of fetal hepatotoxicity because of fetal metabolism. However, reports of third-trimester fetal hepatotoxicity are rare and are only associated with severe maternal toxicity. The factors associated with poor fetal outcome after a large APAP overdose are delayed treatment with NAC and young gestational age.

The decision to treat a pregnant woman with NAC requires evaluation of the known efficacy and beneficial effects as well as the adverse events of NAC for both the fetus and the mother. Data suggests that NAC is both safe and effective in treating the mother, but there are inadequate data to evaluate efficacy in fetuses, although fetal outcome is generally excellent after maternal treatment with NAC. Given that NAC is safely used in many pregnancies and fetal mortality is linked to delays to treatment, NAC should be initiated in pregnant women who meet the same criteria as nonpregnant patients. The 21-hour IV protocol probably is the most commonly recommended NAC protocol used for pregnant women worldwide; however, there is a paucity of published experience supporting oral NAC treatment courses shorter than the 72-hour protocol.

### Ethanol and Risk Determination

Although not entirely consistent, both animal and human data suggest that acute ethanol coingestion with APAP is hepatoprotective. Ethanol coingestion decreases NAPQI formation presumably by inhibiting CYP2E1 in both humans and animals. In large retrospective evaluations of overdoses, acute ethanol ingestion independently decreases the risk of severe hepatotoxicity in chronic heavy ethanol users and in nonchronic heavy ethanol users but did not significantly decrease the risk of hepatotoxicity ([ALT] > 1,000 IU/L) in a smaller prospective study. However, chronic ethanol administration increases the risk of hepatotoxicity from APAP dosing in animals. This is due to induction of CYP2E1 metabolism after the ethanol is metabolized, resulting in increased NAPQI formation, as well as decreased mitochondrial GSH supply impairing hepatocyte protection and regeneration.

After *acute APAP overdose*, chronic heavy alcohol users who have not coingested ethanol are at a slightly increased risk; however, this elevated risk is of little clinical importance given the sensitivity of the treatment line. Thus the 150 treatment line is adequately sensitive for screening after an acute APAP overdose, regardless of the patient's history of chronic ethanol use.

### CYP Inducers and Risk Determination

Isoniazid is an inducer of CYP2E1 that has been theorized to proportionally increase the production of NAPQI from APAP. Similarly, several other medications, including phenytoin, carbamazepine, and phenobarbital, are theorized to increase APAP toxicity because of nonspecific CYP induction or induction of other CYPs. However, clinical experience suggests that there is no need to change the approach to these patients.

### Risk Assessment of Hepatotoxicity When the Diagnosis is Uncertain

In some cases, patients present with, or develop, hepatotoxicity with no clear ingestion history. Because APAP is the most common cause of acute liver failure (ALF), the most reasonable approach to patients with evidence of liver failure or highly elevated aminotransferase concentrations is to consider them at risk of APAP-induced ALF even with an undetectable [APAP]. Other common causes of acute elevations of [aminotransferase] should be considered, including rhabdomyolysis and hepatotoxicity related to hypoperfusion or hypoxemia. The pattern of laboratory tests suggest that ALF is from APAP but are not absolutely diagnostic. Cases of APAP ALF tend to have higher [AST] and [ALT] and lower [bilirubin] than other common causes of ALF. Several biomarkers differentiate APAP ALF from other causes but are not yet clinically available (see below).

### Assessing Actual Toxicity: Critical Components of the Diagnostic Approach

***Initial Testing.*** The [APAP] should be measured in patients with acute APAP overdose and no evident hepatotoxicity, but no other initial laboratory assessment is required. The [AST] should be measured in patients who are considered to be at risk for APAP toxicity according to the nomogram or history (in the case of repeated supratherapeutic dosing) or in those suspected of already having mild hepatotoxicity by history and physical examination. Unless evidence of serious hepatotoxicity is present, the [AST] is a sufficient indication of hepatic conditions, and no additional testing is initially needed.

***Ongoing Monitoring and Testing.*** If no initial elevation of [AST] is noted, then repeated determination of [AST] alone—without other biochemical testing—is sufficient to exclude the development of hepatotoxicity. The [AST] should be determined before the end of the protocol or every 12-24 hours if using a longer protocol. If an elevated [AST] is noted, then PT, INR, and [creatinine] should be measured and repeated every 24 hours or more frequently if clinically indicated. If evidence of hepatic failure is noted, then careful monitoring of blood glucose, pH, PT, INR, [creatinine], [lactate], and [phosphate] is important in assessing extrahepatic organ toxicity and is vital in assessing hepatic function and the patient's potential need for hepatic transplant (see Assessing Prognosis). In addition, meticulous bedside evaluation is necessary to determine and document vital signs, neurologic status, and evidence of bleeding.

### Role of Biomarkers and Risk Determination

Although the risk of hepatotoxicity is generally low when NAC is started in the appropriate time frame, there are cases in which risk assessment is difficult or impossible. In cases with unknown time of ingestions, late presenters, or multiple (staggered) ingestions, it may not be possible to accurately determine risk, and the current practice is to proceed conservatively. However, the conservative practice of treatment with NAC for unclear risk scenarios carries with it a risk of adverse reactions to NAC (which are more common in these scenarios) as well as excessive healthcare resource management. In these cases, use of a biomarker allows for targeted therapy to select individuals at high risk of adverse outcomes or allow early and safe discharge of well and low-risk groups. Although these biomarkers will be mentioned here briefly, none is currently rapidly clinically available for use and data are insufficient to recommend their use.

***Protein Adducts.*** Protein adducts indicate intracellular binding of NAPQI to the hepatocyte. After overexposure to APAP, NAPQI is not immediately bound to GSH and is released within the cell to bind with the cysteine components on proteins. One of these protein-APAP adducts is 3-(cysteinyl-S-yl)-APAP. However, hepatic toxicity from APAP requires not only protein binding, and therefore protein adducts, but an inflammatory cascade to produce cell necrosis. As such, protein adducts are signs of NAPQI binding, but not necessarily of toxicity. In humans with therapeutic dosing of APAP, protein adducts are usually detected in small quantities in the blood (< 0.5 nmol/mL). However, some patients with therapeutic dosing have concentrations of up to 1.0 nmol/mL. Unlike [AST], [protein adduct] remain detectable for up to 2 weeks and a concentration above 1.0 nmol/mL is suggested as being consistent with an acute APAP overdose.

***Micro RNA.*** Micro RNAs (miRNAs) are small, noncoding RNAs that regulate cell proteins by repressing mRNA. In human studies, miRNA-122 increases before other markers, such as [ALT], and is actively released from hepatocytes before cell lysis. The [miRNA-122] correlates with peak [ALT] and peak INR. In patients with acute APAP overdose whose initial [ALT] is normal and in patients who are treated within 8 hours, [miRNA-122] is higher in those who develop hepatic injury, suggesting that it may be useful in differentiating low-risk patients from high-risk patients earlier than other markers.

## MANAGEMENT

### Gastrointestinal Decontamination

In cases of very early presentation or coingestion of xenobiotics that delay gastrointestinal (GI) absorption, gastric emptying is appropriate for some patients. In general, however, gastric emptying is not appropriate for patients with isolated APAP overdose because of the very rapid GI absorption of APAP and the availability of an effective and safe antidote. Administration of oral activated charcoal (AC) shortly after APAP ingestion decreases the number of patients who have an [APAP] above the treatment line. Although AC is most effective when given within the first 1 to 2 hours after APAP ingestion, it is reasonable to give AC at later times provided there are no contraindications. Limited data suggest that delayed AC is associated with a reduced need for NAC and a decrease in the magnitude of rise of hepatic aminotransferases.

### Supportive Care

General supportive care consists primarily of managing the hepatic injury, acute kidney injury, and other manifestations. Treatment of these problems is based on general principles and is not APAP dependent. Discussion of the management of hepatic failure is beyond the scope of this chapter, but certain aspects deserve mention. Monitoring for and treatment of hypoglycemia are critical because hypoglycemia is one of the most readily treatable of the life-threatening effects of hepatic failure. If adequate viable hepatocytes are present, vitamin K produces some improvement in coagulopathy; thus, trial dosing is reasonable as hepatic injury develops and as it resolves. Administration of fresh-frozen plasma (FFP) and prothrombin complex concentrates (PCCs) should be based on specific indications rather than correction of PT and INR alone in the absence of a clinical acute indication. Hemorrhage is rare in APAP-induced hepatic failure, and correction of coagulopathy should only be necessary for procedures and life-threatening bleeding. Supportive therapies for cerebral edema, including cooling, hypertonic saline, elevation of the head, and support of the cerebral perfusion pressure, are all indicated.

### Antidotal Therapy with *N*-Acetylcysteine

Conceptually, it is helpful to think of NAC as serving three distinct roles. During the metabolism of APAP to NAPQI, NAC *prevents toxicity* by limiting the formation of NAPQI. More important, it *increases the capacity to detoxify* NAPQI that is formed (Fig. 6–1). In fulminant hepatic failure, NAC *treats toxicity* through nonspecific mechanisms that preserve multiorgan function (Antidotes in Brief: A3).

*N*-Acetylcysteine prevents toxicity mostly by serving as a GSH precursor and as a GSH substitute, combining with NAPQI and being converted to cysteine and mercaptate conjugates. *N*-Acetylcysteine also supplies cysteine as a substrate for sulfation, allowing less metabolism by oxidation to NAPQI. Based on large clinical trials, NAC efficacy is nearly complete as long as it is initiated within 8 hours of an acute overdose. However, the relationship between the time to administration of NAC and the risk of hepatotoxicity is a continuous variable. The risk of hepatotoxicity begins to increase at 6 hours for patients with an [APAP] greater than 600 μg/mL (3969 μmol/L) and is closer to 8 hours for patients with an [APAP] just over the treatment line. For this reason, NAC therapy should be initiated as soon as possible after 4 hours and not delayed past 8 hours.

*N*-Acetylcysteine is administered via the oral or IV routes and in protocols that have historically varied in duration. The most common regimens are a 12-hour IV infusion, a 21-hour IV infusion, and a 72-hour oral dosing protocol. With the exception of established hepatic failure, for which only the IV route has been investigated, the IV and oral routes of NAC are equally efficacious in preventing or treating APAP toxicity. There are three scenarios in which IV NAC is preferentially recommended: (1) APAP toxicity in pregnant women, (2) APAP-induced hepatic failure, and (3) intractable vomiting preventing oral treatment.

It is important to realize that even in low-risk patients (those treated within 8 hours), regardless of the protocol duration (12, 21, 36, 48, or 72 hours) or route of delivery, NAC therapy should be continued until APAP metabolism is complete (the [APAP] is below detection) and there are no signs of hepatotoxicity. With this concept in mind, it is reasonable to *shorten* a set course of NAC if the patient is at low risk and the above criteria are met ([APAP] undetectable, [AST] normal, PT/INR less than twice normal, and no encephalopathy). However, adequate studies have not definitively confirmed the safety of shortened protocols.

*N*-Acetylcysteine therapy should be continued *beyond* the prescribed "protocol duration" if there is evidence of hepatic injury ([AST] > 1,000 IU/L, PT/INR greater than twice normal, or encephalopathy is present) or APAP metabolism is incomplete the ([APAP] detectable). After NAC therapy is extended beyond a set-duration protocol, the decision to discontinue therapy should be entirely based on the patient's condition. For patients who develop hepatic failure, we recommend continuing IV NAC until the PT or INR is below twice the upper limit of normal values and encephalopathy, if present, is resolved. For patients without hepatic failure but with an elevated [AST], we recommend continuing NAC until hepatic abnormalities improve (eg, [AST] is decreasing and < 1,000 IU/L or the [AST]/[ALT] ratio < 0.4). The [AST] should be used to determine whether to stop NAC, as the [AST] decreases earlier upon recovery than [ALT] (half-life of 15 h for [AST] and 40 h for [ALT]).

***Assessing Risk of Hepatotoxicity.*** In general, both the time from ingestion to the initiation of NAC and the [APAP] are directly proportional to the patient's risk of developing hepatotoxicity and hepatic failure. Even in patients treated early after their ingestion, the risk of hepatotoxicity is significant if their [APAP] is highly elevated. In patients who are treated with NAC, the risk of hepatotoxicity increases from below 5% to about 10% if the [APAP] is over the "300 line" and to 20% to 40% if over the "500 line." Unfortunately, this only predicts the risk of a peak [aminotransferase] above 1,000 IU/L and cannot determine the risk of death or need for transplantation. The multiplicative sum of the [AST] (or [ALT]) and the [APAP] also predicts hepatotoxicity (sensitivity of 91% and specificity of 63% if the sum is > 1,500 mg/L*IU/L).

***NAC Dose Adjustment.*** In rare cases, patients with massive ingestions with or without antimuscarinic coingestants have a highly elevated [APAP] for prolonged periods or secondary elevations of the [APAP]. Several of these patients developed hepatotoxicity despite early (< 6 hours) IV NAC therapy, raising the question of whether the traditional IV NAC infusion (6.25 mg/kg/h) provides enough NAC for these rare patients with a late elevated [APAP] or massive ingestions. In these rare patients, we recommend treating with greater amounts of NAC when prolonged, massive [APAP] is evident. No data exist to determine which, if any, alternative NAC dosing strategy is superior. For a detailed description of increased dosing for massive ingestions, highly elevated [APAP], and prolonged elevations of [APAP], see Antidotes in Brief: A3.

### Hepatic Transplantation

Hepatic transplantation increases survival for a select group of severely ill patients who have APAP-induced fulminant hepatic failure. Tremendous improvements in transplantation and supportive hepatic care have increased immediate survival rates after hepatic transplantation to 69% to 83% with 3- to 5-year survival rates of 50% to 66%, respectively. Patients who meet criteria for transplant but do not receive an organ have survival rates of 25% to 40%. Concerns that patients who receive transplants for APAP-induced fulminant hepatic failure will have lower survival rates and be unable to maintain posttransplant medication regimens have resulted in the majority of patients not being listed for transplant.

### Assessing Prognosis

The most commonly used prognosticator of mortality is the King's College criteria (KCC) (Table 6–1). The survival rate of patients who meet the KCC but are not transplanted is 25% to 40%. Survival rates have significantly increased since the original studies, likely because of the utilization of prolonged NAC therapy and improved supportive care for patients with acute hepatic failure. When determining the KCC, interpretation of PT and INR must include awareness of concurrent NAC therapy as well as therapy with vitamin K, PCCs, factor VII, and FFP. The prognostic importance of monitoring PT

| TABLE 6–1 King's College Criteria |
|---|
| Either of the following historically predicted a survival rate <20% and the need for immediate transplantation; currently, the survival rate for these patients is 25-40% without transplantation. |
| 1. Arterial pH <7.3 or [lactate] >3.0 mmol/L after fluid resuscitation |
| *OR* |
| 2. All of the following: |
| a. [Creatinine] >3.3 mg/dL (292 μmol/L) |
| b. Prothrombin time >100 sec (or international normalized ratio >6.5) |
| c. Grade III or IV encephalopathy (somnolence to stupor, responsive to verbal stimuli, confusion, gross disorientation) |

and INR in this setting suggests that FFP should be given only for evidence of bleeding, with risk of bleeding from known concomitant trauma, or before invasive procedures, and not based merely on the PT or INR. A [lactate] above 3.5 mmol/L at a median of 55 hours after APAP ingestion or [lactate] above 3.0 mmol/L after fluid resuscitation is both a sensitive and specific predictor of patient death without transplant.

Unfortunately, patients often meet the KCC and lactate criteria quite late in their course of disease, so these criteria are not useful as early predictors or as standards for transfer to a facility that performs hepatic transplant. Additional predictors of severity of hepatic toxicity in patients treated with NAC include a rapid doubling of the [AST] or [ALT] (doubling < 8 hours) and an [AST] or [ALT] reaching 1,000 IU/L within 20 hours of NAC treatment. Table 6–2 summarizes the utility of currently used scoring systems for determining death or the need for transplant.

**TABLE 6–2 Prediction of Death or Transplant in 125 Patients With Acetaminophen-Induced Liver Failure**

| *Score* | *Sensitivity (%)* | *Specificity (%)* | *PPV* | *NPV* |
|---|---|---|---|---|
| King's College Criteria | 47 | 83 | 0.70 | 0.65 |
| Acute Physiology and Chronic Health Evaluation II (>12) | 67 | 76 | 0.69 | 0.75 |
| Sequential Organ Failure Assessment (>12) | 67 | 80 | 0.74 | 0.74 |
| Model for End-Stage Liver Disease (>32) | 89 | 25 | 0.49 | 0.77 |
| [Lactate] (>3.3 mmol/L) | 91 | 52 | 0.69 | 0.83 |

NPV = negative predictive value; PPV = positive predictive value.

## ELIMINATION TECHNIQUES

Several clinical scenarios benefit from increasing clearance of APAP from the body. Indications early after APAP overdose include patients with an exceedingly high [APAP] who are at high risk of hepatotoxicity despite NAC therapy as well as those with an elevated lactate and a metabolic acidosis. Later in the course of APAP toxicity, elimination techniques are used to remove the remaining [APAP] in patients who are imminently receiving a hepatic transplant or for removal of toxins related to hepatic failure.

### Hemodialysis

The Extracorporeal Treatments in Poisoning (EXTRIP) workgroup suggests hemodialysis for patients with altered mental status, elevated [lactate], or metabolic acidosis with an [APAP] greater than 700 μg/mL (4,630 μmol/L) or for an [APAP] greater than 900 μg/mL (5,960 μmol/L) if the patient is treated with NAC. Furthermore, hemodialysis is recommended for an [APAP] greater than 1,000 μg/mL (6,620 μmol/L) regardless of therapy. Because hemodialysis also removes NAC, we recommend doubling NAC infusion rates during hemodialysis to compensate. No dosing adjustment is likely necessary during continuous venovenous hemofiltration.

### Plasmapheresis and Plasma Exchange

Plasmapheresis is useful in patients with ALF to correct coagulopathy, but it does not reliably correct encephalopathy. Exchange transfusion was used in one 1.22-kg neonate who had an [APAP] of 75 μg/mL after maternal oral overdose and subsequent delivery with little reduction in [APAP] and is therefore not routinely recommended.

### Liver Dialysis

Liver dialysis devices such as the molecular adsorbent recirculation system (MARS) or fractionated plasma separation and adsorption, and single-pass albumin dialysis (Prometheus) are used as a bridge to transplantation, for hemodynamic stabilization before hepatic transplant, or as a bridge to spontaneous recovery in patients with APAP-induced hepatic failure. Although some surrogate benefits are reported, a meta-analysis concluded that MARS has no effect on mortality in multiple causes of ALF. We recommend treatment with one of these techniques, if available, in patients with fulminant hepatic failure who meet clinical criteria for transplantation or high mortality (eg, KCC) regardless of whether or not they will be transplanted.

# A3 *N*-ACETYLCYSTEINE

## INTRODUCTION

*N*-Acetylcysteine (NAC) is the cornerstone of therapy for patients with potentially toxic acetaminophen (APAP) overdoses. If administered early, NAC can prevent APAP-induced hepatotoxicity. If administered after the onset of hepatotoxicity, NAC improves outcomes and decreases mortality. *N*-Acetylcysteine appears to also limit hepatotoxicity from other xenobiotics that result in glutathione (GSH) depletion and free radical formation, such as cyclopeptide-containing mushrooms, carbon tetrachloride, chloroform, pennyroyal oil, clove oil, and possibly liver failure from chronic valproic acid use.

## HISTORY

Shortly after the first case of APAP hepatotoxicity was reported, Mitchell described the protective effect of GSH. Prescott first suggested NAC for APAP poisoning in 1974 and by 1977 the first treated patients were reported. Several human investigations were performed with oral (PO) and intravenous (IV) NAC starting in the late 1970s. The US Food and Drug Administration (FDA) approved NAC for PO use in 1985 and for IV use in 2004.

## PHARMACOLOGY

### Chemistry

The amino acids cysteine, glycine, and glutamate are used in vivo to synthesize GSH, the primary intracellular antioxidant. *N*-Acetylcysteine is a thiol containing (R-SH) compound that increases intracellular cysteine concentrations when deacetylated (into cysteine) and causes release of intracellular protein- and membrane-bound cysteine.

### Related Xenobiotics

Cysteamine, methionine, and NAC, which are all GSH precursors or substitutes, have been used successfully to prevent hepatotoxicity, but cysteamine and methionine both produce more adverse effects than NAC, and methionine is less effective than NAC. Therefore, NAC emerged as the preferred treatment.

### Mechanism of Action

Early after ingestion when APAP is being metabolized to *N*-acetyl benzoquinoneimine (NAPQI), NAC prevents toxicity by rapidly detoxifying NAPQI. In this preventive role, NAC acts primarily as a precursor for the synthesis of GSH. The availability of cysteine is the rate-limiting step in the synthesis of GSH, and NAC is effective in replenishing diminished supplies of both cysteine and GSH. Additional minor mechanisms of NAC in preventing hepatotoxicity include acting as a substrate for sulfation, as an intracellular GSH substitute by directly binding to NAPQI, and by enhancing the reduction of NAPQI to APAP.

After hepatotoxicity is evident, NAC decreases toxicity through several nonspecific mechanisms, including free radical scavenging, increasing oxygen delivery, increased mitochondrial adenosine triphosphate (ATP) production, antioxidant effects, and alteration of microvascular tone. These nonspecific effects support the use of NAC in nonacetaminophen induced liver injury.

### Pharmacokinetics and Pharmacodynamics

*N*-Acetylcysteine has a relatively small volume of distribution (0.5 L/kg), and protein binding is estimated at 83%. *N*-Acetylcysteine is metabolized to many sulfur-containing compounds such as cysteine, GSH, methionine, cystine, and disulfides, as well as conjugates of electrophilic compounds, that are not routinely measured. Thus, the pharmacodynamic study of NAC is complex.

***Pharmacokinetics of Oral* N*-Acetylcysteine.*** Oral NAC is rapidly absorbed, but its bioavailability is low (10%–30%) because of significant first-pass liver metabolism. The mean time to peak serum concentration is 1.4 ± 0.7 hours. The mean elimination half-life is 2.5 ± 0.6 hours. Interindividual serum NAC concentrations can vary tenfold. The effervescent NAC formulation (when dissolved in water) has a mean time to peak serum concentration of 1.8 hours with similar peak concentration and area under the plasma drug concentration versus time curve (AUC) as an equivalent dose of the PO NAC solution.

Conflicting in vitro and in vivo data regarding the concomitant use of PO NAC and activated charcoal suggest that the resultant bioavailability of NAC is either decreased or unchanged. This interaction is of limited clinical importance, and PO NAC can be initiated without concern for activated charcoal interaction (Chap. 6).

***Pharmacokinetics of Intravenous* N*-Acetylcysteine.*** Serum concentrations after IV administration of an initial loading dose of 150 mg/kg over 15 minutes reach approximately 500 mg/L (3,075 μmol/L). A steady-state serum concentration of 35 mg/L (range 10–90 mg/L) is reached in approximately 12 hours with the standard IV protocol. Several alternative protocols exist with variable kinetics. In general, slower loading doses lead to lower peak [NAC], and shorter protocols (eg, 12-hour protocol) lead to lower 20-hour [NAC] than longer protocols. Approximately 30% of NAC is eliminated renally. When in the blood, IV and PO NAC have a similar half-life (2–2.5 hours). This half-life is increased in the setting of severe liver failure or end-stage kidney disease because of a reduction in clearance.

***Intravenous versus Oral Administration.*** As in the case of many issues related to APAP toxicity, the choice of PO versus IV NAC is complex. Because no controlled studies have compared IV with PO NAC, conclusions about the relative benefit of each are difficult. With the exception of fulminant hepatic failure, for which only the IV route has been investigated, IV and PO NAC administration are essentially equally efficacious in treating patients with APAP toxicity. The route of NAC should not be a factor when considering efficacy.

Nausea and vomiting are more frequent in patients treated with PO NAC, whereas anaphylactoid reactions are more common during the rapid initial bolus of the standard IV protocol. Several alternative IV NAC protocols, mainly modifying the initial bolus dose/time, reported lower rates of anaphylactoid reactions requiring medical treatment when compared with the traditional three-bag protocol. Anaphylactoid reactions are severe in approximately 1% of cases, and in rare instances lead to hypotension and death.

Intravenous NAC is dosed using a complex three-bag preparation system (see Dosing and Administration section later) that has led to an up to 33% error rate, including 19% of patients having a greater than 1-hour interruption of NAC. Attempts at simplifying this system are described but are not adequately studied for general use (Table A3–1). Additional safety concerns involve dosing for both small children and obese adults.

The main disadvantages of the PO NAC formulation are the high rate of vomiting and the concern that vomiting delays therapy. Delays in administration of NAC are correlated with an increased risk of hepatotoxicity. A potential disadvantage of PO NAC is that its systemic absorption takes up to 1 hour compared with the immediate systemic availability of IV NAC. Finally, PO NAC doses are difficult to administer to patients with altered mental status because of aspiration risks; IV NAC offers a distinct advantage in these instances. One theoretical, albeit unproven, advantage of PO NAC early in the course of toxicity is that direct delivery via the portal circulation yields a higher concentration of NAC in the target compartment of toxicity, the liver. However, an elevated serum NAC concentration may be an advantage of IV NAC administration when the liver is not the only target organ of NAC, such as liver failure accompanied by cerebral edema or pregnancy.

Several economic analyses conclude that IV NAC is less expensive than PO NAC, but others conclude the opposite. However, the majority of cost is associated with length of hospital stay, and because none of these studies have taken into account that many patients treated with PO NAC now receive shorter courses than 72 hours, the studies do not represent costs of current use.

***Specific Indications for Intravenous* N*-Acetylcysteine.*** Three situations exist for which the available information suggests IV NAC is preferable to PO NAC: (1) fulminant hepatic failure, (2) inability to tolerate PO NAC, and (3) APAP poisoning in pregnancy. Other common indications for IV NAC include patients with very high [APAP] who are approaching or are more than 6 to 8 hours from the time of ingestion. Use of IV NAC is recommended to prevent further delays and resultant loss of NAC efficacy.

**TABLE A3–1 Three-Bag Method Dosage Guide for *N*-Acetylcysteine by Weight for Patients Weighing ≥ 40 kg[a]**

| Body Weight | | *Loading Dose (150 mg/kg in 200 mL $D_5W$ over 60 minutes)* | *Second Dose (50 mg/kg in 500 mL $D_5W$ over 4 hours)* | *Third Dose (100 mg/kg in 1000 mL $D_5W$ over 16 hours)* |
|---|---|---|---|---|
| *(kg)* | *(lb)* | N-*Acetylcysteine 20% (mL)*[b] | N-*Acetylcysteine 20% (mL)*[b] | N-*Acetylcysteine 20% (mL)*[b] |
| 100 | 220 | 75 | 25 | 50 |
| 90 | 198 | 67.5 | 22.5 | 45 |
| 80 | 176 | 60 | 20 | 40 |
| 70 | 154 | 52.5 | 17.5 | 35 |
| 60 | 132 | 45 | 15 | 30 |
| 50 | 110 | 37.5 | 12.5 | 25 |
| 40 | 88 | 30 | 10 | 20 |

[a]The total volume administered should be adjusted for patients weighing < 40 kg and for those requiring fluid restriction. [b]Acetadote (acetylcysteine) is available in 30-mL (200-mg/mL) single-dose glass vials.

$D_5W$ = 5% dextrose in water.

## ROLE IN ACETAMINOPHEN TOXICITY

In acute overdose, treatment with NAC should be initiated if the serum [APAP] plotted on the Rumack-Matthew nomogram is above the treatment line or the patient's history suggests an acute APAP ingestion of 150 mg/kg or greater and the results of blood tests will not be available within 8 hours of ingestion. In patients with chronic APAP ingestions, treatment with NAC should be initiated if either aspartate aminotransferase (AST) is above normal or the [APAP] is higher than expected given a pharmacokinetic assessment of the dose and time (Chap. 6).

## ROLE IN NONACETAMINOPHEN POISONING

The use of NAC has been studied for a number of xenobiotics associated with free radical or reactive metabolite toxicity such as chloroform, carbon tetrachloride, pennyroyal oil, clove oil, and zidovudine. Human data are insufficient for any of these xenobiotics to definitively recommend NAC as a therapeutic intervention. However, the best evidence supports the use of NAC in cases of acute exposures to cyclopeptide containing mushrooms and carbon tetrachloride. *N*-Acetylcysteine is reasonable in cases of acute pennyroyal oil (ie, pulegone) or clove oil (eg, eugenol) ingestions based on their similarities to APAP-induced hepatotoxicity. Both pulegone and eugenol are converted to reactive metabolites that deplete GSH, leading to centrilobular hepatic necrosis. Given the risk–benefit ratio, we recommend the use of NAC for these indications.

## ADVERSE EVENTS AND SAFETY ISSUES

Although the IV route ensures delivery, rate-related anaphylactoid reactions occur in 14% to 18% of patients, mainly during the initial bolus. Up to one-third of patients have the infusion completely stopped because of reactions, although it can be restarted in most cases. Most reactions are mild (6%) or moderate (10%) such as cutaneous reactions, nausea, and vomiting; severe reactions such as bronchospasm, hypotension, and angioedema are rare (1%). Anaphylactoid reactions

**TABLE A3–2 Three-Bag Method Dosage Guide for *N*-Acetylcysteine by Weight for Patients Weighing < 40 kg[a]**

| Body Weight | | Loading Dose (150 mg/kg over 60 minutes) | | Second Dose (50 mg/kg over 4 hours) | | Third Dose (100 mg/kg over 16 hours) | |
|---|---|---|---|---|---|---|---|
| (kg) | (lb) | N-Acetylcysteine 20% (mL) | $D_5W$ (mL)[b] | N-Acetylcysteine 20% (mL)[b] | $D_5W$ (mL) | N-Acetylcysteine 20% (mL)[b] | $D_5W$ (mL) |
| 30 | 66 | 22.5 | 100 | 7.5 | 250 | 15 | 500 |
| 25 | 55 | 18.75 | 100 | 6.25 | 250 | 12.5 | 500 |
| 20 | 44 | 15 | 60 | 5 | 140 | 10 | 280 |
| 15 | 33 | 11.25 | 45 | 3.75 | 105 | 7.5 | 210 |
| 10 | 22 | 7.5 | 30 | 2.5 | 70 | 5 | 140 |

[a]Acetadote (*N*-Acetylcysteine ) is hyperosmolar (2,600 mOsm/L) and is compatible with $D_5W$, one-half normal saline (0.45% sodium chloride injection), and water for injection.
[b]Acetadote is available in 30-mL (200-mg/mL) single-dose glass vials.
$D_5W$ = 5% dextrose in water.

are more common in patients with lower APAP concentrations because APAP decreases histamine release from mononucleocytes and mast cells in a dose-dependent manner. If hypotension, dyspnea, wheezing, flushing, or erythema occurs, then NAC should be stopped. Adverse reactions, confined to flushing and erythema, are usually transient, and we recommend continuing NAC with meticulous monitoring for systemic symptoms that indicate the need to stop the NAC. Urticaria can be managed with diphenhydramine with the same precautions. After the reaction resolves, we recommend carefully restarting NAC at a slower rate no later than 1 hour after the cessation, assuming NAC is still indicated. If the reaction persists or worsens, IV NAC should be discontinued and a switch to PO NAC is recommended. We recommend against stopping NAC treatment because of mild anaphylactoid reactions because there is evidence of poor outcomes in patients who are undertreated with NAC in these scenarios. Intravenous NAC decreases clotting factors and increases the prothrombin time. International normalized ratio (INR) elevations are typically below 1.5 to 2.0.

Iatrogenic overdoses with IV NAC resulted in severe reactions, including hypotension, hemolysis, cerebral edema, seizures, and death.

## SAFETY IN PREGNANCY AND NEONATES

*N*-Acetylcysteine is FDA Pregnancy Category B. Untreated APAP toxicity is a far greater threat to fetuses than is NAC treatment. *N*-Acetylcysteine traverses the human placenta and produces cord blood concentrations comparable to maternal blood concentrations. For treatment of pregnant patients with APAP toxicity, IV NAC (not PO NAC) has the advantage of assuring sufficient fetal delivery of NAC because of reduction of the first-pass metabolism.

Limited data exist with regard to the management of neonatal APAP toxicity, although IV and PO NAC have been used safely. When treating neonates, IV administration has the advantage of assuring adequate antidotal delivery and has been administered without adverse effects. Caution regarding NAC preparation is paramount to avoid iatrogenic dilution administration errors.

## DOSING AND ADMINISTRATION

The standard IV NAC protocol uses 3 consecutive infusions without interruption (as shown in Tables A3–1 and A3–2). The standard 72-hour oral regimen uses a loading dose of 140 mg/kg followed by 17 maintenance doses of 70 mg/kg (as shown in Tables A3–3 and A3–4). If any dose

**TABLE A3–3 Calculating the Loading Dose of Oral *N*-Acetylcysteine Solution[a]**

| Body Weight (kg) | Body Weight (lb) | N-Acetylcysteine (g) | mL of 20% N-Acetylcysteine Oral Solution | Diluent (mL) | 5% Solution (Total mL) |
|---|---|---|---|---|---|
| 100–109 | 220–240 | 15 | 75 | 225 | 300 |
| 90–99 | 198–218 | 14 | 70 | 210 | 280 |
| 80–89 | 176–196 | 13 | 65 | 195 | 260 |
| 70–79 | 154–174 | 11 | 55 | 165 | 220 |
| 60–69 | 132–152 | 10 | 50 | 150 | 200 |
| 50–59 | 110–130 | 8 | 40 | 120 | 160 |
| 40–49 | 88–108 | 7 | 35 | 105 | 140 |
| 30–39 | 66–86 | 6 | 30 | 90 | 120 |
| 20–29 | 44–64 | 4 | 20 | 60 | 80 |

[a]If the patient weighs < 20 kg (usually patients younger than 6 years), calculate the dose of *N*-acetylcysteine. Each milliliter of 20% *N*-acetylcysteine solution contains 200 mg of *N*-acetylcysteine. The loading dose is 140 mg per kilogram of body weight. Three milliliters of dilluent is added to each milliliter of 20% *N*-acetylcysteine solution. Do not decrease the proportion of diluent.

**TABLE A3–4 Calculating the Mainenance Dose of Oral *N*-Acetylcysteine Solution[a]**

| Body Weight (kg) | Body Weight (lb) | *N-Acetylcysteine (g)* | *20% N-Acetylcysteine Oral Solution (mL)* | *Diluent (mL)* | *5% Solution (Total mL)* |
|---|---|---|---|---|---|
| 100–109 | 220–240 | 7.5 | 37 | 113 | 150 |
| 90–99 | 198–218 | 7 | 35 | 105 | 140 |
| 80–89 | 176–196 | 6.5 | 33 | 97 | 130 |
| 70–79 | 154–174 | 5.5 | 28 | 82 | 110 |
| 60–69 | 132–152 | 5 | 25 | 75 | 100 |
| 50–59 | 110–130 | 4 | 20 | 60 | 80 |
| 40–49 | 88–108 | 3.5 | 18 | 52 | 70 |
| 30–39 | 66–86 | 3 | 15 | 45 | 60 |
| 20–29 | 44–64 | 2 | 10 | 30 | 40 |

[a]If the patient weighs < 20 kg (usually patients younger than 6 years), calculate the dose of *N*-acetylcysteine. Each milliliter of 20% *N*-acetylcysteine solution contains 200 mg of *N*-acetylcysteine. The maintenance dose is 70 mg/kg of body weight. Three milliliters of dilluent is added to each milliliter of 20% *N*-acetylcysteine solution. Do not decrease the proportion of diluent.

is vomited within 1 hour of administration, then we recommend repeating the dose or using the IV route. Several other regimens, including 48-hour IV, 36-hour IV, 12-hour IV, 36-hour PO, and 20-hour PO protocols, are described; however, none of these has been adequately studied for general use (Chap. 6).

Three additional protocols have been developed with the intent of decreasing anaphylactoid reactions. The SNAP protocol infuses an initial 100 mg/kg over 2 hours and then 200 mg/kg over 10 hours. In a randomized controlled trial, this protocol decreased severe anaphylactoid rates from 31% with the traditional IV NAC "three-bag" protocol to 5%. Although the study was not large enough to prove equivalent efficacy, hepatotoxicity rates were similar (2% SNAP protocol versus 3% IV NAC "three-bag" protocol). Another protocol infused 200 mg/kg over 4 hours and then 100 mg/kg over 16 hours and found a lower rate of anaphylactoid reactions (4.3% versus 10%) and no difference in hepatotoxicity. A third group suggested infusing 200 mg/kg at the time of presentation and over a variable time (4–9 h) and then 100 mg/kg over 16 hours but had a high rate of overtreatment. Although these protocols seem to decrease adverse events and severe anaphylactoid reactions, their efficacy has not been studied against the standard protocol.

Conceptually, NAC therapy should be started if the patient is at risk of toxicity, continued as long as is necessary, and stopped when the patient is no longer at risk of toxicity. For a detailed description of the indications for treating APAP toxicity with NAC, see Chap. 6. Briefly, in acute overdoses (from 4–24 h after ingestion), NAC therapy should be initiated if the initial APAP concentration falls above the treatment line of the Rumack-Matthew nomogram. In acute overdoses when the patient arrives more than 24 hours after ingestion, we recommend starting NAC if the APAP concentration is detectable or if the [AST] is greater than the upper limit of normal. In repeated supratherapeutic ingestions, NAC therapy should be initiated if *either* the APAP concentration is detectable *or* the AST is elevated (Chap. 6).

After the protocol is initiated, an [APAP] and [AST] are evaluated before the end of the NAC infusion (<20 h for IV NAC) or at 24 hours (for PO NAC). If a shortened protocol is being used (eg, SNAP), then an [APAP] and [AST] should be evaluated at the end of the infusion. If the [APAP] is undetectable and the [AST] is normal, then we recommend discontinuing NAC. We continue NAC beyond the "protocol length" if the [APAP] remains detectable or the [AST] is significantly elevated. We recommend continuing the NAC protocol until the [APAP] is undetectable; there is no evidence of hepatic failure; and the [AST], if it was elevated, has significantly decreased. There are no validated criteria to define a significant decrease in [AST], but two consecutive decreasing values of an [AST] less than 1,000 IU/L, or an [AST]/[ALT] ratio of 0.4 are reasonable and are commonly used. If hepatic failure intervenes, then IV NAC is recommended at 6.25 mg/kg/h and continued until the patient has a normal mental status (or recovery from hepatic encephalopathy) and the patient's INR decreases below 2.0, or until the patient receives a liver transplant.

For the rare patient who ingests exceptionally large doses of APAP or who has prolonged and significantly elevated [APAP], consideration should be given to treating with greater amounts of NAC when prolonged, massive APAP concentrations are evident. No data exist to determine which, if any, alternative NAC dosing strategy is effective; however, it seems reasonable to increase NAC dosing if the hepatic exposure to APAP (and therefore NAPQI) is prolonged and massive. The following is reasonable: we recommend that any patient who presents with an [APAP] above the 500 mg/L at 4 hour line receive the traditional IV NAC dosing in addition to traditional PO NAC dosing. In the event a patient cannot take the PO NAC (eg, somnolent, caustic coingestion), we recommend that the patient should receive the IV loading dose followed by the 4-hour dose (12.5 mg/kg/h) for the duration of the treatment regimen. In the event a patient presents later than 8 hours and the [APAP] is above the theoretical "500" line, then we recommend that the IV loading dose is followed by 12.5 mg/kg/h (thus doubling the last infusion rate) for the duration of the treatment regimen.

*N*-Acetylcysteine is efficiently removed by hemodialysis, and we suggest doubling NAC infusion rates during hemodialysis to compensate. *N*-Acetylcysteine clearance during continuous venovenous hemodialysis (CVVHD) is much less affected; therefore, we recommend against dosing adjustment during CVVHD. Although there are few studies on NAC dosing in obese patients, it is reasonable to limit PO and IV NAC dosing using a maximum weight of 100 kg, given that patients who are larger than 100 kg have an equivalent hepatic volume and similar ingestion amounts as patients who weigh less than 100 kg.

## FORMULATION

*N*-Acetylcysteine is available as a 20% concentration in 30-mL single-dose vials designed for dilution before IV administration. *N*-Acetylcysteine liquid for PO administration is available in 10-mL vials of 10% and 20% for PO administration and should also be diluted before administration. *N*-Acetylcysteine is also available as 500-mg and 2.5-g PO effervescent tablets, which are dissolved in water before PO ingestion.

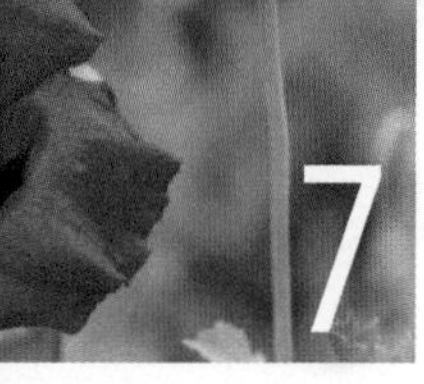

# 7 COLCHICINE, PODOPHYLLIN, AND THE VINCA ALKALOIDS

Colchicine, podophyllotoxin, and the vinca alkaloids exert their primary toxicity by binding to tubulin and interfering with microtubule structure and function. This chapter discusses the history, pharmacology, pharmacokinetics, toxicokinetics, pathophysiology, toxic dose, clinical manifestations, diagnostic testing, and management of toxicity resulting from these xenobiotics both during therapeutic use and in the overdose setting.

## COLCHICINE

### History

The origins of colchicine and its history in poisoning can be traced back to Greek mythology. The use of colchicum for medicinal purposes is reported in an ancient medical text, written in the first century A.D. Benjamin Franklin reportedly had gout and is credited with introducing colchicine in the United States. Colchicine is still used in the acute treatment and prevention of gout and is used in other disorders, including amyloidosis, Behçet syndrome, familial Mediterranean fever, pericarditis, arthritis, pulmonary fibrosis, vasculitis, biliary cirrhosis, pseudogout, certain spondyloarthropathies, calcinosis, and scleroderma. A limited number of cases are caused by intentional suicidal ingestions with colchicine, and therapeutic colchicine administration has contributed to adverse health effects and in some cases death.

### Pharmacology

Colchicine is a potent inhibitor of microtubule formation and function that interferes with cellular mitosis, intracellular transport mechanisms, and maintenance of cell structure and shape. The ubiquitous presence of microtubules in cells comprising various tissues and organs throughout the body presents a wide variety of targets for colchicine in poisoning. Colchicine accumulates in leukocytes and has inhibitory effects on their inflammatory function.

### Pharmacokinetics and Toxicokinetics

Colchicine is rapidly absorbed orally with a bioavailability between 25% and 50%. It is highly lipid soluble with a volume of distribution that ranges from 2.2 to 12 L/kg, and is reported to increase to 21 L/kg in overdose. Colchicine binding to plasma proteins, mostly albumin, approaches 50%. Colchicine is primarily metabolized through the liver (mainly CYP3A4) with up to 20% of the ingested dose excreted unchanged in the urine. Enterohepatic recirculation of colchicine occurs. The terminal elimination half-life ranges from 1.7 to 30 hours. Individuals with end-stage kidney disease and liver cirrhosis have elimination half-lives that are prolonged up to 10-fold. Postmortem examination of colchicine-poisoned patients reveals high concentrations within the bone marrow, testicles, spleen, kidney, lung, brain, and heart.

***Drug Interactions.*** Because colchicine is detoxified by CYP3A4, blood concentrations are susceptible to xenobiotics that alter the function of this enzyme, such as erythromycin, clarithromycin, and grapefruit juice. In particular, coadministration of clarithromycin and colchicine, especially in patients with chronic kidney disease, increases the risk of fatal interaction. P-glycoprotein (P-gp) expels and clears colchicine, and drugs that inhibit P-gp directly affect the amount of colchicine eliminated and hence toxicity. If treatment with a P-gp or a strong CYP3A4 inhibitor is required in patients taking colchicine, a dose reduction or temporary cessation of colchicine treatment is advised.

### Pathophysiology

Microtubules play a vital role in cellular mitosis and possess significant dynamic instability. Xenobiotics that bind to specific regions on tubulin, the building block of microtubules, can interfere with microtubule structure and function, thereby causing mitotic and cellular dysfunction and death. Colchicine also inhibits microtubule-mediated intracellular granule transport.

### Toxic Dose

The acute toxic dose for colchicine is not well established. An early case series suggested that patients with ingestions of greater than 0.8 mg/kg who were not decontaminated uniformly died, whereas those with ingestions between 0.5 mg/kg and 0.8 mg/kg would survive if given supportive care. More recent literature suggests that severe toxicity and even death can occur with smaller doses, and that some patients survive ingestions in excess of 0.8 mg/kg, but toxicity is unlikely at doses <0.3 mg/kg.

### Clinical Presentation

The clinical findings in poisoned patients are commonly described in three phases (Table 7–1).

### Diagnostic Testing

Colchicine concentrations in body fluids are not readily available in a clinically relevant fashion and have no well-established correlation to severity of illness. However, effective steady-state plasma concentrations for treatment of various illnesses are reported as 0.5–3 ng/mL. Concentrations greater than 3 ng/mL are associated with toxicity. Initial laboratory monitoring should include a complete blood count (CBC), serum electrolytes, kidney and liver function tests, creatine kinase, phosphate, calcium, magnesium, prothrombin time, activated partial thromboplastin time, and urinalysis. Other laboratory studies, such as a troponin, arterial or venous blood gases, lactate, fibrinogen, and fibrin split products, are helpful in guiding care if cardiotoxicity, ARDS, or coagulopathies, respectively, are present. If cardiotoxicity is present or suspected, serial troponin concentrations (every 6–12 hours) are recommended. There is an association between increasing troponin concentrations and cardiovascular collapse. A cardiac ultrasound, an electrocardiogram,

**TABLE 7–1 Colchicine Poisoning: Common Clinical Findings, Timing of Onset, and Treatment**

| Phase | Time[a] | Signs and Symptoms | Therapy or Follow-Up |
|---|---|---|---|
| I | 0–24 h | Nausea, vomiting, diarrhea | Antiemetics |
| | | | GI decontamination for early presentation |
| | | Salt and water depletion | IV fluids |
| | | Leukocytosis | Close observation for leukopenia for 24 h |
| II | 1–7 days | Risk of sudden cardiac death (24–48 h) | ICU admission and appropriate resuscitation |
| | | Pancytopenia | G-CSF |
| | | Acute kidney injury | Hemodialysis |
| | | Sepsis | Antibiotics |
| | | ARDS | Oxygen, mechanical ventilation |
| | | Electrolyte imbalances | Repletion as needed |
| | | Rhabdomyolysis | IV fluids, hemodialysis |
| III | > 7 days | Alopecia (sometimes delayed 2–3 wk) | Follow-up within 1–2 mo |
| | | Myopathy, neuropathy, or myoneuropathy | EMG testing, biopsy, and neurologic follow-up as needed |

[a]The interval time course is not absolute, and overlap of symptom presentations occurs.

ARDS = acute respiratory distress syndrome; EMG = electromyography; G-CSF = granulocyte-colony stimulating factor; GI = gastrointestinal; ICU = intensive care unit; IV = intravenous.

and chest radiograph should also be obtained. Serial CBCs are reasonable (at least every 12 h) to evaluate for the development of depression in cell lines.

### Management

Treatment for patients with colchicine poisoning is supportive as no direct antidote has yet to be commercialized. Therapy includes intravenous fluid replacement, vasopressor use, hemodialysis (for renal failure), antibiotics for suspected secondary infection, and adjunctive respiratory therapy (endotracheal intubation, positive end-expiratory pressure), as indicated. Consultation with other specialists should be obtained as needed.

Because most patients with an acute oral colchicine overdose present several hours after their ingestion, vomiting has already begun and the usefulness of gastrointestinal decontamination at this time is inadequately defined. However, given the extensive morbidity and mortality associated with colchicine overdose, orogastric lavage is reasonable in patients who present within 1–2 hours of a potentially lethal ingestion and who have not yet vomited. A dose of activated charcoal should be administered immediately or following lavage if done. Multiple-dose activated charcoal (MDAC) is also suggested because of enterohepatic recirculation. Antiemetics are necessary for good patient care and to facilitate activated charcoal administration. Administration of granulocyte-colony stimulating factor (G-CSF) is recommended if the patient develops leukopenia. Hemodialysis and hemoperfusion are not useful for eliminating colchicine, based on its large volume of distribution and plasma protein binding.

Because of the severe morbidity and mortality associated with colchicine toxicity, all symptomatic patients with suspected or known significant overdose should be admitted to the hospital for observation. Since there is a risk of sudden cardiovascular collapse within the first 24–48 hours, intensive care unit monitoring is recommended for all symptomatic patients for at least this initial time period. All patients should be observed for at least 8–12 hours. Those patients who do not manifest gastrointestinal signs and symptoms within that initial time period following ingestion are unlikely to be significantly poisoned unless a coingestant slowing down gut motility is present.

## PODOPHYLLUM RESIN OR PODOPHYLLIN

### History

Podophyllin is the name often used to refer to a resin extract from the rhizomes and roots of certain plants of the genus *Podophyllum*. Podophyllum resin, or podophyllin, contains at least 16 physiologically active compounds, including podophyllotoxin. Podophyllotoxin is a potent microtubular poison, similar to colchicine, and causes analogous effects in overdose.

Poisoning usually is a result of systemic absorption following topical application, ingestion of the resin or plant, or consumption of a commercial preparation of the extract. Systemic toxicity is described after unintentional dispensing of the incorrect herb, as well as after ingestion of herbal preparations containing podophyllin.

### Pharmacology

Podophyllin is primarily used in modern pharmacopeia as a topical treatment for verruca vulgaris and condyloma acuminatum. The active ingredient is believed to be podophyllotoxin.

### Pharmacokinetics and Toxicokinetics

Very limited information exists regarding the pharmacokinetics of podophyllin. Absorption of podophyllotoxin was measured in seven men after topical application for condylomata acuminata. Peak serum concentrations of 1 to 17 ng/mL were achieved within 1 to 2 hours after topical administration depending on the dose administered.

### Pathophysiology

Podophyllotoxin binds to tubulin subunits and interferes with subsequent microtubule structure and function. Podophyllotoxin also inhibits fast axoplasmic transport similar to colchicine by interference with microtubule structure and function.

### Toxic Dose

The minimum toxic ingested dose of podophyllin is unknown, therefore all ingestions are considered potentially toxic.

### Clinical Presentation

Poisoning is described following ingestion and intravenous administration, as well as after systemic absorption from topical application of podophyllin. Nausea, vomiting, abdominal pain, and diarrhea usually begin within several hours after ingestion. Symptoms of poisoning might be delayed for 12 hours or more after topical exposure to podophyllin and often are caused by improper usage (excessive topical exposure, interruption in skin integrity, or failure to remove the preparation after a short time period). Initial clinical findings are not necessarily dictated by the route of exposure.

Alterations in central and peripheral nervous system function tend to predominate in podophyllin toxicity. Patients present with, or rapidly progress to, confusion, obtundation, and coma. Delirium and both auditory and visual hallucinations are reported during the initial presentation. Patients develop paresthesias, cranial neuropathies, and absent deep tendon reflexes. Patients who recover from the initial event are at risk of developing a peripheral sensorimotor axonopathy. The reported duration for recovery from podophyllin-induced axonopathy is variable but can take several months.

Hematologic toxicity from podophyllin most likely results from its antimitotic effects in a manner similar to colchicine, but is not nearly as consistent in its pattern, severity, and frequency.

### Diagnostic Testing

Podophyllin or podophyllotoxin concentrations are not readily available. Testing for suspected or known podophyllin poisoning should include a complete blood count, electrolytes, and other targeted testing, as needed. Serial complete blood counts should be obtained in cases of poisoning to detect pancytopenia. An electrocardiogram and chest radiograph are also reasonable.

### Management

Management primarily consists of supportive and symptomatic care. Any topically applied podophyllin should be thoroughly removed. If the patient presents within the first several hours of ingestion, a dose of AC is reasonable. Although a few cases report treatment with resin hemoperfusion and charcoal hemoperfusion given the lack of evidence of benefit and potential risk, extracorporeal elimination techniques are not routinely recommended at this time.

Patients with significant ingestions of podophyllin usually develop GI symptoms within a few hours, but patients also present with primarily neurologic symptoms, such as confusion or obtundation. Patients should be observed for the onset of toxicity for at least 12 hours after ingestion and at least 24 hours after dermal exposures. We recommend that asymptomatic patients with unintentional exposures and good follow-up who are discharged after 12 to 24 hours have scheduled follow-up with a primary care physician and a complete blood count within 24 hours.

## VINCRISTINE AND VINBLASTINE

### History

Vincristine and vinblastine, pharmaceuticals derived from the periwinkle plant, are among the most common vinca alkaloid derivatives used in chemotherapy. They are only administered intravenously. Intrathecal administration of vinblastine or vincristine is always an error, is a neurosurgical emergency, and is associated with life-threatening complications (Special Considerations: SC6 and SC7).

### Pathophysiology

Vincristine and vinblastine disrupt microtubule assembly from tubulin subunits by either preventing their formation or depolymerization, both of which are necessary for routine cell maintenance. Mitotic metaphase arrest is commonly observed and cell death quickly ensues as a result of the interruption of basic homeostatic functions.

The mechanism of neurotoxicity is not well understood but is related to inhibition of microtubular synthesis, which leads to axonal degeneration in the peripheral nervous system.

### Pharmacokinetics

After IV administration, vincristine is rapidly distributed and is 50%–80% protein bound. The vinca alkaloids are primarily eliminated through the liver. Vincristine overdose is the most frequently reported chemotherapeutic overdose in the literature. This is because there are at least four different potentially inappropriate ways to dose and administer vincristine, including confusing it with vinblastine, misinterpreting the dose, administering it by the wrong route, and confusing two different-strength vials.

### Drug Interactions

Administration of xenobiotics that inhibit CYP3A subfamily of enzymes or inhibit P-gp–mediated efflux increases the risk for toxicity.

### Toxic Dose

Chemotherapeutic regimens tend to keep single doses at or below 2 mg to decrease the likelihood of peripheral neuropathy. Unfortunately, toxicity occurs with cumulative dosing over time, as that typically occurs with chemotherapeutic regimens. Any acute dose greater than 1.2 mg/m$^2$ in an adult (2 mg/m$^2$ in child) with cancer or any dose delivered in error to a patient not being treated is problematic.

### Clinical Presentation

In therapeutic dosing, vincristine and vinblastine differ in their clinical toxicity. Vincristine produces less bone marrow suppression and more neurotoxicity than does vinblastine. However, myelosuppression is common in overdose with a decrease in cell counts beginning within the first week and lasting for up to 3 weeks. Other manifestations of acute vincristine toxicity are mucositis, central nervous system disorders, and syndrome of inappropriate antidiuretic hormone (SIADH).

Central nervous system disorders are varied and unusual during therapeutic vincristine therapy because of its poor penetrance of the blood–brain barrier. They are, however, more common when there is delayed elimination, damage to the blood–brain–barrier, overdose, or inadvertent intrathecal administration. Generalized seizures from toxicity or secondary effects generally occur from 1 to 7 days after exposure. Other manifestations are depression, agitation, insomnia, and hallucinations. Ascending peripheral neuropathies occur after inadvertent large doses and appear about 2 weeks after overdose. Paresthesias, neuralgia, ataxia, bone pain, wrist drop, foot drop, involvement of cranial nerves III to VII and X, and diminished reflexes are observed.

## Testing

Vincristine and vinblastine testing is not readily available at most hospitals. Organ-specific toxicity is evaluated through the use of routinely available laboratory tests (eg, complete blood count, electrolytes, renal and liver function tests).

## Management

Generalized seizures should be treated with benzodiazepines followed by other antiepileptics as necessary. Supportive and symptomatic care is recommended for organ-specific toxicity as needed. Monitoring daily blood counts is recommended, and G-CSF is used to treat neutropenia.

Nerve conduction studies are helpful in assessing the extent of any clinical signs and symptoms of peripheral neuropathy. In a controlled clinical trial for vincristine-induced peripheral neuropathy, glutamic acid 500 mg orally three times per day had limited efficacy. Other treatments include pain and paresthesia management, including opioids, nonsteroidal antiinflammatory drugs, tricyclic antidepressants, vitamin E, gabapentin, and lamotrigine.

The rapid distribution and high protein binding characteristics of vincristine favor early intervention and methods other than hemodialysis. Based on the pharmacokinetic profile of vincristine and case reports, exchange transfusion is the preferred method of enhanced elimination in children and plasmapheresis is the preferred method in adults when the patient presents soon after the administration of the drug.

Patients receiving an overdose of vincristine intravenously (as defined above) should be admitted to a cardiac-monitored bed and observed for 72 hours. If patients remain asymptomatic during the observation period, they can be discharged with follow-up for bone marrow suppression and SIADH; otherwise, depending on the patient's clinical condition, continual observation for progression of neurologic symptoms is warranted. Table 7–2 compares the manifestations of overdose of the xenobiotics in this chapter.

**TABLE 7–2 Comparison of Antimitotic Overdose**

| | *Colchicine* | *Podophyllum Resin* | *Vincristine* | *Vinblastine* |
|---|---|---|---|---|
| Route of exposure | PO | PO and cutaneous | IV | IV |
| Initial symptoms | GI effects,[a] neurologic effects (obtundation, confusion, delirium, seizures, myoneuropathy, areflexia) | GI effects,[a] fever, neurologic effects (obtundation, confusion, delirium, paresthesias, lost reflexes, cranial nerve involvement) | GI effects,[a] fever, neurologic effects (depression, agitation, delirium, paresthesias, muscle weakness, lost reflexes, cranial nerve involvement) | GI effects,[a] fever, myalgias, neurologic effects (but *less* than vincristine) |
| Initial symptom onset | Several hours after ingestion; delayed onset beyond 12 h very unlikely | Several hours after ingestion; delayed presentation (past 12 h) is possible, especially after cutaneous exposure | Usually within 24–48 h | Usually within 24–48 h |
| Hematologic effects | Leukocytosis (24–48 h after ingestion); pancytopenia (beginning 48–72 h after ingestion) | Similar to colchicine; however, not well characterized and reported less frequently | Occurs but *decreased* severity compared with vinblastine | Myelosuppression; *increased* severity compared with vincristine |
| CNS effects | Late (48–72 h after ingestion); obtundation, confusion, and lethargy secondary to progression of MSD | Can be early (< 12 h after ingestion); typically occur later or secondary to progression of MSD | Variable; cranial neuropathies; seizures; obtundation, confusion, and lethargy; also occur because of progression of MSD | Occur but *decreased* severity compared with vincristine |
| Delayed PNS effects | Myoneuropathy most common (can also occur early); reported most often in chronic colchicine users with kidney dysfunction | Peripheral sensorimotor axonopathy | Autonomic and ascending peripheral neuropathy; *increased* severity compared with vinblastine | Autonomic and peripheral neuropathy; *decreased* severity compared with vincristine |
| Clinical course | Recovery or MSD and death | Recovery or MSD and death | Recovery or MSD and death; SIADH | Recovery or MSD and death; SIADH |
| Management | Supportive; GI decontamination (activated charcoal, orogastric lavage for life-threatening ingestions if within 1–2 h, no contraindications present, and provider is proficient in the procedure); G-CSF for neutropenia | Supportive; GI decontamination (activated charcoal) for oral exposures and skin decontamination for cutaneous exposures | Primarily supportive; G-CSF for neutropenia<br>For treatment of intrathecal overdoses, see Special Considerations: SC6 | Primarily supportive; G-CSF for neutropenia; exchange transfusion, plasmapheresis, or plasma exchange is reasonable for severe toxicity<br>For treatment of intrathecal overdoses, see Special Considerations: SC6 |

[a]Nausea, vomiting, diarrhea, and abdominal discomfort.

CNS = central nervous system; G-CSF = granulocyte colony-stimulating factor; GI = gastrointestinal; IV = intravenous; MSD = multisystem organ dysfunction; PNS = peripheral nervous system; PO = oral; SIADH = syndrome of inappropriate antidiuretic hormone secretion.

# 8 NONSTEROIDAL ANTIINFLAMMATORY DRUGS

## HISTORY AND EPIDEMIOLOGY

Nonsteroidal antiinflammatory drugs (NSAIDs) are a heterogeneous group of chemicals that share similar therapeutic properties. NSAIDs have analgesic, antipyretic, and antiinflammatory effects. Ibuprofen was first introduced in the United States (US) in 1974 and was approved for nonprescription use in 1984. Like ibuprofen, the first-generation NSAIDs inhibit cyclooxygenase (COX) in a nonselective fashion. With the realization that COX inhibition could be separated into COX-1 and COX-2, and that most of the adverse gastrointestinal (GI) effects were mediated by COX-1, selective COX-2 inhibitors were introduced and marketed as having less GI toxicity than the older, less selective NSAIDs. In 2004, the manufacturer of Vioxx (rofecoxib), a COX-2 inhibitor, voluntarily withdrew it from sale when it was discovered that there was an increased cardiovascular mortality associated with its use. In 2005, FDA findings led the manufacturer of Bextra (valdecoxib) to withdraw that COX-2 inhibitor from the market, leaving Celebrex (celecoxib) as the only selective COX-2 inhibitor available in the US.

Nonsteroidal exposures are increasingly common, accounting for more than 3% of all cases reported to poison centers in the US. Reported deaths are extremely uncommon.

## PHARMACOLOGY

The pharmacologic properties of NSAIDS are outlined in Table 8–1. They all share the ability to inhibit prostaglandin (PG) synthesis (Fig. 8–1). Inhibition of COX-1 decreases synthesis of thromboxane $A_2$ in platelets and interferes with their aggregation. COX-2 is induced by inflammatory mediators and produces prostaglandins at the site of inflammation, which are responsible for mediating vasodilation, increasing vascular permeability, and sensitizing pain fibers. Inhibition of COX-2 is associated with both the analgesic and antiinflammatory actions of the NSAIDs, without antiplatelet effects.

## PHARMACOKINETICS AND TOXICOKINETICS

Most NSAIDs are organic acids with extensive protein binding (95%–99%) and small volumes of distribution of approximately 0.1 to 0.2 L/kg. Oral absorption of most NSAIDs occurs rapidly and is near complete, resulting in bioavailabilities above 80%. Time to achieve peak plasma concentrations varies widely (Table 8–1).

## PATHOPHYSIOLOGY

Gastrointestinal toxicity is the most common adverse effect from NSAID use. Normally, the COX-1 enzyme expressed in the gastric epithelial cells leads to the production of PGs ($PGE_2$ and $PGI_2$), which are responsible for maintaining GI mucosal integrity by increasing cytoprotective mucous production, decreasing stomach acid production, and enhancing mucosal blood flow. Antiinflammatory drugs inhibit the production of these cytoprotective PGs, as well as the platelet aggregatory $TXA_2$, and they also have a direct cytotoxic or local irritative effect, increasing the risk of gastric and duodenal ulcers, perforations, and hemorrhage. Selective COX-2 inhibitors decrease the incidence of significant GI toxicity compared with some nonselective NSAIDs. Effects on other organs systems are outlined in Table 8–2.

## CARDIOVASCULAR RISK OF SELECTIVE CYCLOOXYGENASE-2 INHIBITORS AND NONSELECTIVE NONSTEROIDAL ANTIINFLAMMATORY DRUGS

Atherosclerosis is a dynamic process of thrombus formation and inflammation involving numerous tissue factors and inflammatory mediators. Given the ability to inhibit synthesis of proinflammatory PGs, selective COX-2 inhibitors would be expected to be antithrombotic; however, their ability to inhibit endothelial-derived $PGI_2$ combined with their relative inability to inhibit platelet-activating $TXA_2$ (a predominantly COX-1 effect) shifts the balance toward thrombus formation.

In 2004, rofecoxib was withdrawn from the worldwide market given data demonstrating an elevated cardiovascular risk. Several other studies addressing selective COX-2 inhibitors showed similar findings, suggesting a class effect. The current data on nonselective NSAID use support an increased cardiovascular risk, yet this risk varies depending on the nonselective NSAID being used. Some nonselective NSAIDs have an elevated cardiovascular risk (eg, diclofenac, meloxicam, indomethacin, and, to a lesser extent, ibuprofen), but naproxen has a minimal cardiovascular risk.

## CLINICAL MANIFESTATIONS

Initial clinical manifestations are usually mild and predominantly include GI symptoms. More moderate and severe findings are rare and include central nervous system (CNS), metabolic, renal, and cardiac effects. Massive NSAID ingestions lead to multisystem organ failure and death.

### Neurologic Effects

The neurologic effects of NSAID use vary from the mild drowsiness, headache, and dizziness with therapeutic dosing to the more life-threatening CNS depression, coma, and seizures in overdose. The mechanism associated with the decreased level of consciousness is unknown.

### Renal and Electrolyte Effects

Anion gap metabolic acidosis, with and without acute kidney injury (AKI), complicates many acute, massive ibuprofen ingestions and is often severe. The cause of the acidosis is most likely multifactorial, involving profound hypotension and tissue hypoperfusion with elevated lactate concentrations and the accumulation of weak acid metabolites.

**TABLE 8–1 Classes and Pharmacology of Selected Nonsteroidal Antiinflammatory Drugs**

| | *Time to Peak Plasma Concentration (hours)* | *Half-Life (hours)* | *Pharmacokinetics* | *Unique Features* |
|---|---|---|---|---|
| ***CARBOXYLIC ACIDS*** | | | | |
| ***Acetic Acids*** | | | | |
| Diclofenac[a,b] | 2–3 | 1–2 | First-pass effect; hepatic metabolism (CYP2C9) | Decreases leukocyte arachidonic acid concentration; topical activity; hepatotoxic |
| Etodolac | 1 | 7 | Hepatic metabolism | Inhibits leukocyte motility; coronary vasoconstrictor effect |
| Indomethacin | 1–2 | 2.5 | Demethylation (50%) | Poor antiinflammatory effect; topical activity |
| Ketorolac | < 1 | 4–6 | Urinary excretion | Also formulated for parenteral use also |
| Sulindac | 1–2 | 7 | Active metabolite with a half-life of 18 h | Prodrug; hepatotoxic |
| Tolmetin | < 1 | 5 | Hepatic metabolism | Accumulates in synovial fluid |
| ***Fenamic Acids*** | | | | |
| Meclofenamate | 0.5–2.0 | 2–3 | Urinary excretion (~70%); active metabolite | Seizures; GI inflammation |
| Mefenamic acid | 2–4 | 3–4 | Urinary excretion (50%) | Seizures; prostaglandin antagonist |
| ***Propionic Acids*** | | | | |
| Fenoprofen | 2 | 2–3 | Decreased oral absorption (~85%) | Increased CSF concentration |
| Flurbiprofen | 1–2 | 6 | Urinary excretion unchanged (~20%) | Increased CSF concentration |
| Ibuprofen[c,d] | < 0.5 | 2–4 | Hepatic metabolism; urinary excretion | Also formulated for parenteral use |
| Indobufen[e] | 2 | 6–7 | Urinary excretion (70%–80%) | In Europe, used as prophylaxis for thrombus formation |
| Ketoprofen[c] | 1–2 | 2 | Hepatic metabolism; urinary excretion | Bradykinin antagonist; stabilizes lysosomal membranes |
| Naproxen[c] | 1 | 14 | Increased half-life with kidney dysfunction | Inhibitory effect on leukocytes; prolonged platelet inhibition |
| Oxaprozin | 3–6 | 40–60 | Hepatic metabolism | Once-daily administration |
| ***Salicylates (Chap. 10)*** | | | | |
| ***ENOLIC ACIDS*** | | | | |
| ***Oxicams*** | | | | |
| Meloxicam[a] | 5–10 | 15–20 | Hepatic metabolism (CYP2C9) | High COX-2 selectivity |
| Nabumetone | 3–6 | 24 | Hepatic metabolism; active metabolites | Prodrug |
| Piroxicam | 3–5 | 45–50 | Hepatic metabolism (CYP2C9) | Inhibits neutrophil activation |
| ***Pyrazolone*** | | | | |
| Phenylbutazone[e] | 2 | 54–99 | Hepatic metabolism; active metabolites | Irreversible agranulocytosis; aplastic anemia |
| ***CYCLOOXGENASE-2 SELECTIVE INHIBITORS*** | | | | |
| Celecoxib | 2–4 | 6–12 | Hepatic metabolism (CYP2C9) | Inhibits CYP2D6 |
| Nimesulide[e] | 1–3 | 2–5 | Urinary excretion (60%); active metabolites | Inhibits neutrophil activation |

[a]COX-2 preferential. [b]Available in combination with misoprostol. [c]Nonprescription. [d]Available in combination with oxycodone and hydrocodone. [e]Not available in the US for humans.

COX = cyclooxygenase; CSF = cerebrospinal fluid; GI = gastrointestinal.

## Gastrointestinal Effects

Adverse GI effects from acute and chronic NSAID use range from mild dyspepsia to ulcer formation, which can lead to life-threatening GI hemorrhage and perforation.

## Immunologic and Dermatologic Effects

The nonimmunologic anaphylactoid and the IgE-mediated anaphylactic reactions that are reported with the use of NSAIDs are clinically indistinguishable from one another, producing flushing, urticaria, bronchospasm, peripheral edema, and hypotension. The most common skin reactions include angioedema and facial swelling, urticaria and pruritus, bullous eruptions, and photosensitivity. Although rare, toxic epidermal necrolysis and Stevens-Johnson syndrome are reported.

## Hematologic Effects

As a class, NSAIDs are frequently implicated in the development of drug-induced thrombocytopenia and cause

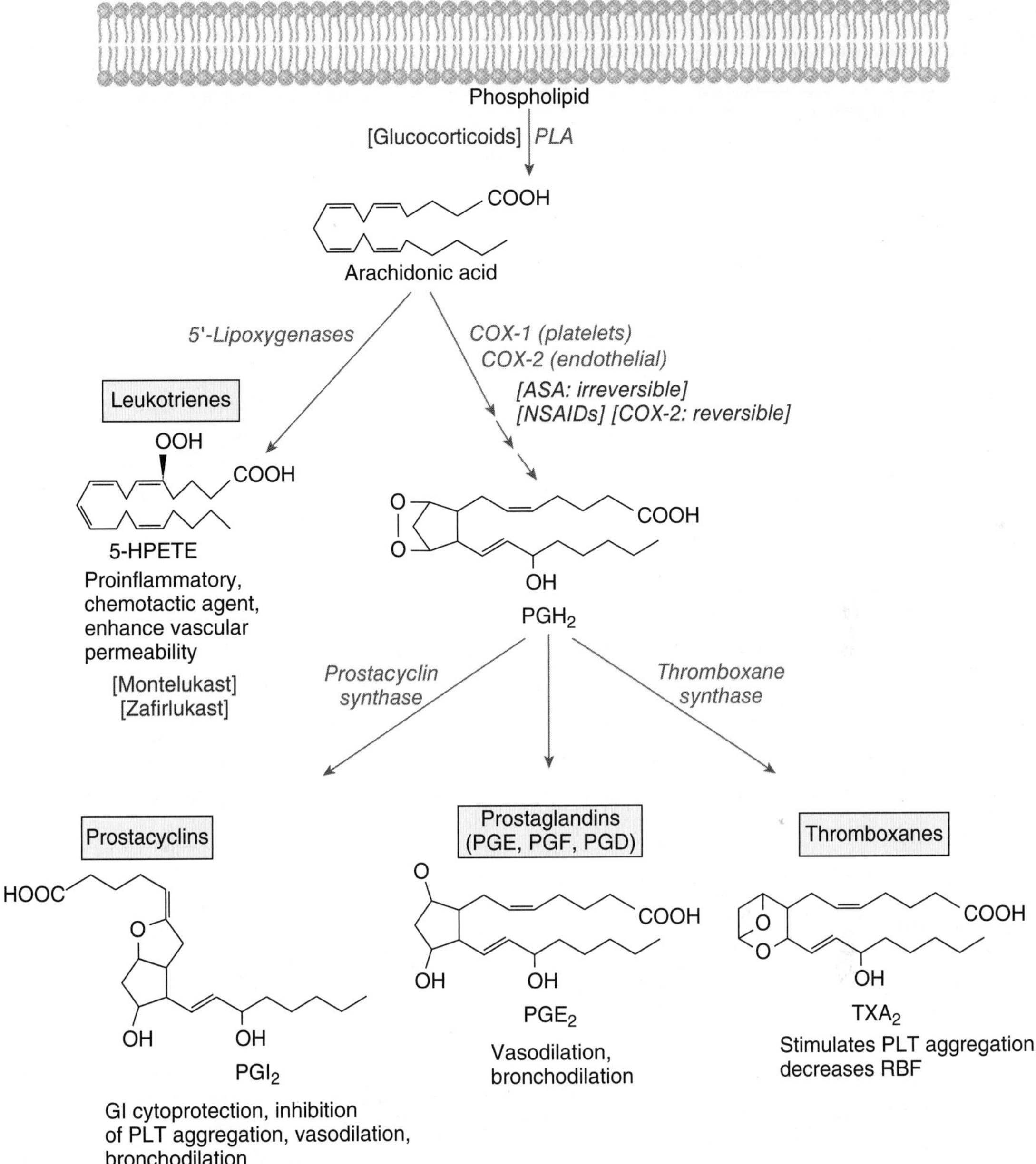


**FIGURE 8–1.** Arachidonic acid (AA) metabolism. This figure also illustrates some of the major differences between cyclooxygenase-1 (COX-1) and cyclooxygenase-2 (COX-2). Phospholipase A (PLA) is stimulated by physical, chemical, inflammatory, and mitogenic stimuli and releases AA from cell membranes. The COX-1 enzyme synthesizes prostaglandins (PGs) that maintain cellular and vascular homeostasis. The COX-2 enzyme produces PGs within activated macrophages and endothelial cells that accompany inflammation. Whereas nonsteroidal antiinflammatory drugs (NSAIDs) reversibly inhibit both COX isoforms, selective COX-2 inhibitors inhibit the COX-2 isoform. Some authors suggest that inhibiting the COX enzymes shunts AA metabolism toward the production of chemotactic-vasoactive leukotrienes. Glucocorticoids inhibit PLA and downregulate induced expression of COX-2. ASA = acetylsalicylic acid; 5-HPETE, hydroperoxy eicosatetraenoic acid; GI = gastrointestinal; $PGI_2$ = prostacyclin; PGD = prostaglandin D; $PGE_2$ = prostaglandin $E_2$; PGF = prostaglandin F; $PGH_2$ = prostaglandin $H_2$; PLT = platelet; RBF = renal blood flow; $TXA_2$ = thromboxane.

adverse effects on most other cell lines and function, including agranulocytosis, aplastic anemia, hemolytic anemia, methemoglobinemia, and pancytopenia. One dose of ibuprofen prolongs the bleeding time within 2 hours and persists for up to 12 hours. Nonsteroidal antiinflammatory drugs potentiate bleeding in patients such as those with thrombocytopenia, coagulation factor deficiencies, or von Willebrand disease and those ingesting alcohol or receiving warfarin therapy.

### Cardiovascular Effects

Although no evidence supports a direct cardiotoxic effect of NSAIDs or their metabolites, acute and massive NSAID overdoses are complicated by persistent and severe hypotension,

**TABLE 8–2 Selected Adverse Effects of Nonsteroidal Antiinflammatory Drugs**

| |
|---|
| ***Gastrointestinal*** |
| Acute: dyspepsia, ulceration, perforation, hemorrhage, elevated hepatic aminotransferases, hepatocellular injury (rare) |
| Chronic: same as above |
| ***Renal*** |
| Acute: acidemia, acute kidney failure, fluid retention, hyperkalemia, hypertension, interstitial nephritis, nephrotic syndrome, papillary necrosis, azotemia |
| Chronic: same as above |
| ***Hypersensitivity or Pulmonary*** |
| Acute: asthma exacerbation, anaphylactoid and anaphylactic reactions, urticaria, angioedema, acute respiratory distress syndrome, drug-induced lupus |
| Chronic: angioedema, drug-induced lupus |
| ***Hematologic*** |
| Acute: increased bleeding time, agranulocytosis, aplastic anemia, thrombocytopenia, neutropenia, hemolytic anemia |
| Chronic: same as above |
| ***Central Nervous System*** |
| Acute: headache, dizziness, lethargy, coma, aseptic meningitis, delirium, cognitive dysfunction, hallucinations, psychosis |
| Chronic: same as above |
| ***Drug Interactions*** |
| Aminoglycosides: increased risk of aminoglycoside toxicity |
| Anticoagulants (eg, warfarin, salicylates, heparins, direct thrombin inhibitors and Xa inhibitors): increased risk of gastrointestinal bleeding |
| Antihypertensives (especially diuretics, β-adrenergic antagonists, angiotensin receptor blockers, and angiotensin-converting enzyme inhibitors): reduced antihypertensive effects |
| Digoxin: increased risk of digoxin toxicity |
| Ethanol: increased bleeding time |
| Lithium: increased risk of lithium toxicity |
| Methotrexate: increased risk of methotrexate toxicity |
| Sulfonylureas: increased hypoglycemic effect |

myocardial ischemia, cardiac conduction abnormalities and dysrhythmias, including bradycardia, ventricular tachycardia or fibrillation, and prolonged QT interval.

### Pulmonary Effects

Although there is no evidence of direct pulmonary toxicity, some case reports describe the development of acute respiratory distress syndrome similar to the clinical manifestations of salicylate toxicity, suggesting an NSAID class mechanism-based process.

## DIAGNOSTIC TESTING

Serum concentrations of most NSAIDs can be determined but usually only by a specialty laboratory requiring several days to report results. Although ibuprofen nomograms were constructed in an attempt to correlate serum concentrations with clinical toxicity, the utility of these nomograms proved limited. We recommend obtaining a complete blood count, serum electrolytes, blood urea nitrogen, and creatinine, for all symptomatic patients, patients with intentional ingestions, ibuprofen ingestion of greater than 400 mg/kg in a child, or ibuprofen ingestion of greater than 6 g in an adult. For patients presenting with significant neurologic effects, such as CNS depression, further evaluation of acid–base and ventilatory status by blood gas, hepatic aminotransferases, and prothrombin time are recommended. An acetaminophen (APAP) concentration should always be determined in patients with intentional ingestions and in patients presenting with an unclear history. People often mistake APAP for NSAIDs and many variably compounded analgesics because of confusing labeling and packaging or unawareness that they are completely different types of analgesics. For similar reasons, obtaining a salicylate concentration is indicated.

## MANAGEMENT

Management is largely supportive and guided by the clinical signs and symptoms. Most asymptomatic patients with intentional overdose and those with normal vital signs require observation for 4 to 6 hours and a serum APAP concentration before being medically cleared. Children with ibuprofen ingestions of less than 100 mg/kg can be observed at home. Those who ingest greater than 400 mg/kg are at high risk for toxicity. We recommend activated charcoal (AC) for asymptomatic patients with the potential for a large ingestion, symptomatic patients, and children with a history of ibuprofen ingestion greater than 400 mg/kg. For patients with massive overdoses of sustained-release preparations, gastric lavage followed by AC and subsequent multiple-dose AC is reasonable.

Airway management and IV fluid therapy are required for severe overdoses. Electrolyte imbalances should be corrected, and sodium bicarbonate therapy administered for life-threatening metabolic acidosis. Given their high protein binding and low volumes of distribution, NSAIDs are not amenable to extracorporeal removal techniques. Although we recommend not to perform hemodialysis to remove an NSAID, hemodialysis or continuous renal replacement therapies are useful in cases of refractory metabolic acidosis or AKI,

# 9 OPIOIDS

## HISTORY AND EPIDEMIOLOGY

The medicinal value of opium, the dried extract of the poppy plant *Papaver somniferum*, was first recorded circa 1500 B.C. in the Ebers papyrus. Raw opium is composed of at least 10% morphine, but extensive variability exists depending on the environment in which the poppy is grown. Over the centuries since the Ebers papyrus, opium and its components have been used in two distinct manners: medically to produce profound analgesia and nonmedically to produce psychoactive effects. Morphine was isolated from opium by Armand Séquin in 1804. Charles Alder Wright synthesized heroin from morphine in 1874. Because of mounting concerns of addiction and overdose in the United States (US), the Harrison Narcotics Tax Act, enacted in 1914, made nonanalgesic use of opioids illegal.

In 2009, deaths from prescription drugs, mainly opioids, first exceeded those from motor vehicle crashes. Current data demonstrate that the US' opioid epidemic includes two distinct but interrelated trends: a 20-year increase in overdose deaths involving prescription opioid analgesics and a more recent surge in illicit opioid overdose deaths, driven largely by heroin and other illicit opioids.

Over the past decade, the realization that opioid analgesics are subject to extensive abuse has led to the development of newer formulations of existing opioids that theoretically reduced abuse potential. The use of "tamper-resistant formulations" was emphasized as an approach to reduce the abuser's ability to crush or dissolve the tablet for insufflation or injection, respectively. Although renamed "abuse deterrent formulations" (ADFs), the true clinical benefit of such formulations in reducing abuse is not known.

The terminology used in this chapter recognizes the broad range of xenobiotics commonly considered to be opiumlike. The term *opiate* specifically refers to the alkaloids naturally derived directly from the opium poppy: morphine and codeine. *Opioids* are a much broader class of xenobiotics that are capable of either producing opiumlike effects or binding to opioid receptors. A *semisynthetic opioid*, such as heroin or oxycodone, is created by chemical modification of an opiate. A *synthetic opioid* is a chemical, not derived from an opiate, that is capable of binding to an opioid receptor and producing opioid effects clinically. The term *opioid* as used hereafter encompasses the opioids and the opiates.

## PHARMACOLOGY

### Opioid-Receptor Subtypes

The current, widely accepted schema postulates the coexistence of three major classes of opioid receptors, each with multiple subtypes, and several poorly defined minor classes. Initially, the reason such an elaborate system of receptors existed was unclear because no endogenous ligand could be identified. However, in 1975 metenkephalin and leuenkephalin were discovered, and β-endorphin and dynorphin were subsequently identified. As a group, these endogenous ligands for the opioid receptors are called *endorphins* (*endo*genous mo*rphine*). Additionally, a minor related endogenous opioid (nociceptin/orphanin FQ) and its receptor ORL are described.

All three major opioid receptors consist of seven transmembrane segments, an amino terminus, and a carboxy terminus. Significant sequence homology exists between the transmembrane regions of opioid receptors and those of other members of the guanosine triphosphate (GTP)–binding protein (G-protein)–binding receptor superfamily. However, the extracellular and intracellular segments differ from one another. These nonhomologous segments probably represent the ligand-binding and signal transduction regions, respectively, which would be expected to differ among the three classes of receptors. The individual receptors have distinct distribution patterns within the central nervous system (CNS) and peripherally on nerve endings within various tissues, mediating unique but not entirely understood clinical effects.

The currently proposed nomenclature suggests the addition of a single letter in front of the OP designation and the elimination of the number. In this schema, the μ receptor is identified as MOP. Binding typically is not limited to one receptor type, and the relative affinity of an opioid for differing receptors accounts for the clinical effects (Table 9–1).

***Mu Receptor ($\mu$, MOP, $OP_3$).*** Experimentally, two subtypes ($\mu_1$ and $\mu_2$) are well defined, although currently no xenobiotics have sufficient selectivity to make this dichotomy clinically relevant. The μ receptors are found in the medullary cough center, peripherally in the gastrointestinal (GI) tract, and on various sensory nerve endings, including the articular surfaces. All of the currently available μ agonists have some activity at the $\mu_2$ receptor and therefore produce some degree of respiratory compromise. Localization of μ receptors to regions of the brain involved in analgesia, euphoria and reward, and respiratory function is expected.

***Kappa Receptor ($\kappa$, KOP, $OP_2$).*** Although dynorphins now are known to be the endogenous ligands for these receptors, originally, they were identified by their ability to bind ketocyclazocine and thus were labeled κ. These receptors exist predominantly in the spinal cords of higher animals, but they also are found in the antinociceptive regions of the brain and the substantia nigra.

***Delta Receptor ($\delta$, DOP, $OP_1$).*** Little is known about δ receptors, although the enkephalins are their endogenous ligands. These receptors do not modulate dopamine in the mesolimbic tracts and have only a slight behavioral reinforcing role.

***Nociceptin/Orphanin FQ Receptor ($ORL_1$, NOP, $OP_4$).*** The $ORL_1$ receptor was identified in 1994 based on sequence homology during screening for opioid-receptor genes with DNA libraries. It has a similar distribution pattern in the brain and uses similar transduction mechanisms as the other opioid-receptor subtypes. It binds many different opioid agonists

**TABLE 9–1 Clinical Effects Related to Opioid Receptors**

| *1996 Conventional Name* | *Proposed IUPHAR Name* | *IUPHAR Name* | *Important Clinical Effects of Receptor Agonists* |
|---|---|---|---|
| $\mu_1$ | $OP_{3a}$ | MOP | Supraspinal analgesia<br>Peripheral analgesia<br>Sedation<br>Euphoria<br>Prolactin release |
| $\mu_2$ | $OP_{3b}$ | MOP | Spinal analgesia<br>Physical dependence<br>Gastrointestinal dysmotility<br>Pruritus<br>Bradycardia<br>Growth hormone release<br>Respiratory depression |
| $\kappa_1$ | $OP_{2a}$ | KOP | Spinal analgesia<br>Miosis<br>Diuresis |
| $\kappa_2$ | $OP_{2b}$ | KOP | Psychotomimesis<br>Dysphoria |
| $\kappa_3$ | $OP_{2b}$ | KOP | Supraspinal analgesia |
| δ | $OP_1$ | DOP | Spinal and supraspinal analgesia<br>Modulation of μ-receptor function<br>Inhibit release of dopamine |
| Nociceptin/ orphanin FQ | $OP_4$ | NOP | Anxiolysis<br>Analgesia |

IUPHAR = International Union of Pharmacology Committee on Receptor Nomenclature.

and antagonists. Its insensitivity to antagonism by naloxone, often considered the sine qua non of opioid character, delayed its acceptance as an opioid-receptor subtype. Simultaneous identification of an endogenous ligand, called *nociceptin* by the French investigators and *orphanin* FQ by the Swiss investigators, allowed the designation $OP_4$.

### Opioid-Receptor Signal Transduction Mechanisms

Figure 9–1 illustrates opioid-receptor signal transduction mechanisms.

## CLINICAL MANIFESTATIONS

Table 9–2 outlines the clinical effects of opioids.

### Therapeutic Effects of Opioids

***Analgesia and Euphoria.*** Although classical teaching attributes opioid analgesia solely to the brain, opioids actually modulate cerebral cortical pain perception at supraspinal, spinal, and peripheral levels. Intraarticular morphine (1 mg) administered to patients after arthroscopic knee surgery produces significant, long-lasting analgesia that is prevented with intraarticular naloxone. Xenobiotics with strong binding affinity for δ receptors in humans, when given intrathecally, produce significantly more analgesia than morphine administered similarly. Blockade of the *N*-methyl-D-aspartate (NMDA) receptor, a mediator of excitatory neurotransmission, enhances the analgesic effects of μ-opioid agonists and reduces the development of tolerance. Even more intriguing is the finding that low-dose naloxone (0.25 μg/kg/h) actually improves the efficacy of morphine analgesia. Although undefined, the mechanism may be related to selective inhibition of $G_s$-coupled excitatory opioid receptors by extremely low concentrations of opioid-receptor antagonist.

***Antitussive.*** Codeine and dextromethorphan are two opioids with cough-suppressant activity. Cough suppression is not likely mediated via the $\mu_1$ opioid receptor because the ability of other opioids to suppress the medullary cough centers is not correlated with their analgesic effect.

### Nontherapeutic and Adverse Effects of Opioids

***Abuse and Addiction.*** Addiction is defined as a maladaptive pattern of substance use leading to clinically significant impairment or distress. Opioid use disorder (OUD, which replaced the term opioid dependence in the *Diagnostic and Statistical Manual of Mental Disorders,* 5th edition) is defined as a problematic pattern of opioid use leading to clinically significant impairment or distress (Table 9–3).

There is an association between opioids prescribed for acute pain and the development of long-term opioid use. The pleasurable effects of many xenobiotics used by humans are mediated by the release of dopamine in the mesolimbic system. This final common pathway is shared by all opioids that activate the μ–δ receptor complex in the ventral tegmental area, which, in turn, indirectly promotes dopamine release in the mesolimbic region. Opioids also have a direct reinforcing effect on their self-administration through μ receptors within the mesolimbic system.

Exogenous opioids do not induce uniform psychological effects. Some of the exogenous opioids, particularly those that are highly lipophilic such as heroin, are euphorigenic, but morphine is largely devoid of such pleasurable effects. Chronic users note that fentanyl produces effects that are subjectively similar to those of heroin. Certain opioids, such as pentazocine, produce dysphoria, an effect that is related to their affinity for κ or Sigma (σ) receptors.

***Hyperalgesia.*** Chronic use of opioid analgesics is associated with hyperalgesia, or a heightened sensitivity to pain. This effect was described decades ago in methadone-maintained patients and is again recognized because of the increased use of chronic opioid therapy for pain. Clinically, hyperalgesia manifests as the need for increasing doses of analgesics to mitigate pain, and it occurs as part of or is confused with the development of tolerance. Conceptually, as opposed to tolerance, which is the progressive failure of a drug to adequately treat the pain, hyperalgesia is the intrinsic increase in the degree of pain in response to an analgesic. The exact mechanisms for the development of opioid-induced hyperalgesia are still not clearly understood. The treatment for hyperalgesia should include weaning from opioids and providing alternative modalities of pain relief.

***Miosis.*** Stimulation of parasympathetic pupilloconstrictor neurons in the Edinger-Westphal nucleus of the oculomotor nerve by morphine produces miosis. Additionally, morphine increases firing of pupilloconstrictor neurons to light, which

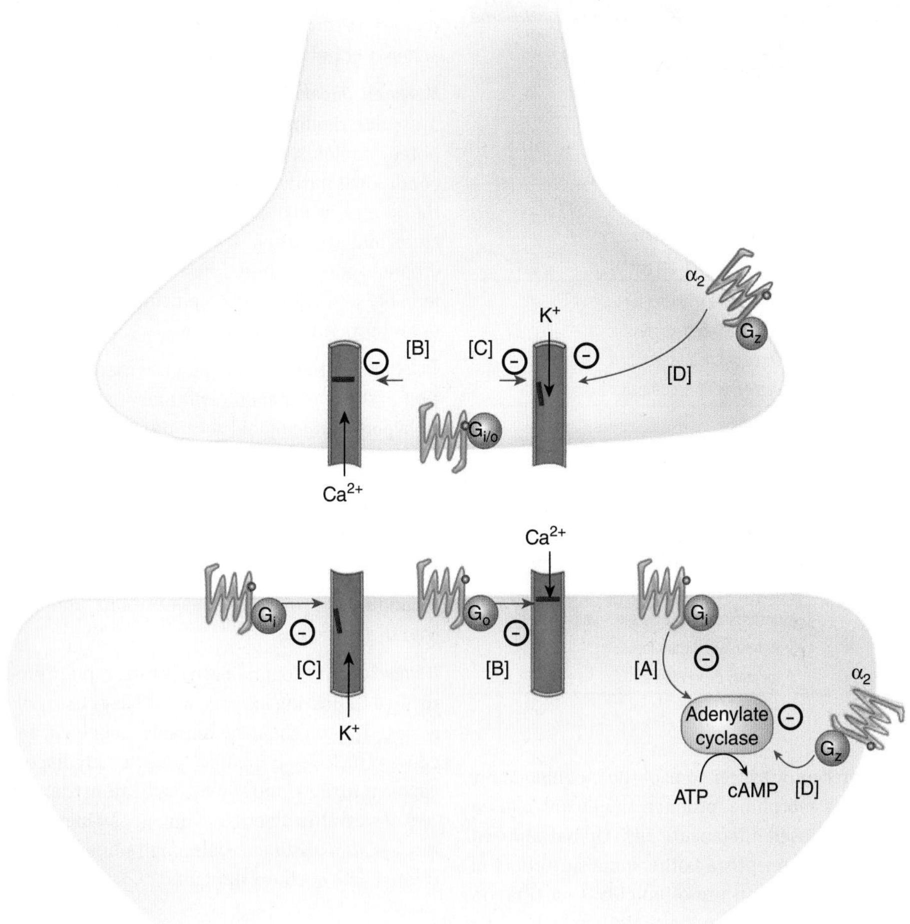


**FIGURE 9–1.** Opioid-receptor signal transduction mechanisms. Upon binding of an opioid agonist to an opioid receptor, the respective G protein is activated. G proteins (**A**) reduce the capacity of adenylate cyclase to produce cyclic adenosine monophosphate (cAMP); (**B**) close calcium channels that reduce the signal to release neurotransmitters; or (**C**) open potassium channels and hyperpolarize the cell, which indirectly reduces cell activity. Each mechanism is found coupled to each receptor subtype, depending on the location of the receptor (pre- or postsynaptic), and the neuron within the brain (see text). Note that $\alpha_2$ receptors (**D**) mediate similar effects using a different G protein ($G_z$).

**Adenylate cyclase/cAMP (A).** Inhibition of adenylate cyclase activity by $G_i$ or $G_o$ is the classic mechanism for postsynaptic signal transduction invoked by the inhibitory μ receptors. However, this same mechanism is identified in cells bearing either δ or κ receptors. Activation of cAMP production by adenylate cyclase, with subsequent activation of protein kinase A, occurs after exposure to very-low-dose opioid agonists and produces excitatory, antianalgesic effects.

**Calcium ($Ca^{2+}$) channels (B).** Presynaptic μ receptors inhibit norepinephrine release from the nerve terminals of cells of the rat cerebral cortex. Adenylate cyclase is not the modulator for these receptors because inhibition of norepinephrine release is not enhanced by increasing intracellular cAMP levels by various methods. Opioid-induced blockade is, however, prevented by increased intracellular calcium concentrations that are induced either by calcium ionophores, which increase membrane permeability to calcium, or by increasing the extracellular calcium concentration. This implies a role for opioid-induced closure of N-type calcium channels, presumably via a $G_o$ protein. Reduced intraterminal concentrations of calcium prevent the neurotransmitter-laden vesicles from binding to the terminal membrane and releasing their contents. Nerve terminals containing dopamine have an analogous relationship with inhibitory κ receptors, as do acetylcholine-bearing neurons with opioid receptors.

**Potassium($K^+$) channels (C).** Increased conductance through a potassium channel, generally mediated by $G_i$, or $G_o$, results in membrane hyperpolarization with reduced neuronal excitability. Alternatively, protein kinase A–mediated reduction in membrane potassium conductance enhances neuronal excitability.

increases the sensitivity of the light reflex through central reinforcement. Because opioids classically mediate inhibitory neurotransmission, hyperpolarization of sympathetic nerves or of inhibitory neurons to the parasympathetic neurons (removal of inhibition) ultimately mediates the classic "pinpoint pupil" associated with opioid use. Not all patients using opioids present with miosis. Meperidine has a lesser miotic effect than other conventional opioids, and propoxyphene use does not result in miosis.

***Gastrointestinal.*** Emesis induced by apomorphine is mediated through agonism at dopamine ($D_2$) receptor subtypes

**TABLE 9–2 Clinical Effects of Opioids**

| | |
|---|---|
| Cardiovascular | Bradycardia<br>Orthostatic hypotension<br>Peripheral vasodilation |
| Dermatologic | Flushing (histamine)<br>Pruritus |
| Endocrinologic | Reduced antidiuretic hormone release<br>Increased prolactin release<br>Reduced gonadotropin release |
| Gastrointestinal | Increased anal sphincter tone<br>Increased biliary tract pressure<br>Reduced gastric acid secretion<br>Reduced motility (constipation) |
| Neurologic | Analgesia<br>Antitussive<br>Euphoria<br>Sedation, coma<br>Seizures (meperidine, propoxyphene) |
| Ophthalmic | Miosis |
| Pulmonary | Acute respiratory distress syndrome<br>Bronchospasm (histamine)<br>Respiratory depression |

within the chemoreceptor trigger zone of the medulla. Many opioids, particularly morphine, produce significant nausea and vomiting when used therapeutically. Opioid-induced constipation (OIC) is frequently a bothersome side effect of both medical and nonmedical use of opioids. Constipation is mediated by $\mu_2$ receptors within the smooth muscle of the intestinal wall. "Peripherally restricted" opioid antagonists that do not cross the blood–brain barrier are useful for OIC and do not induce withdrawal in tolerant patients.

**TABLE 9–3 DSM-5 Criteria for Diagnosis of an Opioid Use Disorder**

Diagnosis requires at least 2 of 11 criteria to be present. Severity is graded by the number of criteria present: mild (2–3 criteria), moderate (4–5 criteria), and severe (6 or more criteria). Criteria can be clustered into the following four groups:

I. ***Impaired control:***
- (1) Taking more or for longer than intended
- (2) Unsuccessful efforts to stop or cut down use
- (3) Spending a great deal of time obtaining, using, or recovering from use
- (4) Craving for substance

II. ***Social impairment:***
- (5) Failure to fulfill major obligations due to use
- (6) Continued use despite problems caused or exacerbated by use
- (7) Important activities given up or reduced because of substance use

III. ***Risky use:***
- (8) Recurrent use in hazardous situations
- (9) Continued use despite physical or psychological problems that are caused or exacerbated by substance use

IV. ***Pharmacologic dependence:***
- (10) Tolerance to effects of the substance
- (11) Withdrawal symptoms when not using or using less.

Reproduced with permission from Azari S, Zevin B, Potter MB. Chronic Pain Management in Vulnerable Populations. In: King TE, Wheeler MB. eds. *Medical Management of Vulnerable and Underserved Patients: Principles, Practice, and Populations,* 2e. McGraw Hill; 2016.

***Movement Disorders.*** Patients infrequently experience acute muscular rigidity with rapid IV injection of certain high-potency opioids, especially fentanyl and its derivatives. This condition is particularly prominent during induction of anesthesia and in neonates. The rigidity primarily involves the trunk and impairs chest wall movement sufficiently to exacerbate hypoventilation. Chest wall rigidity contributes to the lethality associated with epidemics of fentanyl-adulterated or fentanyl-substituted heroin.

***Endocrine.*** Chronic use of opioids is associated with hypofunction of the hypothalamic–pituitary–gonadal axis by binding to hypothalamic opioid receptors and decreasing the secretion of gonadotropin-releasing hormone. Clinical findings include reduced libido, erectile dysfunction, hot flashes, and depression, as well as anemia, hair loss, and osteopenia. Disruption of the hypothalamic–pituitary axis reduces adrenal function, and clinically relevant adrenal insufficiency occurs. In addition, prolactin concentrations commonly rise and lead to gynecomastia.

***Hearing Loss.*** Although relatively rare, rapidly progressive sensorineural hearing loss occurs in heavy users of opioid analgesics. The mechanism remains unknown, and suggested causes include ischemia, genetic predisposition, direct cochlear toxicity, and hypersensitization that manifests upon reexposure after a period of opioid abstinence. Most patients recover after abstinence, although some are only successfully treated with cochlear implants.

### Toxic and Life-Threatening Effects of Opioids

Most adverse or toxic effects are predictable based on opioid pharmacodynamics (eg, respiratory depression), although several opioids produce unexpected "nonopioid" responses. Determining that a patient has opioid toxicity is generally more important than identifying the specific opioid involved. Notwithstanding some minor variations, patients poisoned by all available opioids predictably develop a constellation of signs, known as the *opioid toxic syndrome* (Chap. 1). Mental status depression, hypoventilation, miosis, and hypoperistalsis are the classic elements.

***Respiratory Depression.*** Experimental use of various opioid agonists and antagonists consistently implicates $\mu_2$ receptors in the respiratory depressant effects of morphine. Through these receptors, opioid agonists reduce ventilation by diminishing the sensitivity of the medullary chemoreceptors to hypercarbia. In addition to loss of hypercarbic stimulation, opioids depress the ventilatory response to hypoxia. The combined loss of hypercarbic and hypoxic drive leaves virtually no stimulus to breathe, and apnea ensues.

It is important to recognize that respiratory depression results from a reduction in either respiratory rate or tidal volume. Thus, although respiratory rate is more accessible for clinical measurement, it is not an ideal index of respiratory depression. In fact, morphine-induced respiratory depression in humans initially is related more closely to changes in tidal volume.

***Pulmonary and Acute Respiratory Distress Syndrome.*** Reports linking opioids with the development of acute pulmonary abnormalities became common in the 1960s, although the first report was made by William Osler in 1880. Almost all opioids are implicated, and opioid-related acute respiratory distress syndrome (ARDS) is reported in diverse clinical situations. Typically, the patient regains normal ventilation after a period of profound respiratory depression, either spontaneously or after the administration of an opioid antagonist, and over the subsequent several minutes to hours develops hypoxemia, crackles on auscultation, and classic frothy, pink sputum.

No single mechanism can be consistently invoked in the genesis of opioid-associated ARDS. Based on animal experiments and clinical experience, the most likely mechanism in association with antagonist-induced reversal involves release of inhibition to the catecholamine surge that results from hypercarbia and hypoxia. In animals, ventilation prior to reversal significantly reduces the risk of ARDS. Since ARDS was reported prior to antagonist reversal, other mechanisms are likely also important.

***Cardiovascular.*** Arteriolar and venous dilation secondary to opioid use results in a mild reduction in blood pressure. Bradycardia is unusual with most opioids, although a reduction in heart rate is common as a result of the associated reduction in CNS stimulation. Opioid-induced hypotension is mediated by histamine release, which does not appear to occur through interaction with an opioid receptor. Not all opioids are equivalent in their ability to release histamine. Experimentally meperidine produces the most hypotension and elevation of serum histamine concentrations; fentanyl produces the least.

Certain opioids at therapeutic concentrations, particularly methadone, interfere with normal cardiac repolarization and produce QT interval prolongation, an effect that predisposes to the development of torsade de pointes. Methadone prolongs the QT interval via interactions with cardiac potassium ($I_{Kr}$) channels.

***Seizures.*** Seizures are a rare complication of therapeutic use of most opioids. In patients with acute opioid overdose, seizures most likely are caused by hypoxia. Seizures should be anticipated in patients with meperidine, pentazocine, tapentadol, or tramadol toxicity.

## SPECIFIC OPIOIDS

The vast majority of opioid-poisoned patients follow predictable clinical courses that can be anticipated based on an understanding of opioid receptor pharmacology. However, certain opioids taken in overdose produce atypical manifestations. Therefore, careful clinical assessment and institution of empiric therapy usually are necessary to ensure proper management (Table 9–4).

### Morphine and Codeine

Morphine is poorly bioavailable by the oral route because of extensive first-pass elimination. Morphine is hepatically metabolized primarily to morphine-3-glucuronide (M3G) and, to a lesser extent, to morphine-6-glucuronide (M6G), both of which are cleared renally. Unlike M3G, which is essentially devoid of activity, M6G has μ-agonist effects in the CNS. The relative potency of morphine and M6G in the brain is incompletely defined, but the metabolite is generally considered to be several-fold more potent. This explains why caution is required when administering morphine to patients with kidney failure. Codeine itself is an inactive opioid agonist, and it requires metabolic activation by *O*-demethylation to morphine by CYP2D6 (Fig. 9–2). Approximately 5% to 7% of white patients, who are devoid of CYP2D6 function, cannot derive an analgesic response from codeine. An increasingly recognized phenomenon is that ultrarapid CYP2D6 metabolizers produce unexpectedly large amounts of morphine from codeine, with resulting life-threatening opioid toxicity.

### Heroin

Heroin has a lower affinity for the μ opioid receptor than does morphine, but it is rapidly metabolized to 6-monoacetylmorphine, a more potent μ agonist than morphine (Fig. 9–2). The enhanced euphorigenic effect is likely related to the enhanced blood–brain barrier penetration.

Heroin is available in two distinct chemical forms: base or salt. The high water solubility of hydrochloride salt allows simple IV administration. Heroin base is virtually insoluble in water, and IV administration requires either heating the heroin until it liquefies or mixing it with acid. Alternatively, because the alkaloidal form is heat stable, smoking or "chasing the dragon" is sometimes used as an alternative route. Recognition of the efficacy of intranasal heroin administration, or snorting, has fostered a resurgence of heroin use, particularly in suburban communities.

***Adulterants, Contaminants, and "Heroin" Substitutes.*** Retail (street-level) heroin almost always contains adulterants or contaminants, which are differentiated by the intent of their admixture. Adulterants typically are benign because inflicting harm on the consumer with their addition would be economically and socially unwise, although adulterants occasionally are responsible for epidemic death. Historically, alkaloids, such as quinine and strychnine, were used to adulterate heroin to mimic the bitter taste of heroin and to mislead clients. Quinine adulteration currently is much less common than it was in the past. Trend analysis of illicit wholesale and street-level heroin adulteration over a 12-year period in Denmark revealed that although caffeine, acetaminophen, methaqualone, and phenobarbital all were prevalent adulterants, quinine was not found. Analysis of US heroin samples revealed the presence of procaine, quinine, caffeine, acetaminophen, mannitol, lactose, and diphenhydramine in significant quantities.

Poisoning by scopolamine-tainted heroin reached epidemic levels in the northeastern US in 1995. Exposed patients

**TABLE 9–4 Classification, Potency, and Characteristics of Opioids and Opioid Antagonists**

| *Opioid* | *Type*[a] | *Derivation* | *Analgesic Dose (mg) (via route, equivalent to 10 mg of morphine SC*[b]*)* | *Comments*[a,c] |
|---|---|---|---|---|
| Buprenorphine | PA | Semisynthetic | 0.3 IM | Medication assisted therapy requires 6–16 mg/day (contains naloxone) |
| Butorphanol | AA | Semisynthetic | 2 IM | |
| Codeine | Ag | Natural | 60 PO | Often combined with acetaminophen; requires demethylation to morphine by CYP2D6 |
| Dextromethorphan | NEC | Semisynthetic | Nonanalgesic (10–30 PO) | Antitussive; psychotomimetic via NMDA receptor |
| Diphenoxylate | Ag | Synthetic | Nonanalgesic (2.5 PO) | Antidiarrheal, combined with atropine; difenoxin is potent metabolite |
| Fentanyl | Ag | Synthetic | 0. 075 IM | Very short acting (<1 h) |
| Fentanyl analogs | Ag | Synthetic | Variable, but high potency | Examples include furanyl fentanyl and carfentanil |
| Heroin | Ag | Semisynthetic | 5 SC | Used therapeutically in some countries; Schedule I medication in the US |
| Hydrocodone | Ag | Semisynthetic | 1 IM, 2 PO | |
| Hydromorphone | Ag | Semisynthetic | 1.3 SC | |
| Levorphanol | Ag | Semisynthetic | 2 SC or IM | |
| Loperamide | Ag | Synthetic | Nonanalgesic (2 PO) | Antidiarrheal; abuse; P-glycoprotein substrate, potassium channel blockade |
| Meperidine | Ag | Synthetic | 75 SC or IM | Seizures caused by metabolite accumulation |
| Methadone | Ag | Synthetic | 10 IM | Very long acting (24 h) |
| Methylnaltrexone | Ant | Synthetic | Nonanalgesic (8–12 SC); 15 PO | Peripherally acting antagonist; reverses opioid-induced constipation |
| Morphine | Ag | Natural | 10 SC or IM | |
| Naloxegol | Ant | Synthetic | Nonanalgesic (25 PO) | Peripherally acting antagonist; reverses opioid constipation; P-glycoprotein substrate |
| Nalbuphine | AA | Semisynthetic | 10 IM | |
| Naloxone | Ant | Semisynthetic | Nonanalgesic (0.04 IV or IM) | Short-acting antagonist (0.5 h) |
| Naltrexone | Ant | Semisynthetic | Nonanalgesic (50 PO) | Very long-acting antagonist (24 h) |
| Oxycodone | Ag | Semisynthetic | 5 PO | Often combined with acetaminophen; OxyContin is extended release |
| Oxymorphone | Ag | Semisynthetic | 1 SC | |
| Paregoric | Ag | Natural | 25 mL PO | Tincture of opium (0.4 mg/mL) |
| Pentazocine | AA | Semisynthetic | 50 SC | Psychotomimetic via $\kappa$ receptor |
| Tapentadol | Ag | Synthetic | 50 PO | Seizures |
| Tramadol | Ag | Synthetic | 50–100 PO | Seizures possible with therapeutic dosing |

[a]Agonist–antagonists, partial agonists, and antagonists may cause withdrawal in tolerant individuals. [b]Typical dose (mg) for xenobiotics without analgesic effects is given in parentheses. [c]Duration of therapeutic clinical effect 3–6 h unless noted; likely to be exaggerated in overdose.

AA = agonist antagonist ($\kappa$ agonist, $\mu$ antagonist); Ag = full agonist ($\mu_1$, $\mu_2$, $\kappa$); Ant = full antagonist ($\mu_1$, $\mu_2$, $\kappa$ antagonist); IM = intramuscular; IV = intravenous; NEC = not easily classified; NMDA = *N*-methyl-D-aspartate; PA = partial agonist ($\mu_1$, $\mu_2$ agonist, $\kappa$ antagonist); PO = oral; SC = subcutaneous.

presented with acute psychosis and anticholinergic signs. Several patients were treated with physostigmine, with excellent therapeutic results. Clenbuterol, a $\beta_2$-adrenergic agonist with a rapid onset and long duration of action, was found to be a contaminant in street heroin in the Eastern US in early 2005 (Chap. 36).

***"Chasing the Dragon".*** "Chasing the dragon" defines the practice whereby users inhale the white pyrolysate that is generated by heating heroin base on aluminum foil using a handheld flame. This produces heroin pharmacokinetics similar to those observed after IV administration. In the early 1980s, a group of individuals who smoked heroin in the Netherlands developed spongiform leukoencephalopathy. Since the initial report, similar cases were recognized in other parts of Europe and in the US. Initial findings typically occur within 2 weeks of use and include bradykinesia, ataxia, abulia, and speech abnormalities. Of those whose symptoms did not progress, about half recovered. Progression to spastic paraparesis, pseudobulbar palsy, or hypotonia occurred over several weeks, and death was common.

The syndrome has the characteristics of a point-source toxic exposure, but no culpable contaminants were identified. A component or pyrolysis product unique to certain batches of "heroin" is possible. Treatment is largely supportive. Based on the finding of regional mitochondrial dysfunction on functional brain imaging and an elevated brain lactate concentration, supplementation with coenzyme Q 300 mg four times a day has purported benefit and is a reasonable treatment, but this treatment has not undergone controlled study.

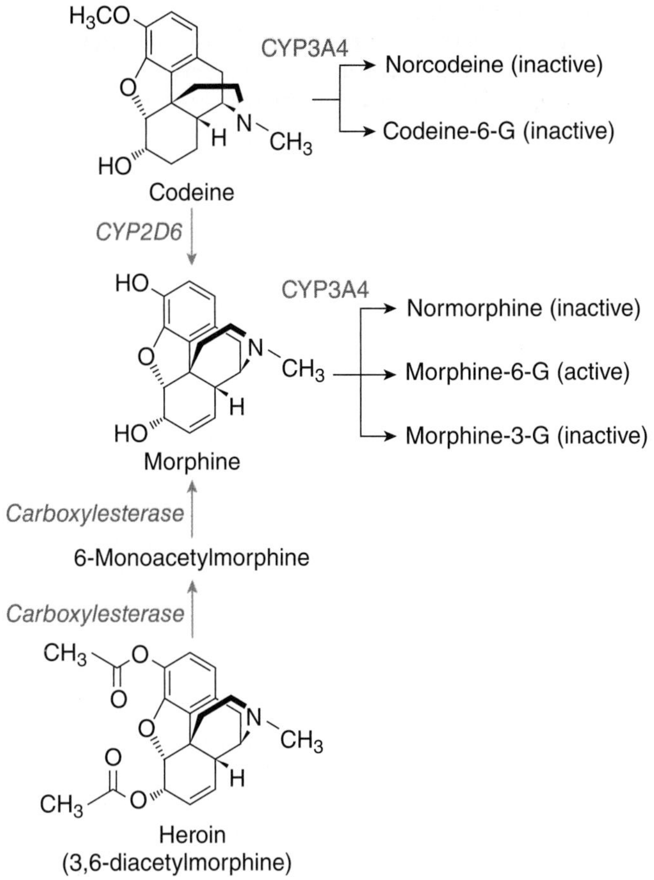

**FIGURE 9–2.** Opiate and opioid metabolism. Codeine is *O*-methylated to morphine, *N*-demethylated to norcodeine, or glucuronidated to codeine-6-glucuronide (codeine-6-G). Morphine is *N*-demethylated to normorphine or glucuronidated to either morphine-3-glucuronide (morphine-3-G) or morphine-6-glucuronide (morphine-6-G). Heroin is converted to morphine by a two-step process involving plasma cholinesterase and two human liver carboxylesterases known as human carboxylesterase-1 and human carboxylesterase-2.

### Oxycodone, Hydrocodone, Hydromorphone, and Oxymorphone

For acute pain, the opioids sold in fixed combination with acetaminophen (eg, Percocet {oxycodone}, Vicodin {hydrocodone}), raising concerns about the complications of acetaminophen hepatotoxicity as the dose of opioid is escalated. Most of these combinations are also available in extended-release formulations.

### Fentanyl and Its Analogs

Fentanyl is a short-acting opioid agonist that has approximately 50 to 100 times the potency of morphine. It is well absorbed by the transmucosal route, accounting for its use in the form of a "lozenge" or spray. Fentanyl is widely abused as a heroin substitute (intentionally or unintentionally because of adulteration). Experienced heroin users cannot easily differentiate fentanyl from heroin. Thousands of deaths are attributed to the illicit use of pharmaceutical fentanyl across North America. In 2015, there was a further sharp increase in opioid fatalities attributable to novel fentanyl analogs, such as acetyl fentanyl, butyryl fentanyl, furanyl fentanyl, and carfentanil. Other novel "research" opioids, including compounds such as MT-45, AH-7921, U-47700, and U-50488, which are not fentanyl derivatives, are also associated with significant public health and medical consequences. The clinical responsiveness of the fentanyl analogs to reversal by naloxone is very difficult to predict. Given the unpredictability of dosing and the extreme potency of the illicit opioids, administration of a large dose, either in absolute or relative terms, should reasonably be expected to require higher than normal doses of naloxone for reversal (Antidotes in Brief: A4).

A transdermal fentanyl patch is widely used by patients with chronic pain syndromes (Special Considerations: SC2). Fentanyl patch misuse and abuse occur either by application of one or more patches to the skin or by withdrawal or extraction of the fentanyl from the reservoir for subsequent administration.

### Xenobiotics Used in Medication-Assisted Therapy (MAT): Methadone and Buprenorphine

Two contrasting approaches to the management of patients with chronic opioid use exist: (1) detoxification and abstinence and (2) maintenance therapy.

***Methadone.*** Methadone is a synthetic μ-opioid–receptor agonist used both for treatment of chronic pain and as MAT for opioid dependence. Although therapeutic use of methadone, whether for pain or MAT, is generally safe, rapid dose escalation during induction of therapy rarely results in toxicity and fatal respiratory depression. This adverse effect is generally the result of the combination of variable pharmacokinetics (unpredictable but generally long half-life) and the time lag for the development of tolerance.

Methadone is administered as a chiral mixture of (*R*,*S*)-methadone. In humans, methadone metabolism is mediated by several cytochrome P450 (CYP) isoenzymes, mainly CYP3A4 and CYP2B6 and to a lesser extent CYP2D6. CYP2B6 demonstrates stereoselectivity toward *(S)*-methadone. In vivo data show that CYP2B6 slow metabolizer status is associated with high *(S)*-, but not serum *(R)*-methadone concentrations.

Methadone predictably produces QT interval prolongation because of blockade of the hERG (human *ether-a-gogo* related gene) channel. Syncope and sudden death caused by ventricular dysrhythmias (eg, torsade de pointes) are the result. Genetic factors in the metabolism of methadone and baseline QT status at the initiation of methadone therapy underlie and potentially predict adverse effects. In clinical trials, QT interval prolongation was greater in individuals who were CYP2B6 slow metabolizers, and this population had higher *(S)*-methadone concentrations.

A major difficulty is identification of individuals who are at risk for life-threatening dysrhythmias from methadone-induced QT interval prolongation. Expert-derived guidelines recommend questioning patients about intrinsic heart disease or dysrhythmias, counseling patients initiating methadone therapy, and obtaining a pretreatment electrocardiogram (ECG) and a follow-up ECG at 30 days and yearly. Patients who receive methadone doses of greater than 100 mg/day necessitate more frequent ECGs, particularly after dose escalation or change in comorbid disease status.

***Buprenorphine.*** Because prescription of methadone for MAT is restricted to federally licensed methadone maintenance treatment programs (MMTPs), it is inaccessible and inconvenient for many patients. Buprenorphine was approved in 2000 for MAT for office-based prescribing in patients with opioid addiction. It is administered daily at home, providing a more attractive alternative for patients than daily MMTP visits, and it substantially broadened the potential for obtaining outpatient MAT. However, because of the initial limitations on patient volume (which was subsequently expanded), the requirement for physician certification, and possibly the hesitation on the part of community physicians to welcome patients with substance use disorders into their practices, many of the benefits of office-based buprenorphine therapy over methadone are not yet realized.

Buprenorphine, a partial μ-opioid agonist, in doses of 8 to 16 mg sublingually, is effective at suppressing both opioid withdrawal symptoms and the use of illicit drugs. Buprenorphine overdose is associated with markedly less respiratory depression than full agonists such as methadone. Because there is no reported effect on the QT interval, patients on methadone with concerning QT interval prolongation are offered the opportunity to switch to buprenorphine.

Buprenorphine is available as sublingual (SL) tablets or sublingual or buccal films containing both buprenorphine and naloxone (Suboxone), which is added to prevent IV use. At therapeutic doses, buprenorphine produces nearly complete occupancy of the μ-opioid receptors, and its receptor affinity is sufficiently strong that it prevents other opioids from binding.

As a partial agonist, buprenorphine has a ceiling effect on respiratory depression in healthy volunteers, with a similar plateau in analgesic effect. However, respiratory depression and deaths are associated with concomitant use of other drugs, most often benzodiazepines, or to the IV injection of crushed buprenorphine tablets. Children are at particularly high risk. Although naloxone prevents the clinical effects of buprenorphine, the reversal of respiratory effects by naloxone appears to be related in a nonlinear fashion. Therefore, it is recommended that the reversal of respiratory depression be treated with a starting dose that is slightly higher than that used to reverse other opioids and increased slowly and titrated to reversal of respiratory depression. For example, a starting dose of naloxone of 0.02 mg/kg, or 1 mg in an adult, is a reasonable initial dose (Antidotes in Brief: A4).

### Other Unique Opioids

***Tramadol and Tapentadol.*** Tramadol and tapentadol are synthetic analgesics with both opioid and nonopioid mechanisms responsible for their clinical effects. Tramadol is a reuptake inhibitor of norepinephrine and serotonin, and it has an active metabolite, *O*-desmethyltramadol catalyzed by CYP2D6, which is a μ opioid receptor agonist. Tapentadol, which does not require activation, has relatively strong μ-opioid receptor agonism and inhibits the reuptake of norepinephrine but not serotonin. Both are available in immediate- and extended-release formulations.

A large number of spontaneous reports to the FDA describe therapeutic use of tramadol resulting in seizures, particularly on the first day of therapy. Tramadol-related seizures are not responsive to naloxone but are suppressed with benzodiazepines. Patients develop typical opioid manifestations after a large overdose. Significant respiratory depression is uncommon and should respond to naloxone. Hypoglycemia is associated with therapeutic use of tramadol, and it is reasonable to admit all patients with tramadol-induced hypoglycemia because of the uncertainty of continuing risk. Patients using monoamine oxidase inhibitors (MAOIs) are at risk for development of serotonin toxicity after use of tramadol.

***Diphenoxylate.*** Although diphenoxylate is structurally similar to meperidine, its extreme insolubility limits absorption from the GI tract. This factor enhances its use as an antidiarrheal, which presumably occurs via a local opioid effect at the GI μ receptor. However, in children, there is significant systemic absorption of the standard adult formulation with resulting toxicity, and all such exposures should be deemed consequential. Diphenoxylate is formulated with a small dose (0.025 mg) of atropine (as Lomotil), both to enhance its antidiarrheal effect and to discourage illicit use.

Because both components of Lomotil are absorbed and their pharmacokinetic profiles differ somewhat, a biphasic clinical syndrome is occasionally noted. Patients typically manifest atropine poisoning (anticholinergic syndrome), either independently or concomitantly with the opioid effects of diphenoxylate. Delayed, prolonged, or recurrent toxicity is common and is classically related to the delayed gastric emptying effects inherent to both opioids and anticholinergics. However, these effects are more likely explained by the accumulation of the hepatic metabolite difenoxin, which is a significantly more potent opioid than diphenoxylate and possesses a longer serum half-life. The relevance of gastroparesis is highlighted by the retrieval of Lomotil pills by gastric lavage as late as 27 hours postingestion.

A review of 36 pediatric reports of diphenoxylate overdoses found that although naloxone was effective in reversing the opioid toxicity, recurrence of CNS and respiratory depression was common. This series included a patient with an asymptomatic presentation 8 hours postingestion who was observed for several hours and then discharged. This patient returned to the ED 18 hours postingestion with marked signs of atropinism. In this same series, children with delayed onset of respiratory depression and other opioid effects were reported, and others describe cardiopulmonary arrest 12 hours postingestion. Because of the delayed and possibly severe consequences, all individuals with potentially significant ingestions should be admitted for monitored observation in the hospital.

***Loperamide.*** Loperamide is another insoluble meperidine analog that is used to treat diarrhea and is available as a nonprescription medication. At therapeutic doses, it inhibits peristaltic activity through agonism of μ-opioid receptors, calcium channel blockade, calmodulin inhibition, and decreasing paracellular permeability in the large intestine. At therapeutic dosing (< 16 mg/day), loperamide is essentially devoid of central opioid effects because transporter protein P-glycoprotein actively facilitates removal of the drug from the gut and the CNS. However, larger than recommended doses overcome these mechanisms, enabling CNS penetration and affording relief of opioid withdrawal symptoms or even opioidlike euphoria. Loperamide was initially placed in Schedule II, down-scheduled to Schedule V in 1977, and descheduled in 1982. Because it is not tracked as a controlled substance, the true extent of use, diversion, and abuse are largely unavailable.

Deaths are reported at the high doses required for CNS effects (70–400 mg) and are associated with respiratory depression and cardiotoxicity. Loperamide inhibits human cardiac sodium and potassium channels and produces prolongation of both the QRS complex and the QT interval. Naloxone should be administered to reverse consequential respiratory depression associated with loperamide overdose. In patients who present with wide complex dysrhythmias and polymorphic ventricular tachycardia, it is reasonable to use sodium bicarbonate and magnesium sulfate as potentially preventive measures, but primary treatment is electrical cardioversion.

***Dextromethorphan.*** Dextromethorphan is devoid of analgesic properties altogether, even though it is the optical isomer of levorphanol, a potent opioid analgesic. At high doses, dextromethorphan produces miosis, respiratory depression, and CNS depression, which are at least partially reversed by naloxone. Binding to the phencyclidine (PCP) site on the NMDA receptor causes sedation. Blockade of presynaptic serotonin reuptake by dextromethorphan causes serotonin toxicity in patients receiving MAOIs or other serotonergics. Movement disorders, described as choreoathetoid or dystonialike, occasionally occur and presumably result from alteration of dopaminergic neurotransmission.

Dextromethorphan is available without prescription in cold preparations, primarily because of its presumed lack of significant addictive potential. Common street names include "DXM," "dex," and "roboshots." Users often have expectations of euphoria and hallucinations, but a dysphoria comparable to that of phencyclidine (PCP) commonly ensues.

***Meperidine.*** Meperidine was previously widely used for treatment of chronic and acute pain syndromes. Its use was dramatically reduced and is either closely monitored in many institutions or eliminated because of its adverse risk–benefit profile. Meperidine produces clinical manifestations typical of the other opioids and may lead to greater euphoria caused by its blockade of presynaptic serotonin reuptake. This most consequential nonopioid-receptor effect causes serotonin toxicity, characterized by muscle rigidity, hyperthermia, and altered mental status, particularly in patients using MAOIs (Chap. 44). Normeperidine, a toxic, renally eliminated hepatic metabolite, causes excitatory neurotoxicity, which manifests as delirium, tremor, myoclonus, or seizures.

## DIAGNOSTIC TESTING

### Laboratory Considerations

Opioid-poisoned patients are particularly appropriate for a rapid clinical diagnosis because of the unique characteristics of the opioid toxic syndrome. Several well-described problems with laboratory testing of opioids are described later.

***Cross-Reactivity.*** Many opioids share significant structural similarities, such as morphine and oxycodone or methadone and propoxyphene. Because most clinical assays depend on structural features for identification, structurally similar xenobiotics are frequently detected in lieu of the desired one. Some cross-reactivities are predictable, such as that of hydrocodone with morphine.

***Congeners and Adulterants.*** Commercial opiate assays, which are usually specific for morphine (a metabolite of heroin), do not readily detect most of the semisynthetic and synthetic opioids. Oxycodone, hydrocodone, and other common morphine derivatives have variable detectability by different opioid screens and generally only when in high concentrations.

***Drug Metabolism.*** A fascinating dilemma often arises in patients who ingest moderate to large amounts of poppy seeds. These seeds, which are widely used for culinary purposes, are derived from poppy plants and contain both morphine and codeine. After ingestion of a single poppy seed bagel, patients infrequently develop elevated serum morphine and codeine concentrations and test positive for morphine. Because the presence of morphine on a drug abuse screen supports illicit heroin use, the implications are substantial. Federal workplace testing regulations thus require corroboration of a positive morphine assay with assessment of another heroin metabolite, 6-monoacetylmorphine, before reporting a positive result. Humans readily deacetylate heroin, which is diacetylmorphine but cannot acetylate morphine and therefore cannot synthesize 6-monoacetylmorphine. Thus the presence of 6-monoacetylmorphine confirms illicit heroin use.

*Forensic Testing.* Decision making regarding the cause of death in the presence of systemic opioids often is complex. Specifics regarding the timing of exposure, the preexisting degree of sensitivity or tolerance, the role of cointoxicants, and postmortem redistribution and metabolism all complicate the assessment.

## MANAGEMENT

The consequential effects of acute opioid poisoning are CNS and respiratory depression. Although early support of ventilation and oxygenation is generally sufficient to prevent death, prolonged use of bag-valve-mask ventilation and endotracheal intubation can often be avoided by cautious administration of an opioid antagonist. Opioid antagonists, such as naloxone, competitively inhibit binding of opioid agonists to opioid receptors, allowing the patient to resume spontaneous respiration. Naloxone is effective at reversing almost all adverse effects mediated through opioid receptors (Antidotes in Brief: A4).

### Antidote Administration

The goal of naloxone therapy is not necessarily complete restoration of normal consciousness; rather, the goal is reinstitution of adequate spontaneous ventilation. Because precipitation of withdrawal is potentially detrimental and often unpredictable, for hospitalized patients we recommend administering the lowest practical naloxone dose initially, with rapid escalation as warranted by the clinical situation. Most patients respond to 0.04 mg of naloxone administered IV, although the requirement for ventilatory assistance is often slightly prolonged because the onset will be slower than with larger doses. We recommend repeating this dose several times at 3-minute intervals, as needed for persistent findings, with escalation up to 0.4-mg and 2-mg doses. Subcutaneous administration allows for smoother arousal than the high-dose IV route, but is unpredictable in onset and prolonged in offset. Patients with recurrent or profound poisoning by long-acting opioids, such as methadone, or patients with large GI burdens (eg, "body packers" or those taking extended-release preparations) often require continuous infusion of naloxone to ensure continued adequate ventilation (Table 9–5). Other routes of administration and other antagonists are discussed in detail in the Antidotes in Brief: A4.

**TABLE 9–5 Recommended Use of Naloxone**

1. Start with 0.04 mg IV. If successful, monitor the patient for recurrence and the need for repeat administration.
2. If respiratory depression is not reversed after the initial bolus dose:
   Increase dose slowly and titrate to reversal of respiratory depression. Administer up to 10 mg of naloxone as an IV bolus.
   If the patient does not respond, do not initiate an infusion.
   AND prepare for
   Intubation of the patient, as clinically indicated.
3. If the patient develops withdrawal after the bolus dose:
   Allow the effects of the bolus to abate.
   If respiratory depression recurs, administer half of the initial bolus dose and begin an IV infusion at two-thirds of the new bolus dose per hour. Frequently reassess the patient's respiratory status.
4. If the patient develops withdrawal signs or symptoms during the infusion:
   Stop the infusion until the withdrawal symptoms abate.
   Restart the infusion at half the initial rate; frequently reassess the patient's respiratory status.
   Exclude withdrawal from other xenobiotics.
5. If the patient develops respiratory depression during the infusion:
   Readminister half of the initial bolus and repeat until reversal occurs.
   Increase the infusion by half of the initial rate; frequently reassess the patient's respiratory status.
   Exclude continued absorption, readministration of opioid, and other etiologies as the cause of the respiratory depression.

IV = intravenous.

The decision to discharge a patient who awakens appropriately after naloxone administration is based on practical considerations. Patients presenting with profound hypoventilation or hypoxia are at risk for development of ARDS or posthypoxic encephalopathy. We recommend observing these patients for at least 24 hours in a medical setting. Based on the pharmacokinetics of naloxone, patients manifesting only moderate signs of opioid poisoning who remain normal for at least 2 hours after a standard parenteral dose of naloxone are likely safe to discharge (Antidotes in Brief: A4). Patients requiring larger doses of parenteral naloxone and those given nasal naloxone in the prehospital setting should be observed longer, although 6 hours should generally be sufficient. Patients with uncontrolled drug use or after a suicide attempt often need psychosocial interventions before discharge from the emergency department. Patients receiving a naloxone infusion should be maintained for 12 to 24 hours and then observed an additional 4 to 6 hours after discontinuation of the naloxone infusion (Antidotes in Brief: A4).

### Body Packers

In an attempt to transport illicit drugs from one country to another, body packers ingest large numbers of multiple-wrapped packages of concentrated cocaine or heroin. When the authorities discover such individuals or when individuals in custody become ill, they may be brought to a hospital for evaluation and management. Although these patients generally are asymptomatic on arrival, they are at risk for delayed, prolonged, or lethal poisoning as a consequence of packet rupture. Assessment and management recommendations are provided in Special Considerations: SC4.

### Rapid and Ultrarapid Opioid Detoxification

The concept of antagonist-precipitated opioid withdrawal is promoted extensively as a "cure" for opioid dependency, particularly heroin and oxycodone, but has fallen out of favor in recent years. Rather than slow, deliberate withdrawal or detoxification from opioids over several weeks, antagonist-precipitated withdrawal occurs over several hours or days. The purported advantage of this technique is a reduced risk of relapse to opioid use because the duration of discomfort is reduced and a more rapid transition to naltrexone maintenance can be achieved. Although most studies find some beneficial short-term results, relapse to drug use is very common. Rapid opioid detoxification techniques typically consist of naloxone- or naltrexone-precipitated opioid withdrawal tempered with varying amounts of clonidine, benzodiazepines, antiemetics, or other drugs. Ultrarapid opioid detoxification (UROD) uses a similar concept but involves the use of deep sedation or general anesthesia for greater patient control and comfort. The risks of these techniques are not fully defined but are of substantial concern. Massive catecholamine release, ARDS, acute kidney injury, and thyroid hormone suppression occurs after UROD, and many patients still manifest opioid withdrawal 48 hours after the procedure. We agree with the professional medical organizations involved in addiction management that have publicly expressed concern for this form of detoxification.

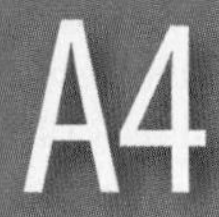

Antidotes in Brief

# A4 OPIOID ANTAGONISTS

## INTRODUCTION

Naloxone, naltrexone, and methylnaltrexone are pure competitive opioid antagonists at the mu (μ), kappa (κ), and delta (δ) receptors. Opioid antagonists prevent the actions of opioid agonists, reverse the effects of both endogenous and exogenous opioids, and may cause opioid withdrawal in opioid-dependent patients. Naloxone is the primary opioid antagonist used to reverse respiratory depression in patients manifesting opioid toxicity.

## HISTORY

*N*-Allylnorcodeine was the first opioid antagonist synthesized (in 1915), and *N*-allylnormorphine (nalorphine) was synthesized in the 1940s. Nalorphine was recognized as having both agonist and antagonist effects in 1954. Naloxone was synthesized in 1960, and naltrexone in 1963. The subsequent synthesis of opioid antagonists that are unable to cross the blood–brain barrier (sometimes called peripherally restricted) allowed patients receiving long-term opioid analgesics to avoid opioid-induced constipation, one of the most uncomfortable side effects associated with opioid therapy.

## PHARMACOLOGY

### Chemistry

Minor structural alterations are used to convert an agonist into an antagonist. Naloxone and naltrexone are antagonists derived from oxymorphone.

### Mechanism of Action

The currently available opioid receptor antagonists are all competitive antagonists of the μ receptor, with higher doses required to affect the κ and δ receptors. When they bind to the opioid receptor they prevent the binding of agonists, partial agonists, or mixed agonist–antagonists without producing any independent action.

### Pharmacokinetics

The oral bioavailability of naloxone is less than 2%. The bioavailability of a concentrated intranasal naloxone formulation is approximately 44% that of naloxone administered by the intramuscular (IM) route. The apparent half-life of 4 mg sprayed into one or both nostrils is approximately 2.1 hours compared with 1.24 hours for 0.4 mg administered IM into the thigh. Naloxone is well absorbed by all parenteral routes of administration. The approximate onset of action with the various routes of administration of the same dose of naloxone are as follows: intralingual, 30 seconds; intravenous (IV), 1 to 2 minutes; endotracheal, 60 seconds; intranasal, 3.4 minutes; inhalational (nebulized), 5 minutes; subcutaneous (SC), 5.5 minutes; and IM, 6 minutes. The distribution half-life is rapid (~5 minutes) because of its high lipid solubility. Protein binding is low, and the volume of distribution ($V_d$) is 0.8 to 2.64 L/kg. The duration of action of naloxone is approximately 20 to 90 minutes and depends on the dose and route of administration, and the relative rates of elimination of the agonist and naloxone. When naloxone is administered intranasally, this results in the delivery of unpredictable doses. In the prehospital setting, the time to onset of clinical effect of intranasal naloxone is comparable to that of IV or IM naloxone, largely because of the delay in obtaining IV access and slow absorption, respectively.

Naltrexone is rapidly absorbed with an oral bioavailability of 5% to 60%, and peak serum concentrations occur at 1 hour. Distribution is rapid, with a $V_d$ of approximately 15 L/kg and low protein binding. Naltrexone is metabolized in the liver to β-naltrexol (major metabolite with 2%–8% activity) and 2-hydroxy,3-methoxy-β-naltrexol and undergoes an enterohepatic cycle. The plasma elimination half-lives are 4 hours for naltrexone and 13 hours for β-naltrexol, with a terminal phase of elimination of 96 hours and 18 hours, respectively.

Methylnaltrexone, a derivative of naltrexone, is peripherally restricted because of its poor lipid solubility and limited ability to cross the blood–brain barrier. After SC administration, peak serum concentrations occur in about 30 minutes. The drug has a $V_d$ of 1.1 L/kg and is minimally protein bound (11%–15%). Although there are several metabolites, 85% of the drug is eliminated unchanged in the urine.

Naloxegol is an orally bioavailable, pegylated derivative of naloxone. Pegylation reduces its ability to cross the blood–brain barrier and allows its removal by the P-glycoprotein efflux pump. Peak serum concentration occurs at about 2 hours. Elimination is primarily through CYP3A4 metabolism, and the half-life is 6 to 11 hours.

### Pharmacodynamics

In the proper doses, pure opioid antagonists reverse all of the effects at the μ, κ, and δ receptors of endogenous and exogenous opioid agonists. Actions of opioid agonists that are not mediated by interaction with opioid receptors, such as direct mast cell liberation of histamine and the potassium channel–blocking effects of methadone, are not reversed by these antagonists. Chest wall rigidity from rapid fentanyl infusion is usually reversed with naloxone.

## ROLE IN OPIOID TOXICITY

Naloxone use by medical personnel for the management of patients with opioid toxicity has evolved over the past 50 years. The goal of reversal of opioid toxicity is to improve the patient's ventilation while avoiding withdrawal. Take-home naloxone distribution and naloxone prescribing for bystander administration in addition to programs for nonmedical first responders continue to significantly expand around the world. The majority of the naloxone available for community-based use is intended for administration by the intranasal route. Higher doses are routinely used in the community.

## ROLE IN MAINTENANCE OF OPIOID ABSTINENCE

Opioid dependence is managed either by substitution of the primary opioid, typically heroin or a prescription opioid, with methadone or buprenorphine or by detoxification and subsequent abstinence. Maintenance of abstinence is facilitated by the administration of daily or depot formulations of naltrexone. Before naltrexone is administered for abstinence maintenance, the patient must be weaned from opioid dependence and be a willing participant. Naloxone should be administered intravenously to confirm that the patient is no longer opioid dependent and is therefore safe for naltrexone administration. With naloxone, opioid withdrawal, if it occurs, will be short lived instead of a prolonged withdrawal following naltrexone administration.

## ROLE IN ETHANOL ABSTINENCE

Naltrexone, particularly the IM depot form, reduces ethanol craving, the number of drinking days, and relapse rates and is thus useful to promote and maintain abstinence.

## OTHER USES

Peripherally restricted opioid antagonists (eg, methylnaltrexone) are used to prevent or treat the constipation occurring as a side effect of opioid use, whether for pain management or medication-assisted therapy. Evacuation from methylnaltrexone occurs within 4 hours, and within 6 hours for naloxegol.

Opioid antagonists are sometimes used in the management of overdoses with nonopioids such as ethanol, clonidine and other imizaolines, captopril, and valproic acid. In none of these instances is the reported improvement as dramatic or consistent as in the reversal of an opioid. The mechanisms for each of these, although undefined, is suggested to relate to reversal of endogenous opioid peptides at opioid receptors.

## ADVERSE EFFECTS AND SAFETY ISSUES

Pure opioid antagonists produce no clinical effects in opioid-naïve or nondependent patients even when administered in massive doses (grams) such as was done in a spinal cord injury study. When patients dependent on opioid agonists are exposed to opioid antagonists, they exhibit opioid withdrawal. Antagonist-precipitated withdrawal also sometimes results in an "overshoot" phenomenon, from a transient increase in circulating catecholamines, resulting in hyperventilation, tachycardia, and hypertension.

In the cardiovascular system, myocardial ischemia and infarction, myocardial stunning (takotsubo, stress cardiomyopathy), heart failure, hypertension, and dysrhythmias are rarely reported. In the CNS, agitation should be expected and is occasionally profound, and seizures, although rare, may occur. Delirium, although rarely reported in patients withdrawing because of opioid abstinence, occurs during precipitated opioid withdrawal. In the lungs, acute respiratory distress syndrome (ARDS) is associated with naloxone administration, almost uniformly in opioid-dependent patients. If the patient's airway is unprotected during withdrawal and vomiting occurs, aspiration pneumonitis may complicate the recovery.

### Observation Period After Antagonist Administration

After IV bolus naloxone at doses less than 2 mg, observation for 2 hours is typically adequate to determine whether sedation and respiratory depression will return as the naloxone effect diminishes and the initial opioid effects return. Patients discontinued from a continuous naloxone infusion or those who received large total initial doses of naloxone by any route, including intranasal, typically necessitate subsequent observation for at least 4 hours, and perhaps 6 hours, to ensure that respiratory depression or sedation does not recur. Observation should be meticulous and include periodic direct assessment of consciousness and ventilatory rate and effort, as well as continuous pulse oximetry off supplemental oxygen. Optimally, continuous capnometry should also be used.

### Management of Iatrogenic Withdrawal

Excessive administration of an opioid antagonist to an opioid-dependent patient will predictably result in opioid withdrawal. When induced by naloxone, all that is generally required is protecting the patient from harm and reassuring the patient that the effects will be short lived. After inadvertent administration of naltrexone, the expected duration of the withdrawal syndrome generally mandates the use of pharmacologic intervention. If only moderate withdrawal is present (ie, a Clinical Opiate Withdrawal Scale (COWS) score $< 25$), the administration of metoclopramide, clonidine, or a benzodiazepine is usually adequate. In more severe cases, we typically use fentanyl in titrated doses. Fentanyl has the advantage over morphine of causing less histamine release. Although the use of buprenorphine was only indirectly studied in this role, it has several potential advantages, including high receptor affinity, long duration of action, low risk of oversedation and the possibility of converting to long-term buprenorphine treatment. At this point, data are insufficient to routinely recommend buprenorphine at this time.

## PREGNANCY AND LACTATION

Naloxone and naltrexone are pregnancy Category C medications. Inducing opioid withdrawal in the mother probably will induce withdrawal in the fetus and should be avoided. Similarly, administering naloxone (or naltrexone) to newborns of opioid-tolerant mothers may induce neonatal withdrawal and should be used cautiously when apnea or severe respiratory depression is present.

## DOSING AND ADMINISTRATION

Before administration of naloxone, the patient should receive adequate ventilation to ensure that the patient is not hypercapnic. Currently, the initial empiric parenteral dose that we recommend in the hospital for all opioid-dependent adult patients is 0.04 mg. Nondependent patients can receive higher doses without concern for precipitating withdrawal. A dose of naloxone of 0.4 mg IV will reverse the respiratory depressant effects of most opioids and is an appropriate starting dose in non–opioid-dependent patients. However, this dose in an opioid-dependent patient usually produces withdrawal, which should be avoided if possible. The goal is to produce a spontaneously and adequately ventilating patient without precipitating significant or abrupt opioid withdrawal. Therefore, 0.04 mg IV is a reasonable starting dose in most patients, with incremental increases by 0.04 mg, while supporting the patient's ventilation and oxygenation, up to a dose of 0.12 mg. In those without response, increasing by 0.2 or 0.4 mg up to a dose of 2 mg is a reasonable approach. In situations in which an ultrapotent opioid, often a fentanyl derivative, has been administered, there are reports of response after very large naloxone doses of 10 mg. Failure of the patient to respond to 8 to 10 mg of naloxone given in rapid boluses suggests that a conventional opioid is not responsible for the respiratory depression and sedation, an additional respiratory depressant is present, or the patient has hypoxic encephalopathy. The dose in children without opioid dependence is essentially the same as for adults (ie, 0.1 mg/kg to the adult dose of 2 mg). The dose in neonates is 0.01 mg/kg given the concerns for withdrawal. However, for those with opioid dependence, we recommend the same strategy discussed for adults above. When intravenous access is not available, intramuscular or intraosseous administration is recommended.

Intranasal naloxone is not recommended as first-line treatment by healthcare providers in hospitals but is reasonable for prehospital providers when other routes of administration are unavailable or undesirable. Nebulized naloxone has similar limitations in dose accuracy and is further limited in patients with severe ventilatory depression, the group most in need of naloxone, and is therefore not recommended.

Evaluation for the redevelopment of respiratory depression after naloxone administration requires nearly continuous monitoring. Resedation should be treated with either periodic repeated dosing of the antagonist or a continuous infusion of naloxone. The continuous infusion should be started immediately following an appropriate bolus and run at two-thirds of the total bolus dose per hour. At approximately 15 minutes into the infusion, a repeat bolus of half the initial dose may be required. Titration upward or downward is easily accomplished as necessary to both maintain adequate ventilation and avoid withdrawal.

Use of longer acting opioid antagonists, such as naltrexone, places the patient at substantial risk for protracted withdrawal syndromes. The use of a long-acting opioid antagonist in acute care situations should be reserved for carefully considered special indications, such as unintentional exposures to short-acting opioids in nondependent patients, together with extended periods of observation or careful follow-up. For the uncommon patient with opioid toxicity for whom naltrexone is indicated, an oral dose of 150 mg generally lasts 48 to 72 hours and should be adequate.

### Buprenorphine

Naloxone reverses the respiratory depressant effects of buprenorphine in a unique dose–response curve. Bolus doses of naloxone of 2 to 3 mg followed by a continuous infusion of 4 mg/h in adults were able to fully reverse the respiratory depression associated with IV buprenorphine administered in a total dose of 0.2 and 0.4 mg over 1 hour. Doses of naloxone greater than 4 mg/h actually led to the redevelopment of respiratory depression. Therefore, excess naloxone should be avoided in adults because it can worsen the respiratory depression. Children do not seem to be susceptible to this effect.

## FORMULATION AND ACQUISITION

Naloxone (Narcan) for IV, IM, or SC administration is available in concentrations of 0.4 and 1 mg/mL, with and without parabens in 1- and 2-mL ampoules, vials, and syringes and in 10-mL multidose vials with parabens. Naloxone is frequently diluted in 0.9% sodium chloride solution or 5% dextrose to facilitate continuous IV infusion.

Naltrexone is available as a 50-mg capsule-shaped tablet. It is also available as a 380-mg vial for reconstitution with a carboxymethylcellulose and polysorbate diluent to form an injectable suspension intended for monthly IM administration. Methylnaltrexone is available as a 12-mg/0.6-mL solution for SC injection. Naloxegol is available as an oral tablet, in 12.5-mg and 25-mg strengths.

Special Considerations

# SC4 INTERNAL CONCEALMENT OF XENOBIOTICS

There are two distinct categories of concealment colloquially known as "body stuffers" and "body packers." The term *body stuffer* refers to an individual who precipitously hides xenobiotics in a body cavity or ingests them in an attempt to avoid imminent discovery. The term *body packer* refers to an individual who intentionally conceals xenobiotics almost exclusively for the purposes of international smuggling.

## BODY PACKERS

Internal concealment of xenobiotics for the purpose of smuggling was first reported in Canada in 1973. Internal xenobiotic smuggling is now a worldwide problem. As screening and detection methods have increased, there has been an unfortunate shift toward the use of pregnant women and children as young as 6 years of age.

### Composition of Packages

Body packers typically swallow large numbers (50–100) of well-prepared packages, each filled with substantial amounts of xenobiotic. Therefore, one person may carry many lethal doses of xenobiotic. Although ingestion is common, packets are also sometimes concealed by insertion into the vagina and rectum. The most frequently smuggled cargo is either heroin or cocaine, but other xenobiotics are also reported.

A number of materials are used for xenobiotic packaging and include latex, carbon paper, aluminum foil, cellophane, wax, tape, surgical ligatures, paraffin, and fiberglass. Although the initial reports suggested a high rate of complications caused by packaging failure, advances in the technology of packet construction have decreased rates of rupture. A typical packet in current use is composed of a core of compacted xenobiotic covered by several layers of latex and encased in an outer wax coating. Transport of xenobiotic in liquid form is also reported.

### Bioavailability

The oral bioavailability of cocaine hydrochloride is approximately 30% to 40%, which is similar to intranasal administration. Rectal and vaginal bioavailability of cocaine hydrochloride and the oral, rectal, and vaginal bioavailability of crack cocaine have not been studied. Ingestion of heroin results in rapid first-pass metabolism to morphine. The peak concentrations after 10 mg of oral heroin are similar to those expected from 10 mg of oral morphine. The rectal bioavailability is about 50% less than the oral bioavailability.

### Clinical Manifestations

Body packers undergoing medical examinations may be asymptomatic or may have classic cocaine or opioid toxidromes (Chaps. 9 and 48). They may also present with mechanical bowel obstruction or perforation. Individuals carrying opioids appear to be at higher risk of gastrointestinal (GI) obstruction, even with intact packets. While it is possible that small amounts of opioid on the packet surface or micro leakage slows gut motility, neither of these theories has been substantiated.

### Laboratory Evaluation

Drug screening results are difficult to interpret. Although generally, a positive result should raise concern for a ruptured packet, positive results may also be due to external contamination of the packet during preparation from a microperforation or from prior xenobiotic utilization. The rate of positive drug screens in asymptomatic patients is reported to be as great as 72%. Screening typically correlates closely with the drug carried, but it is potentially misleading in that some patients transporting any xenobiotic will ingest opioids for the purpose of slowing GI transit time. Additionally, some patients carry packets containing different xenobiotics. An initially negative result that later becomes positive suggests a ruptured packet and is an indication for very close monitoring or surgical removal.

### Radiographic Evaluation

All suspected body packers should undergo radiographic evaluation. Abdominal radiographs have a detection sensitivity of 75% to 95%. Caution must be used when interpreting plain radiographic studies. In one series, 19% of patients had false-negative radiographs, with one patient subsequently passing 135 packets. False-positive results are also reported because of constipation, intraabdominal calcifications, and bladder stones. Oral contrast administration increases the sensitivity of plain radiography. Computed tomography (CT) scanning has a higher sensitivity than plain radiography, and ranges from 96% to 100% (Figs. SC4–1 and SC4–2). Noncontrast CT is the preferred modality because contrast may obscure packets.

Although likely to identify patients with multiple packets, a false-negative contrast CT scan after whole-bowel irrigation (WBI) was reported in a body packer who subsequently passed a single packet per rectum. Although ultrasonography is potentially useful as a screening tool, particularly for patients in whom CT has increased risk, such as pregnant patients, based on existing data it cannot definitively exclude packets. Magnetic resonance imaging (MRI) is used less commonly than CT except in pregnant women and children. However, MRI is able to detect the presence of packets, although it is less reliable in determining the number of packets.

### Management

All patients suspected of internal concealment of drugs should be closely monitored during evaluation. This should include blood pressure, heart rate, temperature, pulse

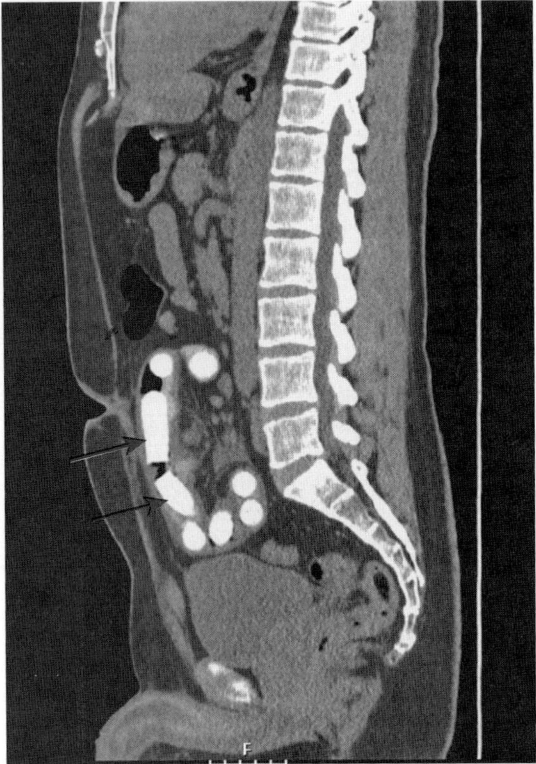

**FIGURE SC4–1.** Computed tomography (sagittal view) of the abdomen showing packets in the intestine. *(Used with permission from The Fellowship in Medical Toxicology, New York University School of Medicine, New York City Poison Center.)*

oximetry, and continuous carbon dioxide monitoring, as well as direct visualization of the patient. Patients should be questioned about the number of packets ingested. While they almost always know the exact count, there may be reasons for them to under- or overestimate the number.

Gastrointestinal decontamination is a vital element in the management of body packers. Currently, we suggest a conservative nonsurgical management for asymptomatic patients supported by several large series (Fig. SC4–3). Whole-bowel irrigation is the mainstay of therapy for asymptomatic body packers. Use of promotility xenobiotics, such as metoclopramide and erythromycin, is reported, but these are unlikely to add significantly to the use of WBI. Activated charcoal (AC) is of questionable value for cocaine packers given the higher risk of the need for surgical intervention. Also, it is not likely to improve the outcome of symptomatic heroin body packers because these patients can be successfully managed with opioid antagonists and mechanical ventilation. Paraffin oil may dissolve some packet wrappers, potentially resulting in drug toxicity.

Patients manifesting opioid toxicity should be treated with the opioid antagonist naloxone by intravenous bolus and infusion and mechanical ventilation if necessary (Antidotes in Brief: A4). Surgical intervention is generally only necessary, however, for mechanical obstruction as long as the patient can be maintained with naloxone. Rupture of a cocaine packet is a life-threatening emergency that requires aggressive medical and surgical therapy (Chap. 48). Benzodiazepines or other sedative–hypnotics such as propofol are recommended as temporizing measures, but surgical intervention for packet removal should be performed emergently

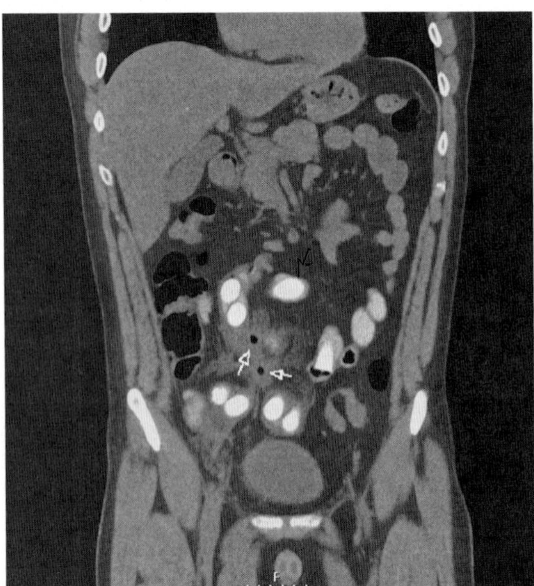

**FIGURE SC4–2.** Computed tomography (coronal view) of the abdomen showing packets associated with free air (lower two arrows) caused by bowel perforation. *(Used with permission from The Fellowship in Medical Toxicology, New York University School of Medicine, New York City Poison Center.)*

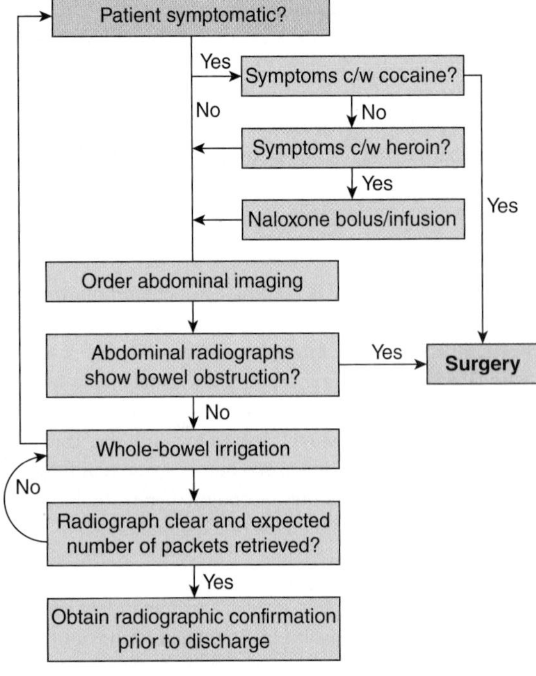


**FIGURE SC4–3.** Algorithm for managing cocaine or heroin body packers.

in body packers with *any* sign of cocaine or amphetamine toxicity. Surgical removal of the packets is also the therapy of choice in the case of mechanical obstruction from any xenobiotic-containing packet.

Endoscopy and proctoscopy have been used successfully for removal of packets. However, caution must be used because attempted endoscopic removal can cause packet rupture and resultant toxicity. Endoscopic removal should be reserved for cases in which a few packets are retained after failure of nonsurgical management. It is essential to ensure the passage of all packets before discharging a patient from medical care. It is therefore recommended that patients be observed for 24 hours after the passage of three packet-free stools and negative confirmatory CT.

## BODY STUFFERS

Body stuffers usually present for health care when they are taken into custody by law enforcement officers. Typically, the person has hastily ingested the xenobiotic or inserted it into the rectum or vagina to hide the evidence from the police. Because the person was not planning to conceal the xenobiotic, the xenobiotic is likely unwrapped, or poorly wrapped in materials intended for distribution.

Pertinent historical information includes time of ingestion, xenobiotic, amount ingested, packaging, and symptoms consistent with xenobiotic ingestion. Unfortunately, an accurate history is often difficult to obtain.

## COMPOSITION OF PACKAGES

Because xenobiotics are typically transported locally in plastic bags, condoms, balloons, glassine envelopes, aluminum foil, or crack vials, these are the most frequently reported wrappers. It is important to obtain a precise history related to packaging material as this correlates with the risk of leakage.

### Clinical Manifestations

After ingestion of drug packets or crack rocks, toxicity is most frequently absent or mild. However, although most case series report low rates of complications, both significant toxicity and death occur. Most body stuffers reported in the literature had symptom onset within 6 hours of ingestion, although there are a few notably delayed cases with onset of symptoms at 10–12 hours.

### Laboratory Evaluation

Laboratory xenobiotic testing is difficult to interpret in body stuffers because these patients are often have substance use disorders. One study of 50 suspected body stuffers found that urine drug screening correctly classified the presence or absence of packets only 57% of the time. Therefore, we do not recommend the use of urine drug assays in this setting.

### Radiographic Evaluation

Although detection of stuffed xenobiotics is possible by diagnostic imaging studies, the sensitivity is very poor. In one series of patients with crack vial ingestions, only 2 of 23 of abdominal radiographs were positive in patients who subsequently passed vials. In two other series of cocaine body stuffers, all plain radiographs were negative. The sensitivity of computed tomography is unknown but expected to be better. Imaging is therefore not likely to be clinically useful in these patients.

### Management

Body stuffers who exhibit xenobiotic toxicity should be managed according to standard principles for managing that xenobiotic or suspected xenobiotic (Chaps. 9 and 48).

Patients with GI complaints should be evaluated for ileus or obstruction. Management of asymptomatic body stuffers has not been rigorously evaluated. Given the theoretical benefit, a dose of AC is recommended in an awake and cooperative patient. WBI may reduce intestinal transit time, but also may provide additional solvent and enhance the leakage and absorption of poorly wrapped packets. Therefore, WBI is not routinely recommended unless life-threatening amounts of xenobiotic (in packages) are ingested.

A therapeutic endpoint has not been established in part because packages are often not recovered from body stuffers. Since a review of more than 1,000 published cases of body stuffers revealed only a few cases in which onset of toxicity occurred more than 6 hours after ingestion, it is reasonable to observe asymptomatic patients for 6 hours. Because rare patients may have more delayed presentations, patients who have ingested large, potentially lethal doses or those who refuse AC should be observed for 12–24 hours in a closely monitored setting. Multiple stools devoid of packages or a lack of symptoms after 24 hours are reasonable endpoints for monitoring those patients.

## LEGAL PRINCIPLES

In the United States, patients have a legal right to refuse care if they are competent to do so. This includes body stuffers and body packers who are under arrest. Patients with decisional capacity cannot be forced to take AC, WBI, or any other form of therapy or diagnostic procedure. If in police custody, however, the individual may be kept in the hospital for an extended observation period. This strategy maintains the patient's medical autonomy and ensures clinical stability. If signs of life-threatening toxicity subsequently develop, the patient will most likely have lost decisional capacity, and therapy and management can proceed as medically necessary.

If a body packer who is not in legal custody presents for medical care, physicians face an ethical dilemma. Calling the authorities is a violation of the patient's right to confidentiality. However, possession of large amounts of drugs may theoretically endanger the hospital staff because criminal elements expect drug delivery. Consultation with hospital legal counsel, risk management, and/or the ethics committee are recommended in this situation.

# SC5 PREVENTION, TREATMENT, AND HARM REDUCTION APPROACHES TO OPIOID OVERDOSES

## INTRODUCTION

In the United States (US), an opioid drug epidemic persists, driven by high rates of per capita opioid analgesic dispensing, paired with a growing availability of illicit heroin, fentanyl, and fentanyl derivatives. In 2012, the Centers for Disease Control and Prevention (CDC) reported that for every unintentional overdose death related to an opioid analgesic, 9 people were admitted for substance abuse treatment, 35 visited EDs, 161 reported drug abuse or dependence, and 461 reported nonmedical uses of opioid analgesics.

The availability and dissemination of core evidence-based interventions that treat and prevent overdose events and fatalities, however, have not kept pace with the number of persons using, suffering harm, and dying from opioids. Evidence for and policies supporting core community-based overdose interventions, which are harm reduction education and counseling, and naloxone distribution and administration, are reviewed here.

## EPIDEMIOLOGY

### Overdose Rates

Opioid use in the US has grown steadily since the 1990s, largely because of widespread and routine opioid analgesic prescribing. Heroin availability and related problems appear to be accelerating, and heroin "markets" have expanded to all large US metropolitan areas as well as a substantial proportion of rural counties. More recently, novel opioids, such as U-47700 and W-18, and illicit fentanyl analogs, such as carfentanil, have entered street heroin formulations.

### Risk Factors

"Opioid overdose" generally refers to oversedation, hypoventilation, and anoxia stemming from an excessive dose of an opioid agonist alone or in combination with other central nervous system depressants. Established risk factors for opioid overdose include:

- People with opioid dependence, particularly after periods of reduced use, resulting in loss of tolerance
- People who inject opioids
- People who use high doses of prescription opioids therapeutically
- People who use opioids in combination with other sedating xenobiotics
- People who use opioids and have medical conditions such as major depression, HIV, liver dysfunction, lung disease, or obstructive sleep apnea
- Household members, including children, of people in possession of opioids

## NALOXONE AND HARM REDUCTION APPROACHES TO OVERDOSE PREVENTION AND OVERDOSE REVERSAL

Naloxone administration is the principal overdose intervention taught to at-risk opioid users, persons in treatment, and family members, as well as first responders. Naloxone pharmacokinetics and naloxone efficacy for overdose are discussed in Chapter 9 and Antidotes in Brief: A4.

### Community-Based Effectiveness

Since most opioid overdoses occur in the setting of a bystander and often in a private location, many educational initiatives aim to reach those most likely to be in first contact with the patient. Education generally consists of overdose prevention; rapid recognition; and appropriate response, including timely administration of naloxone, rescue breathing or cardiopulmonary resuscitation, recovery positioning, and emergency medical services (EMS) activation. Although no randomized controlled trial exists, several cohort studies demonstrate effectiveness of community-based opioid overdose programs in terms of reduced rates of opioid-related deaths.

### Controversies Regarding Naloxone

One common objection to increasing the supply of naloxone is that it will allow users to feel more comfortable with drug use, ultimately leading to paradoxical increased use and risk-taking behavior. This has not occurred in communities where naloxone programs were initiated. In fact, several communities where naloxone programs exist observed decreased drug use.

Another common concern is that when naloxone is given, there is no perceived need to activate 911, a critical component of overdose response. In New York City, EMS was activated 74% of the time by naloxone-trained laypersons, which is similar to a 68% activation rate in a prior New York City study involving those without naloxone education.

Another concern is the inappropriate administration of naloxone by laypersons, especially if under the influence of an opioid or other xenobiotic, but studies have shown that trained laypersons are able to recognize opioid overdose and safely and appropriately administer naloxone.

### Policies Regarding Naloxone

Reforms and efforts are being undertaken to increase the availability, prescribing, and administration of naloxone. One target is decreasing prescriber and dispenser liability. Many states have given prescribers immunity or are allowing third-party or standing prescriptions (ie, prescribing to someone other than the patient). Many states have expanded regulations to include laypersons. Others are moving toward pharmacist dispensing without a prescription or without personal identification. Good Samaritan laws are another effort to increase administration of naloxone and activation of EMS by laypersons without fear of legal repercussions.

### Safe Injection Sites and Medical Heroin Interventions

Although controversial safe injection sites are becoming more prevalent in the US and internationally. Heroin-assisted treatment (HAT) appears to be an effective intervention in terms of higher treatment retention both in European and Canadian studies. In one study HAT had higher retention than methadone, and although 115 out of 70,000 patients experienced an overdose, compared to zero in the methadone group, all resolved with only a minority (10/115) requiring naloxone. HAT was also associated with lower self-reported rates of criminal activity and superior cost-effectiveness.

### Opioid Treatment as Overdose Prevention

Opioid use disorder treatment is itself intended to reduce illicit opioid use and prevent harm and death. Treatment effects associated with methadone, buprenorphine, and to some extent naltrexone include prevention of overdoses; reduced rates of communicable disease transmission and injection drug use; improved function and quality of life; and lower health and societal costs, including reduced criminal behavior and incarceration.

### Methadone and Buprenorphine

μ-Opioid receptor agonist maintenance treatments with methadone (a full agonist) or buprenorphine (a partial agonist) are the evidence-based, first-line treatments for an active opioid use disorders. Maintenance opioid therapy allows the patient to retain acceptable levels of energy, cognition, and daily function, with reduced cravings and urges for illicit opioids. Systematic reviews, meta-analyses, and epidemiologic studies consistently find associations between exposure and retention in methadone maintenance with lower mortality rates compared with opioid-dependent individuals who discontinue such treatment.

### Extended-Release Naltrexone

Extended-release naltrexone (XR-NTX) is a more recently Food and Drug Administration–approved (2010) therapy for opioid use disorder, specifically for the prevention of opioid relapse after detoxification. The monthly intramuscular depot formulation is designed to improve adherence to naltrexone therapy. To qualify for extended-release naltrexone, a patient must be detoxified and opioid free at the time of induction. The naltrexone blockade then renders usual doses of opioid analgesics or heroin ineffective and noneuphoric. This can become problematic if the patient subsequently requires an opioid for an acutely painful condition.

### Counseling-Only Treatments

Contrary to opioid pharmacotherapy treatments, detoxifying from opioids and graduation to further residential or outpatient counseling-only modalities elevate the acute risk of overdose. There are some practical advantages to counseling-only opioid addiction treatments. There are minimal requirements for a licensed medical provider or prescriber to be a member of the program staff, which is often composed primarily of addiction counselors. Patient preference for a "drug-free" recovery is respected. However, many studies show opioid relapse, overdose, and death occur at higher rates in counseling-only treatments compared with medication maintenance approaches. Furthermore, acutely weaning and lowering the tolerance of an opioid-dependent user in a controlled environment followed by return to the community is an important overdose risk factor and arguably worse for patients who relapse than no treatment and continued illicit opioid use.

## OPIOID POLICIES AND PRACTICE REFORMS IN THE UNITED STATES

Overall efforts to reduce the volume and supply of opioid analgesics have important implications for overdose prevention. Prescriber practice reforms and regulatory efforts aimed at reducing individual opioid analgesic prescribing and state prescription monitoring programs may all contribute to lower opioid prescribing and overdose rates. More peripherally, states with regulated medical marijuana and cannabis legalization laws report lower rates of opioid overdose. An overriding public health aim regarding opioid use is to reduce harm and limit overdose risk, and these types of policies will require continuous evaluation and revision. The routine prescription of potent opioid analgesics for nonmalignant chronic pain by US providers should end as described in the 2016 CDC practice guidelines.

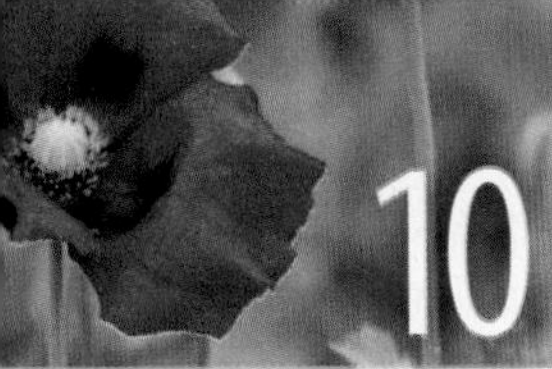

# 10 SALICYLATES

| Therapeutic serum concentration | 15–30 mg/dL |
|---|---|
| | 1.1–2.2 mmol/L |

## HISTORY AND EPIDEMIOLOGY

The Ancient Egyptians recognized the pain-relieving effects of concoctions made from myrtle and willow leaves. Hippocrates was among the first reported to use willow bark and leaves from the *Salix* species to relieve fever, but it was not until 1829 that the glycoside salicin was extracted from the willow bark and used as an antipyretic. From the 1950s to 1970s, salicylates were the leading cause of fatal childhood poisoning. The association with Reye syndrome, safer packaging, and the increased use of nonsteroidal antiinflammatory drugs (NSAIDs), acetaminophen (APAP), and other alternatives to aspirin decreased the incidence of unintentional salicylate poisoning. Despite decline in general use, it is still imperative that clinicians are adept at early recognition and swift management of patients with salicylate overdose.

## PHARMACOLOGY

Aspirin has analgesic, antiinflammatory, and antipyretic properties. Most of the beneficial effects of NSAIDs result from their inhibition of cyclooxygenase (COX). This enzyme enables the synthesis of prostaglandins, which in turn mediate inflammation and fever. Contributing to the antiinflammatory effects and independent of the effects on prostaglandins, salicylates and other NSAIDs also directly inhibit neutrophils. Although there are many different salicylates, most of the studies of salicylate metabolism involve acetylsalicylic acid (aspirin, ASA). Because platelets cannot regenerate COX-1, a daily dose of as little as 30 mg of ASA inhibits COX-1 for the 8- to 12-day lifespan of the platelet. There is an implicit assumption that all members of the salicylate class have similar properties after being converted to salicylic acid.

## PHARMACOKINETICS

ASA is rapidly absorbed from the stomach. The pKa of ASA is 3.5, and the majority is nonionized (ie, acetylsalicylic acid) in the strongly acidic stomach (pH 1–2). Although absorption of ASA is less efficient in the small bowel because of its higher pH, it is substantial and rapid because the large surface area of the small intestine increases the solubility of acetylsalicylate. After ingestion of therapeutic doses of immediate-release ASA, therapeutic serum concentrations are achieved in 30 minutes, and maximum concentrations are often attained in less than 1 hour. The plasma half-life of ASA is about 15 minutes because it is rapidly hydrolyzed to salicylate. The apparent half-life for salicylate is about 2 to 3 hours at antiplatelet doses and increases to 12 hours at antiinflammatory doses demonstrating dose-dependent elimination. ASA undergoes biotransformation in the liver and is then eliminated by the kidneys. The apparent volume of distribution ($V_d$) increases from 0.2 L/kg at low concentrations to 0.3 to 0.5 L/kg at higher concentrations.

## TOXICOKINETICS

In overdose, there is a decrease in protein (albumin) binding from 90% at therapeutic concentrations to less than 75% at toxic concentrations, which is caused by saturation of protein binding sites. Salicylates have substantially longer apparent half-lives at toxic concentrations than at therapeutic concentrations, varying from 2 to 4 hours at therapeutic concentrations to as long as 20 hours at toxic concentrations. Delayed absorption of immediate-release aspirin results from salicylate-induced pylorospasm or pharmacobezoar formation. Therapeutic doses of enteric-coated tablets produce peak serum concentrations at 4 to 6 hours after ingestion, and in overdose, the reported peak is delayed up to 24 hours after ingestion.

Salicylates are conjugated with glycine and glucuronides in the liver and are eliminated by the kidneys (Fig. 10–1). As the concentration of salicylates increases, two of the five pathways of elimination—those for salicyluric acid and the salicylic phenolic glucuronide—become saturated and exhibit zero-order kinetics. As a result of this saturation, overall salicylate elimination changes from first-order kinetics to zero-order kinetics. At very high serum concentrations, salicylate elimination again resembles first-order elimination as an increasing fraction undergoes renal clearance. Free salicylic acid is filtered through the glomerulus and is both passively reabsorbed and actively secreted from the proximal tubules. More than 30% of an ingested salicylate dose is eliminated in alkaline urine and as little as 2% in acidic urine. A rapid rise in elimination occurs when the urine pH is greater than 7.5.

### Other Forms of Salicylate

***Topical Salicylate, Methyl Salicylate (Oil of Wintergreen), and Salicylic Acid.*** Topical salicylates are rarely responsible for salicylate poisoning when used in their intended manner because absorption through intact normal skin is very slow. However extensive application of topical preparations containing methyl salicylate results in poisoning. Heat, occlusive dressings, young age, inflammation, certain body areas with enhanced absorption, cracked skin, and psoriasis may increase topical salicylate absorption.

Ingestion of methyl salicylate is potentially lethal because 1 mL of 98% oil of wintergreen contains an equivalent quantity of salicylate as 1.4 g of ASA. The minimum toxic salicylate dose of approximately 150 mg/kg body weight can almost be achieved with 1 mL of oil of wintergreen, which represents 140 mg/kg of salicylates for a 10-kg child.

***Bismuth Subsalicylate.*** Bismuth subsalicylate, which is available in several nonprescription formulations to relieve dyspepsia, releases salicylate in the gastrointestinal (GI) tract, where it is subsequently absorbed, especially in the setting of

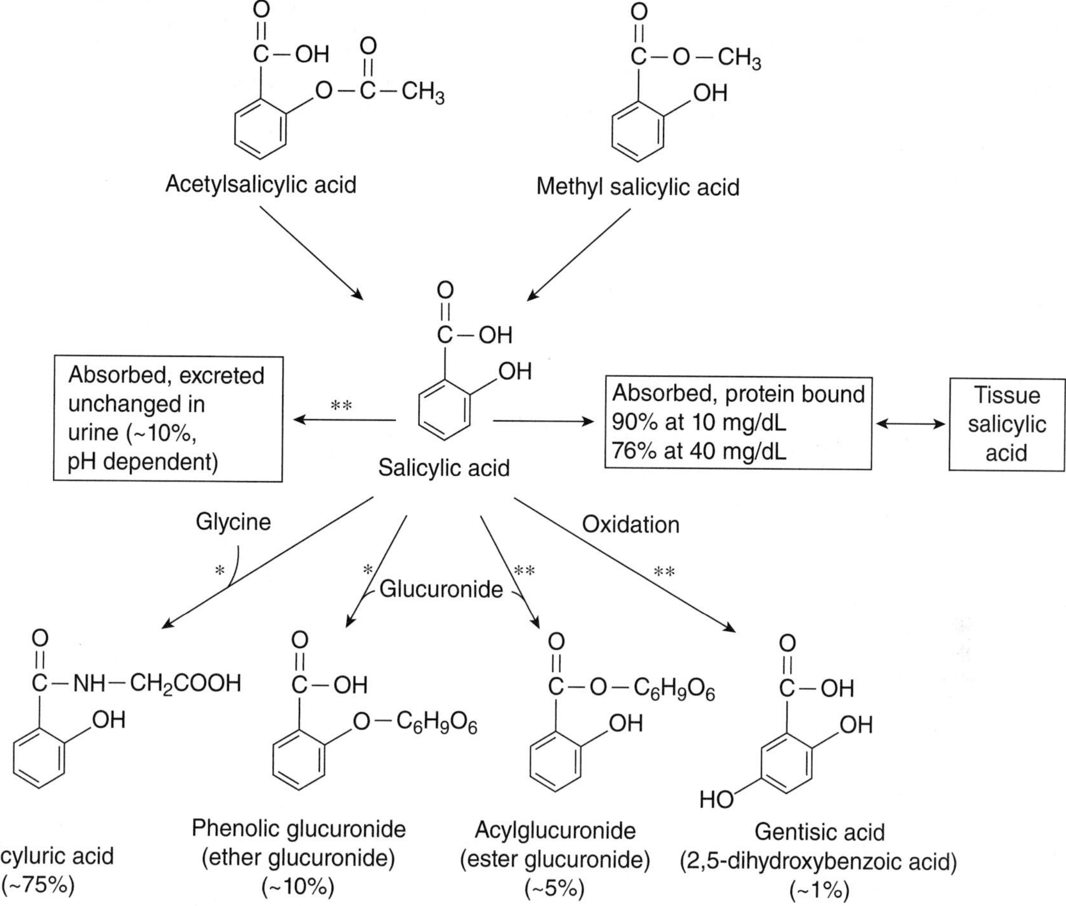


**FIGURE 10–1.** Salicylic acid metabolism. At excessive dose, the four mechanisms of salicylic acid metabolism are overloaded, leading to increased tissue binding, decreased protein binding, and increased excretion of unconjugated salicylic acid. *Asterisk* (*) indicates Michaelis-Menten kinetics; *double asterisk* (**) indicates first-order kinetics.

abnormal mucosa. Patients with diarrhea and infants with colic using large quantities of bismuth subsalicylate are at increased risk for developing salicylate toxicity, and rarely bismuth toxicity.

## PATHOPHYSIOLOGY

ASA has a pKa of 3.5, and is rapidly hydrolyzed to salicylic acid, which has a pKa of 2.97. Salicylic acid at physiologic pH exists predominantly in a charged (ionized) state. But in overdose, as the serum pH falls, more salicylate shifts toward a nonionized (uncharged) salicylic acid form that readily traverses lipid bilayers and cell membranes.

### Acid–Base and Metabolic Effects

Salicylate interferes with the citric acid cycle, which limits the production of adenosine triphosphate (ATP). It also uncouples oxidative phosphorylation, causing accumulation of pyruvic and lactic acids and releasing energy as heat. Salicylate induced increases in fatty acid metabolism generates β-hydroxybutyric acid, acetoacetic acid, and acetone. Toxic concentrations of salicylate impair renal hemodynamics, leading to the accumulation of inorganic acids. The net result of all of these metabolic processes is an anion gap metabolic acidosis in which the unmeasured anions include salicylate and its metabolites, lactate, ketoacids, and inorganic acids. Hypoglycemia results from the combined effect of increased energy demands, depletion of glycogen stores, and decreased gluconeogenesis.

### Neurologic Effects

With increasing CNS salicylate concentrations, neuronal energy depletion develops as salicylate uncouples neuronal and glial oxidative phosphorylation. Despite normal serum glucose concentrations, CSF glucose concentrations decrease. Salicylate also induces neuronal cell apoptosis. These effects ultimately lead to cerebral edema.

### Hepatic Effects

Because hepatic injury is rare, other concurrent coingestants and causes should be evaluated if there is a clinically significant elevation of aminotransferases or bilirubin concentration, or signs of acute liver failure.

### Otolaryngologic Effects

The molecular mechanism of salicylate ototoxicity is not completely understood but appears to be multifactorial.

Likely factors include; inhibition of cochlear COX and prevention of prostaglandin synthesis.

### Pulmonary Effects

Direct stimulation of the medullary respiratory neurons produces hyperpnea and tachypnea even at therapeutic concentrations. Some patients with severe toxicity develop acute respiratory distress syndrome (ARDS). Although the mechanism is unclear and likely multifactorial, risk factors for ARDS include cigarette smoking, chronic overdose, acidemia, and neurologic symptoms at the time of arrival.

### Gastrointestinal Effects

Salicylate disrupts the mucosal barrier that normally protects the gastric lining from the extremely acidic contents of the stomach. Emesis is triggered both by local mucosal irritation and central stimulation of the chemoreceptor trigger zone.

### Renal Effects

The kidneys play a major role in the excretion of salicylate and its metabolites. Volume losses that develop from hyperventilation and hyperthermia also cause prerenal acute kidney injury (AKI). The kidneys also respond to salicylate poisoning by excreting an increased solute load, including large quantities of bicarbonate, sodium, potassium, and organic acids.

### Hematologic Effects

The platelet dysfunction, caused by irreversible acetylation of COX-1, prevents the formation of thromboxane A2, which is normally responsible for platelet aggregation. At supratherapeutic doses, salicylate decreases the plasma concentration of the $\gamma$-carboxyglutamate containing coagulation factors and an accumulation of microsomal substrates for vitamin K–dependent carboxylase in the liver and lung. This results in hypoprothrombinemia (factor II) as well as decreases in factors VII, IX, and X (Chap. 31).

## CLINICAL MANIFESTATIONS OF SALICYLATE POISONING

### Acute Salicylate Poisoning

The earliest signs and symptoms of salicylate toxicity, which include nausea, vomiting, diaphoresis, and tinnitus, typically develop within 1 to 2 hours of acute ingestion. Salicylates are extremely irritating to the GI mucosa; early nausea and vomiting after ingestion are warning signs of a potentially clinically significant ingestion. Pylorospasm, delayed gastric emptying, and decreased GI motility complicate toxicity by altering absorption kinetics. Hemorrhagic gastritis also occurs, likely as a consequence of severe emesis and alteration of protective mucosal GI barriers. Direct stimulation of the respiratory center increases minute volume ventilation, determined by the product of respiratory rate and tidal volume. A primary respiratory alkalosis predominates initially, although an anion gap metabolic acidosis begins to develop early in the course of salicylate toxicity. By the time a symptomatic adult patient presents to the hospital after a salicylate overdose, a mixed acid–base disturbance is often prominent. This latter finding includes two primary processes, respiratory alkalosis and metabolic acidosis. Salicylate-poisoned adults who demonstrate respiratory acidosis should alert the clinician to the fact that systemic toxicity is severe. These patients will likely be late in the clinical course of poisoning and have salicylate-induced ARDS, fatigue from hyperventilating for a prolonged period of time, or CNS depression (from either salicylate itself or coingestants). These broad variations of clinical toxicity can be divided into three general time frames based on rapidly available laboratory testing. The progressive stages of salicylate poisoning are demonstrated in Table 10–1.

| TABLE 10–1 Progressive Acid–Base Stages of Salicylate Poisoning |
|---|
| **Early:** Respiratory alkalosis, alkalemia, and alkaluria |
| **Intermediate:** Respiratory alkalosis, metabolic acidosis, alkalemia, and aciduria |
| **Late:** Metabolic acidosis with either a diminishing respiratory alkalosis or respiratory acidosis, acidemia, and aciduria |

Tinnitus, a subjective sensation of ringing or hissing with or without hearing loss, loss of absolute acoustic sensitivity, and alterations of perceived sounds are the three effects resulting from exposure to large doses of salicylates. Tinnitus is a demonstrable manifestation of CNS toxicity even without alterations in mental status. Patients subsequently develop a spectrum of CNS abnormalities that includes confusion, agitation, and lethargy and then ultimately seizures and coma. The most severe neurologic clinical findings are likely associated with the development of cerebral edema and portend a poor prognosis.

Paratonia, extreme muscle rigidity, is reported in severe salicylate poisoning pre- and postmortem. This excess neuromuscular activity leads to rhabdomyolysis, acute tubular necrosis, and most concerning, hyperthermia, which is typically a preterminal condition.

### Chronic Salicylate Poisoning

Chronic salicylate poisoning most typically occurs in older adults as a result of unintentionally overdosing on salicylates used for secondary prevention of cardiovascular disorders and osteoarthritis in addition to analgesia and as an antipyretic (Table 10–2). Presenting signs and symptoms of chronic salicylate poisoning can be similar to those of acute toxicity and include nausea and vomiting, hearing loss and tinnitus, dyspnea and hyperventilation, tachycardia, hyperthermia, and neurologic manifestations (eg, confusion, delirium, agitation, hyperactivity, slurred speech, hallucinations, seizures, coma). Although there is considerable overlap with acute salicylate poisoning, the slow, insidious onset of chronic poisoning in older adults frequently causes delayed recognition of the true cause of the patient's presentation.

On occasion, ill patients who have chronic salicylate poisoning are misdiagnosed as having delirium, dementia, or encephalopathy of undetermined origin; or diseases such as sepsis (fever of unknown origin), alcoholic ketoacidosis, respiratory failure, or cardiopulmonary disease. A delay in diagnosis is associated with increased morbidity and mortality.

| TABLE 10–2 Differential Characteristics of Acute and Chronic Salicylate Poisoning | | |
|---|---|---|
| | *Acute* | *Chronic* |
| Age | Younger | Older |
| Etiology | Overdose usually intentional | Therapeutic misadventures; iatrogenic |
| Diagnosis | Easily recognized (absent coingestion) | Frequently unrecognized |
| Other diseases | None | Underlying disorders (especially chronic pain conditions) |
| Suicidal ideation | Typical | Atypical |
| Serum concentrations | Marked elevation | Intermediate elevation |
| Mortality | Uncommon when recognized and properly treated | More common due to delayed recognition |

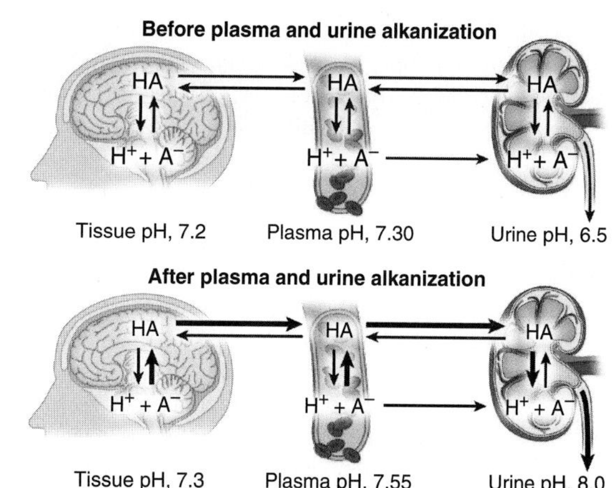


**FIGURE 10–2.** Rationale for alkalinization. Alkalinization of the plasma with respect to the tissues and alkalinization of the urine with respect to plasma shift the equilibrium to the plasma and urine and away from the tissues, including the brain. This equilibrium shift results in "ion trapping" and enhanced urinary elimination.

## EVALUATION AND DIAGNOSTIC TESTING

Systemic toxicity is concerning after the following exposures: ingestion of 150 mg/kg or 6.5 g of aspirin, whichever is less; ingestion of greater than a lick or taste of oil of wintergreen (98% methyl salicylate) by children younger than 6 years of age; and ingestion of more than 4 mL of oil of wintergreen by patients 6 years of age and older. These patients as well as those with significant topical exposures and signs of toxicity should be promptly evaluated for salicylate toxicity.

The initial approach should include a serum salicylate concentration, arterial blood gas (ABG) or venous blood gas (VBG), electrolytes, a urinalysis, and a lactate concentration. Although an anion gap metabolic acidosis is likely found in most cases of salicylate toxicity, severe salicylism is rarely reported to falsely elevate serum chloride, bringing the anion gap closer to a normal range.

### Salicylate Analysis

Serum salicylate concentrations are relatively easy to obtain in most hospital laboratories. Serum salicylate concentrations are commonly reported in mg/dL in the United States, but confusion can arise because values can also be reported in mg/L and μg/mL. It should also be noted that several clinical scenarios and xenobiotic exposures are recognized to cause false-positive or falsely elevated salicylate concentrations. Depending on the assay, medications that reportedly interfered with accurate salicylate measurement include thioridazine, diflunisal, promethazine, prochlorperazine, chlorpromazine, and cysteamine. Hyperbilirubinemia and hyperlipidemia can also cause significant false elevations of serum salicylate concentrations.

### Interpretation of Serum Salicylate Concentrations and Correlation With Toxicity

The recommended therapeutic concentration of salicylate is 15 to 30 mg/dL (1.1-2.2 mmol/L), but this varies by indication. Serum concentrations greater than 30 mg/dL (2.17 mmol/L) are usually not found unless there is a supratherapeutic, acute, or chronic toxic exposure. Unfortunately, the correlation of serum salicylate concentrations and clinical toxicity is often poor and dependent on several factors. A concurrent arterial or venous blood pH should be determined when a serum salicylate concentration is obtained because in the presence of acidemia, more salicylic acid leaves the blood and enters the CSF and other tissues (Fig. 10–2), increasing the toxicity. Animal models demonstrate that CSF concentrations correlate more closely with death than serum concentrations. A decreasing serum salicylate concentration is difficult to interpret in isolation because it may reflect either an increased tissue distribution with increasing toxicity or an increased clearance with decreasing toxicity.

## MANAGEMENT

The management of patients with salicylate poisoning is aimed at supporting vital signs and organ function, preventing or limiting ongoing exposure from the gut or skin, and enhancing elimination of salicylate that has already entered the systemic circulation. It is imperative to understand that there is no true antidote for salicylate toxicity; no xenobiotic can combat the clinical toxicity demonstrated in severe poisoning.

### Gastrointestinal Decontamination and Use of Activated Charcoal

The use of orogastric lavage and activated charcoal (AC) is discussed in Chap. 3 and Antidotes in Brief: A1. Their effects on the absorption and elimination of salicylates have been extensively studied. The sooner AC is given after salicylate ingestion, the more effective it will be in reducing absorption. A 10:1 ratio of AC to ingested salicylate appears to result in maximal efficacy but is often impractical given the fact that ingestions of salicylate often reach 20- to 30-g amounts or more. More than one dose of AC is recommended to achieve desired ratios of AC to salicylate. Overall, the administration of two to four properly timed doses of AC is recommended.

The administration of AC must be balanced against risks of vomiting and aspiration, especially in patients with altered mental status and unprotected airways (Chap. 3). The use of whole-bowel irrigation (WBI) with polyethylene glycol electrolyte lavage solution (PEG-ELS) is reasonable following AC for patients with large ingestions of delayed-release formulations.

### Fluid Replacement

Fluid losses in patients with salicylate poisoning are prominent and can be attributed to hyperventilation, vomiting, fever, a hypermetabolic state, polyuria, and perspiration. For all of these reasons, the patient's volume status must be adequately assessed and corrected if necessary. Increasing fluids beyond restoration is potentially hazardous and unlikely to be beneficial and is therefore not recommended.

### Serum and Urine Alkalinization

The cornerstone of the management of patients with salicylate toxicity is to shift salicylate out of the brain and tissues into the serum, where elimination through the kidneys can then occur. Alkalinization of the serum with respect to the tissues and alkalinization of the urine with respect to the serum accomplishes this goal by facilitating the movement and "ion trapping" of salicylate into the serum and the urine (Fig. 10–2). Renal excretion of salicylate is very dependent on urinary pH. Alkalinizing the urine from a pH of 5 to 8 logarithmically increases renal salicylate clearance from 1.3 to 100 mL/min (Fig. 10–3).

Alkalinization with IV sodium bicarbonate is recommended for all symptomatic patients whose serum salicylate concentrations exceed the therapeutic range and for clinically suspected cases of salicylism until a salicylate concentration is available to guide treatment. Alkalinization is typically achieved with a bolus of 1 to 2 mEq/kg of sodium bicarbonate IV followed by an infusion of 3 ampules of sodium bicarbonate (132 mEq) in 1 L of 5% dextrose in water administered at 1.5 to 2.0 times the maintenance fluid range. Urine pH should be maintained at 7.5 to 8.0, and hypokalemia must be corrected to achieve maximum urinary alkalinization. The volume load should remain modest while previous losses are repleted (Antidotes in Brief: A5).

Hypokalemia is a common complication of salicylate poisoning and sodium bicarbonate therapy and can prevent urinary alkalinization unless corrected. In the presence of hypokalemia, the renal tubules reabsorb potassium ions in exchange for hydrogen ions, preventing urinary alkalinization. If urinary alkalinization cannot be achieved easily, hypokalemia, excretion of organic acids, and salt and water depletion are the likely reasons for failure. Serum potassium concentration should be maintained at 4.0 mEq/L or greater.

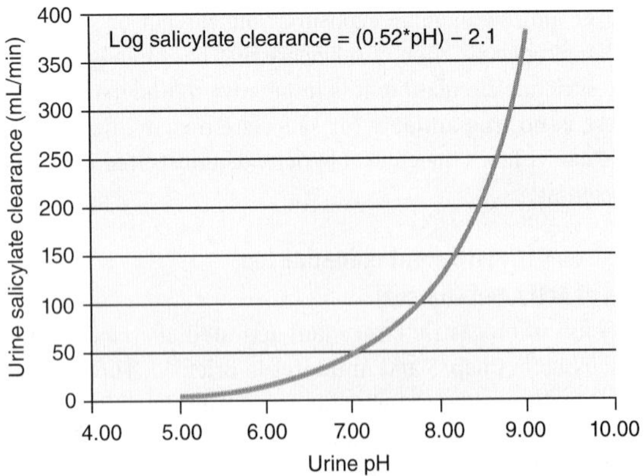


**FIGURE 10–3.** The relationship between urine pH and urine salicylate clearance. This curve was adapted from a logarithmic relationship determined by Kallen in patients with salicylate poisoning. It illustrates the need to substantially increase urine pH above 7 to impact elimination. *(Adapted from: Kallen RJ, et al. Hemodialysis in children: technique, kinetic aspects related to varying body size, and application to salicylate intoxication, acute renal failure and some other disorders. Medicine (Baltimore). 1966;45:1-50.)*

### Glucose Supplementation

Salicylate poisoning significantly alters glucose metabolism, transport, and relative requirements. Clinically, this is relevant in that the presence of a normal serum glucose concentration may not be reflective of a normal CSF glucose concentration. The neurotoxicity of salicylism could be partly caused by this hypoglycorrhachia. Since dextrose administration has reversed acute delirium associated with salicylate toxicity, it is recommended to liberally administer dextrose to all patients with altered mental status and salicylate toxicity regardless of their serum glucose concentration. A bolus of 0.5 to 1 g/kg of dextrose with additional doses or even continuous infusion is recommended for patients being treated for severe salicylate toxicity.

### Extracorporeal Removal

Indications for hemodialysis (HD) are shown in Table 10–3. Hemodialysis will not only remove salicylate but also rapidly correct fluid, electrolyte, and acid–base disorders that will not be corrected by hemoperfusion (HP) alone. Nephrology consultation should be sought early and liberally to

**TABLE 10–3 Indications for Hemodialysis in Patients with Salicylate Poisoning**

**General Recommendation**
- Intermittent hemodialysis is the preferred modality.

**Indications**

Extracorporeal treatment (ECTR) is recommended if *any* of the following are met:
- Salicylate concentration ≥ 100 mg/dL (≥ 7.2 mmol/L)
- Salicylate concentration ≥ 90 mg/dL (≥ 6.5 mmol/L) in the presence of impaired kidney function
- Altered mental status
- New hypoxemia requiring supplemental oxygen
- If standard therapy (eg, supportive measures, bicarbonate) fails and:
  - Salicylate concentration ≥ 90 mg/dL (≥ 6.5 mmol/L)
  - Salicylate concentration ≥ 80 mg/dL (≥ 5.8 mmol/L) in the presence of impaired kidney function
  - If the systemic pH is ≤ 7.20

**Hemodialysis should be continued until**
- There is clear clinical improvement is apparent *and*
- Salicylate concentration < 19 mg/dL (1.4 mmol/L) *or*
- Hemodialysis was performed for a period of at least 4–6 h when salicylate concentrations are not readily available

Reproduced with permission from Juurlink DN, Gosselin S, Kielstein JT, et al. Extracorporeal Treatment for Salicylate Poisoning: Systematic Review and Recommendations From the EXTRIP Workgroup. *Ann Emerg Med.* 2015;66(2):165-181.

anticipate and prevent avoidable morbidity and mortality. Despite the well-recognized benefit of extracorporeal removal of salicylates in severe toxicity, delays in initiating HD remain a potentially preventable cause of death despite repeated calls over many years for prompt HD for patients with salicylate poisoning. While the patient is awaiting HD, alkalinization of serum and urine is recommended using sodium bicarbonate therapy. During HD, it is unnecessary to continue bicarbonate therapy because it will be provided by HD. It is prudent to reinstitute bicarbonate therapy after HD is completed, especially if patients are still symptomatic or serum salicylate concentrations are pending. In Table 10–3, impaired kidney function can be defined as advanced chronic kidney disease, AKI, when baseline not available, elevated creatinine of greater than 2 mg/dL (177 μmol/L) in adults or 1.5 mg/dL (133 μmol/L) in older adults, children with no baseline creatinine concentration, a serum creatinine greater than twice the upper limit of normal for age and sex, or the presence of oligo- or anuria for more than 6 hours, regardless of serum creatinine concentration.

### Sedation, Intubation, and Mechanical Ventilation Risks

Salicylate-poisoned patients have a significantly increased minute ventilation rate brought about by both tachypnea and hyperpnea, often exceeding 20 to 30 L/min. Any decrease in minute ventilation increases the $PCO_2$ and decreases the pH. This shifts salicylate into the CNS, exacerbating toxicity. Thus, extreme caution must be used during sedation, intubation, and initiation of mechanical ventilation.

Although early endotracheal intubation to maintain hyperventilation will aid in the management of patients whose respiratory efforts are faltering, healthcare providers must maintain appropriate hypocarbia through hyperventilation. Ventilator settings that result in an increase in the patient's $PCO_2$ relative to premechanical ventilation will produce relative respiratory acidosis even if serum pH remains in the alkalemic range. Inadequate mechanical ventilation of patients with salicylate poisoning is associated with respiratory acidosis, a decrease in the serum pH, and an abrupt clinical deterioration.

If sedation is required, although there is no clear choice of preferred sedative, the goals are to minimize respiratory depression and use the minimum amount required for desired sedation. If intubation is deemed necessary, which it often is in severe toxicity or multidrug ingestions, the following steps should be taken to optimize before, during, and after intubation conditions. The goal should be to maintain or exceed minute ventilation rates that were present before intubation. Before intubation, an attempt should be made to optimize serum alkalinization by administering a 2 mEq/kg bolus of sodium bicarbonate. Preparations should be made to minimize the time the patient will spend with apnea or decreased ventilation by considering an awake intubation. The provider most experienced in intubation should be present as well as any adjunct materials to increase first-pass success. An intensivist, respiratory technician, or other mechanical ventilator expert should be consulted to help match preintubation minute ventilation. After mechanical ventilation has begun, frequent blood gas monitoring should be obtained and ventilator settings adjusted as needed. If mechanical ventilation has already occurred or is planned in patients with salicylate toxicity, emergent nephrology consult is indicated for HD if not previously obtained.

### Serum Salicylate Concentration and pH Monitoring

Careful observation of the patient, correlation of the serum salicylate concentrations with blood pH, and repeat determinations of serum salicylate concentrations every 2 to 4 hours are essential until the patient is clinically improving and has a low serum salicylate concentration in the presence of a normal or high blood pH. In all cases, after a presumed peak serum salicylate concentration is reached, at least one additional serum concentration should be obtained several hours later. Analyses should be obtained more frequently in managing seriously ill patients to assess the efficacy of treatment and the possible need for HD.

### Pediatric Considerations

The predominant primary respiratory alkalosis that initially characterizes salicylate poisoning in adults either does not occur or is often transient in young children. This likely results from the limited ventilatory reserve of small children that prevents the same degree of sustained hyperpnea as occurs in adults. Although after a significant salicylate exposure, some children present with a mixed acid–base disturbance and a normal or high pH, most present with acidemia, suggesting the need for more urgent intervention because the protective effect of alkalemia on CNS penetration of salicylate is already lost. Although not routinely recommended, exchange transfusion effectively removes large quantities of salicylate in infants too small to undergo emergent HD without extensive delays.

### Pregnancy

Salicylate poisoning during pregnancy poses a particular hazard to fetuses because of the acid–base and hematologic characteristics of fetuses and placental circulation. Salicylates cross the placenta and are present in higher concentrations in a fetus than in the mother. The respiratory stimulation that occurs in the mother after toxic exposures does not occur in the fetus, which has a decreased capacity to buffer acid. The ability of a fetus to metabolize and excrete salicylates is also less than in the mother. This raises concerns that a fetus is at greater risk from salicylate exposures than is the mother. The need for emergent delivery of near-term fetuses of salicylate-poisoned mothers should be evaluated on a case-by-case basis. For salicylate-poisoned pregnant women who cannot undergo emergent delivery, decontamination and elimination strategies should be performed in a critical care setting with consultation from medical toxicology, nephrology, and obstetrics.

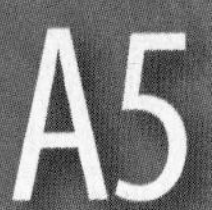

# A5 SODIUM BICARBONATE

## INTRODUCTION

Sodium bicarbonate is a nonspecific antidote that is effective in the treatment of a variety of poisonings by means of a number of distinct mechanisms (Table A5–1).

## PHARMACOLOGY

The onset of action of intravenous (IV) sodium bicarbonate is rapid, with a duration of action of 8 to 10 minutes. Sodium bicarbonate increases plasma bicarbonate and buffers excess hydrogen ion. The apparent bicarbonate space (ABS, or volume of distribution) proportionally increases in severe acidemia. In human studies, the ABS in liters = $(0.36 + 2.44/[HCO_3^-]) \times$ weight (kg).

## ALTERED INTERACTION BETWEEN XENOBIOTIC AND SODIUM CHANNEL

The most important role of sodium bicarbonate in toxicology is the ability to reverse potentially fatal cardiotoxic effects of myocardial $Na^+$ channel blockers such as cyclic antidepressants (CAs) and other type IA and IC antidysrhythmics. Sodium bicarbonate has a crucial antidotal role in myocardial $Na^+$ channel blocker poisoning by increasing the number of open $Na^+$ channels, thereby partially reversing fast $Na^+$ channel blockade. This decreases QRS complex prolongation and reduces life-threatening cardiovascular toxicity such as ventricular dysrhythmias and hypotension. The animal evidence supports two distinct and additive mechanisms for this effect: a pH-dependent effect and a sodium-dependent effect. The pH-dependent effect increases the fraction of the more freely diffusible nonionized xenobiotic. Both the ionized xenobiotic and the nonionized forms are able to bind to the $Na^+$ channel, but approximately 90% of the block results from the ionized form. Increase in the nonionized fraction limits the quantity of xenobiotic available to bind to the $Na^+$ channel. The sodium-dependent effect increases the availability of $Na^+$ ions to pass through the open channels. While both hyperventilation (respiratory alkalosis) and hypertonic saline improve conduction, hypertonic sodium bicarbonate was shown to be superior in both animal models and in vitro studies.

Prospective validation of treatment criteria for use of sodium bicarbonate after CA overdose has not been performed. Recommended indications are conduction delays (QRS complex duration greater than 100 ms), wide-complex tachydysrhythmias, and hypotension. Because studies demonstrate a critical threshold QRS complex duration (160 ms or greater) at which ventricular dysrhythmias significantly increase in propensity, it seems reasonable that narrowing the QRS complex duration through use of sodium bicarbonate or hyperventilation prevents the development of dysrhythmias. Although sodium bicarbonate has no proven efficacy in either the treatment or prophylaxis of CA-induced seizures, seizures often produce acidemia, which rapidly increases the risks of conduction disturbances and ventricular dysrhythmias. Administering sodium bicarbonate when the QRS complex duration is 100 ms or greater establishes a theoretical margin of safety in the event the patient suddenly deteriorates without adding significant immediate risk.

Because cardiotoxicity often worsens during the first few hours after ingestion, we recommend sodium bicarbonate therapy be initiated immediately if the QRS complex is greater than 100 ms. Because CA-induced hypotension responds to sodium bicarbonate, we recommend hypotension be treated with prompt sodium bicarbonate therapy. In CA-poisoned patients who present with altered mental status or seizures without QRS complex widening or hypotension, we recommend **not** to give sodium bicarbonate. It is reasonable to discontinue sodium bicarbonate upon hemodynamic improvement and resolution of cardiac conduction abnormalities and altered mental status, although controlled data supporting such an approach are lacking.

Sodium bicarbonate is useful to alkalinize the serum of patients with cardiotoxicity from other myocardial $Na^+$ channel blockers who present with widened QRS complexes, dysrhythmias, and hypotension as listed in Table A5–1. For all these indications, we recommend IV administration of 1 to 2 mEq of sodium bicarbonate per kilogram of body weight as a bolus followed by a continuous sodium bicarbonate infusion of 150 mEq in 1 L of 5% dextrose in water ($D_5W$) at 150 to 200 mL/h (or about twice the maintenance requirements in a child).

## ALTERED XENOBIOTIC IONIZATION TO ALTER DISTRIBUTION AND ENHANCE ELIMINATION

### Salicylates

Alkalinizing the urine with sodium bicarbonate is recommended in the treatment of salicylate toxicity. Through its ability to alter the concentration gradient of the ionized and nonionized fractions of salicylates, sodium bicarbonate decreases tissue (eg, CNS) concentrations of salicylates and enhances urinary elimination of salicylates (Fig. 10–2). Salicylate lethality is directly related to primary CNS dysfunction, which in turn corresponds to a critical brain salicylate concentration. At physiologic pH, at which a very small proportion of the salicylate is in the nonionized form, a small change in pH is associated with a significant change in amount of nonionized molecules. For example, as the pH decreases from 7.40 to 7.20, the percent of salicylate molecules in the nonionized form doubles. In experimental models, lowering the blood pH produced a shift of salicylate into the tissues and increasing the blood pH with sodium bicarbonate produced a shift in salicylate out of the tissues and into the

**TABLE A5–1 Sodium Bicarbonate: Mechanisms, Site of Action, and Uses in Toxicology**

| *Mechanism* | *Site of Action* | *Uses* |
|---|---|---|
| Alters interaction between the xenobiotic and $Na^+$ channel | Heart | β-Adrenergic antagonists with MSA<br>Amantadine<br>Bupropion<br>Carbamazepine<br>Chloroquine<br>Citalopram<br>Cocaine<br>Cyclic antidepressants<br>Dimenhydrinate<br>Diphenhydramine<br>Disopyramide<br>Encainide<br>Flecainide<br>Fluoxetine<br>Hydroxychloroquine<br>Lamotrigine<br>Mesoridazine<br>Orphenadrine<br>Procainamide<br>Propafenone<br>Propoxyphene<br>Quinidine<br>Quinine<br>Thioridazine<br>Venlafaxine |
| Alters xenobiotic ionization leading to altered tissue distribution | Retina<br>Brain | Formic acid<br>Phenobarbital<br>Salicylates |
| Alters xenobiotic ionization leading to enhanced xenobiotic elimination | Kidneys | Chlorophenoxy herbicides<br>Chlorpropamide<br>Diflunisal<br>Fluoride<br>Formic acid<br>Methotrexate<br>Phenobarbital<br>Salicylates<br>Uranium |
| Corrects life-threatening acidemia | Metabolic | Cyanide<br>Ethylene glycol<br>Metformin<br>Methanol |
| Increases xenobiotic solubility | Kidneys | DAMPA<br>Methotrexate |
| Neutralization | Lungs | Chlorine gas, HCl |
| Maintenance of chelator effect | Kidneys | Dimercaprol (BAL)–metal |
| Prevents ferrihemate release from myoglobin | Kidneys | Drug-induced rhabdomyolysis |
| Shifts potassium into cells | | Drug-induced hyperkalemia |

BAL = British anti-Lewisite; DAMPA = methotrexate metabolite 4-amino-4-deoxy-10-methylpteroic acid; MSA = membrane-stabilizing activity: acebutolol, betaxolol, carvedilol, metoprolol, oxprenolol, propranolol.

blood. Enhancing the elimination of salicylate by trapping ionized salicylate in the urine is also beneficial. The relationship between salicylate clearance and urine pH suggests that increasing urine pH from 5.0 to 8.0 could increase the amount of salicylate cleared by almost 40-fold.

We recommend sodium bicarbonate in the treatment of salicylate poisoning for most patients with evidence of significant systemic toxicity or toxic serum concentrations. Relative contraindications to sodium bicarbonate use include severe acute kidney injury (AKI) or chronic kidney disease (CKD) and acute respiratory distress syndrome. We recommend alkalinization be started with a continuous sodium bicarbonate infusion of 150 mEq in 1 L of dextrose in water ($D_5W$) at 150 to 200 mL/h (or about twice the maintenance requirements in a child). Continued titration with sodium bicarbonate over 4 to 8 hours is recommended until the urinary pH reaches 7.5 to 8.0. For patients with and initial low serum bicarbonate, we recommend an IV bolus of 1 to 2 mEq of sodium bicarbonate per kilogram of body weight. The addition of the dextrose is important because salicylate toxicity causes hypoglycemia. Fastidious attention to the patient's changing acid–base status is required. Blood pH should not rise above 7.55 to prevent complications of alkalemia. It is important to maintain a normal potassium concentration because in hypokalemic patients, the kidneys preferentially reabsorb potassium in exchange for hydrogen ions. Urinary alkalinization will be unsuccessful as long as hydrogen ions are excreted into the urine.

## Phenobarbital

Although cardiopulmonary support is the most critical intervention for the treatment of patients with severe phenobarbital overdose, sodium bicarbonate is a useful adjunct. As in the case of salicylates, alkalinization of the urine reduces the severity and duration of toxicity. Given relatively high pKa of phenobarbital, significant urinary phenobarbital accumulation is evident only when urinary pH is increased above 7.5. As the pH approaches 8.0, a threefold increase in urinary elimination occurs. In humans, urinary alkalinization with sodium bicarbonate was associated with a decrease in phenobarbital elimination half-life from 148 to 47 hours. However, this beneficial effect was less than the effect achieved by multiple-dose activated charcoal (MDAC), which reduced the half-life to 19 hours. Interestingly, the combination of MDAC and urine alkalinization proved inferior to MDAC alone but was better than alkalinization alone.

We do not currently recommend sodium bicarbonate therapy for the treatment of patients with ingestions of other barbiturates, such as pentobarbital and secobarbital, which either have a pKa above 8.0 or are predominantly eliminated hepatically. The dosing recommendations are the same as for salicylates, although a bolus is rarely needed.

## Methotrexate

Urinary alkalinization with sodium bicarbonate in addition to hydration is routinely used during high-dose methotrexate cancer chemotherapy to achieve a urine pH of 7.0 or greater prior to methotrexate administration. Methotrexate is predominantly eliminated unchanged in the urine. Unfortunately, methotrexate, as well as its metabolites DAMPA (4-amino-4-deoxy-10-methylpteroic acid) and 7-hydroxymethotrexate, are poorly water soluble in acidic urine. Under these conditions, tubular precipitation of the methotrexate occurs, leading to AKI and decreased elimination, increasing the likelihood of methotrexate toxicity. Administration of sodium bicarbonate (as well as intensive hydration) during high-dose methotrexate infusions increases methotrexate solubility and the elimination of methotrexate and its metabolites.

In practice, urine alkalization is typically maintained with intravenous sodium bicarbonate 50 to 150 mEq/L to achieve adequate urine flow and alkalinization until leucovorin administration ceases. In the setting of methotrexate toxicity, it is reasonable to provide sodium bicarbonate 150 mEq in 1 L of $D_5W$ at 150 to 250 mL/h in a manner similar to salicylate toxicity to prevent precipitation of methotrexate in the kidney; clearance is confirmed with serial methotrexate concentrations.

### Chlorophenoxy Herbicides

Urinary alkalinization is recommended in the treatment of patients with poisonings from herbicides that contain chlorophenoxy compounds, such as 2,4-dichlorophenoxyacetic acid (2,4-D) or 2-(4-chloro-2-methylphenoxy) propionic acid (MCPP). These compounds are weak acids (pKa of 2.6 and 3.8 for 2,4-D and MCPP, respectively) that are excreted largely unchanged in the urine. In an uncontrolled case series of 41 patients poisoned with a variety of chlorophenoxy herbicides, 19 of whom received sodium bicarbonate, alkaline diuresis significantly reduced the half-life of each by enhancing renal elimination. Dosing recommendations are the same as for salicylates.

## CORRECTION OF LIFE-THREATENING METABOLIC ACIDOSIS

Some toxins cause an accumulation of acid byproducts leading to metabolic acidosis. Unchecked, metabolic acidosis leading to acidemia has important physiologic consequences. When blood pH decreases from 7.40 to 7.20, cardiac output increases because of increased catecholamine concentrations, but when below 7.10 to 7.20, a decrease in cardiac output ensues. Other cardiovascular effects include increased propensity for dysrhythmias, decreased systemic vascular tone, and pulmonary vasoconstriction. The respiratory system suffers from increased respiratory stimulus and increased work of breathing. Additionally, 2,3-BPG (2,3-bisphosphoglycerate) decreases, leading to a rightward shift of the oxygen dissociation curve and decreased release of oxygen to the tissues. Further consequences include cerebral vasodilation, hyperkalemia, hypercalcemia, increased renal oxygen demand and diuresis, decreased splanchnic perfusion with delayed gastric emptying, impaired platelet aggregation, and coagulopathy.

Treatment of metabolic acidosis is largely aimed at treating the underlying cause. However, because the effects of persistent acidemia are severe, sodium bicarbonate is reasonable to administer to correct the acidemia in select poisonings such as toxic alcohols and metformin toxicity, pending the institution of more definitive therapy.

## TOXIC ALCOHOLS

Sodium bicarbonate has two important roles in treating patients with toxic alcohol ingestions. As an immediate temporizing measure, it is reasonable to administer sodium bicarbonate to treat the life-threatening acidemia associated with toxic alcohol ingestions. In rats poisoned with ethylene glycol, the administration of sodium bicarbonate alone resulted in a fourfold increase in the median lethal dose. The second role of bicarbonate in the treatment of toxic alcohol poisoning involves its ability to favorably alter the distribution and elimination of certain toxic metabolites. In cases of methanol poisoning, the proportion of ionized formic acid is increased by administering bicarbonate, thereby trapping formic acid in the blood compartment. Consequently, this results in the removal of the toxic metabolite from the ocular compartment and decreases visual toxicity.

Early treatment with sodium bicarbonate is recommended in cases of methanol and ethylene glycol poisoning. Sodium bicarbonate therapy should be administered to toxic alcohol-poisoned patients with an arterial pH below 7.30. More than 400 to 600 mEq of sodium bicarbonate may be required in the first few hours. In cases of ethylene glycol toxicity, sodium bicarbonate administration worsens hypocalcemia, so the serum calcium concentration should be monitored. Treating the acidemia, however, is not the mainstay of therapy, but rather a temporizing measure while evaluating the need to administer IV fomepizole or ethanol, and if indications for hemodialysis are present.

### Metformin

Metformin toxicity, either from overdose or therapeutic use in the setting of AKI or CKD, causes severe, life-threatening metabolic acidemia with an elevated lactate concentration. The use of high-dose sodium bicarbonate to correct the metabolic acidosis, as well as extracorporeal removal of the metformin, is recommended in these cases. Although an exact threshold for initiating sodium bicarbonate therapy is not well-defined, it would be reasonable to initiate therapy in severe acidemia, similar to that of other metabolic causes of acidemia (pH < 7.10, serum bicarbonate < 10 mmol/L).

## NEUTRALIZATION

### Chlorine Gas

Inhaled dilute sodium bicarbonate neutralizes the hydrochloric acid that is formed when the chlorine gas reacts with the water in the respiratory tree. In a sheep model of chlorine inhalation, animals treated with 4% nebulized sodium bicarbonate solution demonstrated a higher $PO_2$ and lower $PCO_2$ than did the 0.9% sodium chloride–treated animals. There was no difference, however, in 24-hour mortality rate or pulmonary histopathology. Patients exposed to chlorine gas who received nebulized sodium bicarbonate had significantly higher forced expiratory volume in 1 second ($FEV_1$) values at 120 and 240 minutes and scored significantly higher on a posttreatment quality of life questionnaire than those who were not treated with nebulized sodium bicarbonate. It is reasonable to treat with a nebulized solution of 4 mL of sodium bicarbonate solution (diluted to approximately 4%)

in addition to humidified oxygen and inhaled $\beta_2$-adrenergic agonists. Nebulized sodium bicarbonate failed to demonstrate a benefit in the treatment of chloramine gas exposure.

## OTHER INDICATIONS

Adverse effects and safety concerns are associated with the dissociation of the dimercaprol (British anti-Lewisite {BAL}) metal binding that occurs in acid urine. Because dissociation of the BAL–metal chelate occurs in acidic urine, it is recommended to alkalinize the urine of patients receiving BAL with hypertonic sodium bicarbonate to a pH of 7.5 to 8.0 to prevent renal liberation of the metal. Sodium bicarbonate also provides a renal protective benefit in animals after exposure to depleted uranium.

## ADVERSE EFFECTS AND SAFETY ISSUES

The use of sodium bicarbonate has associated risks. Excessive alkalemia (with adverse effects upon respiratory physiology), hypernatremia, fluid overload, hypokalemia, and hypocalcemia can occur with prolonged infusion. Extravasation can cause local tissue damage. Dobutamine and norepinephrine, among other medications are incompatible with sodium bicarbonate solutions. If mixed with sodium bicarbonate calcium solutions precipitate.

## PREGNANCY AND LACTATION

According to the US Food and Drug Administration (FDA), sodium bicarbonate is a Category C drug and is compatible with breastfeeding.

## DOSING AND ADMINISTRATION

### Serum Alkalinization

For the treatment of QRS complex prolongation in the setting of myocardial sodium channel poisoning, we recommend administration of 1 to 2 mEq/kg of sodium bicarbonate IV as a bolus over a period of 1 to 2 minutes. Greater amounts, totaling as much as 35 mEq/kg over hours of resuscitation, are sometimes required to treat patients with recurrent unstable ventricular dysrhythmias. Similar boluses should be repeated as needed to achieve a blood pH of 7.50 to 7.55. Because sodium bicarbonate has a brief duration of effect, a continuous infusion usually is required after the initial IV boluses especially with ingestion of xenobiotics with a long duration of action. The treatment endpoint is the narrowing of the QRS complex. Excessive alkalemia (pH > 7.55) and hypernatremia should be avoided. To prepare a sodium bicarbonate infusion, three 50-mL ampules of 8.4% or 7.5% solution should be placed in 1 L of $D_5W$ and run at twice maintenance with frequent evaluation of the QRS duration, potassium concentration, and pH, depending on the fluid requirements and blood pressure of the patient. Frequent evaluation of the fluid status should be performed to avoid precipitating pulmonary edema. An optimal duration of therapy has not been established.

### Urine Alkalinization

For the treatment of patients with salicylate poisoning or other poisonings requiring urinary alkalinization, sodium bicarbonate should be administered by bolus or infusion using the dosing strategies described earlier to achieve a serum pH of 7.45 to 7.55, with a goal of a urinary pH of 8.0. Careful and frequent monitoring of the urinary pH and serum potassium concentration is critical to ensure optimal treatment. In salicylate-poisoned patients with altered mental status, administration of sodium bicarbonate is required to ensure that the serum pH is greater than at least 7.40 to 7.45.

## FORMULATIONS

The most commonly used sodium bicarbonate preparations are an 8.4% solution (1 M) containing 1 mEq each of sodium and bicarbonate ions per milliliter (calculated osmolarity of 2,000 mOsm/L) and a 7.5% solution containing 0.892 mEq each of sodium and bicarbonate ions per milliliter (calculated osmolarity of 1,786 mOsm/L). The common infant formulation is a 4.2% solution packaged as a 10-mL injectable ampule. This yields 5 mEq per ampule (0.5 mEq/mL each of sodium and bicarbonate ions).

# 11 BOTULISM

## HISTORY AND EPIDEMIOLOGY

Botulism, a potentially fatal neuroparalytic illness, results from exposure to botulinum neurotoxin (BoNT), which is produced by the bacterium *Clostridium botulinum* and other *Clostridium* species. The earliest cases of botulism were described in Europe in 1735 and were attributed to improperly preserved German sausage; the name of the disease alludes to this association because *botulus* is the Latin word for *sausage*. In adults, most cases result from ingestion of toxin in contaminated food, but in infants, most cases result from consumption of bacterial spores that proliferate and produce toxin in the gastrointestinal (GI) tract. Less common forms of botulism include wound botulism, in which spores are inoculated into a wound and locally produce toxin, and inhalational botulism caused by aerosolized BoNT, which potentially can be used as a weapon of bioterrorism.

Botulism outbreaks occur throughout the world. In 2016, a total of 150 laboratory-confirmed cases and 10 probable cases of botulism were reported to the United States (US) Centers for Disease Control and Prevention (CDC). In the past 50 years, home-processed food has accounted for 65% of outbreaks, with commercial food processing constituting only 7% of reported cases; in the remaining outbreaks, the origin is unknown. Of 29 laboratory-confirmed cases of foodborne botulism in 2016, there were three multicase outbreaks, each involving two or three patients. Among hundreds of reports of botulism from 1975 to 1988 involving more than 400 persons, approximately 70% involved only one person, 20% involved two persons, and only 10% involved more than two persons, yielding a mean of 2.7 cases per outbreak. Single affected patients were more severely ill, presumably because diagnosis in the index case leads to more rapid therapeutic intervention for associated cases.

## BACTERIOLOGY

The genus *Clostridium* comprises a group of four spore-forming anaerobic gram-positive bacillary species that produce eight different neurotoxic proteins. *C. botulinum* produces all BoNT serotypes A through H, *C. baratii* produces toxin type F, *C. butyricum* produces tunioxin type E, and *C. argentinense* (sometimes considered a subgroup of *C. botulinum*) produces toxin type G. Most cases of botulism result from BoNT types A, B, E, or F.

Clostridial species are ubiquitous, and the bacteria and spores are present in soil, seawater, and air. In the US, toxin type A is found in soil west of the Mississippi; type B is found east of the Mississippi; and type E is found in the Pacific northwest and the Great Lakes states. Toxin types A and B typically are found in poorly processed meats and vegetables. Toxin type E is commonly found in raw or fermented marine fish and mammals.

All botulinum spores are dormant and highly resistant to damage. They withstand boiling at 212°F (100°C) for hours, although they usually are destroyed by 30 minutes of moist heat at 248°F (120°C). Factors that promote germination of spores in food are pH greater than 4.5, sodium chloride content less than 3.5%, and low nitrite concentration. Unlike the spores, the toxin itself is heat labile and is destroyed by heating to 176°F (80°C) for 30 minutes or to 212°F (100°C) for 10 minutes.

Foods contaminated with *C. botulinum* toxin types A and B often look or smell putrefied because of the action of proteolytic enzymes. In contrast, because toxin type E organisms are saccharolytic and not proteolytic, foods contaminated with toxin type E typically look and taste normal.

## PHARMACOKINETICS AND TOXICOKINETICS

BoNT is the most potent toxin known. The $LD_{50}$ for mice is 3 million molecules injected intraperitoneally. The human oral lethal dose is 1 μg. Foodborne botulism results from ingestion of preformed BoNT from food contaminated with *Clostridium* spores. The median incubation period for all patients is 1 day, but it ranges from 0 to 7 days for toxin type A, 0 to 5 days for toxin type B, and 0 to 2 days for toxin type E.

Infant botulism results from ingestion of *C. botulinum* spores, which germinate in the GI tract and produce toxin. The immaturity of the bacterial flora in the infant GI tract facilitates colonization by the organisms. Adults with altered GI tracts (eg, those who have undergone gastric bypass or are taking proton pump inhibitors or $H_2$ antagonists) also rarely develop botulism in the same way, with the onset of symptoms typically following ingestion by 1 or 2 months. In wound botulism, spores proliferate in a wound or abscess and locally elaborate toxin. The incubation period is typically less than 2 weeks, but delays as long as 51 days are reported.

## PATHOPHYSIOLOGY

Botulinum neurotoxin is produced as a protein consisting of a single polypeptide chain. To become fully active, the single-chain polypeptide undergoes proteolytic cleavage to generate a dichain structure consisting of a heavy chain linked by a disulfide bond to a light chain. The ingested toxin binds to serotype-specific receptors on the mucosal surfaces of gastric and small intestinal epithelial cells, where endocytosis is followed by transcytosis, permitting release of the toxin on the serosal (basolateral) cell surface. The dichain form travels intravascularly to peripheral cholinergic nerve terminals, where it binds rapidly and irreversibly to the cell membrane and is taken up by endocytosis. The heavy chain is responsible for cell-specific membrane binding to acetylcholine-containing neurons where it is rapidly moved intracellularly and the light chain is released into the cytosol. Once inside the cell, the light chain inhibits acetylcholine release (Fig. 11–1).

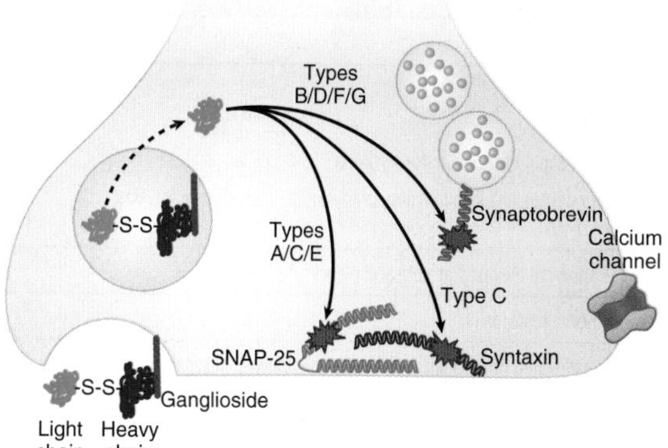


**FIGURE 11–1.** Botulinum toxins consist of two peptides linked by disulfide bonds. The heavy chain is responsible for specific binding to acetylcholine (ACh)-containing neurons. After binding to the cell surface, the entire complex undergoes endocytosis and subsequent translocation of the light chain into the nerve cell cytoplasm. The light chain contains a zinc-requiring endopeptidase that cleaves soluble *N*-ethylmaleimide sensitive factor (NSF) attachment protein receptor (SNARE) proteins belonging to the docking-fusion complex required for neuroexocytosis of ACh. These proteins may be associated with the synaptic vesicles (v-SNARE) or with their targets on the presynaptic membrane (t-SNARE). Botulinum neurotoxin types A and E proteolyze the t-SNARE protein known as synaptosomal-associated protein (SNAP)-25, and BoNT type C cleaves both SNAP-25 and syntaxin, which is attached to SNAP-25 and to the presynaptic membrane. Botulinum neurotoxin types B, D, F, and G target the v-SNARE protein VAMP/synapto synaptobrevin. As a result of cleavage of these components of the docking complex by the endopeptidase, ACh is not released and neuromuscular transmission is impaired.

## CLINICAL MANIFESTATIONS

### Foodborne Botulism

The onset of symptoms typically occurs the day after ingestion. Early GI signs and symptoms of botulism include nausea, vomiting, abdominal distension, and pain. However, the initial phase of the disease often is so subtle that it is often misdiagnosed on the first visit to a healthcare provider. A time lag (from 12 hours to several days but usually not more than 24 hours) typically occurs before neurologic signs and symptoms appear. Common findings include diplopia (often horizontal); blurred vision with impaired accommodation; and bilaterally symmetric flaccid paralysis, which typically begins in cranial muscles and descends to the limbs. Constipation caused by smooth muscle involvement is frequent, and urinary retention and ileus also occur. Anticholinergic-like effects such as dry mouth, dysphagia, and dysarthria or dysphonia (manifested by a nasal quality to the voice) occur, and many patients exhibit fixed mydriatic pupils with ptosis. Deep tendon reflexes are usually reduced or absent. Hypotension and bradycardia sometimes develop, but temperature regulation is normal. Severe weakness of respiratory muscles necessitates intubation and mechanical ventilation. Importantly, mental status and sensation remain normal. The differential diagnosis of botulism includes a variety of toxicologic and nontoxicologic conditions (Table 11–1). The most difficult and frequently encountered diagnostic challenge is differentiating between botulism and the Miller Fisher variant of Guillain-Barré syndrome (Table 11–2).

### Infant Botulism

Cases of infant botulism have now been confirmed from all inhabited continents. Interestingly, 95% of reported cases occur in the US and infant botulism is the most common form of botulism in the US. Affected children are younger than 1 year (median, 15 weeks). The first signs of infant botulism are constipation; difficulty with feeding, sucking, and swallowing; a feeble cry; and diffusely decreased muscle tone

**TABLE 11–1A Toxicologic Differential Diagnosis of Botulism**

| *Xenobiotic Exposure* | *Typical Associated Findings* |
|---|---|
| Aminoglycosides | Paralysis (usually in a patient with myasthenia gravis or other neuromuscular disorders) |
| Anticholinergics | Mydriasis, vasodilation, fever, tachycardia, ileus, dry mucosa, urinary retention, altered mental status |
| Batrachotoxin (eg, poison dart frog) | Paralysis is rapid, cardiac arrest |
| Buckthorn (*Karwinskia humboldtiana*) | Rapidly progressive ascending paralytic neuropathy with quadriplegia |
| Carbon monoxide | Headache, nausea, altered mental status, tachypnea, elevated carboxyhemoglobin level |
| Conotoxin (cone snails) | Burning, itching, and edema at site of sting; circumoral paresthesias; nausea; facial muscle paralysis, ptosis, sialorrhea; respiratory and cardiac arrest |
| Depolarizing and nondepolarizing neuromuscular blockers (eg, curare, succinylcholine, rocuronium, vecuronium) | Paralysis without sedation or sensory involvement |
| Diphtheria | Exudative pharyngitis, cardiac manifestations, hypotension, demyelinating neuropathy with cranial nerve involvement (late) |
| Bungarotoxin (Elapids: kraits, coral snakes, sea snakes) | Cramps, fasciculations, tremor, salivation, nausea, vomiting followed by bulbar palsy and paralysis including slurred speech, diplopia, ptosis, dysphagia, dyspnea, respiratory compromise |
| Organic phosphorus compounds, carbamates | Salivation, lacrimation, urination, defecation, miosis, fasciculations, bronchorrhea, delayed neuropathy |
| Paralytic shellfish poisoning (saxitoxin, neosaxitoxin) | Incubation < 1 h, dysesthesias, paresthesias, dysphagia, respiratory paralysis |
| Tetrodotoxin (pufferfish, blue-ringed octopus, *Taricha spp* newts) | Nausea, diarrhea; circumoral paresthesias, dizziness, hypotension, bradycardia<br>When severe: hypersalivation, cyanosis, diaphoresis, dysphagia, anarthria |
| Thallium | Alopecia, painful ascending sensory neuropathy, constipation, cranial neuropathy, Mees lines |

**TABLE 11–1B Nontoxicologic Differential Diagnosis of Botulism**

| *Condition* | *Typical Associated Findings* |
|---|---|
| Electrolyte abnormalities | |
| • Hyperkalemia | Fatigue, dyspnea, palpitations, nausea, vomiting, paresthesias |
| • Hypokalemia | Fatigue, exercise intolerance, myalgia, dyspnea, palpitations or dysrhythmia |
| • Hypermagnesemia | Hyporeflexia, facial paresthesias, respiratory depression, hypotension, bradycardia, ileus, diffuse flushing, nausea, vomiting |
| Encephalitis | Fever, altered mental status, seizures; CSF showing elevated protein and pleocytosis |
| Food "poisoning" (other bacterial) | Rapid onset of disease; absence of cranial nerve findings |
| Guillain-Barré syndrome or acute inflammatory demyelinating polyneuropathy (and Miller Fisher variant) | Areflexia, paresthesias, ataxia, CSF showing elevated protein without pleocytosis, slowed nerve conduction velocity; ophthalmoparesis in Miller Fisher syndrome |
| Hypokalemic periodic paralysis | Proximal muscle weakness; no cranial nerve involvement or sensory findings |
| Inflammatory or infectious myelopathy and polyradiculopathy | Complete (transverse) or incomplete spinal syndrome with paraparesis or sensory level or sensory signs; possible sphincter dysfunction or back pain; may be preceded by viral illness; CSF pleocytosis and elevated protein |
| Lambert-Eaton myasthenic syndrome | Neoplasm (especially small cell lung cancer), limb weakness exceeding ocular or bulbar weakness, increased strength after sustained contractions; postexercise facilitation on repetitive nerve stimulation; antibodies to voltage-gated calcium channels |
| Myasthenia gravis | Aggravation of fatigue with exercise, fluctuating weakness, acetylcholine receptor or muscle-specific (MuSK) antibodies, positive edrophonium test, decremental response on high-frequency repetitive nerve stimulation |
| Poliomyelitis | Fever, GI symptoms, asymmetric weakness; CSF showing elevated protein and pleocytosis |
| Polymyositis | Insidious onset; proximal limb weakness; dysphagia; muscle tenderness sometimes present; elevated creatine kinase, aldolase, C-reactive protein, and ESR; fibrillations and sharp waves on electromyography |
| Stroke | Asymmetric weakness, abnormal brain imaging |
| Tetanus | Rigidity; cranial nerves usually normal |
| Tick paralysis (*Dermacentor spp*) | Rapidly evolving paralysis, ptosis, absence of paresthesias; normal CSF analysis, presence of an embedded tick with resolution upon removal |

CSF = cerebrospinal fluid; ESR = erythrocyte sedimentation rate; GI = gastrointestinal.

("floppy baby"). The hypotonia is particularly apparent in the limbs and neck. Ophthalmoplegia, loss of facial grimacing, dysphagia, diminished gag reflex, poor anal sphincter tone, and respiratory failure are often present, but fever does not occur. Mydriasis typically is present. Because the toxin in infant botulism is absorbed gradually as it is produced, the onset of clinical manifestations commonly is less abrupt than in severe cases of foodborne botulism.

Infant botulism results from ingestion of *C. botulinum* organisms in food or following the inhalation or ingestion of organism-laden aerosolized dust. Many cases occur near construction sites or soil disruption for other reasons, or in children of parents who work in construction, farming, plant nursery, or plumbing. Honey is the only food generally considered likely to be a risk factor for infant botulism. Although bile acids and gastric acid in the GI tract inhibit clostridial growth in older children and adults, gastric acidity is reduced in the infant during the first few months of life. Approximately 70% of infant botulism cases occur in breastfed infants, even though only 45% to 50% of all infants are breastfed. Formula-

**TABLE 11–2 Differentiating Botulism from Guillain-Barré Syndrome**

| | *Botulism* | *Guillain-Barré Syndrome* | *Miller Fisher Variant of Guillain-Barré Syndrome* |
|---|---|---|---|
| Fever | Absent (except in wound botulism) | Occasionally present | Occasionally present |
| Pupils | Dilated or unreactive (50%) | Normal | Normal |
| Ophthalmoparesis | Present (early) | May be present (late) | Present (early) |
| Paralysis | Descending | Ascending (classically, but not necessarily) | Descending |
| Deep tendon reflexes | Diminished | Absent | Absent |
| Ataxia | Absent | Often present | Present |
| Paresthesias | Absent | Present | Present |
| CSF protein | Normal | Elevated (late) | Elevated (late) |

CSF = cerebrospinal fluid.

fed infants are rapidly colonized with organisms that inhibit *C. botulinum* multiplication.

Patients with infant botulism must be managed in the hospital, preferably in a pediatric intensive care unit, at least for the first week, when the risk of respiratory arrest is greatest. In one series, younger patients were more likely to require mechanical ventilation. Airway complications of intubation such as stridor, granuloma formation, and subglottic stenosis are common, yet tracheotomy is infrequently required. The survival rate in infant botulism is approximately 98% with treatment and most patients are discharged home from the hospital.

### Wound Botulism

Classic presentation of wound botulism involves a motor vehicle crash resulting in a deep muscle laceration, crush injury, or compound fracture treated with open reduction. The wound typically is dirty and associated with inadequate débridement, subsequent purulent drainage, and local tenderness, although in some cases, the wound appears clean and uninfected. Four to 18 days later, cranial nerve palsies and other neurologic findings typical of botulism appear. Other manifestations characteristic of food-related botulism, such as GI symptoms, usually are absent.

### Adult Intestinal Colonization Botulism

Prior to 1997, only 15 cases were reported. Patients invariably have anatomic or functional GI abnormalities. Risk factors favoring organism persistence and *C. botulinum* colonization include achlorhydria (surgically or pharmacologically induced), previous intestinal surgery, and probably recent antibiotic therapy. These factors compromise the gastric and bile acid barrier, gut flora, and motility, thus allowing spore germination, altered bacterial growth, and toxin development. In such hosts, botulism results from the ingestion of food contaminated with *C. botulinum* organisms and no preformed toxin, with intraluminal elaboration of toxin occurring in vivo.

### Iatrogenic Botulism

Botulinum toxins are used therapeutically in the treatment of a variety of disorders such as. cervical dystonia, upper or lower limb spasticity, blepharospasm, strabismus, chronic migraine, severe axillary hyperhidrosis, and for cosmetic purposes. Botulinum neurotoxin is thought to exert its therapeutic effect in most cases by temporarily weakening muscles whose overactivity results in the clinical condition. Although one early marketing assumption was that the neurotoxin does not diffuse from the injection site, BoNT can diffuse into adjacent tissues and produce local adverse effects. Systemic manifestations are of concern when an inadvertent, excessive, or misdirected dose of toxin is administered or in the setting of a neuromuscular disorder that may be previously undiagnosed. In addition, a number of studies demonstrate that even appropriately injected doses result in neuromuscular junction abnormalities throughout the body, occasionally producing autonomic dysfunction without muscle weakness. Several cases of iatrogenic botulism-like symptoms, including diplopia and severe generalized muscle weakness with widespread electromyographic (EMG) abnormalities, resulted from therapeutic or cosmetic use of intramuscular BoNT injections. In 2009, the FDA mandated changes to the prescribing information for the BoNT products, requiring a Boxed Warning highlighting the possibility of potentially life-threatening effects distant from the injection site.

### Inhalational Botulism

Inhaled BoNT is estimated to be 100 times more potent than ingested BoNT. A 1962 report from West Germany described three veterinary workers who inhaled BoNT type A from the fur of animals they were handling. On the third day after exposure, they developed mucus in the throat, dysphagia, and dizziness, and on the next day, they developed ophthalmoparesis, mydriasis, dysarthria, gait dysfunction, and weakness. Use of aerosolized BoNT as a bioweapon has been attempted by terrorists and state-sponsored biological warfare programs (Chap. 99).

## DIAGNOSTIC TESTING

The CDC case definition for foodborne botulism is established in a patient with a neurologic disorder manifested by diplopia, blurred vision, bulbar weakness, or symmetric paralysis in whom:

- Botulinum neurotoxin is detected in serum, stool, or implicated food samples *or*
- *C. botulinum* is isolated from stool *or*
- A clinically compatible case is epidemiologically linked to a laboratory-confirmed case of botulism

Routine laboratory studies, including cerebrospinal fluid analysis, are normal in patients with botulism but are usually performed to exclude other etiologies. Specific tests can be helpful in diagnosing botulism.

### Edrophonium Testing

Edrophonium is a rapidly acting cholinesterase inhibitor of short duration that is useful in the diagnosis of myasthenia gravis. It is occasionally used to differentiate myasthenia gravis from botulism. This drug inhibits the metabolism of acetylcholine located in synapses, permitting continued binding with the reduced number of postsynaptic acetylcholine receptors in myasthenia gravis. Because release of acetylcholine is impaired in botulism, preventing its catabolism with an anticholinesterase medication typically has little clinical benefit, but a weaker effect is occasionally observed if some neurons maintain the ability to release acetylcholine. Thus, in rare cases, early in the course of botulism, injection of edrophonium results in limited improvement in strength, but this is far less dramatic than the improvement that occurs in patients with myasthenia gravis.

### Electrophysiologic Testing

In all forms of botulism, sensory nerve action potentials are normal. Motor potentials in severely affected muscles typically are reduced in amplitude, but conduction velocity is not affected. The needle EMG examination in botulism is characterized by low-amplitude, short-duration motor unit action potentials (MUAPs) caused by blockade of neuromuscular

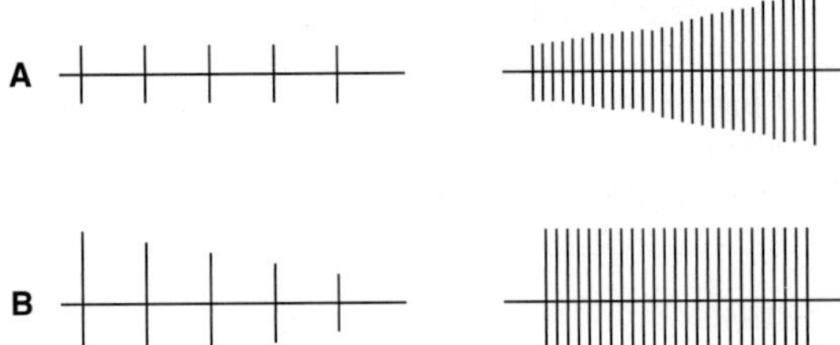


**FIGURE 11–2.** Schematic representations of repetitive nerve stimulation at low (5/sec) and high (50/sec) frequencies. In botulism (**A**), stimulation produces a small muscle action potential that is facilitated (increases in amplitude) by repetitive stimulation at higher frequencies. This effect (which, although classic, is not found in all cases of botulism) results from increased acetylcholine release with high-frequency stimulation because of intracellular calcium accumulation. In contrast, myasthenia gravis (**B**) is associated with a normal muscle action potential amplitude and a decremental response at low-frequency stimulation with a normal response at high-frequency stimulation. Myasthenia gravis, a disorder of the muscle endplate, produces this decremental response at low frequencies because the natural reduction in acetylcholine response with subsequent stimulation falls below threshold.

transmission in many muscle fibers (Fig. 11–2). Although these electrodiagnostic abnormalities support the diagnosis of botulism, there are no pathognomonic electrophysiologic findings. Nerve conduction studies and EMG are most useful for excluding alternative diagnoses, including Guillain-Barré syndrome and other neuropathies (both demyelinating and axonal), poliomyelitis, myasthenia gravis, and myopathies.

### Laboratory Testing

If foodborne botulism is suspected, samples of serum, stool, vomitus, gastric contents, and suspected foods should be subjected to anaerobic culture (for *C. botulinum*) and mouse bioassay (for BoNT) (Table 11–3). When wound botulism is considered, serum, stool, exudate, débrided tissue, and swab samples should be collected. For infant botulism, feces and serum samples also should be obtained. In infants who are constipated, an enema with nonbacteriostatic sterile water will facilitate collection. All enema fluid and stool should be sent for analysis. Detailed information on specimen collection and examination is available online from the CDC (https://www.cdc.gov/mmwr/volumes/70/rr/rr7002a1.htm).

## MANAGEMENT

### Supportive Care

Respiratory compromise is the usual cause of death from botulism. To prevent or treat this complication, hospital admission of the patient and of all individuals with suspected exposure is mandatory. Careful continuous monitoring of respiratory status using parameters such as vital capacity, peak expiratory flow rate, negative inspiratory force (NIF), pulse oximetry, end-tidal $CO_2$, and the presence or absence of a gag reflex is essential to determine the need for intubation if a patient begins to manifest signs of bulbar paralysis. The NIF is the most reliable, readily obtainable test for determining the need for intubation. When suspicion of botulism is high and the vital capacity is less than 20 mL/kg or the NIF is poorer than −30 cm $H_2O$, intubation is generally indicated. In addition to attention to respiratory issues, patients require nutrition (enteral or parenteral), prompt recognition and treatment of secondary infections, and prophylaxis against deep vein thromboses.

### Gastrointestinal Decontamination

Removal of the spores and toxin from the gut should be attempted. Activated charcoal is recommended as a routine part of supportive care because in vitro it adsorbs BoNT type A and probably also the other BoNT types. If a cathartic is chosen, sorbitol is preferable because other cathartics such as magnesium salts potentially exacerbate neuromuscular blockade.

### Wound Care

Thorough wound débridement is the most critical aspect in the management of wound botulism and should be performed promptly. Antibiotic therapy alone is inadequate. We recommend against using medications that interfere with neuromuscular transmission, such as aminoglycosides, fluoroquinolones, and clindamycin.

### Guanidine, Dalfampridine, and 3,4-Diaminopyridine

Guanidine is no longer recommended for treatment of botulism because its merits were not substantiated. Evidence for dalfampridine (4-aminopyridine) and 3,4-diaminopyridine is insufficient to recommend their routine use at this time.

**TABLE 11–3** Epidemiologic and Laboratory Assessment of Botulism[a]

| *Classification* | *Foodborne* | *Infant* | *Wound* | *Adult Intestinal Colonization* |
|---|---|---|---|---|
| BoNT type | A, B, E, F, G in humans; C, D in animals | A, B, C, F, H | A, B | A |
| Route | Ingestion of toxin | Ingestion of bacteria and spores | Wound, abscess (sinusitis) | Ingestion of bacteria and spores |
| Specimens | Stool: positive for bacteria/spores and toxin | Stool: positive for bacteria/spores and toxin for up to 8 wk after recovery | Wound site: Gram stain, aerobic and anaerobic cultures; positive for bacteria/spores | Stool: positive for bacteria/spores and toxin |
| BoNT in serum | Yes | Yes (but low sensitivity) | Yes | Yes |
| Bacteria/spores[a] in food | Yes | Yes | Not applicable | Yes |
| BoNT in food | Yes | No | Not applicable | No |

[a]"Bacteria/spores" refers to *C. botulinum*.

BoNT = botulinum toxin.

### Botulinum Antitoxin

In the US, botulinum antitoxin (BAT) is available for adults and children older than 1 year through the CDC. State public health officials can obtain the antitoxin through the CDC by calling 770-488-7100. In 2013, the FDA approved a heptavalent BAT containing equine-derived antibody to botulinum toxin types A through G. It currently is the only BAT available in the US for the treatment of botulism in adults and for cases of infant botulism caused by nerve toxins other than types A and B. In a CDC analysis of an open-label observational study involving 109 patients with suspected or confirmed botulism, treatment with BAT within 2 days of symptom onset was associated with a shorter length of hospitalization (13.7 days less), shorter duration in intensive care unit (6.6 days less), and shorter duration of mechanical ventilation (11.8 days less) compared with patients treated later. In a review of 132 cases of type A foodborne botulism from 1984 (when only trivalent antitoxin was available), a lower fatality rate and a shorter course of illness were demonstrated for patients who received the antitoxin, even after controlling for age and incubation period. Because of the benefit of earlier treatment, physicians should contact their state health department at the time the diagnosis of botulism is first suspected to expedite obtaining antitoxin from the CDC.

The antitoxin neutralizes only unbound toxin; consequently, it can prevent paralysis but does not affect already paralyzed muscles. Because of the potential lethality of foodborne botulism, the antitoxin should be given to patients in whom the diagnosis is suspected; treatment should not be delayed while awaiting laboratory confirmation of the diagnosis. In the event of a potential outbreak of foodborne botulism, asymptomatic individuals should be closely monitored for early signs of illness so that antitoxin can be administered promptly (Antidotes in Brief: A6).

### Treatment of Infant Botulism

Similar to adults, infants with botulism require intensive care, with meticulous monitoring for respiratory compromise and autonomic dysfunction. Constipation can be severe. Human-derived botulism antitoxin antibodies known as botulism immune globulin (BabyBIG) are US FDA approved for treatment of infant botulism types A and B. A randomized trial of 122 cases of infant botulism showed that treatment with intravenous BIG significantly reduced the length of hospital stay and intensive care, duration of mechanical ventilation and tube or intravenous feeding, and cost of hospitalization relative to placebo without causing serious adverse effects. BabyBIG is available from the California Department of Health Services Infant Botulism Treatment and Prevention Program (510-231-7600; http://www.infantbotulism.org).

### Prevention

The most important measures used to prevent infant botulism include limiting exposure to spores by thoroughly washing foods and objects that might be placed in a child's mouth. In addition, honey should not be given to infants younger than 6 months of age.

## PROGNOSIS

The prolonged and variable period of recovery that occurs after exposure to BoNT is directly related to the extent of neuromuscular blockade and neurogenic atrophy as well as the regeneration rates of nerve endings and presynaptic membranes. If the patient has excellent respiratory support during the acute phase and receives adequate parenteral nutrition, residual neurologic disability may not occur. Although the initial course sometimes is protracted, near-total functional recovery can follow within several months to 1 year. Common long-term sequelae include dysgeusia, dry mouth, constipation, dyspepsia, arthralgia, exertional dyspnea, tachycardia, and easy fatigability.

## PREGNANCY

At least eight cases of botulism occurring during pregnancy have been reported. None of the neonates had neurologic evidence of botulism. The large molecular weight of the neurotoxin makes passive diffusion through the placenta unlikely, and experimental results in rabbits attest that this does not take place. Appropriate care of the affected mother and preparation for maternal complications of delivery appear to ensure the best potential outcome for the infant.

All commercially available BoNT products are US FDA Pregnancy Category C. It is unknown whether BoNT is excreted in breast milk.

## EPIDEMIOLOGIC AND THERAPEUTIC ASSISTANCE

Whenever botulism is suspected or proven, the local health department should be contacted. The health department should report to the CDC Emergency Operations Center at 770-488-7100. All foods that are potentially responsible for the illness should be refrigerated and preserved for epidemiologic investigation.

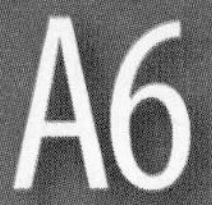

# A6 BOTULINUM ANTITOXIN

## INTRODUCTION

Antidotal therapies for adult and infant *Clostridium botulinum* infection are available as equine- and human-derived immunoglobulin antitoxins.

## HISTORY

Beginning in the 1930s, a formalin-inactivated toxoid against botulinum neurotoxin was first tested in humans, and in 1946, a bivalent (against types A and B) formaldehyde-inactivated toxoid was deployed by the US Department of Defense. Over the years, many new preparations have come in and out of use. In 2013, the US Food and Drug Administration (FDA) approved H-BAT, equine Botulism Antitoxin Heptavalent (A, B, C, D, E, F, G), which is currently available.

Botulism Immune Globulin Intravenous (Human) (BIG-IV), or BabyBIG was created by the California Department of Health Services (CDHS) in 1991 to treat infants affected by type A or type B botulism; it received US FDA approval in 2003.

## PHARMACOLOGY

### Chemistry and Preparation

An antitoxin is an antibody or antibody fragment capable of neutralizing a toxin. Each antibody has two sites that recognize antigens, known as the highly variable (Fv) ends. Opposite those sites is the Fc portion, which binds to the surface of mast cells and basophils. Heptavalent botulism antitoxin is produced by pooling plasma from horses immunized with seven specific botulinum toxoid types (A–G) followed by pepsin digestion to remove the Fc fragment portion and blending of the seven unique serotype antitoxins into a heptavalent product. Removal of the horse Fc portion essentially eliminates the immunogenicity of the antitoxin thereby limiting allergic reactions. The antitoxin potencies for botulism serotypes A to G in H-BAT are provided in Table A6–1. By convention, 1 IU of BAT neutralizes 10,000 mouse intraperitoneal median lethal doses ($MIPLD_{50}$) of toxin types A, B, C, D, and F and 1,000 $MIPLD_{50}$ of toxin type E (the IU for type G remains undefined).

BabyBig is derived from cold ethanol precipitation of pooled adult plasma from persons who were immunized with a recombinant botulinum vaccine for serotypes A and B, followed by a number of purification steps to inactivate and/or remove infectious agents. The product contains greater than or equal to 15 IU/mL anti-type A toxin activity and greater than or equal to 4 IU/mL anti-type B toxin activity.

### Mechanism of Action

Current antitoxins (whether equine or human derived) bind to and neutralize only the circulating botulinum toxin. Thus, antitoxins are ineffective against toxin bound to presynaptic acetylcholine release sites.

### Pharmacokinetics and Pharmacodynamics

Antidotal antibody fragments and single-chain variable fragments demonstrate shortened half-lives in vivo compared with whole immunoglobulins. Improved renal clearance and uptake by vascular endothelium and surrounding tissues contribute to this effect. The specific pharmacokinetic parameters are listed in Table A6–1. The neutralization parameters provided by botulism antitoxin (BAT) produce serum concentrations of BAT sufficient to bind toxin concentrations in excess of those typically reported in patients with foodborne botulism. A second vial would provide even greater protection. This might be warranted in particularly severe exposures because circulating neutralizing antibody concentrations and botulinum toxin interactions are nonlinear. When antibody concentrations are increased, there is a disproportionate, more efficacious increase in botulinum toxin neutralization.

## ANTITOXIN ROLE IN ADULT BOTULISM

Simian experiments demonstrate reduced mortality with antitoxin administration. The decision to administer H-BAT is often made on the basis of empirical clinical and epidemiologic grounds. Earlier disease recognition and an organized public health approach consisting of surveillance, emergency notification, stocking, a release and distribution system, and laboratory confirmation appear to be responsible for decreasing morbidity and increasing survival after typical foodborne botulism. Early antitoxin administration appears to be a critical factor affecting clinical course and outcome. In multiple studies, early administration of BAT (especially prior to mechanical ventilation) is associated with improved clinical outcomes. However, the absolute time frame for efficacy remains undetermined. In one review, toxin could be recovered in patients' sera up to 11 days after ingestion, suggesting that even delayed administration may be clinically useful. In fact, significant improvement (weaning from mechanical ventilation and resumption of feeding) was documented in a case of BIG-IV first administered 13 days after onset of infant botulism.

## ANTITOXIN ROLE IN INFANT BOTULISM

BabyBIG is approved for treatment of patients younger than 1 year of age with infant botulism caused by toxin type A or B. In a double-blind and subsequent open-label trial, treatment with BabyBIG-IV significantly reduced the overall length of hospital and intensive care stay, the duration of mechanical ventilation, tube and intravenous (IV) feeding, and the cost of hospitalization. Because babyBIG is derived from human donors only immunized with recombinant botulinum vaccine for serotypes A and B, it will be ineffective in infants

**TABLE A6–1 Botulinum Antitoxin Parameters**

| | *Antitoxin Serotype* | | | | | | |
|---|---|---|---|---|---|---|---|
| | *A* | *B* | *C* | *D* | *E* | *F* | *G* |
| ***Heptavalent Botulinum Antitoxin (H-BAT)*** | | | | | | | |
| Antitoxin potency (IU per vial) | 4,500 | 3,300 | 3,000 | 600 | 5,100 | 3,000 | 600 |
| Anticipated neutralization ($MIPLD_{50}$) | $4.5 \times 10^7$ | $3.3 \times 10^7$ | $3.0 \times 10^7$ | $6.0 \times 10^6$ | $5.1 \times 10^6$ | $3.0 \times 10^7$ | Undefined |
| Maximum concentration values (IU/mL), one-vial administration | 2.69 | 1.90 | 2.26 | 0.81 | 0.94 | 2.37 | 0.59 |
| Maximum concentration values ($MIPLD_{50}$/mL) | $2.69 \times 10^4$ | $1.90 \times 10^4$ | $2.26 \times 10^4$ | $8.1 \times 10^3$ | $9.4 \times 10^2$ | $2.37 \times 10^4$ | Undefined |
| Maximum concentration values (IU/mL), 1-vial administration | 6.23 | 4.28 | 4.89 | 1.60 | 1.75 | 4.29 | 1.19 |
| Maximum concentration values ($MIPLD_{50}$/mL) | $6.23 \times 10^4$ | $4.28 \times 10^4$ | $4.89 \times 10^4$ | $1.60 \times 10^4$ | $1.75 \times 10^3$ | $4.29 \times 10^4$ | Undefined |
| Half-life (h), one-vial administration | 8.64 | 34.2 | 29.6 | 7.51 | 7.75 | 14.1 | 11.7 |
| Half-life (h), two-vial administration | 10.2 | 57.1 | 45.6 | 7.77 | 7.32 | 18.2 | 14.7 |
| Volume of distribution, one-vial administration | 3,637 | 9,607 | 6,066 | 1,465 | 14,172 | 3,413 | 2,372 |
| Volume of distribution, two-vial administration | 3,993 | 14,865 | 8,486 | 1,653 | 11,596 | 4,334 | 3,063 |
| ***Botulism Immune Globulin Intravenous (Human) (BabyBIG-IV)*** | | | | | | | |
| Potency (IU/mL)[a] | 15 | 4 | | | | | |
| Anticipated neutralization ($MIPLD_{50}$) | $1.5 \times 10^5$ | $4 \times 10^4$ | | | | | |
| Half-life (days) | 28 | 28 | | | | | |
| ***Bivalent botulinum antitoxin AB (BAT-AB) (for historical comparison)*** | | | | | | | |
| Antitoxin potency (IU) | 7,500 | 5,500 | | | | | |
| ***Monovalent serotype E botulinum antitoxin (BAT-E) (for historical comparison)*** | | | | | | | |
| Antitoxin potency (IU) | | | | | 5,000 | | |
| ***Equine trivalent antitoxin (BAT-ABE) (for historical comparison)*** | | | | | | | |
| Antitoxin potency (IU) | 7,500 | 5,500 | | | 8,500 | | |

[a]The reconstituted vial contains a total of 2 mL.
$MIPLD_{50}$ = mouse intraperitoneal median lethal dose.

poisoned with other serotypes. Thus, H-BAT is required to treat infants with confirmed non–type A or B botulism.

## ADVERSE EFFECTS AND SAFETY ISSUES

Despite purification, inactivation, and filtration measures, potential transmission of bloodborne infectious agents from animal or human donors (pooled equine or human plasma) may still occur. There is also a risk of allergy and serum sickness. Healthy participants administered H-BAT in clinical trials (56 subjects, of whom 20 received two vials) reported headache, pruritus, nausea, and urticaria at rates of 9%, 5%, 5%, and 5%, respectively. Two subjects with moderate allergic reactions required treatment. The open-label CDC observation study revealed the following adverse reactions in 10% of 228 assessable patients: pyrexia (4%), rash (2%), chills (1%), nausea (1%), and edema (1%). There were no immediate hypersensitivity reactions, one cardiac arrest, and one episode of serum sickness. Heptavalent botulism antitoxin contains maltose, which can interfere with certain non–glucose-specific blood glucose monitoring systems and falsely elevate glucose readings.

Hypersensitivity reactions might also occur to human BIG-IV, although this was not reported in clinical trials. The most commonly reported adverse reaction was a mild, transient erythematous rash on the face or trunk. Administration of live-virus vaccines (ie, measles, mumps, rubella, and varicella) should be delayed for 3 or more months after BabyBIG-IV treatment because of concerns of reduced immunization efficacy.

## PREGNANCY AND LACTATION

Although there is limited information regarding H-BAT use in pregnancy, whole equine bivalent and trivalent antitoxins have been previously administered without apparent harm to the mother or the fetus. Pregnancy is not a contraindication to H-BAT. Given the morbidity and mortality of botulism, maternal treatment benefits presumably exceed risks of harm, although all decisions are ultimately made on a case-by-case basis. The breast milk distribution of heptavalent botulism antitoxin is unknown.

## DOSING AND ADMINISTRATION

Because of the risk of severe allergic reactions administration should occur in a critical care setting with clinicians skilled in airway management present. Epinephrine, corticosteroids, antihistamines should be immediately available.

**TABLE A6–2 Dosing and Administration of Hepatavalent Botulism Antitoxin**

| *Patient* | *Dose* | *Starting Infusion Rate (first 30 min)* | *Incremental Infusion Rate (every 30 min if tolerated)* | *Maximal Infusion Rate* |
|---|---|---|---|---|
| Adult ≥ 17 year | One vial | 0.5 mL/min | Double the rate | 2 mL/min |
| Child 1-17 year | *20–100% of adult dose | **0.01 mL/kg/min | 0.01 mL/kg/min | **0.03 mL/kg/min |
| Infant < 1 year | 10% of the adult dose | 0.01 mL/kg/min | 0.01 mL/kg/min | 0.03 mL/kg/min |

*For children ≤30 kg or less, the percentage of the adult dose is equal twice the body weight (in kg); for children >30 kg, the percentage of the adult dose is the weight (in kg) + 30, not to exceed the adult dose.

**Not to exceed the adult rate

### Botulism Antitoxin Heptavalent (A, B, C, D, E, F, and G)

The adult dose is one vial. The vial is diluted 1:10 in 0.9% sodium chloride and administered intravenously via an optional 15-micron in-line filter (Table A6–2).

### Botulism Immune Globulin Intravenous (Human)

The lyophilized product is reconstituted with 2 mL of Sterile Water for Injection USP, to obtain a 50 mg/mL human BIG-IV solution. The vial should not be shaken because this causes foaming. A dedicated IV line using low-volume tubing and a constant infusion pump are used to provide 75 mg/kg (1.5 mL/kg of reconstituted 50 mg/mL BIG-IV solution) at an initial rate of 25 mg/kg/h (0.5 mL/kg/h of reconstituted 50 mg/mL BIG-IV solution) for the first 15 minutes, which is then increased to 50 mg/kg/h (1 mL/kg/h of reconstituted 50 mg/mL BIG-IV solution), for a total infusion time of 97.5 minutes at the recommended dose.

### Other Immunoglobulins

In regions outside the US where whole, equine-derived antitoxins are still available, these products require sensitivity testing and potential desensitization, and the package inserts should be consulted for specific procedural details for dosing and administration, particularly because titers and volumes may differ by brand.

## FORMULATION AND ACQUISITION

Heptavalent botulism antitoxin is supplied in either 20-mL or 50-mL single-dose vials that are stored frozen at or below 5°F (−15°C) until used. Rapid thawing can be achieved by placing vials at room temperature for 1 hour followed by a water bath at 98.6°F (37°C) until thawed. Reconstituted H-BAT may be stored refrigerated for use within 8 to 10 hours. BabyBIG is formulated as a single-use, solvent-detergent-treated, sterile vial containing 100 ± 20 mg of lyophilized immunoglobin (primarily IgG with trace amounts of IgA and IgM), stabilized with 5% sucrose and 1% albumin (human), without preservative and supplied with 2 mL of Sterile Water for Injection USP for reconstitution.

Clinicians who suspect botulism should immediately call their local or state health department's emergency 24-hour telephone service to request release of BAT and comply with legal reporting requirements; a single case is a public health emergency. When local and state public health authorities are unavailable, the CDC Emergency Operations Center telephone contact is 770-488-7100. The California Infant Botulism Treatment and Prevention Program (510-231-7600) maintains the supply of BabyBIG for infant botulism treatment.

# 12 FOOD POISONING

Each year in the United States (US) known foodborne pathogens are responsible for approximately 30.7 million illnesses, 228,144 hospitalizations, and 2,612 deaths. It is estimated that foodborne illness costs an annual burden to the American society of 36 billion dollars. Worldwide food distribution, large-scale national food preparation and distribution networks, limited food regulatory practices, and corporate greed place everyone at risk. This chapter is organized into four major types of food poisoning: foodborne poisoning with neurologic effects, food poisoning with gastrointestinal (GI) symptoms, foodborne poisoning with anaphylaxis-like effects, and food poisoning used for bioterrorism.

## HISTORY AND EPIDEMIOLOGY

The estimated annual number of episodes of foodborne pathogen–related illness, hospitalization, and death in the US is shown in Table 12–1. Globally, researchers estimated foodborne pathogens were found to cause 582 million cases of illnesses annually. The leading cause of foodborne illness was norovirus (125 million cases) followed by *Campylobacter* (96 million). Most important, around 43% of the disease burden from contaminated food occurred in children younger than 5 years of age, who make up 9% of the population.

**TABLE 12–1** Estimated Annual Number of Episodes of Illness, Hospitalizations, and Death Caused by Pathogens Transmitted Commonly by Food in the US (2014)

| Pathogen | *Total Mean Episodes* | *Total Mean Hospitalizations* | *Total Mean Deaths* |
|---|---|---|---|
| **BACTERIA** | | | |
| *Bacillus cereus* | 62,623 | 20 | 0 |
| *Campylobacter* spp | 1,322,137 | 13,240 | 119 |
| *Clostridium botulinum* | 56 | 42 | 9 |
| *Clostridium perfringens* | 969,342 | 439 | 26 |
| STEC 0157* | 96,534 | 3,268 | 31 |
| *Listeria monocytogenes* | 1,662 | 1,520 | 266 |
| *Salmonella* spp | 1,229,007 | 23,128 | 452 |
| *S. enterica* | 5,752 | 623 | 0 |
| *Shigella* spp | 494,908 | 5,491 | 38 |
| *Staphylococcus* spp | 241,994 | 1,067 | 6 |
| *Streptococcus* group A | 11,257 | 1 | 0 |
| *Vibrio vulnificus* | 207 | 202 | 77 |
| *Vibrio parahaemolyticus* | 44,950 | 129 | 5 |
| *Yersinia enterocolitica* | 116,706 | 637 | 34 |
| **PARASITES** | | | |
| *Cryptosporidium* spp | 748,123 | 210 | 46 |
| *Giardia intestinalis* | 1,221,564 | 225 | 34 |
| *Trichinella* | 162 | 6 | 0 |
| **VIRUSES** | | | |
| Astrovirus | 3,090,384 | 17,430 | 5 |
| Hepatitis A | 35,769 | 2,255 | 171 |
| Norovirus | 20,865,958 | 56,013 | 571 |
| *Rotavirus* | 3,090,384 | 69,721 | 32 |

*STEC = shiga toxin–producing *Escherichia coli*.

## FOODBORNE POISONING WITH NEUROLOGIC SYMPTOMS

The differential diagnosis of patients with foodborne poisoning presenting with neurologic symptoms is vast (Tables 12–2 and 12–3). In cases of ciguatera poisoning, the major symptoms usually are neurotoxic, and the GI symptoms are minor. Knowing where the food was caught or harvested often helps establish a diagnosis, but refrigerated transport of foods and rapid worldwide travel can complicate the assessment. Travelers to Caribbean, Pacific, and Canary Islands, as well as those traveling within the US, have experienced ciguatera poisoning. In geographically disparate regions of Canada, individuals have experienced domoic acid poisoning caused by ingestion of cultivated mussels from Prince Edward Island.

### Ciguatera Poisoning

Ciguatera poisoning is one of the most commonly reported forms of vertebrate fishborne poisonings in the US, accounting for almost half of the reported cases. Ciguatera poisoning is endemic to warm water, bottom-dwelling reef fish living around the globe between 35° North and 35° South latitude, which includes tropical areas such as the Indian Ocean, the South Pacific, and the Caribbean. Hawaii and Florida report 90% of all cases occurring in the US, most commonly from May through August. The incidence and geographical distribution of ciguatera are increasing because of increased fish trade and consumption, international tourism, and climate changes.

More than 500 fish species have caused human cases of ciguatera poisoning. Ciguatoxin is found in blue-green algae, protozoa, and the free algae dinoflagellates. Photosynthetic dinoflagellates such as *Gambierdiscus toxicus* and bacteria within the dinoflagellates are the origins of ciguatoxin. Dinoflagellates are the main nutritional source for small herbivorous fish, which, in turn, are the major food source for larger carnivorous fish, thereby increasing the ciguatoxin concentrations in larger fish.

**TABLE 12–2** Differential Diagnosis of Possible Foodborne Poisoning Presenting with Neurologic Findings[a]

| |
|---|
| Anticholinergic poisoning |
| Bacterial food poisoning |
| Botulism |
| Dinoflagellates (brevetoxin, saxitoxin) |
| Marine food poisoning (ciguatoxin, tetrodotoxin) |
| Metals (arsenic, lead, mercury) |
| Monosodium glutamate |
| Mushrooms (*Amanita* spp, *Gyromitra* spp) |
| Organic phosphorus compounds |

[a]Altered mental status, motor weakness, and sensory changes.

**TABLE 12–3 Foodborne Neurologic Toxicity (Primary Presenting Symptoms)**

| *Disease* | *Toxin* | *Toxin Source and Mechanism*** | *Onset* | *Duration* | *Findings* | *Therapy* | *Diagnosis* |
|---|---|---|---|---|---|---|---|
| Ciguatera | Ciguatoxin | Large reef fish: amber jack, barracuda, snapper, parrot, sea bass, moray<br>**Increased sodium channel permeability | 2–24 h | Days-weeks | Paresthesias, nausea; vomiting, diarrhea, temperature reversal | Mannitol, amitriptyline | Clinical, mouse bioassay, immunoassay |
| Tetrodotoxin | Tetrodotoxin | Puffer fish, fugu, blue-ringed octopus, newts, horseshoe crab<br>**Blocks sodium channel | Minutes to hours | Days | Paresthesias, respiratory depression, hypotension | Respiratory support | Clinical |
| Neurotoxic shellfish poisoning | Brevetoxin | Mussels, clams, scallops, oysters, *Ptychodiscus brevis*: "red tide"<br>**Increased sodium channel permeability | 15 min to 18 h | Days | Bronchospasm, temperature reversal, nausea, vomiting, diarrhea, paresthesias | Bronchodilators | Clinical, mouse bioassay of food, HPLC |
| Paralytic shellfish poisoning | Saxitoxin | Mussels, clams, scallops, oysters, *Protogonyaulax catanella, Protogonyaulax tamarensis*<br>**Decreases sodium channel permeability | 30 min | Days | Respiratory depression, paresthesias, nausea, vomiting, diarrhea | Respiratory support | Clinical, mouse bioassay of food, HPLC |
| Amnestic shellfish poisoning | Domoic acid | Mussels, possibly other shellfish; *Nitzschia pungens*<br>**Excitatory neurotoxicity | 15 min to 38 h | Years | Amnesia, nausea, vomiting, diarrhea, paresthesias, respiratory depression | Respiratory support | Clinical, mouse bioassay of food, HPLC |
| Botulism | Botulinum toxin | Home-canned foods, honey, corn syrups, *Clostridium botulinum*<br>**Binds presynaptically, blocks acetylcholine release | 12–72 h | Weeks | Vomiting, diarrhea, respiratory depression, initial cranial nerve paralysis followed by a symmetric descending paralysis of the motor and autonomic nerves | Antitoxin, respiratory support | Clinical, immunoassay, serologic, bacteriologic |

HPLC = high-pressure liquid chromatography.

Ciguatoxin is heat stable, lipid soluble, acid stable, odorless, and tasteless. The toxin binds to voltage-sensitive sodium channels in diverse tissues and increases the sodium permeability of the channel. The ciguatoxins cause hyperpolarization and a shift in the voltage dependence of channel activation, which opens the sodium channels. Multiple ciguatoxins are identified in the same fish, perhaps explaining the variability of symptoms and differing severity.

People can be affected after eating fresh or frozen fish that was prepared by all common methods: boiling, baking, frying, stewing, or broiling. The appearance, taste, and smell of the ciguatoxic fish are usually unremarkable. The majority of symptomatic episodes begin 2 to 6 hours after ingestion, 75% within 12 hours, and 96% within 24 hours. Symptoms include diaphoresis, headaches, abdominal pain with cramps, nausea, or vomiting; profuse watery diarrhea, and a constellation of dramatic neurologic symptoms. A sensation of loose or painful teeth is reported. Typically, peripheral dysesthesias and paresthesias predominate. Watery eyes, tingling, and numbness of the tongue, lips, throat, and perioral area occur. A strange metallic taste is frequently reported as is a reversal of temperature discrimination, the pathophysiology of which remains to be elucidated. Myalgias, most often in the lower extremities, arthralgias, ataxia, and weakness are commonly experienced. Dysuria and symptoms of dyspareunia and vaginal and pelvic discomfort are reported to occur in some women after sexual intercourse with men who are ciguatoxic and whose semen contains the toxin. Vertigo, seizures, and visual disturbances (eg, blurred vision, scotomata, and transient blindness) are reported. Bradycardia and orthostatic hypotension are described. The GI symptoms usually subside within 24 to 48 hours. However, cardiovascular and neurologic symptoms typically persist for several days to weeks. Although deaths are reported, internationally, none have been documented in the US.

The US Food and Drug Administration's (FDA's) and ciguatoxin fish testing procedure is performed in an analytical laboratory setting. To date, there is no commercially available, rapid, cost-effective, fish-testing product that has been demonstrated to provide ciguatoxin detection in seafood with adequate reliability or accuracy.

In most patients, elimination of the toxin is accelerated if vomiting (40%) and diarrhea (70%) have occurred. Administration of activated charcoal has benefit for patients who are not vomiting. In patients with significant GI fluid loss, intravenous (IV) fluid and electrolyte repletion are essential. The orthostatic hypotension responds to IV fluids and α-adrenergic agonists. Symptomatic bradycardia is treated with atropine. Intravenous mannitol (1 g/kg IV) is reasonable in the first 24 h to attempt to alleviate neurologic and muscular dysfunctional symptoms associated with ciguatera; however, GI symptoms are not ameliorated. Admission to the hospital for cautious supportive care is essential when the diagnosis is uncertain or when volume depletion or any consequential manifestations are present (Tables 12–2 and 12–3). Late in the course of ciguatera poisoning, amitriptyline 25 mg orally twice daily helps alleviate symptoms. Patients recovering from ciguatera should avoid alcohol and nuts for 3 to 6 months if their consumption exacerbates symptoms.

### Ciguateralike Poisoning

Moray, conger, and anguillid eels carry a ciguatoxinlike neurotoxin in their viscera, muscles, and gonads that does not affect the eel itself. The toxin is a complex ester that is structurally very similar to ciguatoxin and is heat stable. Individuals who eat these eels can infrequently manifest neurotoxic symptoms similar to ciguatoxin or show signs of cholinergic toxicity, such as hypersalivation, nausea, vomiting, and diarrhea. Shortness of breath, mucosal erythema, and cutaneous eruptions also occur. These findings are present in addition to the neurotoxic symptoms. Management is supportive. Death is related to the complications of neurotoxicity, such as seizures and respiratory paralysis.

### Shellfish Poisoning

Healthy mollusks living between 30° North and 30° South latitude ingest and filter large quantities of dinoflagellates. During warmer months these dinoflagellates are responsible for "red tides." The number of toxic dinoflagellates in these "red tides" is often so overwhelming that birds and fish die, and humans who walk along the beach experience respiratory symptoms caused by aerosolized toxin.

Ingestion of contaminated shellfish causes neurotoxic, paralytic, and amnestic syndromes. The dinoflagellates most frequently implicated are *Karenia brevis* (originally named *Gymnodinium breve* in 1948, renamed *Ptychodiscus brevis* in 1979, and reclassified again to the current nomenclature in 2000). The diatoms causing neurotoxic shellfish poisoning (NSP) include *Protogonyaulax catanella* and *Protogonyaulax tamarensis*, which cause paralytic shellfish poisoning, and *Nitzschia pungens*, which causes amnestic shellfish poisoning.

*Paralytic shellfish poisoning* is caused by saxitoxin. Saxitoxin blocks the voltage-sensitive sodium channel in a manner identical to tetrodotoxin (TTX). The higher the number of affected shellfish consumed, the more severe the symptoms. Symptoms usually occur within 30 minutes of ingestion. Neurologic effects predominate and include paresthesias and numbness of the mouth and extremities, a sensation of floating, headache, ataxia, vertigo, muscle weakness, paralysis, and cranial nerve dysfunction manifested by dysphagia, dysarthria, dysphonia, and transient blindness. Gastrointestinal symptoms are less common. Fatalities occur as a result of respiratory failure, usually within the first 12 hours after symptom onset. Muscle weakness often persists for weeks. Treatment is supportive. Early intervention for respiratory failure is indicated. Orogastric lavage and cathartics are not recommended. Activated charcoal is reasonable if vomiting has not occurred.

*Neurotoxic shellfish poisoning* is caused by brevetoxin. Brevetoxin, which is produced by *K. brevis*, is a lipid-soluble, heat-stable polyether toxin similar to ciguatoxin. It acts by stimulating sodium flux through the sodium channels of both nerve and muscle. Gastrointestinal symptoms include abdominal pain, nausea, vomiting, diarrhea, and rectal burning. Neurologic features include paresthesias, reversal of hot and cold temperature sensation, myalgias, vertigo, and ataxia. Other effects include headache, malaise, tremor, dysphagia, bradycardia, decreased reflexes, and mydriasis. Paralysis does not occur. The incubation period is 3 hours (range, 15 minutes–18 hours). Gastrointestinal and neurologic symptoms appear simultaneously. Treatment is supportive, and severe respiratory depression is very uncommon.

*Amnestic shellfish poisoning* is caused by domoic acid, which is produced by the diatom a *N. pungens*. Domoic acid, which is structurally similar to glutamic acid, kainic acid, and aspartic acid, interacts with the glutamate receptors on nerve cell terminals. Amnestic shellfish poisoning is characterized by GI symptoms of nausea, vomiting, abdominal cramps, and diarrhea, and neurologic symptoms of memory loss and, less frequently, coma, seizures, hemiparesis, ophthalmoplegia, purposeless chewing, and grimacing. Other signs and symptoms include hemodynamic instability and cardiac dysrhythmias. Symptoms typically begin 5 hours (range, 15 minutes–38 hours) after ingestion of mussels. The mortality rate is 2%, with death most frequently occurring in older patients, who experience more severe neurologic symptoms. Ten percent of victims have long-term antegrade memory deficits, as well as motor and sensory neuropathy. Postmortem examinations revealed neuronal damage in the hippocampus and amygdala.

### Tetrodotoxin Poisoning

This type of fish poisoning involves only the order Tetraodontiformes. Approximately 100 freshwater and saltwater species exist in this order, including a number of pufferlike fish such as the globe fish, balloon fish, blowfish, and toad fish. Tetrodotoxin (TTX) found in these fish is also isolated from the blue-ringed octopus, the gastropod mollusk, and horseshoe crab eggs. Certain TTX-containing newts (*Taricha, Notophthalmus, Triturus*, and Cyanops) are also found in Oregon, California, and southern Alaska. In Japan, fugu (a local variety of puffer fish) is considered a delicacy, but special licensing is required to prepare this exceedingly toxic fish.

Tetrodotoxin is a heat-stable, water-soluble nonprotein found mainly in the fish skin, liver, ovary, intestine, and possibly muscle. Similar to saxitoxin, TTX is produced by marine bacteria and likely accumulate in animals higher on the food chain that consume these bacteria. Neurotoxicity is produced by inhibition of sodium channels and blockade of neuromuscular transmission.

Effects of TTX poisoning typically occur within minutes of ingestion. Headache, diaphoresis, dysesthesias, and paresthesias of the lips, tongue, mouth, face, fingers, and toes evolve rapidly. Buccal bullae and salivation develop. Dysphagia, dysarthria, nausea, vomiting, and abdominal pain ensue. Generalized malaise, loss of coordination, weakness, fasciculations, and an ascending paralysis occur in 4 to 24 hours. In more severe toxicity, hypotension is present. In some studies, the mortality rate approaches 50%. Therapy is supportive.

### *Clostridium botulinum*

Home-canned fruits and vegetables, as well as commercial fish products, are among the common foods causing botulism (Chap. 11 and Antidotes in Brief: A6).

## PREVENTION OF MARINE FOODBORNE DISEASE

Careful evaluation of the symptoms and meticulous reporting to local and state health departments, as well as to the US Centers for Disease Control and Prevention (CDC), will allow for more precise analysis of epidemics of poisoning from contaminated or poisonous food or fish. Many states and countries have developed rigorous health codes with regard to harvesting certain species of fish in certain areas at certain times.

### Less Common Poisonings

***Echinoderms.*** The sea urchin usually causes toxicity by contact with its spinous processes, but this Caribbean delicacy is also toxic upon ingestion. When the sea urchin is prepared as food, the venom-containing gonads should be removed because they contain an acetylcholine-like substance that causes the cholinergic syndrome of profuse salivation, abdominal pain, nausea, vomiting, and diarrhea.

***Haff Disease.*** The consumption of cooked seafood can potentially lead to a syndrome of myalgias and rhabdomyolysis. This syndrome is termed Haff disease, after an outbreak that occurred in persons living along the Koenigsberg Haff, an inlet of the Baltic Sea. The actual etiology of Haff disease is unknown, but it is suspected that the causative agent is similar to a palytoxin, which is a potent vasoconstrictor. Treatment is hydration with intravenous fluids.

## FOOD POISONING ASSOCIATED WITH DIARRHEA

The initial differential diagnosis for acute diarrhea involves several etiologies: infectious (bacterial, viral, parasitic, and fungal), structural (including surgical), metabolic, functional, inflammatory, toxin induced, and food induced. An elevated temperature is caused by invasive organisms, including *Salmonella* spp, *Shigella* spp, *Campylobacter* spp, invasive *E. coli*, *Vibrio parahaemolyticus*, and *Yersinia* spp. Episodes of acute gastroenteritis not typically associated with fever are caused by organisms producing toxins, including *S. aureus*, *Bacillus cereus*, *Clostridium perfringens*, enterotoxigenic *E. coli*, and most viruses. The timing of diarrheal onset is summarized in Table 12–4.

Fecal leukocytes typically are found in patients with invasive shigellosis, salmonellosis, *Campylobacter* enteritis, typhoid fever, invasive *E. coli* colitis, *V. parahaemolyticus*, *Yersinia enterocolitica*, and inflammatory bowel disease. In

**TABLE 12–4** Foodborne Infections: Gastrointestinal (Time of Onset and Primary Presenting Symptom)

| *Etiology* | *Symptoms* *Onset* | *A* | *V* | *Di* | *Dy* | *F* | *Source* | *Pathogenesis* | *Therapy* |
|---|---|---|---|---|---|---|---|---|---|
| *Staphylococcus* spp | 2–6 h | + | + | + | – | – | Prepared foods: meats, pastries, salads | Heat-stable enterotoxin | Fluid and electrolyte resuscitation |
| *Bacillus cereus* | | | | | | | | | |
| Type I | 1–6 h | + | + | + | – | – | Fried rice | Heat-labile toxin | Fluid and electrolyte resuscitation |
| Type II | 12 h | + | – | + | – | – | Meats, vegetables | Heat-labile toxin | |
| Anisakiasis | 1–12 h | + | + | – | – | – | Raw fish, sushi (*Eustrongylides*), minnows, salmon, cod, herring, squid, tuna | Intestinal larvae | Endoscopy, laparotomy removal |
| *Clostridium perfringens* | 8–24 h | + | ± | + | ± | – | Poultry, heat-processed meats | Heat-labile enterotoxin | Fluid and electrolyte resuscitation |
| *Salmonella* spp | 8–24 h | ± | ± | + | ± | + | Poultry, eggs | Bacteria, endotoxin (bacteremia) | Antibiotics |
| *Escherichia coli* | | | | | | | | | |
| Enterotoxigenic | <6 h | + | ± | + | – | + | Enteric contact | | Fluid and electrolyte resuscitation |
| Invasive | 24–72 h | + | – | + | + | + | Raw produce | Bacteria (invasive) | Antibiotics |
| Hemorrhagic | 24–72 h | + | + | + | + | ± | Under cooked beef, unpasteurized milk | Shiga toxin heat stable | Fluid and electrolyte resuscitation and hematologic (blood transfusion) support |
| *Vibrio cholerae* | 24–72 h | ± | ± | + | – | ± | Water, food, enteric contact | Heat labile enterotoxin | Fluid and electrolyte resuscitation, antibiotics |
| *Shigella* spp | 24–72 h | + | ± | + | + | ± | Institutional food handler, household, preschool, enteric contact | Endotoxin Shiga toxin | Antibiotics |
| *Campylobacter jejuni* | 1–7 d | + | + | + | ± | + | Milk, poultry, unchlorinated water | Bacteria, heat labile enterotoxin | Antibiotics |
| *Yersinia* spp | 1–7 d | + | + | + | ± | + | Pork, milk, pets | Bacteria, enterotoxin | Antibiotics |

A = abdominal pain; Di = diarrhea; Dy = dysentery; F = fever; V = vomiting.

**TABLE 12–5 Epidemiologic Analysis of Gastrointestinal Disease**

1. Is the occurrence of the disease in a large group significant enough to be consistent with foodborne disease (two or more cases)?
2. Is the symptomatology in affected individuals well defined and similar?
3. Are the onset, time, and duration of illness similar among affected group members (incubation)?
4. What are the possible modes of transmission (eg, contact, food, water)?
5. Is there a relationship between the time of exposure of the group and the mode of transmission?
6. Do attack rates differ for age, gender, or occupation?
7. Can it be determined which foods were served and to whom? Can the items that were not eaten by those who did not become ill be identified?
8. What is the food-specific attack rate?
9. How was the food procured? How was it stored?
10. Was cooking technique adequate?
11. Was personal hygiene acceptable?
12. Was there animal contamination?

all of these conditions, except typhoid fever, the leukocytes are primarily polymorphonuclear; in typhoid fever, they are mononuclear. No stool leukocytes are noted in cholera, viral diarrheas, noninvasive *E. coli* diarrhea, or nonspecific diarrhea.

### Epidemiology

Epidemiologic analysis is of immediate importance, particularly when GI diseases strike more than one person in a group (Table 12–5). If available, an infectious disease consultant or infection control officer should be called for assistance. Alternatively, assistance from state and local health departments should be sought. Often, only the CDC or state health department has the resources to investigate and confirm a presumptive diagnosis in an outbreak.

**Salmonella *Species.*** *Salmonella enterica* infections are of great concern in the US. The contamination of food that is widely distributed places thousands at risk. Outbreaks of *Salmonella* food poisoning are commonly associated with eggs, milk, and peanut butter. Additional concern developed over the widespread use of antibiotics in animal feed, responsible for meats, poultry, and manure-fertilized vegetables now frequently containing resistant bacterial strains to which virtually the entire population is exposed. The diagnosis of *Salmonella* infection is made through culture of the stool. The treatment of *Salmonella* is fluid and electrolyte resuscitation and antibiotics (ciprofloxacin or azithromycin).

## FOODBORNE POISONING ASSOCIATED WITH MULTIORGAN SYSTEM DYSFUNCTION

Hemolytic uremic syndrome (HUS) begins with a prodrome of diarrhea in 90% of cases. The diarrhea lasts for 3 to 4 days and frequently becomes bloody. Abdominal pain caused by colitis is common, and vomiting, altered mental status (irritability or lethargy), pallor, and low-grade fever frequently occur. At presentation, many patients have oliguria or anuria, and 10% of children have a generalized seizure at HUS onset. Typical laboratory findings in HUS include microangiopathic hemolytic anemia, thrombocytopenia, and acute kidney injury (AKI).

Hemolytic uremic syndrome is frequently associated with enterohemorrhagic *E. coli* (EHEC) or *E. coli* O157:H7, which produces a toxin similar to that produced by *Shigella dysenteriae* type I, referred to as Shigalike toxin (SLT) or verotoxin. Detection of *E. coli* O157:H7 through stool culture early in the course of disease is useful. Treatment of HUS should focus on meticulous supportive care, with fluid and electrolyte balance as the priority. Hemodialysis should be instituted early for azotemia, hyperkalemia, acidemia, and fluid overload. Red blood cells and platelet transfusions are often required. There is some evidence that early treatment with antibiotics increases the risk of development HUS in children with *E. coli* O157:H7 infections. Because of this concern, it is not typically recommended to initiate antibiotics in patients with clinical or epidemiologic presentations consistent with *E. coli* O157:H7 infections (crampy abdominal pain, bloody diarrhea, regional outbreak) until a definitive pathogen can be identified.

### *Staphylococcus* Species

In cases of suspected food poisoning with a short incubation period, the physician should first assess the risk for staphylococcal causes. The usual foods associated with staphylococcal toxin production include milk products and other proteinaceous foods, cream-filled baked goods, potato and chicken salads, sausages, ham, tongue, and gravy. A routine assessment must be made for the presence of lesions on the hands or nose of any food handlers involved. Unfortunately, carriers of enterotoxigenic staphylococci are difficult to recognize because they usually lack lesions and appear healthy.

Although patients with staphylococcal food poisoning rarely have significant temperature elevations, 16% of 2,992 documented cases in a published review had a subjective sense of fever. Abdominal pain, nausea followed by vomiting, and diarrhea dominate the clinical findings. Diarrhea does not occur in the absence of nausea and vomiting.

Most enterotoxins are produced by *S. aureus* coagulase–positive species. The enterotoxins initiate an inflammatory response in GI mucosal cells and lead to cell destruction. The enterotoxins also result in sudden effects on the emesis center in the brain and diverse other organ systems. The illness usually lasts for 24 to 48 hours. The treatment is supportive care with hydration and electrolyte repletion.

### *Bacillus cereus*

Another foodborne toxin that produces GI effects is associated with eating reheated fried rice. *Bacillus cereus* type I is the causative organism, and bacterial overgrowth and toxin production cause consequential early-onset nausea and vomiting. *Bacillus cereus* type II has a delayed onset of similar GI effects including diarrhea. The diagnosis of *B. cereus* infection is made through culture of the stool. The treatment of *B. cereus* is fluid and electrolyte resuscitation and antibiotics (eg, ciprofloxacin or vancomycin).

### *Campylobacter jejuni*

*Campylobacter jejuni* is a major cause of bacterial enteritis. The organism is most commonly isolated in children younger than 5 years and in adults 20 to 40 years of age. *Campylobacter* enteritis outbreaks are more common in the summer months in temperate climates and the most frequent sources are raw or undercooked poultry products and unpasteurized milk. The incubation period for *Campylobacter* enteritis varies from 1 to 7 days (mean, 3 days). Typical symptoms include diarrhea, abdominal cramps, and fever. Other symptoms include headache, vomiting, excessive gas, and malaise. The diarrhea contains gross blood, and leukocytes are frequently present on microscopic examination. Illness usually lasts 5 to 6 days (range, 1–8 days). Treatment is supportive and consists of volume resuscitation and antibiotics for the more severe cases.

#### *Yersinia enterocolitica*

*Yersinia enterocolitica* causes enteritis most frequently in children and young adults. Typical clinical features include fever, abdominal pain, and diarrhea, which usually contains mucus and blood. Less common features include prolonged enteritis, reactive polyarthritis, pharyngeal and hepatic involvement, and rash. Sources of human infection include milk products, raw pork products, infected household pets, and person-to-person transmission. Patients receiving the chelator deferoxamine (Antidotes in Brief: A7) acquire *Yersinia* infections because the deferoxamine–iron complex acts as a siderophore for organism growth. Therapy is usually supportive, but patients with invasive disease (eg, bacteremia, bacterial arthritis) should be treated with IV antibiotics.

#### *Listeria monocytogenes*

Listeriosis transmitted by food usually occurs in pregnant women and their fetuses, older adults, and immunocompromised individuals using corticosteroids or with malignancies, diabetes mellitus, kidney disease, or HIV infection. Typical food sources include undercooked chicken and unpasteurized milk as well as soft cheeses. Symptoms of fever, severe headache, muscle aches, and pharyngitis develop. Treatment with IV ampicillin and an aminoglycoside or trimethoprim–sulfamethoxazole is indicated for systemic *Listeria* infections.

### Xenobiotic-Induced Diseases

In addition to the aforementioned toxins, many other xenobiotics contaminate our food sources. Careful assessment for possible foodborne pesticide poisoning is essential. Also, the possibility of unintentional acute metal salt ingestion must also be evaluated. This type of poisoning most typically occurs when very acidic fruit punch is served in metal-lined containers. Antimony, zinc, copper, tin, or cadmium in a container is dissolved in an acidic food or juice medium.

### Mushroom-Induced Disease

Some species produce major GI effects (Chap. 90).

### Intestinal Parasitic Infections

*Anisakis simplex* and *Pseudoterranova decipiens* are Anisakidae that are found in several types of consumed raw fish, including mackerel, cod, herring, rockfish, salmon, yellow fin tuna, and squid. The popularity of eating raw fish, or sushi, led to an increase in reported intestinal parasitic infections. Etiologic agents are roundworms (*Eustrongyloides anisakis*) and fish tapeworms (*Diphyllobothrium* spp). Symptoms of anisakiasis are either upper intestinal (occur 1–12 hours after eating) or lower intestinal (delayed for days or weeks). Typical symptoms include nausea, vomiting, and severe crampy abdominal pain; intestinal perforation, severe pain, rebound, and guarding can also occur. A dietary history of eating raw fish is needed to establish diagnosis and therapy. Visual inspection of the larvae (on endoscopy, laparotomy, or pathologic examination) is useful. Treatment of intestinal infection involves surgical or laparoscopic removal.

Diphyllobothriasis (fish tapeworm disease) is caused by eating uncooked fish such as herring, salmon, pike, and whitefish that harbor the parasite. The symptoms are less acute than with intestinal roundworm ingestions and usually begin 1 to 2 weeks after ingestion. Signs and symptoms include nausea, vomiting, abdominal cramping, flatulence, abdominal distension, diarrhea, and megaloblastic anemia due to vitamin $B_{12}$ deficiency. The diagnosis is based on a history of ingesting raw fish and on identification of the tapeworm proglottids in stool. Treatment with niclosamide, praziquantel, or paromomycin usually is effective.

### Monosodium Glutamate

This clinical presentation resulting from the ingestion of monosodium glutamate (MSG) consists of a burning sensation of the upper torso, facial pressure, headache, flushing, chest pain, nausea and vomiting, and, infrequently, life-threatening bronchospasm and angioedema. The intensity and duration of symptoms are generally dose related but with significant variation in individual responses to the amount ingested. Monosodium glutamate causes "shudder attacks" or a seizurelike syndrome in young children. Absorption is more rapid after fasting and only lasts approximately 1 hour. There is evidence that humans have a unique taste receptor for glutamate. This explains its ability to act as a flavor enhancer for foods. Glutamate is also an excitatory neurotransmitter that can stimulate central nervous system neurons through activation of glutamate receptors and be the explanation for some of the neurologic symptoms described with ingestion.

### Anaphylaxis and Anaphylactoid Presentations

Some foods and foodborne toxins cause allergic or anaphylacticlike manifestations, also sometimes referred to as "restaurant syndromes" (Table 12–6).

### Scombroid Poisoning

Scombroid poisoning originally was described with the Scombridae fish (including the large dark-meat marine tuna, albacore, bonito, mackerel, and skipjack). However, the most commonly ingested vectors identified by the US CDC are nonscombroid fish, such as mahi mahi, amber jack, bluefish, and tilapia. Scombroid poisoning can result from eating cooked, smoked, canned, or raw fish. The implicated fish all have a high concentration of histidine in their dark meat. *Morganella morganii, E. coli,* and *Klebsiella pneumoniae,* commonly found on the surface of the fish, contain a histidine decarboxylase enzyme that acts on a warm (not refrigerated), freshly killed fish, converting histidine to histamine.

The appearance, taste, and smell of the fish are usually unremarkable. Rarely, the skin has an abnormal "honeycombing" character or a pungent, peppery taste that is a clue to

**TABLE 12–6 Symptoms of Foodborne Toxicity**

| | Onset | Symptoms or Signs | Cause | Therapy |
|---|---|---|---|---|
| Anaphylaxis (anaphylactoid) | Minutes to hours | Urticaria, angioedema, bronchospasm, hypotension, cardiorespiratory arrest | Allergens—nuts, eggs, milk, fish, shellfish, peanuts, soy | Oxygen, epinephrine, $\beta_2$-adrenergic agonists, corticosteroids, fluid and electrolyte resuscitation, $H_1$ histamine antagonists, avoidance |
| Monosodium glutamate (MSG) | Minutes | Flushing, hypotension, palpitations, facial pressure, headaches, rhinitis, bronchospasm, shivering | Flavor enhancer of foods | Oxygen, $\beta_2$-adrenergic agonists, fluid and electrolyte resuscitation, avoidance |
| Metabisulfites | Minutes | Flushing, hypotension, bronchospasm | Preservative in wines, salad (bars), fruit juice, shrimp | See Anaphylaxis; avoidance |
| Scombroid | Minutes to hours | Flushing, hypotension, urticaria, headache, pruritus, gastrointestinal symptoms | Large fish—poorly refrigerated; tuna, bonito, albacore, mackerel, mahi mahi (histamine) | Histamine ($H_1$, $H_2$) antagonists |
| Tyramine | Minutes to hours | Headache, hypertension | Wines, aged cheeses that contain tyramine (INH or MAOI) increase risk | Avoidance |
| Tartrazine | Hours | Urticaria, angioedema, bronchospasm | Yellow coloring food additive | See Anaphylaxis; avoidance |

INH = isoniazid; MAOI = monoamine oxidase inhibitor.

its toxicity. Within minutes to hours after eating the fish, the individual experiences numbness, tingling, or a burning sensation of the mouth; dysphagia; headache; and, of particular significance for scombroid poisoning, a unique flush characterized by an intense diffuse erythema of the face, neck, and upper torso. Rarely, pruritus, urticaria, angioedema, or bronchospasm ensues. Nausea, vomiting, dizziness, palpitations, abdominal pain, diarrhea, and prostration may develop.

The prognosis is good with appropriate supportive care and parenteral antihistamines such as diphenhydramine. Histamine ($H_2$)-receptor antagonists are also reasonable to administer because they can be useful in alleviating GI symptoms. Inhaled $\beta_2$-adrenergic agonists and epinephrine are recommended if bronchospasm is prominent. Patients should be reassured that they are not allergic to fish if other individuals experience a similar reaction while eating the same fish at the same time. If any remaining fish can be preserved, it should be tested for elevated histamine concentrations. If this information is not available, then an anaphylactic reaction to the fish cannot be excluded.

### Global Food Distribution: Illegal Food Additives

The US imports food from all over the world, year-round. Approximately 19% of the food consumed in the US is imported. The number of outbreaks associated with an imported food has increased from an average of 3 per year (1996–2000) to an average of 18 per year (2009–2014). Xenobiotics are given to animals to increase their health and growth.

Clenbuterol, a $\beta_2$-adrenergic agonist, was administered to cattle raised for human consumption. Clenbuterol causes toxicity in humans who eat contaminated animal meat, producing tachycardia, tremors, nausea, epigastric pain, headache, muscle pain, and diarrhea. The globalization of food supplies and international agricultural trade have created a new global threat—the apparent purposeful contamination of food for profit. In 2008, almost 300,000 children in China were affected by melamine contamination of milk. Additional cases were found outside of China because melamine was used in candy, chocolate, cookies, and biscuits ultimately sold in the US. Melamine is a nonnutritious, nitrogen-containing compound added to falsify the protein content of milk. Melamine and its metabolite cyanuric acid are excreted in the kidneys leading to kidney stones and acute kidney injury.

## FOOD POISONING AND BIOTERRORISM

The threat of terrorist assaults is discussed in Chaps. 98 and 99. The use of food as a vehicle for intentional contamination with the intent of causing mass suffering or death has already occurred. Outbreaks of *Shigella dysenteriae* type II and *Salmonella typhimurium* are linked to intentional events. In another case, a disgruntled employee contaminated 200 lb of meat at a supermarket with a nicotine-containing insecticide resulting in 92 people becoming ill and four seeking medical care. Signs and symptoms included vomiting, abdominal pain, rectal bleeding, and one case of atrial tachycardia. There are multiple reports of deliberate food poisoning with tetramine resulting in status epilepticus.

## PREVENTION OF FOODBORNE ILLNESS

The incidence of foodborne disease has increased over the years and has resulted in a major global public health problem. The current methods for detecting foodborne pathogens are inefficient. This has led to the research and development of rapid detection methods. The three major types of rapid detection methods are biosensor-based, nucleic acid–based, and immunological-based methods. Biosensor detection methods use an analytical device that contains a bioreceptor and transducer. The transducer converts the biological interactions into a measurable electrical signal. Examples of biosensor-based methods are optical, electrochemical, and mass-based biosensors. Nucleic acid–based detection methods work by detecting specific DNA or RNA in the pathogen. An example of this test is polymerase chain reaction.

Immunological-based methods detect foodborne pathogens based on antibody–antigen interactions, whereby a particular antibody binds to the specific antigen. An example of an immunological-based detection method is enzyme-linked immunosorbent assay.

In general, the rapid detection methods are more efficient and sensitive than the conventional detection methods. Rapid detection methods may be a very useful way of preventing foodborne disease in the future. Implementing special equipment and training personnel, along with high costs, have thwarted comprehensive application of rapid detection methods at this time.

# 13 DIETING XENOBIOTICS AND REGIMENS

## INTRODUCTION AND HISTORY

Obesity is a worldwide epidemic, and the United States (US) has the largest proportion of a national population of overweight and obese individuals. Some estimates predict that nearly 38% of the world's adult population will be overweight and 20% will be obese by 2030. Even more alarming, the incidence of obesity in children between the ages of 6 and 19 years has tripled in the past 30 years.

Americans spend upward of $60 billion per year on weight loss therapies. Pharmacologic interventions typically result in a 5% to 10% weight loss, although a return to baseline upon drug cessation is common. Surgical interventions consistently achieve substantial weight loss, causing up to a 30% reduction in weight, but they are associated with numerous and varied complications. Weight loss xenobiotics (Table 13–1) are available as prescription medications, nonprescription dietary supplements, and nonprescription diet aids. Numerous other prescription medications, including thyroid medications and metformin, have been used on an off-label basis for weight loss. Numerous xenobiotics are promoted as weight loss aids, many with no proven efficacy and some with serious toxicity. The history of dieting xenobiotics is checkered. A number of weight loss therapies were withdrawn or banned by the US Food and Drug Administration (FDA) because of serious adverse health effects (Table 13–2).

Since 2012, the US FDA has approved numerous new medications that show modest promise, at best, in the weight loss drug armamentarium. There is ongoing research both for existing and novel pharmaceutical approaches for weight loss. Despite numerous innovative pharmacologic approaches and advancements, there will likely be no perfect weight loss drug.

## PHARMACOLOGY

Dieting xenobiotics can be divided into classes based on one or more of the following mechanisms of action: (1) appetite suppression (*anorectics*), (2) alteration of food absorption or elimination, or (3) increased energy expenditure. The hypothalamus is the key site in the brain that regulates food intake, energy expenditure, satiety, and metabolism. It also integrates endocrine signaling to meet the energy demand. The pathways and sites of action of xenobiotics are shown in Figure 13–1. The individual xenobiotics are discussed below.

## SYMPATHOMIMETICS

Although controversial, certain sympathomimetic amines still carry official indications for short-term weight reduction. Regardless of their source and legal status, sympathomimetics generally share a spectrum of toxicity and produce adverse effects similar to amphetamines (Chap. 46).

### Pharmacology

Sympathomimetic amines that act at α- and β-adrenergic receptors are clinically effective in promoting weight loss. The weight loss effect of amphetamine was readily apparent in early animal studies (Chap. 46). The primary mechanism of action of the weight loss effects of sympathomimetics is central nervous system (CNS) stimulation, resulting from increased release of norepinephrine and dopamine. The effects include direct suppression of the appetite center in the hypothalamus and reduced taste and olfactory acuity, leading to decreased interest in food. Increased energy and euphoriant effects of the stimulants also contribute to weight loss. However, tachyphylaxis occurs, and the rate of weight loss diminishes within a few weeks of initiating therapy. Significant side effects and abuse potential severely limit the therapeutic use of this class.

### Adverse Effects

Mild cardiovascular and CNS stimulant effects include headache, tremor, sweating, palpitations, and insomnia. More severe effects that occur after overdose include anxiety, agitation, psychosis, seizures, palpitations, and chest pain.

Hypertension is common after overdose and occasionally after therapeutic use. Patients present with confusion and altered mental status as a result of hypertensive encephalopathy. Other manifestations include chest pain, palpitations, tachycardia, hypertension, syncope, coronary vasospasm, mania, psychosis, and convulsions. Clinically significant hypertension should be treated with a rapid acting, easily titratable vasodilator such as nicardipine or phentolamine. Analogous to the management of cocaine toxicity, we recommend against the use of β-adrenergic antagonists because the resultant unopposed α-adrenergic agonist effects may lead to greater vasoconstriction and hypertension. Agitation, tachycardia, and seizures should be treated initially with benzodiazepines.

### Herbal Sympathomimetic Products

Since ephedra was banned, herbal weight loss supplements have been reformulated. Many now contain an extract of bitter orange (*Citrus aurantium*), a natural source of the sympathomimetic amine synephrine, often in combination with caffeine, guarana, theophylline, willow bark (containing salicylates), diuretics, and other constituents. The predominant constituents, *p*-synephrine and octopamine, are structurally similar to epinephrine and norepinephrine. The isomer *m*-synephrine (phenylephrine) is used extensively as a vasopressor and nasal decongestant. Although the physiologic actions of synephrine are not fully characterized, it appears to interact with amine receptors in the brain and acts at peripheral $\alpha_1$-adrenergic receptors, resulting in vasoconstriction and increased blood pressure. Some evidence indicates

**TABLE 13–1 Weight Loss Xenobiotics**

| *Drug or Supplement*[a] | *Mechanism of Action* | *Regulation Status, DEA Schedule* | *Adverse Effects or Contraindications*[b] |
|---|---|---|---|
| ***Sympathomimetics*** | | | |
| Bitter orange extract (*Citrus aurantium*) | Contains synephrine and octopamine; increases thermogenesis and lipolysis | Dietary supplement | Hypertension, cerebral ischemia, myocardial ischemia, prolonged QT interval |
| Bupropion/naltrexone | Increased release of norepinephrine; synergistic effect of midbrain dopamine | Nonscheduled prescription drug | Tachycardia, hypertension, seizures<br>Opioid withdrawal in tolerant patients |
| Diethylpropion | Increased release of norepinephrine and dopamine | Schedule IV | Dry mouth, tremor, insomnia, headache, agitation, palpitations, hypertension, stroke, dysrhythmias; contraindications: monoamine oxidase inhibitor use within 14 days, glaucoma, hyperthyroidism |
| Guarana (*Paullinia cupana*) | Contains caffeine, which may increase thermogenesis | Dietary supplement | Nausea, vomiting, insomnia, diuresis, anxiety, palpitations |
| Mazindol | Increased release of norepinephrine and dopamine | Schedule IV | Dry mouth, tremor, insomnia, headache, agitation, palpitations, hypertension, stroke, dysrhythmias; contraindications: monoamine oxidase inhibitor use within 14 days, glaucoma, hyperthyroidism |
| Phentermine | Increased release of norepinephrine and dopamine | Schedule IV | Similar to diethylpropion |
| Phentermine/topiramate | Increased release of norepinephrine and dopamine (phentermine); exact mechanism of action for topiramate remains speculative | Schedule IV | Phentermine: similar to diethylpropion<br>Topiramate: central nervous system depression, ataxia, non–anion gap metabolic acidosis, kidney stones<br>Contraindication: first trimester pregnancy |
| Raspberry ketone | Structurally similar to synephrine; increases thermogenesis and lipolysis | Dietary supplement | Nausea, vomiting, insomnia, hypertension, tachycardia, anxiety, palpitations |
| ***Serotonergics*** | | | |
| Lorcaserin (Belviq) | Selective agonist at $5\text{-HT}_{2C}$ | Schedule IV | Dizziness, headache, nausea; serotonin toxicity possible after overdose |
| ***GLP-1 Agonists*** | | | |
| Albiglutide<br>Dulaglutide<br>Exenatide<br>Liraglutide | GLP-1 analog | Nonscheduled prescription medication | Nausea, diarrhea<br>Potential: hypoglycemia |
| ***GI Agents*** | | | |
| Chitosan | Insoluble marine fiber that binds dietary fat | Dietary supplement | Decreased absorption of fat-soluble vitamins<br>Contraindications: shellfish allergy |
| Orlistat | Inhibits gastric and pancreatic lipases | Prescription and nonprescription medication | Abdominal pain, oily stool, fecal urgency or incontinence; fat-soluble vitamin loss<br>Contraindications: cholestasis, chronic malabsorption |
| ***Fibers and Other Supplements*** | | | |
| Chromium picolinate | Improves blood glucose and lipids; produces fat loss (unproven) | Dietary supplement | Dermatitis, hepatitis, possibly mutagenic in high doses |
| *Garcinia cambogia* | Increases fat oxidation (unproven) | Dietary supplement | None reported |
| Glucomannan | Expands in stomach to increase satiety | Dietary supplement | GI obstruction with tablet form<br>Contraindications: abnormal GI anatomy |

[a]Trade names and botanical names are given in parentheses. [b]All weight loss xenobiotics are contraindicated during pregnancy and lactation.
GI = gastrointestinal; GLP-1 = glucagon-like peptide-1; MAOI = monamine oxidase inhibitor; $5\text{-HT}_{2c}$ = serotonin receptor subtype 2c.

that synephrine also has both $\beta_2$- and $\beta_3$-adrenergic agonist activity, which could increase lipolysis. Numerous case reports describe *C. aurantium* toxicity. Tachydysrhythmias, cerebral ischemia, QT interval prolongation, and myocardial infarction are all reported.

Raspberry ketone, which is structurally similar to synephrine, is promoted to induce weight loss and is available as a supplement. There has been only one report of toxicity described in the literature, and clinical effects are consistent with other sympathomimetics.

**TABLE 13–2 High-Risk Xenobiotics Unapproved or Withdrawn by the US Food and Drug Administration**

| *Drug or Supplement*[a] | *Mechanism of Action* | *Regulation Status, DEA Schedule, or Withdrawal Date* | *Adverse Effects or Contraindications* |
|---|---|---|---|
| Amphetamine | Increased release of norepinephrine and dopamine | Schedule II | Sympathomimetic effects, psychosis, dependence |
| Benzphetamine | Increased release of norepinephrine and dopamine | Schedule III | Sympathomimetic effects, psychosis, dependence |
| Caffeine | $\beta_2$-Adrenergic agonist activity; increased energy expenditure | Not approved, available without prescription | Nausea, vomiting, tachycardia, wide pulse pressure, hypokalemia, hyperglycemia, anion gap metabolic acidosis |
| Clenbuterol | $\beta_2$-Adrenergic agonist activity | Never approved | Tachycardia, headache, nausea, vomiting; may be prolonged |
| Dexfenfluramine | Promotes central serotonin release and inhibits its reuptake | Withdrawn September 1997 | Valvular heart disease, primary pulmonary hypertension |
| Dieter's teas (senna, cascara, aloe, buckthorn) | Stimulant laxative herbs that promote colonic evacuation | FDA required label warning, June 1995 | Diarrhea, vomiting, nausea, abdominal cramps, electrolyte disorders, dependence |
| Dinitrophenol | Alters metabolism by uncoupling oxidative phosphorylation | Never approved; available on the Internet | Hyperthermia, cataracts, hepatotoxicity, skin rash, peripheral neuropathy |
| Ephedra sinica (Ma-huang) | Increased release of NE and dopamine | Banned by FDA, April 2004 | Sympathomimetic effects, psychosis |
| Fenfluramine | Increased release and decreased reuptake of serotonin | Withdrawn September 1997 | Valvular heart disease, primary pulmonary hypertension |
| Guar gum | Hygroscopic polysaccharide swells in stomach, producing early satiety | Banned by FDA, July 1990 | Esophageal and small bowel obstruction, fatalities |
| β-Human chorionic gonadotrophin | Unknown | Never approved | Coronary artery dissection |
| LipoKinetix (sodium usniate, norephedrine, 3,5-diiodothyronine, yohimbine, caffeine) | Unknown | FDA warning, November 2001 | Acute hepatitis |
| Phendimetrazine | Increased release of NE and dopamine | Schedule III | Sympathomimetic effects, psychosis |
| Phenylpropanolamine | $\alpha_1$-Adrenergic agonist | Withdrawn November 2000 | Sympathomimetic effects, headache, hypertension, myocardial infarction, intracranial hemorrhage |
| Rimonabant | Endocannabinoid receptor inverse partial agonist | Never approved in the US; withdrawn from European market in 2011 | Anxiety, nausea, diarrhea, dizziness; increased suicidality and depression |
| Salicylate (willow bark) | Uncoupler of oxidative phosphorylation | Never approved | Nausea, vomiting, tinnitus, tachycardia, altered mental status, anion gap metabolic acidosis (see Chapter 10) |
| Sibutramine | Inhibits reuptake of serotonin and norepinephrine | Withdrawn October 2010 | Increase in cardiovascular toxicity; increase in nonfatal myocardial infarction; increase in nonfatal stroke |

[a]Trade names or botanical names as appropriate are given in parentheses.

DEA = Drug Enforcement Administration; FDA = Food and Drug Administration; NE = norepinephrine.

### Phentermine/Topiramate

Phentermine is a sympathomimetic that retains an FDA indication for short-term weight loss. It increases release of norepinephrine, which serves as an appetite suppressant via the effects on the hypothalamus. Topiramate is available for a variety of conditions, including seizure disorders and migraine headaches. Weight loss is a demonstrated side effect of topiramate when used for these indications. The mechanism of weight loss induced by topiramate remains speculative and is likely a combination of decreased caloric intake, increased energy expenditure, and decreased energy efficiency. Phentermine/topiramate controlled release is approved by the US FDA for long-term management of weight loss.

Cardiovascular effects reveal mild increases in heart rate at therapeutic dosing. Topiramate is a carbonic anhydrase inhibitor. Electrolyte abnormalities are commonly associated with its use; hyperchloremia, hypokalemia, and decreased bicarbonate result in non–anion gap metabolic acidosis. Overdose of topiramate causes CNS depression, ataxia, seizures, and the laboratory abnormalities noted above. Although there have been no documented cases of overdose of this combination product, its toxicity can be extrapolated from the known toxicities of the individual components.

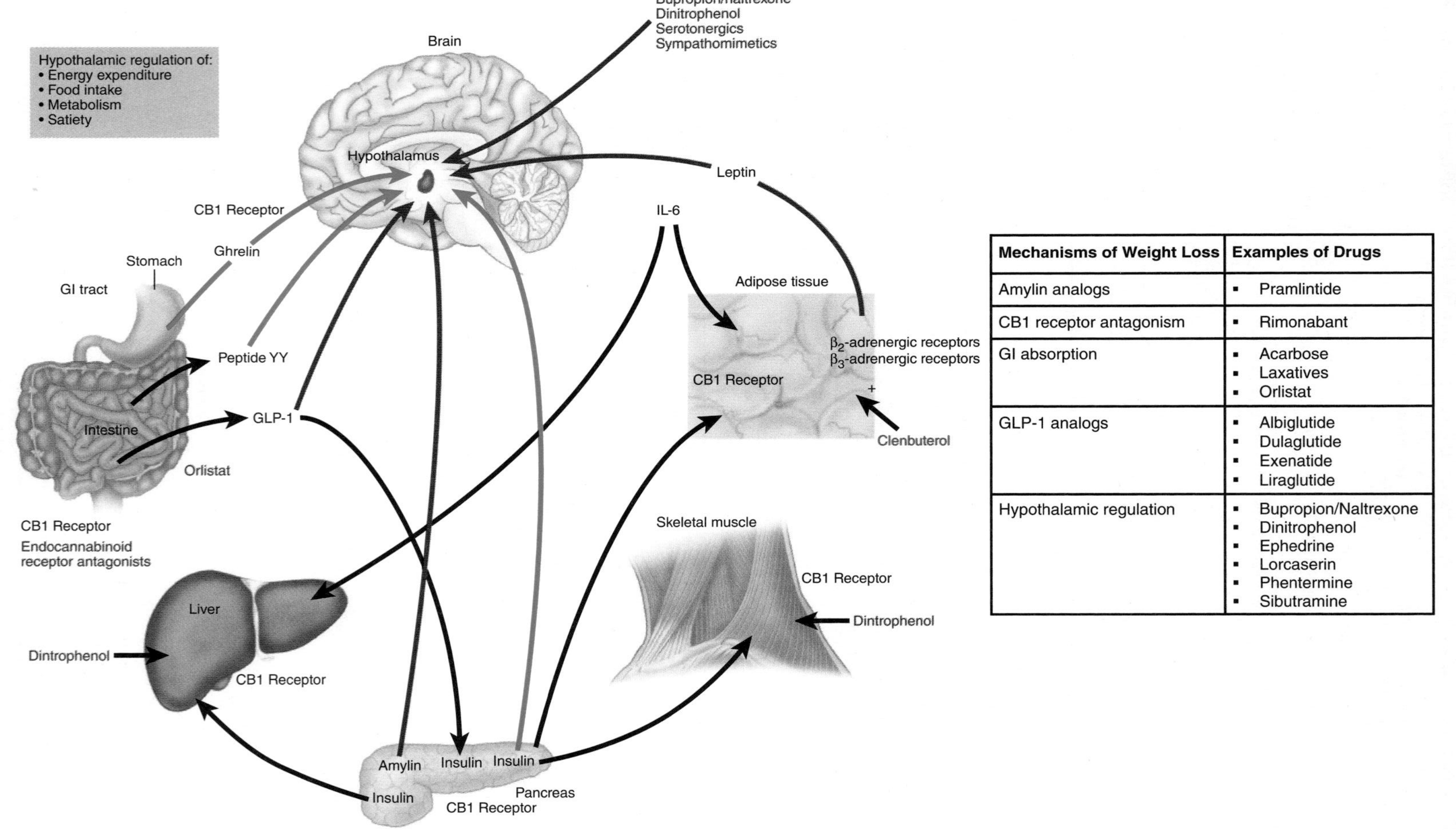


| Mechanisms of Weight Loss | Examples of Drugs |
|---|---|
| Amylin analogs | ▪ Pramlintide |
| CB1 receptor antagonism | ▪ Rimonabant |
| GI absorption | ▪ Acarbose<br>▪ Laxatives<br>▪ Orlistat |
| GLP-1 analogs | ▪ Albiglutide<br>▪ Dulaglutide<br>▪ Exenatide<br>▪ Liraglutide |
| Hypothalamic regulation | ▪ Bupropion/Naltrexone<br>▪ Dinitrophenol<br>▪ Ephedrine<br>▪ Lorcaserin<br>▪ Phentermine<br>▪ Sibutramine |

**FIGURE 13–1.** Endocrine and neuroendocrine pathways of obesity and weight loss regimens. Systems regulating food ingestion and energy balance are interconnected and regulated. The hypothalamus regulates food intake, satiety, energy expenditure, and metabolism. Adipose tissue functions for glucose uptake and conversion; lipogenesis and lipolysis; β oxidation of fatty acids; and release of leptin, adiponectin, and interleukin-6 (IL-6), all of which regulate energy balance. CB1 = endocannabinoid receptor; GI = gastrointestinal; GLP-1 = glucagon-like peptide 1; Red text: *Suggests a negative effect or antagonist effect;* Green text: *Suggests a positive effect or agonist effect;* Red arrow: *promotes satiety;* Green arrow: *increases hunger;* Black arrow: *normal cause/effect and + if promotes positive effects and - if promotes negative effects.*

## SEROTONERGICS

Serotonin is believed to have a role in appetite suppression, which is due to the effect on the hypothalamic serotonin 5-$HT_{2C}$ receptor, as well as the 5-$HT_{1A}$, 5-$HT_{1B}$, and 5-$HT_6$ receptors. Serotonin receptor effects also enhance energy expenditure. Use of serotonin agonists for weight loss is associated with cardiac valvulopathy (5-$HT_{2B}$ receptor), hallucinations (5-$HT_{2A}$ receptor), pulmonary hypertension (5-$HT_{1B}$), and serotonin toxicity.

Lorcaserin is a selective agonist at the 5-$HT_{2C}$ receptor. A recent case series of lorcaserin exposures reported agitation or irritability, diaphoresis, drowsiness, tachycardia, and muscle rigidity consistent with serotonergic toxicity. Benzodiazepines are recommended for tachycardia and hypertension that occurs in the setting of psychomotor agitation. Rapid identification and management of serotonin toxicity are essential to prevent associated morbidity and mortality (Chap. 42).

## XENOBIOTICS THAT ALTER FOOD ABSORPTION, METABOLISM, AND ELIMINATION

### Fat Absorption Blockers

Orlistat is the only US FDA-approved drug that alters the absorption and metabolism of food. Orlistat is a potent inhibitor of gastric and pancreatic lipase, thus reducing lipolysis and increasing fecal fat excretion. The drug is not systemically absorbed but exerts its effects locally in the GI tract. Adverse effects correlate with the amount of dietary fat consumption and include abdominal pain, oily stool, fecal incontinence, fecal urgency, flatus, and increased defecation. Systemic effects are rare because of the lack of systemic absorption. Liver toxicity manifesting as cholestatic, jaundice, and centrilobular necrosis is rarely reported. Because orlistat reduces absorption of fat-soluble food constituents, daily ingestion of a multivitamin supplement containing vitamins A, D, and K, and β-carotene is advised to prevent resultant deficiency. There are no reported intentional overdoses of orlistat.

### Dietary Fibers

Glucomannan, a dietary fiber consisting of glucose and mannose, is derived from konjac root, a traditional Japanese food. Purified glucomannan is available in capsule form and is found in various proprietary products marketed for weight loss. On contact with water, glucomannan swells to approximately 200 times its original dry volume, turning into a viscous liquid. Following several reports of esophageal obstruction, glucomannan tablets were withdrawn from the market in Australia in 1985. Serious adverse effects are not described with encapsulated glucomannan, presumably because slower dissolution allows for GI transit before expansion.

### Dinitrophenol

Dinitrophenol is readily available in capsules or tablets and can be purchased online. Dinitrophenol increases metabolic work by uncoupling oxidative phosphorylation in the mitochondria. Through this mechanism, the hydrogen ion gradient that facilitates adenosine triphosphate (ATP) synthesis is disrupted, and ATP production is arrested, although oxidative metabolism in the citric acid cycle continues. This mechanism results in inefficient substrate utilization, and the resulting energy loss is dissipated as heat. This wastes calories but also increases temperature and, occasionally, life-threatening hyperthermia occurs.

Symptoms related to dinitrophenol toxicity include malaise, rashes, headache, diaphoresis, thirst, peripheral neuropathy, and dyspnea. Acute toxic effects include hyperthermia, hepatotoxicity, agranulocytosis, respiratory failure, coma, and death. Management should emphasize rapid cooling. Benzodiazepines should also be used as an adjunct therapy for management of agitation and seizures.

## ENDOCANNABINOID RECEPTOR ANTAGONISTS AND INVERSE AGONISTS

In the past 15 years, the endocannabinoid system (ECS) and its involvement in weight loss sparked excitement and potential for novel xenobiotics. It has long been known that tetrahydrocannabinol, the active principle in marijuana (*Cannabis sativa*), stimulates appetite and is an effective antiemetic (Chap. 47). Several $CB_1$ receptor antagonists and inverse agonists showed promise in both animal and human studies of weight loss. Rimonabant was approved for therapeutic use in Europe, and clinical trials in the US were performed. Unfortunately, there was a significant increase in adverse events, including anxiety and depression, and rimonabant was never approved by the US FDA. Other studies involving other endocannabinoid receptor inverse agonists (eg, taranabant) were terminated early because of a range of dose-related GI, nervous, psychiatric, cutaneous, and vascular side effects.

## NALTREXONE/BUPROPION

Bupropion/naltrexone was US FDA approved in late 2014. The mechanisms by which naltrexone/bupropion cause weight loss are incompletely understood. Adverse events from this product result from the known toxicity of each individual xenobiotic. Naltrexone is generally expected to be safe and well tolerated in opioid-naïve patients; however, it will cause prolonged opioid withdrawal symptoms in opioid-tolerant patients and will significantly reduce the efficacy of opioids if they are required (Antidotes in Brief: A4). Bupropion toxicity is well described in the literature. Seizures occur with bupropion doses greater than 450 mg/day. Bupropion toxicity is discussed in detail in Chap. 42.

## LIRAGLUTIDE

Glucagon-like peptide-1 (GLP-1) is produced in the brain and distal intestine. During a meal, GLP-1 concentrations increase and remain elevated for several hours. Glucagon-like peptide-1 inhibits food intake, inhibits glucagon secretion, decreases gastric acid secretion, and delays gastric emptying. There are currently four GLP-1 analogs available in the US (liraglutide, exenatide, dulaglutide, and albiglutide). Only liraglutide has an approved indication for weight loss. The drug was well tolerated, with nausea and diarrhea being the most common adverse events. In one case of intentional overdose of 72 mg liraglutide, mild GI toxicity predominated, and significant hypoglycemia was absent.

## ALTERNATIVE PHARMACEUTICAL APPROACHES

In an attempt to find the "perfect" therapeutic alternative for weight loss, there is a desire to use currently approved xenobiotics for weight loss. Similar to topiramate, xenobiotics that are known to cause weight loss at therapeutic doses such as metformin, bupropion, and zonisamide continue to be investigated for both labeled and off-label use. Combination therapy aimed at multiple systems may prove efficacious. Although these xenobiotics provide a beneficial weight loss, each of them has its own inherent toxicities. Metformin can cause a metabolic acidosis with elevated lactate concentration (MALA), particularly in patients with underlying kidney dysfunction and after large intentional overdoses (Chap. 20). Zonisamide, an adjunct antiepileptic that is not used commonly, is associated with adverse events, including CNS depression and hypersensitivity (Chap. 21).

## HYPOCALORIC DIETS AND CATHARTIC OR EMETIC ABUSE

Starvation, as well as abuse of laxatives, syrup of ipecac, diuretics, and anorectics, has led to morbidity and mortality, often in young patients. The potential for fad diets and laxative abuse should be evaluated in young people with unexplained salt and water depletion, syncope, hypokalemia, and metabolic alkalosis. A variety of extreme calorie-restricted diets resulting in profound weight loss were very popular in the late 1970s but reports of a possible association between these diets and sudden death followed. Myocardial atrophy was a consistent finding on autopsy. Torsade de pointes and other ventricular dysrhythmias may have occurred as a result of hypokalemia, and protein-calorie malnutrition is proposed as a cause of death.

Dieter's teas that contain combinations of herbal laxatives, including senna and *Cascara sagrada*, can produce profound diarrhea, salt and water depletion, and hypokalemia. They are associated with sudden death, presumably as a result of cardiac dysrhythmias. Chronic laxative use can result in an atonic colon ("cathartic bowel") and the development of tolerance, with the subsequent need to increase dosing to achieve catharsis. The combination of misuse or abuse of laxatives in conjunction with orlistat has the potential to cause severe diarrhea and subsequent fluid and electrolyte imbalances.

Syrup of ipecac was chronically used to induce emesis by patients with eating disorders, such as bulimia nervosa, leading to the development of cardiomyopathy, subsequent dysrhythmias, and death. Emetine, a component of syrup of ipecac, was the alkaloid responsible for the severe cardiomyopathy.

## OTHER HERBAL REMEDIES

Several herbal approaches for weight loss have resulted in serious toxicity. In France, germander (*Teucrium chamaedrys*) supplements taken for weight loss resulted in seven cases of hepatotoxicity. A "slimming regimen" first prescribed in a weight loss clinic in Belgium produced an epidemic of progressive kidney disease, known as Chinese herb nephropathy, when botanical misidentification led to the substitution of *Stephania tetrandra* with the nephrotoxic plant *Aristolochia fangji*. A case of profound digitalis toxicity occurred with a laxative regimen contaminated with *Digitalis lanata*. Until regulation of herbal products is improved and manufacturing practices worldwide are standardized, sporadic reports of herb-related toxicity likely will continue (Chap. 16).

## NONPHARMACOLOGIC INTERVENTIONS

Although not a specific toxicologic concern, surgical modifications of the GI tract alter the pharmacokinetic properties of orally administered medications and nutrients. Gastric modifications have emerged as an absolute contraindication to orogastric lavage, a new risk factor for Wernicke encephalopathy, and a potential risk for adult botulism.

# 14 ATHLETIC PERFORMANCE ENHANCERS

## HISTORY AND EPIDEMIOLOGY

Interest in extraordinary athletic achievement fuels the modern-day science of performance enhancement in sports. The desire to improve athletic performance in a scientific manner is a relatively recent development. Today, "sports doping" refers to the use of a prohibited xenobiotic to enhance athletic performance. The word *doping* comes from the Dutch word *doop*, a viscous opium juice used by the ancient Greeks.

Controversy surrounding the systematic use of performance-enhancing xenobiotics by the participating athletes has marred many sporting events. Since the International Olympic Committee (IOC) began testing during the 1968 Olympic games, prominent athletes have been sanctioned and stripped of their Olympic medals because they tested positive for banned xenobiotics. However, from a public health perspective, the use of performance-enhancing xenobiotics among athletes of all ages and abilities is a far more serious concern than the highly publicized cases involving world-class athletes. Studies of high school students document that 6.6% of male seniors have used anabolic steroids.

## PRINCIPLES

Performance enhancers are classified in several ways. According to the 2017 World Anti-Doping Agency (WADA) World Anti-Doping Code, a xenobiotic or method constitutes doping and can be added to the Prohibited List if it is a masking xenobiotic or if it meets two of the following three criteria: it enhances performance, its use presents a risk to the athlete's health, and it is contrary to the spirit of sport (Table 14–1). Some of the prohibited xenobiotics are used to treat legitimate medical conditions of athletes. Athletes with documented medical conditions requiring the use of a prohibited substance or method may request a therapeutic use exemption (TUE).

**TABLE 14–1 Abbreviated Summary of World Anti-Doping Agency 2017 Prohibited List**

**Substances (S) and Methods (M) Prohibited at All Times (In and Out of Competition)**

- S0. Any pharmacological substance with no current approval for therapeutic use
- S1. Anabolic Agents
  - Anabolic androgenic steroids
  - Other anabolic agents
    - Clenbuterol
    - Selective androgen receptor modulators
- S2. Peptide Hormone, Growth Factors, Related Agents, and Mimetics
  - Erythropoiesis stimulation agents
  - Chorionic gonadotropin and luteinizing hormone
  - Corticotropins
  - Growth hormone

Additional prohibited growth factors: affecting muscle, tendon, or ligament protein synthesis/degradation, energy utilization, regenerative capacity, or fiber type switching

- S3. $\beta_2$-Adrenergic Agonists
  - Except inhaled salbutamol, formoterol, and salmeterol with urinary concentration limits
- S4. Hormone Antagonists and Metabolic Modulators
  - Aromatase inhibitors
  - Selective estrogen receptor modulators
  - Antiestrogens
  - Myostatin modulators
  - Metabolic modulators
    - Insulins
    - Peroxisome proliferator activated receptor delta agonist and AMP activate protein kinase axis agonists
    - Meldonium
- S5. Diuretics and Other Masking Agents
  - Desmopressin, probenecid, plasma expanders, glycerol, intravenous administration of albumin, dextran, hydroxyethyl starch, and mannitol
  - Exception: ophthalmic use of carbonic anhydrase inhibitors

**Prohibited Methods**

- M1. Manipulation of Blood and Blood Components
- M2. Chemical and Physical Manipulation
  - Tampering with samples
  - Intravenous infusions
- M3. Gene Doping: The transfer of polymers of nucleic acids or analogues, the use of normal or genetically modified cells

**Substances (S) and Methods (M) Prohibited in Competition**

In addition to the above, the following categories are prohibited only in competition:

- S6. Stimulants
- S7. Narcotics
- S8. Cannabinoids: natural (marijuana) or cannabimimetics, eg, "spice," JWH-018, JWH-073, HU-210
- S9. Glucocorticosteroids; all are prohibited when administered by oral, intravenous, intramuscular, or rectal routes

**Substances Prohibited in Particular (P) Sports**

- P1. Alcohol in competition. Detection by analysis of breath and/or blood. Threshold is 0.10 g/L (air sports, archery, automobile, powerboating).
- P2. β-Adrenergic Antagonists

## ANABOLIC XENOBIOTICS

### Anabolic Androgenic Steroids

Anabolic-androgenic steroids (AASs) increase muscle mass and lean body weight and cause nitrogen retention. The androgenic effects of steroids are responsible for male appearance and secondary sexual characteristics such as increased growth of body hair and deepening of the voice. Testosterone is the prototypical androgen, and most AASs are synthetic testosterone derivatives. In this chapter, the term *anabolic steroid* means any xenobiotic, chemically and pharmacologically related to testosterone, other than estrogens, progestins, corticosteroids, and dehydroepiandrosterone (DHEA).

The United States (US) Congress enacted the Anabolic Steroid Control Act of 1990, which placed anabolic steroids in Schedule III. Schedule III implies that a drug has a currently accepted medical use in the US and has less potential for abuse than the drugs categorized as Schedule I or II. The Anabolic Steroid Control Act of 2004 added certain steroid precursors, such as androstenedione and dihydrotestosterone, to the list of controlled substances that are considered illegal without a prescription. Nevertheless, AASs are

**TABLE 14–2 Synthetic Testosterone Derivatives/Anabolic Androgenic Steroids: Generic Nomenclature**

| *17α-Alkyl Derivatives (Oral)* | *17β-Ester Derivatives (Parenteral)* | *Testosterone Preparations (Topical)* |
|---|---|---|
| Ethylestrenol | Boldenone | Buccal gel, sublingual |
| Fluoxymesterone | Nandrolone decanoate | Dermal gel, ointment |
| Methandrostenolone | Nandrolone phenpropionate | Transdermal reservoir patch |
| Methyltestosterone | | |
| Oxandrolone | Testosterone esters | |
| Oxymetholone | Testosterone cypionate | |
| Stanozolol | Testosterone enanthate | |
| | Testosterone ester combination | |
| | Testosterone propionate | |
| | Trenbolone | |

still available illicitly via the Internet from international marketers, veterinary pharmaceutical companies, and legitimate US manufacturers (Table 14–2).

## Antiestrogens and Antiandrogens

In male athletes using androgens, avoiding the unwanted side effects of feminization, such as gynecomastia, or in female athletes, avoiding masculinization and features such as facial hair and deepening voice, requires manipulation of the metabolic pathways of androgen metabolism. Xenobiotics capable of manipulating metabolic pathways associated with undesirable side effects are divided into four main groups.

1. Aromatase inhibitors such as anastrozole and aminoglutethimide prevent the conversion of androstenedione and testosterone into estrogen.
2. The antiestrogen clomiphene blocks estrogen receptors in the hypothalamus, opposing the negative feedback of estrogen, causing an increase in gonadotropin-releasing hormone, thereby increasing testosterone release.
3. Selective estrogen receptor modulators (SERMs) such as tamoxifen and raloxifene bind to estrogen receptors and exhibit agonist or antagonist effects at the estrogen receptors. By indirectly increasing gonadotropin release, SERMs restore endogenous testosterone production upon discontinuation of AASs.
4. Selective androgen receptor modulators (SARMs) are nonsteroidal tissue-selective *anabolic* xenobiotics. Selective androgen receptor modulators are neither aromatized nor substrates for 5α-reductase, nor do they undergo the same metabolic pathways as testosterone. Therefore, they have fewer unwanted androgenic side effects compared with testosterone.

## Administration

AASs are either taken orally or administered by intramuscular injection. Unlike therapeutically indicated regimens, which consist of fixed doses at regular intervals, athletes typically use AASs in cycles of 6 to 8 weeks. For example, the athlete may use steroids for 2 months and then abstain for 2 months. This *cycling* of steroid use is based on the athlete's individual preferences and not on any validated protocol. *Stacking* implies combining the use of several AASs at one time, often with both oral and IM administration. To prevent *plateauing,* or developing tolerance, to any one AAS, some athletes use an average of five different AASs simultaneously on a cycle. *Pyramiding* implies starting the AASs at a low dose, increasing the dose many times, and then tapering once again. *Bridging* refers to the practice of halting the administration of long-lasting alkylated testosterone formulations so that urine analyses at a specific time offer no evidence of use, but injections of shorter acting testosterone esters are used to replace the orally administered alkylated formulations.

## Clinical Manifestations of Anabolic-Androgenic Steroid Use

***Cancer.*** Testicular and prostatic carcinomas are reported in more frequent users of AASs. Hepatocellular carcinoma, cholangiocarcinoma, Wilms tumor, and renal cell carcinoma are also reported in young AAS users.

***Cardiovascular.*** Cardiac complications include acute myocardial infarction, venous thromboembolism, and sudden cardiac arrest due to lethal dysrhythmias. Autopsy examination of the heart often reveals biventricular hypertrophy, extensive myocardial fibrosis, and contraction-band necrosis. There is a dose-dependent association with the coronary atheroscslerotic burden. Growth hormone (GH) potentiates the effects of AASs and further increases concentric remodeling of the left ventricle. In addition to direct myocardial injury, vasospasm or thrombosis occurs. Alkylated androgens lower concentrations of high-density lipoprotein (HDL) cholesterol and increase platelet aggregation. Thromboembolic complications include pulmonary embolus, stroke, carotid arterial occlusion, cerebral sinus thrombosis, poststeroid balance disorder, and popliteal artery entrapment.

***Dermatologic and Gingival.*** Cutaneous side effects are common and include keloid formation, sebaceous cysts, comedones, seborrheic furunculosis, folliculitis, and striae. A common triad of acne, striae, and gynecomastia occurs.

***Endocrine.*** Conversion of AASs to estradiol in peripheral tissues results in feminization of male athletes. Gynecomastia and testicular atrophy result. In women, menstrual irregularities and breast atrophy are reported.

***Hepatic.*** Hepatic subcapsular hematoma with hemorrhage is reported. Peliosis hepatis, a condition of blood-filled sinuses in the liver that results in fatal hepatic rupture, occurs most commonly with the use of alkylated androgens and often does not improve when androgen use is stopped.

***Infectious.*** Local complications from injection include septic joints, cutaneous abscess, and *Candida albicans* endophthalmitis. Injection of AASs using contaminated needles has led to transmission of infectious diseases such as human immunodeficiency virus and hepatitis B and C.

***Musculoskeletal.*** Supraphysiologic doses of testosterone, when combined with strength training, increase muscle strength and size. The most common musculoskeletal complications of steroid use are tendon and ligament rupture.

***Neuropsychiatric.*** Distractibility, depression or mania, delirium, irritability, insomnia, hostility, anxiety, mood lability, and

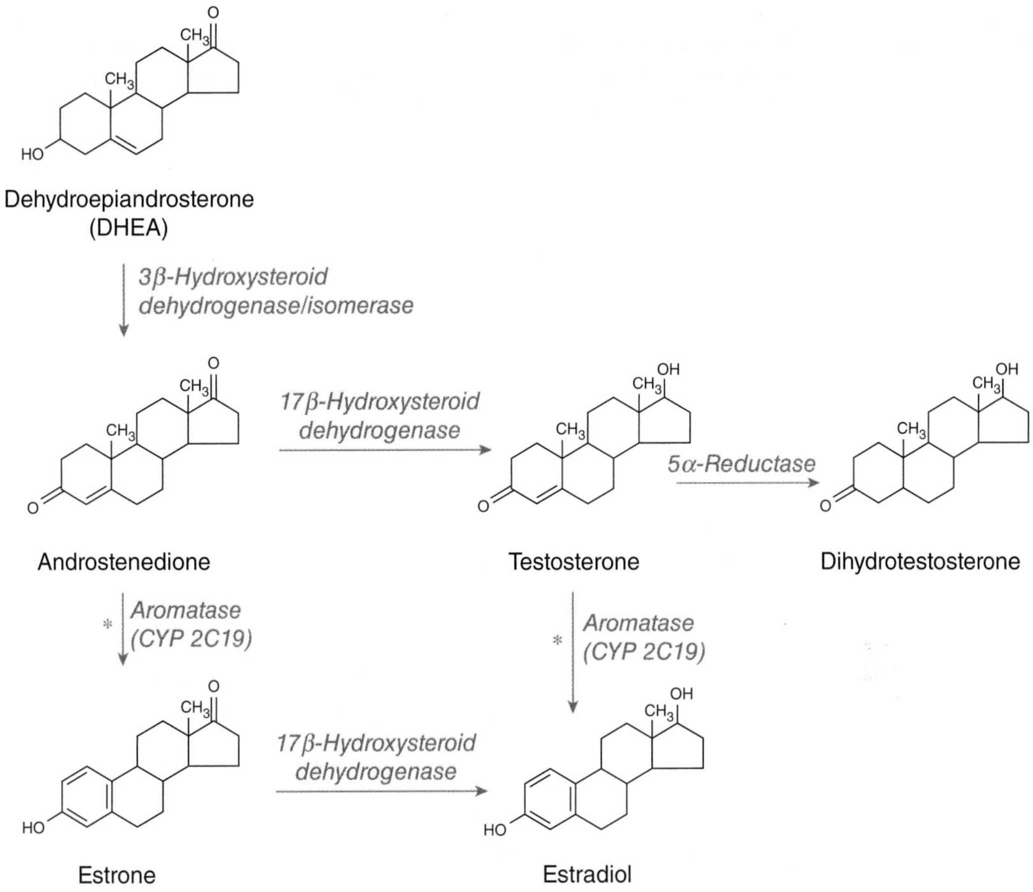

**FIGURE 14–1.** Metabolic pathway of the transformation of dehydroepiandrosterone (DHEA) to androgens and estrogens. Anastrozole and aminogluthemide inhibit aromatase *(asterisk)*, thus blocking feminization after the utilization of androgens.

aggressiveness ("roid rage") may occur. Withdrawal symptoms from AAS include decreased libido, fatigue, and myalgias.

### Specific Anabolic Xenobiotics

***Dehydroepiandrosterone.*** Dehydroepiandrosterone (DHEA) is a precursor to testosterone (Fig. 14–1). Because it is produced endogenously, DHEA most commonly is not categorized as an AAS. However, DHEA is weakly anabolic and weakly androgenic. Although banned by the US FDA in 1996, this xenobiotic subsequently was marketed as a nutritional supplement and is available for purchase without a prescription.

***Clenbuterol.*** Clenbuterol is a $\beta_2$-adrenergic agonist that decreases fat deposition and prevents protein breakdown in animal models. Clenbuterol increases the glycolytic capacity of muscle and causes hypertrophy, enhancing the growth of fast-twitch fibers.

## PEPTIDES AND GLYCOPROTEIN HORMONES

### Creatine

Creatine is an amino acid formed by combining the amino acids methionine, arginine, and glycine. It is synthesized naturally by the liver, kidneys, and pancreas. Creatine is found in protein-containing foods such as meat and fish. In its phosphorylated form, it is involved in the rapid resynthesis of adenosine triphosphate (ATP) from adenosine diphosphate (ADP) by acting as a substrate to donate phosphorus. Because ATP is the immediate source of energy for muscle contraction, creatine is used by athletes to increase energy during short, high-intensity exercise. Numerous studies demonstrate improved performance with creatine supplementation, particularly in sports requiring short, high-intensity effort. Consuming carbohydrates with creatine supplements increase total creatine and phosphorylated creatine stores in skeletal muscle. Creatine supplementation is most commonly accomplished with creatine monohydrate. A dose of 20 to 25 g/day can increase the skeletal muscle total creatine concentration by 20%.

One adverse effect of creatine supplementation is weight gain, which is thought to result primarily from water retention, but also a net protein increase results. Diarrhea was the most commonly reported side effect of creatine use in one study of 52 male college athletes. Creatine supplementation increases urinary creatine and creatinine excretion and may increase serum creatinine concentrations by 20%. Long- and short-term creatine supplementation, however, does not have an adverse effect on kidney function.

### Human Growth Hormone

Human growth hormone (hGH) is an anabolic peptide hormone secreted by the anterior pituitary gland. It stimulates protein synthesis and increases growth and muscle mass in children. Growth hormone secretion is stimulated by GH-releasing hormone and is inhibited by somatostatin. Release of hGH, which occurs mainly during sleep in a pulsatile manner. Exercise stimulates hGH release, and more intense exercise causes proportionately more hGH release. Growth hormone receptors are found in many tissues, including the liver. Binding of hGH to hepatic receptors causes secretion of insulinlike growth factor-1 (IGF-1), which has potent anabolic effects and is the mediator for many of the actions of hGH.

Growth hormone is used by athletes for its anabolic potential. It is particularly attractive because laboratory detection is difficult. Administration of hGH often causes myalgias, arthralgias, carpal tunnel syndrome, and edema. The effects of hGH on skeletal growth depend on the user's age. In preadolescents, excessive hGH causes increased bony growth and gigantism. In adults, excessive hGH causes acromegaly. Growth hormone causes glucose intolerance and hyperglycemia. High-density lipoprotein concentrations are decreased, a change associated with increased risk of coronary artery disease.

The detection of GH relies primarily on the identification of hGH-dependent factors through which hGH exerts its effects, such as IGF-1 and IGF binding proteins, as well as other markers of bone growth and turnover, such as the *N*-terminal extension peptide of procollagen type III. In athletes using recombinant hGH (rhGH), endogenous hGH with its multiple isoforms is suppressed through negative feedback on the pituitary. Therefore, the 22-kDa form characteristic of rhGH becomes predominant while the ratio of isoforms, as measured by immunoassay, changes.

### Insulinlike Growth Factor-1

Insulinlike growth factor-1 is a peptide chain structurally related to insulin. A recombinant form is available. Parenteral administration of IGF-1 is approved for clinical treatment of dwarfism and insulin resistance. Children who develop antibodies to rhGH often respond to IGF-1. The actions of IGF-1 can be classified as either anabolic or insulinlike. Few studies on the efficacy of IGF-1 in improving the conditioning of athletes are available. Insulinlike growth factor-1 is preferred by female athletes because it does not cause virilization.

Side effects are similar to those associated with use of GH and include acromegaly. Other effects include headache, jaw pain, edema, and alterations in lipid profiles. A potentially serious side effect of IGF-1 is hypoglycemia.

### Insulin

Insulin is used by body builders for its anabolic properties. Insulin inhibits proteolysis and promotes growth by stimulating movement of glucose and amino acids into muscle and fat cells. It increases the synthesis of glycogen, fatty acids, and proteins (Chap. 20). As expected, hypoglycemia is reported in body builders using insulin.

### Meldonium

Meldonium inhibits the carnitine transporter type 2, thereby reducing L-carnitine biosynthesis and transport. Long-term meldonium treatment may be beneficial by improving energy metabolism during hypoxia. Meldonium improves glucose utilization.

### Human Chorionic Gonadotropin

In men, hCG stimulates testicular steroidogenesis. Administration of hCG causes an increase in the total testosterone and epitestosterone produced. In women, hCG is secreted by the placenta during pregnancy. It is sometimes used by male athletes to prevent testicular atrophy during and after androgen administration. Very small amounts of hCG are normally present in men and nonpregnant women. Currently, measurement is made by immunoassay. The decision limit, the concentration at which the test result is considered positive, is set at 5 IU/mL urine.

## OXYGEN TRANSPORT

### Erythropoietin

Human erythropoietin (EPO) induces erythropoiesis by stimulating stem cells. Human EPO is secreted primarily by the kidney, although some is produced by the liver. Erythropoietin has been available since 1988 as recombinant human EPO (rhEPO), and its use in international competition has been prohibited since 1990. Because EPO increases exercise capacity and hemoglobin production, it is used by athletes, often with additional iron supplementation. The mean apparent half-lives of rhEPO are 4.5 hours after intravenous (IV) administration and 25 hours after subcutaneous administration. The clinical effects of increased hemoglobin occur several days after administration. Erythropoietin increases maximal oxygen uptake by 6% to 7%, an effect that lasts approximately 2 weeks after rhEPO administration is completed. Erythropoietin analogs such as darbepoetin are *erythropoiesis-stimulating proteins*, differing from EPO by five amino acids. Darbepoetin has a much longer half-life and can be injected weekly. Another protein, known as *synthetic erythropoiesis protein,* has a similar protein structure to EPO.

Erythropoietin enhances endothelial activation and platelet reactivity and increases systolic blood pressure during submaximal exercise. These effects, in addition to the increase in hemoglobin, increase the risk of thromboembolic events, hypertension, and hyperviscosity syndromes. EPO overdose is rarely reported but associated with hematocrits of 70% or higher and complications of hyperviscosity. Treatment is with phlebotomy, IV hydration and erythrophereis.

***Testing for Erythropoietin.*** Erythropoietin is directly measured by a monoclonal anti-EPO antibody test, which does not distinguish between endogenously produced and exogenously administered recombinant EPO. Therefore, tracking indirect methods of EPO detection are used, such as measurement of hemoglobin or hematocrit. State-of-the-art detection of EPO doping is accomplished by two techniques: isoelectric focusing and immunoblotting performed on urine samples. The two isoforms of EPO, recombinant and endogenous, have different glycosylation patterns and glycan sizes, resulting in differing molecular charges. An immunoblotting procedure takes advantage of these different net charges, and the proteins can be separated by their charges when they are placed in an electric field. Subsequently, by isoelectric focusing, this method obtains an image of EPO patterns in the urine. Because of the structural similarity of darbepoetin to EPO, these detection techniques also are effective for darbepoetin.

## STIMULANTS

### Caffeine

Caffeine is a central nervous system stimulant that causes a feeling of decreased fatigue and increases endurance performance (Chap. 36).

### Amphetamines

The beneficial effects of amphetamines in sports result from their ability to mask fatigue and pain. Initial studies done in soldiers showed that they could march longer and ignore pain when taking amphetamines (Chap. 46). However, although the perception of fatigue decreased, lactic acid accumulates, and maximal oxygen consumption is unchanged.

### Sodium Bicarbonate

Sodium bicarbonate loading, known as "soda loading," has a long history of use in horse racing. Sodium bicarbonate buffers the metabolic acidosis associated with an elevated lactate caused by exercise, thereby delaying fatigue and enhancing performance. Several studies demonstrated improved performance in running when sodium bicarbonate was ingested 2 to 3 hours before competition. Adverse effects of bicarbonate loading include diarrhea, abdominal pain, and the possibility of hypernatremia.

## DIURETICS

Diuretics are used in sports in which the athlete must achieve a certain weight to compete in discrete weight classes. Diuretics also result in increased urine production, thereby diluting the urine and making the detection of other banned xenobiotics more difficult.

## LABORATORY DETECTION

Enormous amounts of energy and money are expended to determine the presence or absence of performance-enhancing xenobiotics. Analysis of samples on the international level is performed by a limited number of accredited laboratories. The majority of tests are performed on urine, with careful procedural requirements regarding handling of samples. Attention must be paid to proper storage of specimens because bacterial metabolism may increase urinary steroid concentrations. Upon arrival of a sample at the testing laboratory, the integrity of the sample is checked, including the code, seal, visual appearance, density, and pH. Registration of the sample is completed, and the sample is divided into two aliquots. All testing is done on the first aliquot, and any positive results are confirmed on the second aliquot. Sample preparation is difficult and time consuming.

### Capillary Gas Chromatography–Mass Spectrometry

Capillary gas chromatography allows the determination of approximately 95% of all doping positive results. Gas chromatography typically is combined with mass spectrometry for detection of the majority of substances. Analysis of the urine by gas chromatography–mass spectrophotometry (GC-MS) is the current standard for detection of AASs. Such analysis relies on a large amount of previously derived reference data.

### Testosterone-to-Epitestosterone Ratio

Gas chromatography–mass spectrophotometry cannot distinguish endogenous testosterone from pharmaceutically derived exogenous testosterone. Therefore, other methods of detection are needed. One way of detecting the use of exogenous testosterone is to measure the testosterone-to-epitestosterone (T/E) ratio. Epitestosterone is not a metabolite of testosterone, but it is a 17-$\alpha$ epimer, differing from testosterone only in the configuration of the hydroxyl group on C-17. Men produce 30 times more testosterone than epitestosterone; however, 1% of testosterone and 30% of epitestosterone are excreted unchanged in the urine. Therefore, the normal T/E ratio in the urine is about 1:1. A T/E ratio less than 4:1 is considered acceptable; a T/E ratio greater than 4:1 is considered evidence of doping using testosterone. To maintain a normal T/E ratio, athletes self-administer both testosterone and epitestosterone.

### Isotope Ratio Mass Spectrometry

Carbon is made up of six protons and six neutrons, giving it an atomic weight of 12 ($^{12}C$). Sometimes carbon has an extra neutron, giving it an atomic weight of 13 ($^{13}C$). Warm climate plants, such as soy, process carbon dioxide differently than other plants, using different photosynthetic pathways for carbon dioxide fixation, causing the depletion of $^{13}C$. Pharmaceutical testosterone is made from plant sterols, primarily soy plants, and therefore has less $^{13}C$ isotope than endogenous testosterone, made in the body from a typical human diet based in corn and not soy. This difference in isotope ratios is measured by isotope ratio mass spectrometry and compared to an international standard.

### Insulin

The technology for testing for insulin uses immunoaffinity purification followed by liquid chromatography–tandem mass spectrometry to identify analytes including urinary metabolites of insulin. When insulin is modified to improve its receptor selectivity or give it other favorable properties, the change in molecular weight or amino acid profile from human insulin makes it detectable by GC-MS.

### Masking Xenobiotics

Any chemical or physical manipulation done with the purpose of altering the integrity of a urine is called masking. Some xenobiotics are added to the urine for the sole purpose of interfering with urine testing and are easily detected. Niacin is used to alter urine test results, although there is no evidence it is effective for this purpose. There are reports of niacin toxicity, including skin reactions such as itching, flushing, and burning, when niacin is used for this purpose. More serious effects, including nausea, elevated liver enzymes, hypoglycemia, and anion gap metabolic acidosis, are reported as a result of ingesting niacin in large amounts, in the 2.5 to 5.5 g range over 1 to 2 days.

A significant issue in the analysis of urine for the presence of prohibited peptides such as rhEPO is the masking potential of proteases surreptitiously added to urine specimens slated for doping analysis. The proteases are packaged in "grains" known as protease granules or "rice grains" and placed in the urethra. Upon urination for the purpose of providing a specimen for doping analysis, the grain flows with urine into the specimen cup. The proteases, including trypsin, chymotrypsin, and papain, quickly degrade renally excreted peptides, most notably EPO, making them undetectable. By the process of autolysis, proteases themselves become undetectable over time. Normally, the presence of urinary proteins creates the image of a visible band by gel electrophoresis. However, the urine with elevated protease activity will demonstrate something called *trace of burning*, a term indicating an absence of proteins.

The list of prohibited masking xenobiotics includes diuretics; epitestosterone; probenecid; plasma expanders such as albumin, dextran, and hydroxymethyl starch; and α-reductase inhibitors such as finasteride and dutasteride. Probenecid blocks urinary excretion of the glucuronide conjugates of AAS.

### Gene Doping

The discovery of the genetic codes for some diseases has made gene therapy of medical conditions, such as muscular dystrophy, a reality. Gene doping is defined as "the non-therapeutic use of cells, genes, genetic elements, or of the modulation of gene expression, having the capacity to enhance athlete performance."

***Athlete's Biological Passport.*** A significant development in the detection of blood transfusion, known as blood doping, is the development of a longitudinal record of an athlete's RBC parameters called the *athlete's biological passport.* This is individualized longitudinal monitoring that tests blood for markers of doping.

### Neurocognitive Enhancement

Improvement in brain function and mental agility is an element of performance enhancement receiving increasing study. Students report improving academic productivity as the motivation for use of stimulants. Nutritional studies are reported to demonstrate the positive effects of fruit flavonoid supplementation. Blueberries and other berries in the diet are suggested to enhance memory both with acute and chronic diet inclusion in both animals and human subjects. Enhancement of neurocognitive performance using vitamins and minerals is a new area of study.

## PERFORMANCE ENHANCEMENT AND SUDDEN DEATH IN ATHLETES

Many unexpected deaths in certain groups of young competitors have occurred in the absence of obvious medical or traumatic causes. In some of these cases, the use of performance-enhancing drugs was linked to the deaths. The use of EPO is suggested to have contributed to the large number of deaths in young European endurance athletes. Nevertheless, the leading cause of nontraumatic sudden death in young athletes is most often associated with cardiac anomalies. In autopsy studies of athletes in the US with congenital sudden death, hypertrophic cardiomyopathy is the most common structural abnormality, accounting for more than one-third of the cardiac arrests followed by coronary artery anomalies. In Italy, dysrhythmogenic right ventricular cardiomyopathy is implicated in one-fourth of these deaths.

# 15 ESSENTIAL OILS

## INTRODUCTION

Essential oils are a class of volatile oils that are extracted through steam distillation or are cold pressed from the leaves, flowers, bark, wood, fruit, or peel of a single parent plant. The term *essential* refers to the essence of a plant rather than an indispensable component of the oil or a vital biologic function.

## HISTORY AND EPIDEMIOLOGY

Therapeutic use of essential oils can be traced back thousands of years in history to the ancient Greeks and ancient Egyptians, and it is also described in biblical writings. The first documents detailing an actual distillation process date back to the ninth century, when such oils were imported into Europe from the Middle East. By the 16th century, concepts of separating fatty oils and essential oils from aromatic water became more defined, and oils were used frequently for fragrance, flavoring, and medicinal purposes. By the 19th century, these processes became industrialized, and specific chemicals could be identified and mass produced. Currently, these oils are not regulated by the United States (US) Food and Drug Administration (FDA) creating the potential for variability in active ingredients and adulterants with each producer. This chapter highlights some of the most commonly used oils for medicinal purposes that also have the greatest potential for toxicity.

### Absinthe

***History.*** *Artemisia absinthium* is more commonly known as wormwood because of its use as an anthelmintic in ancient times. The earliest recorded use of wormwood is found in the Ebers papyrus, which covers writings circa 1550 B.C. in Egypt. Absinthe is a liqueur composed of ethanol, oil of wormwood, and various other herbs, and it is known for its green color and bitter taste. It was first distilled in Switzerland but came to prominence during the early 19th century, with Pernod's distillery in France. As early as 1850, descriptions of toxicity were documented. By the 1910s, many countries had made it illegal. In the 20th century, thujone was discovered to be the toxic component of absinthe.

***Pharmacology.*** The bitter taste and anthelmintic properties come from the lactones absinthin and anabsinthin. However, the toxicity of wormwood is due to its thujone content. After absorption, thujone is metabolized primarily to 7-hydroxy α-thujone by CYP3A4 in humans. This metabolite achieves a higher concentration in the brain, but it is less potent in binding the γ-aminobutyric acid (GABA) A receptor and is less toxic compared with its parent compound.

***Pathophysiology.*** α-Thujone is a noncompetitive $GABA_A$ receptor antagonist, similar to picrotoxin. This antagonism causes neuroexcitation, which results in hallucinations or seizures in a dose-dependent fashion. The psychotropic effects are mediated by the ability of α-thujone to desensitize the $5\text{-}HT_3$ receptor.

***Clinical Features.*** Clinical features of acute toxicity are similar to those of ethanol intoxication, including euphoria and confusion, which can progress to restlessness, visual hallucinations, and delirium. Seizures have also occurred. Rhabdomyolysis and acute kidney injury (AKI) are also reported after ingestion of oil of wormwood intended for preparation as absinthe. The etiology of the rhabdomyolysis is unknown.

### Camphor

***History.*** Originally derived from the bark of the camphor tree (*Cinnamomum camphora*), camphor has been widely used for centuries. It was described in writings from Marco Polo's visits to China, and in the 16th century, it was referred to as the "balsam of disease." Camphor has been used as an abortifacient, a contraceptive, a cold remedy, an aphrodisiac, an *anti*aphrodisiac, a lactation suppressor, an antiseptic, a moth repellant, and a cardiac stimulant. In the 20th century, camphor was predominantly used as a topical rubefacient to provide local analgesia and antipruritic effects. It also became a key ingredient in paregoric (camphorated tincture of opium), a common household remedy for diarrhea and cough used until 1970. Throughout the 20th century, camphor was also available as a nonprescription remedy and toxicity occurred in cases in which camphorated oil was mistaken for castor oil and ingested in large amounts. In 1982, the US FDA limited any product from containing more than 11% camphor and banned camphorated oil. Despite these restrictions concentrated camphor products are still found in the US. Today, camphor is most commonly found in topical products.

***Pharmacology.*** Camphor is rapidly absorbed from the gastrointestinal (GI) tract. Serum concentrations are detected within 15 minutes of ingestion. It is also readily absorbed from the skin and mucous membranes. Camphor is very lipophilic with a large volume of distribution. It is metabolized in the liver by CYP2A6 and excreted in the urine after glucuronidation.

***Pathophysiology.*** The mechanism for seizures is still unknown. Topical effects of camphor result from desensitization of the transient receptor potential vanilloid subtype 1 (TRPV1) channel, a nonspecific cation channel that mediates thermosensation and nociception in the peripheral nervous system (Fig. 15–1). Currently, there are several known transient receptors (Fig. 15–2). Camphor's antitussive effects are presumed to be through the desensitization of TRPV1 and antagonism of TRPA1. Hepatotoxicity is also reported and can range from a mild elevation in aminotransferase concentrations to fulminant hepatic failure.

***Clinical Features.*** Camphor toxicity is reported after nasal, topical, inhalational, and oral administration. Two grams of camphor can cause significant toxicity in adults when ingested, and children have died from as little as 0.7 to 1 g of 20% camphorated oil (1 tsp). Gastrointestinal signs and symptoms such as nausea and vomiting usually develop within 5 to

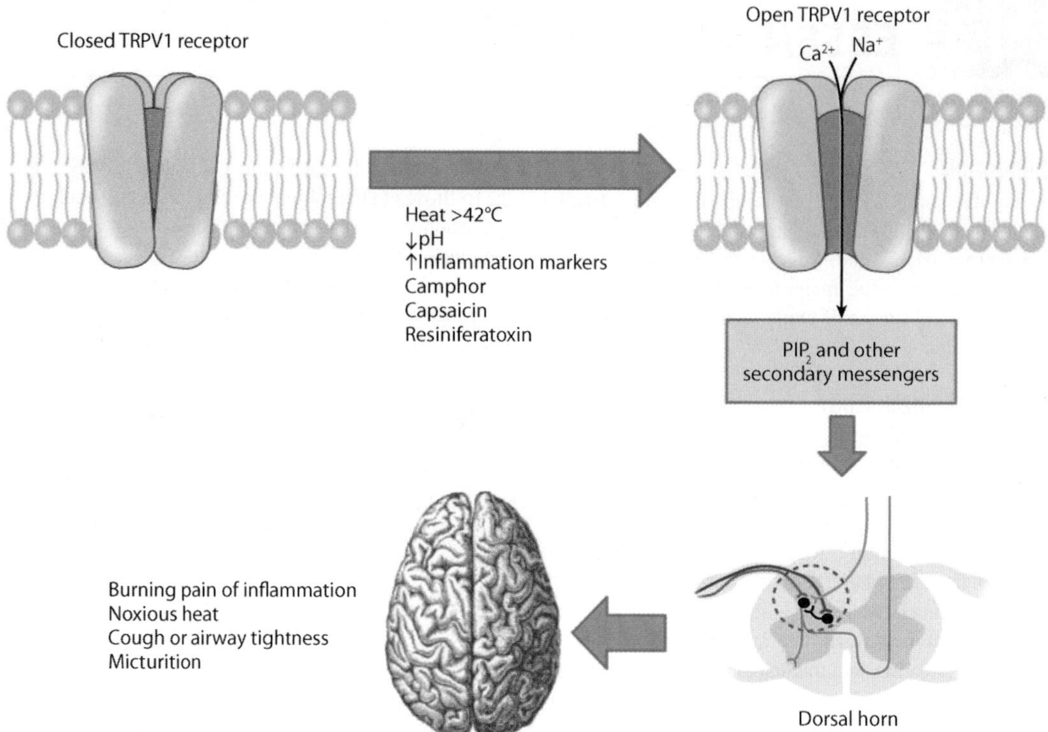


**FIGURE 15–1.** The transient receptor potential vanilloid subtype 1 (TRPV1) receptor is a nonspecific cation channel that is located on the skin and bladder, in the peripheral nociceptors and the dorsal horn of the spinal cord, and in the airway. Stimulation by heat, acidemia, and inflammation increases its activity; camphor, capsaicin, and resiniferatoxin are direct agonists. When open, TRPV1 stimulates intracellular signaling via $PIP_2$ to relay sensation of burning pain, noxious heat, airway tightness, and the need for micturition.

90 minutes after ingestion. Patients complain of feeling warm, faint, and vertiginous and have headaches. Severe effects and findings include confusion, agitation, delirium, and hallucinations. Seizures are common and usually develop within minutes to a few hours of exposure. Status epilepticus is reported.

## Clove Oil

***History.*** Clove oil is extracted from the plant *Syzygium aromaticum*, also known as *Eugenia aromatica*. In medieval and Renaissance Europe, cloves were considered to be a valuable commodity. They were used for flavoring and fragrance, as well as for medicinal purposes, and that tradition remains intact today. Today, clove oil is commonly mixed with zinc oxide as a sealant in dentistry, a practice that dates as early as 1873. Clove oil is also used to alleviate toothaches.

***Pharmacology.*** Typically, clove oil contains 60% to 90% eugenol, which is the primary active component. Eugenol undergoes sulfonation and glucuronidation in the liver, with a minor pathway involving the CYP enzymes to form a reactive intermediate that requires glutathione for proper elimination.

***Pathophysiology.*** The anesthetic properties of eugenol are mediated by blockade of various ion currents in nerves. In rodent studies, eugenol acts in both a capsaicin receptor mediated pathway and by an independent pathway. Eugenol also inhibits voltage-gated sodium channels independently of TRPV1, and this likely mediates its anesthetic effects. In rat hepatocytes, eugenol causes glutathione depletion and subsequent hepatotoxicity in a dose- and time-dependent manner. Eugenol also inhibits prostaglandin synthetase, which would support the claims for its use as an antiinflammatory xenobiotic in dentistry.

***Clinical Features.*** Infants and children ingesting clove oil develop depressed mental status, anion gap metabolic acidosis, and hepatotoxicity complicated by coagulopathy and hypoglycemia. Acute respiratory distress syndrome (ARDS) is reported with intravenous (IV) administration of clove oil.

## Eucalyptus Oil

***History.*** Oil of eucalyptus is derived primarily from *Eucalyptus globulus*, a tree native to Australia. Eighteenth-century British explorers noted that the aboriginal people traditionally used eucalyptus as a fever remedy. In the 19th and early 20th centuries, eucalyptus oil was a common household remedy for coughs and fevers, and it was also used as an antiseptic.

***Pharmacology.*** Eucalyptus oil contains almost 70% eucalyptol. It is rapidly absorbed from the GI tract and metabolized by CYP3A4 and CYP3A5 to the 2-hydroxy and 3-hydroxy metabolites.

***Pathophysiology.*** Eucalyptus inhibits potassium-induced contractions of airway smooth muscles causing a myorelaxant effect, thus alleviating upper respiratory irritation. However, eucalyptus also potentiates acetylcholine-induced contractions of the trachea in vitro, possibly by inhibiting

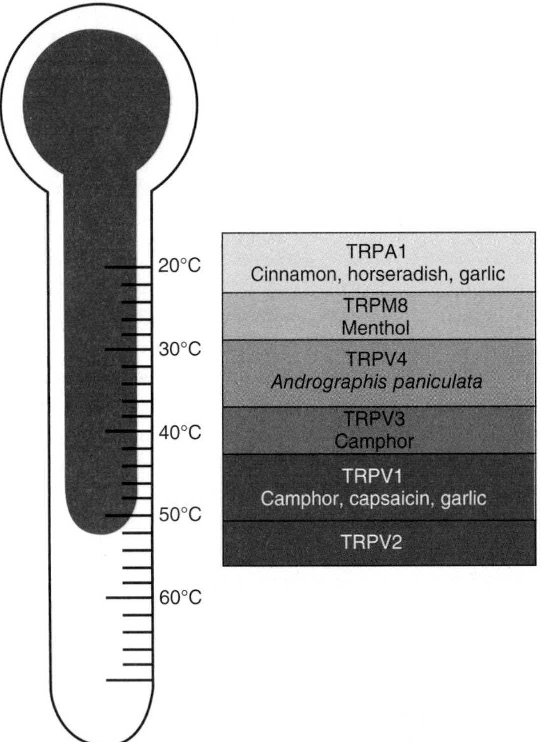


**FIGURE 15–2.** Schematic of six mammalian thermo–transient receptor potential (TRP) channels based on their temperature threshold for activation. Certain natural xenobiotics can activate these receptors, which may lead to burning or heat sensation. Transient receptor potential A1 cation channel subfamily M member 8 (TRPM8) mediates cold sensation in sensory neurons. Menthol and eucalyptus's cooling and analgesic effects are thought to be caused by TRPM8 activation. Camphor desensitizes TRP vanilloid subtype 1 (TRPV1), which could explain the initial hot and then cool sensation when applied to skin. Camphor antagonizes TRPA1, which may mediate its antitussive effects.

acetylcholinesterase. This finding would explain the upper respiratory irritation that commonly plagues workers who process eucalyptus trees for papers and other materials. Eucalyptol inhibits monocytes from producing several cytokines and also suppresses arachidonic acid metabolism. These findings underlie the ability of eucalyptol to control mucous hypersecretion, making it a potential adjunct in controlling asthma and chronic obstructive pulmonary disease, for which it is frequently used as an alternative medicine. The cooling effects of eucalyptus are likely mediated by TRPM8. The mechanism of toxicity has yet to be elucidated.

***Clinical Features.*** In children, significant toxicity is reported after ingesting as little as a teaspoon. Fatalities are reported in adults who have ingested as little as a tablespoon. Typical effects and findings of eucalyptus toxicity include drowsiness, slurred speech, ataxia, nausea, and vomiting. Rarely, seizures and coma occur. Symptom onset is usually within minutes to hours and rarely exceeds 4 hours.

### Lavender Oil

***History.*** Lavender is one of the most commonly used essential oils for fragrance and aromatherapy. It was used by the ancient Romans and Greeks for its believed antimicrobial, carminative, sedative, and antidepressive properties. The oil is produced by steam distillation of the flower heads and foliage of the *Lavandula* species. Lavender oil is most commonly used in aromatherapy to enhance mood, decrease anxiety, or control pain. Silexin is an oral preparation of *Lavandula angustifolia* that is sold as an anxiolytic in Germany. Studies show it be noninferior to lorazepam or paroxetine in treatment of various anxiety disorders.

***Pharmacology.*** The main components of lavender oil are linalool, linalyl acetate, 1,8-cineole, β-ocimene, terpinen-4-ol, and camphor. Linalool and linalyl acetate are the components believed to be responsible for the sedative and narcotic effects of lavender oil. These compounds are rapidly absorbed through the skin and can reach peak serum concentrations as soon as 19 minutes postexposure. Studies in mice show that lavender oil acts on serotonin receptors, rather than GABA receptors, and this underlies its anxiolytic effects. Linalool inhibits both nicotinic receptor–mediated acetylcholine release and glutamate release.

***Pathophysiology.*** Lavender oil is very allergenic. Several case series report the development of gynecomastia in prepubertal boys using lavender oil. In vitro data showed that lavender oil elicits a dose-dependent increase in estrogen responsivity and antiandrogenic activity in breast cancer cell cultures, similar to the effects of estradiol.

***Clinical Features.*** The predominant clinical feature of exposure is contact dermatitis. Unexplained or "idiopathic" gynecomastia in prepubertal boys with negative endocrine evaluations should prompt questions regarding the use of these essential oils.

### Nutmeg Oil

***History.*** Nutmeg and mace originate from the evergreen tree *Myristica fragans*. The name *nutmeg* refers to the seed of the tree, which looks like a glossy brown nut. Mace is derived from the scarlet-colored aril that encloses the seed. Although nutmeg is a common household spice and flavoring agent, it has been used for centuries for various ailments, including digestive disorders, cholera, rheumatic disease, psychiatric disorders, and pain. Mace was used as an aphrodisiac, and nutmeg was commonly used in Europe and North America, albeit ineffectually, as an emmenagogue and abortifacient. Indeed, most of the cases of nutmeg poisoning in the early 20th century were due to women attempting to terminate pregnancies or induce menses. However, most cases of toxicity today are caused by people using nutmeg as a natural high.

***Pharmacology.*** The nutmeg seed yields 7% to 16% volatile oil, 4% to 8% of which is myristicin. Elemicin is another main ingredient of the volatile oil. Extensive liver metabolism is theorized in animals. Human data are lacking.

***Pathophysiology.*** Studies in mice suggest that nutmeg and fresh myristicin are monoamine oxidase inhibitors (MAOIs). Data from an in vitro study show that nutmeg stimulates the cannabinoid system by inhibiting enzymes that degrade the body's own endocannabinoids. Animal data show that nutmeg can induce tachycardia and increase the speed of conduction through the atrioventricular node in the acute setting, but chronic exposure caused bradycardia. The exact mechanism for this is unknown.

*Clinical Features.* Tachycardia, nausea, and dry mouth are common in acute exposures. Some patients develop GI distress and vomiting. Central nervous system effects and findings range from giddiness to a sense of detachment or impending doom to hallucinations and delusions. Nutmeg ingestion rarely causes significant morbidity or mortality, although deaths are reported. A single report describes seizures and altered mental status requiring intubation in a patient who intentionally ingested 39 g of ground nutmeg as a suicide attempt.

### Pennyroyal Oil

*History.* Oil of pennyroyal is derived from the plant *Mentha pulegium* and has a mintlike odor. Its initial use was as a flea repellant. Pennyroyal has been used for centuries as an emmemagogue and abortifacient, and most reported toxicities are from women ingesting large quantities to induce these effects. Pennyroyal is still used as a flavoring and fragrance agent in foods and cosmetics.

*Pharmacology.* Pulegone, the active ingredient, is metabolized by the CYP450 enzymes into several metabolites, including menthofuran, which is thought to be the metabolite primarily responsible for hepatotoxicity, although other reactive intermediates are also implicated.

*Pathophysiology.* In animal studies, pulegone depletes glutathione and causes centrilobular hepatic necrosis. An unknown reactive metabolite is implicated because blocking the CYP450 system prevents glutathione depletion. *R*(+)-Pulegone also causes necrosis in lung epithelium, but the mechanism remains unknown. In addition, *R*(+)-pulegone decreases inward current from L-type calcium channels and blocks the inward rectifying potassium channels on the rat myocardium.

*Clinical Features.* Common initial signs and symptoms are nausea, abdominal pain, and vomiting, often occurring within a few hours of exposure. Central nervous system toxicity, including seizures and coma, develop in severe cases. Fatal cases develop liver failure, kidney failure, and disseminated intravascular coagulation. Most cases of severe toxicity involve women ingesting large amounts of the herb to induce an abortion; however, two cases involved confusing the leaves of *M. pulegium* for nontoxic mint leaves to make tea.

### Peppermint Oil

*History.* Menthol or peppermint oil is one of the most commonly used flavoring agents in the world. It is derived from the distillation of leaves of the *Mentha piperita*. Peppermint flavor is common in oral care products, candies, cosmetics, pharmaceuticals, and beverages. Menthol is also sold as an herbal remedy for pruritus, GI disorders such as irritable bowel syndrome, and cough and cold symptoms, as well as a topical analgesic.

*Pharmacology.* Peppermint oil typically contains 30% to 55% menthol. Menthol is very lipid soluble and easily absorbed through the skin. Menthol is rapidly metabolized by the CYP450 system primarily to *p*-menthane-3,8 diol and then glucuronidated and eliminated in the urine. In human pharmacokinetic studies, only glucuronidated menthol is detected in urine in ranges of 45% to 46% of the menthol ingested. The plasma half-life of menthol glucuronide was determined to be 56.2 minutes and 42.6 minutes, respectively, when mint teas and candies were used.

*Pathophysiology.* Menthol activates the TRP cation channel subfamily M member 8 (TRPM8), which usually responds to thermal stimuli in the cool to cold range of 46° to 82°F (8°–28°C) (Fig. 15–2). Menthol and cold stimuli increase intracellular calcium, which leads to depolarization and generation of an action potential. In vitro data with isolated animal ileum and jejunum tissue show that menthol reduces contractions by reducing calcium influx. Menthol and peppermint oil both inhibit 5-$HT_3$ receptors in vitro as well as reduce serotonin-induced contractions of rat ileum, which could mediate some of the antiemetic effects. Menthol is also commonly used to relieve the symptoms of upper respiratory infections, in particular rhinitis. However, despite the sensation of improved airflow and decreased congestion, menthol actually causes increased nasal congestion.

*Clinical Features.* Case reports regarding menthol toxicity are rare. A case report describes acute respiratory distress syndrome (ARDS) developing in a patient after an intentional IV injection of 5 mL of peppermint oil in a suicide attempt. Symptoms began within 2 hours of the exposure.

### Pine Oil

*History.* Pine oil is commonly used as a household cleaner, varnish, and polish. The cleaning products typically include 20% pine oil, 6% to 10% isopropyl alcohol, and other hydrocarbons.

*Pharmacology.* Pine oil is readily absorbed following ingestion. The major terpene is α-pinene. The major metabolite is bornyl acetate, which is produced by the enzymatic processes of hydration, hydroxylation, rearrangement, acetylation, and reduction in the liver. The metabolites are excreted through the kidneys and lungs.

*Pathophysiology.* Pine oil is a volatile hydrocarbon compound with low viscosity. Aspiration and inhalational injury are common (Chap. 78). Animals injected with pine oil develop ARDS, but the mechanism is unknown.

*Clinical Features.* The lethal dose is in the range of 60 to 120 g in adults and clinical effects usually occur within 2 to 3 hours postingestion. The most common reported symptoms are impaired mentation, psychomotor agitation, delirium, headache, nausea, ataxia, and GI distress. Gastrointestinal irritation and gastritis are reported, but actual perforation or high-grade lesions have not been found. Acute kidney injury is also reported. The most severe outcomes involve an aspiration pneumonitis that can progress to ARDS or a secondary pneumonia.

### Tea Tree Oil

*History.* Tea tree oil is derived from the distillation of leaves of *Melaleuca alternifolia*, a plant that is native to Australia and is also known as melaleuca oil. The first reported use of *M. alternifolia* was in Australian Aborigines. Crushed leaves were inhaled to treat cough and cold symptoms, and poultices of the leaves were applied to wounds. The oil itself was not distilled until the 20th century, at which time it was touted as antibacterial.

***Pharmacology.*** Pharmacokinetic and pharmacodynamic data are limited. Tea tree oil is composed of terpene hydrocarbons and contains more than 100 components. An international standard stipulates that tea tree oil should contain at least 30% terpinen-4-ol, which is believed to be the primary antimicrobial and less than 15% 1,8-cineole, which is believed to be primarily responsible for the irritating properties.

***Pathophysiology.*** Tea tree oil is bactericidal, but its mechanism of action is only partly elucidated. Tea tree oil also has antiinflammatory effects. Specifically, it inhibits lipopolysaccharide-induced production of the inflammatory mediators TNF-$\alpha$, IL-1$\alpha$, IL-10, and prostaglandin E2 by monocytes in vitro.

***Clinical Manifestations.*** Skin irritation and allergic reactions are common effects with topical exposure. Case reports of children unintentionally ingesting a 100% concentration of tea tree oil show ataxia and other neurologic symptoms developing within 30 minutes of exposure that usually resolve within a day. A case report describes using surfactant to treat an 18-month-old boy who developed ARDS after an unintentional ingestion of 100% tea tree oil.

### Oil of Wintergreen

***History.*** Oil of wintergreen was originally derived from *Gaultheria procumbens*, or the Eastern teaberry, which is a fragrant ground cover plant found in North America. The active ingredient in oil of wintergreen is methyl salicylate, which has a pleasant, minty smell and taste, posing a significant hazard to children. Pure oil of wintergreen contains at least 98% methyl salicylate, but most commercial preparations of methyl salicylate contain far less. The US FDA regulations require that any drug containing more than 5% methyl salicylate have a warning against using it other than as a topical agent and keeping it out of the reach of children. Oil of wintergreen has been used as a fragrance and flavoring agent in foods and household products. It is also found in topical preparations worldwide, such as Tiger Balm and Ben-Gay, which are used to treat inflammation and myalgias. The first reported case of toxicity occurred in 1832, when six soldiers used the oil to flavor their tea. The seminal case series was reported in the 1930s in which 43 exposures were tabulated; 20 exposures involved children younger than the age of 4 years and had a 75% fatality rate.

***Pharmacology.*** Methyl salicylate is absorbed both from the GI tract and transdermally. Normally, only 12% to 20% of topical salicylate is absorbed from the skin after 10 hours of application. Heat, inflamed or broken skin, and prolonged use of occlusive dressings increase absorption. Children are presumed to be at greater risk for toxicity because of their higher surface area–to–weight ratio and more permeable skin. After it has been absorbed, methyl salicylate enters the circulation and is transported to the liver, where it undergoes hydrolysis to form salicylic acid. The salicylic acid undergoes conjugation with glycine and glucuronic acid, forming salicyluric acid, salicyl acyl, and phenolic glucuronide. Salicylates are then renally eliminated in the forms of salicyluric acid (75%), free salicylic acid (10%), salicylic phenol (10%), acyl glucuronides (5%), and gentisic acid (<1%).

***Pathophysiology.*** Five milliliters (1 tsp) of oil of wintergreen is equivalent in salicylate content to 7 g of aspirin, which has been a fatal amount in some reported cases. An extensive discussion of salicylate pathophysiology is given in Chap. 10.

***Clinical Features.*** An overdose of methyl salicylate presents similarly to that of other salicylates. Salicylate poisoning is characterized by diaphoresis, nausea, vomiting, tinnitus, hyperpnea, and tachypnea. Mental status changes represent severe toxicity. Symptom onset is typically within a few hours given rapid absorption of the oil. Severe toxicity is associated with seizures, cerebral edema, ARDS, coma, and death.

## DIAGNOSTIC TESTING

Laboratory testing is of little utility in most essential oil toxicity, and the patient's clinical status will determine which tests are indicated. Some essential oil exposures require specific studies, and they are listed below. Generally, blood or urine concentrations of the active ingredients are not available in a meaningful time frame and cannot and should not guide management. Patients who present with altered mental status or seizures warrant a complete evaluation that includes a rapid assessment of glucose, basic metabolic studies, a head computed tomography scan, and lumbar puncture for serious potential structural, infectious, or metabolic etiologies as guided by the history and examination. In patients who present with respiratory symptoms, chest radiographs and continuous pulse oximetry are warranted.

- **Absinthe:** Laboratory studies should include a complete blood count (CBC), chemistry panel, creatine phosphokinase concentration, and glucose monitoring in patients who present with seizures. Urinalysis should be performed to evaluate for myoglobinuria.
- **Pennyroyal Oil:** A CBC and liver function studies, including the aminotransferases, bilirubin, prothrombin time, and partial thromboplastin time, and a $\beta$-human chorionic gonadotropin in women are indicated because many women ingest pennyroyal oil to terminate unwanted pregnancies.
- **Oil of wintergreen:** Serum salicylate concentrations, blood gas, serum potassium concentration, and urine pH initially should be sent every 1 to 2 hours to determine extent of toxicity and need for treatment (Chap. 10).

## TREATMENT

The mainstay of treatment of patients with symptomatic essential oil toxicity is supportive care, including monitoring of vital signs, IV fluids, and supplemental oxygen as needed. A dose of activated charcoal is reasonable in alert patients with an intact airway, but if there is a concern for seizures or vomiting, activated charcoal should be withheld or deferred until the airway is protected. Dermal exposures should be properly decontaminated to prevent further absorption. Benzodiazepines are the mainstay of treatment in patients who present with agitation and seizures. A few of the essential oils require specific treatment:

- **Absinthe:** Rhabdomyolysis should be treated with IV fluids.
- **Camphor:** Most patients need supportive care with a focus on airway and circulatory management as well as treatment of seizures. The molecular weight and lipophilic nature of camphor indicates that it would likely be adsorbed by activated charcoal. Activated charcoal should only be administered in patients with massive life-threatening ingestions and protected airways.
- **Clove oil:** In patients who exhibit signs of hepatotoxicity, it is reasonable to administer *N*-acetylcysteine (NAC).
- **Pennyroyal oil:** One case of ingestion of a potentially fatal amount of pennyroyal was successfully treated with NAC. Given in vitro studies showing glutathione depletion, it is recommended to administer NAC in cases of pennyroyal-induced hepatotoxicity. Because there is no established dosing regimen, using the same regimen used for acetaminophen toxicity would be reasonable.
- **Oil of wintergreen:** Alkalization with sodium bicarbonate and hemodialysis are indicated in cases of severe salicylate toxicity (Chap. 10).

# 16 PLANT- AND ANIMAL-DERIVED DIETARY SUPPLEMENTS

## INTRODUCTION

Dietary supplements include vitamins, minerals, plant- and animal-derived preparations, amino acids, and a variety of other "natural" and "traditional" remedies with established history of use. Within the United States (US) regulatory context, dietary supplements are distinct from *medications* because this term is reserved for drugs approved by the US Food and Drug Administration (FDA), which are regulated more rigorously in terms of safety and effectiveness. Although these products are distinct from medications, they contain xenobiotics that have many physiologic effects on the human body. This chapter discusses the history, epidemiology, and regulation of plant- and animal-derived dietary supplements.

## HISTORY AND EPIDEMIOLOGY

Since ancient times, people of nearly all cultures have used plant- and animal-derived dietary supplements to treat disease and promote health. A 60,000-year-old Iraqi burial site contained eight different medicinal plants. The Egyptian Ebers papyrus, written circa 1500 B.C., lists 160 medicinal plants and their intended uses. During the Scientific Revolution, scientists began to isolate purified extracts of plant products for use as medicinals, and many modern pharmaceuticals are still derived from plant products. In the current era, naturopaths, traditional healers, shamans, and a multitude of sometimes dubious websites offer plant- and animal-derived dietary supplements for medicinal purposes. The products they sell are unfortunately often highly unreliable and potentially injurious. An estimated 5% of children and 18% of adults in the US use nonvitamin, nonmineral dietary supplements, many of which are plant- and animal-derived dietary supplements.

## REGULATION OF DIETARY SUPPLEMENTS

In the US, all dietary supplements are loosely regulated by the FDA. They are classified as a type of dietary supplement, meaning that they are considered nutrients with nondrug status and are therefore are not subject to the same rigorous standards as pharmaceutical products. There is no requirement to show effectiveness, a typical expectation associated with approval of pharmaceuticals. The burden of proof regarding safety is on the FDA and relies heavily on a postmarketing surveillance.

Although dietary supplements are not to be advertised for the treatment of disease without the approval of the FDA, research suggests that they often are. A study determined that 81% of websites marketing dietary supplements made one or more health claims without approval from the FDA, and of these sites, 55% made specific claim to treat, prevent, or cure a specific disease. In addition, two studies suggest that many dietary supplements do not even contain appreciable quantities of the listed herb. In one study of 54 ginseng products, 60% of those analyzed contained pharmacologically insignificant amounts of ginseng, and 25% contained no ginsenosides. A study of echinacea preparations determined that 10% of preparations contained no measurable echinacea, the assayed species was consistent with labeled content in 52% of the sample, and only 43% met the quality standard described by the label. Perhaps more concerning than the insufficient quantities of herbs are the unlisted ingredients that contaminate and adulterate some dietary supplements.

Many hospitals do not have formal policies governing the use of dietary supplements in their facilities. Some hospitals ban dietary supplements, but most allow them as long as they were ordered by an authorized prescriber. Some concerns include difficulties in identifying products (particularly "home supply" products) and uncertainty about appropriate dosing, efficacy, safety, and consistency, as well as the potential for herb–xenobiotic interactions. Facilities struggle to balance patient-centered care with the legal, medical, and ethical concerns about the efficacy, safety, and cost of dietary supplements.

## PHARMACOLOGIC PRINCIPLES

The pharmacologic activity of dietary supplements is classified by five active constituent classes: volatile oils, resins, alkaloids, glycosides, and fixed oils.

**Volatile oils** are aromatic plant ingredients (Table 16–1). They are also called ethereal or essential oils because they evaporate at room temperatures and have an odor, which is generally pleasant. Many are mucous membrane irritants and have central nervous system (CNS) activity.

**Resins** are complex chemical mixtures of acrid resins, resin alcohols, resinol, tannols, esters, and resenes. These substances are often strong gastrointestinal (GI) irritants.

**Alkaloids** are a heterogeneous group of alkaline and nitrogenous compounds. The alkaloid compound usually is found throughout the plant. This class consists of many pharmacologically active and toxic compounds

**Glycosides** are esters that contain a sugar component (glycol) and a nonsugar (aglycone), which yields one or more sugars during hydrolysis.

**Fixed oils** are esters of long-chain fatty acids and alcohols. Herbs containing fixed oils are generally used as emollients, demulcents, and bases for other products. Generally, they are the least active and least dangerous of all plant- and animal-derived dietary supplements.

## PHARMACOKINETICS AND TOXICOKINETICS

For many dietary supplements, the details of absorption, distribution, metabolism, and excretion are poorly characterized. Many dietary supplements simply have not been studied rigorously. This section describes considerations related to the pharmacokinetics and toxicokinetics of xenobiotics derived from complex, living organisms.

**TABLE 16–1 Selected Dietary Supplements, Popular Use, and Potential Toxicities**

| *Herbal* | *Scientific Name* | *Other Common Names* | *Traditional and Popular Usage* | *Active or Toxic Ingredient(s)* | *Adverse Effects* |
|---|---|---|---|---|---|
| Aconite | *Aconitum napellus, Aconitum kusnezoffii, Aconitum carmichaelii* | Monkshood, wolfsbane caowu, chuanwu, bushi | Topical analgesic, neuralgia, asthma, heart disease, arthritis | Aconite alkaloids (C19 diterpenoid esters), aconitine | GI upset, dysrhythmias |
| Alfalfa | *Medicago sativa* | | Arthritis, diabetes | L-Canavanine | Lupus, pancytopenia |
| Aloe | *Aloe vera* and other species | Cape, Zanzibar, Socotrine, Curacao, Carrisyn | Heals wounds, emollient, laxative, abortifacient | Anthraquinones, barbaloin, isobarbaloin | GI upset, dermatitis, hepatitis |
| Apricot pits | *Prunus armeniaca* | — | (Laetrile) cancer remedy | Amygdalin | Cyanide poisoning |
| Aristolochia | *Aristolochia clematis, Aristolochia reticulata, Aristolochia fangchi* | Birthwort, heartwort, fangchi | Uterine stimulant, cancer treatment, antibacterial | Aristolochic acid | Nephrotoxicity, renal cancer, bladder cancer, retroperitoneal fibrosis |
| Astragalus | *Astragalus membranaceus* | Huang qi, milk vetch root | Immune booster, HIV, cancer, antioxidant, increase endurance | Astrogalasides, trigonoside, and flavonoid constituent | Alters effectiveness of immunosuppressives (eg, steroids, cyclosporine) |
| Atractylis | *Atractylis gummifera* | Piney thistle | Chewing gum, antipyretic, diuretic, gastrointestinal remedy | Potassium atractylate and gummiferin | Hepatotoxicity, altered mental status, seizures, vomiting, hypoglycemia |
| Autumn crocus | *Colchicum autumnale* | Crocus, fall crocus, meadow saffron, mysteria, vellorita | Gout, rheumatism, prostate, hepatic disease, cancer, gonorrhea | Colchicine | GI upset, kidney disease, agranulocytosis |
| Bee pollen, royal jelly | Derived from *Apis mellifera* | — | Increase stamina, athletic ability, longevity | Pollen mixture containing hyperallergenic plant pollen or fungi contamination | Allergic reactions |
| Bee venom | Derived from *Apis mellifera* | — | Immunomodulator | Phospholipase $A_2$ and mellitin, hyaluronidases | Allergic reactions |
| Betel nut | *Areca catechu* | Areca nut, pinlang, pinang | Stimulant | Arecoline | Bronchospasm; chronic use associated with leukoplakia and oropharyngeal squamous cell carcinoma |
| Bitter orange | *Citrus aurantium* | Changcao, *Fructus aurantii*, green orange, kijitsu, Seville orange, sour orange, Zhi shi | Dyspepsia, increase appetite, weight loss | Synephrine | Myocardial infarction, stroke, ephedrine-like effects |
| Black cohosh | *Cimicifuga racemosa* | Black snakeroot, squawroot, bugbane, baneberry | Abortifacient, menstrual irregularity, astringent, dyspepsia | Triterpene glycosides | Dizziness, nausea, vomiting, headache |
| Blue cohosh | *Caulophyllum thalictroides* | Squaw root, papoose root, blue ginseng | Abortifacient, dysmenorrhea, antispasmodic | *N*-methylcytisine (2.5% the potency of nicotine) | Nicotinic toxicity |
| Boneset | *Eupatorium perfoliatum* | Thoroughwort, vegetable antimony, feverwort | Antipyretic | Pyrrolizidine alkaloids | Hepatotoxicity, dermatitis, milk sickness |
| Borage | *Borago officinalis* | Bee plant, bee bread | Diuretic, antidepressant, antiinflammatory | Pyrrolizidine alkaloids, amabiline | Hepatotoxicity |
| Boron | | Boron | Topical astringent, wound remedy | Boron | Dermatitis, GI upset, kidney toxicity and hepatotoxicity, seizures, coma |
| Broom | *Cytisus scoparius* | Scotch broom, Bannal, broom top | Cathartic, diuretic, induce labor, drug of abuse | L-Sparteine | Nicotinic toxicity |
| Buchu | *Agathosma betulina* | Bookoo, buku, diosma, bucku, bucco | Diuretic, stimulant, carminative, urine infections, insect repellent | Diosmin, hesperidin, pulegone | Hepatotoxicity |
| Buckthorn | *Rhamnus frangula* | | Laxative | Anthraquinones | Diarrhea, weakness |
| Burdock root | *Arctium lappa, Arctium minus* | Great burdock, gobo, lappa, beggar's button, hareburr, niu bang zi | Diuretic, choleretic, induce sweating, skin disorders, burn remedy, diabetes treatment | Atropine (contamination with belladonna alkaloids during harvesting) | Anticholinergic toxicity |

(*Continued*)

**TABLE 16–1 Selected Dietary Supplements, Popular Use, and Potential Toxicities (*Continued*)**

| *Herbal* | *Scientific Name* | *Other Common Names* | *Traditional and Popular Usage* | *Active or Toxic Ingredient(s)* | *Adverse Effects* |
|---|---|---|---|---|---|
| Caapi | *Banisteriopsis caapi* | Ayahuasca, yage | Used to increase bioavailability of DMT in other plants as part of ayahuasca ritual | Harmine, harmaline, tetrahydroharmine | Serotonin toxicity, hallucinations |
| Cantharidin | *Cantharis vesicatoria* beetle | Spanish fly, blister beetles | Aphrodisiac, abortifacient, blood purifier | Terpenoid: cantharidin | GI upset, urinary tract and skin irritant, kidney toxicity |
| Carp bile (raw) | *Ctenopharyngodon idellus, Cyprinus carpio* | Grass carp, common carp | Improve visual acuity and health | Cyprinol, C27 bile alcohol | Hepatitis, kidney failure |
| Cascara | *Rhamnus purshiana* | Cascara sagrada | Laxative | Anthraquinones | Diarrhea, weakness |
| Catnip | *Nepeta cataria* | Cataria, catnep, catmint | Indigestion, colic, sedative, euphoriant, headaches, emmenagogue | Nepetalactone | Sedation |
| Chacruna | *Psychotria viridis* | Chacruna | Ingested as part of ayahuasca ritual | DMT | Serotonin toxicity |
| Ch'an Su | *Bufo bufo gargarizans, Bufo bufo melanosticus* | Stone, lovestone, black stone, rock hard, chuan wu, kyushin | Topical anesthetic, aphrodisiac, cardiac disease | Bufodienolides, bufotenin | Dysrhythmias, hallucinations |
| Chamomile | *Matricaria chamomilla, Chamaemelum nobile* | Manzanilla | Digestive disorders, skin disorders, cramps | Allergens | Contact dermatitis, allergic reactions |
| Chaparral | *Larrea tridentata* | Creosote bush, greasewood, hediondilla | Bronchitis, analgesic, anti-aging, cancer | Nondihydroguaiaretic acid | Hepatotoxicity (chronic) |
| Chuen-Lin | *Coptis chinensis, Coptis japonicum* | Golden thread, Huang-Lien, Ma-Huang | Infant tonic | Berberine: displaces bilirubin from protein | Neonatal hyperbilirubinemia |
| Cinchona bark | *Cinchona succirubra, Cinchona calisaya, Cinchona ledgeriana* | Red bark, Peruvian bark, Jesuit bark, China bark, Cinchona bark, quinaquina, fever tree | Malaria, fever, indigestion, cancer, hemorrhoids, varicose veins, abortifacient | Quinine | Cinchonism: GI complaints, tinnitus, visual symptoms, cardiovascular toxicity, CNS toxicity |
| Clove | *Syzygium aromaticum* | Caryophyllum | Expectorant, antiemetic, counterirritant, antiseptic, carminative, euphoriant | Eugenol (4-allyl-2-methoxyphenol) | Pulmonary toxicity (cigarettes) |
| Coltsfoot | *Tussilago farfara* | Coughwort, horsehoof, kuandong hua | Throat irritation, asthma, bronchitis, cough | Pyrrolizidine alkaloids: tussilagin, senkirkine | Allergy, hepatotoxicity |
| Comfrey | *Symphytum officinale, Symphytum* spp, *S. x uplandicum* | Knitbone, bruisewort, blackwort, slippery root, Russian comfrey | Ulcers, hemorrhoids, bronchitis, burns, sprains, swelling, bruises | Pyrrolizidine alkaloids: symphytine, echimidine, lasiocarpine | Hepatotoxicity |
| Compound Q | *Trichosanthes kirilowii* | Gualougen, GLQ-223, Chinese cucumber root | Fevers, swelling, expectorant, abortifacient, diabetes, AIDS | Trichosanthin | Pulmonary injury (ARDS), cerebral edema, cerebral hemorrhage, seizures, fevers |
| Dong quai | *Angelica polymorpha* | Tang kuei, dang gui | Blood purifier, dysmenorrhea, improve circulation | Coumarin, psoralens, safrole in essential oil | Anticoagulant effects, photodermatitis, possible carcinogen in oil |
| Echinacea | *Echinacea angustifolia, Echinacea purpurea* | American cone flower, purple cone flower, snakeroot | Infections, immunostimulant | Echinacoside | CYP1A2 inhibitor |
| Elder | *Sambucus* spp | Elderberry, sweet elder, sambucus | Diuretic, laxative, astringent, cancer | Isoquercitrin cyanogenic glycoside: sambunigrin in leaves | GI upset, weakness if uncooked leaves ingested |
| Ephedra | *Ephedra* spp | Ma-huang, Mormon tea, yellow horse, desert tea, squaw tea, sea grape | Stimulant, bronchospasm | Ephedrine, pseudoephedrine | Headache, insomnia, dizziness, palpitations, seizures, stroke, myocardial infarction |
| Evening primrose | *Oenothera biennis* | Oil of evening primrose | Coronary disease, multiple sclerosis, cancer, diabetes, rheumatoid arthritis, premenstrual syndrome | Cis-γ-linoleic acid | Seizures |

(*Continued*)

**TABLE 16–1 Selected Dietary Supplements, Popular Use, and Potential Toxicities (*Continued*)**

| *Herbal* | *Scientific Name* | *Other Common Names* | *Traditional and Popular Usage* | *Active or Toxic Ingredient(s)* | *Adverse Effects* |
|---|---|---|---|---|---|
| Fennel | *Foeniculum vulgare* | Common, sweet, or bitter fennel | Gastroenteritis, expectorant, emmenagogue, stimulate lactation | Volatile oils: transanethole, fenchone; estrogens: dianethole, photoanethole | Ingestion of volatile oils: vomiting, seizures, pulmonary injury (ARDS), dermatitis, estrogen effects |
| Fenugreek | *Trigonella foenumgraecum* | Bird's foot, Greek hay seed | Expectorant, demulcent, antiinflammatory, emmenagogue, galactogogue, diabetes | 4-Hydroxyisoleucine | Hypoglycemia, hypokalemia |
| Feverfew | *Tanacetum parthenium* | Featherfew, altamisa, bachelor's button, featherfoil, febrifuge plant, midsummer daisy, nosebleed, wild quinine | Migraine headache, menstrual pain, asthma, dermatitis, arthritis, antipyretic, abortifacient | Parthenolide | Oral ulcerations, "post-feverfew syndrome:" rebound of migraine symptoms, anxiety, insomnia following cessation of chronic use |
| Fo-Ti | *Polygonum multiflorum* | Climbing knotwood, he shou-wu | Scrofula, cancer, constipation therapy, promote longevity | Anthraquinones: chrysophanol, emodin, rhein | Cathartic |
| Foxglove | *Digitalis purpurea, Digitalis lanata, Digitalis lutea, Digitalis* spp | Purple foxglove, throatwort, fairy finger, fairy cap, lady's thimble, scotch mercury, witch's bells, dead man's bells | Asthma, sedative, diuretic or cardiotonic, wounds and burns (India) | Cardioactive steroids (eg, digitoxin, gitoxin, digoxin, digitalin, gitaloxin) | Blurred vision, GI upset, dizziness, muscle weakness, tremors, dysrhythmias |
| Garcinia | *Garcinia cambogia* | Brindleberry, hydroxycitric acid | Weight loss | Hydroxycitric acid | Hypoglycemia in diabetics |
| Garlic | *Allium sativum* | Allium, stinking rose, rustic treacle, nectar of the gods, da suan | Infections, coronary artery disease, hypertension | Alliin, ajoene | Contact dermatitis, gastroenteritis, antiplatelet effects |
| Germander | *Teucrium chamaedrys* | Wall germander | Antipyretic, abdominal disorders, wounds, diuretic, choleretic | Furano neoclerodane diterpenes | Hepatotoxicity |
| Ginger | *Zingiber officinale* | | Carminative, diuretic, antiemetic, stimulant, motion sickness | Volatile oil, phenol, zingerone | Anticoagulant and antiplatelet effects |
| Ginkgo | *Ginkgo biloba* | Maidenhair tree, kew tree, tebonin, tanakan, rokan, kaveri | Asthma, chilblain, digestive aid, cerebral dysfunction | Ginkgo flavone glycosides and terpene lactones (ginkgolides and bilobalide) | Extracts: GI upset, headache, skin reaction; leaf: antiplatelet: allergic reactions |
| Ginseng | *Panax ginseng, Panax quinquefolius, Panax pseudoginseng* | Ren shen | Respiratory illnesses, gastrointestinal disorders, impotence, fatigue, stress, adaptogenic, external demulcent | Ginsenosides: panaxin, ginsenin | Ginseng abuse syndrome: elevated blood pressure, insomnia, anxiety, and diarrhea |
| Glucomannan | *Amorphophallus konjac* | Konjac, konjac mannan | Weight-reducing agent: "grapefruit diet," increase viscosity, decrease gastric emptying | Polysaccharides | Esophageal and lower GI obstruction |
| Glucosamine | 2-Amino-2-deoxyglucose | Chitosamine | Wound-healing polymer, antiarthritic | Glucosamine | Hepatotoxicity |
| Goat's rue | *Galega officinalis* | French lilac, French honeysuckle | Antidiabetic | Galegine, paragalegine | Hypoglycemia |
| Goji | *Lycium barbarum, chinense* | Wolfberry, gou qi zi | Protect liver, improve eyesight, enhance immune system | Carotenoids, lutein, atropine | Interaction with warfarin likely due to CYP2C9 inhibition |
| Goldenseal | *Hydrastis canadensis* | Orange root, yellow root, turmeric root | Astringent, GI disorders, dysmenorrhea | Berberine, hydrastine | GI upset, paralysis, and respiratory failure |
| Gordolobo yerba | *Senecio longiloba, Senecio aureu, Senecio vulgaris, Senecio spartoides* | Groundsel, liferoot | Gargle, cough, emmenagogue | Pyrrolizidine alkaloids | Hepatotoxicity |

(*Continued*)

**TABLE 16–1 Selected Dietary Supplements, Popular Use, and Potential Toxicities (*Continued*)**

| *Herbal* | *Scientific Name* | *Other Common Names* | *Traditional and Popular Usage* | *Active or Toxic Ingredient(s)* | *Adverse Effects* |
|---|---|---|---|---|---|
| Gotu kola | *Centella asiatica* | Hydrocotyle, Indian pennywort, talepetrako | Wound healing, tonic, antibacterial | Asiaticoside, asiatic acid, madecassic acid | Contact dermatitis |
| Green tea | *Camillia sinensis* | Green tea | Antioxidant, weight loss, reduce cholesterol | Polyphenols (catechins and epigallocatechin gallate) | Hepatoxicity from green tea extracts |
| Hawthorn | *Crataegus oxyacantha, Crataegus laevigata, Crataegus monogyna* | English hawthorn, haw, maybush, whitethorn | Hypertension, CHF, dysrhythmias, antispasmodic, sedative | Hyperoside, vitexin, procyanidin | Hypotension, sedation |
| Heliotrope | *Crotalaria specatabilis, Heliotropium europaeum* | Rattlebox, groundsel, viper's bugloss, bush tea | Cancer | Pyrrolizidine alkaloids | Hepatotoxicity |
| Henbane | *Hyoscyamus niger* | Fetid nightshade, poison tobacco, insane root, stinky nightshade | Sedative, analgesic, antispasmodic, asthma | Hyoscyamine, hyoscine | Anticholinergic toxicity |
| Holly | *Ilex aquifolium, Ilex opaca, Ilex vomitoria* | English holly, American holly, and yaupon | Tea, emetic, CNS stimulant, coronary artery disease | Saponins | GI upset |
| Horse chestnut | *Aesculus hippocastanum* | Horse chestnut, California buckeye, Ohio buckeye, buckeye | Arthritis, rheumatism, varicose veins, hemorrhoids | Esculin, nicotine, quercetin, quercitrin, rutin, saponin, shikimic acid | Fasciculations, weakness, incoordination, GI upset, paralysis, stupor |
| Hydrangea | *Hydrangea arborescens, Hydrangea paniculata* | Seven bark, wild hydrangea | Diuretic, stimulant, carminative, cystitis, renal calculi, asthma | Hydrangin, saponin | Dizziness, chest pain, GI upset |
| Iboga | *Tabernanthe iboga* | Ibogaine | Aphrodisiac, stimulant, hallucinogen, addiction treatment | Ibogaine | Hallucinations, prolonged QT interval, torsade de pointes |
| Impila | *Callilepsis laureola* | | Zulu traditional remedy | Potassium atractylate-like compound | Vomiting, hypoglycemia, centrilobular hepatic necrosis |
| Jalap | *Ipomoea purga* | | Cathartic | Convolvulin | Profuse watery diarrhea |
| Jimsonweed | *Datura stramonium* | Datura, stramonium, apple of Peru, Jamestown weed, thornapple, tolguacha | Asthma | Atropine, scopolamine, hyoscyamine, stramonium | Anticholinergic toxicity |
| Kava kava | *Piper methysticum* | Awa, kava-kava, kew, tonga | Relaxation beverage, uterine relaxation, headaches, colds, wounds, aphrodisiac | Kava lactones, flavokwain A and B | Mild euphoria, muscle weakness, skin discoloration, liver failure |
| Khat | *Catha edulis* | Qut, kat, chaat, Kus es Salahin, Tchaad, Gat | CNS stimulant, depression, fatigue, obesity, ulcers | Cathine, cathinone | Euphoria, dysphoria, stimulation, sedation, psychological dependence, leukoplakia |
| Kola nut | *Cola acuminata* | Botu cola, cola nut | Digestive aid, tonic, aphrodisiac, headache, diuretic | Caffeine, theobromine, kolanin | CNS stimulant |
| Kombucha | Mixture of bacteria and yeast | Manchurian tea | Memory loss, premenstrual syndrome, cancer | Unknown bacteria | Hepatotoxicity, metabolic acidosis |
| Kratom | *Mitragyna speciosa* | Ketum | Pain, opioid replacement, psychoactive effects | Mitragynine | Intrahepatic cholestasis, seizure, dysrhythmias, impaired memory, coma |
| Licorice | *Glycyrrhiza glabra* | Spanish licorice, Russian licorice, gancao | Gastric irritation | Glycyrrhizin | Flaccidity weakness, dysrhythmias, hypokalemia, lethargy |
| Lipoic acid | | α-Lipoic acid, thioctic acid | Antioxidant, diabetes, neuropathy, AIDS | Lipoic acid | Hypoglycemia |
| Lobelia | *Lobelia inflata* | Indian tobacco | Antispasmodic, respiratory stimulant, relaxant | Lobeline | Nicotine toxicity |

(*Continued*)

**TABLE 16–1** Selected Dietary Supplements, Popular Use, and Potential Toxicities (*Continued*)

| *Herbal* | *Scientific Name* | *Other Common Names* | *Traditional and Popular Usage* | *Active or Toxic Ingredient(s)* | *Adverse Effects* |
|---|---|---|---|---|---|
| Mace | *Myristica fragrans* | Mace, muscade, seed cover of nutmeg | Diarrhea, mouth sores, insomnia, rheumatism | Myristicin (methoxysafrole) | Hallucinations, GI upset |
| Mandrake | *Mandragora officinarum* | | Hallucinogen | Atropine, scopolamine, hyoscyamine | Anticholinergic toxicity |
| Mate | *Ilex paraguayensis* | Paraguay tea | Stimulant | Caffeine | Methylxanthine toxicity |
| Mayapple | *Podophyllum peltatum, P. hexandrum* | Mayapple, podophyllum | Emetic, cathartic, warts | Podophyllotoxin | GI upset, delirium, hallucinations, coma, cranial nerve abnormalities, peripheral sensorimotor axonopathy, hematologic toxicity, microtubule toxin |
| Mistletoe | *Viscum album, Phoradendron leucarpum* | Iscador | Antispasmodic, calmative, cancer, HIV | Viscotoxins, lectins | GI upset, bradycardia, delirium |
| Morning glory | *Ipomoea purpurea, Ipomoea violacea* | Heavenly blue, blue star, flying saucers | Hallucinogen | D-Lysergic acid amide (ergine) | Hallucinations |
| Mugwort | *Artemisia vulgaris, Artemisia dracunculus, Artemisia lactiflora* | Felon herb, moxa, guizhou | Depression, dyspepsia, menstrual disorder, abortifacient | Lactones (sesquiterpenes) | Hallucinations allergic reaction (skin, pulmonary), vivid dreams |
| Nutmeg | *Myristica fragrans* | Mace, rou dou kou | Hallucinogen, abortifacient, aphrodisiac, GI disorders | Myristicin | Hallucinogen, GI upset |
| Oleander | *Nerium oleander* | Adelfa, laurier rose, rosa laurel, rose bay, rose francesca | Cardiac disorders, asthma, corns, cancer, epilepsy | Oleandrin, neriin, gentiobiosyl-oleandrin, odoroside A | GI upset, diarrhea, dysrhythmias |
| Ostrich fern | *Matteuccia struthipteris* | Fiddlehead fern | Laxative | Flavonoids | GI upset if eaten undercooked |
| Parsley | *Petroselinum crispum* | Rock parsley, garden parsley | Diuretic, uterine stimulant, abortifacient | Myristicin, apiol, furocoumarin, psoralen | Uterine stimulant, photosensitization |
| Passion flower | *Passiflora incarnata* | Passiflora, maypop | Insomnia, analgesic, stimulant | Harmala alkaloids | Sedation |
| Pau d'Arco | *Tabebuia* spp | Ipe roxo, lapacho, taheebo tea | Tonic, "blood builder," cancer, HIV | Napthoquinone derivative: lapachol | GI upset, anemia, bleeding |
| Pennyroyal oil | *Hedeoma pulegioides, Mentha pulegium* | American pennyroyal, Squawmint, mosquito plant | Abortifacient, regulate menstruation, digestive tonic | Cyclohexanone: pulegone | Hepatotoxicity |
| Periwinkle | *Catharanthus roseus* | Red periwinkle, Madagascar or Cape periwinkle, old maid, church-flower, ram-goat rose, "myrtle," magdalena | Hallucinogen, ocular inflammation, diabetes, hemorrhage, insect stings, cancers | Vincristine, vinblastine, indole alkaloid | GI upset, altered mental status, peripheral neuropathy, microtubule toxin |
| Pokeweed | *Phytolacca americana, Phytolacca decandra* | American nightshade, Cancer jalap, inkberry, poke, scoke | Arthritis, emetic, purgative | Saponins: phytolaccigenin, jaligonic acid, phytolaccagenic acid, pokeweed mitogen | Gastroenteritis, blurry vision, weakness, respiratory distress, seizures, leukocytosis |
| Rue | *Ruta graveolens* | Herb of grace, herb grass | Emmenagogue, antispasmodic, abortifacient | Furocoumarins, bergapten, xanthoxanthin | Photosensitization |
| Sage | *Salvia officinalis* | Garden sage, true sage, scarlet sage, meadow sage | Antiseptic, astringent, hormonal stimulant, carminative, abortifacient | Camphor, thujone | Seizures |
| St. John's wort | *Hypericum perforatum* | Klamath weed, John's wort, goatweed, sho-rengyo | Anxiety, depression, gastritis, insomnia, promote healing, HIV | Hyperforin, hypericin | Occasional photosensitization; interacts with many different drugs via induction of CYP3A4, CYP2B6, P-glycoprotein activity, as well as inhibition of monoamine oxidase |

(*Continued*)

**TABLE 16–1 Selected Dietary Supplements, Popular Use, and Potential Toxicities (*Continued*)**

| *Herbal* | *Scientific Name* | *Other Common Names* | *Traditional and Popular Usage* | *Active or Toxic Ingredient(s)* | *Adverse Effects* |
|---|---|---|---|---|---|
| Salvia | *Salvia divinorum, Salvia miltiorrhizae* | Sierra mazateca, diviner's sage, magic mint, Maria pastora | Hallucinogen, renal disease | Salvinorum A, lithospermate B | Hallucinations |
| Sassafras | *Sassafras albidum* | Lauraceae | Stimulant, antispasmodic, purifier | Sassafras oil (80% Safrole) | Hepatotoxicity, carcinogen |
| Saw palmetto | *Serenoa repens* | Sabal, American dwarf palm tree, cabbage palm | Genitourinary disorders, increase sperm production, sexual vigor | 5α-Reductase inhibitor | Diarrhea |
| Senna | *Cassia acutifolia, Cassia angustifolia* | Alexandrian senna | Stimulant, laxative, diet tea | Anthraquinone, glycosides (sennosides) | Diarrhea, CNS effects |
| Slippery elm | *Ulmus rubra, Ulmus fulva* | Elm, elm bark, red elm | Acne, boils, indigestion, abortifacient | Polysaccharide mucilage, oleoresin | Contact dermatitis |
| Soapwort | *Saponaria officinalisxs* | Bruisewort, bouncing bet, dog cloves, fuller's herb, latherwort | Acne, psoriasis, eczema, boils, natural soaps | Saponins | Intravenous: highly toxic<br>Oral: none |
| Soy isoflavone | *Glycine max* | | Menopausal symptoms, heart disease | Phytoestrogens: genistein, daidzein, glycitein | Carcinogen |
| Squill | *Urginea maritima, Urginea indica* | Sea onion, red squill | Diuretic, emetic, cardiotonic, expectorant | Cardioactive steroid, scillaren A | Emesis, dysrhythmias |
| Syrian rue | *Peganum harmala* | Harmal, Espand, African rue, Mexican rue, Turkish rue | Antibiotic, anxiolytic, analgesic, emmenagogue, abortifacient, ayahuasca substitute, and as a protector against evil eye | Harmala alkaloids, quinazoline alkaloids | Serotonin toxicity, tremor, abortion |
| T'u-san-chi | *Gynura segetum* | | Tea | Pyrrolizidine alkaloids | Hepatotoxicity |
| Tonka bean | *Dipteryx odorata, Dipteryx oppositifolia* | Tonquin bean, cumaru | Food, cosmetics | Coumarin | Anticoagulant effect |
| Tung seed | *Aleurites moluccana, Aleurites fordii* | Tung, candlenut, candleberry, barnish tree, balucanat, otaheite | Wood preservative (oil), purgative (oil), asthma treatment (seed) | Saponins, phytotoxins | GI upset, hyporeflexia, latex: dermatitis |
| Valerian | *Valeriana officinalis* | Radix valerianae, Indian Valerian, red valerian | Anxiety, insomnia, antispasmodic | Valepotriates, valerenic acid | Sedation |
| White cohosh | *Actaea alba, Actaea rubra* | Baneberry, snakeberry, doll's eyes, coralberry | Emmenagogue | Protoanemonin | Headache, GI upset, delirium, circulatory failure |
| White willow bark | *Salix alba* | Common willow, European willow | Fever, pain, astringent | Salicin | Salicylate toxicity: GI upset, tachypnea, anion gap metabolic acidosis, tinnitus, CNS toxicity, hyperthermia, cerebral edema, ARDS, coagulopathy |
| Wild lettuce | *Lactuca virosa, Lactuca sativa* | Lettuce opium, prickly lettuce | Sedative, cough suppressant, analgesic | Unknown | Sedative, potentiates other sedatives |
| Woodruff | *Galium odoratum* | Sweet woodruff | Wound healing, tonic, varicose veins, antispasmodic | Coumarin | Hepatotoxicity, bleeding |
| Wormwood | *Artemisia absinthium* | Absinthes | Sedative, analgesic, antihelminthic | Thujone | Psychosis, hallucinations, seizures |
| Yarrow | *Achillea millefolium* | Bloodwort, carpenter's grass, dog daisy, nosebleed | Heal wounds, viral symptoms, digestive disorder, diuretic | Unknown | Contact dermatitis |
| Yew | *Taxus baccata* | Yew | Antispasmodic, cancer remedy | Taxine | Dizziness, dry mouth, bradycardia, cardiac arrest |
| Yohimbe | *Pausinystalia yohimbe* | Yohimbi, yohimbehe | Body building, aphrodisiac, stimulant | Yohimbine | Hypertension, abdominal pain, weakness |

ADHD = attention-deficit/hyperactivity disorder; ARDS = acute respiratory distress syndrome; CHF = congestive heart failure; CNS = central nervous system; DMT = dimethyltryptamine; GI = gastrointestinal; HIV = human immunodeficiency virus; LSD = lysergic acid diethylamide.

Dietary supplements are prepared using a variety of techniques, which introduces variation in the resulting product. The American Botanical Council describes a variety of methods for processing plants into dietary supplements, including decoction, infusion, tincture, liniment, poultice, essential oils, herbal infused oils, and percolation. Herbalists extract xenobiotics from raw materials using water, oils, alcohols, or other solvents at different temperatures for varying lengths of time, leading to variation in content and concentration of xenobiotics that are available to be absorbed in the final product.

Some of the unique considerations relevant to understanding toxicokinetics and toxicodynamics of living organisms are illustrated through the example of the hepatotoxic pyrrolizidine alkaloids (PAs). The concentration of PA within a single species differs greatly depending on the environment in which a plant is grown. The concentration of PA varies widely in different parts of the plant and is often higher in the roots and young shoots. The PA concentration of pepsin–comfrey capsules was found to vary from 270 mg/kg to 2,900 mg/kg, depending on whether leaves or roots were used as a source. More than 600 different PA are recognized, and an individual plant typically produces several different PAs, which vary greatly in toxicity. While a plant is alive, it bioconverts from one PA to another PA in response to environmental conditions, for example, in response to predation by herbivores. Because certain PAs are much more toxic than others, the toxicity of an individual plant can change dynamically throughout the day. The production of PA also changes throughout the life cycle of a plant, often reaching peak shortly before flowering. This variation makes it difficult to predict the exact xenobiotic contents without extensive testing of every individual dietary supplement product. After they have been absorbed, PAs are metabolized by cytochrome P450 monooxygenases in the liver to form highly reactive electrophilic metabolites that quickly adduct with nucleophilic groups in DNA and protein, explaining the predominance of hepatoxicity. However, a smaller amount of PAs are metabolized to less immediately reactive metabolites or bind to less nucleophilic groups and then are slowly released to act in other parts of the body. Therefore, some PAs are more likely to cause immediate liver damage and others more likely to persist over time and cause indolent damage to a variety of tissues. Hydrolysis of ester bonds in PAs leads to a nontoxic metabolite that is excreted by the kidney. Pyrrolizidine alkaloid toxicity is discussed in more detail later.

## PHARMACOLOGIC INTERACTIONS

A major concern related to the use of dietary supplements is the potential for interactions with pharmaceutical products (Table 16–2). Research suggests that 15% of patients taking pharmaceutical products use herbal preparations concurrently, and many of these products pose a risk for pharmacologic interactions. The risk is highest in pharmaceutical products with a narrow therapeutic index, such as warfarin and digoxin.

Pharmacologic interactions with dietary supplements occur via a variety of pharmacokinetic and pharmacodynamic mechanisms. Concurrent use of dietary supplements and pharmaceutical products causes pharmacokinetic interactions that affect absorption, distribution, metabolism, and elimination of various pharmaceuticals by competing for binding at drug transport sites and drug metabolism enzymes. Herbal preparations also cause pharmacodynamic interactions through action at end-organ receptors. Therefore, some dietary supplements acutely amplify or attenuate the effects of pharmaceutical products. St. John's wort (*Hypericum perforatum*) is a common herbal preparation that exemplifies numerous pharmacokinetic and pharmacodynamic interactions (Fig. 16–1).

## PHARMACOLOGIC SYNERGY

Herbalists and traditional healers often suggest that the healing properties of plant- and animal-derived dietary supplements operate according to synergistic effects of multiple constituents that cannot be understood through a reductionist paradigm that focuses on the effects of a single active compound. Therefore, a whole plant is considered by some healers to be greater than the sum of its parts because the parts (ie, various xenobiotics) interact with one another to alter one another's pharmacologic effect. Herbalists also often coadminister herbs, reasoning that different herbs work together in concert to have a greater effect or less toxicity than when administered alone. A well-described example of herbal synergy is the ayahuasca brew, which contains *Banisteriopsis caapi* and *Psychotria viridis* (See Harmala Alkaloids below).

## ADULTERATION WITH PHARMACEUTICAL PRODUCTS

The US FDA released reports of more than 80 sexual enhancement dietary supplements that were adulterated with unlisted ingredients such as pharmaceuticals. The US FDA has also found that many plant- and animal-derived dietary supplements contain unlisted and potentially harmful ingredients. Weight loss, sexual enhancement, and body building products are most commonly implicated in cases of unlisted pharmaceutical adulterants. Patent medications are ready-made preparations used by traditional Chinese herbalists. Patent medications sometimes contain combinations of herbs and pharmaceuticals, such as acetaminophen, aspirin, antihistamines, or corticosteroids. Many of these adulterant pharmaceuticals are not listed on the packaging and sometimes are not even approved for use in the US.

## CONTAMINATION WITH METALS AND MINERALS

Metal and mineral poisonings from lead, cadmium, mercury, copper, selenium, zinc, and arsenic are associated with plant- and animal-derived dietary supplement usage. In one study, 20% of surveyed Ayurvedic products produced in South Asia and sold on a nonprescription basis in stores in the Boston area contained potentially harmful concentrations of lead, mercury, or arsenic. A follow-up study determined that a similar 21% of Ayurvedic products sold through the Internet also contained potentially harmful concentrations of these metals irrespective of whether manufacture occurred in the US or India. In some cases, these ingredients are intentionally included for purported medicinal benefit.

**TABLE 16–2 Selected Dietary Supplement–Drug Interactions**

| *Herbal Preparation* | *Scientific Name* | *Reported Drug Interactions* | *Proposed Mechanisms* |
|---|---|---|---|
| Danshen | *Salvia miltiorrhiza* | Increased risk of bleeding in patients on warfarin | Pharmacokinetic and pharmacodynamic mechanisms |
| Garlic | *Allium sativum* | Increased clotting time and INR in patients taking warfarin<br>Decreased concentration of saquinavir | Pharmacokinetic effects via inhibition of CYP2E1 and induction of P-glycoprotein |
| Gingko | *Ginkgo biloba* | Enhanced sedative effects of trazadone and benzodiazepines; increased risk of bleeding in patients taking aspirin, warfarin, and NSAIDs<br>Increased concentration of digoxin<br>Increases or decreases effects of antihypertensives, depending on dose, duration, and xenobiotic<br>Lowers seizure threshold, decreasing effectiveness of antiepileptics or increasing risk of seizure in drugs with proconvulsant effects<br>Enhances the efficiency and reduces the extrapyramidal side effects of the classic antipsychotic haloperidol in patients with schizophrenia | Pharmacokinetic effects via induction of CYP2C19 activity and inhibition of intestinal and hepatic CYP3A4 activity<br>Pharmacodynamic effects |
| Ginseng | *Panax ginseng* | Decreased INR in patients on warfarin<br>Case reports of headache, tremulousness, and manic episodes in patients taking phenelzine | Both pharmacokinetic and pharmacodynamic effects |
| Kava | *Piper methysticum* | Enhances sedative effects of alcohol and benzodiazepines<br>Increased "off" periods in patient on levodopa for Parkinson disease | Pharmacodynamic effects via GABA agonism and dopamine antagonism<br>Pharmacokinetic effects via inhibition of CYP2E1, CYP1A2, CYP2C9, CYP2C19, CYP2D6, CYP3A4, CYP4A9, and CYP4A11 |
| Licorice | *Glycyrrhiza glabra* | Modulates metabolism of corticosteroids, leading to mineralocorticoid excess | Pharmacokinetic effects via both inhibition and/or induction of CYP3A activity depending on dose or duration; also inhibits 5α-, 5β-reductase, and 11β-dehydrogenase |
| Piperine | *Piper nigrum Linn,*<br>*Piper longum Linn* | Increased concentrations of propranolol, rifampin, spartein, theophylline, phenytoin | Pharmacokinetic effects via inhibition of P-glycoprotein and CYP3A4 in enterocytes and hepatocytes |
| St. John's wort | *Hypericum perforatum* | Decreases concentration of amitriptyline, nortriptyline, alprazolam, midazolam, cyclosporine, digoxin, imatinib, irinotecan, methadone, indinavir, nevirapine, quazepam, simvastatin, tacrolimus, irinotecan, finasteride<br>Decreases effectiveness of oral contraceptives<br>Decreases INR in patients taking warfarin<br>Increases or decreases fexofenadine concentration depending on duration of treatment<br>Increased risk of serotonin toxicity in patients taking SSRIs or other serotonergic agents<br>Increased effect of clopidogrel on platelet aggregation in clopidogrel-resistant patients | Pharmacokinetic effects via induction of CYP3A4, CYP2E1, CYP2C19, and P-glycoprotein<br>Pharmacodynamic effect via inhibition of monoamine reuptake, leading to interactions with antidepressants<br>Also pharmacodynamic effects via inhibition of COX-1, leading to decreased platelet aggregation |

COX = cyclooxygenase; GABA = γ-aminobutyric acid; INR = international normalized ratio; NSAID = nonsteroidal antiinflammatory drug; SSRI = selective serotonin reuptake inhibitor.

Ayurvedic remedies are either herbal only or *rasa shastra,* which, based on ancient traditional healing of India, deliberately combines metals such as gold, silver, copper, zinc, iron, lead, tin, and mercury, and are used by the majority of the Indian population.

## PATHOPHYSIOLOGY AND CLINICAL MANIFESTATIONS

### Amygdalin

Amygdalin is a cyanogenic glycoside that is contained in many different plants, and it is most abundant in the seeds of several fruits from the Rosaceae family. The highest concentrations of amygdalin have been found in the seeds of familiar fruits such as green plums (10 mg/g), apricots (14 mg/g), peaches (7 mg/g), and red cherries (4 mg/g). Amygdalin is also known as laetrile and "vitamin $B_{17}$," although it is not a vitamin. Amygdalin is enzymatically metabolized to form glucose, benzaldehyde, and hydrogen cyanide. Cyanide poisoning leads to metabolic acidosis with hyperlactatemia and cardiovascular collapse (Chap. 96).

### Aconites

Aconites are derived from the roots of plants from the genus *Aconitum.* In China, aconite usually is derived from *Aconitum carmichaelii* (chuan wu) or *A. kuznezoffii* (caowu). In Europe and the US, aconite is derived from *A. napellus,* commonly known as *monkshood* or *wolfsbane.* Aconites are

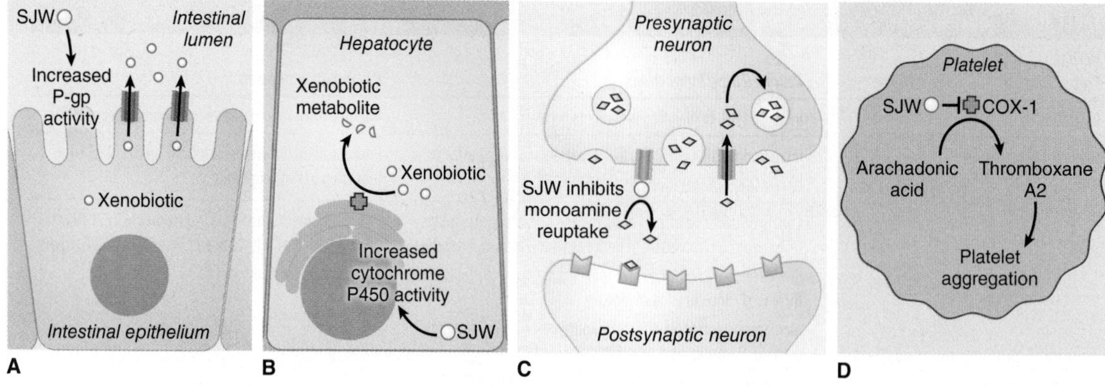


**FIGURE 16–1.** Mechanisms of pharmacokinetic and pharmacodynamic iteractions involving St. John's wort (SJW). (**A**) Induction of P-glycoprotein (P-gp) in the intestinal mucosa. St. John's wort induces activity of the efflux transporter P-gp, leading to decreased absorption and increased excretion of a variety of xenobiotics along the intestinal mucosa. (**B**) Induction of CYP enzymes in hepatocytes. St. John's wort induces activity of CYP2E1 and CYP2C19. Increased activity of CYP enzymes leads to increased metabolism of many different xenobiotics. (**C**) Inhibition of monoamine reuptake in synapse. St. John's wort inhibits reuptake of monoamines serotonin, norepinephrine, and dopamine, increasing the amount of these neurotransmitters in the synapse and increasing risk of serotonin toxicity when combined with other xenobiotics that act on the serotonin system. (**D**) Inhibition of cyclooxygenase-1 (COX-1) in platelets. St. John's wort inhibits COX-1, decreasing conversion of arachidonic acid to thromboxane A2 and inhibiting platelet aggregation, especially in combination with other antiplatelet agents.

traditionally used to treat fever and pain and to induce diuresis and diaphoresis. Aconitine binds to the open state of voltage-sensitive sodium channels in the heart, nervous system, and muscles, leading to increased and prolonged sodium influx through these channels. Paresthesias of the oral mucosa and entire body may be followed by nausea, vomiting, diarrhea, and hypersalivation and then by progressive skeletal muscle weakness. In the heart, the sodium channel effects of aconite poisoning lead to increased inotropy, delayed afterdepolarization, and early afterdepolarization, all of which cause a variety of dysrhythmias, including torsade de pointes, ventricular ectopic beats, ventricular tachycardia, and ventricular fibrillation.

## Aristolochic Acids

The *Aristolochia* genus contains more than 500 species, many of which are used as herbal remedies by a variety of healing traditions. Traditional indications include treatment of infections and cancer and as a weight loss agent. *Aristolochia* plants contain toxic aristolochic acids, which cause aristolochic acid nephropathy (AAN) and urothelial cancer in a dose-dependent fashion. Patients with AAN typically present with elevated serum creatinine, hypertension, anemia, glucosuria, proteinuria, white blood cell casts in the urine, and small kidneys with irregular cortical outlines on imaging.

## Artemisia, Absinthe, and Artesunate

Wormwood (*Artemisia absinthium*) extract has a long history of use for a variety of traditional medical indications, most prominently as an antihelmintic, and it is also the main ingredient in absinthe liquor. This volatile oil is a mixture of $\alpha$- and $\beta$-thujone, which are monoterpene ketones. Chronic absinthe use was formerly believed to cause "absinthism," characterized by psychosis, hallucinations, intellectual deterioration, and seizures, although now it is believed that these symptoms more likely resulted from alcoholism than wormwood itself. Thujone causes seizures in research animals in a dose-dependent fashion, possibly through effects on $\gamma$-aminobutyric acid (GABA) receptors.

## Betel Nut and Other Nicotinics

Betel (*Areca catechu*) is chewed by an estimated 200 million people worldwide for its euphoric effect. As an herb, it is used as a digestive aid and as a treatment for cough and sore throat. Its active ingredient is arecoline, a direct-acting nicotinic agonist that is a bronchoconstrictor. The betel leaf also contains a phenolic volatile oil and an alkaloid capable of producing sympathomimetic reactions. Long-term use of betel nut is associated with leukoplakia and squamous cell carcinoma of the oral mucosa.

## Bufadienolides and Other Cardioactive Steroids

Ch'an Su, Kyushin, and "Love Stone" contain the secretions of the parotid and sebaceous glands of the toad *Bufo bufo gargarizans* or *Bufo melanostictus.* Ch'an Su and Kyushin are traditional Chinese medicines used for the treatment of tonsillitis, sore throat, furuncles, palpitations, and cardiovascular diseases. "Love Stone," also known as "Black Stone" and "Rock Hard," is an "aphrodisiac" intended for topical use. Bufo toad extracts contain two groups of toxic compounds: digoxin-like cardioactive steroids consisting of bufadienolides and the tryptamine alkaloid bufotenin. Clinical findings after ingestion are similar to those after cardioactive steroid poisoning, including GI effects and dysrhythmias (Chap. 35 and Antidotes in Brief: A22).

## Ephedra, Ephedrine, and Pseudoephedrine

Members of the genus *Ephedra* generally consist of erect evergreen plants resembling small shrubs. *Ephedra* species have a long history of use as stimulants and for the management of bronchospasm. They contain the alkaloids ephedrine and pseudoephedrine, among others. In large doses, ephedrine causes nervousness, headache, insomnia, dizziness, hypertension, palpitations, skin flushing, tingling, vomiting, anxiety, restlessness, mania, and psychosis. In 2004, the US FDA banned the sale of ephedra-containing dietary supplements. However, other herbal preparations, such as bitter orange (*Citrus aurantia*), contain ephedralike alkaloids (synephrine), are still widely available, and may pose risk for cardiovascular events (Chap. 22).

### Glycyrrhizin and Other Endocrine Disruptors

Licorice root from the *Glycyrrhiza glabra* plant is widely used as an ingredient in candies, lozenges, teas, and herbal preparations. The root contains glycyrrhizin, which inhibits 11-β-hydroxysteroid dehydrogenase, decreasing conversion of cortisol to cortisone. Chronic licorice consumption increases cortisol concentrations, which then act on renal mineralocorticoid receptors. Repeated consumption of licorice root causes a syndrome of mineralocorticoid excess with hypokalemia, sodium and water retention, peripheral edema, hypertension, and weakness.

### Harmala Alkaloids

*Peganum harmala* and *Banisteriopsis caapi* contain various pharmacologically active alkaloids; the most toxicologically relevant are the β-carboline alkaloids (also known as harmala alkaloids), such as harmine and harmaline. *Peganum harmala* is used in the Middle East and northern Africa for numerous traditional indications such as an antibiotic, anxiolytic, analgesic, emmenagogue, and abortifacient and as a protector against evil eye. *Banisteriopsis caapi* is used in combination with plants containing dimethyltryptamine (DMT) (eg, *Psychotria viridis*) to produce a hallucinogenic state as part of ethnobotanical hallucinogenic rituals, or ayahuasca ceremonies. The monoamine oxidase inhibition of β-carboline alkaloids prevents first-pass metabolism of ingested tryptamines such as DMT. It also poses risks for more severe serotonin toxicity when combined with other xenobiotics or drugs with serotonergic effects (Chaps. 42 and 44). For more information on psychoactive dietary supplement usage, see Table 16–3.

### Kratom

Kratom (*Mitragyna speciosa*) is used as an analgesic, antidepressant, antidiarrheal, euphoriant, stimulant, and opioid replacement. Kratom contains the alkaloids mitragynine and 7-hydroxymitragynine, which are μ-opioid receptor agonists and additionally have activity on adrenergic, serotonergic, and dopaminergic receptors. The toxic and lethal doses of mitragynine are not well-defined. Kratom has potential for abuse due to the μ-opioid activity and sometimes produces a withdrawal syndrome when discontinued after chronic use. Kratom use is associated with hepatotoxicity, psychosis, seizure, coma, and death.

### Pyrrolizidine Alkaloids and Other Hepatotoxins

The PAs are potent hepatotoxins that are estimated to be present in 3% of the world's flowering plants, among various diverse plant families. Plants in the genera *Senecio, Crotalaria, Heliotropium,* and *Symphytum* are found throughout the world. Common names include bush tea and comfrey tea. Acute exposure to PAs causes a highly characteristic syndrome of hepatic sinusoidal hypertrophy and venous occlusion, resulting in hepatic sinusoidal obstruction syndrome, hepatomegaly, and cirrhosis. Chronic low-level exposure causes cirrhosis with a pathological profile that is difficult to distinguish from cirrhosis resulting from other causes, as well as pulmonary artery hypertension.

### Strychnine

The Chinese herbal preparation maqianzi is derived from the dried seeds of the *Strychnos nux vomica* plant and is traditionally used in China to treat rheumatism and other musculoskeletal complaints. Maqianzi contains the alkaloids strychnine and brucine that compete with glycine for binding to glycinergic chloride channels, resulting in a loss of inhibition from the ventral horn of the spinal cord. Strychnine poisoning is characterized by involuntary generalized muscle contractions, respiratory and metabolic acidosis, rhabdomyolysis, and hyperthermia (Chap. 87).

### Tropane Alkaloids, Anticholinergics

Many plants contain the tropane alkaloids atropine (D,L-hyoscyamine), hyoscyamine, and scopolamine (L-hyoscine). They are sometimes used therapeutically for treatment of asthma and occasionally are mistakenly included in herbal teas. Signs and symptoms of anticholinergic poisoning include mydriasis, diminished bowel sounds, urinary retention, dry mouth, flushed skin, tachycardia, and agitation. Mildly poisoned patients usually require only supportive care and sedation with IV benzodiazepines. More severe cases are treated with IV physostigmine (Antidotes in Brief: A11).

**TABLE 16–3 Constituent Psychoactive Xenobiotics in Herbal Preparations**

| *Labeled Ingredient* | *Scientific Name* | *Usage* | *Active Ingredients* | *Classification of Effect* |
|---|---|---|---|---|
| Broom | *Cytisus scoparius* | Smoked for relaxation | L-Sparteine | Sedative |
| Caapi | *Banisteriopsis caapi* | Ingested in combination with other plants as part of ayahuasca ritual | Harmala alkaloids | Inhibits monoamine oxidase to increase bioavailability of DMT |
| California poppy | *Eschscholzia californica* | Smoked | Protopine, escholtzine, allocryptopine, californidine, chelirubine, sanguinarine, and macarpine | Euphoriant, sedative |
| Catnip | *Nepeta cataria* | Smoked or tea | Nepetalactone | Euphoriant |
| Ch'an Su | *Bufo bufo gargarizans, Bufo melanostictus* | Smoked or licked | 5-Methoxy-DMT | Hallucinogen |
| Cinnamon | *Cinnamomum camphora* | Smoked, essential oil | Cinnamaldehyde | Stimulant |

(*Continued*)

**TABLE 16–3 Constituent Psychoactive Xenobiotics in Herbal Preparations (*Continued*)**

| *Labeled Ingredient* | *Scientific Name* | *Usage* | *Active Ingredients* | *Classification of Effect* |
|---|---|---|---|---|
| Chacruna | *Psychotria viridis* | Ingested as part of ayahuasca ritual | DMT | Hallucinogen |
| Clove | *Syzgium aromaticum* | Smoked in cigarette or "kreteks" | Eugenol | Euphoriant |
| Damiana | *Turnera diffusa* | Smoked | Unknown | Stimulant, hallucinogen |
| Hops | *Humulus lupulus* | Smoked or tea | Humulone, lupulone ⟶ methylbutenol | Sedative |
| Hydrangea | *Hydrangea paniculata* | Smoked | Hydrangin, saponin | Stimulant |
| Ibogaine | *Tabernanthe iboga* | Ingested | Ibogaine | Hallucinogen |
| Juniper | *Juniperus macropoda* | Smoked as hallucinogen | Unknown | Hallucinogen |
| Jurema | *Mimosa hostilis* | Smoked, tea or used as source for extraction DMT | DMT | Hallucinogen |
| Kava kava | *Piper methysticum* | Smoked or tea | Kava lactones | Hallucinogen |
| Kola nut | *Cola acuminata* | Smoked, tea, or capsules | Caffeine, theobromine, kolanin | Stimulant |
| Kratom | *Mitragyna speciosa* | Smoked, tea, or capsules | Mitragynine | Euphoriant, stimulant, opioid |
| Lobelia | *Lobelia inflata* | Smoked or tea | Lobeline | Euphoriant |
| Mandrake | *Mandragora officinarum* | Tea | Atropine, scopolamine | Hallucinogen |
| Mate | *Ilex paraguayensis* | Tea | Caffeine | Stimulant |
| Mormon tea | *Ephedra nevadensis* | Tea | Ephedrine | Stimulant |
| Morning glory | *Ipomoea violacea* | Ingested seeds | D-Lysergic acid amide (ergine) | Hallucinogen |
| Nutmeg | *Myristica fragrans* | Tea | Myristicin | Hallucinogen |
| Passion flower | *Passiflora incarnata* | Smoked, tea, or capsules | Harmala alkaloids | Sedative |
| Periwinkle | *Catharanthus roseus* | Smoked or tea | Indole alkaloids | Hallucinogen |
| Prickly poppy | *Argemone mexicana* | Smoked | Protopine, bergerine, isoquinolones | Analgesic |
| Salvia | *Salvia divinorum* | Smoked, chewn | Salvinorum A | Hallucinogen |
| Snakeroot | *Rauwolfia serpentina* | Smoked or tea | Reserpine | Tranquilizer |
| Syrian rue | *Peganum harmala* | Smoked, ingested | Harmala alkaloids, quinazoline alkaloids | Serotonin toxicity, abortifacient |
| Thorn apple | *Datura stramonium* | Smoked or tea | Atropine, scopolamine | Hallucinogen |
| Tobacco | *Nicotiana* spp | Smoked | Nicotine | Stimulant |
| Valerian | *Valeriana officinalis* | Tea or capsules | Chatinine, velerine alkaloids | Sedative |
| Wild lettuce | *Lactuca sativa* | Smoked | Unknown | Analgesic, sedative |
| Wormwood | *Artemisia absinthium* | Smoked, tea, spirits | Thujone | Analgesic |
| Yohimbe | *Pausinystalia yohimbe* | Smoked or tea | Yohimbine | Hallucinogen |

DMT = dimethyltryptamine.

# 17 VITAMINS

Vitamins are essential for normal human growth and development. By definition, a vitamin is a substance present in small amounts in natural foods and is necessary for normal metabolism, and the lack of vitamins in the diet causes a deficiency disease. A standard North American diet is sufficient to prevent overt vitamin deficiency diseases. However, suboptimal vitamin status is common in Western populations and is a risk factor for chronic diseases such as cardiovascular disease, cancer, and osteoporosis. Groups at risk include older adults, hospitalized patients, alcohol-dependent individuals, pregnant women, those with gastrointestinal disorders, those following gastric bypass interventions, and other patients with poor nutritional status. The American Dietetic Association posits that the best strategy for promoting optimal health and reducing chronic disease is to choose a wide variety of nutrient-rich foods, and the use of supplements can help some people meet their nutritional needs.

Unfortunately, many individuals share the mistaken beliefs that vitamin preparations provide extra energy or promote muscle growth and regularly ingest quantities of vitamins in great excess of the recommended dietary allowances (RDAs) (Table 17–1). Some vitamins are associated with consequential adverse effects when ingested in very large doses. Adverse effects also are associated with the use of some vitamins at the RDA or at amounts less than or approaching the established tolerable upper intake level (UL) in certain populations. For example, individuals taking medications to reduce blood clotting, such as warfarin, should not take supplemental vitamin K because it is involved in blood clotting and reduces the effectiveness of warfarin and similar medications.

Vitamins can be divided into two general classes. Most of the vitamins in the *water-soluble* class have minimal toxicity because they are stored to only a limited extent in the body. Thiamine, riboflavin, pantothenic acid, folic acid, $B_{12}$, and biotin are not reported to cause any toxicity after ingestion. Ascorbic acid (vitamin C), nicotinic acid (vitamin $B_3$), and pyridoxine (vitamin $B_6$) are water-soluble vitamins with associated toxicity syndromes. The *fat-soluble* vitamins bioaccumulate and therefore have toxic potentials that greatly exceed those of the water-soluble group. Vitamins A, D, and E (but not K) are associated with toxic syndromes after very large overdose or chronic overuse.

## VITAMIN A

### History and Epidemiology

Two independent groups discovered vitamin A in 1913. They reported that animals fed an artificial diet with lard as the sole source of fat developed a nutritional deficiency characterized by xerophthalmia. They found that this deficiency could be corrected by adding to the diet a factor contained in butter, egg yolks, and cod liver oil. They named the substance "fat-soluble vitamin A." Vitamin A is also found naturally in liver, fish, cheese, and whole milk. In the United States (US) and other parts of the world, including some developing countries, many cereal, grain, dairy, and other products, as well as infant formulas, are fortified with vitamin A.

Vitamin A toxicity occurs in people who ingest large doses of preformed vitamin A in their daily diets. Inuits in the 16th century recognized that ingestion of large amounts of polar bear liver caused a severe illness characterized by headaches and prostration. Most modern reported cases of vitamin A toxicity result from inappropriate use of vitamin supplements.

Vitamin A is present in two forms. Preformed vitamin A as retinol is derived from retinyl esters, its storage form, in animal sources of food. Provitamin A carotenoids are vitamin A precursors and are found in plants. Among the carotenoids, β-carotene is most efficiently made into retinol. The term *vitamin A* was classically only used to refer to the compound retinol. Currently, it is used to describe all retinoids, compounds chemically related to retinol that exhibit the biological activity of retinol. Vitamin A activity is expressed in retinol activity equivalents (RAEs). One RAE corresponds to 1 μg of retinol or 3.33 IU of vitamin A activity as retinol. One RAE also corresponds to 12 μg of β-carotene.

As a group, retinoids have specific sites of action and varying degrees of biologic potency. Retinoic acid is primarily responsible for maintaining normal growth and differentiation of epithelial cells in mucus-secreting or keratinizing tissue. Vitamin A deficiency results in the disappearance of goblet mucous cells and replacement of the normal epithelium with a stratified, keratinized epithelium. Dermal manifestations are the earliest to develop and include dry skin and hair and broken fingernails. In the cornea, hyperkeratization is called *xerophthalmia* and leads to permanent blindness. Alterations in the epithelial lining of other organ systems leads to increased susceptibility to respiratory infections, diarrhea, and urinary calculi. Vitamin A, in the form of 11-*cis*-retinal, plays a critical role in retinal function. Deficiency results in *nyctalopia*, which is decreased vision in dim lighting, more commonly known as *night blindness*.

Vitamin A is prescribed for patients with specific dermatologic and ophthalmic conditions. Vitamin A toxicity often occurs in adults who continue to use the vitamin without medical supervision. Isotretinoin, 13-*cis*-retinoic acid, is prescribed for treatment of severe cystic acne. Of concern is the teratogenicity associated with its use by pregnant women; therefore, it is contraindicated. All-*trans*-retinoic acid (ATRA), or tretinoin, is used as a differentiating chemotherapeutic in the treatment of acute promyelocytic leukemia (APL).

### Pharmacology, Pharmacokinetics, and Toxicokinetics

Absorption of vitamin A in the small intestine is nearly complete. The majority of vitamin A is ingested as retinyl esters, the storage form of retinol. Retinyl esters undergo enzymatic

**TABLE 17–1 Recommended Dietary Daily Allowances or Adequate Daily Intakes**

| Age (years) | Vitamin A (μg RAE/IU) | Vitamin D (μg/IU) | Vitamin E (mg α-TA/IU) | Vitamin C (mg) | Vitamin $B_6$ (mg) | Niacin (mg NE)[a] |
|---|---|---|---|---|---|---|
| **Infants** | | | | | | |
| 0.0–0.5 | 400/1,300[a] | 5/200[a] | 4/4[a] | 40[a] | 0.1[a] | 2[a] |
| 0.5–1.0 | 500/1,700[a] | 5/200[a] | 5/5[a] | 50[a] | 0.3[a] | 4[a] |
| **Children** | | | | | | |
| 1–3 | 300/990 | 5/200[a] | 6/6 | 15 | 0.5 | 6 |
| 4–8 | 400/1,300 | 5/200[a] | 7/7 | 25 | 0.6 | 8 |
| **Males** | | | | | | |
| 9–13 | 600/2,000 | 5/200[a] | 11/11 | 45 | 1 | 12 |
| 14–18 | 900/3,000 | 5/200[a] | 15/15 | 75 | 1.3 | 16 |
| 19–50 | 900/3,000 | 5/200[a] | 15/15 | 90 | 1.3 | 16 |
| 51–70 | 900/3,000 | 10/400[a] | 15/15 | 90 | 1.7 | 16 |
| > 70 | 900/3,000 | 15/600[a] | 15/15 | 90 | 1.7 | 16 |
| **Females** | | | | | | |
| 9–13 | 600/2,000 | 5/200[a] | 11/11 | 45 | 1.0 | 12 |
| 14–18 | 700/2,300 | 5/200[a] | 15/15 | 65 | 1.2 | 14 |
| 19–50 | 700/2,300 | 5/200[a] | 15/15 | 75 | 1.3 | 14 |
| 51–70 | 700/2,300 | 10/400[a] | 15/15 | 75 | 1.5 | 14 |
| > 70 | 700/2,300 | 15/600[a] | 15/15 | 75 | 1.5 | 14 |
| **Pregnant Women** | | | | | | |
| ≤ 18 | 750/2,500 | 5/200[a] | 15/15 | 80 | 1.9 | 18 |
| 19–50 | 770/2,500 | 5/200[a] | 15/15 | 85 | 1.9 | 18 |
| **Lactating Women** | | | | | | |
| ≤ 18 | 1,200/4,000 | 5/200[a] | 19/19 | 115 | 2 | 17 |
| 19–50 | 1,300/4,300 | 5/200[a] | 19/19 | 120 | 2 | 17 |

[a]These values represent the adequate daily intakes. Values without an [a]represent the recommended dietary daily allowances.

NE = niacin equivalent; RAE = retinol activity equivalents; α-TA = α-tocopherol acetate.

Data from Dietary Reference Intakes for Calcium, Phosphorous, Magnesium, Vitamin D, and Fluoride (1997); Dietary Reference Intakes for Thiamin, Riboflavin, Niacin, Vitamin B6, Folate, Vitamin B12, Pantothenic Acid, Biotin, and Choline (1998); Dietary Reference Intakes for Vitamin C, Vitamin E, Selenium, and Carotenoids (2000); Dietary Reference Intakes for Vitamin A, Vitamin K, Arsenic, Boron, Chromium, Copper, Iodine, Iron, Manganese, Molybdenum, Nickel, Silicon, Vanadium, and Zinc (2001); Dietary Reference Intakes for Water, Potassium, Sodium, Chloride, and Sulfate (2005); and Dietary Reference Intakes for Calcium and Vitamin D (2011). These reports may be accessed via www.nap.edu.

hydrolysis to retinol by digestive enzymes in the intestinal lumen and brush border of the intestinal epithelial wall. A small portion of retinol is absorbed directly into the circulation, where it is bound to retinol-binding protein (RBP) and transported to the liver. Most of the retinol is taken into intestinal epithelial cells by RBP. Subsequently, retinol is reesterified and incorporated into chylomicrons, which are released into the blood and taken up by the Ito cells of the liver. After large oral doses, significant amounts of retinyl esters coupled to chylomicrons circulate in association with low-density lipoprotein (LDL) and are delivered to the liver. The liver releases vitamin A into the bloodstream to maintain a constant plasma retinol concentration and is thus delivered to tissues as needed.

Carotenoid absorption requires bile and absorbable fat in the stomach or intestine. These components combine with carotenoids to form mixed lipid micelles that move into the duodenal mucosal cells via passive diffusion. Most β-carotene that is metabolized undergoes central cleavage via oxidation to form retinal, which is then reduced to retinol. Massive doses of β-carotene are rarely associated with vitamin A toxicity because of saturation of absorption.

The normal serum retinol concentration is approximately 30 to 70 μg/dL. These concentrations are maintained at the expense of hepatic reserves when insufficient amounts of vitamin A are ingested. A normal adult liver contains enough vitamin A to fulfill the body's requirements for approximately 2 years. Vitamin A has a half-life of 286 days.

### Pathophysiology

Retinoic acid influences gene expression by combining with nuclear receptors. Retinoids also influence expression of receptors for certain hormones and growth factors. Thus, they can influence the growth, differentiation, and function of target cells.

Excessive concentrations of retinoids where goblet cells are present lead to the production of a thick mucin layer and inhibition of keratinization. In addition, lipoprotein membranes have increased permeability and decreased stability, resulting in extreme thinning of the epithelial tissue. In vitro studies in bone demonstrate that high doses of vitamin A are capable of directly stimulating bone resorption and inhibiting bone formation leading to osteoporosis.

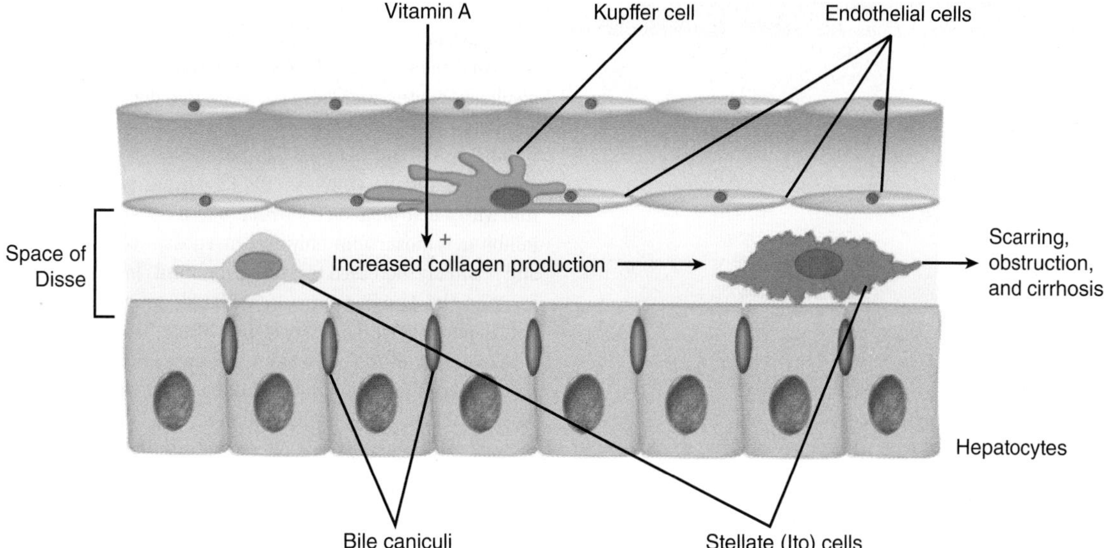


**FIGURE 17–1.** Schematic demonstration of hepatotoxicity resulting from excessive deposition of vitamin A in the Ito cells of the liver.

Hepatotoxicity develops secondary to a single large acute overdose or ingestion of smaller doses if taken over a prolonged time. A total of 90% of hepatic vitamin A stores are in the Ito, or fat-storing, cells of the liver, which are in the perisinusoidal space of Disse and are responsible for maintaining normal hepatic architecture. Ito cells undergo hypertrophy and hyperplasia as vitamin A storage increases. This results in transdifferentiation of the Ito cell into a myofibroblast-like cell that secretes a variety of extracellular matrix components, leading to narrowing of the perisinusoidal space of Disse, obstruction to sinusoidal blood flow, and noncirrhotic portal hypertension (Fig. 17–1). Continued ingestion of vitamin A and hepatic storage leads to obliteration of the space of Disse, sinusoidal barrier damage, perisinusoidal hepatocyte death, fibrosis, and cirrhosis.

Vitamin A toxicity has long been thought to be the cause of the severe headaches and papilledema associated with idiopathic intracranial hypertension (IIH). However, the mechanisms by which vitamin A leads to increased intracranial pressure (ICP) in IIH are not definitively known.

## Clinical Manifestations

Clinical toxicity correlates well with total body vitamin A content, which is a function of both dose and duration of administration. The minimal dose required to produce toxicity in humans is not established. However, an animal study demonstrated a median lethal acute dose in monkeys of 560,000 IU (168,000 RAE) per kilogram of body weight. Vitamin A toxicity occurs more frequently secondary to chronic ingestions of vitamin A. Hepatotoxicity typically requires vitamin A ingestions of at least 50,000 to 100,000 IU/day (15,000–30,000 RAE/day) for months or years.

Symptoms of an acute massive overdose of vitamin A often develop within hours to 2 days after ingestion and include headache, papilledema, scotoma, photophobia, seizures, anorexia, drowsiness, irritability, nausea, vomiting, abdominal pain, liver damage, and desquamation. Chronic toxicity of vitamin A affects the skin, hair, bones, liver, and brain. The most common skin manifestations include xerosis, which is associated with pruritus and erythema, skin hyperfragility, and desquamation. Retinoid toxicity causes hair thinning and even diffuse hair loss in 10% to 75% of patients with characteristic curly or kinky hair change after regrowth, which is sometimes permanent. Nail changes include a shiny appearance, brittleness, softening, and loosening. Dryness of mucous membranes develops with chapped lips and xerosis of nasal mucosa, which sometimes is associated with nasal bleeding.

Hypercarotenemia develops when massive doses of β-carotenes are ingested over several weeks. It manifests as a yellow-orange skin discoloration that can be differentiated from jaundice by the absence of scleral icterus and usually is not associated with morbidity.

Findings from epidemiologic studies are consistent with bone loss and a resulting increase in fracture risk. Hypercalcemia, with low or normal parathyroid hormone (PTH) concentrations, likely results from increased osteoclast activity and bone resorption. Other musculoskeletal findings include skeletal hyperostoses, most commonly affecting the vertebral bodies of thoracic vertebrae, extraspinal tendon and ligament calcifications, soft tissue ossification, cortical thickening of bone shafts, periosteal thickening, and bone demineralization. Many of these findings are apparent on radiographs. Patients often complain of bone and joint pain and muscle stiffness or tenderness.

The degree of hepatotoxicity appears to correlate with the dose of vitamin A and chronicity of use. Hepatotoxicity occurs in humans after an acute ingestion of a massive dose of vitamin A (>600,000 IU or 180,000 RAE). With large doses, cirrhosis develops and leads to portal hypertension, esophageal varices, jaundice, and ascites.

**TABLE 17–2 Xenobiotics Associated with Intracranial Hypertension**

| |
|---|
| Antibiotics |
| Ampicillin |
| Minocycline |
| Metronidazole |
| Nalidixic acid |
| Nitrofurantoin |
| Sulfamethoxazole |
| Tetracycline |
| Corticosteroid therapy (oral and intranasal) and cessation |
| Enflurane |
| Griseofulvin |
| Halothane |
| Ketamine |
| Lead |
| Lithium |
| Oral contraceptives and progestins |
| Phenothiazines |
| Phenytoin |
| Tubocurarine |
| Vitamin A |

Idiopathic intracranial hypertension is characterized by elevated ICP in the absence of a structural anomaly. Although excessive vitamin A is implicated, other etiologies should be considered (Table 17–2). Patients typically present with headache and visual disturbances, including sixth nerve palsies, visual field deficits, and blurred vision, and have a normal mental status. Despite severe papilledema, visual loss often is minimal.

Acute promyelocytic leukemia differentiation syndrome (DS), previously known as ATRA syndrome, is the main adverse effect of treatment with ATRA. The pathophysiology of DS is not well understood but involves an inflammatory response. The onset of symptoms and manifestations is typically 2 to 21 days after initiation of ATRA. The hallmarks of DS are fever and respiratory distress. Other common signs and symptoms include an elevated white blood count, dyspnea, pulmonary edema, pulmonary infiltrates, and pleural and pericardial effusions. Weight gain, bone pain, headache, hypotension, congestive heart failure, acute kidney injury, and hepatotoxicity occur less commonly.

### Diagnostic Testing

The diagnosis of vitamin A–associated hepatotoxicity is supported by histologic evidence of Ito cell hyperplasia with fluorescent vacuoles on liver biopsy. Laboratory testing should include serum electrolytes, including calcium, hepatic enzymes, a complete blood cell count, and a vitamin A concentration. Because the liver has a large storage capacity for excess vitamin A, hepatotoxicity occurs before an elevation in the serum concentration of vitamin A, which may be normal or even low, in the setting of an acute overdose.

### Treatment

Management of a patient with a recent acute, large overdose of vitamin A should begin with 50 g of oral activated charcoal. Discontinuation of vitamin A and supportive care are the mainstays of treatment. Hypercalcemia should be treated in the usual manner with IV fluids, loop diuretics, calcitonin, bisphosphonates, and steroids, as needed depending on the severity.

Idiopathic intracranial hypertension requires more aggressive therapy, which should be performed in consultation with a neurologist. Acetazolamide, a carbonic anhydrase inhibitor, is most commonly used at a dosage of 0.5 to 1 g/day and gradually increased to 3 to 4 g/day until clinical improvement occurs. Lumbar puncture with CSF drainage is reasonable in patients with extremely high ICP.

Treatment of APL DS involves prompt administration of corticosteroids, commonly dexamethasone 10 mg IV twice daily until symptoms resolve followed by a 2-week taper. In patients with severe DS, an oncology consultation should be obtained.

## VITAMIN D

### History and Epidemiology

Vitamin D is the name given to both ergocalciferol (vitamin $D_2$) and cholecalciferol (vitamin $D_3$). In humans, both forms of vitamin D have the same biologic potency, although vitamin $D_3$ is typically recommended. One microgram of vitamin D is equivalent to 40 IU of vitamin D.

Rickets, a disease of urban children living in temperate zones, was thought to result from the lack of a dietary factor or adequate sunshine. In 1919, two independent groups demonstrated that rickets could be prevented or cured by either the addition of cod liver oil to the diet or exposure to sunlight. Vitamin D is found in cod liver oil and other foods, including butter, cheese, and cream, eggs, and fatty fish. Some foods typically are fortified with vitamin D, including cereals, bread, and milk.

Vitamin D deficiency should not occur in individuals who eat a well-balanced diet and are exposed to adequate sunlight. Casual exposure of cutaneous tissues to ultraviolet light during the summer months should produce adequate vitamin D storage for winter months. Breastfed infants require supplemental vitamin D if they have limited exposure to sunlight because the vitamin D content of human milk is extremely low.

The use of vitamin D supplements in an attempt to prevent and treat a variety of illnesses has increased substantially over the past decade. Vitamin D toxicity secondary to excessively fortified food and supplements is a continuing problem.

### Pharmacology, Pharmacokinetics, and Toxicokinetics

Vitamin D itself is not biologically active and must go through extensive metabolism to an active form (Fig. 17–2). Vitamin D might be more appropriately called a hormone rather than a vitamin because it is synthesized in the body, circulates in the blood, and then binds to receptors to evoke its biologic action. The primary role of vitamin D is regulation of calcium homeostasis via interactions with the intestines and bones. Protein-bound calcitriol is taken up by cells and then binds to a specific nuclear vitamin D receptor protein that, in turn, binds to regulatory sequences on chromosomal DNA.

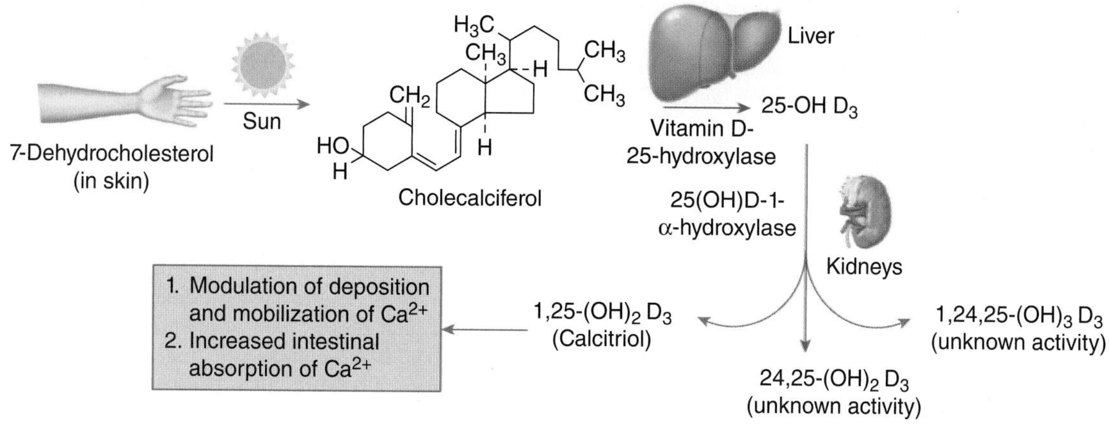

**FIGURE 17–2.** Schematic representation of the synthesis and physiologic response to vitamin D.

The result is induction of gene transcription and translation of proteins that carry out the cellular functions of vitamin D. In the intestines, calcitriol increases the production of calcium binding proteins and plasma membrane calcium pump proteins, thereby increasing calcium absorption through the duodenum. In the bone, calcitriol stimulates osteoclastic precursors to differentiate into mature osteoclasts. Mature osteoclasts, together with PTH, lead to mobilization of calcium stores from bone, thereby raising serum concentrations of calcium. Given sufficient serum concentrations of calcium, calcitriol promotes bone mineralization by osteoblasts, resulting in increased deposition of calcium hydroxyapatite into the bone matrix. Calcitriol also binds to a vitamin D receptor in the parathyroid glands, which leads to decreased synthesis and secretion of PTH.

Vitamin D deficiency results in hypocalcemia, leading to increased secretion of PTH, which acts to restore plasma calcium concentrations at the expense of bone. In children, this situation leads to rickets in which newly formed bone is not adequately mineralized and results in bone deformities and growth defects. Adults develop osteomalacia, a disease characterized by undermineralized bone matrix. Patients typically present with bone pain and tenderness and proximal muscle weakness. Bone deformities are limited to the advanced stages of disease.

The literature varies regarding the toxic dose of vitamin D, with little scientific data available for corroboration. Case reports describe toxicity in the setting of vitamin D intake of 50,000 to 600,000 IU or, simply, doses in the milligram range, daily for prolonged periods.

## Pathophysiology

The hallmark of vitamin D toxicity is hypercalcemia.

## Clinical Manifestations

Patients with vitamin D toxicity present with signs and symptoms characteristic of hypercalcemia. Early manifestations include weakness, fatigue, somnolence, irritability, headache, dizziness, muscle and bone pain, nausea, vomiting, abdominal cramps, and diarrhea or constipation. As the calcium concentration increases, hypercalcemia induces polyuria and polydipsia. Diuresis results in salt and water depletion, further impairing calcium excretion. Severe hypercalcemia presents with ataxia, confusion, psychosis, seizures, coma, and acute kidney injury. In addition, cardiac dysrhythmias result from a shortened refractory period and slowed conduction. Findings on electrocardiography include increased PR intervals, widening of QRS complexes, QT interval shortening, and flattened T waves. Patients can develop metastatic calcification of the kidneys, blood vessels, myocardium, lung, and skin.

## Diagnostic Testing

Vitamin D toxicity should be considered in patients presenting with signs and symptoms of hypercalcemia. In addition to an elevated serum calcium concentration, laboratory results reveal hyperphosphatemia given that vitamin D facilitates phosphate absorption in the small intestine, enhances its mobilization from bone, and decreases its excretion by the kidney. Serum 25(OH)D is measurable, but it is unlikely that results will be available quickly.

## Management

Treatment of hypercalcemia in patients with vitamin D toxicity should include discontinuation of both vitamin D and calcium supplementation, maintenance of a low calcium diet, and administration of adequate volumes of oral or IV fluid to overcome dehydration and increase renal calcium clearance. Many cases of hypercalcemia will respond to such supportive care. When patients are euvolemic, it is reasonable to add a loop diuretic in moderate cases of hypercalcemia requiring ongoing IV fluid administration. This helps prevent fluid overload and increases renal calcium clearance. Moderate to severe cases of hypercalcemia require additional treatment and should be managed like cases of moderate to severe hypercalcemia from other causes. Calcitonin reduces the serum calcium concentration by increasing renal calcium excretion. Salmon calcitonin is recommended at a dosage of 4 units/kg intramuscularly every 12 hours for up to 48 hours. Calcitonin is more efficacious when administered with bisphosphonates, which also inhibit bone resorption via an effect on osteoclasts. Pamidronate 90 mg

IV over 2 hours or zoledronic acid 4 mg IV over 15 minutes is recommended. Glucocorticoids decrease calcitriol production, thereby reducing serum calcium concentrations via a decrease in intestinal calcium absorption or inhibition of bone resorption. It is reasonable to administer hydrocortisone 100 mg/day or prednisone 40 mg/day over 5 days to treat severe cases of hypercalcemia. Hemodialysis is reasonable in refractory cases of hypercalcemia.

## ANTIOXIDANTS (VITAMINS E AND C)

The antioxidants include vitamins E and C and β-carotene. During the 1990s, the concept that antioxidants had a protective effect against atherosclerosis and carcinogenesis was widely promoted. However, several prospective, randomized, placebo-controlled clinical trials, designed to test for the effect of antioxidant vitamins on cardiovascular disease and cancer, demonstrated that commonly used antioxidant regimens do not significantly reduce or prevent overall cardiovascular events or cancer.

## VITAMIN E

### History and Epidemiology

The existence of vitamin E was first demonstrated in 1922 by researchers noting that female rats deficient in a dietary principle were unable to sustain a pregnancy. Testicular lesions in male rats were described in deficiency states, and vitamin E was referred to as the "anti-sterility vitamin." Vitamin E was first isolated from wheat-germ oil in 1936. The richest sources of vitamin E include nuts, wheat germ, whole grains, and vegetable and seed oils, including soybean, corn, cottonseed, and safflower, and the products made from these oils. In general, animal products are poor sources of vitamin E. Human milk, in contrast to cow's milk, has sufficient vitamin E in the form of α-tocopherol to meet the needs of breastfed infants.

Vitamin E is an essential nutrient that is necessary for normal functioning of the nervous, reproductive, muscular, cardiovascular, and hematopoietic systems. Vitamin E includes eight naturally occurring compounds in two classes—tocopherols and tocotrienols—that have differing biologic activities. The most biologically active form is RRR-α-tocopherol, previously known as D-α-tocopherol, which is the most widely available form of vitamin E in food. One IU is equivalent to 1 mg of α-tocopherol acetate (α-TA).

Vitamin E deficiency is found in patients with malabsorption syndromes, which occur in the presence of pancreatic insufficiency or hepatobiliary disease, such as biliary atresia. Patients with abetalipoproteinemia are at risk for vitamin E deficiency. The clinical syndrome of deficiency is primarily manifested by a peripheral neuropathy and spinocerebellar syndrome that improves with supplemental vitamin E. Clinical findings include ophthalmoplegia, hyporeflexia, gait disturbances, and decreased sensitivity to vibration and proprioception.

### Pharmacology, Pharmacokinetics, and Toxicokinetics

Vitamin E absorption is dependent on the ingestion and absorption of fat. The presence of bile also is essential. Vitamin E is passively absorbed in the intestinal tract into the lymphatic circulation by a nonsaturable process. Approximately 45% of a dose is absorbed in this manner and subsequently enters the bloodstream in chylomicrons, which are taken up by the liver. Vitamin E then is secreted back into the circulation, where it is primarily associated with low-density lipoprotein (LDL) cholesterol. Vitamin E is distributed to all tissues, with the greatest accumulation in adipose tissue, liver, and muscle.

The primary biologic function of vitamin E is as an antioxidant. It prevents damage to biologic membranes by protecting polyunsaturated fats within membrane phospholipids from oxidation. It accomplishes this task by preferentially binding to peroxyl radicals and forming the corresponding organic hydroperoxide and tocopheroxyl radical, which, in turn interacts with other antioxidant compounds, such as ascorbic acid, thereby regenerating tocopherol.

Large amounts of vitamin E, ranging from 400 to 800 IU/day (400–800 mg/day) for months to years, were previously thought to be without apparent harm. Vitamin E supplementation results in few obvious adverse effects, even at dosages as high as 3,200 mg/day (3,200 IU/day). However, a meta-analysis reveals that all-cause mortality increases at doses equal to or greater than 400 IU/day (400 mg/day).

### Pathophysiology

In vitro studies demonstrate that in high doses vitamin E may have a paradoxical prooxidant effect. High doses of vitamin E displace other antioxidants, thereby disrupting the natural balance of the antioxidant system and increasing vulnerability to oxidative damage. High doses of vitamin E inhibit human cytosolic glutathione *S*-transferases, enzymes that are active in the detoxification of xenobiotics and endogenous toxins.

### Clinical Manifestations

Gastrointestinal symptoms, including nausea and gastric distress, were reported in patients who had received vitamin E 2,000 to 2,500 IU/day (2,000–2,500 mg/day). Diarrhea and abdominal cramps were reported in patients who received a dosage of 3,200 IU/day (3,200 mg/day). The most significant toxic effect of vitamin E, at dosages exceeding 1,000 IU/day (1,000 mg/day), is its ability to antagonize the effects of vitamin K. Although high oral doses of vitamin E typically do not produce a coagulopathy in normal humans with adequate vitamin K stores, coagulopathy develops in vitamin K–deficient patients and patients taking warfarin.

## VITAMIN C

### History and Epidemiology

Vitamin C is used to prevent scurvy. In 1747, James Lind, a physician in the British Royal Navy, analyzed the relationship between diet and scurvy and confirmed the protective and curative effects of citrus fruits. Vitamin C was isolated from cabbage in 1928 and subsequently shown in 1932 to be the active antiscorbutic factor in lemon juice. It was given the name *ascorbic acid* to indicate its role in preventing scurvy. Today, those at risk for developing scurvy include older adults, alcoholics, chronic drug users, and others with inadequate diets, including infants fed formula diets with insufficient concentrations of vitamin C. Symptoms include gingivitis, poor wound healing, bleeding, and perifollicular hemorrhage and ecchymoses. Musculoskeletal signs and symptoms consisting of arthralgias, myalgias, hemarthroses, and muscular hematomas develop in 80% of cases. Children experience severe pain in their lower limbs secondary to subperiosteal bleeding.

Vitamin C is commonly employed as a preventive for the common cold despite an absence of scientific support. Its function as an antioxidant led to its use for the prevention and treatment of cardiovascular disease and cancer. Human data from clinical trials do not demonstrate that vitamin C significantly reduces or prevents overall cardiovascular events or cancer. Vitamin C is popularly used to promote wound healing, treat cataracts, combat chronic degenerative diseases, counteract the effects of aging, increase mental attentiveness, and decrease stress. However, little, if any, objective data demonstrate a benefit of treatment for any of these indications. Vitamin C dietary supplements are commonly taken in dosages of 500 mg/day.

### Pharmacology, Pharmacokinetics, and Toxicokinetics

After ingestion, intestinal absorption of vitamin C occurs via an active transport system that is saturable at about 3 g/day. Vitamin C is distributed from the plasma to all cells in the body. Metabolic degradation of vitamin C forms oxalate. Because absorption and metabolic conversion are saturable, large ingestions of vitamin C should not significantly increase oxalate production.

Plasma concentrations of vitamin C typically are maintained at approximately 1 mg/dL. The kidney efficiently eliminates excess vitamin C as unchanged ascorbic acid.

Vitamin C is a cofactor in several hydroxylation and amidation reactions by functioning as a reducing agent. As a result, vitamin C plays an important role in the synthesis of collagen, carnitine, folinic acid, and norepinephrine. Vitamin C reduces iron from the ferric to the ferrous state in the stomach, thereby increasing intestinal absorption of iron.

### Clinical Manifestations

The possibility of oxalate nephrolithiasis should not be a significant clinical concern. Nevertheless, conflicting studies and reports exist regarding the association between vitamin C overdose and the development of oxalosis. Oxalosis also is more likely to develop in patients with chronic kidney disease. Gastrointestinal effects of high doses of vitamin C include localized esophagitis, given prolonged mucosal contact with ascorbic acid, and an osmotic diarrhea.

## VITAMIN $B_6$

### History

Pyridoxine, pyridoxal, and pyridoxamine are related compounds that have the same physiologic properties. Although all three compounds are included in the term *vitamin $B_6$*, the vitamin is assigned the name *pyridoxine.* This vitamin was discovered in 1936 as the water-soluble factor whose deficiency was responsible for the development of dermatitis in rats. Pyridoxine is found in several foods, including meat, liver, whole-grain breads and cereals, soybeans, and vegetables. In humans, deficiency is characterized by cheilosis, stomatitis, glossitis, blepharitis, and a seborrheic dermatitis around the eyes, nose, and mouth. More important, pyridoxine deficiency is associated with seizures. Pyridoxine deficiency should not occur in people who eat normal diets.

Today, the most common use of pyridoxine is in combination with doxylamine for nausea and vomiting in pregnancy. In toxicology, $B_6$ is used an antidote for seizures that result from ingestions of isoniazid or gyromitin-containing mushrooms (Antidotes in Brief: A15). Other historical uses of pyridoxine have included treatment of premenstrual syndrome and carpal tunnel syndrome.

### Pharmacology

All forms of vitamin $B_6$ are well absorbed from the intestinal tract. Pyridoxine is rapidly metabolized to pyridoxal phosphate (PLP). Pyridoxal phosphate accounts for approximately 60% of circulating vitamin $B_6$ and is the primary form that crosses cell membranes. Most vitamin $B_6$ is renally excreted as 4-pyridoxic acid, with only 7% excreted unchanged in the urine.

Pyridoxal phosphate is the active form of vitamin $B_6$. It is a coenzyme required for the synthesis of γ-aminobutyric acid (GABA), an inhibitory neurotransmitter. Decreased GABA formation in the setting of pyridoxine deficiency contributes to seizures. Isoniazid and other hydrazines inhibit the enzyme responsible for conversion of pyridoxine to PLP (Chap. 29). In addition, isoniazid enhances the elimination of pyridoxine, leading to neuropathy. Therefore, pyridoxine should be administered concomitantly with isoniazid to limit the development of peripheral neuropathy. Seizures resulting from isoniazid overdose often are successfully treated with pyridoxine (Antidotes in Brief: A15).

### Pathophysiology

Ironically, both pyridoxine deficiency and pyridoxine toxicity are characterized by neurologic effects. In 1942, pyridoxine was recognized to cause severe weakness and pathological changes in peripheral nerves and dorsal root ganglia in dogs and rats. Administration of IV pyridoxine 2 g/kg in two patients for the treatment of mushroom poisoning resulted in permanent dorsal root and sensory ganglia deficits. Similar findings were described in patients who were taking pyridoxine 2 to 6 g/day for 2 to 40 months for premenstrual syndrome.

### Clinical Manifestations

Chronic overdoses are associated with progressive sensory ataxia and severe distal impairment of proprioception and vibratory sensation. Reflexes are diminished or absent. Touch, pain, and temperature sensation are minimally impaired. Nerve conduction and somatosensory studies show dysfunction in the distal sensory peripheral nerves. Nerve biopsy shows widespread, nonspecific axonal degeneration. The most common findings reported are numbness (96%), burning pain (49.9%), tingling (57.7%), balance difficulties (30.7%), and weakness (7.8%). In most cases, symptoms gradually improved over several months with abstinence from pyridoxine. However, clinical manifestations sometimes progress for 2 to 3 weeks after pyridoxine discontinuation.

## NICOTINIC ACID

### History

Nicotinic acid, or niacin, was discovered as an essential dietary component in the early 1900s. A deficiency of this vitamin, also known as vitamin $B_3$, causes pellagra, which is characterized by dermatitis, diarrhea, and dementia. Food sources of nicotinic acid include eggs, milk, meet, fish, poultry, nuts, legumes, and whole-grain and enriched breads and cereals. Supplementation of flour with nicotinic acid in 1939 probably is responsible for the near eradication of this disease in the US. Chronic alcohol users still develop pellagra, likely secondary to malnutrition.

Niacin was introduced as a treatment for hyperlipidemia in 1955. Nicotinic acid reduces triglyceride synthesis, with a resultant drop in very-low-density lipoprotein cholesterol and LDL cholesterol and a rise in high-density lipoprotein cholesterol. More recently, the nonmedicinal ingestion of niacin for altering or masking the results of urine testing for illicit drugs was noted. However, there is no evidence that ingestion of niacin is capable of this effect.

### Pharmacology, Pharmacokinetics, and Toxicokinetics

Nicotinic acid is well absorbed from the intestinal tract and is distributed to all tissues. With therapeutic dosing, little unchanged vitamin is excreted in the urine. When extremely high doses are ingested, the unchanged vitamin is the major urinary component. Nicotinic acid ultimately is converted to nicotinamide adenine dinucleotide ($NAD^+$) and nicotinamide adenine dinucleotide phosphate ($NADP^+$), which are the physiologically active forms of this vitamin. The reduced forms of $NAD^+$ and $NADP^+$, NADH and NADPH, respectively, act as coenzymes for proteins that catalyze oxidation-reduction reactions that are essential for tissue respiration.

### Clinical Manifestations

The most common adverse effect associated with niacin use is a vasodilatory cutaneous flushing described as a sense of warmth in the face, ears, neck, trunk, and less frequently in the extremities, lasting less than 1 to 2.5 hours. Other symptoms include erythema, itching, and tingling. Symptoms commence within 15 to 30 minutes after ingestion of immediate-release niacin, 30 to 120 minutes after ingestion of extended-release niacin, and at more variable times after ingestion of sustained-release niacin. In addition, niacin induces hetapotoxicity with dosages as low as 1 g/day, but signs of hepatic dysfunction occur at dosages of 2 to 3 g/day. These patients have elevated serum bilirubin and ammonia concentrations and a prolonged prothrombin time. They develop fatigue, anorexia, nausea, vomiting, and jaundice. In most cases, liver function improves after niacin withdrawal. Severe cases progress to fulminant hepatic failure and hepatic encephalopathy. Niacin also causes amblyopia, hyperglycemia, hyperuricemia, coagulopathy, myopathy, and hyperpigmentation.

### Management

A dose of 325 mg of aspirin taken 30 minutes before ingestion of niacin diminishes flushing. Treatment for hepatotoxicity is largely supportive.

# 18 IRON

| | |
|---|---|
| Normal serum concentration | 80–180 μg/dL<br>14–32 μmol/L |

## INTRODUCTION

Iron poisoning has become uncommon. Regulatory controls and education of parents and healthcare professionals have led to a great decline in iron-related morbidity. However, when significant iron poisonings do occur, clinicians must be aware of the nuances of presentation and diagnosis, and be prepared to intervene if gastrointestinal (GI) toxic effects, acid–base disturbances, altered mental status, or hemodynamic compromise arises.

## HISTORY AND EPIDEMIOLOGY

Despite its long history of use, the first reports of iron toxicity only occurred in the mid-20th century. In the 1990s, iron became the leading cause of poisoning deaths in children younger than 6 years of age. In 1997, the United States (US) Food and Drug Administration (FDA) mandated the placement of warning labels on all iron salt-containing preparations regarding the dangers of pediatric iron poisoning. Other preventive initiatives instituted in 1997 included US FDA-mandated warning labels and limiting the number of pills dispensed (ie, maximum 30-day supply). These efforts to prevent unintentional exposure dramatically decreased the incidence of morbidity and mortality associated with iron poisoning.

## PHARMACOLOGY, PHARMACOKINETICS, AND TOXICOKINETICS

Iron is critical to organ function because it is able to accept and donate electrons easily as it shifts from ferric ($Fe^{3+}$) to ferrous ($Fe^{2+}$) states. This reduction-oxidation (redox) interchange gives iron an essential role in multiple protein and enzyme complexes, including cytochromes, myoglobin, and hemoglobin. Insufficient iron results in anemia, whereas excess total-body iron results in hemochromatosis.

Iron stores are regulated by controlling its absorption from the gastrointestinal tract. In iron deficiency, iron uptake increases from a normal of 10% to 35% to as much as 80% to 95%. Following uptake, iron is either stored as ferritin and lost when the cell is sloughed or released to transferrin, a serum iron-binding protein. In therapeutic doses, some of these processes become saturated and absorption is limited. However, in overdose the destructive effects of iron on GI mucosal cells leads to dysfunction of this regulatory balance and increases passive absorption of iron.

Iron supplements are available as the iron salts and as the nonionic preparations carbonyl iron and polysaccharide iron. Additional sources of significant quantities of iron are vitamin preparations, especially prenatal vitamins. Toxicity is based on the amount of elemental iron in each preparation (Table 18–1). Iron polysaccharide and carbonyl iron are safer formulations than iron salts despite high elemental iron content. Carbonyl iron is a form of elemental iron that is highly bioavailable. Toxicity is limited in overdose because carbonyl iron must be solubilized to be absorbed. The slow oxidation of carbonyl iron to ferrous ($Fe^{2+}$) ion in stomach acid serves as a rate-limiting step.

**TABLE 18–1 Common Iron Formulations and Their Elemental Iron Content**

| *Iron Formulation: Oral* | *Elemental Iron (%)* |
|---|---|
| *Ionic* | |
| Ferrous chloride | 28 |
| Ferrous fumarate | 33 |
| Ferrous gluconate | 12 |
| Ferrous lactate | 19 |
| Ferrous sulfate | 20 |
| *Nonionic*[a] | |
| Carbonyl iron | 98 |
| Polysaccharide iron | 46 |
| *Iron Formulation: Parenteral* | |
| Ferric carboxymaltose | 5 |
| Ferric gluconate | 1.25 |
| Ferumoxytol | 3 |
| Iron dextran (low molecular weight) | 5 |
| Iron sucrose | 2 |

[a]Although the nonionic iron formulations contain higher elemental iron content than ionic formulations, carbonyl iron and iron polysaccharide have better therapeutic-to-toxic ratios because of their limited gastrointestinal absorption rates.

## PATHOPHYSIOLOGY

The participation of iron in redox reactions such as the Fenton reaction and Haber-Weiss cycle causes oxidative stress. Generation of reactive oxygen species oxidizes membrane-bound lipids and results in the loss of cellular integrity with subsequent tissue injury. Oxidative damage to the GI epithelium enhances iron entry into the systemic circulation. Iron ions are rapidly bound to circulating binding proteins, particularly transferrin. Once transferrin is saturated with iron, "free" iron (iron not bound safely to a transport protein) is widely distributed to the various organ systems where it promotes damage. Iron ions disrupt mitochondrial oxidative phosphorylation leading to a metabolic acidosis. In addition, as iron is absorbed from the gastrointestinal tract, ferrous iron ($Fe^{2+}$) is converted to ferric iron ($Fe^{3+}$). Ferric iron ions exceed the binding capacity of plasma, leading to formation of ferric hydroxide and production of three protons ($Fe^{3+} + 3H_2O \rightarrow Fe\{OH\}_3 + 3\,H^+$).

In animals, decreased cardiac output contributes to hemodynamic shock. Although significant volume loss is contributory, iron also has a direct negative inotropic effect on the myocardium. Free iron inhibits thrombin and the effect of thrombin on fibrinogen, with coagulopathy occurring independently of hepatotoxicity.

## CLINICAL MANIFESTATIONS

Toxic GI effects of iron poisoning occur at doses of 10–20 mg/kg elemental iron. Above 50 mg/kg, metabolic acidosis and hemodynamic instability should be expected. Doses greater than 100 mg/kg should be considered potentially life-threatening. Although five stages of iron toxicity are described, a clinical stage should never be assigned based on the number of hours postingestion, as patients do not necessarily follow the same temporal course through these stages.

The first stage of iron toxicity is characterized by nausea, vomiting, abdominal pain, and diarrhea. The "local" toxic effects of iron predominate, and subsequent salt and water depletion contribute to the patient's condition. Intestinal ulceration, edema, transmural inflammation, and, in some extreme cases, small-bowel infarction and necrosis occur. Hematemesis, melena, or hematochezia contribute to hemodynamic instability. Gastrointestinal symptoms always follow significant overdose, and, conversely, the absence of vomiting in the first 6 hours following ingestion essentially excludes serious iron toxicity.

The "latent" or second stage of iron poisoning commonly refers to the period 6 to 24 hours following the resolution of GI symptoms and before overt systemic toxicity develops. This second stage is not a true quiescent phase, as during this phase there is ongoing cellular toxicity. Gastrointestinal complaints resolve, but patients in the latent phase generally have lethargy, tachycardia, and metabolic acidosis.

Patients who progress to the third or shock stage of poisoning manifest as early as the first few hours after a massive ingestion or 12 to 24 hours after a more moderate ingestion. The etiology of shock is multifactorial, resulting from hypovolemia, vasodilation, and poor cardiac output. Coagulopathy worsens bleeding and hypovolemia. Systemic toxicity produces CNS effects with lethargy, hyperventilation, seizures, or coma.

The fourth stage of iron poisoning is characterized by hepatic failure, which occurs 2 to 3 days following the ingestion. The hepatotoxicity is directly attributed to uptake of iron by the reticuloendothelial system in the liver, where it causes oxidative damage.

The fifth stage of iron toxicity rarely occurs. Gastric outlet obstruction, secondary to strictures and scarring from the initial GI injury, can develop 2 to 8 weeks following ingestion.

## DIAGNOSTIC TESTING

### Radiography

Finding radiopaque pills on an abdominal radiograph is most useful as a guide for evaluating the success of GI decontamination (see Figure 5–2). However, the absence of the radiographic evidence of pills is not a reliable indicator to exclude potential toxicity. Liquid iron formulations and chewable iron tablets are typically not radiopaque. Because adult iron preparations have a higher elemental iron content and do not readily disperse, they tend to be more consistently radiopaque.

### Laboratory

A high anion gap metabolic acidosis with an elevated lactate concentration is common in serious iron poisonings. Anemia results from GI blood loss but may not be evident initially because of hemoconcentration secondary to plasma volume loss. Although frequently discussed, the elevated white blood cell count and glucose concentration actually have very little predictive value, and decisions based on these results can be erroneous.

Although iron poisoning remains a clinical diagnosis, serum iron concentrations can be used effectively to gauge toxicity and the success of treatment. Peak serum iron concentrations occur 4 to 6 hours postingestion. Serum iron concentrations greater than 300 μg/dL (53.7 μmol/L) are generally consistent with GI symptoms. Serum iron concentrations between 300 and 500 μg/dL (53.7–89.5 μmol/L) usually correlate with significant GI toxicity and modest systemic toxicity. Concentrations between 500 and 1,000 μg/dL (89.5–179 μmol/L) are associated with pronounced systemic toxicity and shock, and concentrations greater than 1,000 μg/dL (179 μmol/L) are associated with significant morbidity and mortality. Lower concentrations cannot be used to exclude the possibility of serious toxicity, as a single value may not represent a peak concentration. Total iron-binding capacity (TIBC) is not valuable for comparison to serum iron concentration, as TIBC factitiously increases as a result of iron poisoning and the method of laboratory determination.

## MANAGEMENT

### Initial Approach

The overall management of patients is summarized in Figure 18–1. Patients who appear well and have had only one or two brief episodes of vomiting can be observed for 6 hours and then safely dispositioned. A serum iron concentration and most other laboratory testing are not indicated in patients who have minimal symptoms and normal vital signs. Following a significant ingestion, initial stabilization must include airway assessment and establishment of IV access. In the absence of coingestants, evidence of hematemesis or lethargy after an iron exposure is a manifestation of significant toxicity. Intravenous volume repletion should begin in any patient with a history of massive exposure (> 60 mg/kg) or tachycardia, lethargy, or metabolic acidosis. In any lethargic patient at risk for further deterioration, early endotracheal intubation facilitates controlled GI decontamination. Abdominal radiography is recommended to estimate the iron burden in the GI tract given the caveats discussed earlier. Laboratory values, including chemistries, hemoglobin, iron concentration, coagulation, and hepatic profiles, should be obtained. An arterial or venous blood gas and a lactate concentration rapidly identify a metabolic compromise.

### Limiting Absorption

Adequate gastric emptying is critical as iron is not well adsorbed to activated charcoal. Orogastric lavage is often of limited value because of the large size and poor solubility of

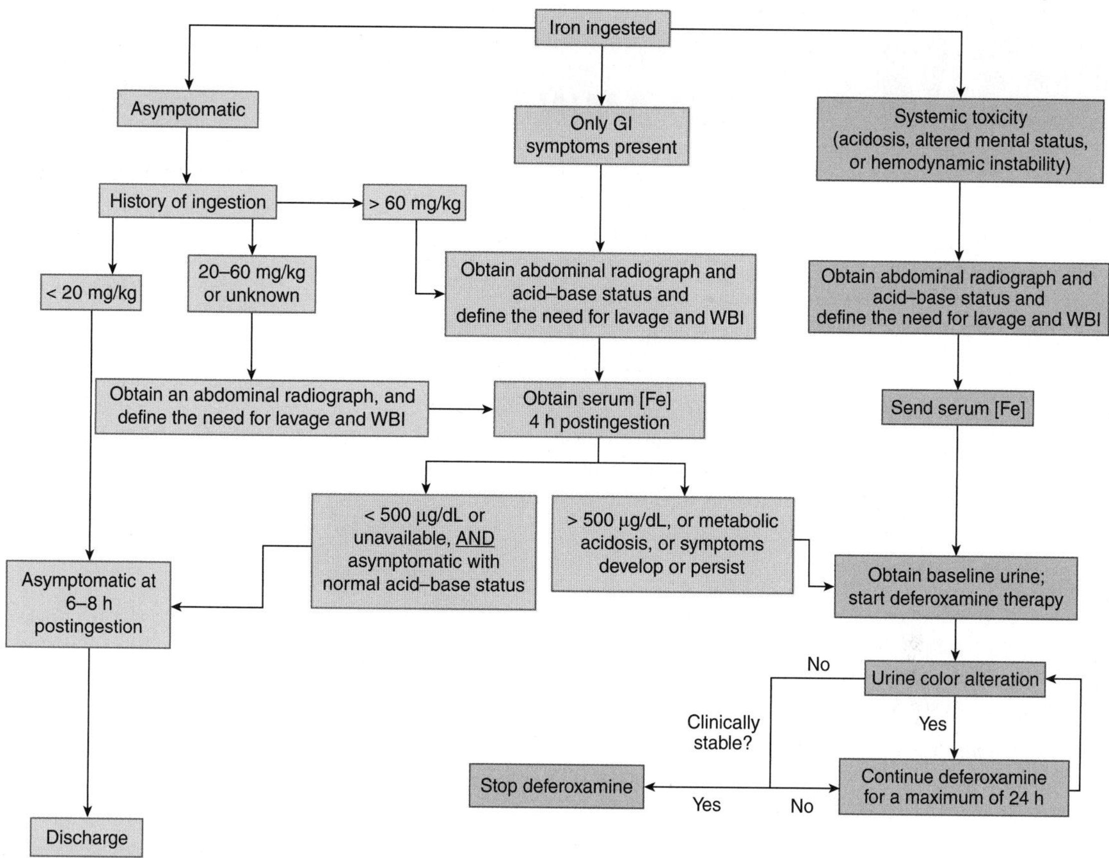


**FIGURE 18–1.** Algorithm for decision analysis after iron salt ingestion. GI = gastrointestinal; WBI = whole-bowel irrigation; 500 µg/dL = 89.5 µmol/L.

most iron tablets. The presence and location of radiopaque tablets on abdominal radiography can help guide early orogastric lavage in patients with suspected significant poisoning. Whole-bowel irrigation is recommended in severe cases using polyethylene glycol electrolyte lavage solution (PEG-ELS) as described in Antidotes in Brief: A2. For patients with life-threatening toxicity who demonstrate persistent iron in the GI tract despite orogastric lavage and whole-bowel irrigation, it is reasonable to pursue upper endoscopy or gastrotomy and surgical removal of iron tablets adherent to the gastric mucosa.

## Deferoxamine

Intravenous administration of deferoxamine (DFO) is recommended in all iron-poisoned patients with any of the following findings: metabolic acidosis, repetitive vomiting, toxic appearance, lethargy, hypotension, or signs of shock. Deferoxamine administration should also be considered in any patient with serum iron concentrations greater than 500 µg/dL. In patients manifesting serious signs and symptoms of iron poisoning, an intravenous infusion of DFO should be initiated slowly and gradually increasing to a dose of 15 mg/kg/h. Most authors agree that DFO therapy should be discontinued when the patient appears clinically well, the anion gap acidosis has resolved, and there is no further urine color change. In patients with persistent signs and symptoms of serious toxicity following 24 hours of intravenous DFO, continuing therapy should be undertaken cautiously and perhaps at a lower dose if at all because of the risk of acute respiratory distress syndrome (Antidotes in Brief: A7).

## Pregnant Patients

The frequent diagnosis of iron-deficiency anemia during pregnancy is associated with access to iron preparations with resultant serious, and even fatal, iron ingestions in pregnant women. Neither iron nor DFO is transferred to the fetus in appreciable quantities. Fetal demise presumably results from maternal iron toxicity and not from direct iron toxicity to the fetus. Consequently, DFO should be used to treat serious maternal iron poisoning and never withheld because of unfounded concern for fetal exposure to DFO.

## Adjunctive Therapies

An iron-poisoned toddler was treated with DFO and venovenous hemofiltration. Also, in toddlers with severe poisoning, exchange transfusion is reasonable early in the clinical course to help physically remove all iron from the blood while replacing it with normal blood. However, removal of blood volume must be performed cautiously because it can worsen hypotension in iron-poisoned patients with hemodynamic instability.

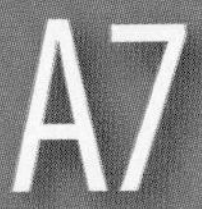

# A7 DEFEROXAMINE

## INTRODUCTION

Deferoxamine (DFO) is the chelator of choice for treatment of acute iron poisoning. Deferoxamine is also used for chelation of aluminum in patients with chronic kidney disease.

## HISTORY

Ferrioxamine is a brownish-red compound containing trivalent iron (ferric, $Fe^{3+}$) isolated from the organism *Streptomyces pilosus.* Deferoxamine is the colorless compound that results when the trivalent iron is chemically removed from ferrioxamine B.

## CHEMISTRY

One mole of DFO binds 1 mole of $Fe^{3+}$; therefore, 100 mg of DFO binds 8.5 mg of $Fe^{3+}$. Because DFO has a far greater affinity for iron than for zinc, copper, nickel, magnesium, or calcium, it complexes almost exclusively with iron.

**FIGURE A7–1.** Ferrioxamine.

### Related Chelators

Deferiprone is approved by the United States Food and Drug Administration (FDA) for the treatment of iron overload in patients with thalassemia major. Three moles of deferiprone bind 1 mole of $Fe^{3+}$ to form a stable complex, which is excreted in the urine. Animal studies of the use of deferiprone in acute iron toxicity are contradictory. Adverse events include elevation of hepatic enzymes, gastrointestinal (GI) effects, arthralgia, and chromaturia. Deferiprone also carries a boxed warning for neutropenia and agranulocytosis. Deferiprone is listed as category D in pregnancy.

Deferasirox is an oral iron chelator that is indicated to treat chronic iron overload caused by blood transfusions or in patients with thalassemia major and elevated hepatic iron concentrations. Deferasirox binds $Fe^{3+}$ in a 2:1 ratio, which is then predominantly eliminated in the feces. In a human model of a modest supraphysiologic iron ingestion (only 5 mg/kg), deferasirox reduced serum iron concentrations compared with placebo. Concerns about achieving the effective dose ratio of deferasirox to iron of 2:1 and the effects of acidemia on the binding of deferasirox to iron in a large overdose limit its use. In addition, concerns exist about increasing oral absorption of the deferasirox-iron complex and the toxicity of this complex in an acute iron overdose. Adverse events include boxed warnings for GI hemorrhage, kidney failure, and hepatic failure, but since this antidote is rarely used in acute iron overdose, these risks are unquantified.

## MECHANISM OF ACTION

Deferoxamine binds $Fe^{3+}$ forming a stable octahedral iron complex (Fig. A7–1). Deferoxamine chelates free iron (non-transferrin bound plasma iron) and iron in transit between transferrin and ferritin (chelatable labile iron pool), while not directly affecting the iron of hemoglobin, hemosiderin, or ferritin. Additionally, deferoxamine chelates and inactivates cytoplasmic iron, preventing cellular disruption.

## PHARMACOKINETICS

The volume of distribution of DFO ranges from 0.6 to 1.33 L/kg, with an initial distribution half-life of 5 to 10 minutes and a terminal elimination half-life of approximately 6 hours in healthy patients. Deferoxamine is metabolized in the plasma to several metabolites, one of which is believed to be toxic. Unmetabolized DFO is renally eliminated. In comparison, ferrioxamine has a smaller volume of distribution than DFO, which implies that DFO has a more extensive tissue distribution. Ferrioxamine is entirely eliminated by the kidney within 5 hours. Because DFO is hemodialyzable, it can be administered during hemodialysis to remove ferrioxamine. Hemodialysis, particularly high-flux hemodialysis, is recommended in patients with kidney failure.

## ROLE IN IRON TOXICITY

Because only a limited amount of iron can be chelated by DFO, GI decontamination and supportive measures are always recommended (Chap. 18).

### Animal Studies

Studies of iron poisoning in a variety of animal models show dramatic improvement in survival rates after DFO is administered. Mortality rates correlate directly with the delay to DFO administration. However, because dogs given an iron-DFO complex orally had an increased mortality, oral DFO should not be used.

### Early Human Use and History of Dosing Recommendations

In an early case series, 1 g of DFO was administered intravenously at a maximum of 15 mg/kg/h every 4 to 12 hours to 28 patients who were in shock or severely ill. Only three of these patients died, one of whom received late treatment with DFO.

### Parenteral Administration

Prior to 1976, IM DFO was the preferred route of administration and IV DFO was reserved for patients in shock. However, because IV DFO significantly enhances urinary iron elimination over IM DFO, the IV route is preferred in all patients.

### Duration of Dosing

The optimum duration of DFO administration is unknown. In canine models, serum iron concentrations peak within 3 to 5 hours and then fall quickly as iron is transported into the tissues. In one human study, patients with initial iron concentrations of about 500 μg/dL decreased to approximately 100 μg/dL within 12 hours. Other reports suggest that by 24 hours most of the easily chelatable iron is distributed out of the blood compartment. Given that prolonged DFO is associated with toxicity, treatment for more than 24 hours is not routinely recommended.

## ROLE IN ALUMINUM TOXICITY

Deferoxamine binds aluminum to form aluminoxamine, which is excreted renally. In patients with kidney disease, hemodialysis (HD) effectively removes aluminoxamine. The dosing of DFO should be tailored to the patient's serum aluminum concentrations, symptoms, and response. For acute toxicity in patients with stage 5 chronic kidney disease, 3 to 4 hours of HD is performed 6 to 8 hours after chelation with 15 mg/kg of DFO intravenously. Patients with normal kidney function and urine output do not require HD. For patients with chronic aluminum toxicity, the National Kidney Foundation guidelines recommend 4 months of once-weekly DFO at 5 mg/kg over 1 hour given 5 hours before a regularly scheduled HD session when the serum aluminum concentration is greater than 300 μg/L. When the serum aluminum concentration is between 50 and 300 μg/L, DFO at 5 mg/kg is recommended during the last hour of HD, once a week for 2 months. Therapy is repeated as needed based on kidney function and neurologic symptoms.

## ADVERSE EFFECTS

In acute iron overdose, DFO is associated with rate-related hypotension and delayed-onset pulmonary toxicity. The mechanism for the rate-related hypotension is not fully understood, although histamine release is implicated, and hypotension is exacerbated by volume depletion. Acute respiratory distress syndrome (ARDS) occurs in patients with iron overdoses given IV DFO for longer than 24 hours. Deferoxamine therapy rarely leads to infection with unusual organisms, including *Yersinia enterocolitica*, *Zygomycetes* spp., and *Aeromonas hydrophila*, because they thrive on DFO-bound iron.

When administered to patients with chronic iron overload, DFO is associated with auditory, ophthalmic, and pulmonary toxicity and infection. Ophthalmic toxicity is characterized by decreased visual acuity, night blindness, color blindness, and retinal pigmentary abnormalities. Ototoxicity documented by abnormal audiograms indicating partial or total deafness is reported. These complications are not expected in the treatment of acute iron overdose.

## PREGNANCY AND LACTATION

Iron toxicity is associated with spontaneous abortion, preterm delivery, and maternal death. There is no evidence that DFO is teratogenic. Neither iron nor DFO crosses the ovine placenta. A review of 40 pregnant patients with thalassemia treated extensively with DFO found no evidence of teratogenicity. Deferoxamine is listed as FDA pregnancy category C and should be administered to pregnant women with acute iron overdose for the same indications as for nonpregnant women. Excretion in breast milk is unknown.

## DOSING AND ADMINISTRATION

The indications and dosage schedules for DFO administration are largely empiric and the duration of therapy should be limited to 24 hours in most cases to maximize effectiveness while minimizing the risk of pulmonary toxicity. An intravenous infusion is started at 5 mg/kg/h and increased every 15 minutes, as long as the blood pressure is maintained, up to maximal rate of 15 mg/kg/h. The total daily parenteral dose is limited by the infusion rate in children. In adults, conservative recommendations limit the dose to 6 to 8 g/day, although doses as high as 16 g/day have been administered without incident.

## URINARY COLOR CHANGE

Most data suggest that the absence of a urine color change, often referred to as a *vin rosé*, after DFO administration indicates very little renal excretion of ferrioxamine. However, unless a baseline urine color is obtained, post–DFO administration comparisons of urine color are unreliable. No relationship between urinary iron excretion, clinical iron toxicity, and the effectiveness of DFO is established.

## FORMULATION AND ACQUISITION

Deferoxamine mesylate is available in vials containing 500 mg or 2 g of sterile, lyophilized powder. Addition of 5 mL or 20 mL of sterile water for injection to either the 500-mg or the 2-g vials, respectively, results in a solution of 100 mg/mL that is isotonic. The resulting solution can be further diluted with 0.9% NaCl solution, dextrose in water, or lactated Ringer solution for intravenous administration.

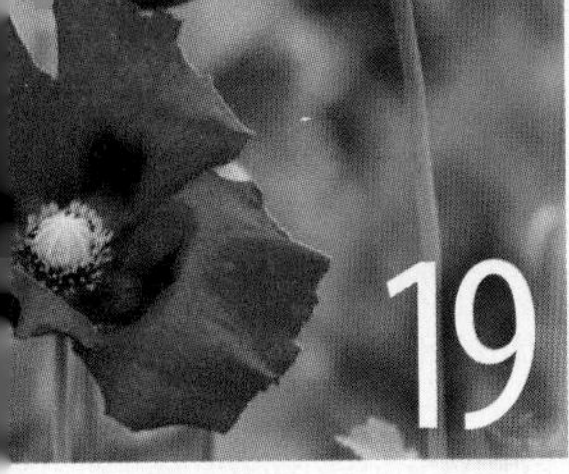

C. Pharmaceuticals

# 19 PHARMACEUTICAL ADDITIVES

Additives, or excipients as they are more properly termed, are necessary to act as vehicles, to add color, to improve taste, to provide consistency, to enhance stability and solubility, and to impart antimicrobial properties to medicinal formulations. Most cases of excipient toxicity involve exposure to large quantities or to prolonged or improper use (Table 19–1).

During the last two centuries, there were several outbreaks of toxicity associated with pharmaceutical additives in the United States (US). The Massengill sulfanilamide disaster in 1937, the most notorious of these epidemics, involved diethylene glycol. More recently, there was concern over potential mercury toxicity and a link to autism from the preservative thimerosal, a mercury derivative that has been used in parenteral vaccines for 70 years. No evidence has yet shown toxicity to result from routine vaccination. Although these additive-related occurrences are rare relative to the frequency of pharmaceutical additive use, they illustrate the potential of pharmaceutical additive toxicity. Unlike active ingredients, there is no specific US Food and Drug Administration (FDA) approval system for pharmaceutical excipients.

## BENZALKONIUM CHLORIDE

Benzalkonium chloride (BAC) or alkyldimethyl (phenylmethyl) ammonium chloride is a quaternary ammonium cationic surfactant composed of a mixture of alkyl benzyl dimethyl ammonium chlorides. Although it is the most widely used ophthalmic preservative in the US, it is also considered the most cytotoxic (Table 19–2). Benzalkonium chloride is also used in otic and nasal formulations and in some small-volume parenterals.

**TABLE 19–2 Benzalkonium Chloride Concentrations of Common Ophthalmic Medications**

| *Medication* | *Percent* |
|---|---|
| Apraclonidine | 0.01 |
| Artificial tears | 0.005–0.01 |
| Betaxolol | 0.01 |
| Brimonidine/timolol | 0.005 |
| Carteolol | 0.005 |
| Ciprofloxacin | 0.006 |
| Cyclopentolate | 0.01 |
| Dexamethasone | 0.01 |
| Dorzolamide/timolol | 0.0075 |
| Gentamicin | 0.01 |
| Ketorolac | 0.01 |
| Levobunolol | 0.004 |
| Naphazoline | 0.01 |
| Ofloxacin | 0.005 |
| Phenylephrine | 0.01 |
| Pilocarpine | 0.01 |
| Polymyxin B sulfate/trimethoprim | 0.004 |
| Tetrahydrozoline | 0.01 |
| Timolol | 0.01 |
| Tobramycin | 0.01 |
| Tropicamide | 0.01 |

### Ophthalmic Toxicity

Following exposure to BAC, mitotic activity ceases and degenerative changes are noted in harvested corneal epithelium. Patients with continued use develop visual abnormalities associated with punctate corneal erosions or more severe breakdown of the corneal epithelium. Although some patients improve upon cessation of exposure, injury can be permanent.

**TABLE 19–1 Potential Systemic Toxicity of Various Pharmaceutical Excipients**

| | |
|---|---|
| Cardiovascular | Ophthalmic |
| Chlorobutanol | Benzalkonium chloride |
| Propylene glycol | Chlorobutanol |
| Fluid and electrolyte | Renal |
| Polyethylene glycol | Polyethylene glycol |
| Propylene glycol | Propylene glycol |
| Sorbitol | |
| Gastrointestinal | |
| Sorbitol | |
| Neurologic | |
| Benzyl alcohol | |
| Chlorobutanol | |
| Polyethylene glycol | |
| Propylene glycol | |

### Nasopharyngeal and Oropharyngeal Toxicity

Benzalkonium chloride decreases the viscosity of the normal protective mucous lining of the naso- and oropharynx, resulting in cytotoxicity. Human adenoidal tissue exposed to oxymetazoline nasal spray preserved with BAC developed irregular and fractured epithelial cells.

## BENZYL ALCOHOL

Benzyl alcohol (benzene methanol) is a colorless, oily liquid with a faint aromatic odor that is most commonly added to pharmaceuticals as a bacteriostatic agent (Table 19–3). In 1982, a "gasping" syndrome, which included hypotension, bradycardia, gasping respirations, hypotonia, progressive metabolic acidosis, seizures, cardiovascular collapse, and death, was first described in low-birth-weight neonates in intensive care units. All the infants had received either

**TABLE 19–3 Benzyl Alcohol Concentrations of Common Medications**

| *Medication (concentration)* | *Percent* | *Benzyl Alcohol Dose (mg/dose volume)* |
|---|---|---|
| Amiodarone (50 mg/mL) | 2.0 | 60.6 mg/3 mL |
| Atracurium (10 mg/mL) | 0.9 | 45 mg/5 mL |
| Bacteriostatic saline for injection | 0.9 | 9 mg/mL |
| Bacteriostatic water for injection | 0.9 | 9 mg/mL |
| Bumetanide (0.25 mg/mL) | 1.0 | 40 mg/4 mL |
| Diazepam (5 mg/mL) | 1.5 | 30 mg/2 mL |
| Enalaprilat (1.25 mg/mL) | 0.9 | 9 mg/mL |
| Etoposide (20 mg/mL) | 3.0 | 150 mg/5 mL |
| Glycopyrrolate (0.2 mg/mL) | 0.9 | 9 mg/mL |
| Lorazepam (2 mg/mL, 4 mg/mL) | 2.0 | 20 mg/mL |
| Methotrexate (25 mg/mL) | 0.9 | 9 mg/mL |
| Midazolam (1 mg/mL, 5 mg/mL) | 1.0 | 10 mg/mL |
| Prochlorperazine (5 mg/mL) | 0.75 | 7.5 mg/mL |

bacteriostatic water or sodium chloride containing 0.9% benzyl alcohol to flush intravenous catheters or in parenteral medications reconstituted with bacteriostatic water or saline. The World Health Organization (WHO) currently estimates the acceptable daily intake of benzyl alcohol to be not more than 5 mg/kg body weight.

### Pharmacokinetics

In adults, benzyl alcohol is oxidized to benzoic acid, conjugated in the liver with glycine, and excreted in the urine as hippuric acid. The immature metabolic capacities of infants diminish their ability to metabolize and excrete benzyl alcohol resulting in metabolic acidosis.

### Neurologic Toxicity

Benzyl alcohol is believed to have a role in the increased frequency of cerebral intraventricular hemorrhages and mortality reported in very-low-birth-weight (VLBW) infants (weight < 1000 g) who received flush solutions preserved with benzyl alcohol. Transient paraplegia occurred following the intrathecal or epidural administration of chemotherapeutics or analgesics containing benzyl alcohol as a preservative. The local anesthetic effects are most likely responsible for the immediate paraparesis, although chronic intrathecal exposure causes demyelinization.

## CHLOROBUTANOL

Chlorobutanol has antibacterial and antifungal properties and is widely used as a preservative in injectable, ophthalmic, otic, and cosmetic preparations at concentrations up to 0.5% (Table 19–4). Chlorobutanol also has mild sedative and local anesthetic properties and was formerly used therapeutically as a sedative–hypnotic. The lethal human chlorobutanol dose is estimated to be 50 to 500 mg/kg.

### Central Nervous System Depression

Because chlorobutanol has a chemical structure similar to trichloroethanol, the active metabolite of chloral hydrate, this is believed to be the mechanism for its sedating property.

**TABLE 19–4 Chlorobutanol Concentrations of Common Medications**

| *Medication (concentration)* | *Percent* | *Chlorobutanol Dose (mg/dose volume)* |
|---|---|---|
| Epinephrine injection (1 mg/mL) | 0.5 | 1.5 mg/0.3 mL |
| Isoniazid injection (100 mg/mL) | 0.25 | 7.5 mg/3 mL |
| Methadone injection (10 mg/mL) | 0.5 | 5 mg/mL |
| Thiamine injection (100 mg/mL) | 0.5 | 5 mg/mL |
| Pyridoxine (100 mg/mL) | 0.5 | 5 mg/mL |
| Tobramycin ophthalmic ointment | 0.5 | — |
| Vasopressin (20 U/mL) injectable | 0.5 | 2.5 mg/0.5 mL |
| Vitamin A injection (50,000 IU/mL) | 0.5 | 5 mg/mL |

### Ophthalmic Toxicity

Chlorobutanol is a commonly used preservative in ophthalmic preparations and is less toxic to the eye than benzalkonium chloride. However, an in vitro experiment using corneal epithelial cells harvested from human cadavers demonstrated arrested mitotic activity following chlorobutanol exposure. At the commonly formulated concentration of 0.5%, chlorobutanol can cause eye irritation, and degeneration of human corneal epithelial cells specifically manifested as membranous blebs, cytoplasmic swelling, and occasional breaks in the external cell membrane.

## LIPIDS

There are three types of commercial intravenous lipid drug-delivery systems available: lipid emulsion, liposomal, and lipid complex (Table 19–5). Lipid emulsions are immiscible lipid droplets dispersed in an aqueous phase stabilized by an emulsifier (eg, egg or soy lecithin). Liposomes differ from emulsion lipid droplets in that they are vesicles comprised of one or more concentric phospholipid bilayers surrounding an aqueous core. Lipophilic drugs are formulated for intravenous administration by partitioning them into the lipid phase of either an emulsion or liposome. Liposomes are capable of encapsulating hydrophilic xenobiotics within their aqueous core to exploit lipid pharmacokinetic properties. Attaching a therapeutic drug to a lipid to form a lipid complex is another way to take advantage of lipid pharmacokinetics.

Lipid drug-delivery systems are biocompatible because of their similarity to endogenous cell membranes. The

**TABLE 19–5 Lipid Carrier Formulations of Common Medications**

| *Medication* | *Lipid Carrier* |
|---|---|
| Amphotericin B | Lipid complex |
| Amphotericin B | Liposome |
| Bupivacaine | Liposome |
| Cytarabine | Liposome |
| Doxorubicin | Liposome (stealth) |
| Morphine sulfate | Liposome |
| Propofol | Emulsion |

biodistribution, and the rate of release and metabolism of a drug incorporated in a lipid drug-delivery system, is regulated by the type and concentration of oil and emulsifier used, pH, drug concentration dispersed in the medium, the size of the lipid particle, and the manufacturing process. The rate of clearance of a lipid drug-delivery system from the blood depends on its physicochemical properties and the molecular weight of the emulsifier.

For a therapeutic drug available in more than one lipid drug-delivery systems (eg, amphotericin B), it is important to note that any change in the lipid formulation can alter the pharmacokinetic, pharmacodynamic, and safety parameters of the drug; consequently, they are not equivalent dosage formulations (Chap. 27).

## PARABENS

The parabens, or parahydroxybenzoic acids, are a group of compounds widely employed as preservatives in cosmetics, food, and pharmaceuticals (Table 19–6). Methylparaben and propylparaben are most commonly used. The parabens have a relatively low order of toxicity; however, because of their allergenic potential, they are now considered less suitable for injectable and ophthalmic preparations.

In addition to allergic reactions, parabens have the potential to cause other adverse effects. Bilirubin displacement from albumin binding sites occurred with administration of methyl and propyl paraben. Spermicidal activity is also demonstrated.

## PHENOL

Phenol (carbolic acid, hydroxybenzene, phenylic acid, phenylic alcohol) is a commonly used preservative in injectable medications (Table 19–7). Phenol is well absorbed from the gastrointestinal tract, skin, and mucous membranes and is excreted in the urine as phenyl glucuronide and phenyl sulfate metabolites. Although there are numerous reports of phenol toxicity following intentional ingestions or unintentional dermal exposures, adverse reactions to its use as a pharmaceutical excipient are uncommon, most likely because of the small quantities used.

**TABLE 19–6 Parabens Concentrations of Common Medications and Doses**

| *Medication (concentration)* | *Percent* | *Parabens Dose (mg/dose volume)* |
|---|---|---|
| Bupivacaine HCl injection[a] | 0.1 | 1 mg/mL |
| Flumazenil injection (0.1 mg/mL) | 0.2 | 4 mg/2 mL |
| Labetalol injection (5 mg/mL) | 0.09 | 3.6 mg/4 mL |
| Lidocaine injection[a] | 0.1 | 1 mg/mL |
| Methyldopa injection (50 mg/mL) | 0.17 | 8.5 mg/5 mL |
| Naloxone injection (0.4 mg/mL) | 0.2 | 2 mg/mL |
| Ondansetron injection (2 mg/mL) | 0.14 | 2.7 mg/2 mL |
| Pentazocine injection (30 mg/mL) | 0.1 | 1 mg/mL |
| Sulfacetamide ophthalmic solution (100 mg/mL) | 0.06 | 0.03 mg/drop |

[a]Multidose vials of all strengths contain 0.1% parabens.

**TABLE 19–7 Phenol Concentrations of Common Medications**

| *Medication* | *Percent* | *Phenol Dose (mg/dose volume)* |
|---|---|---|
| Antivenom (Crotaline) | 0.25 | 25 (per vial) |
| Antivenom (*Micrurus fulvius*) | 0.25 | 25 (per vial) |
| Pneumococcal 23 vaccine | 0.25 | 1.25 mg/0.5 mL |
| Neostigmine methylsulfate injection[a] | 0.45 | 4.5 mg/mL |
| Quinidine gluconate injection 80 mg/mL | 0.25 | 25 mg/10 mL |
| Typhoid Vi vaccine | 0.25 | 1.25 mg/0.5 mL |

[a]Multidose vials of all strengths contain 0.45% phenol.

### Cutaneous Absorption

Systemic toxicity from cutaneous absorption of phenol is reported. Ventricular tachycardia was observed in an 11-year-old boy following application of a chemical peel solution containing 88% phenol in water and liquid soap. A urinary phenol concentration confirmed absorption. In a case series of 181 patients undergoing chemical face peeling with phenol-based solutions, 12 demonstrated cardiac dysrhythmias.

## POLYETHYLENE GLYCOL

Polyethylene glycols (PEGs; Carbowax, Macrogol) include several compounds with molecular weights (MWs) varying from 200 to 40,000 daltons. They are typically available as mixtures designated by a number denoting their average molecular weight. Polyethylene glycols are stable, hydrophilic substances, making them useful excipients for cosmetics and pharmaceuticals of all routes of administration (Table 19–8). Commercially available products used for whole-bowel irrigation are solutions of PEG 3350 combined with electrolytes (PEG-ELS) (Antidotes in Brief: A2). Low-molecular-weight PEG exposures have caused adverse effects similar to the chemically related toxic alcohols ethylene and diethylene glycol (Special Considerations: SC8).

### Pharmacokinetics

High-molecular-weight PEGs (> 1,000 daltons) are not significantly absorbed from the gastrointestinal tract; however, low-molecular-weight PEGs are absorbed when taken orally. Once in the systemic circulation, PEGs are mainly excreted unchanged in the urine, although low-molecular-weight PEGs are metabolized by alcohol dehydrogenase to hydroxyacid and diacid metabolites.

**TABLE 19–8 Common Medications Containing PEG**

| *Medication* | *PEG Molecular Weight (Da)* |
|---|---|
| Etoposide injection | 300 |
| Lorazepam injection | 400 |
| Medroxyprogesterone depot | 3,350 |
| Mupirocin ointment | 400, 3,350 |
| PEG electrolyte lavage solution | 3,350 |
| Peginterferon $\alpha$-2a | 40,000 |

PEG = polyethylene glycol.

### Nephrotoxicity and Related Disturbances

Acute tubular necrosis with oliguria and azotemia can occur after oral and topical exposures to low-molecular-weight PEGs (200 and 300 daltons). Serum hyperosmolality and anion gap metabolic acidosis are reported.

### Neurotoxicity

There are reports of neurologic complications, such as paraplegia and transient bladder atony, following intrathecal steroidal injections containing 3% PEG as a vehicle.

### Fluid, Electrolyte, and Acid–Base Disturbances

Hyperosmolality was reported in three patients with burn surface areas ranging from 20% to 56% following repeated applications of a topical antibiotic dressing containing a mixture of PEGs.

Metabolism of the lower-molecular-weight PEGs by alcohol dehydrogenase to hydroxyacid and diacid metabolites likely explains the metabolic acidosis that is rarely reported following intravenous or topical PEG preparations.

## PROPYLENE GLYCOL

Propylene glycol (PG), or 1,2-propanediol, is a clear, colorless, odorless, sweet viscous liquid employed in numerous pharmaceuticals, foods, and cosmetics (Table 19–9).

### Pharmacokinetics

Propylene glycol is rapidly absorbed from the gastrointestinal (GI) tract following oral administration and has a volume of distribution of approximately 0.6 L/kg. Percutaneous absorption occurs following application to damaged skin. Most absorbed PG is hepatically metabolized sequentially by alcohol dehydrogenase and aldehyde dehydrogenase to lactic acid. The terminal half-life of PG is reported to be between 1.4 and 5.6 hours in adults, and as long as 16.9 hours in neonates.

### Cardiovascular Toxicity

Intravenous preparations containing 40% PG (eg, phenytoin) are associated with hypotension, bradycardia, widening of the QRS duration, increased amplitude of T waves with occasional inversions, and transient ST elevations.

**TABLE 19–9 Propylene Glycol Concentrations of Common Medications**

| *Medication (concentration)* | *Percent* | *Propylene Glycol Dose (g/dose volume)* |
|---|---|---|
| Diazepam injection (5 mg/mL) | 40 | 0.8 g/2 mL |
| Digoxin injection (250 mcg/mL) | 40 | 0.8 g/2 mL |
| Etomidate (2mg/mL) | 35 | 7 g/20 mL |
| Lorazepam injection (2 mg/mL, 4 mg/mL) | 80 | 0.8 g/mL |
| Multivitamin injection | 30 | 3 g/10 mL |
| Nitroglycerin injection (5 mg/mL) | 30 | 3 g/10 mL |
| Pentobarbital sodium injection (50 mg/mL) | 40 | 0.8 g/2 mL |
| Phenobarbital sodium injection (65 mg/mL, 130 mg/mL) | 67.8 | 0.7 g/mL |
| Phenytoin injection (50 mg/mL) | 40 | 0.8 g/2 mL |
| Trimethoprim-sulfamethoxazole injection (16–80 mg/mL) | 40 | 2 g/5 mL |

### Neurotoxicity

Smaller infants have a decreased ability to clear PG when compared to older children and adults. An increased frequency of seizures was reported in low-birth-weight infants who received 3 g of PG daily in a parenteral multivitamin preparation. Propylene glycol possesses inebriating properties similar to ethanol. Central nervous system depression was reported following an intentional ingestion of a PG-containing product.

### Ototoxicity

The effects of PG in the human middle ear have not been studied, but toxicity in animals occurs. Nearly all medications developed for application to the external ear canal are contraindicated in patients with perforated tympanic membranes.

### Fluid, Electrolyte, and Acid–Base Disturbances

Patients receiving continuous or large quantities of medications containing PG can develop high PG concentrations, particularly those with renal or hepatic insufficiency. Propylene glycol-induced electrolyte and metabolic disturbances are manifested by hyperosmolality and an elevated osmol gap attributed to the osmotically active properties of PG. In most cases, both an anion gap metabolic acidosis and an elevated lactate concentration are present, which result from PG metabolism.

Hemodialysis is effective in removing PG and correcting acidemia. The administration of fomepizole is reasonable with elevated PG concentrations to prevent further metabolism to lactic acid.

### Nephrotoxicity

Human proximal tubular cells exposed in vitro to PG exhibit significant cellular injury. Chronic administration of PG contributes to proximal tubular cell damage and subsequent decreased kidney function. Patients with chronic kidney disease are at greater risk for accumulating PG because up to 45% of PG is eliminated unchanged by the kidneys.

## SORBITOL

Sorbitol (D-glucitol) is widely used in the pharmaceutical industry as a sweetener, moistening agent, and a diluent (Table 19–10). Sorbitol occurs naturally in the ripe berries of many fruits, trees, and plants. It is particularly useful in chewable tablets because of its pleasant taste.

### Pharmacokinetics

Unlike sucrose, sorbitol is not readily fermented by oral microorganisms and is poorly absorbed from the GI tract. Any absorbed sorbitol is metabolized in the liver to fructose and glucose. Sorbitol has a caloric value of 4 kcal/g and is better tolerated by diabetics than sucrose; however, some of it is metabolized to glucose. Individuals with hereditary fructose intolerance (HFI) receiving sorbitol-containing agents are at risk of toxicity.

### Gastrointestinal Toxicity

In large dosages, sorbitol can cause abdominal cramping, bloating, flatulence, vomiting, and diarrhea. Sorbitol exerts

**TABLE 19–10 Common Medications Containing Sorbitol**

| Medication (concentration) | Percent | Sorbitol Dose (g/dose volume) |
|---|---|---|
| Amantadine syrup (10 mg/mL) | 64 | 6.4 g/10 mL |
| Calcium carbonate suspension (250 mg/mL) | 28 | 1.4 g/5 mL |
| Carbamazepine syrup (20 mg/mL) | 17 | 0.85 g/5 mL |
| Cimetidine syrup (60 mg/mL) | 46 | 2.3 g/5 mL |
| Digoxin elixir (50 μg/mL) | 21 | 1 g/5 mL |
| Ferrous sulfate infant drops (15 mg/mL) | 31 | 0.3 g/mL |
| Furosemide solution (8 mg/mL) | 35 | 1.75 g/5 mL |
| Methadone HCl solution (1 mg/mL, 2 mg/mL) | 14 | 0.7 g/5 mL |
| Potassium chloride solution (1.33 mEq/mL) | 17.5 | 2.6 g/15 mL |
| Pseudoephedrine liquid (3 mg/mL, 6 mg/mL) | 35 | 1.75 g/5 mL |

its cathartic effects by its osmotic properties, resulting in fluid shifts within the GI tract. Ingestion of large quantities of sorbitol (> 20 g/day in adults) is not recommended (Antidotes in Brief: A2).

## THIMEROSAL

Thimerosal (Merthiolate, Mercurothiolate), or sodium ethylmercurythiosalicylate, is an organic mercury compound that is approximately 49% elemental mercury (Hg) by weight. Thimerosal has been widely used as a preservative since the 1930s in contact lens solutions, biologics, and vaccines, particularly those in multidose containers (Table 19–11). High-dose thimerosal results in neurotoxicity and nephrotoxicity. Although concerns exist regarding infant exposure to low-dose thimerosal through vaccinations and its effects on neurodevelopment, including possible links to causes of autism, these concerns are unfounded (Chap. 68). Regardless, thimerosal was removed from most US-licensed immune globulin product single-dose vaccines. Multidose vials requiring thimerosal preservative remain important for immunization programs in developing countries. When a thimerosal-containing vaccine is the only alternative, the benefits of vaccination far exceed any theoretical risk of mercury toxicity.

**TABLE 19–11 Thimerosal Concentration of Common Medications**

| Medication | Percent | Dose (mg) |
|---|---|---|
| **Injectable** | | |
| Antivenom (crotaline polyvalent immune) Fab | 0.005 | 0.03 (per vial) |
| Antivenom (*Latrodectus mactans*) | 0.01 | 0.25 (per vial) |
| Antivenom (*Micrurus fulvius*) | 0.005 | 0.5 (per vial) |
| Diphtheria and tetanus toxoids[a] | Trace | <0.3 μg |
| Influenza virus vaccine[b] (various) | 0.01 | 0.025 |
| Meningococcal vaccine-A/C/Y/W-135[b] | 0.01 | 0.025 |
| **Topical** | | |
| Flurbiprofen ophthalmic solution | 0.005 | — |
| Neosporin (triple antibiotic) ophthalmic solution | 0.001 | — |
| Thimerosal tincture | 0.1 | — |

[a]Trace defined by the US Food and Drug Administration as < 1 μg mercury each dose.
[b]Multidose vials only.

### Pharmacokinetics

Limited pharmacokinetic data exist for thimerosal and ethylmercury. Once absorbed, thimerosal breaks down to form ethylmercury and thiosalicylate. Some ethylmercury further decomposes into inorganic mercury in the blood, and the remainder distributes into kidney and, to a lesser extent, brain tissue. Because of its longer organic chain, ethylmercury is less stable and decomposes more rapidly than methylmercury, leaving less ethylmercury available to enter the kidney and brain tissue. Ethylmercury crosses the blood–brain barrier by passive diffusion. Once intracellular, ethylmercury decomposes into inorganic mercury and bioaccumulates. The half-life of thimerosal is estimated to be about 18 days. Thimerosal is eliminated in the feces as inorganic mercury (Chap. 68).

### Mercury or Thimerosal Toxicity

***Oral Administration.*** A case report described a 44-year-old man who ingested 5 g (83 mg/kg) of thimerosal in a suicide attempt; within 15 minutes, he began vomiting spontaneously. Gastroscopy revealed a hemorrhagic gastritis. Acute kidney injury was noted on the day of admission and persisted for 40 days. The patient also developed an autonomic and ascending peripheral polyneuropathy that persisted for 13 days. Oral absorption of thimerosal resulted in the fatal poisoning of an 18-month-old girl from the otic instillation of a solution containing 0.1% thimerosal and 0.14% sodium borate. Tympanostomy tubes placed 1 year earlier allowed the irrigation solution to flow through the auditory tube into the nasopharynx and subsequently to be swallowed and absorbed through the oral mucosa and gastrointestinal tract.

***Intramuscular Administration.*** Urine mercury concentrations were elevated in 19 of 26 patients with hypogammaglobinemia, who received weekly intramuscular immunoglobulin G (IgG) replacement therapy preserved with 0.01% thimerosal. Six cases of severe mercury poisoning resulting in four deaths were reported following the intramuscular administration of chloramphenicol preserved with thimerosal. A manufacturing error produced vials containing 510 mg of thimerosal (250 mg Hg) instead of 0.51 mg per vial.

***Topical Administration.*** Thirteen infants were exposed to applications of a 0.1% thimerosal tincture for the treatment of exomphalos. Analysis showed elevated mercury concentrations in organs of some infants who unexpectedly died, suggesting percutaneous absorption from these repeated topical applications.

***Ophthalmic Administration.*** Nine patients undergoing keratoplasty were exposed to a contact lens stored in a solution containing 0.002% thimerosal. After 4 hours, the lens was removed and mercury concentrations of the aqueous humor and excised corneal tissues were determined. Mercury concentrations were elevated in both aqueous humor and corneal tissues as compared with eyes that had not been fitted with contact lenses. No adverse effects were noted. A possible drug interaction between orally administered tetracyclines and thimerosal resulted in varying degrees of eye irritation in contact lens wearers using thimerosal-containing contact lens solutions who started treatment with tetracycline.

# 20 ANTIDIABETICS AND HYPOGLYCEMICS/ANTIGLYCEMICS

## HISTORY AND EPIDEMIOLOGY

Insulin first became available for use in 1922 after Banting and Best successfully treated diabetic patients using pancreatic extracts. The hypoglycemic activity of a sulfonamide derivative used for typhoid fever was noted during World War II. The sulfonylureas in use today are chemical modifications of that original sulfonamide compound. The biguanides metformin and phenformin were developed as derivatives of *Galega officinalis*, the French lilac, recognized in medieval Europe as a treatment for diabetes mellitus. Exenatide, a synthetic form of a compound found in the saliva of the Gila monster, is an incretin mimetic. Incretin is a hormone that stimulates insulin secretion in response to meals. Liraglutide, dulaglutide, and albiglutide are synthetic analogs of human incretin. Other newer xenobiotics include the gliptins, the amylin analog pramlintide, and the sodium glucose co-transporter 2 ($SGLT_2$) inhibitors.

In a study of 99,628 emergency hospitalizations for adverse drug events in adults older than 65 years, 14% were due to insulin and 11% were due to oral hypoglycemics. The majority (95%) of the hospitalizations related to insulin and oral hypoglycemics were due to hypoglycemia. Other causes of hypoglycemia are listed in Table 20–1.

## PHARMACOLOGY

Insulin is synthesized as a precursor polypeptide in the β-islet cells of the pancreas. Proteolytic processing results in the formation of proinsulin, which is cleaved, giving rise to C-peptide and insulin itself. Glucose concentration plays a major role in the regulation of insulin release (Fig. 20–1). After release, insulin binds to specific receptors on cell surfaces in insulin-sensitive tissues, particularly the hepatic, muscle, and adipose cells. The action of insulin on these cells involves various phosphorylation and dephosphorylation reactions. All the sulfonylureas bind to receptors on the pancreatic β-cell membrane, resulting in closure of $K^+$ channels. This mimics the effect of naturally elevated intracellular ATP and results in insulin release. Repaglinide and nateglinide are representatives of the meglitinide class that also bind to $K^+$ channels on pancreatic cells, resulting in increased insulin secretion.

Metformin acts by several mechanisms, the most important of which involves the inhibition of mitochondrial complex I, which subsequently leads to activation of adenosine monophosphate activated protein kinase (AMPK). Adenosine monophosphate activated protein kinase activation is postulated to mediate antihyperglycemic effects. Metformin also inhibits glycerol-3-phosphate dehydrogenase, which results in inhibition of gluconeogenesis. Alteration of intestinal microbiota by metformin impairs the uptake and utilization of glucose by the intestines. Finally, metformin increases concentrations of glucagonlike peptide-1 (GLP-1), an incretin that is released in response to an oral glucose load and induces GLP-1 receptors. Incretins enhance the release of insulin, delay gastric emptying, and reduce food intake. Glucose lowering by metformin can be summarized to occur by a combination of effects, which include inhibition of gluconeogenesis, decreased hepatic glucose output, enhanced peripheral glucose uptake, decreased fatty acid oxidation, and increased intestinal use of glucose.

Acarbose and miglitol are oligosaccharides that inhibit α-glucosidase enzymes such as glucoamylase, sucrase, and maltase in the brush border of the small intestine. As a result,

**TABLE 20–1 Xenobiotic and Non-toxicologic Causes of Hypoglycemia**

| | | | |
|---|---|---|---|
| **Artifactual** | **Medical Conditions** | **Neoplasms** | Hypoglycin (ackee) |
| Chronic myelogenous leukemia | Acquired immunodeficiency syndrome (AIDS) | Carcinomas (diverse extrapancreatic) | Indomethacin |
| Polycythemia vera | Alcoholism | Hematologic | Methylenecyclopropylglycine (litchi) |
| **Endocrine Disorders** | Anorexia nervosa | Insulinoma | Pentamidine |
| Addison disease | Autoimmune disorders | Mesenchymal | Propoxyphene |
| Glucagon deficiency | Burns | Multiple endocrine adenopathy type 1 | Quinidine |
| Graves disease | Diarrhea (childhood) | Sarcomas (retroperitoneal) | Quinine |
| Panhypopituitarism (Sheehan syndrome) | Leucine sensitivity | **Reactive Hypoglycemia** | Ritodrine |
| **Hepatic Disease** | Muscular activity (excessive) | **Xenobiotics** | Salicylates |
| Acute hepatic atrophy | Postgastric surgery (including gastric bypass) | β-Adrenergic antagonists | Streptozocin |
| Carcinoma | Pregnancy | Alloxan | Sulfonamides |
| Cirrhosis | Protein-calorie malnutrition | Antidiabetics | Vacor |
| Galactose or fructose intolerance | Rheumatoid arthritis | Cibenzoline | Valproic acid |
| Glycogen storage disease | Septicemia | Disopyramide | Venlafaxine |
| Neoplasia | Shock | Ethanol | |
| **Kidney Disease** | Systemic lupus erythematosus | Gatifloxacin | |
| Chronic hemodialysis | | | |
| Chronic kidney disease | | | |

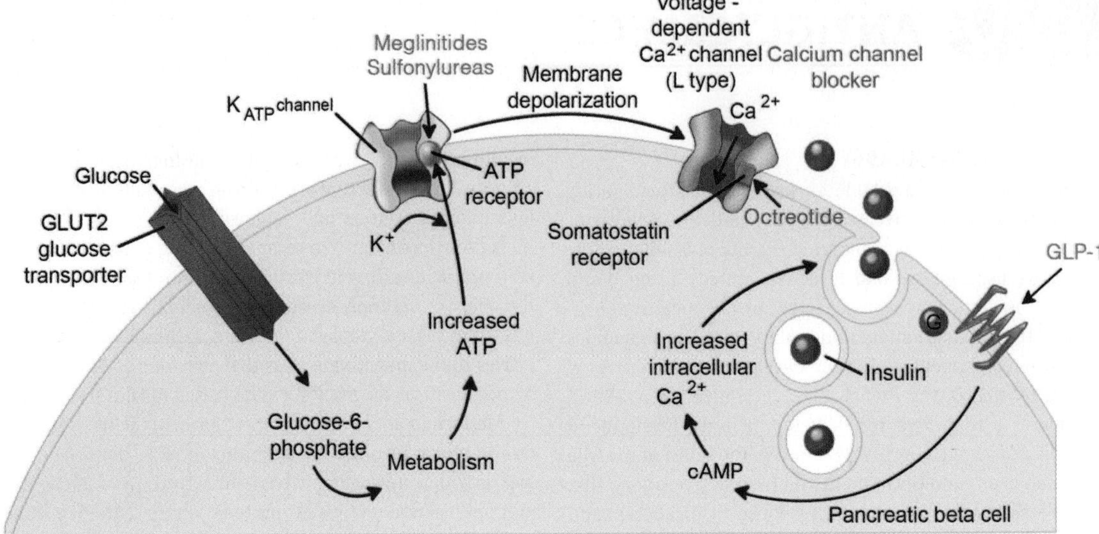


**FIGURE 20–1.** Under normal conditions, cells release insulin in response to elevation of intracellular ATP concentrations. Sulfonylureas potentiate the effects of ATP at its "sensor" on the ligand-gated $K^+$ channels and prevent efflux of $K^+$. The subsequent rise in intracellular potential opens voltage-gated $Ca^{2+}$ channels, which increases intracellular calcium concentration through a series of phosphorylation reactions. The increase in intracellular calcium results in the release of insulin. Release of insulin is also caused by binding of sulfonylureas to postulated receptor sites on regulatory exocytosis kinase and insulin granular membranes. Octreotide inhibits calcium entry through the $Ca^{2+}$ channel, thereby inhibiting insulin release. GLP-1 acts on a G-protein coupled receptor, which results in accumulation of cAMP, and subsequent increased intracellular calcium-stimulated insulin release. GLUT = membrane-bound glucose transporter. GLP-1 = glucagonlike peptide-1; cAMP = cyclic adenosine monophosphatase.

postprandial elevations in blood glucose concentrations are blunted. The thiazolidinedione derivatives decrease insulin resistance by potentiating insulin sensitivity in the liver, adipose tissue, and skeletal muscle. Uptake of glucose into adipose tissue and skeletal muscle is enhanced, whereas hepatic glucose production is reduced.

Exenatide, liraglutide, dulaglutide, and albiglutide are structurally similar to GLP-1. Sitagliptin, saxagliptin, linagliptin, and alogliptin inhibit dipeptidyl peptidase-4 (DPP-4), the enzyme responsible for the inactivation of GLP-1. Pramlintide is an amylin analog. Amylin is produced in the pancreatic β-cell and acts in conjunction with insulin to inhibit gastric emptying, decrease postprandial glucagon secretion, and promote satiety.

The kidneys contribute significantly to glucose homeostasis. The $SGLT_2$ are located mainly in the proximal tubules and account for up to 90% of glucose absorption. The $SGLT_2$ inhibitors, such as canagliflozin, block the reabsorption of glucose, with subsequent excretion into the urine.

## PHARMACOKINETICS AND TOXICOKINETICS

Pharmacokinetic parameters of the hypoglycemics are given in Table 20–2 and Table 20–3. Because there are a finite number of insulin receptors, insulin overdoses of varying amounts probably are equivalent in terms of the degree of resultant hypoglycemia once receptor saturation occurs, but not in terms of its duration. As with insulin overdose, the sulfonylureas cause delayed onset of hypoglycemia following overdose. The reason for the potential delayed onset of effects with sulfonylureas cannot be simply explained by known kinetic principles but could be related to counterregulatory mechanisms that fail over time.

## PATHOPHYSIOLOGY OF HYPOGLYCEMIA

With variable risk, the antidiabetics all produce a nearly identical clinical condition of hypoglycemia. The etiologies of hypoglycemia are divided into three general categories: physiologic or pathophysiologic conditions (Table 20–1), direct effects of various hypoglycemics (Tables 20–2 and 20–3), and potentiation of hypoglycemics by interactions with other xenobiotics (Table 20–4). Hypoglycemia usually results in decreased insulin secretion, with production of alternate fuels, particularly ketones. Ketone production occurs as a result of fatty acid metabolism.

Central nervous system (CNS) symptoms predominate in hypoglycemia because the brain relies almost entirely on glucose as an energy source. However, during prolonged starvation, the brain can utilize ketones derived from free fatty acids. In contrast to the brain, other major organs such as the heart, liver, and skeletal muscle often function during hypoglycemia because they can use various fuel sources, particularly free fatty acids.

The autonomic nervous system regulates glucagon and insulin secretion, glycogenolysis, lipolysis, and gluconeogenesis. β-Adrenergic antagonists affect all of these mechanisms and can result in hypoglycemia. β-Adrenergic antagonist–induced hypoglycemia is a particular risk secondary to increased insulin half-life and reduced renal gluconeogenesis in the presence of renal dysfunction. In addition, the clinical presentation of hypoglycemia may be muted when

**TABLE 20–2 Characteristics of Noninsulin Antidiabetics**

| *Xenobiotic* | *Duration of Action* | *Active Hepatic Metabolite* | *Active Urinary Excretory Product* | *Likelihood of Hypoglycemia in Overdose* |
|---|---|---|---|---|
| **I. Sulfonylureas** | | | | |
| *First-generation* | | | | |
| Acetohexamide | 12–18 h | (++) | (++) | H |
| Chlorpropamide | 24–72 h | (+) | (++) | H |
| Tolazamide | 10–24 h | (++) | (++) | H |
| Tolbutamide | 6–12 h | (+) | (++) | H |
| *Second-generation* | | | | |
| Glimepiride | 24 h | (++) | (++) | H |
| Glipizide | 16–24 h | (–) | (+) | H |
| Glyburide | 18–24 h | (++) | (++) | H |
| **II. Biguanides** | | | | |
| Metformin | 12–24 h | (–) | (++) | L |
| Phenformin | 6–8 h | (–) | (++) | L |
| **III. α-Glucosidase Inhibitors** | | | | |
| Acarbose | 2 h | (–) | (+) | L |
| Miglitol | 2 h | (–) | (++) | L |
| **IV. Thiazolidinedione Derivatives** | | | | |
| Pioglitazone | 16–24 h | (++) | (++) | L |
| Rosiglitazone | 12–24 h | (–) | (–) | L |
| **V. Meglitinides** | | | | |
| Nateglinide | 4–6 h | (++) | (+) | H |
| Repaglinide | 1–3 h | (–) | (–) | H |
| **VI. GLP-1 Analogs** | | | | |
| Exenatide | 6–8 h | (–) | (–) | L |
| Liraglutide | 24 h | (–) | (–) | L |
| Dulaglutide | 1 wk | (–) | (–) | L |
| Albiglutide | 1 wk | (–) | (–) | L |
| **VII. DPP-4 Inhibitors** | | | | |
| Sitagliptin | 24 h | (–) | (++) | L |
| Saxagliptin | 24 h | (++) | (++) | L |
| Linagliptin | 24 h | (–) | (+) | L |
| Alogliptin | 24 h | (++) | (++) | L |
| **VIII. Amylin Analog** | | | | |
| Pramlintide | 3 h | (–) | (–) | L |
| **IX. $SGLT_2$ Inhibitors** | | | | |
| Canagliflozin | 24 h | (–) | (–) | L |
| Dapagliflozin | 24 h | (–) | (–) | L |
| Empagliflozin | 24 h | (–) | (++) | L |

(++) = Substantial; (+) = Limited; (–) = None/Negligible; H = High Likelihood; L = Low Likelihood.
GLP-1 analogs = glucagonlike peptide-1 analogs; $SGLT_2$ = sodium-glucose cotransporter; DPP-4 inhibitor = dipeptidyl peptidase-4 inhibitor.

β-adrenergic antagonists are present because the expected autonomic responses of tachycardia, diaphoresis, and anxiety may not occur. As glucose concentrations fall, normal sensing mechanisms result in decreased insulin secretion and increased glucagon and epinephrine secretion. These counterregulatory defenses against hypoglycemia are defective in most people with type 1 diabetes mellitus and in many with type 2 diabetes mellitus. This autonomic failure results in hypoglycemic unawareness.

## CLINICAL MANIFESTATIONS

Hypoglycemia and its secondary effects on the CNS (neuroglycopenia) are the most common adverse effects related to insulin and the sulfonylureas. It is essential to remember that hypoglycemia is primarily a clinical, not a numerical, disorder. Clinical hypoglycemia is the failure to maintain a CSF glucose concentration that prevents signs or symptoms of glucose deficiency. The clinical presentations of patients with hypoglycemia are extremely variable, and hypoglycemia must

**TABLE 20–3 Characteristics of Various Forms of Insulin**

| Insulin | *Onset of Action (hours)* | *Duration of Action (hours)* | *Peak Glycemic Response (hours)* |
|---|---|---|---|
| **Rapid Acting** | | | |
| Aspart | 0.25 | 3–5 | 0.75–1.5 |
| Glulisine | 0.5 | < 5 | 1.5–2 |
| Lispro | 0.25–0.5 | < 5 | 0.5–2.5 |
| **Short Acting** | | | |
| Regular | 0.5–1 | 5–8 | 2.5–5 |
| **Intermediate Acting** | | | |
| Lente | 1–3 | 18–24 | 6–14 |
| NPH | 1–2 | 18–24 | 6–14 |
| **Long Acting** | | | |
| Detemir | 1.5 | 24 | No true peak |
| Glargine | 1.1 | 24 | No true peak |
| Ultralente | 4–6 | 20–36 | 8–20 |

be excluded as an etiology of any neuropsychiatric abnormality, whether persistent or transient, focal or generalized. The cerebral cortex usually is most severely affected. These findings are categorized below:

- Delirium with subdued, confused, or agitated behavior.
- Coma with multifocal brainstem abnormalities, including decerebrate spasms and respiratory abnormalities, with preservation of the oculocephalic (doll's eyes), oculovestibular (cold-caloric), and pupillary responses.
- Focal neurologic deficits simulating a cerebrovascular accident (CVA) with or without the presence of coma.
- Seizure activity (single, multiple, or status epilepticus).

These neuropsychiatric symptoms are usually reversible if the hypoglycemia is corrected promptly. The morbidity

**TABLE 20–4 Xenobiotics Known to React with Hypoglycemics Resulting in Hypoglycemia**

| |
|---|
| β-Adrenergic antagonists |
| Angiotensin-converting enzyme (ACE) inhibitors |
| Allopurinol |
| Anabolic steroids |
| Chloramphenicol |
| Clofibrate |
| Disopyramide |
| Ethanol |
| Fluoroquinolones |
| Haloperidol |
| Methotrexate |
| Monoamine oxidase inhibitors |
| Pentamidine |
| Phenylbutazone |
| Probenecid |
| Quinine |
| Salicylates |
| Sulfonamide |
| Trimethoprim-sulfamethoxazole |
| Warfarin |

resulting from undiagnosed hypoglycemia is related partly to the etiology and partly to the duration and severity of the hypoglycemia. In one tertiary care medical center, 1.2% of all admitted patients had numerical hypoglycemia; defined as a glucose concentration < 50 mg/dL (< 2.8 mmol/L). Their overall mortality was 27%.

The glycemic threshold is the glucose concentration below which clinical manifestations develop, a threshold that is host variable. In one study, the mean glycemic threshold for hypoglycemic symptoms was 78 mg/dL (4.3 mmol/L) in patients with poorly controlled type 1 diabetes compared to 53 mg/dL (2.9 mmol/L) in those without the disease.

Sinus tachycardia, atrial fibrillation, and ventricular premature contractions are the most common dysrhythmias associated with hypoglycemia. An outpouring of catecholamines in a response to hypoglycemia, transient electrolyte abnormalities, and underlying heart disease appear to be the most likely etiologies. Increased release of catecholamines during hypoglycemia increases myocardial oxygen demand and decreases supply by causing coronary vasoconstriction. Hypoglycemia leads to catecholamine release, which also causes cardiac repolarization abnormalities that contribute to atrial and ventricular dysrhythmias. The same mechanism is responsible for tremor, diaphoresis, and anxiety. Hypothermia is common and usually mild; 90°F–95°F (32°C–35°C).

Besides decreasing glucose concentrations, the hypoglycemics can produce a number of adverse effects, both in overdose and in therapeutic doses. Older sulfonylureas, predominantly chlorpropamide, cause a syndrome of inappropriate antidiuretic hormone secretion and disulfiram-ethanol reactions. These adverse effects are exceedingly uncommon with the newer second-generation sulfonylureas.

Hypoglycemia is at times delayed until 18 hours after lente insulin overdose, persists for up to 53 hours after subcutaneous insulin glargine overdose, and is reported to persist up to 6 days after ultralente insulin overdose. Similarly, in patients with sulfonylurea overdoses, the time from ingestion to the onset of hypoglycemia is variable. The longest delay is 21 hours after ingestion of glyburide and 48 hours after ingestion of chlorpropamide. In a retrospective poison control center review of 93 cases of sulfonylurea exposures in children, 25 patients (27%) developed hypoglycemia, with a time of onset ranging from 0.5 to 16 hours and a mean of 4.3 hours. In a prospective poison control center study of sulfonylurea exposures in children, 56 of 185 (30%) patients developed hypoglycemia, with a time of onset ranging from 1 to 21 hours and a mean of 5.3 hours. Single-tablet ingestions of chlorpropamide 250 mg, glipizide 5 mg, and glyburide 2.5 mg result in hypoglycemia in young children. Hypoglycemia did not occur until 45 hours after ingestion of a 10-mg extended-release glipizide tablet in a 6-year-old child. Hypoglycemia is also reported in a few cases of metformin overdose.

Despite limited overdose data, acarbose and miglitol are not likely to cause hypoglycemia based on their mechanism of action of inhibiting α-glucosidase. The most common adverse effects associated with therapeutic use of these xenobiotics are gastrointestinal, including nausea, bloating, abdominal pain, flatulence, and diarrhea.

Hypoglycemia would not be expected after thiazolidinedione overdose, despite limited overdose data. The most serious adverse effect of troglitazone is the development of liver toxicity with therapeutic doses, which in some cases was severe enough to require liver transplantation. Therapeutic use of pioglitazone and rosiglitazone leads to fluid retention in some patients with congestive heart failure. A meta-analysis concluded that rosiglitazone therapy is associated with an increased risk of myocardial infarction and death from cardiovascular causes.

Hypoglycemia should be anticipated after repaglinide and nateglinide overdose and is reported in one case to be delayed 14 hours postingestion. Hypoglycemia is uncommonly reported after ingest of GLP-1 analogs and gliptins. "Severe hypoglycemia" was reported in a phase III clinical trial after inadvertent administration of 10 times the normal dose of exenatide. Nausea, vomiting, and diarrhea are other common adverse reactions. There are limited overdose data with regard to amylin analogs. Pramlintide is used therapeutically in conjunction with insulin, and hypoglycemia in this setting is more likely than with insulin use alone.

Therapeutic use of $SGLT_2$ inhibitors results in euglycemic ketoacidosis. This is one of the newest classes of drugs used for diabetes, with limited overdose data. Based on their pharmacology, inhibition of renal glucose reabsorption would not be expected to occur to a degree that would result in hypoglycemia.

## DIAGNOSTIC TESTING

Suspicion of hypoglycemia, particularly neuroglycopenia, is important in any patient with an abnormal neurologic examination. The most frequent reasons for failure to diagnose hypoglycemia and mismanaging patients are the erroneous conclusions that the patient is not hypoglycemic but rather is psychotic, epileptic, experiencing a CVA, or intoxicated because of an "odor of alcohol" on the breath (Chap. 49). Compounding the problem of misdiagnosis is the erroneous assumption that a single bolus of 0.5 to 1 g/kg of hypertonic dextrose will always be sufficient.

Glucose reagent strip testing can be performed at the bedside. The sensitivity of these tests for detecting hypoglycemia is excellent, but these tests are not perfect. Several interfering substances may cause false elevations of bedside glucose reagent strip concentrations, including maltodextrin, acetaminophen, bilirubin, triglyceride, and uric acid. Bedside glucose testing is discussed in more detail in Antidotes in Brief: A8. Analysis of blood urea nitrogen, creatinine, and eGFR (estimated glomerular filtration rate) indicates the presence of renal dysfunction as a causative factor of hypoglycemia. This commonly occurs in patients with diabetes taking insulin, who often develop renal dysfunction after they have had the disease for several years, with insulin half-life increasing as eGFR decreases.

In the majority of overdose cases, laboratory testing for specific antidiabetics is not helpful. Exceptions might include malicious, surreptitious, or unintentional overdoses. Metformin concentrations vary and do not necessarily correlate with the clinical condition.

## EVALUATION OF MALICIOUS, SURREPTITIOUS, OR UNINTENTIONAL INSULIN OVERDOSE

The physical examination will often provide helpful clues to the evaluation of a suspected malicious, surreptitious, or unintentional insulin overdose. A meticulous search will reveal a site that is erythematous, hemorrhagic, atypically boggy in nature, or even painful if the subcutaneous or intramuscular injection of insulin was particularly large. A simple unexplained needle puncture mark in the appropriate clinical setting suggests insulin injection. Table 20–5 provides a framework for analyzing blood concentrations in the setting of suspected overdose.

## MANAGEMENT

Treatment centers on the correction of hypoglycemia and the anticipation that hypoglycemia may recur. Symptomatic patients with hypoglycemia require immediate treatment with 0.5 to 1 g/kg hypertonic intravenous dextrose in the form of $D_{50}W$ in adults, $D_{25}W$ in children, and $D_{10}W$ in neonates. Occasionally, patients require a larger dose to achieve an initial response (Antidotes in Brief: A8). We recommend not to use glucagon as an antihypoglycemic except in the

**TABLE 20–5 Laboratory Assessment of Fasting Hypoglycemia**

| *Clinical State* | *Insulin[a] (Serum) (μU/mL)* | *C-Peptide (Serum) (nmol/L)* | *Proinsulin Serum (pmol/L)* | *Antiinsulin Antibodies[b]* |
|---|---|---|---|---|
| Normal | < 6 | < 0.2 | < 5 | – |
| Exogenous insulin | Very high | Low (suppressed) | Absent | Present[c] |
| Insulinoma | High | High | Present | Absent |
| Sulfonylurea ingestion[d] | High | High | Present | Absent |
| Autoimmune | Very high (artifact) | Low (or) high (artifact) | Present | Present |
| Decreased glucose production | Low | Low | Present | Absent |
| Neoplasia (non–β-cell) | Low | Low | Present | Absent |

[a]Insulin concentrations are determined during fasting-induced hypoglycemia at low concentrations, preferably < 60 mg/dL (3.3 mmol/L) of plasma glucose. [b]The antiinsulin antibodies produced spontaneously differ from those of treated (exposed to exogenous insulin) and those of untreated insulin-dependent diabetic patients. [c]The presence of antiinsulin antibodies occurs less frequently in those exposed only to human insulin. [d]Sulfonylurea ingestion is diagnosed by detection of the parent compound metabolites in serum or urine.

uncommon situation in which intravenous access cannot be obtained. Glucagon has a delay to onset of action and is ineffective in patients with depleted glycogen stores, as in the malnourished elderly patients with cancer or those with alcoholism.

A common occurrence involves symptomatic hypoglycemic patients who receive intravenous dextrose in the prehospital setting and subsequently refuse transport to the hospital. Although most patients do well, some develop recurrent hypoglycemia, posthypoglycemic encephalopathy, and even death. We therefore recommend that all hypoglycemic patients should be transported to the emergency department (ED).

Emesis, lavage, and catharsis are of limited benefit in the management of patients who overdose on hypoglycemics. Single-dose activated charcoal should be beneficial in the management of these overdoses.

In patients who overdose on insulin, case reports describe the use of surgical excision of the injection site. However, this technique has not been studied in a systematic fashion and we recommend against excision. Needle aspiration of a depot site is less invasive and can be performed, but intravenous dextrose should be sufficient in most cases.

## MAINTAINING EUGLYCEMIA AFTER INITIAL CONTROL

After the patient is awake and alert, further therapy depends on the pharmacokinetics of the xenobiotic involved and pancreatic islet cell function. One problem associated with dextrose administration occurs in individuals who can produce insulin via glucose-stimulated insulin release (nondiabetic patients and those with type 2 diabetes mellitus), placing them at substantial risk for recurrent hypoglycemia. This complication occurs with insulin overdose but is particularly problematic with overdoses of sulfonylurea or meglitinide because these hypoglycemics stimulate insulin release. Treatment with hypertonic dextrose solutions can be expected to result in dramatic yet only transient increases in glucose concentrations, with a subsequent fall in plasma glucose concentration, possibly back to hypoglycemic concentrations.

For patients with diabetes who unintentionally inject an excessive amount of insulin and are not neuroglycopenic, feeding (carbohydrates and proteins) should be initiated and intravenous access maintained while avoiding routine dextrose infusion. In the event of recurrent symptomatic hypoglycemia, a hypertonic intravenous dextrose bolus followed by an infusion of $D_5W$ is recommended. Overdose in the setting of suicidal or homicidal intent likely involves significant quantities of insulin. Nondiabetic patients are particularly prone to significant hypoglycemia because they lack insulin resistance. Feeding is recommended with a target of maintaining glucose concentrations in the 100 to 150 mg/dL (5.6–8.3 mmol/L) range using a hypertonic dextrose infusion ($D_{10}W$ or greater) as needed. Central venous lines should be used when a $D_{20}W$ or greater infusion is instituted, because hypertonic dextrose solutions are venous irritants and sclerosing to the vasculature. Phosphate concentrations should be monitored because dextrose loading may lead to hypophosphatemia. Potassium concentrations should be monitored because dextrose administration leads to hypokalemia in nondiabetic patients and rarely hyperkalemia in patients with impaired insulin secretion.

The therapeutic approach differs for patients who overdose on sulfonylureas or meglitinides. After initial control of hypoglycemia with hypertonic dextrose, feeding is again recommended. Intravenous access is necessary, but routine continuous dextrose infusion should be avoided. As with insulin overdose, frequent monitoring of glucose concentrations and mental status is critical. We recommend use of octreotide for recurrent hypoglycemia in this setting because of the significant risk of glucose-stimulated insulin release. Our suggested adult octreotide dose is 50 μg subcutaneously every 6 hours (Antidotes in Brief: A9). The patient should be monitored for 12 to 24 hours after the last dose of octreotide. This observation will ensure that recurrence of hypoglycemia does not occur.

## ADMITTING PATIENTS TO THE HOSPITAL

The decision to admit a patient is complex, but several guidelines can be followed. Admission is usually required for hypoglycemia related to sulfonylureas, ethanol, starvation, hepatic failure, renal dysfunction, and for hypoglycemia of unknown etiology. In most cases, if a diabetic patient on therapeutic doses of insulin develops hypoglycemia after a missed meal, the patient can be discharged after a 4- to 6-hour observation period during which the individual eats a meal and remains asymptomatic with no evidence of hypoglycemia. Patients receiving therapeutic doses of insulin usually require inpatient evaluation of recurrent and unexplained hypoglycemic episodes. Patients with hypoglycemia after unintentional overdose with long-acting insulin should generally be admitted. Hospitalization is usually recommended after unintentional overdose with ultrashort-acting, short-acting, or intermediate-acting insulin if hypoglycemia is persistent or recurrent during a 4- to 6-hour observation period in the ED.

Admission is also indicated for any patient, regardless of serum glucose concentration or presence or absence of symptoms, who intentionally overdoses on a sulfonylurea or any form of injected insulin, because delayed, profound, and protracted hypoglycemia is expected. Hypoglycemia related to sulfonylurea use in any setting including a missed meal or a viral illness typically necessitates hospitalization.

A 6-hour observation period is recommended after metformin overdose. Further observation or hospital admission is usually not required for patients who remain asymptomatic during this period with no evidence of metabolic acidosis, elevated lactate concentration, renal dysfunction, emesis, or hypoglycemia.

Patients who overdose on α-glucosidase inhibitors are not expected to have delayed or serious systemic toxicity, and routine medical admission is unnecessary. There are limited data regarding the risk of hypoglycemia and other adverse events after thiazolidinedione ingestion. Based on the mechanism of action and existing clinical experience, hypoglycemia is possible but uncommon after unintentional thiazolidinedione overdose. Delayed onset of hypoglycemia or other serious clinical manifestations is unlikely. A 4- to 6-hour observation period after thiazolidinedione overdose is recommended. Meglitinides are expected to behave pharmacologically like sulfonylureas. For this reason alone, hospital admission after meglitinide overdose is generally advisable, even when the patient is asymptomatic. A 4- to 6-hour observation period is recommended after overdose of GLP-1 analogs, gliptins, amylin analogs, and $SGLT_2$ inhibitors. Delayed onset of clinical manifestations is unlikely.

Children who unintentionally ingest one or more sulfonylurea tablets should generally be hospitalized for 24 hours. Although this recommendation may be controversial and some authors suggest shorter observation periods or even home monitoring in some cases, we believe that delayed hypoglycemic effects of sulfonylurea ingestion in children are well documented and convincing enough to support admission in most cases. Asymptomatic children with single-tablet exposures to sulfonylureas are best managed without prophylactic intravenous dextrose, which could contribute to delayed onset of hypoglycemia.

## METABOLIC ACIDOSIS WITH AN ELEVATED LACTATE CONCENTRATION

Throughout this chapter, the term *metabolic acidosis with an elevated lactate concentration* (MALA) is used rather than *metformin-associated lactic acidosis* or *metformin-induced metabolic acidosis.* The biochemical and pathophysiologic processes involving lactate are complex, but a few points are worth summarizing. An elevated lactate concentration occurs in various diseases and can be present in the absence of acidosis. The production of lactic acid does not result in a net increase in hydrogen ion concentration unless there is associated impairment of oxidative metabolism. Impaired oxidative metabolism leads to an increase in hydrogen ion production through the hydrolysis of ATP. Figure 20–2 summarizes the mechanism of action of metformin.

Metabolic acidosis with an elevated lactate concentration related to metformin usually occurs in the presence of an underlying condition, particularly renal dysfunction. In this setting, increased tissue burden of metformin, which is renally eliminated, occurs. Metabolic acidosis with an elevated lactate concentration also occurs after acute metformin overdose even in patients without diabetes or previous metformin use.

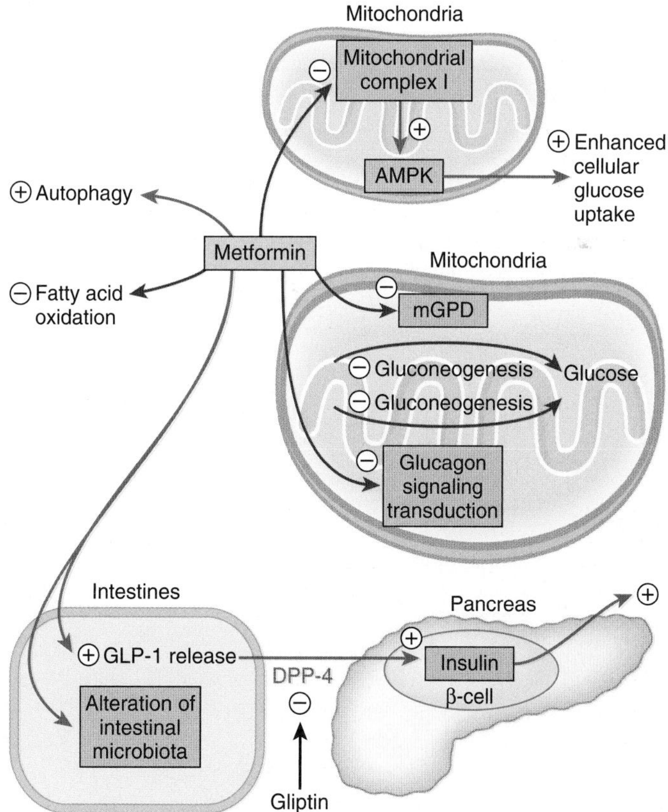


**FIGURE 20–2.** Metformin inhibits mitochondrial complex I, which activates adenosine monophosphate activated protein kinase (AMPK), resulting in enhanced cellular glucose uptake. Metformin also causes inhibition of mitochondrial glycerol-3-phosphate dehydrogenase (mGPD), leading to inhibition of gluconeogenesis. Inhibition of glucagon signaling transduction also leads to inhibition of gluconeogenesis. Metformin enhances glucagonlike peptide-1 (GLP-1) release from the intestines and stimulates GLP-1 receptors on pancreatic β islet cells, leading to enhanced insulin release. Gliptins enhance the effect of GLP-1 by inhibition of its inactivation by dipeptidyl peptidase-4. Other mechanisms of metformin include induction of autophagy, inhibition of fatty acid oxidation, and favorable alteration of intestinal microbiota.

It is difficult to predict outcome after metformin overdose. A retrospective literature review found no deaths in cases with a nadir serum pH greater than 6.9, a peak serum lactate concentration less than 25 mmol/L, or a peak serum metformin concentration less than 50 μg/mL. However, a retrospective review of intensive care unit patients with MALA found no association between metformin concentrations in survivors and nonsurvivors.

MALA is, however, a potentially lethal condition. Recognition and awareness of this disorder are important. Symptoms are nonspecific and include abdominal pain, nausea, vomiting, malaise, myalgia, and dizziness. More severe clinical manifestations include confusion, blindness, mental status depression, hypothermia, respiratory insufficiency, and hypotension. Aggressive airway management and vasopressor therapy should be given as clinically indicated. Indications for use of intravenous sodium bicarbonate in critically ill patients with metabolic acidosis with an elevated lactate concentration of various etiologies are poorly defined and controversial. Rather than using an arterial pH cutoff, we recommend using sodium bicarbonate given evidence of impaired buffering capacity based on a serum bicarbonate threshold concentration of less than 5 mEq/L.

Metformin would be expected to be dialyzable based on its small size and limited protein binding. However, it has a large volume of distribution. The Extracorporeal Treatments in Poisoning (EXTRIP) workgroup concluded that metformin is moderately dialyzable, and extracorporeal treatment is recommended if either the blood lactate concentration is greater than 20 mmol/L or the pH is less than or equal to 7.00, or standard therapies, including sodium bicarbonate, are not effective. Even if metformin removal is inadequate, clinical improvement may occur due to correction of acid–base status.

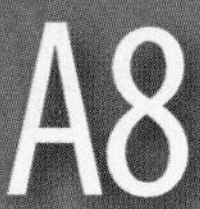

# A8 DEXTROSE (D-GLUCOSE)

## INTRODUCTION

Hypoglycemia is a common cause of altered mental status. Although classically associated with tachycardia, tremor, and diaphoresis, the predictive value of these manifestations is too low to be relied on. As a result, all patients with altered consciousness require either rapid point-of-care glucose testing or empiric treatment for presumed hypoglycemia. When rapidly diagnosed and treated, hypoglycemic patients typically recover without sequelae. Delayed or incomplete therapy may lead to permanent neurologic dysfunction.

## HISTORY

This chapter will use *dextrose* as the term for the antidote and *glucose* as the general term for actual molecule aldohexose.

### Chemistry and Physiology

*Sugar* is the general term used for sweet carbohydrates that are used as food. Simple sugars are called monosaccharides and include glucose (also known as dextrose, as the L-isomer is hardly found in nature), fructose (also known as fruit sugar, the sweetest of them all), and galactose. The disaccharides include maltose, lactose, and sucrose (also known as table or granulated sugar).

In humans, carbohydrates are absorbed and transported via two main systems. Sodium-dependent glucose transporters ($SGLT_1$–$SGLT_6$) are responsible for the intestinal and renal glucose absorption. Glucose uptake transporters include $GLUT_1$–$GLUT_{14}$ and HMIT ($H^+$/myoinositol transporter). Movement of glucose through GLUT and HMIT is by facilitative diffusion, which means that it is an energy-independent process.

Glucose delivered hematogenously to the liver, adipose tissue, and muscle cells is absorbed and stored as glycogen—under the influence of insulin—or used by all cells to produce adenosine triphosphate (ATP) and pyruvate via glycolysis. Hepatic glycogen can later be converted to glucose and returned to the blood when insulin concentrations are low or absent. In contrast, glycogen found in muscle and adipose cells is used internally and not released into the systemic circulation. Some glucose is converted to lactate by astrocytes in the brain and then utilized as an energy source. Finally, glucose is also directly used by intestinal cells and red blood cells.

### Pharmacokinetics

At equilibrium, 25 g of dextrose distributed in total body water in a 70-kg adult is calculated to increase the serum glucose concentration by about 60 mg/dL. However, in actuality, the value obtained is unpredictable. In one study, 25 g (50 mL) of $D_{50}W$ administered to both diabetic and nondiabetic adults resulted in a mean blood glucose elevation of 166 mg/dL (9.21 mmol/L) when measured in the opposite extremity 3 to 5 minutes after the bolus; however, the range of this elevation was between 37 and 370 mg/dL (2.05–20.5 mmol/L) above baseline. Two prehospital studies also evaluated the magnitude of glucose elevation in hypoglycemic patients after a 10 g dextrose bolus (100 mL of $D_{10}W$). Pretreatment mean serum glucose concentrations were 37 and 38 mg/dL, respectively. After the bolus, the median glucose concentrations were 91 and 98 mg/dL, respectively. Thus, the median rise in serum glucose concentration was between 54 and 60 mg/dL 3.0–3.33 mmol/L).

### Pharmacodynamics

Adenosine triphosphate provides the energy that fuels all critical cellular processes. In adult brains, the anaerobic and aerobic metabolism of glucose occurring through glycolysis and the citric acid cycle, respectively, are the primary sources of ATP. Although the adult brain can use fatty acids, amino acids, lactate, and ketones as alternate substrates for ATP synthesis, these are neither adequate nor sufficient to sustain normal cerebral function in the setting of glucose deprivation. In contrast, in fetal and neonatal brains, glucose is the only substrate for ATP production.

Although a blood or serum glucose less than 60 mg/dL (3.33 mmol/L) defines hypoglycemia, clinical hypoglycemia cannot be entirely predicted by strict numerical values. Rather, it is best defined by central nervous system dysfunction in the setting of inadequate glucose concentrations. An important study of diabetic patients demonstrated that the mean blood glucose concentration for symptomatic hypoglycemia in poorly controlled diabetic patients was 78 mg/dL (4.33 mmol/L) compared with 53 mg/dL (2.94 mmol/L) in well-controlled patients. Additionally, a report described two patients with salicylate toxicity who presented with altered mentation that resolved after treatment with $D_{50}W$, despite normal serum glucose concentrations. The etiology was attributed to salicylate-induced neuroglycopenia. The occurrence of low brain glucose concentrations despite normal serum glucose concentration is described in a rat model of salicylate toxicity. Diabetic patients with repeated episodes of hypoglycemia—usually those subjected to tight control—will have neuroglycopenia *before* the appearance of autonomic warning signs such as sweating, palpitations, and anxiety. This condition, known as hypoglycemia-associated autonomic failure, often termed "hypoglycemia unawareness," results in prolonged exposure to low serum glucose concentrations.

## ROLE IN HYPOGLYCEMIA

### Empiric Treatment Considerations

Tachycardia, diaphoresis, pallor, hypertension, tremor, hunger, and restlessness tend to predominate when the decline in blood glucose concentration is rapid. However, neuroglycopenia, even when severe, will not always trigger autonomic responses. Signs and symptoms are further blunted or absent in the setting of concurrent use of β-adrenergic antagonists. Central nervous system signs of neuroglycopenia are also nonspecific. Hypoglycemia causes a myriad of neuropsychiatric sequelae that are clinically indistinguishable from those of other toxic metabolic, infectious, and structural brain injuries. In a case series, presenting signs and symptoms of hypoglycemia included dizziness and tremulousness (8%); focal stroke syndromes (2%); movement disorders or seizures (7%); irritability, confusion, or bizarre behavior (30%); delirium, stupor, or coma (52%); and irreversible encephalopathy. Hypoglycemic hemiplegia is a well-recognized, although rare, entity, and therein lies the relevance of a serum glucose concentration in patients with focal neurologic symptoms. In children, sometimes the only sign of neuroglycopenia is lethargy or irritability. The heart is partially dependent on glucose as an energy substrate. Hypoglycemia causes myocardial stress that manifests as angina and/or dysrhythmias.

The bedside diagnosis of hypoglycemia is limited by the sensitivity and specificity of reagent strips, which range between 92% and 97%. The accuracy of these point-of-care testing methods is affected by the source of blood, whether arterial, venous, or capillary, and by the poor perfusion associated with shock and cardiac arrest. The "safe" number at which no cases of symptomatic hypoglycemia are missed by reagent strip testing is a subject of debate because of the inherent risk of error from lack of sensitivity. In one study in which hypoglycemia was defined as a blood glucose concentration less than 60 mg/dL (3.33 mmol/L), 2 of 33 hypoglycemic patients were not detected at the bedside. A cutoff of 90 mg/dL (5.0 mmol/L) would have detected 100% of numerically hypoglycemic patients. Based on these studies, it can be argued that a bedside reagent measurement of 90 mg/dL is a conservative cutoff for assurance of euglycemia in all patients.

With reagent strip testing, variations in hematocrit and the presence of isopropyl alcohol in the sample and a number of interfering substances and xenobiotics lead to potential errors. Notably, icodextrin, an absorbable ingredient in peritoneal dialysis, results in overestimation of glucose measurements because it is metabolized to maltose. In several case reports and at least 18 cases reported in a review, this resulted in excess insulin administration and subsequent hypoglycemia. Table 20–1 summarizes xenobiotics and nontoxicologic conditions that are associated with hypoglycemia.

## ROLE IN ETHANOL DISORDERS

Alcoholic ketoacidosis (AKA) is a metabolic emergency (Chap. 49). The management of AKA consists of rehydration using isotonic, dextrose-containing solutions; parenteral thiamine administration; potassium replacement; and addressing the underlying medical problem that led to AKA.

## ROLE IN SALICYLATE POISONING

Rare patients with salicylate toxicity demonstrate symptoms of neuroglycopenia despite normal serum glucose concentrations. Dextrose administration reverses these signs and symptoms of neuroglycopenia. Chapter 10 provides an in-depth discussion of salicylate toxicity and its management.

## ROLE IN CARDIOVASCULAR TOXICITY

High-dose insulin (HDI) is one of the cornerstones of management of patients with drug-induced cardiovascular toxicity. Insulin improves carbohydrate utilization by the cells and restores calcium flux. This improves cardiac contractility and allows for improved vascular tone. The administration of HDI must be supplemented with sufficient dextrose to maintain euglycemia. The use of continuous dextrose infusions with HDI is reviewed in Antidotes in Brief: A21. One common error, which is stopping insulin therapy because of hypoglycemia, can be avoided by proper glucose monitoring and administration. It is exceedingly rare for a patient on HDI therapy to require more than 0.5 to 1 g/kg/h of dextrose. An increase in glucose requirement may also indicate a resolution of the cardiotoxic effect especially with non-dihydropyridine calcium channel blockers.

## ROLE IN HYPERKALEMIA

Intravenous insulin is used to redistribute potassium inside the cell. A dose of 0.1 unit/kg of regular insulin is usually followed by 25 g of IV 50% dextrose to avoid hypoglycemia. Extra care must be taken to avoid delayed hypoglycemia in patients with kidney disease because of impaired insulin clearance.

## ADVERSE EFFECTS AND SAFETY ISSUES

The most serious complications associated with hypoglycemia are directly attributable to the failure to diagnose and treat hypoglycemia. Phlebitis and sclerosis of veins occur with concentrated solutions above 10% dextrose. Tissue necrosis is reported after soft tissue extravasation of $D_{50}W$ and after inadvertent intraarterial injection. Iatrogenic exacerbation of Wernicke encephalopathy with acute glucose or carbohydrate loading in the absence of adequate thiamine replacement was a once popular myth stemming from a single article reporting a handful of patients who had unrecognized Wernicke encephalopathy before prolonged periods of glucose administration. A single acute administration of dextrose has never been reported to cause this effect. Therefore, correction of hypoglycemia should never be delayed in order to administer thiamine (Antidotes in Brief: A27).

An important consideration is the development of rebound hypoglycemia when dextrose is used typically to treat sulfonylurea-induced hypoglycemia, although this also occurs in other patients who received concentrated dextrose solutions as a bolus (Chap. 20). As mentioned above, serial measurements of glucose and close patient monitoring should follow any dextrose boluses.

## PREGNANCY AND LACTATION

Dextrose is a pregnancy category C (IV) and A (oral), as studies do not exist regarding its safety to the fetus. Hypoglycemia is a serious concern for fetal and neonatal well-being, and the best evidence suggests that hypoglycemia in a pregnant woman should be approached in the same manner as in a nonpregnant patient. Although there are no data regarding the use of hypertonic dextrose in lactation, it is unlikely to be a concern, because even if the concentration of glucose in subsequent breast milk is significantly increased, the effect will be transient.

## DOSING AND ADMINISTRATION

Patients with asymptomatic or minimally symptomatic hypoglycemia should be treated with oral carbohydrates (juice, milk, candy, or glucose tablets). For adults, we recommend a dose of 20 g of dextrose orally, which should result in symptomatic improvement in 15 to 20 minutes. Because this improvement is transient and can result in reactive hypoglycemia, we also recommend that the initial glucose intake be followed by a more substantial meal whenever feasible. For the patient unable (coma, seizures) or unwilling (from neuroglycopenia) to receive oral glucose, the IV route must be used. In most cases, the rapid correction of hypoglycemia by the administration of 0.5 to 1.0 g/kg of concentrated IV dextrose (Table A8–1) immediately reverses the neurologic and cardiac effects caused by hypoglycemia. Similarly, the improvement in serum glucose concentration is transient, and the patient should be monitored closely for recurrence of hypoglycemia. In common practice, a dextrose infusion follows the initial dextrose bolus, with the recognition that this supplies very little caloric content and is insufficient in most cases in which glucose is being rapidly redistributed and utilized.

**TABLE A8–1 Dosing of Dextrose for Symptomatic Hypoglycemia**

| *Age* | *Concentration* | *Bolus* | *Dose in mL/kg* |
|---|---|---|---|
| Adult | $D_{50}W$ (50% = 0.5 g/mL) | 0.5–1.0 g/kg | 1–2 |
| Child | $D_{25}W$ (25% = 0.25 g/mL) | 0.5–1.0 g/kg | 2–4 |
| Infant | $D_{10}W$ (10% = 0.1 g/mL) | 0.5–1.0 g/kg | 5–10 |

Rapid increases in serum glucose are sufficient to stimulate insulin release from the pancreas and result in reactive (or rebound) hypoglycemia. Therefore, glucose concentrations must be closely followed after a bolus of concentrated dextrose solution. This effect is exaggerated in patients, particularly those with normally functioning pancreatic islet cells, who have ingested sulfonylureas, which increase the glucose-responsive release of insulin by the islet cells.

### Formulation and Acquisition

Dextrose is available in multiple formulations between 2.5% and 70% for intravenous use. Concentrations greater than 10% should be infused rapidly via a central venous catheter, except in emergencies when a large peripheral catheter or intraosseous access is acceptable.

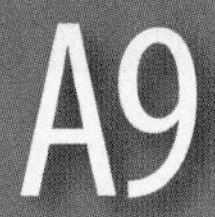

# OCTREOTIDE

## INTRODUCTION

Octreotide is a long-acting, synthetic octapeptide analog of somatostatin, a hormone that inhibits the release of numerous anterior pituitary and gastrointestinal hormones, including pancreatic insulin. It is the essential complement to dextrose (Antidotes in Brief: A8) for the treatment of refractory hypoglycemia induced by overdoses of inhibitors of insulin secretagogues such as sulfonylureas (and rarely the meglitinides), quinine (and rarely other quinolones), and other overdoses such as venlafaxine.

## HISTORY

"Somatostatin" is a collective term for several shorter fragments cleaved from preprosomatostatin and prosomatostatin. In addition to its effects on growth hormone and insulin secretion, somatostatin has far-reaching effects as a central nervous system (CNS) neurotransmitter and as a modulator of hormonal release. Unfortunately, the role for somatostatin is limited because of its short duration of action. Octreotide was synthesized as a longer-acting analog of somatostatin.

## PHARMACOLOGY

### Mechanism of Action on Insulin Secretion

The effects of somatostatin are mediated by high-affinity binding to five different membrane receptors, numbered SSTR 1–5, on target tissues. Octreotide has high binding affinity for SSTR 2 and 5 subtypes, low binding affinity for SSTR 1 and 4 subtypes, and intermediate binding affinity for SSTR 3 subtype. SSTR 2 is found in the pancreas, brain, pituitary, stomach, and kidney, whereas SSTR 5 is found in the brain, pituitary, heart, adrenal glands, placenta, small intestine, and skeletal muscle.

Somatostatin inhibits insulin secretion by a G-protein–mediated decrease in calcium entry through voltage-dependent $Ca^{2+}$ channels. Experiments with somatostatin, both in healthy human volunteers and in an isolated perfused canine pancreas model, demonstrate that somatostatin inhibits glucose-stimulated insulin release. Additionally, somatostatin inhibits the insulin response to glucagon.

### Related Xenobiotics

Lanreotide, vapreotide, and pasireotide are long-acting, United States Food and Drug Administration–approved somatostatin receptor ligands. Use of these pharmaceuticals in insulin secretagogue-induced hypoglycemia is unstudied in humans at this time and therefore cannot be recommended.

## PHARMACOKINETICS

Following IV administration, the distribution half-life of octreotide in human volunteers averages 12 minutes, and the elimination half-life ranges from 72 to 98 minutes. The volume of distribution is 18 to 30 L. Renal elimination accounts for approximately 30% of the elimination and is reduced in the elderly and in those with severe chronic kidney disease.

After subcutaneous administration, bioavailability is 100% and peak concentrations are achieved within 30 minutes. The elimination half-life is 88 to 102 minutes. Peak concentrations are approximately half of the intravenously administered concentration.

### Pharmacodynamics

The duration of action for inhibition of insulin secretion is unknown but presumed to be somewhere between 6 and 12 hours.

## ROLE OF OCTREOTIDE FOR INSULIN SUPPRESSION

Octreotide was studied in several clinical conditions, including insulinomas and hypoglycemia of infancy. In most instances, octreotide suppressed insulin concentrations and glucose concentrations rose. Occasionally, worsening or refractory *hypoglycemia* was observed when suppression of α cell glucagon release outlasted suppression of β cell insulin release, despite appropriate catecholamine and cortisol counterregulatory responses. Octreotide is currently used for the treatment of drug-induced endogenous secretion of insulin. Although the most common setting is sulfonylurea overdose, meglitinides and quinine and related antimalarials also produce hypoglycemia that clinically responds to octreotide therapy.

## ADVERSE EFFECTS

Octreotide is generally well tolerated, but experience in the toxicologic setting is limited. Adverse reactions occurring with short-term administration are usually local or gastrointestinal in nature. Stinging at the site of injection occurs in approximately 7% of patients but rarely lasts more than 15 minutes. In volunteers, no significant side effects occur with intravenous doses of 25 or 50 μg, or with subcutaneous doses of 50 or 100 μg. At higher doses, early transient nausea and later appearing, but longer lasting, diarrhea and abdominal pain frequently occur. Healthy volunteers were given IV bolus doses as high as 1000 μg and infusion doses of 30,000 μg over 20 minutes and 120,000 μg over 8 hours without serious adverse effects.

## PREGNANCY AND LACTATION

Octreotide is considered a category B drug. Maternal to fetal transfer of exogenous octreotide is documented. Studies of octreotide excretion in breast milk are not reported.

## DOSING AND ADMINISTRATION

In adults, a dose of 50 μg octreotide SC given every 6 hours is recommended. In children, a dose of 1 to 1.25 μg/kg SC every 6 hours, up to the adult dose, is recommended for initial therapy. When compromised peripheral blood flow is expected, octreotide is recommended to be administered IV in the same dose but every 4 hours instead of every 6 hours. The available pharmacokinetic, animal, and human data suggest that one or two octreotide doses are likely to be insufficient and that 24 hours to several days of therapy and/or observation will be required, depending on the type and quantity of xenobiotic ingested, coingestants, caloric intake, and individual patient factors. Regardless of the dosing strategy utilized, it is recommended that during octreotide therapy and for 12 to 24 hours following termination of octreotide therapy all patients be carefully monitored for recurrent hypoglycemia. The ability to consume sufficient calories should be ensured as well as a period of observed fasting to monitor for recurrent hypoglycemia.

## FORMULATION AND ACQUISITION

Octreotide acetate injection is available in ampules and multidose vials ranging in concentration from 50 to 1,000 μg/mL. The multidose vials contain phenol. It should not be confused with long-acting depot formulations.

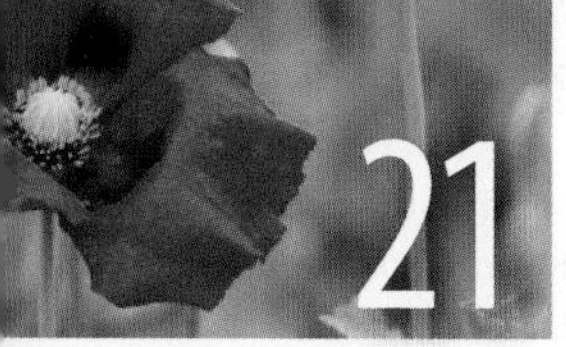

# 21 ANTIEPILEPTICS

## HISTORY AND EPIDEMIOLOGY

Epilepsy affects 6 per 1,000 population in the United States. The first truly effective antiepileptic therapy was introduced in 1857, when the administration of bromides was noted to sedate patients and significantly reduce their seizures. Phenobarbital, a sedative–hypnotic, was first used to treat seizures in 1912. The search for nonsedating antiepileptics led to the introduction of phenytoin in 1938 and benzodiazepines, carbamazepine, and valproic acid (VPA) in the 1960s. There are now a wide variety of antiepileptics with varying mechanisms of action and toxicities. This chapter reviews the toxicity and management of overdoses with antiepileptics other than the benzodiazepines and barbiturates, which are discussed in Chap. 45.

## PHARMACOLOGY

The mechanisms of action of antiepileptics include (1) sodium channel blockade; (2) calcium channel blockade; (3) blockade of excitatory amines; (4) GABA (γ-aminobutyric acid) potentiation; and (5) binding to synaptic vesicle glycoprotein 2A (SV2A). Some antiepileptics have multiple mechanisms of action. Table 21–1 and Figs. 21–1 and 21–2 summarize these effects.

## CARBAMAZEPINE

Carbamazepine is approved for the management of seizures and trigeminal neuralgia. It is a pregnancy category D medication associated with kinked ribs and cleft palate.

### Pharmacokinetics and Toxicokinetics

Carbamazepine is lipophilic, with slow and unpredictable absorption after oral administration and rapid distribution to all tissues. Peak concentrations can be delayed postingestion up to 100 hours. Carbamazepine is unique because it induces its own metabolism after 2 to 4 weeks. The elimination half-life is 25 to 65 hours at initiation of therapy and decreases to 12 to 17 hours with continued dosing. Zero-order elimination kinetics are observed following large overdoses (Tables 21–2 and 21–3).

### Clinical Manifestations

Acute carbamazepine toxicity is characterized by neurologic and cardiovascular effects. The neurologic disturbances include nystagmus, ataxia, seizures, and coma. Status epilepticus is reported. Cardiovascular effects include sinus tachycardia, hypotension, myocardial depression, and, rarely, cardiac conduction abnormalities such as QRS complex and

**TABLE 21–1 Comparison of Mechanisms of Action of Antiepileptics**

| | *$Na^+$ Channel* | *$Ca^{2+}$ Channel* | *GABA* | *GABA Transaminase* | *GABA Reuptake* | *NMDA, AMPA, Kainate* | *Synaptic Vesicle Glycoprotein 2A* | *$K^+$ Channel* | *Carbonic Anhydrase* |
|---|---|---|---|---|---|---|---|---|---|
| Carbamazepine | Blocks | | | | | | | Potentiates? | |
| Eslicarbazepine acetate | Blocks | Blocks (T-type) | | | | | | | |
| Ezogabine | | | | | | | | Potentiates | |
| Gabapentin | | Blocks (N-type) | | | | | | | |
| Lacosamide | Blocks | | | | | | | | |
| Lamotrigine | Blocks | Blocks (N-, P/Q-type) | | | | | | | |
| Levetiracetam | | Blocks (N-type) | | | | | Binding | | |
| Oxcarbazepine | Blocks | | | | | | | | |
| Perampanel | | | | | | Blocks (AMPA) | | | |
| Phenytoin/fosphenytoin | Blocks | | | | | | | | |
| Pregabalin | | Blocks (N-type) | | | | | | | |
| Rufinamide | Blocks | | | | | | | | |
| Stiripentol | | | Potentiates | | | | | | |
| Tiagabine | | | | | Blocks | | | | |
| Topiramate | Blocks | Blocks (L-type) | Potentiates | | | Blocks (kainate) | | | Blocks |
| Valproic acid | Blocks | | | Blocks | | Blocks (NMDA) | | | |
| Vigabatrin | | | | Blocks | | | | | |
| Zonisamide | Blocks | Blocks (T-type) | | | | | | | Blocks |

GABA = γ-aminobutyric acid; NMDA = *N*-methyl-D-aspartate; AMPA = α-amino-3-hydroxyl-5-methyl-4-isoxazolepropionate.

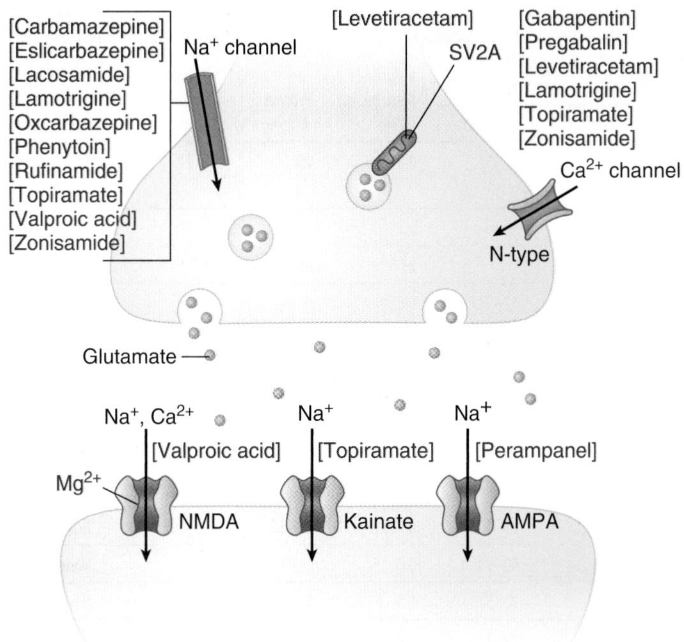


**FIGURE 21–1.** Excitatory neurons. In presynaptic neurons, carbamazepine, eslicarbazepine, lamotrigine, oxcarbazepine, phenytoin, rufinamide, topiramate, valproic acid, and zonisamide all inhibit the $Na^+$ channel, preventing the release of the excitatory neurotransmitter glutamate. Lacosamide binds differently and enhances slow inactivation, ie, inhibitory effect. Gabapentin, lamotrigine, levetiracetam, pregabalin, topiramate, and zonisamide all inhibit the $Ca^{2+}$ channel, preventing the release of glutamate. In postsynaptic neurons, perampanel, topiramate, and valproic acid each inhibits a different excitatory receptor. AMPA = α-amino-3-hydroxy-5-methyl-4-isoxazolepropionic acid; NMDA = *N*-methyl-D-aspartate; $SV2_A$ = synaptic vesicle protein $2_A$.

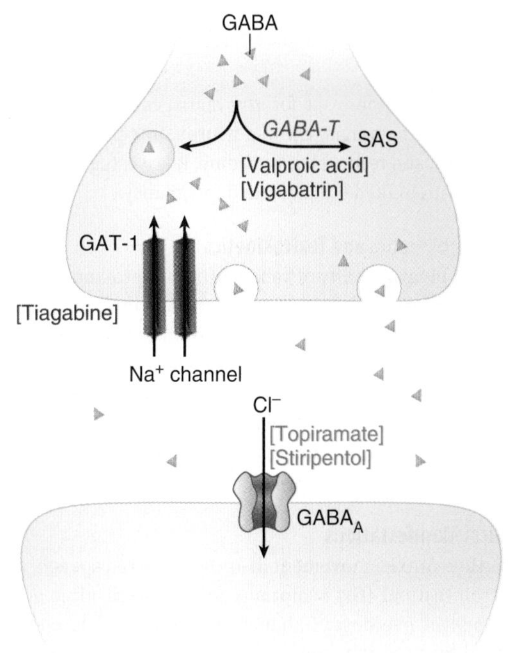


**FIGURE 21–2.** Inhibitory neurons. In presynaptic neurons, valproic acid and vigabatrin inhibit GABA metabolism; tiagabine inhibits its transporter; the end result is increased GABA in the synaptic cleft. In postsynaptic neurons; stiripentol and topiramate modulate $GABA_A$ receptors. GABA = γ-aminobutyric acid; GABA-T = GABA transaminase; GAT1= GABA transporter; SAS = succinic acid semialdehyde.

QT interval prolongation. Children experience a higher incidence of dystonic reactions, choreoathetosis, and seizures and have a lower incidence of electrocardiogram (ECG) abnormalities. The incidence of carbamazepine-induced hyponatremia ranges from 1.8% to 40%. Increased antidiuretic hormone secretion (SIADH) and increased sensitivity of peripheral osmoreceptors to antidiuretic hormone are suggested mechanisms.

## Diagnostic Testing

Therapeutic serum concentrations of carbamazepine are 4 to 12 mg/L. Carbamazepine-10,11-epoxide concentrations are 1 to 10 mg/L and can exceed 10 mg/L with therapeutic use of lamotrigine or VPA, secondary to epoxide hydrolase inhibition (Table 21–4). Electrolytes should be checked in patients with altered mental status because of the risk of hyponatremia. Carbamazepine cross-reacts with some toxicology screening for tricyclic antidepressants (Chap. 41).

## Management

Multiple-dose activated charcoal is associated with improved outcomes in several studies and is recommended for patients presenting with large overdoses, if there are no contraindications. Seizures should be treated with benzodiazepines. Sodium bicarbonate is recommended if the QRS complex duration exceeds 100 milliseconds (ms). Serial serum concentrations should be obtained owing to delays in peak concentrations. Hemodialysis (HD) is reasonable in cases of severe poisonings associated with intractable seizures or life-threatening dysrhythmias.

**TABLE 21–2 Pharmacokinetics of Antiepileptics After Oral Administration**

| | Time to Max Serum Concentration (hours) | Therapeutic Serum Concentration (mg/L) | Therapeutic Serum Concentration (μmol/L) | Volume of Distribution (L/kg) | Protein Binding (%) | Urinary Elimination Unchanged (%) | Active Metabolite | Elimination Half-Life (hours) |
|---|---|---|---|---|---|---|---|---|
| Carbamazepine | 6–8 IR<br>4–26 ER | 4–12 | 17–51 | 0.8–1.8 | 75 | 1–2 | CBZ10–11 epoxide | Acute 6–20; chronic 5–12 |
| Eslicarbazepine | 1–4 | 10–35 | | 2.7 | 35 | 1 | S-licarbazepine | 20–40 |
| Ezogabine | 0.5–2 | [a] | [a] | 2–6 | 80 | 20 | None | 8 |
| Gabapentin | 2–3 | 2–20 | 12–117 | 0.6–08 | 0 | 100 | None | 5–9 |
| Lacosamide | 0.5–4 | 5–10 | 20–40 | 0.6 | 15 | 40 | None | 12–13 |
| Lamotrigine | 1–3 | 3–15 | 12–58 | 0.1–1.4 | 55 | 10 | None | 15–35 |
| Levetiracetam | 1–2 | 10–46 | 60–240 | 0.6 | 0 | 95 | None | 6–8 |
| Oxcarbazepine | 1–5 | 10–35 | 4–12 | 0.7 | 67 | 1 | 10-hydroxy carbazepine | 1–2 |
| Perampanel | 0.5–1.5 | [a] | [a] | 77 | 96 | 2 | None | 70–110 |
| Phenobarbital | 1–6 | 15–40 | 65–172 | 0.7 | 35–50 | 20–50 | None | 53–140 |
| Phenytoin[b] | 5–24 | 10–20 | 40–79 | 0.6 | > 90 | < 5 | None | 6–60 |
| Pregabalin | 1–2 | 2–5 | 18–52 | 0.5 | 0 | > 90 | None | 5–7 |
| Rufinamide | 5–6 | 5–35 | 20–140 | 0.7–1.1 | 30 | 2 | None | 8–12 |
| Tiagabine | 0.5–2 | 0.02–0.2 | 0.027–0.27 | 1–1.3 | 95 | < 5 | None | 5–9 |
| Topiramate | 2–4 | 5–20 | 15–74 | 0.6–0.8 | 15 | 60 | None | 20–30 |
| Valproic acid | 1–24 in overdose | 50–120 | 347–832 | 0.1–0.4 | > 90[b] | < 5 | None | 5–18 |
| Vigabatrin | 1–2 | 0.8–36 | 155–619 | 0.8 | 0 | 100 | None | 6–8 |
| Zonisamide | 2–5 | 10–40 | 47–189 | 1.45 | 50 | 30 | None | 50–70 |

IR = immediate release; ER = extended release; CBZ = carbamazepine. [a]Not yet established. [b]Saturable.

**TABLE 21–3 Metabolism of Antiepileptics and Effects on CYP Enzymes**

| | Metabolized by | Induction | Inhibition |
|---|---|---|---|
| Carbamazepine | 3A4; 1A2; 2C8; 2C9; | 2C9; 3A family | None |
| Eslicarbazepine acetate | Hydrolysis; UGT | Weak 3A4 | 2C9, 2C19 |
| Ezogabine | *N*-acetylation | None | None |
| Gabapentin | None | None | None |
| Lacosamide | 3A4, 2C9, 2C19 | None | None |
| Lamotrigine | UGT | None | None |
| Levetiracetam | None | None | None |
| Oxcarbazepine | UGT | None | 2C19, 3A4 |
| Perampanel | 3A4; UGT | Weak 3A4; 2B6 | Weak 2C8; UGT |
| Phenobarbital | 2C9; 2C19, 2E1 | 3A family | None |
| Phenytoin | 2C9; 2C19; 3A4 | 2C family; 3A family | None |
| Pregabalin | None | None | None |
| Rufinamide | Hydrolysis; UGT | None | None |
| Tiagabine | 3A4 | None | None |
| Topiramate | None | None | 2C19 |
| Valproic acid | 2C9; 2C19; UGT | None | 2C19 |
| Vigabatrin | None | None | None |
| Zonisamide | 3A4; acetylation | None | None |

UGT = uridine-diphosphate-glucuronosyltransferase.

## GABAPENTIN

Gabapentin is approved for the management of seizures, postherpetic neuralgia, chronic neuropathic pain, migraine headaches, and restless leg syndrome. It is a category C medication with limited human data in pregnancy.

### Pharmacokinetics and Toxicokinetics

The oral bioavailability of gabapentin is approximately 60% in the therapeutic dose range. Absorption kinetics are dose-dependent, with decreasing bioavailability at increased dosage. Dosage adjustments are necessary in patients with an estimated glomerular filtration rate (eGFR) of 60 mL/min or less. It is not metabolized by and does not affect the CYP450 system and has no significant interactions with other antiepileptics (Tables 21–2 and 21–3).

### Clinical Manifestations

Sedation, ataxia, movement disorders, slurred speech, and gastrointestinal (GI) symptoms are reported after acute gabapentin overdose. Gabapentin withdrawal is characterized by agitation, confusion, tachycardia, and possibly seizures.

### Diagnostic Testing

Therapeutic serum concentrations of gabapentin are 2 to 20 mg/L. Because of its large therapeutic index, monitoring of serum gabapentin concentrations is not routinely necessary.

TABLE 21–4 Antiepileptic Drug Interactions

| | *Toxicity Increased by* | *Anticonvulsant Effect Decreased by* | *Increases Concentrations of* | *Decreases Concentrations of* |
|---|---|---|---|---|
| Carbamazepine | Allopurinol, amiodarone, cimetidine, danazol, diltiazem, fluoxetine, fluvoxamine, gemfibrozil, INH, ketoconazole, lamotrigine, macrolides, nefazodone, nicotine, propoxyphene, protease inhibitors, stiripentol, verapamil | Benzodiazepines, felbamate, isotretinoin, phenobarbital, phenytoin, primidone, succinimides, VPA | None | Doxycycline, felbamate, haloperidol, lamotrigine, OCPs, phenytoin, primidone, tiagabine, VPA, warfarin |
| Eslicarbazepine | None | CBZ, phenobarbital, phenytoin, topiramate | Phenytoin | CBZ, lamotrigine, topiramate, VPA |
| Ezogabine | None | CBZ, lamotrigine, phenobarbital, phenytoin | Phenobarbital | Lamotrigine |
| Gabapentin | Cimetidine | Antacids | Felbamate | None |
| Lamotrigine | Sertraline, VPA | CBZ, phenobarbital, phenytoin | CBZ epoxide | None |
| Levetiracetam | None | None | Phenytoin | None |
| Oxcarbazepine | None | CBZ, phenobarbital, phenytoin | Phenytoin | Lamotrigine, OCPs |
| Perampanel | None | CBZ, phenobarbital, phenytoin, oxcarbazepine, topiramate | Oxcarbazepine | CBZ, lamotrigine, VPA |
| Phenytoin | Allopurinol, amiodarone, chloramphenicol, chlorpheniramine, clarithromycin, cloxacillin, cimetidine, disulfiram, ethosuximide, felbamate, fluconazole, fluorouracil, fluoxetine, fluvoxamine, imipramine, INH, methylphenidate, metronidazole, miconazole, omeprazole, phenylbutazone, sulfonamides, ticlopidine, trimethoprim, tolbutamide, tolazamide, topiramate, VPA, warfarin | Antacids, antineoplastics CBZ, calcium, diazepam, diazoxide, ethanol (chronic), folic acid, influenza vaccine, loxapine, nitrofurantoin, phenobarbital, phenylbutazone, pyridoxine, rifampin, salicylates, sulfisoxazole, sucralfate, theophylline, tolbutamide, VPA, vigabatrin | Phenobarbital, primidone, warfarin | Amiodarone, CBZ, cardioactive steroids, corticosteroids, cyclosporine, disopyramide, dopamine, doxycycline, furosemide, haloperidol, influenza vaccine, levodopa, methadone, mexiletine, OCPs, phenothiazines, quinidine, tacrolimus, theophylline, tiagabine, tolbutamide, VPA |
| Pregabalin | None | Gabapentin, oxcarbazepine | None | Tiagabine |
| Rufinamide | VPA | CBZ, phenobarbital, phenytoin | Phenytoin | CBZ, lamotrigine |
| Tiagabine | None | CBZ, phenobarbital, phenytoin | None | VPA |
| Topiramate | None | CBZ, phenobarbital, phenytoin | Phenytoin | OCPs, cardioactive steroids |
| Valproic acid | Cimetidine, felbamate, ranitidine | Antacids, CBZ, chitosan, chlorpromazine, felbamate, INH, methotrexate, phenobarbital, phenytoin, primidone, salicylates | Felbamate, lamotrigine, phenobarbital, primidone | CBZ, tiagabine |
| Vigabatrin | None | None | None | Phenytoin |
| Zonisamide | None | CBZ, phenobarbital, phenytoin | CBZ | CBZ |

CBZ = carbamazepine; INH = isoniazid; OCP = oral contraceptive pill; VPA = valproic acid.

### Management

Treatment is largely supportive. Gabapentin withdrawal does not respond well to administration of benzodiazepines and should be treated with tapering doses of gabapentin.

## LACOSAMIDE

Lacosamide is a category C medication with limited data in human pregnancy.

### Pharmacokinetics and Toxicokinetics

Lacosamide is almost 100% bioavailable orally. Enzyme inducers such as carbamazepine and phenytoin can significantly reduce serum lacosamide concentrations (Tables 21–2 and 21–3).

### Diagnostic Testing

The therapeutic serum concentration of lacosamide is 5 to 10 mg/L. Monitoring of concentration is not routinely recommended in overdose.

### Clinical Manifestations

Gastrointestinal effects, QRS complex prolongation, dysrhythmias, intractable hypotension, and death are reported following acute overdose. Prolongation of the QRS complex is reported following overdose of a mix of lacosamide and other $Na^+$ channel blockers.

### Management

Electrocardiographic monitoring and supportive care are recommended. QRS complex prolongation responds to administration of sodium bicarbonate, and hypotension responds to administration of vasopressors, making these reasonable therapeutics.

## LAMOTRIGINE

Lamotrigine is an antiepileptic also approved for maintenance treatment of bipolar mood disorder. It is a category C medication with limited human data in pregnancy.

### Pharmacokinetics and Toxicokinetics

The oral bioavailability of lamotrigine approaches 100%. It is predominantly glucuronidated to lamotrigine-2-*N*-glucuronide. The elimination half-life is approximately 25 hours but is significantly reduced (12 hours) in the presence of phenytoin and carbamazepine and increased by VPA (Tables 21–2 and 21–3).

### Clinical Manifestations

Neurologic and cardiovascular manifestations predominate following lamotrigine overdose. Seizures including status epilepticus, central nervous system depression, agitation, myoclonus, and hyperreflexia are reported. Tachycardia, hypertension, and tachypnea are also frequently present along with QRS complex prolongation.

### Diagnostic Testing

Therapeutic serum concentrations of lamotrigine are 2 to 15 mg/L. Monitoring of concentration is not routinely recommended in overdose.

### Management

Lamotrigine-induced seizures respond to benzodiazepines, and treatment of QRS complex prolongation with hypertonic sodium bicarbonate is recommended.

## LEVETIRACETAM

Levetiracetam is a category C medication with limited human data in pregnancy.

### Pharmacokinetics and Toxicokinetics

The bioavailability of levetiracetam approaches 100%, and metabolism is not dependent on hepatic CYP450 activity. Dosage adjustments are necessary in patients with an eGFR of 80 mL/min or less (Tables 21–2 and 21–3).

### Clinical Manifestations

Mild central nervous system (CNS) depression, ataxia, and respiratory depression are reported.

### Diagnostic Testing

Therapeutic serum concentrations of levetiracetam are 10 to 46 mg/L. Because of its large therapeutic index, routine monitoring of serum levetiracetam concentrations is not necessary.

### Management

Supportive care should be provided.

## OXCARBAZEPINE

Oxcarbazepine is an analog of carbamazepine that is a category C medication in human pregnancy.

### Pharmacokinetics and Toxicokinetics

Oxcarbazepine has 100% orally bioavailability. Rate-limited presystemic ketoreduction rapidly metabolizes oxcarbazepine to licarbazepine. Licarbazepine concentrations are reduced by 25% in the presence of enzyme inducers such as carbamazepine and phenytoin (Tables 21–2 and 21–3).

### Clinical Manifestations

Central nervous system effects (lethargy, nystagmus, dizziness) and cardiovascular effects (tachycardia, hyper-/hypotension) are reported after overdose. In severe cases, coma, respiratory depression, and seizures are noted.

### Diagnostic Testing

Therapeutic serum concentrations of oxcarbazepine are 10 to 35 mg/L. Licarbazepine (monohydroxycarbazepine) serum concentrations are 3 to 35 mg/L. Monitoring of concentrations is not routinely recommended in overdose. Electrolytes should be checked in patients with altered mental status because of the risk of hyponatremia.

### Management

Rigorous supportive care underlies management.

## PHENYTOIN AND FOSPHENYTOIN

Phenytoin is a pregnancy category D medication, associated with the fetal hydantoin syndrome and cerebral hemorrhage in neonates. Fosphenytoin is a water-soluble phosphate ester prodrug of phenytoin. Advantages include more rapid administration, availability for intramuscular (IM) administration, and low potential for tissue injury at injection sites.

### Pharmacokinetics and Toxicokinetics

Oral loading doses of 20 mg/kg yield therapeutic (> 10 mg/L) serum concentrations at 5.6 ± 0.2 hours. In cases of very large oral overdoses, GI absorption is altered and peak serum concentrations can be delayed for days. Phenytoin is extensively bound to serum proteins, mainly albumin. Only the *un*bound free fraction is pharmacologically active. Its rate of elimination varies as a function of its concentration (ie, rate is nonlinear; Michaelis–Menten kinetics). At phenytoin concentrations below 10 mg/L, elimination usually is first-order, and half-life is 6 and 24 hours. At higher concentrations, zero-order elimination occurs because of saturation of the hydroxylation reaction, and the apparent half-life increases to 20 to 105 hours (Tables 21–2 and 21–3). Fosphenytoin is metabolized by tissue and blood phosphatases to phenytoin, phosphate, and formaldehyde.

### Clinical Manifestations

Acute phenytoin toxicity produces predominantly neurologic dysfunction, affecting the cerebellar and vestibular systems. Phenytoin concentrations greater than 15 mg/L are associated with nystagmus; concentrations greater than 30 mg/L are associated with ataxia and poor coordination; and concentrations exceeding 50 mg/L are associated with lethargy, slurred speech, and pyramidal and extrapyramidal manifestations. Ophthalmoplegia, opsoclonus, and other focal neurologic deficits are also reported. Cardiovascular instability, de novo seizures, and death following oral overdoses are rare. Intravenous overdose produces the same symptoms as oral overdose, with the addition of cardiotoxicity, hypotension, and dysrhythmias. These manifestations are usually attributed to the diluents propylene glycol (40%) and ethanol (10%). Iatrogenic overdoses of fosphenytoin are associated with hyperphosphatemia, hypocalcemia (which can result in QT interval prolongation), bradycardia, hypotension, and asystole.

The purple glove syndrome is a serious complication of IV phenytoin or fosphenytoin administration whose incidence ranges from 1% to 6%. Pathophysiology is unclear but appears to be related either to micro-extravasation or an unidentified procoagulant mechanism. Symptoms begin 2 to 12 hours after administration and include discoloration and edema distal to the site of administration. Mild symptoms typically resolve over days, but when severe, lead to necrosis, possibly necessitating amputation. The risk of purple glove syndrome associated with fosphenytoin is lower because of its water solubility.

### Diagnostic Testing

Serum phenytoin concentrations are 10 to 20 mg/L. Therapeutic free phenytoin concentrations are 1.0 to 2.1 mg/L.

### Management

The treatment of patients with oral phenytoin overdoses is largely supportive. Oral multidose activated charcoal (MDAC) is recommended in severe overdoses presenting with profound coma. Hemodialysis is reasonable in severe cases with life-threatening cardiovascular instability or profound neurologic impairment.

Intravenous phenytoin is associated with hypotension, cardiac dysrhythmias, and dyskinesias. These are usually transient and resolve in 60 minutes. Stopping the phenytoin infusion for a few minutes and administering a bolus of 250 to 500 mL of 0.9% sodium chloride solution generally is sufficient to treat the hypotension. Restarting the infusion at half the initial rate is recommended.

The management of extravasation is discussed in Special Considerations: SC7.

## PREGABALIN

Pregabalin is an antiepileptic developed as a more potent analog of gabapentin. It is indicated in the management of seizures and neuropathic pain. Pregabalin is a category C medication in pregnancy.

### Pharmacokinetics and Toxicokinetics

Pregabalin, unlike gabapentin, does not have a saturable GI transporter protein and is highly bioavailable, with rapid absorption. It is not protein-bound, and more than 90% is excreted unchanged in the urine. Dose adjustments are necessary in patients with an eGFR less than 60 mL/min (Tables 21–2 and 21–3).

### Clinical Manifestations

Cerebellar dysfunction (including dizziness, ataxia, and nystagmus), tremors, twitching, and seizures are described after overdose. Third-degree atrioventricular block, QT interval prolongation, encephalopathy, and respiratory failure are observed. Peripheral edema, weight gain, and decompensated congestive heart failure occur with chronic therapy.

### Diagnostic Testing

Therapeutic concentrations of pregabalin are 2.8 to 8.3 mg/L. Monitoring of concentration is not routinely recommended in overdose.

### Management

Rigorous supportive care underlies management. Cardiac monitoring is recommended. It is reasonable to utilize HD in patients with severe chronic kidney disease.

## TIAGABINE

Tiagabine is a category C medication in human pregnancy.

### Pharmacokinetics and Toxicokinetics

Tiagabine is quickly absorbed and has 90% oral bioavailability (Tables 21–2 and 21–3).

### Clinical Manifestations

Lethargy, confusion, and tachycardia are observed following acute overdose. Facial myoclonus (grimacing) and seizures are also reported.

### Diagnostic Testing

Therapeutic tiagabine concentrations are 0.02 to 0.2 mg/L. Monitoring of concentration is not routinely recommended in overdose.

### Management

Supportive care should be provided. Seizures respond to administration of benzodiazepines.

## TOPIRAMATE

Topiramate is an antiepileptic approved for mood stabilizing and migraine prophylaxis. It is a weak inhibitor of carbonic anhydrase. Topiramate is a pregnancy category D medication because of the risk of oral clefts.

### Pharmacokinetics and Toxicokinetics

Topiramate is 80% orally bioavailable (Tables 21–2 and 21–3).

### Clinical Manifestations

Lethargy, ataxia, nystagmus, myoclonus, hallucinations, coma, seizures, and status epilepticus are all reported following topiramate overdose. A hyperchloremic non–anion gap metabolic acidosis results from inhibition of carbonic anhydrase and typically appears within hours of ingestion.

### Diagnostic Testing

Therapeutic concentrations of topiramate are 5 to 20 mg/L. Electrolytes should be evaluated for the presence of a hyperchloremia and metabolic acidosis. Monitoring of concentration is not routinely recommended in overdose.

### Management

Meticulous supportive care should be provided. Severe hyperchloremic metabolic acidosis (pH $< 7.2$) should be treated with sodium bicarbonate 1 to 2 mEq/kg bolus intravenously and an infusion. Sodium bicarbonate impairs the antiepileptic effect of topiramate. It is reasonable to consider intermittent HD in patients with life-threatening topiramate toxicity presenting with significant neurologic impairment, intractable electrolyte abnormalities, or anuria.

## VALPROIC ACID

Valproic acid (VPA) is a simple branched-chain carboxylic acid antiepileptic that is also approved for treatment of mania associated with bipolar disorder and in migraine prophylaxis. It is a category D drug in pregnancy and is associated with neural tube and facial defects.

### Pharmacokinetics, Toxicokinetics, and Pathophysiology

Valproic acid is well absorbed from the GI tract with an oral bioavailability of 90%. Peak concentrations usually are reached in 6 hours, except for enteric-coated and extended-release preparations, for which peak concentrations can be delayed up to 24 hours. Valproic acid is 90% protein bound at therapeutic concentrations. Protein binding can decrease to 15% when VPA concentrations increase as a result of saturation of binding sites (Tables 21–2 and 21–3).

Valproic acid is predominantly metabolized in the liver, with less than 3% excreted unchanged in the urine. β-Oxidation occurs in the mitochondrial matrix and starts with passive diffusion of VPA across the mitochondrial membrane and ends with the transport of metabolites in the opposite direction using acetyl-CoA and carnitine as transporters (Fig. 21–3 and Table 21–5). The result is failure to metabolize ammonia causing hyperammonemia. Hyperammonemia can injure muscle and brain tissue. Mitochondrial dysfunction, inhibition of β-oxidation, depletion of carnitine, depletion of acetyl-CoA, and possibly depletion of glutathione stores impair lipid metabolism and lead to fatty acid accumulation, steatosis, lysosomal leakage, formation of reactive oxygen species, and cytotoxicity histologically similar to Reye syndrome.

### Clinical Manifestations

Valproic acid toxicity is associated with neurologic symptoms and metabolic disturbances. Ataxia and lethargy are common. Patients with serum VPA concentrations greater than 850 mg/L often have coma, respiratory depression, and hypotension. Hypernatremia, hypocalcemia, and hyperammonemia are reported. Anion gap metabolic acidosis is a poor prognostic sign. It results from accumulation of ketoacids, carboxylic acid, and propionic acid. Valproate-induced hyperammonemic encephalopathy is characterized by impaired consciousness with lethargy, focal or bilateral neurologic signs, seizures, and hyperammonemia. It is not always accompanied by elevated VPA concentrations or hepatotoxicity.

### Diagnostic Testing

Therapeutic serum concentrations of VPA are 50 to 120 mg/L. Electrolytes should be monitored because of the risk of hypernatremia, hypocalcemia, elevated serum lactate, and hyperammonemia.

### Management

Activated charcoal is recommended in the initial management. Repetitive doses are reasonable in massive overdoses. L-Carnitine is recommended to treat hyperammonemia or hepatotoxicity. A loading dose of 100 mg/kg IV is administered over 30 minutes (maximum, 6 g) followed by 15 mg/kg IV over 10 to 30 minutes every 4 hours until clinical improvement occurs (Antidotes in Brief: A10). Hemodialysis is recommended in cases of severe poisoning associated with VPA serum concentrations greater than 900 mg/L, coma, respiratory depression requiring intubation, or pH < 7.1.

## VIGABATRIN

Vigabatrin is a category C medication in pregnancy.

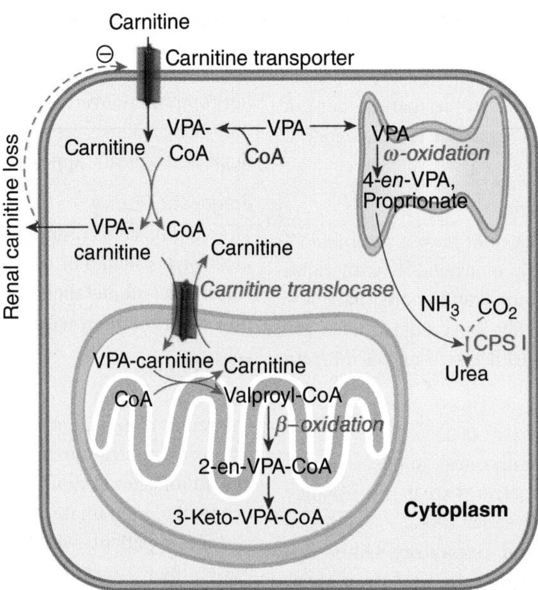


**FIGURE 21–3.** Valproic acid (VPA) metabolism by the hepatocyte. Valproic acid is linked to coenzyme A (CoA) by acyltransferase I and subsequently transferred to carnitine. Valproylcarnitine (VPA-carnitine) is shuttled into the mitochondrion, where, after transfer back to CoA by acyltransferase II, it undergoes β-oxidation, yielding several metabolites. These metabolites sequester CoA, preventing its use in the β-oxidation of other fatty acids. This process may lead to a Reye-like syndrome of hepatic steatosis. Alternatively, valproylcarnitine may diffuse from the cell and be renally eliminated, or it may inhibit cellular uptake of carnitine. In either case, the cellular depletion of carnitine shifts valproate metabolism toward microsomal ω-oxidation, which occurs in the endoplasmic reticulum. This pathway forms 4-*en*-valproate, a putative hepatotoxin. ω-Oxidation products and reduced *N*-acetylglutamate also interfere with carbamoylphosphate synthase I (CPS I), the initial step in the urea cycle, resulting in hyperammonemia.

**TABLE 21–5 Adverse Events Associated With Therapy**

| | *Common* | *Serious* | *DRESS Syndrome* |
|---|---|---|---|
| Carbamazepine | Dizziness, sedation, blurred vision, ataxia, weight gain, nausea, leukopenia | Agranulocytosis (1/200,000), aplastic anemia (1/500,000), rash (10%), SJS (rare), hyponatremia (1.8%–40%) | Yes |
| Eslicarbazepine | Dizziness, sedation, nausea, ataxia, diplopia | Rash | Yes |
| Ezogabine | Skin and nail discoloration, dizziness, sedation, ataxia | Maculopathy, urinary disorders, QT interval prolongation | No |
| Gabapentin | Sedation, dizziness, mild weight gain, ataxia, behavioral effect (children) | None | No |
| Lamotrigine | Dizziness, blurred vision, insomnia, headache | Rash, SJS (1–3/1,000), hypersensitivity (rare), hepatotoxicity (rare) | Yes |
| Lacosamide | Dizziness, sedation, ataxia, nausea | Rash | No |
| Levetiracetam | Fatigue, irritability, anxiety, asthenia | Psychosis (rare) | Yes |
| Oxcarbazepine | Fatigue, dizziness, ataxia, diplopia, nausea, headache | Rash, SJS or TEN (0.5–6/million), hyponatremia (2.5%), anaphylaxis (rare) | Yes |
| Perampanel | Dizziness, sedation, ataxia | Psychiatric and behavioral problems | No |
| Phenytoin | Fatigue, dizziness, ataxia, nausea, headache, gingival hypertrophy, hirsutism, osteopenia | Rash, SJS or TEN (2–4/10,000), megaloblastic anemia (rare), hepatotoxicity (rare), lupuslike syndrome | Yes |
| Pregabalin | Sedation, weight gain, peripheral edema | Peripheral edema | No |
| Rufinamide | Sedation, dizziness, nausea, headache, diplopia | Rash | Possible |
| Tiagabine | Fatigue, dizziness, ataxia, somnolence, anxiety | Seizures | No |
| Topiramate | Sedation, ataxia, word-finding difficulty, slowed speech, difficulty concentrating, anorexia, weight loss, paresthesias, oligohidrosis (children) | Metabolic acidosis (3%), nephrolithiasis (1.5%), acute glaucoma (rare), heat stroke | No |
| Valproic acid | Sedation, ataxia, weight gain, nausea, tremor, hair loss | Hepatotoxicity (1/20,000), pancreatitis (1/3,000), thrombocytopenia, hyperammonemia, aplastic anemia (rare) | No |
| Vigabatrin | Fatigue, headache, dizziness, weight gain | Peripheral vision loss, psychosis | No |
| Zonisamide | Sedation, ataxia, difficulty concentrating, irritability, nausea, headache | Aplastic anemia, nephrolithiasis (0.2%–4%), rash (1%–2%), SJS or TEN (rare), heat stroke (rare) | No |

DRESS = drug reaction with eosinophilia and systemic symptoms; SJS = Stevens–Johnson syndrome; TEN = toxic epidermal necrolysis.

### Pharmacokinetics, Toxicokinetics

Vigabatrin is rapidly absorbed and has a 60% to 80% oral bioavailability (Tables 21–2 and 21–3).

### Clinical Manifestations

Agitation, coma, and psychosis are reported following acute ingestion.

### Diagnostic Testing

Therapeutic serum concentrations of vigabatrin are 0.8 to 36 mg/L. Monitoring of concentration is not routinely recommended in overdose.

### Management

Supportive care should be provided. Benzodiazepines are recommended for severe agitation.

## ZONISAMIDE

Similarly to topiramate, zonisamide inhibits carbonic anhydrase enzymes. It is a category C medication in pregnancy.

### Pharmacokinetics and Toxicokinetics

Zonisamide is 65% orally bioavailable (Tables 21–2 and 21–3).

### Clinical Manifestations

Symptoms include lethargy, coma, seizures, and hyperchloremic metabolic acidosis. QT interval prolongation, hypotension, and cardiac arrest are reported.

### Diagnostic Testing

Therapeutic serum concentrations of zonisamide are 10 to 40 mg/L. Low serum bicarbonate is occasionally present. Monitoring of concentration is not routinely recommended in overdose.

### Management

Supportive care is the mainstay of management. Zonisamide is cleared via HD in chronically hemodialyzed patients. There are no data in overdose and HD is not recommended.

## DRUG-INDUCED HYPERSENSITIVITY SYNDROME

Drug-induced hypersensitivity syndrome (DIHS) is a severe adverse drug event previously known as the anticonvulsant hypersensitivity syndrome or drug reaction with eosinophilia and systemic symptoms (DRESS). The syndrome occurs in approximately one of every 1,000 to 10,000 uses of antiepileptics. The most commonly implicated antiepileptics are carbamazepine, phenytoin, phenobarbital, and lamotrigine, but oxcarbazepine, levetiracetam, and rufinamide are also involved. The etiology of DIHS remains unknown but data suggest a genetic defect in drug or epigenetic disruption leading to reactivation of T cells that harbor latent herpesviruses.

Drug-induced hypersensitivity syndrome occurs most frequently within the first 2 months of therapy and is not related to dose or serum concentration. The pathophysiology is related to the accumulation of reactive arene oxide metabolites resulting from decreased epoxide hydrolase enzyme activity. These metabolites bind to macromolecules and cause cellular apoptosis and necrosis.

Initial symptoms include fever (38°C–40°C) for 1 to 2 weeks followed by a diffuse, pruritic macular exanthem that spreads from face to trunk to extremities. Facial edema is common. Mucositis is present in 30%, and tender lymphadenopathy in 75% of cases. Multiorgan involvement usually occurs 1 to 2 weeks into the syndrome. The liver is the most frequently affected organ (> 80% of cases), although involvement of the CNS (encephalitis), heart (myocarditis), lungs (pneumonitis), kidney (nephritis), and thyroid is possible. Liver disturbances range from mildly elevated aminotransferase concentrations to fulminant hepatic failure. Eosinophilia (> $2.0 \times 10^9$ eosinophils/L) and mononucleosis-type atypical lymphocytosis are common.

There is no reliable standard for the diagnosis of this syndrome. Prompt discontinuation of the offending antiepileptic is essential, and benzodiazepines should be used temporarily to control seizures. Patients should be admitted to the intensive care unit or burn unit for fluid replacement, correction of electrolytes, warming environment, high caloric intake diet, prevention of bacterial or viral superinfection, and appropriate skin care. Topical steroids should be applied for symptomatic relief. Methylprednisolone 30 mg/kg is recommended. Intravenous immunoglobulin 2 g/kg over 5 days is recommended if patient fails to respond quickly to methylprednisolone. The major cause of death is hepatic necrosis.

In one case series, 90% of patients with this syndrome showed in vitro cross-reactivity to other aromatic antiepileptics. Based on this evidence, avoidance of phenytoin, carbamazepine, phenobarbital, primidone, lamotrigine, oxcarbazepine, and rufinamide is recommended; benzodiazepines, VPA, gabapentin, levetiracetam, topiramate, and tiagabine are safe alternatives.

# A10 L-CARNITINE

L-Carnitine (levocarnitine), an amino acid vital to the mitochondrial use of fatty acids, is approved by the United States (US) Food and Drug Administration (FDA) for the treatment of L-carnitine deficiency. L-Carnitine deficiency may result from valproic acid toxicity, inborn errors of metabolism, hemodialysis, or the treatment of zidovudine (AZT)-induced mitochondrial myopathy. Although carnitine can exist as either the D or L form, only the L isomer is active and found endogenously; thus, only the L isomer should be used therapeutically.

## HISTORY

Carnitine was first discovered in 1905 in extracts of muscle. Its name is derived from *carnis*, the Latin word for flesh. Subsequently, its chemical formula and structure were identified, and in 1997, its enantiomeric properties were confirmed.

## PHARMACOLOGY

### Mechanism of Action

Fatty acids provide 9 kcal/g and are an important source of energy for the body. The utilization of fatty acids requires L-carnitine–mediated passage through both the outer and inner mitochondrial membranes to reach the mitochondrial matrix where β-oxidation occurs (Fig. 21–3). Enzymes in the outer and inner mitochondrial membranes (carnitine palmitoyltransferase and carnitine acylcarnitine translocase) catalyze the synthesis, translocation, and regeneration of L-carnitine.

### L-Carnitine Homeostasis

Approximately 54% to 87% of endogenous L-carnitine is derived from the diet, while the remainder is synthesized. Meat and dairy are the primary dietary sources, and although most plants supply very little, avocado and fermented soy products are exceptionally rich in L-carnitine. The remainder of the carnitine needed by the body is synthesized.

## PHARMACOKINETICS OF EXOGENOUS L-CARNITINE

L-Carnitine is not bound to plasma proteins. The volume of distribution is 0.7 L/kg and the terminal elimination half-life averages 10 to 23 hours. Baseline plasma values for L-carnitine are 40 μmol/L but increase to 1,600 μmol/L following administration of 40 mg/kg IV. Whereas 2 g administered IV produces a peak plasma concentration of 1,000 μmol/L, oral administration of 2 g only produces peaks of 15 to 70 μmol/L. The time to peak concentrations following oral administration occurs at 2.5 to 7 hours, indicating a slow uptake by intestinal mucosal cells. The kidneys rapidly eliminate L-carnitine, and as the dose increases, renal clearance increases, reflecting saturation of renal reuptake by organic cation/carnitine transporter.

## ROLE IN VALPROIC ACID AND HYPERAMMONEMIA

Valproic acid causes hyperammonemia without necessarily causing symptoms or hepatic dysfunction. Hyperammonemia and hepatic toxicity are both associated with therapeutic dosing and acute overdose. In the absence of hepatic dysfunction, the postulated mechanisms for hyperammonemia are unclear but are likely to result from interference with hepatic synthesis of urea or a small increase in ammonia production by the kidney (Chap. 21). In human case reports of valproic acid therapy, L-carnitine supplementation reduced ammonia concentrations.

## ROLE IN VALPROIC ACID–ASSOCIATED HEPATOTOXICITY

Valproic acid therapy is commonly associated with a transient dose-related asymptomatic increase in liver enzyme concentrations and a rare symptomatic, life-threatening, idiosyncratic hepatotoxicity similar to Reye syndrome. This presumably results from either L-carnitine or acetyl-CoA deficiency, which inhibits mitochondrial β-oxidation of valproic acid and other fatty acids, causing hepatocellular accumulation. In animal studies when valproate was coadministered with L-carnitine, microvesicular steatosis was reduced. The strongest evidence for the benefit of L-carnitine treatment in improving survival from valproic acid–induced hepatotoxicity comes from the retrospective analysis of patients identified by the International Registry for Adverse Reactions to Valproic Acid. L-Carnitine was associated with an increase survival rate from 10% in untreated patients to 48% in L-carnitine–treated patients. Early diagnosis, prompt discontinuance of valproic acid, and administration of intravenous (IV) rather than oral (PO) L-carnitine were associated with the greatest survival rate.

We recommend the administration of L-carnitine for patients with valproic acid–induced hepatotoxicity. It is reasonable to also give L-carnitine to those with encephalopathy, with or without hepatotoxicity, and in the setting of an acute overdose if the patient develops a metabolic acidosis. There is not enough evidence to recommend routine L-carnitine administration based solely on a supratherapeutic or toxic valproic acid concentrations.

## ADVERSE EFFECTS AND CONTRAINDICATIONS TO L-CARNITINE

L-Carnitine administration is very well tolerated. Transient nausea and vomiting are the most common side effects reported, with diarrhea and a fishy body odor noted at higher doses. The manufacturer of L-carnitine received case reports of convulsive episodes following L-carnitine use by patients with or without a preexisting seizure disorder. No reports of seizures related to L-carnitine can be found in the human literature. The only data suggesting carnitine-related seizures are found in a rat model.

There are no known contraindications to the use of L-carnitine. However, only the L isomer and not DL-carnitine should be used because the DL mixture may interfere with the mitochondrial utilization of L-carnitine.

## OVERDOSE OF L-CARNITINE

No cases of toxicity from overdose are reported, although large oral doses infrequently cause diarrhea.

## PREGNANCY AND LACTATION

L-Carnitine is considered US FDA pregnancy category B. There is no information on excretion into breast milk.

## DOSAGE AND ADMINISTRATION

For patients with valproic acid–induced symptomatic hepatotoxicity, symptomatic hyperammonemia, metabolic acidosis, or encephalopathy, IV L-carnitine is recommended at a dose of 100 mg/kg up to 6 g administered over 30 minutes as a loading dose followed by 15 mg/kg every 6 hours administered over 10 to 30 minutes. The oral dosing of L-carnitine is 50 to 100 mg/kg/day up to 3 g/day and should be reserved for patients who are not acutely ill.

## FORMULATION AND ACQUISITIONAVAILABILITY

L-Carnitine is available as a sterile injection for intravenous use in 1 g/5 mL single-dose vials. L-Carnitine is supplied without a preservative, and once opened, the unused portion should be discarded. The IV formulation is compatible and stable when mixed with normal saline or lactated Ringer solution in concentrations as high as 8 mg/mL for as long as 24 hours. L-Carnitine is also available as a 330-mg tablet and as an oral solution at a concentration of 100 mg/mL.

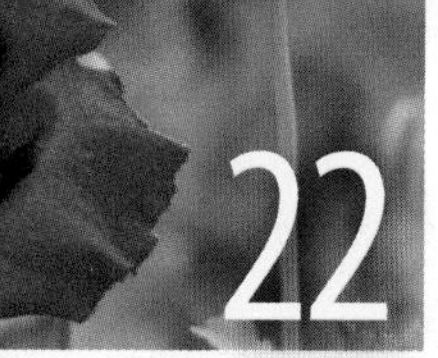

# 22 ANTIHISTAMINES AND DECONGESTANTS

Antihistamines and decongestants rank among the highest prescription and nonprescription xenobiotics used in the United States (US). Despite their widespread use, many reviews of nonprescription medications for cough in adults and children found no evidence for the effectiveness. Unwanted effects associated with their use poses significant public health problems, particularly in children. Fatality studies associated with nonprescription cough and cold medicines report that although uncommon, most deaths involved nontherapeutic dosages, administration for sedation purposes, and use in children primarily younger than 2 years of age. In early 2008, the US Food and Drug Administration (FDA) Public Health Advisory announced that cough and cold products were not recommended for children younger than 2 years. Despite many consumer-directed newsletter and media campaigns, the overall use in the general population seems constant.

Recreational use of antihistamines and decongestants was reported as early as the 1970s. Nonprescription sympathomimetics, such as pseudoephedrine, are also used as precursors in the illicit synthesis of methamphetamine. Dextromethorphan-containing products are widely used for recreational purposes (Chap. 9).

## ANTIHISTAMINES

### History

After the discovery of histamine, Bovet and other researchers at the Pasteur Institute attempted to synthesize antagonists to better understand its physiological role. In 1941, phenbenzamine was the first antihistamine deemed suitable for clinical use. Diphenhydramine was synthesized in 1943, and shortly after, in 1947, orphenadrine was derived. Searle and Company modified diphenhydramine to reduce drowsiness. Dimenhydrinate, the resulting 8-chlorotheophylline salt, serendipitously cured a patient of her long-standing motion sickness. This benefit was proven in a clinical trial in 1949, in which 25% of the troops crossing the Atlantic from New York who received a placebo experienced seasickness compared with only 4% of those receiving dimenhydrinate. Reports of adverse effects and toxicity were soon published. The first report of a death associated with diphenhydramine occurred in 1948.

In the following decade, more than 5,000 compounds were synthesized by more than 500 chemists and tried for human use. In the 1970s, terfenadine was synthesized as a tranquilizer, but it lacked central nervous system (CNS) penetration. However, its peripheral antihistaminic effects proved useful. In 1989, more than 773 reactions to terfenadine were reported ranging from prolonged QT intervals to convulsions in supratherapeutic ingestions. In 1992, the FDA issued a warning for the risk of torsade de pointes with terfenadine when administered with CYP3A4 inhibitors. Fexofenadine, its active metabolite, was marketed instead.

None of the initial xenobiotics could antagonize histamine-induced gastric acid secretion, leading to the determination of the existence of more than one type of histamine receptors. The histamine receptor subtypes were identified as $H_1$ and $H_2$. Cimetidine was synthesized in 1972, but its binding to the heme moiety of the cytochrome P450 with resultant inhibition caused medication interactions as well as altered mental status. Ranitidine, a less polar molecule, did not enter the CNS and did not interfere with the P450 cytochromes. It rapidly became one of the best-selling drugs and remained so until its recent removal for contamination.

### Epidemiology

Antihistamines are available worldwide, and many do not require a prescription. These medications find widespread application in the treatment of conditions such as anaphylaxis, benign positional vertigo, dystonic reactions, hyperemesis gravidarum, gastroesophageal reflux disease, stress gastritis, and other histamine-mediated disorders. Additionally, they are used for symptomatic relief of allergy symptoms as in allergic rhinitis, conjunctivitis, or urticaria and are included in many combination cough and cold preparations as discussed previously. First-generation antihistamines are widely available without prescription and are also marketed as sleep aids. These two factors contribute to their common ingestion in suicide attempts. Second- and third-generation $H_1$ antihistamines are less frequently implicated in suicide attempts. The $H_2$ antihistamines have a better safety profile in therapeutic and overdose situations.

Children are at increased risk for antihistamine toxicity, and most of the reported deaths in this age group involve diphenhydramine. Perhaps this is due to the ease of obtaining a toxic dose in milligrams per kilogram of body weight with very few tablets or very few tablespoons of liquid formulations available in commercial products.

### Pharmacology

***Histamine Receptor Physiology.*** The $H_1$ receptors are located in the CNS, heart, vasculature, airways, sensory neurons, gastrointestinal (GI) smooth muscle, immune system, and adrenal medulla. Stimulation of $H_1$ receptors results in increased synthesis by phospholipases $A_2$ and C, inositol-1,4,5-triphosphate, and several diacylglycerols (DAGs) from phospholipids located in cell membranes. Inositol-1,4,5-triphosphate causes release of calcium, which then activates calcium-calmodulin–dependent myosin light-chain kinase, resulting in enhanced cross-bridging and smooth muscle contraction.

The **$H_1$ receptors** are most commonly associated with mediation of inflammation. The other functions include control of the sleep–wake cycle, cognition, memory, and endocrine homeostasis. The $H_1$ receptor stimulation also causes vasodilation, increases vascular permeability, and increases bronchoconstriction. Cardiac $H_1$ receptor stimulation increases atrioventricular nodal conduction time.

The **$H_2$ receptors** are located in cells of the gastric mucosa, heart, lung, CNS, and uterus and in immune cells.

Stimulation of the $H_2$ receptor results in increased gastric acidity. The cardiac action of histamine on the $H_2$ receptor increases sinus node automaticity, ventricular contraction force, and coronary flow as well as vascular permeability and mucus production in the airways.

The **$H_3$ receptors** are found in neurons of the central and peripheral nervous systems, airways, and GI tract. Stimulation of CNS $H_3$ receptors decreases further release of histamine, acetylcholine, dopamine, and serotonin.

The **$H_4$ receptors** are located in leukocytes, bone marrow, spleen, lung, liver, colon, and hippocampus and play a role in the differentiation of myeloblasts and promyelocytes and in eosinophil chemotaxis.

## Histamine Receptors: Inverse Agonists Versus Antagonists

All known $H_1$ antagonists function as inverse agonists and are not simply reversible competitive antagonists. Rather than preventing the binding of histamine to its receptor as in a classical competitive antagonist model, these xenobiotics stabilize the inactive form of the histamine receptor and shift the equilibrium to this inactive conformation (Fig. 22–1). However, for consistency with the medical

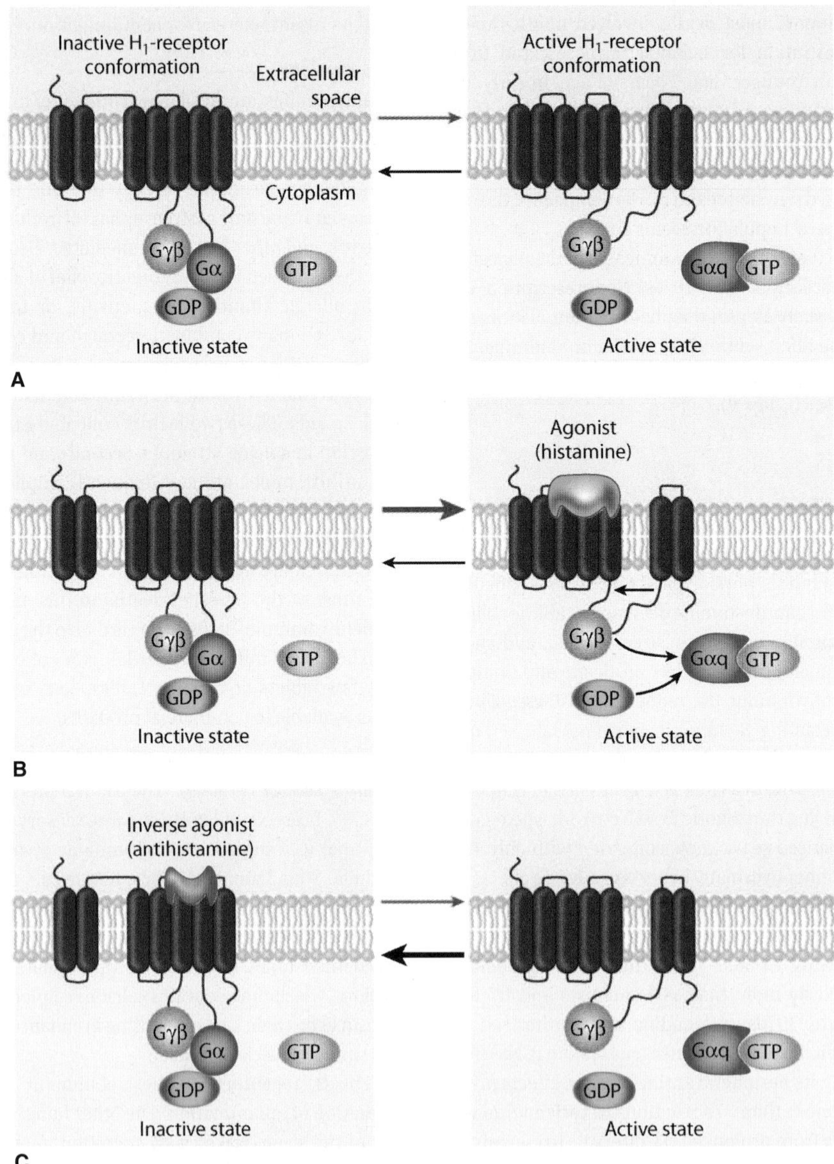


**FIGURE 22–1.** Action of histamine and antihistamines on the $H_1$ receptor. Molecular basis of action of histamine and antihistamines. (**A**) The inactive state of the histamine $H_1$ receptor is in equilibrium with the active state. (**B**) The agonist, histamine, has preferential affinity for the active state, stabilizes the receptor in this conformation, and shifts the equilibrium toward the active state. (**C**) An $H_1$ antihistamine (inverse agonist) has preferential affinity for the inactive state, stabilizes the receptor in this conformation, and shifts the equilibrium toward the inactive state. GDP = guanosine diphosphate; GTP = guanosine triphosphate. (*Reproduced with permission from Simons FE, Simons KJ. Histamine and $H_1$-antihistamines: celebrating a century of progress. J Allergy Clin Immunol. 2011 Dec;128(6):1139-1150.*)

literature and the current terminology for these xenobiotics, the terms *antihistamine* or *histamine antagonist* rather than *inverse agonist* are used.

***$H_1$ Antihistamines.*** Antiallergic and antiinflammatory activities of the $H_1$ antihistamines result from inhibition of the release of mediators from mast cells and basophils and inhibition of the expression of cell adhesion molecules and eosinophil chemotaxis. Another classification system of $H_1$ antihistamines stratifies them by sedating properties and ability to cross the blood–brain barrier.

**First-generation $H_1$ antihistamines** readily penetrate the blood–brain barrier and produce CNS effects, including sedation and performance impairment. Central effects likely result from their high lipophilicity or lack of recognition by the P-glycoprotein efflux pump. First-generation $H_1$ antihistamines also bind to muscarinic, serotonin, and α-adrenergic receptors as well as cardiac ion channels. Their binding to the voltage-gated $Na^+$ channels produces use-dependent block, and their binding to the $K^+$ channels alters repolarization.

**Second-generation $H_1$ antihistamines** are peripherally selective and have a higher therapeutic index. They do not penetrate the CNS well because of their hydrophilicity, their relatively high molecular weight, and recognition by the P-glycoprotein efflux pump. Using recommended doses of antihistamines, positron emission tomography (PET) scanning shows that first-generation antihistamines occupy more than 70% of the $H_1$ receptors in the CNS compared to less than 20% to 30% occupancy by the second-generation antihistamines. Thus, cautious prescribing practices lead to a preference for second-generation $H_1$ antihistamines in patients whose activities are "safety critical" and would be affected by any psychomotor impairment (eg, those who operate motor vehicles). In a randomized placebo-controlled driving simulator trial, 60 mg of fexofenadine did not interfere with driving performance but 50 mg of diphenhydramine produced poorer driving performance than ethanol (100 mg/dL). Overall, the relative incidence of anticholinergic and CNS adverse effects caused by second-generation $H_1$ antihistamines are similar to those produced by placebo.

***$H_2$ Antihistamines.*** These structural analogs of histamine are highly selective inhibitors of the $H_2$ receptor site. The effectiveness of $H_2$ antihistamines in the treatment of diseases caused by excessive gastric acid secretion is shown in Fig. 22–2. Of note, $H_2$ antihistamines have little pharmacologic effect elsewhere in the body, and they have weak CNS penetration secondary to their hydrophilic properties.

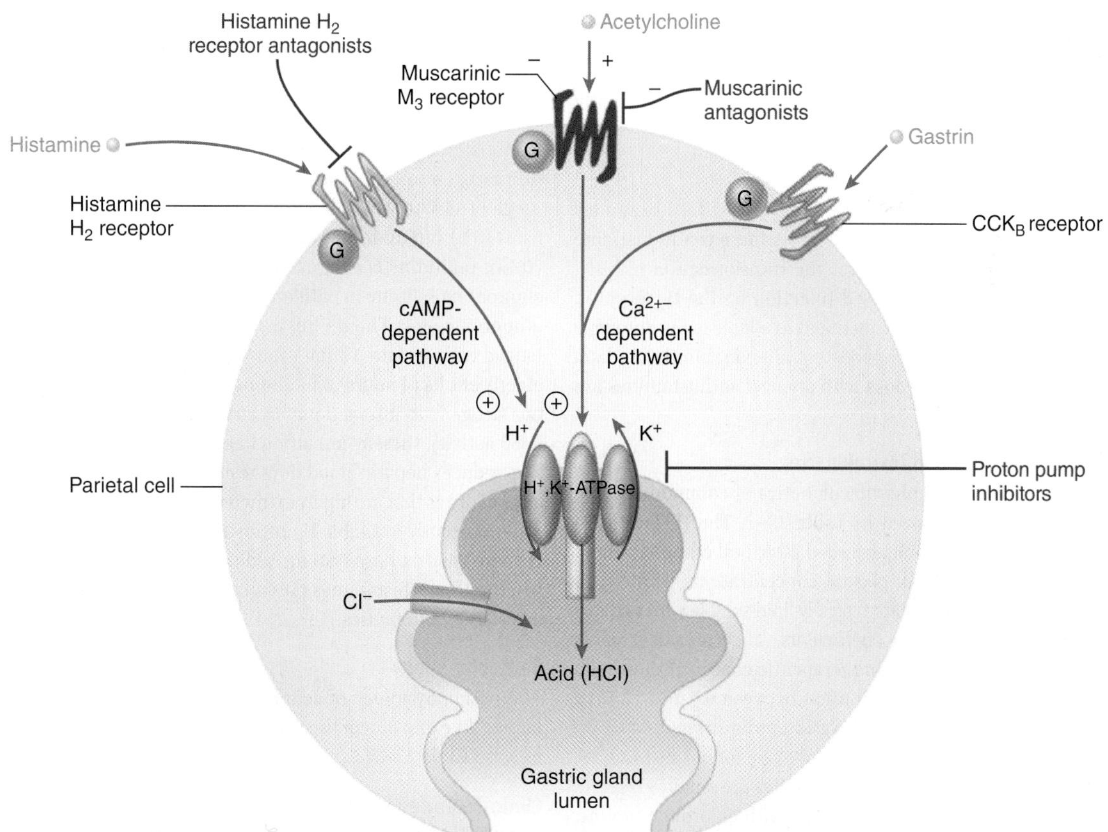


**FIGURE 22–2.** Schematic representation of a gastric parietal cell demonstrating the mechanism of hydrogen ion secretion into the lumen. Gastric acid is modulated by both the calcium-dependent and cyclic adenosine monophosphate (cAMP)–dependent pathway. Histamine binding to the $H_2$ receptor increases gastric acidity by increasing cAMP. Both acetylcholine and gastrin increase gastric acidity by increasing the influx of calcium. Whereas acetylcholine binds at the muscarinic 3 ($M_3$) receptor, gastrin binds the cholecystokinin B ($CCK_B$) receptor.

**TABLE 22–1 Pharmacokinetics Properties of Used Antihistamines in the US**

| *Antihistamine* | | *Half-Life (h)*[b] | *Duration of Action (h)*[a] | *Hepatic Metabolism* | *Log D*[c] | *$V_d$ (L/kg)*[b] | *Urinary Elimination (%)* |
|---|---|---|---|---|---|---|---|
| $H_1$ antihistamines | Chlorpheniramine | 12—43 (urine pH dependent) | 24 | Yes | 1.13 | 5–7 | 30 |
| First-generation | Cyproheptadine | N/A | 4–6 | Yes | 4.93 | N/A | 72 |
| | Diphenhydramine | 3–14 | 12 | Yes | 1.92 | 3–4 | 4 |
| | Doxylamine | 10–11 | N/A | Yes | 1.15 | 2.7 | N/A |
| | Hydroxyzine | 13–27 | 24 | Yes | 2.21 | 13–31 | 15 |
| | Promethazine | 9–16 | 4–6 | Yes | 2.73 | 9–19 | < 1 |
| Second-generation | Cetirizine | 6.5–10 | 12–24 | < 40% | −0.02 | 0.58 | 70 |
| | Desloratadine | 21–27 | > 24 | Yes | 2.95 | 10–30 | 41 |
| | Fexofenadine | 9–20 | 12–24 | < 8% | 2.68 | 12 | 11 |
| | Levocetirizine | N/A | > 24 | < 15% | −0.83 | 0.41 | 85 |
| | Loratadine | 3–20 | 24 | Yes | 6.23 | 26–32 | |
| $H_2$ antihistamines | Cimetidine | 2 | 6–10 | | | 1.4 | 35–60 |
| | Ranitidine | 2.1 | 12 | | | 1.6–2.4 | 69 |
| | Nizatidine | 1.3 | 24 | Yes | N/A | 1.2–1.8 | 61 |
| | Famotidine | 2.6 | 12 | | | 0.9–1.4 | 67 |

[a]Brunton LB, et al., eds: *Goodman & Gilman's The Pharmacological Basis of Therapeutics.* 11th ed. New York: McGraw-Hill; 2005. [b]Baselt RC. *Disposition of Toxic Drugs and Chemicals in Man.* 7th ed. Foster City, CA: Biomedical Publications; 2004. [c]Log D is the octanol/water partition coefficient at a pH of 7.

$V_d$ = volume of distribution.

Data from Wilson CO, Beale JM, Block JH. *Wilson and Gisvold's Textbook of Organic Medicinal and Pharmaceutical Chemistry*, 12th ed. Baltimore, MD: Lippincott Williams & Wilkins; 2011.

***$H_3$ Antihistamines.*** These xenobiotics are the focus of much research; however, none is currently commercially available.

***$H_4$ Antihistamines.*** No xenobiotics of this class are currently commercially available.

## Atypical Antihistamines

Other xenobiotics are named atypical antihistamines because of their inhibitory effect on the enzyme histidine decarboxylase, which catalyzes the transformation of histidine to histamine as opposed to action on the $H_1$ receptor. Tritoqualine has been commercially available in Europe since the 1960s and is used for persistent allergic rhinitis. To date, no case reports of overdose with atypical antihistamines are published.

## Pharmacokinetics and Toxicokinetics

***$H_1$ Antihistamines.*** The pharmacokinetics of common antihistamines are summarized in Table 22–1. The $H_1$ antihistamines are generally well absorbed after oral administration, and most achieve peak plasma concentrations within 2 to 3 hours. Antihistamines are typically lipid soluble with variable octanol/water partition coefficients. They are also highly bound to plasma protein in therapeutic concentrations with an average volume of distribution between 0.5 and 12 L/kg but extending to 30 L/kg with desloratadine. Hepatic metabolism is the primary route of metabolism for antihistamines. All antihistamines and their metabolites are renally excreted. Elimination half-life is quite varied, with chlorpheniramine, hydroxyzine, azelastine, and levocabastine exhibiting the longest termination half-lives up to 24 hours. The duration of action ranges from 3 to 24 hours, which is much longer than predicted from the serum elimination half-lives of the antihistamines.

***$H_2$ Antihistamines.*** Cimetidine is rapidly and completely absorbed after oral administration, but only 40% to 50% of ranitidine and famotidine are bioavailable with a peak concentration within 3 hours. All have reduced absorption when administered concomitantly with food. Volumes of distribution range from 1 to 4 L/kg. All have protein binding in the range of 15% to 25%. Cimetidine has some hepatic metabolism (15%), but ranitidine and famotidine do not (< 5%). Up to 70% of ranitidine is eliminated unchanged in the urine. The elimination half-life in patients with normal kidney function is approximately 2 hours, but the half-life is substantially prolonged with impaired kidney function (up to 10 hours) and in elderly adults (4 hours). Cimetidine is responsible for numerous drug–drug interactions because it inhibits cytochrome P450 activity, thereby impairing hepatic drug metabolism. It also reduces hepatic blood flow, resulting in decreased clearance of drugs that are highly extracted by the liver. None of the other currently available $H_2$ antihistamines inhibit the cytochrome P450 oxidase system. Additionally, by altering gastric pH, the $H_2$ antihistamines potentially alter the absorption of acid-labile xenobiotics.

## Pathophysiology

The pathophysiology of acute $H_1$ antihistamine overdose is largely an extension of the expected therapeutic and adverse effects (Table 22–2).

## Clinical Manifestations

***$H_1$ Antihistamines.*** The toxic doses for each antihistamine are not well defined. The commonly cited threshold of toxicity of 3 to 5 times the therapeutic dose for first-generation antihistamines as well as cetirizine, loratadine, and fexofenadine originating from algorithms in various articles is not validated.

**TABLE 22–2 Effects of $H_1$ Antihistamines**

| *Effects* | *Clinical Result* | *First Generation* | *Second Generation* |
|---|---|---|---|
| Mast cell histamine inhibition | Decreased itching<br>Decreased vascular permeability<br>Vasodilation | Therapeutic | Therapeutic |
| Calcium channel blockade | Decreased mediator release | Therapeutic | Therapeutic |
| CNS antihistamine receptor occupancy | Sedation<br>Impaired psychomotor performance | Marked effect in therapeutic and overdose | Minimal or no effect reported with cetirizine in overdose |
| CNS serotonin receptor antagonism | Increased appetite<br>Weight gain | Occurs in therapeutic doses; no significance in overdose | No effect |
| Peripheral muscarinic receptor antagonism | Dry mucosa<br>Decreased peristalsis<br>Urinary retention<br>Sinus tachycardia<br>Mydriasis | Marked effect in overdose; minimal effect can occur at therapeutic doses | Minimal or no effect |
| Central muscarinic receptor antagonism | Agitation<br>Delirium<br>Hallucinations | Marked effect in overdose | No effect |
| α-Adrenergic receptors | Dizziness<br>Hypotension | Marked effect in overdose; minimal effect can occur at therapeutic doses | No effect |
| Cardiac sodium and potassium channel blockers | Prolonged QRS complex<br>Prolonged QT interval | Marked effect in overdose on $Na^+$ channel | Minimal or no effect at therapeutic doses except terfenadine, astemizole on $K^+$ channel |

CNS = central nervous system.

*Neurologic.* Acute overdose of first-generation $H_1$ antihistamine usually results in the onset of toxicity within 2 hours. Drowsiness that occurs in milder poisoning rapidly progresses to obtundation and seizures with larger ingestions. Compared with adults, children more commonly present with excitation, irritability, or ataxia as well as being more prone to having hallucinations or seizures. Patients typically exhibit an anticholinergic syndrome, including mydriasis, tachycardia, hyperthermia, dry mucous membranes, urinary retention, diminished bowel sounds, and altered mental status such as disorientation and hallucinations. Both vertical and horizontal nystagmus occur in patients with diphenhydramine overdose. The skin appears flushed, warm, and dry. Hyperthermia occurs in severe cases and correlates with the extent of agitation, ambient temperature and humidity, and length of time during which the patient cannot dissipate heat because of anticholinergic-mediated reduction in sweating. Seizures occur at any point in time in the course of the poisoning but typically begin in the first few hours and represent severe toxicity.

Some patients with high therapeutic dosing or after overdose develop a central anticholinergic syndrome in which CNS anticholinergic effects, such as hallucinations, outlast peripheral anticholinergic effects. At a later stage of ingestion, the lack of tachycardia, skin changes, or other peripheral anticholinergic manifestations complicates establishment of the correct diagnosis for antihistamine-poisoned patients unless there is a clear exposure history.

Ingestion of second-generation $H_1$ or $H_2$ antihistamines usually does not result in significant CNS depression or anticholinergic effects except perhaps in pediatric patients or in adults with altered pharmacokinetic parameters. Although dry mouth and mydriasis are common adverse therapeutic effects, sedation is of the greatest concern.

*Cardiovascular.* Sinus tachycardia is a consistent finding after overdose with an $H_1$ antihistamine with anticholinergic effects and can persist after other toxic manifestations and delirium have resolved. Sodium channel blockade results in prolongation of both the QRS complexes and QT intervals and is reported with most first-generation $H_1$ antihistamines at doses that are supratherapeutic.

*Other.* Rhabdomyolysis occurs in patients with extreme agitation or seizures after an $H_1$ antihistamine overdose. Nontraumatic rhabdomyolysis is commonly noted in patients who overdose with doxylamine.

Unless complications such as aspiration or kidney failure develop, most patients are symptomatic for 24 to 48 hours with resolution of cardiac symptoms occurring before neurologic recovery. Anticholinergic delirium and residual sinus tachycardia can last a few days, but generally neither requires cardiac monitoring in intensive care settings.

*Special populations.* Elderly patients are more susceptible to adverse events because kidney and liver dysfunction delay antihistamine metabolism. All $H_1$ antihistamines cross the placenta, and some are teratogenic in animals. First- and second-generation antihistamines fall into FDA categories B and C.

***$H_2$ Antihistamines.*** These xenobiotics are well tolerated in overdose even after large ingestions. Patients uncommonly develop tachycardia, dilated and sluggishly reactive pupils, slurred speech, and confusion. Severe dysrhythmias, including ventricular fibrillation and bradycardia leading to fatal cardiac arrest, are reported following rapid IV infusion of cimetidine. Deaths are reported in rare instances of large ingestion of cimetidine.

### Diagnostic Testing

The bedside diagnosis of antihistamine toxicity is a clinical one. Antihistamines cause false-positive results on several rapid urine drug screens by immunoassay for amphetamines (ranitidine), methadone (diphenhydramine, doxylamine), and phencyclidine (diphenhydramine, doxylamine). Cyproheptadine, diphenhydramine, and hydroxyzine also produce false-positive results for tricyclic antidepressants (TCAs) in serum immunoassays only. Such results are of concern, particularly in children, and should always be confirmed if malicious intent is suspected.

### Management

*General Management.* Guidelines are published and validated with regard to the evidence-based out-of-hospital management of unintentional diphenhydramine and dimenhydrinate exposure and allow for home observation for any ingestion under 7.5 mg/kg in children younger than 6 years or under 300 mg or 7.5 mg/kg for adults and older children. Other criteria for medical evaluation for other antihistamines vary according to local practices, but in general, ingestions of less than 5 times the maximal therapeutic dose are rarely toxic.

Patients presenting to hospitals after exposure of any antihistamine must be triaged and medically assessed quickly, generally within 30 minutes of arrival, because those who will develop severe complications are initially indistinguishable from those who will have a benign course, and the window for GI decontamination may soon elapse. The individual should be attached to a cardiac monitor and observed for signs of $Na^+$ channel blockade (increased QRS complex duration), potassium channel blockade (prolonged QT interval), and related dysrhythmias, as well as for seizures. Intravenous access should be established and airway protection ensured.

Gastrointestinal decontamination is recommended with care to avoid aspiration in patients with large ingestions of first-generation $H_1$ antihistamines or early presentations but is generally not needed for $H_2$ antihistamines. The use of oral activated charcoal (AC) is reasonable, and multiple-dose AC or whole-bowel irrigation (WBI) is usually not indicated. Enhanced elimination techniques do not benefit the toxicity of these xenobiotics because of their large volumes of distribution, extensive protein binding, and absence of enterobiliary circulation. Assessment of the serum acetaminophen concentration is important because of its inclusion in many cough and cold products. Other laboratory studies should be obtained as indicated by history or physical signs and symptoms. Kidney function and creatine kinase should be obtained on all patients, particularly in patients with seizures or doxylamine overdose. Serum pregnancy tests should be obtained in women of childbearing age. An ECG should be obtained on all patients during the initial assessment and repeated at regular intervals, particularly if physostigmine use is considered. Continuous ECG monitoring is preferable for high-risk patients such as those with altered mental status or large ingestions.

Serial assessments of the patient's vital signs, particularly temperature, and mental status should be made. The potential for clinical deterioration necessitates management of symptomatic patients in a monitored environment.

*Specific Treatments.* Sedation can increase the risk for aspiration. Intubation to secure the airway is recommended when excessive sedation compromises ventilation. Seizures should be treated with an IV benzodiazepine such as 2 to 4 mg (0.05–0.1 mg/kg in children) of lorazepam, 2 to 5 mg (0.02 mg/kg in children) of midazolam, or 10 mg (0.2–0.5 mg/kg in children) of diazepam with repeated dosing as necessary. Recurrent seizures refractory to benzodiazepines or hypertonic sodium bicarbonate (see below) should be treated with propofol or general anesthesia.

Hypotension generally responds to isotonic fluids (0.9% sodium chloride solution or lactated Ringer solution). If the desired increase in blood pressure is not attained, hypertonic sodium bicarbonate therapy or vasopressors should be titrated to achieve an acceptable blood pressure. The $Na^+$ channel blockade (type IA antidysrhythmic) properties of diphenhydramine and other antihistamines lead to wide-complex dysrhythmias that resemble those that occur after cyclic antidepressant overdose (Chap. 41). Hypertonic sodium bicarbonate reverses diphenhydramine or other antihistamine-associated conduction abnormalities (Antidotes in Brief: A5). Type IA (quinidine, procainamide, disopyramide), IC (flecainide), and III (amiodarone, sotalol) antidysrhythmics are contraindicated because of their capacity to prolong the QRS complex and the QT interval. The successful use of IV lipid emulsion is reported in several case reports, but its efficacy is debated because of other reports with no change in the patient's clinical condition. Because of the current equipoise in its possible efficacy and known adverse effects, its use is reasonable in cases of cardiovascular compromise refractory to standard treatments. The use of lipid emulsion is explained in more detail in Antidotes in Brief: A23. Extracorporeal life support techniques are rarely needed for refractory shock.

Rhabdomyolysis-associated nephrotoxicity should be prevented by early use of IV fluid, 0.9% sodium chloride, to produce a urine output of 1 to 3 mL/kg/h. Once established, antihistamine-induced rhabdomyolysis is treated with IV fluids. Although urinary alkalinization is reportedly helpful to prevent myoglobin-induced nephrotoxicity, its usefulness is controversial and might be best reserved when urinary pH is lower than 6.5 (Antidotes in Brief: A5).

Hyperthermic patients should be monitored for the development of disseminated intravascular coagulation and other complications. Cooling via evaporative methods (tepid mist or cooling blanket or fan) is generally sufficient, but patients with severe hyperthermia should receive more rapid cooling using an ice bath.

Agitation or psychosis generally responds readily to titration of a benzodiazepine. Although most commonly a direct central effect, other frequent causes of agitation such as urinary retention or bright lights shone into dilated eyes unable to react should not be forgotten. Physostigmine effectively reverses the peripheral or central anticholinergic syndrome and is recommended as a benzodiazepine-sparing strategy but should only be administered after the initial cardiovascular toxicity, if present, has resolved or is unlikley to be of concern. It should be used with caution in an attempt to reverse coma or sedation caused by anticholinergic toxicity (Antidotes in Brief: A11). In a retrospective comparison of physostigmine and benzodiazepines, physostigmine was safer and more effective for treating anticholinergic agitation and delirium.

Before physostigmine is administered, the patient should be attached to a cardiac monitor, and secure IV access should be established. Physostigmine (1–2 mg in adults; 0.5 mg in children) should be administered by slow IV bolus over 5 to 10 minutes with continuous monitoring of vital signs, ECG, breath sounds, and oxygen saturation by pulse oximetry. The initial dose of physostigmine can be repeated at 5- to 10-minute intervals if anticholinergic symptoms are not reversed and cholinergic symptoms such as salivation, diaphoresis, bradycardia, lacrimation, urination, or defecation do not develop. When improvement occurs as a result of physostigmine, repeated doses of physostigmine at 30- to 60-minute intervals are often necessary, taking into account the fact that metabolism of the offending xenobiotic is occurring and that subsequent doses might need to be lowered to avoid cholinergic symptoms.

## DECONGESTANTS

### History and Epidemiology

***History.*** Decongestants are xenobiotics acting on α-adrenergic receptors, producing vasoconstriction, decreasing edema of mucous membranes, and improving bronchiolar air movement. Ma Huang was used in China for at least 2,000 years before it was introduced into Western medicine. Amphetamines were later synthesized to palliate a shortage of *Ephedra* plant availability. Pseudoephedrine is a natural stereoisomer of ephedrine, and phenylephrine was introduced into clinical medicine in the 1930s and in 1949 to replace amphetamines in several compounds. Imidazoline decongestants were derived from piperazine compounds while investigating their use as uric acid remedies to combat gout. Naphazoline was introduced in the 1940s as a decongestant. In the decades that followed, many imidazoline decongestants have been developed and tried for clinical use.

***Epidemiology.*** Despite many years of widespread decongestant use in the US and sporadic case reports of adverse effects, the magnitude and public health significance of adverse effects of this class of medications were only relatively recently appreciated. From 1991 to 2000, the US FDA received 22 spontaneous reports of hemorrhagic stroke associated with phenylpropanolamine (PPA) use. Statistical analysis published in 2000 confirmed that PPA was an independent risk factor for hemorrhagic stroke in women prompting the FDA to recommend removal of PPA from the market. Similarly, in response to studies reporting an association between fatalities in children younger than 2 years and pseudoephedrine-containing cough and cold medications, the US FDA required labeling changes warning of this risk.

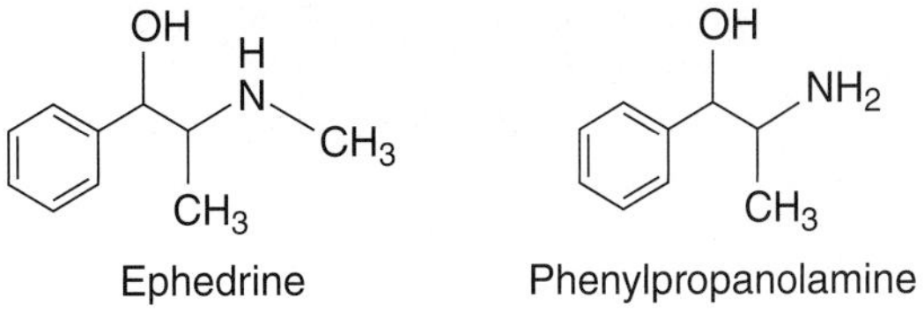

Ephedrine Phenylpropanolamine

**FIGURE 22–3.** Structure of ephedrine and phenylpropanolamine decongestants.

Recreational use of ephedrine-containing stimulants is common, and combinations of these xenobiotics with caffeine or other herbs may be marketed as "herbal ecstasy" (Chap. 16). The sale of dietary supplements containing ephedra was banned by the US FDA in 2004 because of concerns over their cardiovascular effects, including hypertension, seizures, stroke, and dysrhythmias. Since then, many manufacturers have substituted *Citrus aurantium*, whose principal ingredient is *p*-synephrine, and are marketing products as being "ephedra free."

### Pharmacology

Decongestants are divided into two categories: sympathomimetic amines and imidazolines.

***Sympathomimetics.*** The decongestants phenylephrine, pseudoephedrine, ephedrine, and PPA (Fig. 22–3) reduce nasal congestion by stimulating the α-adrenergic receptor sites on vascular smooth muscle (Fig. 22–4). This process constricts dilated arterioles and reduces blood flow to engorged nasal vascular beds. Prolonged topical administration produces rebound congestion upon discontinuation. Some decongestants such as pseudoephedrine and ephedrine are also β-adrenergic receptor agonists.

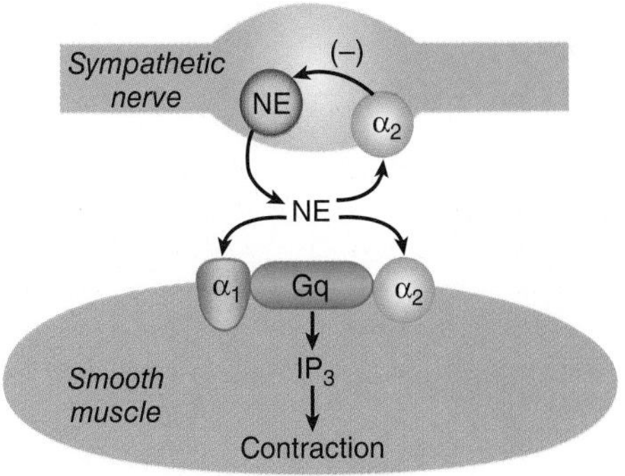


**FIGURE 22–4.** Mechanism of action of the α-adrenergic decongestants. The α-adrenergic decongestants stimulate postsynaptic $\alpha_1$- and $\alpha_2$-adrenergic receptors to increase the concentration of inositol triphosphate ($IP_3$), which mediates vasoconstriction of blood vessels and reduces swollen mucosa. The imidazoline decongestants also bind to postsynaptic $\alpha_2$-adrenergic receptors on these blood vessels.

**TABLE 22–3 Effects of Decongestants**

| | Therapeutic | Duration of Action (h) | Toxic |
|---|---|---|---|
| **Imidazolines** | | | |
| Naphazoline | Nasal decongestant | 8 | Acute: hypertension followed by hypotension, bradycardia, hypoventilation, hypotonia, CNS depression, hallucinations |
| Oxymetazoline | Otorrhea reduction | > 8 | |
| Tetrahydrozoline | Nasal decongestant | 4–8 | |
| Xylometazoline | Nasal decongestant | 5–6 | Chronic: mydriasis from ocular administration |
| **Sympathomimetic** | | | |
| Ephedrine | Nasal decongestant | 3–5 | Hypertension, tachycardia, insomnia, psychosis |
| Phenylephrine | Nasal decongestant, vasopressor | 1 | Hypertension, reflex bradycardia |
| Pseudoephedrine | Nasal decongestant | 3–4 | Hypertension, tachycardia, insomnia, psychosis |

***Imidazolines.*** The imidazolines bind to $\alpha_2$-adrenergic receptors on blood vessels. In addition, these medications have high affinity for imidazoline receptors, which are located in the ventrolateral medulla and some peripheral tissues. Three classes of imidazoline receptors are recognized. Imidazoline$_1$ ($I_1$) receptors mediate the inhibitory actions of imidazoline xenobiotics to lower blood pressure. The imidazoline$_2$ ($I_2$) receptor is an important binding site for monoamine oxidase, and the imidazoline$_3$ ($I_3$) receptor regulates insulin secretion from pancreatic cells. Table 22–3 summarizes the pharmacologic and toxic effects of available decongestants.

The imidazoline (I) category of direct sympathomimetic receptor agonists is generally reserved for topical application in the nasal passages and the eyes. The more common medications include oxymetazoline, tetrahydrozoline, and naphazoline (Fig. 22–5).

## Pharmacokinetics and Toxicokinetics

***Sympathomimetics.*** Absorption from the GI tract is rapid, with peak blood concentrations occurring within 2 to 4 hours of ingestion. They have variable hepatic metabolism via monoamine oxidase and mainly renal elimination. Urinary elimination of pseudoephedrine is pH dependent. Toxic symptoms are an extension of the adverse effects and follow a similar dose–response curve.

***Imidazolines.*** The imidazolines are rapidly absorbed from the GI tract and mucous membranes. Despite their use for many decades, their metabolism is poorly studied. Their elimination half-lives are from 2 to 4 hours. All imidazoline preparations have a relatively rapid onset of action, with 60% of maximum effectiveness occurring after only 20 minutes. Oxymetazoline is the only medication with a duration of action more than 8 hours. The other preparations have an average duration of action of approximately 4 hours. The toxicity of these medications follows a dose–response curve and accentuates the action on receptors.

## Pathophysiology

***Sympathomimetic.*** Sympathomimetic decongestants cause their toxic effects via excessive stimulation of the adrenergic system and in effect produce signs and symptoms associated with the sympathomimetic toxidrome. Excessive vasoconstriction can result in end-organ damage to the brain, retina, heart, and kidneys.

***Imidazolines.*** Imidazolines stimulate imidazoline receptors and produce a sympatholytic effect that in supratherapeutic conditions results in marked bradycardia and hypotension.

## Clinical Manifestations

***Sympathomimetics.*** Ingestions of less than 1 mg/kg of pseudoephedrine in children are reported to produce almost no toxicity and are generally managed conservatively without the need for hospital evaluation. Following an overdose of this class, most patients present with a sympathomimetic syndrome with CNS stimulation, hypertension, tachycardia, or reflex bradycardia in response to pure $\alpha_1$-adrenergic agonist induced hypertension (Chap. 46). In a study of patients with severe manifestations of PPA overdose, headache was the

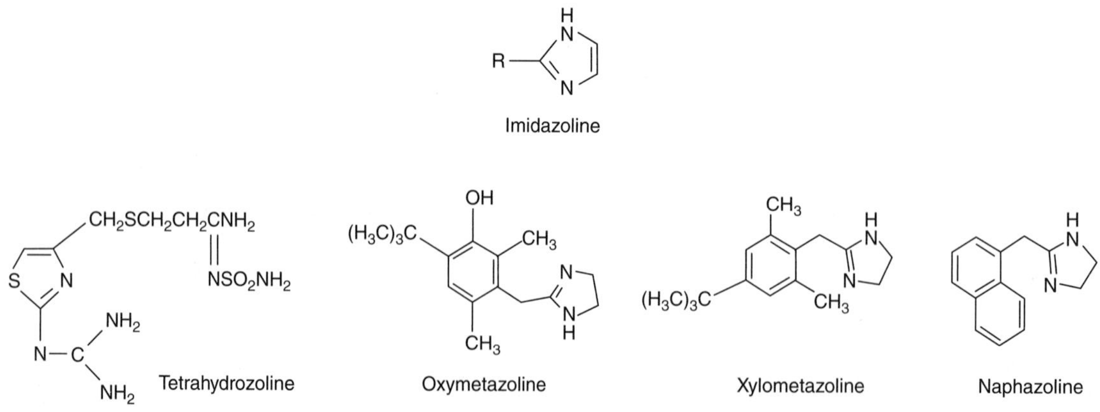

**FIGURE 22–5.** Structure of imidazoline and the imidazoline decongestants.

most common initial symptom (39%). Among the 45 patients who developed hypertensive encephalopathy from PPA ingestion, 24 patients developed intracranial hemorrhages, 15 developed seizures, and 6 died. Seizures, myocardial infarction, bradycardia, atrial and ventricular dysrhythmias, ischemic bowel infarction, and cerebral hemorrhages are reported, even with therapeutic dosing. Psychosis, agitation, and manic behavior are also reported with acute ingestion.

***Imidazolines.*** When ingested, the imidazoline decongestants are potent central and peripheral $\alpha_2$-adrenergic and imidazoline receptor agonists. In overdose, they cause CNS depression, and initial brief hypertension followed by hypotension, bradycardia, and respiratory depression similar to clonidine (Chap. 34). Toxic effects usually resolve within 8 to 16 hours.

## Diagnostic Testing

The bedside diagnosis of decongestant toxicity is a clinical one. Sympathomimetic decongestants cause false-positive results for amphetamines on several rapid urine drug screens by immunoassay.

## Management

Patients presenting after an exposure to decongestants should be triaged promptly and brought to a monitored environment. A cardiac monitor should be attached to the patient and observed for dysrhythmias. Intravenous access should be established, and airway protection ensured. Gastrointestinal decontamination with AC is recommended in patients with large ingestions of pseudoephedrine if no contraindications are present. The decision to give AC in these instances should be made individually because liquid formulations are rapidly absorbed and might not be amenable to AC adsorption by the time of presentation. Activated charcoal administration is reasonable even several hours after ingestion of sustained-release decongestant preparations. More than one dose of AC is reasonable to complete GI decontamination in massive ingestion of oral preparations, but multidose AC for enhanced elimination purposes has no role. Whole-bowel irrigation and renal-enhanced elimination techniques are not indicated.

## Specific Treatment

*Neurologic toxicity.* Patients with extreme agitation, seizures, and psychosis should initially be treated with administration of oxygen and IV benzodiazepines, titrated upward to effect. A patient with a persistent headache, focal neurologic deficits, or abnormal neuropsychiatric findings after decongestant ingestion should be evaluated for cerebral hemorrhage by noncontrast head CT. If the timing of the imaging is delayed, reducing the sensitivity of this modality, subsequent lumbar puncture to exclude subarachnoid hemorrhage is reasonable based on clinical suspicion.

*Respiratory toxicity.* Children presenting with respiratory depression from imidazoline decongestants have responded to naloxone. These case reports are too few to establish the efficacy of this therapy. Nevertheless, the use of naloxone in imidazoline toxicity is reasonable and low risk in non–opioid-dependent patients.

*Cardiovascular toxicity.* Tachycardia, palpitations, and hypertension that occur in mild sympathomimetic poisonings usually respond to benzodiazepines. For a patient who remains hypertensive or is believed to have chest pain of ischemic origin, treatment with phentolamine, an α-adrenergic antagonist, or nicardipine is recommended. β-Adrenergic antagonists should be avoided because of concern for unopposed α-adrenergic effects. An ECG is required, and any ST segment elevation warrants immediate consultation with a cardiologist. Patients with ventricular dysrhythmias from sympathomimetic decongestants should be treated with standard doses of lidocaine or sodium bicarbonate if the QRS complex is prolonged. Phenylpropanolamine causes hypertension with a reflex bradycardia and atrioventricular block that is responsive to standard doses of atropine. Atropine must be used with caution because it can cause a dangerous increase in blood pressure as the reflex bradycardia reverses. Therefore, a vasodilator such as phentolamine is recommended because the stimulus for the bradycardia is corrected with reversal of the hypertension.

Imidazoline-induced hypertension rarely requires therapy, but in the setting of symptomatic hypertension, a short-acting α-adrenergic antagonist such as phentolamine is reasonable. The hypertension is generally transient and followed by hypotension. Initial antihypertensive therapy could exacerbate toxicity and should only be reserved for cases in which severe hypertension represents a true urgency for end-organ damage.

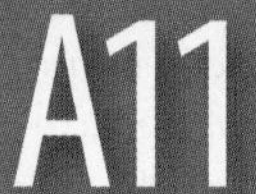

# A11 PHYSOSTIGMINE SALICYLATE

## INTRODUCTION

Physostigmine is a carbamate that reversibly inhibits cholinesterases in both the peripheral and central nervous system (CNS). The tertiary amine structure of physostigmine permits CNS penetration and differentiates it from neostigmine and pyridostigmine, which are quaternary amines that have limited ability to enter the CNS. The inhibition of cholinesterases prevents the metabolism of acetylcholine, allowing acetylcholine to accumulate and antagonize the antimuscarinic effects of xenobiotics.

## HISTORY

The history of physostigmine dates to antiquity and the Efik people of Old Calabar in Nigeria where the chiefs used the poisonous beans in a ritual to test the innocence or guilt of an accused person. Innocent people quickly swallowed the beans, vomited resulting in decontamination. The guilty people hesitated and developed severe toxicity from sublingual absorption. Physostigmine, the active ingredient of these beans, was subsequently instrumental in the development of a bioassay for acetylcholine, concepts of neurohumoral transmission, mapping of cholinergic nerves, the concept of antagonism, the kinetics of enzyme inhibition, and an improved understanding of the blood–brain barrier. Physostigmine was first used as an antidote in 1864 to counteract severe atropine poisoning.

## PHARMACOLOGY

### Chemistry

Physostigmine salicylate is the salicylate salt of physostigmine, a carbamate cholinesterase inhibitor. Naturally occurring physostigmine consists of a racemic mixture with the (−) isomer being greater than 100 times more potent in inhibiting acetylcholinesterase. Physostigmine is a tertiary amine, unlike other medicinal carbamate cholinesterase inhibitors (such as neostigmine), which allows it to effectively cross the blood–brain barrier.

### Mechanism of Action

Physostigmine is both a substrate and a reversible inhibitor of acetylcholinesterase. Whereas following acetylcholine metabolism enzyme reactivation is extremely rapid, the process is much slower for physostigmine, resulting in short-term inhibition. Newer xenobiotics used in the treatment of Alzheimer disease show selectivity for the CNS and for acetylcholinesterase. This group includes tacrine, donepezil, and galantamine, which are reversible cholinesterase inhibitors, and rivastigmine, considered a pseudo-irreversible or slowly reversible inhibitor. These pharmaceuticals have undergone limited study for reversal of patients with anticholinergic poisoning.

## PHARMACOKINETICS AND PHARMACODYNAMICS

Physostigmine is poorly absorbed orally, with a bioavailability of less than 5% to 12%. Mean pharmacokinetic parameters following IV administration demonstrate the following: $V_d$ 2.4 ± 0.6 L/kg; $t_{1/2}$ 16.4 ± 3.2 minutes; peak plasma concentration 3 ± 0.5 ng/mL; and clearance 0.1 L/min/kg. Plasma cholinesterases are inhibited within 2 minutes of initiating the physostigmine infusion; the half-life of inhibition is 83.7 ± 5.2 minutes, with full recovery within 3 hours of the termination of the physostigmine infusion. Thus, the effects on plasma cholinesterase inhibition last about 5 times longer than the half-life of physostigmine.

## ROLE IN ANTIMUSCARINIC TOXICITY

Because of its ability to cause CNS arousal, physostigmine was used in the 1970s to reverse the CNS effects of a large number of anticholinergic xenobiotics appropriately as well as inappropriately to treat toxicity from nonanticholinergic xenobiotics. More than 600 xenobiotics were reported to respond to physostigmine. However, its major limitation was best defined when asystole was reported to follow physostigmine administration in patients with tricyclic antidepressant overdose. A reevaluation concluded that the risks of physostigmine use for xenobiotics that are not primarily antimuscarinic outweigh any benefit. In contrast, in the case of anticholinergic overdose, the use of physostigmine is clearly beneficial.

When compared with benzodiazepines, physostigmine was better at controlling agitation and reversing delirium, as well as shortening recovery time. A study of 52 patients showed that whereas benzodiazepines controlled agitation in 24% of patients and were ineffective in reversing delirium, physostigmine controlled agitation and reversed delirium in 96% and 87% of patients, respectively.

We recommend the use of physostigmine in the presence of peripheral or central antimuscarinic manifestations without evidence of significant QRS complex prolongation. Peripheral manifestations of antimuscarinic toxicity include dry mucosa, dry skin, flushed face, mydriasis, hyperthermia, decreased bowel sounds, urinary retention, and tachycardia. Central manifestations include agitation, delirium, hallucinations, seizures, and coma. The peripheral and central clinical findings are usually both present. Rarely, the central findings may persist longer than the peripheral findings or be more prominent.

## ADVERSE EFFECTS AND SAFETY ISSUES

An excess of physostigmine results in the accumulation of acetylcholine at peripheral muscarinic receptors, nicotinic receptors (skeletal muscle, autonomic ganglia, adrenal glands), and CNS sites. Muscarinic effects produce the stimulation of smooth muscle and glandular secretions in the respiratory, gastrointestinal, and genitourinary tracts and the inhibition of contraction of most vascular smooth musculature. Nicotinic effects are stimulatory at low doses and depressant at high doses. For example, acetylcholine excess at the neuromuscular junction produces fasciculations followed by weakness and paralysis. The effect on the CNS results in anxiety, dizziness, tremors, confusion, ataxia, coma, and seizures. Because of this, we do not recommend administering physostigmine to patients with reactive airway disease, peripheral vascular disease, intestinal or bladder obstruction, intraventricular conduction defects, and atrioventricular block or in patients receiving succinylcholine as they are at great risk for clinically significant adverse effects. In the event that a patient becomes clinically cholinergic due to an excess of physostigmine, they should be managed with intravenous atropine titrated to reverse bronchial secretions and intensive supportive care including mechanical ventilation if needed.

## PREGNANCY AND LACTATION

Physostigmine is United States (US) Food and Drug Administration pregnancy category C. Transient muscular weakness occurred in 10% to 20% of neonates whose mothers received anticholinesterase treatment for myasthenia gravis. Physostigmine should only be given when the benefit clearly outweighs the risk. Safety in lactation is not established.

## DOSING AND ADMINISTRATION

The dose of physostigmine is 1 to 2 mg in adults and 0.02 mg/kg (maximum: 0.5 mg) in children, intravenously infused over at least 5 minutes. The onset of action is usually within several minutes. This dose can be repeated in 10 to 15 minutes if an adequate response is not achieved and muscarinic effects are not noted. Although a total of 4 mg in divided doses is usually sufficient in most clinical situations, significant interindividual variability exists. Rapid administration may cause bradycardia, hypersalivation leading to respiratory difficulty, and possibly seizures. Atropine should be at the bedside and should be titrated to effect should excessive cholinergic toxicity develop. If atropine is needed, we recommend a starting dose of one-half the physostigmine dose. At the present time, physostigmine is unavailable in the US and many clinicians are using rivastigmine.

## FORMULATION AND ACQUSITION

Physostigmine is available in 2-mL ampules with each milliliter containing 1 mg of physostigmine salicylate. The vehicle contains sodium bisulfite and benzyl alcohol.

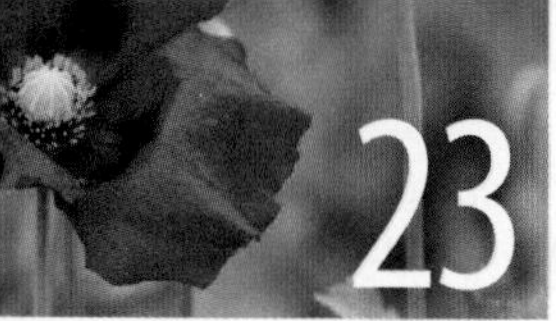

# 23 CHEMOTHERAPEUTICS

Chemotherapeutics or antineoplastics are a unique class of pharmaceuticals commonly used to kill cancer cells. In the last several years, the use of chemotherapeutics has changed as therapeutic indications now include other nonneoplastic diseases, and many medications are administered orally or through novel delivery techniques. Although overdoses of chemotherapeutics are infrequent, these events are of greater consequence than overdoses of many other xenobiotics because many of these drugs have a narrow therapeutic index.

## PATIENT-SPECIFIC FACTORS CONTRIBUTING TO TOXICITY

Aside from unintentional exposures, factors leading to increased toxicity associated with chemotherapeutics include age, sex, comorbidities, compromised host condition, and diminished kidney or liver function. Differences in sex contribute to varying pharmacokinetic parameters, including bioavailability, distribution, metabolism, and elimination. Women treated with 5-fluorouracil (5-FU) for colon cancer had a twofold higher frequency of drug-related toxicity than men. At an individual level, genetic polymorphisms can contribute to differences in xenobiotic responses with resultant toxicity by altering targets, transporters, and enzyme complexes. Two examples of this type of toxicity include irinotecan used for the treatment of metastatic colon cancer and 5-FU used for the treatment of certain types of gastrointestinal (GI) and breast cancers. Irinotecan is a topoisomerase I inhibitor that works through its active metabolite, SN-38, which causes diarrhea and neutropenia at elevated concentrations. A genetic variant of uridine diphosphate glucuronosyltransferase (UGT1A1) glucuronidates SN-38 at a slower rate than other variants, which increases SN-38 concentrations and toxicity. 5-FU, which is an antagonist to uracil, is inactivated by dihydropyrimidine dehydrogenase (DPD) in the liver. Low or absent activity of this enzyme results in hematologic and GI toxicities from treatment with 5-FU or its prodrug capecitabine. A genetic variant produces an inactive enzyme, and patients homozygous for this allele are at risk for severe toxicity and advised to seek an alternative therapeutic.

## CLASSES OF CHEMOTHERAPEUTICS

Most chemotherapeutics are grouped into one of five categories as shown in Table 23–1. Some newer chemotherapeutics target specific proteins located on the cell membrane, such as growth factor receptors, to inhibit the proliferation of tumor cells (Fig. 23–1). These chemotherapeutics are categorized as monoclonal antibodies and protein kinase inhibitors based on their mechanisms of action.

## MECHANISMS OF ACTION

The mechanisms responsible for the cytotoxic effects of the chemotherapeutics are the disruption of cellular growth and proliferation, which impairs DNA function by causing strand breaks, inhibiting strand relaxation, and serving as inhibitory analogs of essential cofactors and nitrogenous bases of nucleic acids (Fig. 23–2).

## MANIFESTATIONS OF TOXICITY

The chemotherapeutics are primarily toxic to cells, with a high level of mitotic activity, such as hematopoietic and intestinal epithelial cells. This characteristic feature accounts for their common clinical manifestations of toxicity, including mucositis, alopecia, and bone marrow suppression. They also cause protracted vomiting because they stimulate the chemoreceptor trigger zone in the medulla by vagal and sympathetic pathways either directly or indirectly through the GI tract. Although the onset of emesis typically occurs within 6 hours and lasts for 24 hours, delayed or persistent (> 24 hours since administration) emesis occurs with cisplatin, cyclophosphamide, carboplatin, and doxorubicin. The onset of other manifestations is typically in the first week following treatment, with mucositis preceding leukopenia.

Dermatologic manifestations caused by chemotherapeutics include hypersensitivity reactions, extravasations (Special Considerations: SC7), and cytotoxicity from the use of tyrosine kinase inhibitors for the epidermal growth factor receptor (EGFR) (eg, gefitinib, erlotinib). Patients commonly develop pruritus, xerosis, erythema, and folliculitis or an acneiform rash that can desquamate during therapy. These reactions develop within the first week of treatment and continue for several weeks. The folliculitis is a dose-dependent response and typically resolves within weeks after treatment. The dermal response is more intense with monoclonal antibodies than the kinase inhibitors for the EGFR. The other kinase inhibitors (ie, sunitinib, sorafenib) involved with growth factor receptors for angiogenesis (ie, vascular endothelial growth factor receptor {VEGFR}, platelet-derived growth factor receptor {PDGFR}) are associated with a "hand-foot" skin reaction, which is a painful erythema and edema of the palm and sole that leads to desquamation.

The common cardiovascular manifestations include congestive heart failure (CHF), dysrhythmias, and hypertension. The anthracyclines, cyclophosphamide, 5-FU, and arsenic trioxide are examples of chemotherapeutics that cause cardiac toxicity (Table 23–2). Arsenic trioxide ($As_2O_3$), which is used for the treatment of acute promyelocytic leukemia, causes dose-dependent prolongation of the QT interval and ventricular tachydysrhythmias, including torsade de pointes, during the course of treatment.

The neurologic toxicities of chemotherapeutics include alterations in mental status and seizures, which occur from the systemic administration of high doses of nitrogen mustards (cyclophosphamide, ifosfamide, and chlorambucil), nitrosoureas (lomustine), methotrexate, and vincristine. L-Asparaginase, 5-FU, and procarbazine. Cerebellar dysfunction is described in 5% of patients treated with 5-FU, and

**TABLE 23–1 Classification of Chemotherapeutics, Their Adverse Effects, and Antidotal Therapy**

| *Class* | *Antineoplastic* | *Adverse Effects* | *Overdose* | *Antidotes* |
|---|---|---|---|---|
| Alkylating agents | Busulphan | Hyperpigmentation, pulmonary fibrosis, hyperuricemia | Myelosuppression | |
| | Dacarbazine | Hypotension, hepatocellular toxicity, influenzalike illness | | |
| | Nitrogen mustards | | | |
| | Chlorambucil, cyclophosphamide, ifosfamide, mechlorethamine, melphalan | Hemorrhagic cystitis, encephalopathy, pulmonary fibrosis | Seizures, encephalopathy, myocardial necrosis, acute kidney injury, hyponatremia | MESNA; methylene blue |
| | Nitrosoureas | | | |
| | Carmustine, lomustine, semustine, streptozocin | Pulmonary fibrosis, hepatocellular toxicity, acute kidney injury | Myelosuppression (delayed onset and prolonged duration) | |
| | Procarbazine | Inhibition of monoamine oxidase (MAOI) | | |
| | Temozolomide | | Myelosuppression | |
| Antibiotics | Anthracycline | | | |
| | Daunorubicin, doxorubicin, epirubicin, idarubicin | Dilated congestive cardiomyopathy | Dysrhythmias, cardiomyopathy, CHF, myelosuppression | Dexrazoxane |
| | Bleomycin | Pulmonary fibrosis | | |
| | Dactinomycin | Hepatocellular toxicity | | |
| | Mitomycin C | Hemolytic uremic syndrome | | |
| | Mitoxantrone | Dilated cardiomyopathy | Cardiomyopathy, CHF | None |
| Antimetabolites | Methotrexate | Mucositis, nausea, diarrhea, hepatocellular toxicity | Mucositis, myelosuppression, acute kidney injury | Folinic acid; glucarpidase (carboxypeptidase-$G_2$) |
| | Purine analogs | | | |
| | Fludarabine | Encephalopathy, muscle weakness | | |
| | Mercaptopurine | Hyperuricemia, pancreatitis, cholestasis | Myelosuppression, hepatocellular toxicity | |
| | Pentostatin | Hepatocellular toxicity | | |
| | Thioguanine | Hyperuricemia | | |
| | Pyrimidine analogs | | | |
| | Cytarabine | Acute respiratory distress syndrome, neuropathy, cerebellar ataxia | | |
| | Fluorouracil, capecitabine | Cardiogenic shock, cardiomyopathy, cerebellar ataxia, diarrhea, mucositis, myelosuppression, neuropathy | Mucositis, myelosuppression, myocardial ischemia, cardiac conduction disorders | Uridine triacetate |
| Antimitotics | Taxanes | | | None |
| | Docetaxel, paclitaxel | GI perforation, peripheral neuropathy, dysrhythmias | | |
| | Vinca alkaloids | | | |
| | Vinblastine, vincristine, vindesine | Peripheral neuropathy, hyponatremia (SIADH) | Encephalopathy, seizures, autonomic instability, paralytic ileus, myelosuppression | |
| Enzyme | L-Asparaginase | Hypersensitivity, pancreatitis, and coagulopathy | No reports | None |
| Monoclonal antibodies | Many: Gemtuzumab, trastuzumab | Hypersensitivity, specific to the site of action, and infection | No reports | None |
| Platinum-based complexes | Cisplatin, carboplatin, oxaliplatin | Acute kidney injury, peripheral neuropathy, hypomagnesemia, hypocalcemia, hyponatremia, ototoxicity, myelosuppression | Seizures, encephalopathy, ototoxicity, retinal toxicity, myelosuppression, peripheral neuropathy | Amifostine; thiosulfate |
| Protein kinase inhibitors | Many: Gefitinib, sorafenib, erlotinib | GI (nausea, diarrhea), acneiform rash (folliculitis), nail fragility, and xerosis (EGFR inhibitor), interstitial lung disease (erlotinib, gefitinib), hypertension (inhibitors of VEGF and PDGFR), hypothyroidism (sunitinib), and infection | Nausea, vomiting, facial rash, and edema | None |

*(Continued)*

| TABLE 23–1 Classification of Chemotherapeutics, Their Adverse Effects, and Antidotal Therapy (*Continued*) | | | | |
|---|---|---|---|---|
| ***Class*** | ***Antineoplastic*** | ***Adverse Effects*** | ***Overdose*** | ***Antidotes*** |
| Topoisomerase inhibitor | Camptothecins | Neutropenia, mucositis, diarrhea, early onset cholinergic syndrome (irinotecan) | Myelosuppression | None |
| | Irinotecan | | | |
| | Topotecan | | | |
| | Epipodophyllotoxins | | | |
| | Etoposide, teniposide | CHF, hypotension | | |

CHF = congestive heart failure; EGFR = epidermal growth factor receptor; GI = gastrointestinal; MESNA= mercaptoethane sulfonate; MAOI = monoamine oxidase inhibitor; PDGFR = platelet-derived growth factor receptor; SIADH = syndrome of inappropriate antidiuretic hormone; VEGF = vascular endothelial growth factor.

high-frequency ototoxicity occurs with cisplatin toxicity. The delayed-onset manifestations of neurotoxicity from chemotherapeutics include leukoencephalopathy and peripheral neuropathies. Leukoencephalopathy from methotrexate typically presents as behavioral and progressive dementia and is irreversible. Peripheral neuropathy involving both sensory and motor findings occurs with the vinca alkaloids (vincristine) and bortezomib, whereas only sensory involvement is noted with cisplatin and paclitaxel.

Kidney failure occurs from methotrexate, cisplatin, ifosfamide, or nitrosoureas in a dose-dependent manner. The nitrosoureas such as semustine can cause glomerular injury leading to sclerosis. Kidney damage is attributed to the formation of insoluble intratubular precipitates of drug metabolites (methotrexate) or reactive intermediates (cisplatin, nitrosoureas) that lead to cell death.

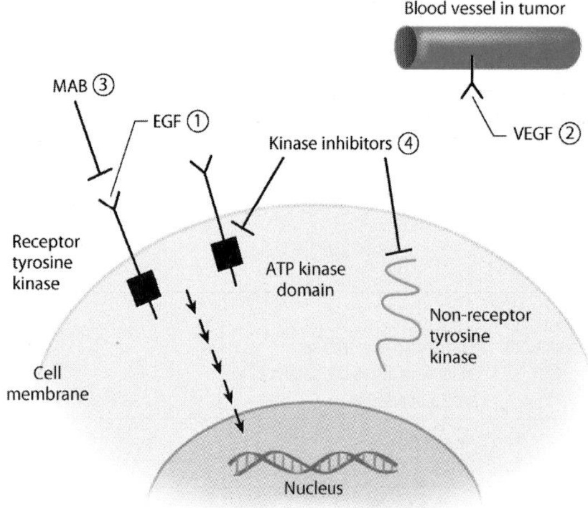


**FIGURE 23–1.** Sites of action of selected targeted agents. Tyrosine kinases initiate signal transduction pathways and production of transcription factors that are responsible for cellular processes, including proliferation, survival, angiogenesis, and progression. Growth factors, such as endothelial growth factor (EGF) and vascular endothelial growth factor (VEGF), bind and activate transmembrane tyrosine kinases by causing receptor dimerization and phosphorylation (1). VEGF promotes endothelial cell mitogenesis and migration, which leads to vascular proliferation (2). Tyrosine kinases are inhibited by monoclonal antibody (MAB) binding at the cell surface receptor site (3) or by kinase inhibitors at the adenine triphosphate (ATP) binding site or substrate-binding site, or by causing a change in the conformation of the enzyme (NIB) (4).

## DIAGNOSTIC TESTING

The determination of a chemotherapeutic concentration in a clinical specimen is not routinely available, except for methotrexate. For certain chemotherapeutics, the presence of typical clinical manifestations strongly suggests their toxicity, for example, cisplatin (acute kidney injury and ototoxicity), vinca alkaloids (peripheral neuropathy, central autonomic instability), anthracyclines (CHF and dilated cardiomyopathy), ifosfamide (encephalopathy and seizures), and methotrexate (acute kidney injury, mucositis, and pancytopenia). The diagnosis of a patient with toxicity from these xenobiotics is therefore based on historical evidence for exposure, clinical manifestations, and laboratory findings that support toxicity or exposure. For patients presenting with delayed symptoms, the association between toxicity and exposure requires an increased level of awareness to establish the causation.

## GENERAL MANAGEMENT

The initial management of these patients includes stabilization of the hemodynamic status, decontamination, institution of antidotal therapy, and enhanced elimination. Maximal benefits from antidotes and enhanced elimination can be obtained through their timely institution. Hypotension typically results from salt and water depletion, cardiac dysfunction, or sepsis. It is reasonable to treat patients with myocardial ischemia from 5-FU with coronary vasodilators, such as nitrates and calcium channel blockers. Seizures are treated with benzodiazepines and propofol. Encephalopathy from high-dose ifosfamide has been treated with methylene blue (Antidotes in Brief: A43). Patients with blood dyscrasias, including neutropenia and thrombocytopenia, should be evaluated for GI bleeding and infections. Those at risk for overwhelming sepsis should be started on broad-spectrum antibiotics and granulocyte colony-stimulating factor as indicated. Oral activated charcoal is recommended for patients who present soon after an oral exposure to limit the GI bioavailability of the chemotherapeutic.

Patients with chemotherapeutic-related vomiting are typically difficult to manage. Combination therapy involving multiple antiemetics is needed to treat patients exposed to chemotherapeutics with high emetogenic potential (eg, cisplatin, doxorubicin, cyclophosphamide, lomustine) or excessive doses of chemotherapeutics with low emetogenic

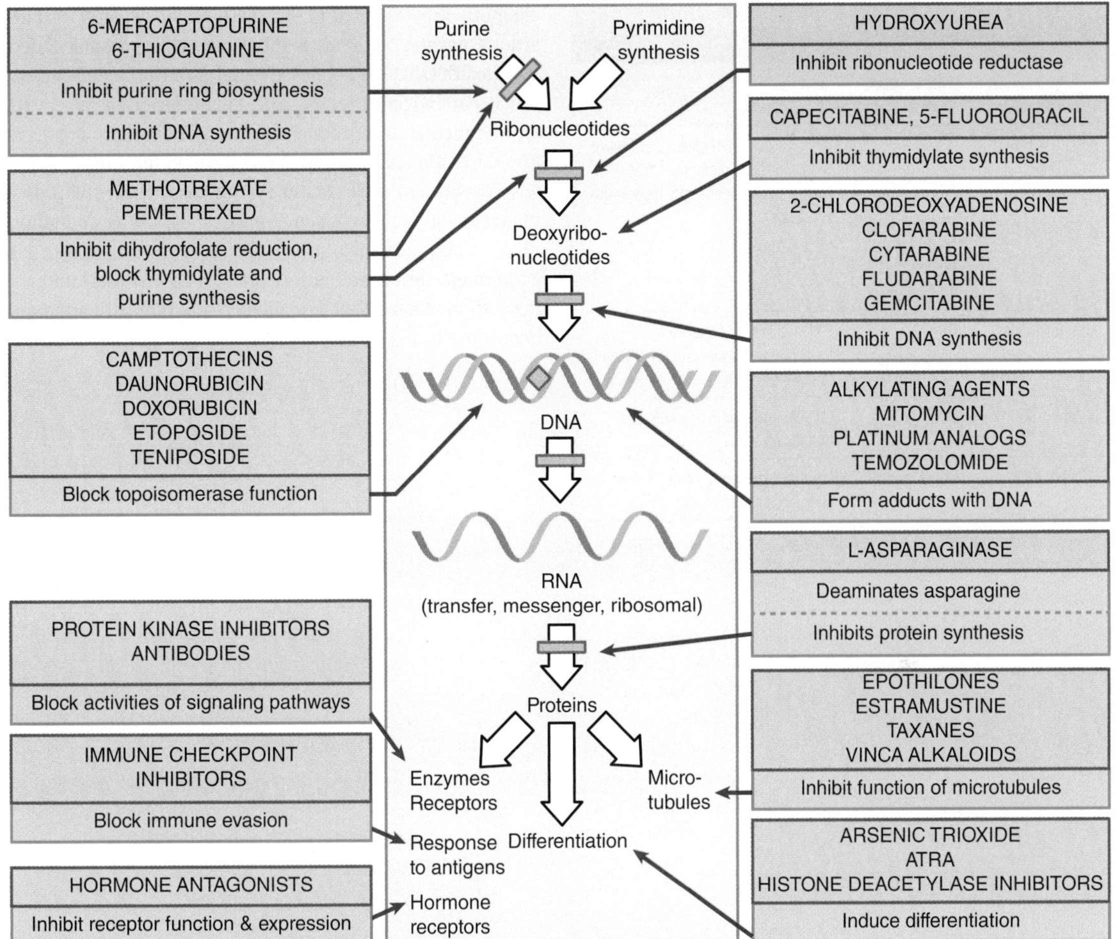


**FIGURE 23–2.** Summary of the mechanisms and sites of action of some chemotherapeutics useful in neoplastic disease. ATRA = all-*trans* retinoic acid. *(Reproduced with permission from Brunton LL, Hilal-Dandan R, Knollmann BC. Goodman & Gilman's: The Pharmacological Basis of Therapeutics, 13th ed. New York, NY: McGraw Hill Education; 2018.)*

potential (eg, vinca alkaloids, 5-FU). Recommended therapies include serotonin receptor antagonists, corticosteroids, dopamine receptor antagonists, NK1 receptor antagonists, or a benzodiazepine.

A basic chemistry panel, complete blood count, urinalysis, and ECG should be obtained for patients with a significant overdose to evaluate toxicity and to establish baseline values. Pregnant women exposed to chemotherapeutics require individualized care that includes consultations with an obstetrician-gynecologist, neonatologist, or a medical oncologist. The patient's peripheral blood count should be followed for up to 2 weeks after a chemotherapeutic is administered because of the delayed onset of myelosuppression.

Gastrointestinal fluid losses can lead to salt and water depletion, which should be treated with intravenous fluids. Patients with cisplatin toxicity should be treated with 0.9% sodium chloride and an osmotic diuretic to maintain an adequate chloride gradient to promote the renal elimination of cisplatin. Urinary alkalinization is recommended for patients with methotrexate toxicity to limit the precipitation of drug metabolites in the renal tubules.

Antidotal therapy is available for only a few xenobiotics, including anthracyclines (dexrazoxane), methotrexate (leucovorin, glucarpidase), cisplatin (amifostine, thiosulfate), 5-FU or capecitabine (uridine triacetate), and ifosfamide (methylene blue, mercaptoethane sulfonate). Additional information regarding these antidotes is found in Chap. 24 and Antidotes in Brief: A12, A13, A14, and A43. Consultation with a hematologist, oncologist, and/or toxicologist is always reasonable to assist with these uncommon cases.

## CHEMOTHERAPEUTICS IN THE WORKPLACE

Pharmacists, nurses, physicians, and others involved in the preparation and dispensing of chemotherapeutics, and those who may be exposed to the body fluids of patients treated with chemotherapeutics, are at increased risk for toxicity. Absorption of these xenobiotics occurs by either the dermal, inhalational, or GI route. The workplace guidelines for

**TABLE 23–2 Cardiovascular Manifestations of Toxicity of Selected Chemotherapeutics**

| *Chemotherapeutic* | *Time of Onset Since Treatment* | *Manifestation* |
|---|---|---|
| Anthracycline | < 24 hours | Dysrhythmias, ST-segment and T-wave changes on ECG; diminished LVEF leading to CHF, pericarditis, myocarditis, and sudden death |
| | Months to years, typically at 1–4 months | Dilated congestive cardiomyopathy |
| Arsenic trioxide | Days | Prolongation of QT interval on ECG leading to ventricular tachydysrhythmias (torsade de pointes) |
| Cyclophosphamide | Days | CHF, hemorrhagic pericarditis, and tamponade |
| 5-Fluorouracil | Hours to days | Myocardial ischemia, cardiac conduction disorders, and cardiogenic shock |

CHF = congestive heart failure, ECG = electrocardiogram; LVEF = left ventricular ejection fraction.

chemotherapeutics fall under the broader category of hazardous agents. National Institute for Occupational Safety and Health (NIOSH) defines a "drug" as a "hazardous agent" if it is carcinogenic, teratogenic, genotoxic, associated with developmental or reproductive toxicity, or toxic to organs at low dose. The current recommendations for worker safety with these xenobiotics at the workplace include the proper management of the work environment (eg, storage, handling, preparation, administration, use of personal protection equipment, decontamination, and waste disposal) and the institution of a medical surveillance program with approved laboratory testing.

# 24 METHOTREXATE, 5-FLUOROURACIL, AND CAPECITABINE

Methotrexate and the fluoropyrimidines (5-fluorouracil and capecitabine) are antimetabolite chemotherapeutics that produce significant and potentially fatal toxicity. Clinicians must rapidly recognize poisoned patients and be prepared to provide immediate interventions that include specific antidotal therapies. The oral formulations of methotrexate and capecitabine present a risk for intentional or unintentional chemotherapeutic ingestions in the home.

## METHOTREXATE

Methotrexate (MTX) is used for many malignant conditions, for termination of pregnancy, and as an immunosuppresant for rheumatoid arthritis, organ transplantation, psoriasis, and trophoblastic diseases. Risk factors for MTX toxicity include impaired kidney function, third compartment spacing, folate deficiency, and concurrent infection. Methotrexate toxicity depends on the dose but even more on the duration of exposure.

### Pharmacology

The chemotherapeutic and toxic effects of MTX are based on its ability to limit DNA and RNA synthesis by inhibiting dihydrofolate reductase (DHFR) and thymidylate synthetase (Fig. 24–1). Methotrexate, a structural analog of folate, competitively inhibits DHFR by binding to the enzymatic site of action. The antiinflammatory effect of MTX likely involves the following mechanisms: (1) inhibition of trans-methylation (by depletion of intracellular folate stores), which causes the death of T cells and inhibits the formation of polyamines (spermine and spermidine) that are involved in the inflammatory cascade; (2) reduction in the intracellular concentration of glutathione; and (3) inhibition of intracellular 5-aminoimidazole-4-carboxamide ribonucleotide (AICAR) transformylase, which ultimately leads to an increased extracellular concentration of adenosine.

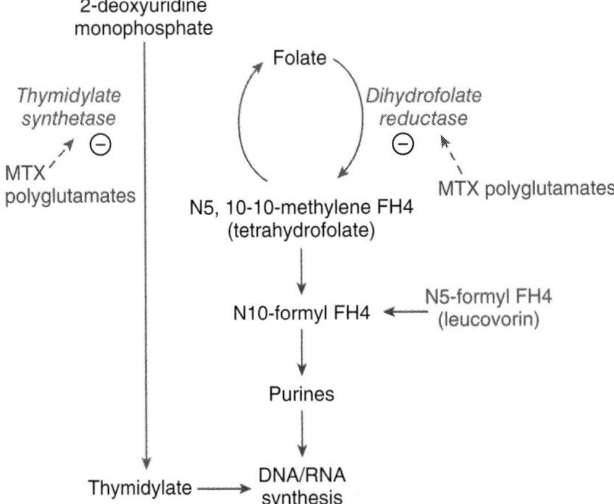


**FIGURE 24–1.** Mechanism of MTX toxicity. Methotrexate inhibits dihydrofolate reductase activity, which is necessary for DNA and RNA synthesis. Leucovorin bypasses blockade to allow for continued synthesis. MTX = methotrexate.

The bioavailability of MTX is limited by a saturable intestinal absorption mechanism. At oral doses less than 30 mg/m$^2$, the absorption is 90% and the peak plasma MTX concentration is achieved at 1 to 2 hours. At oral doses greater than 30 mg/m$^2$, bioavailability significantly decreases. For example, at doses greater than 80 mg/m$^2$, the absorption is less than 20%. Intravenous therapy is required when high concentrations of the drug are indicated. The volume of distribution is 0.6 to 0.9 L/kg and protein binding is 50%. Healthy kidneys eliminate 50% to 80% of MTX unchanged within 48 hours of administration. When the creatinine clearance is less than 60 mL/min, MTX clearance is delayed. Ten percent to 30% of MTX is eliminated unchanged in the bile, which contributes to enterohepatic circulation of the chemotherapeutic. In the setting of kidney failure, the half-life of MTX is prolonged by the recirculation of MTX in the gut.

Hepatic aldehyde oxidase metabolizes a minor portion (< 10%) of MTX to 7-hydroxy methotrexate (7-OH-MTX), which inhibits DHFR but to a lesser extent than MTX. Another metabolite is 2,4-diamino-*N*(10)-methylpteroic acid (DAMPA), and it accounts for less than 5% of MTX. In the gut, bacterial carboxypeptidase acts on MTX to form DAMPA, which is reabsorbed into the blood compartment. Approximately 50% of DAMPA is eliminated unchanged by the kidneys.

### Pathophysiology

At high doses, MTX and the insoluble drug metabolites 7-OH-MTX and DAMPA accumulate and precipitate in the renal tubules, causing reversible acute tubular necrosis. Methotrexate is one-tenth as soluble at a pH of 5.5 as it is at a pH of 7.5. Thus, patients who are either inadequately hydrated or not alkalinized are at risk for acute kidney failure. The threshold concentration for MTX in plasma that inhibits DNA synthesis is lower for intestinal epithelial cells (0.005 μmol/L) than for hematopoietic cells (0.01 μmol/L) by one order of magnitude. Thus, patients with a significant exposure to MTX will develop gastrointestinal (GI) toxicity before bone marrow toxicity.

The decreased production of reduced folates and diminished folate content in the hepatocyte likely contribute to injury, which leads to hepatic fibrosis from the stimulation of hepatic stellate cells by adenosine. Patients on long-term therapy with MTX who also have elevated aminotransferases can develop hepatic fibrosis from persistent injury to the liver.

### Clinical Manifestations

The clinical manifestations of MTX toxicity include stomatitis, esophagitis, kidney failure, myelosuppression, hepatitis, and central neurologic system dysfunction. Nausea and vomiting, considered rare from cancer therapy with MTX at 40 mg/m$^2$, typically begin 2 to 4 hours after high-dose therapy (1,000 mg/m$^2$) and last for about 6 to 12 hours. Mucositis, characterized by mouth soreness, stomatitis, or diarrhea, usually occurs in the first week of therapy and can last for 4 to 7 days. Hepatocellular toxicity, is usually associated with high-dose regimens, and aspartate aminotranferase (AST) and alanine aminotransferase (ALT) will begin to rise within 1 to 3 days following an exposure. Laboratory abnormalities improve within 1 to 2 weeks of discontinuation of MTX. Pancytopenia usually occurs within the first 2 weeks after an acute exposure. At IV doses greater than 5,000 mg/m$^2$ (approximately 130 mg/kg for an adult), severe kidney injury with oliguria, azotemia, and kidney failure is reported. Patients at risk for nephrotoxicity include the elderly, those with underlying kidney disease defined as a glomerular filtration rate of less than 60 mL/min, and those who receive concurrent drug therapy that can delay MTX excretion, which includes xenobiotics that reduce renal blood flow such as nonsteroidal antiinflammatory drugs (NSAIDs), the nephrotoxins such as cisplatin, and the aminoglycosides, or weak organic acids such as salicylates and piperacillin that inhibit renal secretion. The incidence of neurologic toxicity from high-dose MTX therapy is approximately 5% to 15%. Manifestations usually occur from hours to days after the initiation of therapy and include hemiparesis, paraparesis, quadriparesis, seizures, and dysreflexia. Clinical findings usually occurring within 12 hours of intrathecal therapy are attributed to chemical arachnoiditis, and they include acute onset of fever, meningismus, pleocytosis, and increased cerebrospinal fluid (CSF) protein concentration. Leukoencephalopathy is associated with the onset of behavioral disorders and progressive dementia from months to years after treatment. Patients with leukoencephalopathy have findings consistent with edema and demyelination or necrosis of the white matter on computed tomography (CT) and magnetic resonance imaging (MRI) of the brain.

### Diagnostic Testing

Plasma MTX concentrations are monitored during therapy to limit clinical toxicity. Patients with a plasma concentration greater than 1.0 μmol/L at 48 hours posttreatment are considered at risk for bone marrow and GI mucosal toxicities. There are several analytical methods available to measure the serum concentration of MTX. The primary advantage of the high-performance liquid chromatography with ultraviolet detection (HPLC-UVD) is its ability to measure MTX independent of DAMPA. This is especially important when patients are treated with glucarpidase (carboxypeptidase $G_2$) (Antidotes in Brief: A13). An elevated cerebrospinal fluid (CSF) methotrexate concentration (> 100 μmol/L) is indicative of an excessive intrathecal dose or CSF outflow obstruction.

### Management

The initial approach to the patient exposed to MTX is to determine whether the exposure is acute or chronic because the priorities are different for these patients. A patient with chronic MTX toxicity is more likely to die from overwhelming sepsis than the patient with an acute exposure because the former patient typically presents with bone marrow suppression and severe gastroenteritis. The patient with an acute exposure to MTX typically presents early after an oral exposure and is asymptomatic. The essential steps during the evaluation of this patient are limiting further gut absorption of MTX and rapid administration of leucovorin.

Activated charcoal adsorbs MTX, and administration is recommended as soon as possible to limit absorption in the setting of oral exposure. Multiple-dose activated charcoal is recommended for patients with evidence of delayed MTX clearance, such as kidney injury or prolonged half-life (based on blood MTX concentration). Activated charcoal should be withheld in patients with GI hemorrhage. Hydration with 0.9% sodium chloride solution as well as urinary alkalinization with IV sodium bicarbonate (to urine pH 7 to 8) (Antidotes in Brief: A5) is recommended to prevent or limit kidney injury from the precipitation of MTX and its metabolites. Serial measurements of serum creatinine and blood MTX concentration will determine the duration of urinary alkalinization.

The complete blood count (CBC) should be monitored at least as frequently as days 7, 10, and 14. Colony-stimulating factor is recommended for patients with febrile neutropenia and who are at high risk for complications from an infection or are likely to have a poor outcome (eg, absolute neutrophil count < 100 cells/μL, prolonged neutropenia {> 10 days}, age 65 years or older, and hypotension with multiorgan dysfunction). Patients presenting with meningismus or altered mental status following MTX therapy should receive an initial MRI of the brain and then CSF analysis for infection.

### Antidotes

The available antidotes for MTX toxicity are leucovorin (folinic acid) (Antidotes in Brief: A12) and glucarpidase (carboxypeptidase $G_2$) (Antidotes in Brief: A13). The effectiveness of these therapies depends on both the timing of administration and the dose, which warrants the monitoring of serum MTX concentrations during the use of these antidotes. Leucovorin rescue therapy limits the bone marrow and GI toxicity of MTX by allowing for the continuation of essential biochemical processes that are dependent on reduced folates. Glucarpidase (carboxypeptidase $G_2$) inactivates MTX by hydrolyzing it to DAMPA and glutamate. Glucarpidase can also be successfully administered intrathecally to reduce elevated MTX concentrations in the cerebrospinal space (Special Considerations: SC6).

### Extracorporeal Elimination

The patient with delayed renal clearance of a toxic concentration of MTX and who is not a candidate for glucarpidase therapy can benefit the most from extracorporeal elimination of MTX when the procedure is instituted early during the patient's course. Once MTX distributes into the cell and peripheral tissue compartments, extracorporeal procedures cannot remove intracellular polyglutamate derivatives of MTX, and multiple sessions can be required with limited ability to clear additional MTX stored at peripheral sites. Although the volume of distribution (0.6–0.9 L/kg) and protein binding (50% that is not concentration dependent) suggest that MTX is cleared by hemodialysis, clinical evidence suggests otherwise.

In vitro studies indicate that the toxic effects of 100 μmol/L of MTX cannot be reversed by 1,000 μmol/L of leucovorin. This suggests a potential need for extracorporeal elimination, such as high-flux hemodialysis or glucarpidase (or both), to lower persistent plasma MTX concentrations of greater than 100 µmol/L. Patients who are at the greatest risk for developing MTX toxicity despite leucovorin treatment should receive glucarpidase (Antidotes in Brief: A13). If the patient with diminished renal clearance and a toxic MTX concentration is not a candidate for glucarpidase therapy, it is reasonable to use hemodialysis early in the patient's course. Current standard hemodialysis can offer the additional benefit of correcting fluid and electrolyte disorders resulting from kidney failure. Other treatment options to limit additional organ toxicity, including leucovorin and urinary alkalinization, should be continued during extracorporeal MTX removal. Leucovorin needs to be replaced after hemodialysis because it is water-soluble and will be removed by hemodialysis.

## 5-FLUOROURACIL AND CAPECITABINE

The fluoropyrimidines 5-fluorouracil (5-FU), capecitabine, tegafur, and floxuridine are competitive analogs to uridine, and as such, they disrupt the syntheses of DNA (during the S-phase of the cell cycle) and RNA synthesis (Chap. 23). Although floxuridine is metabolized to 5-FU, it has limited systemic toxicity because it is administered to the target organ by the arterial route. Common risk factors for toxicity include genetic polymorphisms (ie, dihydropyrimidine dehydrogenase {DPD} deficiency) and underlying liver, kidney, and coronary artery diseases.

### Pharmacology

Capecitabine is an oral prodrug of 5-FU; it is well absorbed by the gut and then metabolized to 5-FU. The plasma protein binding for capecitabine is 60%. The time to peak blood concentration for capecitabine is 1.5 to 2 hours. Because capecitabine and its metabolites are eliminated primarily by the kidneys (84% in the first 24 hours), it is contraindicated when the creatinine clearance is less than 30 mL/min. In comparison, 5-FU has an erratic oral absorption and needs to be administered intravenously. 5-Fluorouracil has an apparent volume of distribution of 8 to 11 L/m$^2$, distributes to third spaces or compartments, such as peritoneal and pleural fluids, and is approximately 10% protein bound. The terminal half-lives for 5-FU and capecitabine in the blood compartment are about 15 and 45 minutes, respectively. Toxicity is dependent on a balance between the enzymatic formation of active metabolites and the enzymatic degradation of these metabolites and the parent compound (Fig. 24–2). Hepatic metabolism by DPD converts approximately 80% of 5-FU to inactive metabolites that are excreted in the urine. Patients with a significant genetic DPD deficiency will present with early-onset and severe manifestations of toxicity from 5-FU or capecitabine. Similarly, patients with elevated cytidine deaminase activity can develop capecitabine toxicity.

### Pathophysiology

The therapeutic and toxic effects of 5-FU (and capecitabine) are based on its ability to limit DNA and RNA synthesis by serving as an antagonist to the pyrimidine uracil in these macromolecules (Fig. 24–2). The specific sites of action and consequence are as follows: (1) 5-FU (as FdUMP) replaces

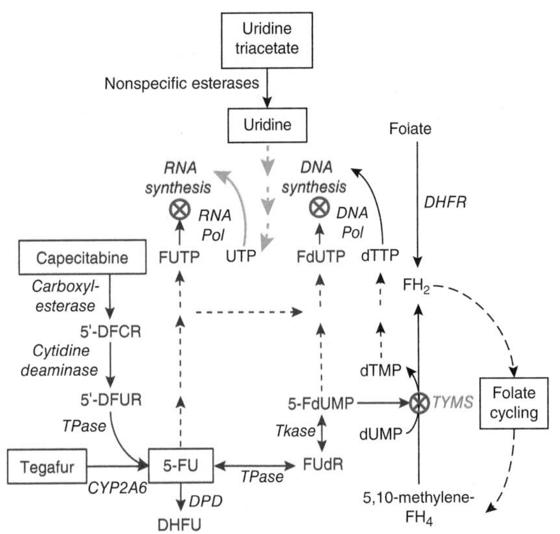


**FIGURE 24–2.** 5-Fluorouracil, capecitabine, and tegafur chemotherapeutic mechanisms of action and uridine triacetate antidotal rescue. 5′-DFCR = 5′-deoxy-5-fluorocytidine; 5′-DFUR = 5′-deoxy-5-fluorouridine; 5-FdUMP = fluorodeoxyuridine monophosphate; 5-FU = 5-fluorouracil; 5,10-methylene-FH4 = 5,10-methylenetetrahydrofolate; CYP2A6 = cytochrome P450, family 2, subfamily A, polypeptide 6; DHFR = dihydrofolate reductase; DHFU = 5,6-dihydrofluorouracil; DNA Pol = DNA polymerase; DPD = dihydropyrimidine dehydrogenase; dTMP = deoxythymidine monophosphate; dTTP = deoxythymidine triphosphate; dUMP = deoxyuridine monophosphate; FdUTP = fluorodeoxyuridine triphosphate; FH2 = dihydrofolate; FUdR = floxuridine; FUTP = fluorouridine triphosphate; RNA Pol = RNA polymerase; TKase = thymidine kinase; TPase = thymidine phosphorylase; TYMS = thymidylate synthase; UTP = uridine triphosphate. *(Reproduced with permission from Silas W. Smith, MD.)*

dUMP and it irreversibly inhibits thymidylate synthetase with the cofactor 5,10-methylenetetrahydrofolate (affects DNA synthesis and repair), (2) FdUTP replaces dUTP and it inhibits DNA replication (because of depleted thymidine triphosphate), and (3) fluorouridine triphosphate (FUTP) replaces UTP and inhibits RNA and protein syntheses. Although the primary mechanism of action in chemotherapy for 5-FU is inhibition of thymidylate synthetase, the impairment of RNA synthesis causes significant toxicity.

### Clinical Manifestations

The clinical manifestations of toxicity from 5-FU or capecitabine are primarily gastroenteritis and bone marrow suppression. Cardiac and central nervous system (CNS) manifestations of toxicity are uncommon in patients treated with these chemotherapeutics. Nausea and diarrhea present early (< 3 days) after the completion of the administration of the chemotherapeutic. Patients at genetically increased risk present with the same findings, only typically after the administration of the first course of treatment. Hand-and-foot syndrome (palmar-plantar erythrodysesthesia) presents with erythema, edema, and pain on the palms and soles. The skin desquamates and blisters, and the lesions can appear at other locations on the body. The dermatitis is more common with capecitabine than 5-FU therapy. It has a variable time of onset (from 11 to 360 days) and is reversible upon discontinuation of the chemotherapeutic. The manifestations of CNS toxicity include confusion, encephalopathy, and coma.

## Diagnostic Testing

Clinical laboratory tests for 5-FU or capecitabine and their metabolites fluoro-beta-alanine (FBAL), and the type of genetic variant or level of activity for selected enzymes, such as DPD or cytidine deaminase, are not routinely available.

## Management

It is reasonable to administer activated charcoal as soon as possible to a patient presenting early after an oral overdose of capecitabine because it can limit gut absorption of the chemotherapeutic. Initiate supportive management with IV fluids for dehydration and an antiemetic for vomiting (as needed) and assess for electrolyte disorders, cardiac and kidney injuries, neutropenia, and sepsis. If the patient presents with an acute coronary syndrome, conservative antianginal therapy (eg, nitrates and calcium channel blockers) should be initiated. The patient will require a cardiac monitored setting and serial ECGs and cardiac enzymes. Patients with a new-onset altered mental status should receive a computed tomography scan of the brain and possibly a lumbar puncture to assess for CNS infection.

## Antidotes

Timely uridine triacetate improves the survival of patients adversely affected by 5-FU or capecitabine. When uridine triacetate was administered within 96 hours of the last dose of the chemotherapeutic to patients with early onset of severe toxicity, all 18 patients survived. However, only three of eight patients survived when uridine acetate was administered after 96 hours.

Uridine triacetate is recommended for patients with (1) an overdose of 5-FU or capecitabine regardless of the presence of clinical toxicity, (2) an early onset (< 96 hours) of severe or life-threatening manifestations of toxicity (cardiovascular, CNS), or (3) an early onset of an unusually severe adverse reaction, such as gastroenteritis or neutropenia, within 96 hours of the administration of 5-FU or capecitabine during the course of chemotherapy. Uridine triacetate is not recommended for the treatment of patients with common or anticipated manifestations of these chemotherapeutics during therapy.

For adults, the dose of uridine triacetate is 10 g administered orally every 6 hours for 20 doses for a total of 5 days. For children, a single dose of uridine triacetate is 6.2 $g/m^2$ of body surface area up to a maximum of 10 g per dose. The dose and schedule for uridine triacetate are not adjusted by sex, amount of 5-FU or capecitabine, or hepatic or renal clearance (Antidotes in Brief: A14)

It is important to remember that leucovorin in not an antidote for patients with 5-FU or capecitabine toxicity as it will enhance toxicty (Antidotes in Brief: A12).

Antidotes in Brief

# A12 FOLATES: LEUCOVORIN (FOLINIC ACID) AND FOLIC ACID

Folates refer to the metabolically active reduced forms of folic acid, including dihydrofolate and tetrahydrofolate, that are vital to the synthesis of purines and DNA. Folic acid must be reduced in vivo by dihydrofolate reductase to tetrahydrofolate. Dihydrofolate reductase inhibitors such as methotrexate (MTX), pyrimethamine, and pemetrexed prevent this reduction. Leucovorin (folinic acid) and levoleucovorin do not require dihydrofolate reductase for activation. Therefore, either leucovorin or levoleucovorin is the primary antidote for a patient who receives an overdose of MTX or another dihydrofolate reductase inhibitor.

## HISTORY

In 1930–1931, Lucy Wills, while studying pregnant textile workers with macrocytic anemia in Mumbai, India, discovered that a yeast extract provided to these nutritionally deficient individuals cured and prevented their anemia. Mitchell isolated the active ingredient from spinach in 1941 and named it folic acid from the Latin *folium*, meaning leaf. In 1950, leucovorin (folinic acid) successfully reversed aminopterin and MTX toxicity, which had previously resisted folate therapy.

## PHARMACOLOGY

Folic acid is the most common of the many folate congeners that exist in nature and is essential for normal cellular metabolic functions. After absorption, folic acid is reduced by dihydrofolic acid reductase (DHFR) to dihydrofolic acid and then tetrahydrofolic acid (THF), which accepts one-carbon groups. Tetrahydrofolic acid serves as the precursor for folinic acid, which is also known as leucovorin or citrovorum factor. Biologically active forms of folate function as cofactors, providing the one-carbon groups necessary for many intracellular metabolic reactions, including the synthesis of thymidylate and purine nucleotides, which are essential precursors of DNA.

Leucovorin is a racemic mixture, and the active isomer is available as levoleucovorin. After a DHFR inhibitor such as MTX inhibits the formation of THF, the intracellular machinery for the synthesis of thymidylate and purine nucleotides comes to a halt, and DNA production ceases. Leucovorin and levoleucovorin are biologically active forms of folic acid and bypass the inhibition of DHFR caused by MTX to restore intracellular DNA production.

Folate also catalyzes the formation of carbon dioxide and water from formic acid, the final metabolic step in methanol elimination. Because there is no inhibition of the formation or recycling of active folate, either folic acid or leucovorin is beneficial in patients with methanol poisoning (Chap. 79).

### Leucovorin Pharmacokinetics

Leucovorin has a volume of distribution ($V_d$) of 13.6 L and a half-life of 35 minutes. The bioavailability of orally administered leucovorin decreases from 100% for a 20-mg dose to 78% for a 40-mg dose and ultimately to 31% for a 200-mg dose, necessitating IV administration when higher doses are desired. Intrathecal administration of leucovorin and levoleucovorin is contraindicated, as it can lower seizure threshold and is associated with fatal neurotoxicity. After IV administration of both leucovorin and levoleucovorin, l-5-methyl-THF enters the cerebrospinal fluid (CSF).

## ROLE IN METHOTREXATE TOXICITY

Methotrexate binds to the active site of DHFR, rendering it incapable of reducing folic acid to its biologically active forms and incapable of regenerating the necessary active forms required for the synthesis of purine nucleotides and thymidylate (Chap. 24). Since leucovorin is already a reduced, active form of folate, it does not require enzymatic interconversion to the form required for purine nucleotide and thymidylate formation. Leucovorin rescue describes the practice of limiting the toxic effects associated with high-dose MTX, by providing leucovorin after the initial MTX infusion and in cases of diminished MTX elimination, which can be due to MTX toxicity itself or other factors.

## ROLE IN METHANOL AND FORMATE TOXICITY

The formate produced from methanol is metabolized to 10-formyltetrahydrofolate in the presence of tetrahydrofolate, which is converted by 10-formyltetrahydrofolate dehydrogenase to carbon dioxide, and regenerated tetrahydrofolate. Higher folate activity correlates with a faster formate elimination half-life across multiple species. Folic acid supplementation in multiple studies of animals poisoned with methanol demonstrates reduced formate accumulation and improved metabolic acidosis.

In a methanol-poisoned patient, the formate half-life was 3.9 hours, which decreased to 1.2 hours after leucovorin treatment. In a patient with an intentional ingestion of formic acid, low plasma formic acid concentrations were present during leucovorin administration but rose significantly after leucovorin cessation. The sum of the animal, human, and ex vivo data supports the continued recommendation of folate or leucovorin in addition to definitive therapy with fomepizole or ethanol (Antidotes in Brief: A33 and A34) and/or hemodialysis.

## ROLE IN ARSENIC TOXICITY

Arsenic contamination of drinking water has plagued millions, causing increased manifestations of chronic arsenic toxicity, including cancer and cardiovascular, dermatologic, and neurologic disorders. In a folate-dependent mechanism, arsenic undergoes methylation to monomethylarsonic acid (MMA) and then to dimethylarsinic acid (DMA), which facilitates urinary arsenic excretion. Patients with higher intake of folate had lower percentages of inorganic arsenic and higher ratios of MMA to inorganic arsenic. Folate deficiency is associated with decreased arsenic methylation capacity, which is a risk factor for arsenic-induced skin lesions. In animal models, folic acid supplementation decreased the embryotoxicity, such as malformations, abnormal cardiac, and abnormal neural development. In randomized controlled trials, folic acid supplementation enhanced arsenic methylation and lowered blood arsenic concentrations.

## ROLE IN TOXICITY FROM DIHYDROFOLATE REDUCTASE INHIBITOR ANTIBIOTICS

Pyrimethamine is a dihydrofolate reductase competitive inhibitor used to treat infections from *Toxoplasma*, *Isospora*, and *Pneumocystis*. In a dose-dependent fashion, leucovorin significantly reduces cytogenetic aberrations associated with pyrimethamine in vitro. Leucovorin is routinely added to pyrimethamine therapy for toxoplasmosis.

## ADVERSE EFFECTS AND SAFETY ISSUES

Reports of adverse reactions to parenteral injections of folic acid and folinic acid are uncommon but include allergic or anaphylactoid reactions and seizures. The calcium content of folinic acid warrants a slow IV infusion at a rate not faster than 160 mg/min in adults. Neither leucovorin nor levoleucovorin should be administered intrathecally.

Leucovorin and levoleucovorin are not antidotes for 5-fluorouracil and its prodrugs capecitabine and tegafur, as they enhance their chemotherapeutic and toxic effects.

Leucovorin is a substrate for glucarpidase. As such, if glucarpidase is used to treat MTX toxicity, it is recommended to separate the administration of leucovorin and glucarpidase by 2 hours (Antidotes in Brief: A13). The order of administration depends on availability and timing. If MTX has already entered the cells, folinic acid should be given first. In the event of an early discovery of an MTX error (such as administration to the wrong patient), glucarpidase should be given first if available. If time is required to obtain glucarpidase, folinic acid should be given immediately.

## PREGNANCY AND LACTATION

Folic acid is a United States (US) Food and Drug Administration (FDA) category A drug and is safe and essential during pregnancy and compatible with breastfeeding. Leucovorin and levoleucovorin are US FDA pregnancy category C drugs. Breast milk excretion is unstudied, but leucovorin is considered compatible with breastfeeding.

## DOSING AND ADMINISTRATION

### Methotrexate Overdose

After MTX overdose, a dose of leucovorin estimated to produce the same plasma concentration as achieved by the MTX should be given as soon as possible, preferably within 1 hour. Because of the safety of leucovorin and because of the toxicity of MTX, underdosing leucovorin should be avoided. Although serum MTX concentrations are often closely followed in patients on diverse oncologic regimens, in the overdose setting, or in MTX toxicity related to treatment for tubal pregnancies, it is ***inappropriate*** to wait for a serum concentration before initiating treatment with leucovorin. An empirical intravenous leucovorin dose of 150 mg/m$^2$ every 3 to 6 hours should be effective in all but the most severe overdoses. This dose should be continued until the serum MTX concentration is less than 0.01 μmol/L, preferably zero.

### Therapeutic Methotrexate Therapy

Leucovorin rescue strategies after high-dose MTX are aligned in the leucovorin, levoleucovorin, and MTX package inserts, with 15 mg leucovorin (7.5 mg of levoleucovorin) provided at baseline every 6 hours for 10 doses beginning 24 hours after MTX administration, so as not to compromise chemotherapeutic efficacy. In the setting of early or delayed MTX elimination or acute kidney injury, leucovorin dosing must be increased to counteract the persistent adverse effects of therapeutic MTX (Table A12–1 and Figure A12–1).

The dose of leucovorin for "leucovorin rescue" after "high-dose" therapeutic MTX treatment (doses of 500 mg/m$^2$ or greater) ranges from 10 to 25 mg/m$^2$ IM or IV every 6 hours for 72 hours up to 1,000 mg/m$^2$ every 6 hours in patients with renal compromise and delayed elimination. Although the dose of leucovorin can be as high as 1,000 mg/m$^2$ every 6 hours, this is rarely warranted and cannot adequately compete with serum concentrations of MTX above 100 μmol/L. Thus when the MTX concentration exceeds this concentration and leucovorin rescue may fail, it is recommended to administer glucarpidase (Antidotes in Brief: A13).

A transition to oral administration of leucovorin depends on the serum concentration of MTX and whether adequate serum concentrations of leucovorin can be achieved orally.

In addition to leucovorin, other modalities to treat patients with MTX overdoses include activated charcoal (AC) (Antidotes in Brief: A1), urinary alkalinization (Antidotes in Brief: A5), and glucarpidase (Antidotes in Brief: A13).

**TABLE A12–1 Leucovorin Dosage and Administration with Chemotherapeutic Methotrexate Use**[a]

| *Clinical Situation* | *Laboratory Findings* | *Leucovorin Dosage* |
|---|---|---|
| Normal methotrexate elimination | Serum [methotrexate] ~10 μmol/L at 24 hours after administration, 1 μmol/L at 48 hours, and < 0.2 μmol/L at 72 hours | 15 mg PO, IM, or IV every 6 hours for 60 hours (10 doses starting at 24 hours after the start of methotrexate infusion) |
| Delayed late methotrexate elimination | Serum [methotrexate] remaining > 0.2 μmol/L at 72 hours and > 0.05 μmol/L at 96 hours after administration | Continue 15 mg PO, IM, or IV every 6 hours until [methotrexate] is < 0.05 μmol/L |
| Delayed early methotrexate elimination or evidence of acute kidney injury | Serum [methotrexate] of ≥ 50 μmol/L at 24 hours or ≥ 5 μmol/L at 48 hours after administration or a ≥ 100% increase in serum [creatinine] at 24 hours after methotrexate administration (eg, an increase from 0.5 to ≥ 1 mg/dL) | 150 mg IV every 3 hours until [methotrexate] is < 1 μmol/L; then 15 mg IV every 3 hours until [methotrexate] is < 0.05 μmol/L |

[a]Leucovorin should not be administered intrathecally. IM = intramuscular; IV = intravenous; PO = oral.

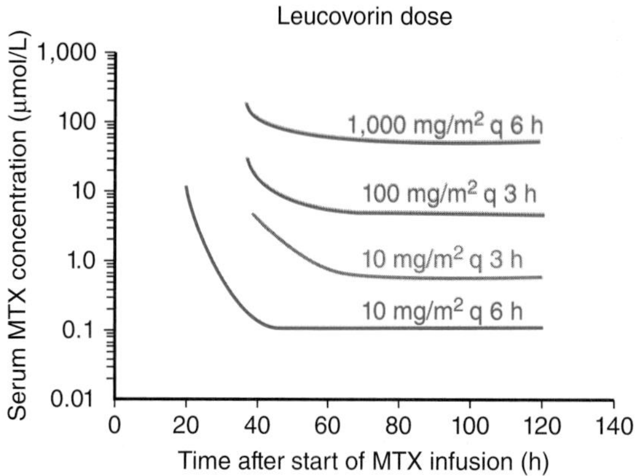


**FIGURE A12–1.** Example of a nomogram developed by Bleyer for pharmacokinetically guided leucovorin rescue after high-dose methotrexate (MTX) administration.

### Intrathecal Methotrexate Overdose

Unintentional overdose with intrathecal MTX is dose dependent and critically important. In these cases, IV leucovorin ***and not intrathecal leucovorin*** should be administered. Although some cases have been managed with IV leucovorin with or without additional drainage procedures, it is reasonable to administer intrathecal glucarpidase in cases of significant intrathecal MTX overdose or signs of neurotoxicity. In intrathecal MTX overdoses, consultation with experienced hematologists/oncologists and medical toxicologists is warranted (Special Considerations: SC6).

### Pemetrexed Toxicity

Pemetrexed toxicity is similar to that of MTX. Toxicity is attenuated initially with a low dose of vitamin $B_{12}$ and leucovorin 100 mg/m$^2$ IV once, followed by 50 mg/m$^2$ IV every 6 hours for 8 days.

### Methanol Toxicity

Either folic acid or leucovorin (folinic acid) parenterally is recommended at the first suspicion of methanol poisoning. Folic acid is most commonly used. The precise dosage necessary is unknown, but 1 to 2 mg/kg every 4 to 6 hours is probably sufficient. Because the first dose is usually administered before hemodialysis, a second dose is recommended at the completion of hemodialysis because this highly water-soluble vitamin will be removed in the dialysate.

## FORMULATION AND ACQUISITION

Leucovorin (folinic acid) powder for injection is available in 50-, 100-, 200-, and 350-mg vials.

Leucovorin is also available in a single-use vial as a solution for injection at a concentration of 10 mg/mL in a 50-mL vial. Because of the calcium content, the rate of IV administration should not be faster than 160 mg/min in adults. Leucovorin is also available orally in a variety of strengths, including 5-, 10-, 15-, and 25-mg tablets.

Levoleucovorin lyophilized powder for injection is available in a single-use 50-mg vial containing the equivalent of 50 mg of levoleucovorin. Because of the calcium content, the rate of IV administration should not be faster than 160 mg/min. It is dosed at half the dose of leucovorin.

Folic acid is available parenterally in 10-mL multidose vials with 1.5% benzyl alcohol in concentrations of 5 or 10 mg/mL from a variety of manufacturers. Once opened, the vial must be kept refrigerated. If administration to neonates is necessary, a benzyl alcohol–free preparation must be used because of the toxicity of benzyl alcohol in neonates (Chap. 19).

Antidotes in Brief

# A13 GLUCARPIDASE (CARBOXYPEPTIDASE $G_2$)

## INTRODUCTION

Glucarpidase (carboxypeptidase $G_2$, $CPDG_2$) is indicated for the management of methotrexate (MTX) toxicity. When given intravenously or intrathecally, it rapidly enzymatically inactivates MTX, folates, and folate analogs. It does not substitute for, and must be used in conjunction with, leucovorin (Antidotes in Brief: A12). Leucovorin should not be administered within 2 hours before or after a dose of glucarpidase.

## HISTORY

Soon after the description of the structure and synthesis of folate, a *Flavobacterium* species capable of removing the glutamate moiety of folate was discovered. Purification of "carboxypeptidase G," a pseudomonad-derived zinc-dependent enzyme responsible for MTX cleavage, was reported in 1967. The carboxypeptidase currently used in clinical practice ($CPDG_2$) was cloned from a *Pseudomonas* strain and expressed in *Escherichia coli* in the early 1980s. The United State (US) Food and Drug Administration (FDA) designated glucarpidase an Orphan Product in 2003 and granted marketing approval in 2012.

## PHARMACOLOGY

### Mechanism of Action

Glucarpidase is a peptidase that hydrolyzes the C-terminal glutamate residues of folate and folate analogs such as MTX, leaving them inactive (Fig. A13–1).

### Pharmacokinetics

When 50 units/kg of glucarpidase was given IV, patients with normal kidney function achieved a mean maximum serum concentration of glucarpidase of 3.1 μg/mL, with a mean half-life of 9.0 hours. Findings were similar in patients with impaired glomerular filtration rates (GFRs). The volume of distribution was 3.6 L. The large size (83-kDa dimer) of glucarpidase precludes traversing the blood–brain barrier or crossing cell membranes to act intracellularly or acting on MTX within the gut lumen or urinary collecting system. It is thus unable, when administered IV, to treat MTX extravasation or intrathecal overdoses.

### Pharmacodynamics

One unit of glucarpidase activity catalyzes the hydrolysis of 1 μmol of MTX per minute at 37°C. The mean enzymatic activity half-life of glucarpidase was 5.6 hours in normal volunteers and 8.2 hours in volunteers with impaired GFRs. Glucarpidase rapidly decreases serum MTX concentrations by greater than 97% within 15 minutes.

## ROLE IN METHOTREXATE TOXICITY

Patients receiving high-dose MTX therapy are routinely "rescued" with leucovorin (eg, 10–15 mg every 6 hours) to prevent systemic toxicity (Antidotes in Brief: A12). However, at MTX concentrations above 100 μmol/L ($1 \times 10^{-4}$ mol/L), adequate leucovorin concentrations cannot be achieved for complete reversal of toxicity. Urine alkalinization and diuresis, which are also helpful with enhancing MTX elimination, are often limited by serum pH, sodium, and fluid administration maximums once patients develop toxicity. Thus, despite adequate leucovorin rescue, alkalization, diuresis, and supportive care, additional antidotal strategies are required in the setting of persistently elevated MTX concentrations. Chemotherapeutic regimens that combine MTX with renal toxic medications such as cisplatin also increase the risk. Thus, it is reasonable to anticipate the need for glucarpidase in approximately 1% to 4% of patients receiving high-dose MTX.

Glucarpidase is labeled for patients with serum MTX concentrations greater than 1 μmol/L in the setting of impaired kidney function (as evidenced by an MTX concentration not falling within 2 standard deviations of the mean MTX excretion curve for the specific administered MTX protocol) (Fig. A12–1). In the absence of an MTX concentration to guide the clinicians, significant mucositis, gastrointestinal distress, myelosuppression, hepatitis, or neurotoxicity should prompt administration of glucarpidase in addition to aggressive leucovorin therapy, while awaiting a confirmatory MTX concentration. Although no fully reported trial has yet demonstrated the superiority of glucarpidase as adjuvant therapy to leucovorin and supportive care alone, the pharmacodynamic efficacy is clear: glucarpidase immediately decreases serum MTX concentrations by greater than 97%. Delaying glucarpidase more than 96 hours after MTX initiation, once intracellular MTX is established, is associated with failure to prevent significant MTX toxicity. This emphasizes the need for close monitoring of MTX concentration to ensure early administration of glucarpidase as soon as indicated.

Persistent intracellular or otherwise inaccessible MTX requires ongoing leucovorin therapy, which is continued until the MTX concentration is below the leucovorin treatment threshold (50–0.05–0.1 × $10^{-6}$ molar) for a minimum of 3 days.

Leucovorin is contraindicated for IT administration as it is toxic to the central nervous system (CNS). Human case reports demonstrate that IT glucarpidase provides an effective means to rapidly lower cerebrospinal fluid (CSF) MTX concentrations in cases of overdose or prolonged CNS persistence. Reductions in CSF range from 72% to 99.8%.

## ADVERSE EFFECTS AND SAFETY ISSUES

### Antidotal Compromise

Because glucarpidase also cleaves active leucovorin, glucarpidase will compromise leucovorin rescue if both antidotes are administered contemporaneously. Leucovorin

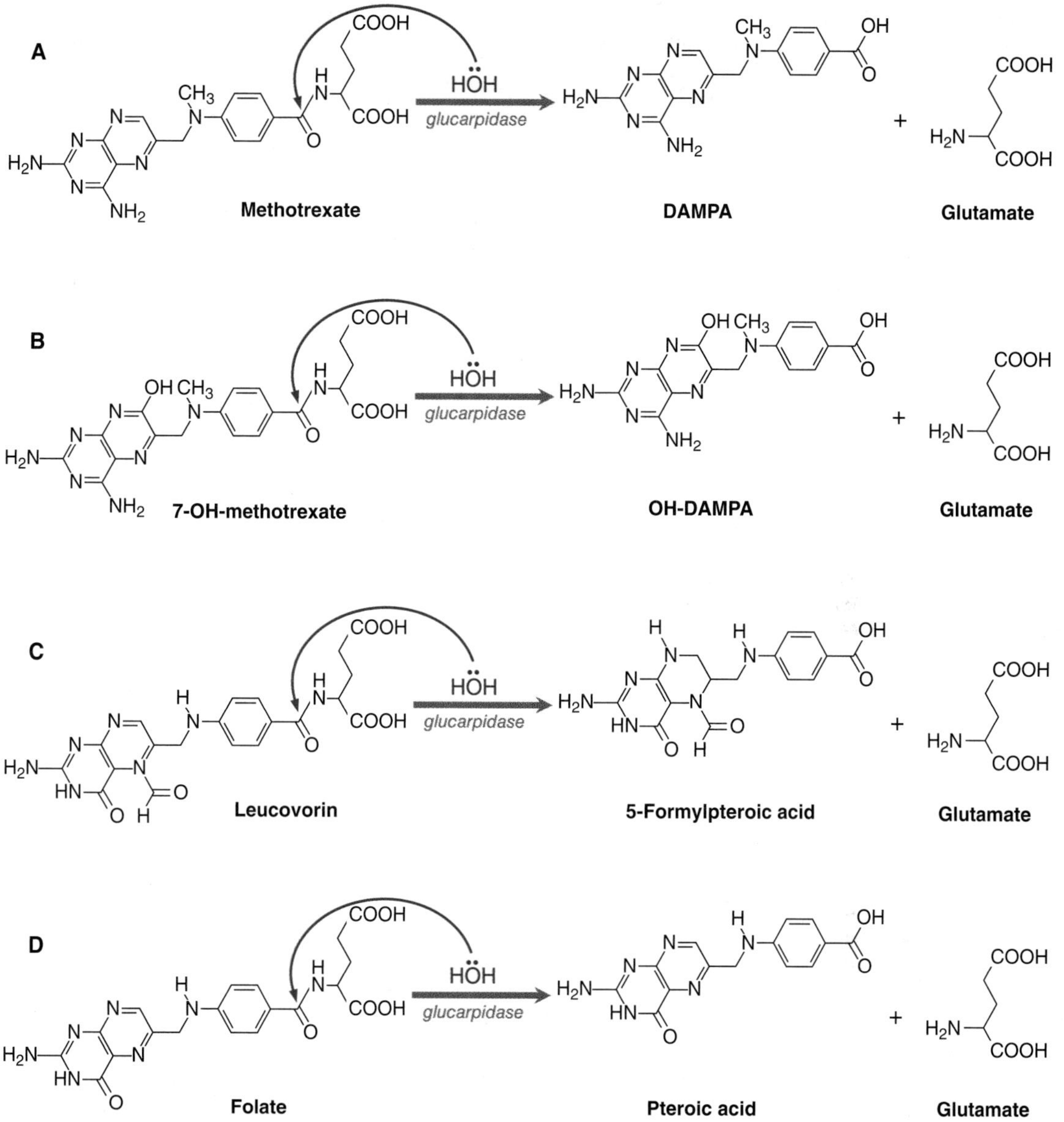

**FIGURE A13–1.** The catalytic domain of glucarpidase permits hydrolysis of the C-terminal glutamate residue of folate and folate analogs such as MTX via hypothesized nucleophilic attack of a zinc-bound water molecule. (**A**, **B**) MTX and its metabolite 7-hydroxy-MTX are split into inactive DAMPA (2,4-diamino-*N*(10)-methylpteroic acid) and hydroxy-DAMPA plus glutamate. Glucarpidase similarly inactivates (**C**) leucovorin (folinic acid) and (**D**) folate by cleavage of terminal glutamate residues.

concentrations decreased in volunteers given leucovorin 2 hours after glucarpidase. Studies confirmed the recommendation that leucovorin should not be administered for at least 2 hours before or after glucarpidase and that the ongoing leucovorin dose should be based on the pre-glucarpidase MTX concentration.

## Immunogenicity

In an evaluation of 205 patients treated with glucarpidase, antiglucarpidase antibodies developed in 32 of 176 (18%) patients following a single glucarpidase dose in 11 of 29 (37.9%) after two or more doses; 14 of 176 (8.0%) single-dose patients had neutralizing antibodies, which increased to 8 of 29 (27.6%) after two or more doses. Although antiglucarpidase antibodies might decrease clinical efficacy or predispose to allergic reaction upon re-exposure, many patients have been successfully treated with more than one dose of glucarpidase for persistently elevated MTX concentrations.

## Other Considerations

Alkalinization and saline diuresis should be continued to prevent toxicity from precipitation of the otherwise inactive methotrexate metabolite (DAMPA) resulting in further renal compromise.

## PREGNANCY AND LACTATION

Glucarpidase carries a pregnancy category C designation, although formal human and animal data are lacking. The excretion of glucarpidase in breast milk is unknown.

## DOSING AND ADMINISTRATION

A single dose of 50 units/kg is administered immediately by IV injection over 5 minutes. Although clinical trials permitted additional glucarpidase doses 24 to 48 hours later in cases of persistent elevated MTX concentrations, repeat administration has not demonstrated significant efficacy and is not recommended. The substantial cost of glucarpidase and the apparent glucarpidase efficacy at lower doses has led some authors to advocate rounding the glucarpidase doses down (eg, to the nearest vial size) or capping glucarpidase doses (eg, at 2,000 units), although this practice is not consistent with the US FDA-approved dose (50 units/kg). Although this approach awaits further formal study, it would be reasonable in cases of glucarpidase shortage or the need to triage dosing. In cases of intrathecal MTX overdose, a fixed dose of glucarpidase (2,000 units) reconstituted in sterile 0.9% sodium chloride has been administered intrathecally (off label) over 5 minutes and is recommended in this scenario.

### Monitoring and Analytical Considerations

False elevations of MTX concentrations are reported with all of the various immunoassay techniques after glucarpidase administration. The DAMPA metabolite significantly cross-reacts with both the MTX radioimmunoassay and competitive dihydrofolate reductase–binding assays. Both MTX metabolites (7-OH-MTX and DAMPA) appreciably interfere with fluorescence polarization immunoassay (FPIA) and enzyme-multiplied immunoassay technique (EMIT) assays. Thus, only high-performance liquid chromatography should be used to determine actual MTX concentration when glucarpidase is given.

## FORMULATION AND ACQUISITION

Glucarpidase is available in single-use glass vials each containing lyophilized glucarpidase (1,000 units). The manufacturer's website details acquisition information for inside and outside of the US (http://www.btgplc.com/products/specialty-pharmaceuticals/voraxazeandhttp://www.btgplc.com/contact-us/contacts, respectively).

Antidotes in Brief

# A14 URIDINE TRIACETATE

## INTRODUCTION

Uridine triacetate is used to treat toxicity from fluoropyrimidines (fluorouracil, capecitabine, tegafur, and floxuridine).

## HISTORY

Fluorouracil (5-FU) synthesis and its antitumor activity were reported in 1957. Studies in 1982 reported successful use of uridine to rescue mice from lethal 5-FU doses and the ability to deliver higher 5-FU chemotherapeutic doses with concomitant uridine. After failures with intravenous and oral uridine, uridine triacetate was given United States Food and Drug Administration (FDA) approval in 2015 to treat patients with 5-FU or capecitabine overdose and early-onset, severe or life-threatening toxicity.

## PHARMACOLOGY

### Mechanism of Action

Uridine as uridine triphosphate is an essential component of RNA, while uridine as uridine diphosphate glucose is an important precursor to glycogen synthesis. Mechanisms of toxicity by the fluoropyrimidines are reviewed in Chap. 24 and summarized in Fig. 24–2. The 5-FU metabolite fluorouridine triphosphate (FUTP) is incorporated in RNA. Uridine triacetate, once absorbed and metabolized, supplies uridine, which can serve as a source for uridine triphosphate to compete with FUTP for RNA incorporation.

### Related Agents

Various uridine formulations that are marketed as dietary supplements are available but they are not recommended to treat fluoropyrimidine toxicity because of a lack of quality control. Uridine triacetate is also packaged as branded Xuriden for treatment of hereditary orotic aciduria (HOA), at a dose that is different than for fluoropyrimidine toxicity.

### Pharmacokinetics and Pharmacodynamics

The goal of therapy is to produce sustained plasma uridine concentrations higher than 70 μmol/L, which are needed to expand intestinal and bone marrow nucleotide pools and to prevent toxicity. The significant pharmacokinetic limitations of rapid uridine plasma clearance and poor bioavailability, as well as poor oral tolerance and the safety issues surrounding intravenous administration, prompted evaluation of uridine delivery as a uridine triacetate prodrug. Uridine triacetate is more lipophilic than uridine and does not require the pyrimidine transporter for absorption, which results in enhanced transport across the gastrointestinal mucosa. In clinical trials with current labeled dosing, the maximum uridine concentrations occurred after 2 to 3 hours, with a half-life of 2 to 2.6 hours. Plasma uridine concentrations were 99 to 119 μmol/L after the first dose and rose to 153 to 160 μmol/L after the final dose.

## ROLE IN FLUOROPYRIMIDINE TOXICITY

Despite supportive measures, fluoropyrimidine toxicity is often severe and includes bone marrow suppression (with neutropenia, infection, and sepsis), gastrointestinal toxicity (with mucositis, stomatitis, vomiting, hepatic enzyme elevation, and severe diarrhea), volume depletion, acute kidney injury, cardiotoxicity (dysrhythmias, congestive heart failure, and hemorrhagic pericarditis), neurotoxicity, multisystem organ failure, and death. Uridine triacetate rescue offers an antidotal mechanism to mitigate fluoropyrimidine toxicity. Hematopoietic and gastrointestinal mucosal progenitors efficiently incorporate exogenous uridine by the salvage pathway, compared to solid tumors, which favor de novo synthesis, providing an explanation for the effectiveness of exogenous uridine in competing with FUTP in normal tissues.

### Animal Studies

In the first mice studies, intraperitoneal (IP) uridine at 1, 5, or 10 g/kg/day produced 100% survival from previously lethal doses of 5-FU. With two doses of uridine 3.5 g/kg IP, the median lethal dose ($LD_{50}$) of 5-FU was increased by 68%. Furthermore, in mice with tumors given uridine rescue, the maximum tolerated dose of 5-FU was doubled with improved efficacy and without attendant toxicity. In an attempt to shift to oral regimens, doses of 4 g/kg oral uridine in mice were shown to be comparable to IP rescue of 5-FU, which was an increase by more than 50% of the maximum tolerated weekly dose. Both immediate (at 2 hours) and delayed (as late as 48 hours) administration of uridine triacetate were evaluated, with successful doubling of the maximum tolerated 5-FU dose. The time window of efficacy of oral uridine triacetate resuscitation was evaluated in mice given a lethal dose of 5-FU IP followed by uridine triacetate at 24, 48, 72, and 96 hours. Survival rates were 90% at 24 hours, which declined to 60%, 30%, and 20% with each subsequent day's delay in administration.

Because many cases of 5-FU toxicity are associated with dihydropyrimidine dehydrogenase (DPD) deficiency and delayed 5-FU clearance, an animal model was created to mimic DPD deficiency. In mice given the lethal combination of 5-FU and the DPD dehydrogenase inhibitor 5-ethynyluracil, survival was 80%, 40%, 50%, and 20% after rescue at 24, 48, 72, and 96 hours after 5-FU, respectively. This demonstrated efficacy even in the setting of compromised 5-FU elimination.

### Human Studies

In the first phase 1 trial of uridine triacetate, in which 38 patients were rescued at 24 hours, the tolerated 5-FU dose could be increased from 0.6 to 1 g/m². In a phase 2 trial, 65 patients with gastric carcinoma were administered 1.2 g/m² of 5-FU (twice the usual dose) with leucovorin, followed by uridine triacetate rescue. This normally toxic 5-FU dose was tolerated with no episodes of severe stomatitis or diarrhea and only a 20% incidence of moderate or severe neutropenia. The pivotal efficacy trials of uridine triacetate were two compassionate-use studies in which 142 patients had documented overdose of 5-FU or capecitabine and an additional 26 patients had rapid onset of toxicity (severe or life-threatening toxicities within 96 hours following the end of 5-FU administration). Survival to 30 days or chemotherapy resumption was achieved in 94% of patients treated with uridine triacetate compared to only 16% of the historical controls that received only supportive care. There are no data on uridine triacetate efficacy in overdose of tegafur, a 5-FU prodrug, although it would be reasonable to provide uridine triacetate in this circumstance.

## ADVERSE EFFECTS AND SAFETY ISSUES

The most common adverse events observed in the clinical trials of uridine triacetate were vomiting (8.1%), nausea (4.6%), and diarrhea (3.5%). Although potassium channel inhibition was reported in vitro with uridine triacetate, this did not occur at physiologically relevant concentrations. No cardiac toxicity was observed in dog or rat studies. In vitro, no significant CYP450 enzyme interactions were found with uridine or uridine triacetate. Uridine triacetate is a weak P-glycoprotein substrate and inhibitor in vitro, and the potential for local inhibition at the gut level cannot be excluded.

## PREGNANCY AND LACTATION

There are insufficient data on the use of uridine triacetate during pregnancy to inform the risks of birth defects or miscarriage. Animal studies did not demonstrate toxicity when uridine triacetate was provided at one-half the human dose. The presence of uridine triacetate in human milk is unstudied.

## DOSING AND ADMINISTRATION

Uridine triacetate dosing in adults is 10 g (1 packet) orally every 6 hours for a total of 20 doses, without regard to meals. The pediatric dose is 6.2 $g/m^2$ up to the adult maximum. Uridine triacetate is mixed with 3 to 4 ounces of soft foods (eg, applesauce, pudding, or yogurt) and ingested within 30 minutes, along with 4 ounces of water. We recommend that a 5-$HT_3$-receptor antagonist such as ondansetron be given as an antiemetic 20 to 30 minutes prior to each dose to prevent vomiting. If vomiting occurs within 2 hours of the last dose, the entire dose is repeated, and the next dose is given at the next scheduled interval.

Nasogastric administration is recommended if the patient cannot tolerate the oral route. If provided via this route, then 4 ounces of a food starch–based thickening product in water should be stirred briskly until the thickener has dissolved, and the contents of one 10-g packet that has been crushed to a fine powder should be added to the reconstituted food starch–based thickening product. For pediatric patients receiving less than 10 g, the mixture should be prepared at a ratio of no greater than 1 g per 10 mL of reconstituted food starch–based thickening product and mixed thoroughly.

## FORMULATION AND ACQUISITION

Uridine triacetate is available in 10-g single-dose packets and is supplied as a full course of therapy with 20 single-dose packets per carton, as well as a "24-Hour Pack" containing four single-dose packets per carton. The manufacturer's contact number for ordering uridine triacetate is 1-844-293-0007.

Special Considerations

# SC6 INTRATHECAL ADMINISTRATION OF XENOBIOTICS

Cerebrospinal fluid (CSF) is produced by the choroid plexus at a rate of 15 to 30 mL/h, or approximately 500 mL/day in adults. Cerebrospinal fluid flows in a rostral to caudal direction and is reabsorbed through the arachnoid villi directly into the venous circulation. The estimated total volume of CSF is 130 to 150 mL in healthy adults and 35 mL in infants.

For more than 100 years, a variety of xenobiotics have been delivered directly into the CSF. Medications are usually administered via a spinal needle or an indwelling intrathecal catheter. The xenobiotic moves by both diffusion and convection, and depending on the lipophilicity, the xenobiotic reaches the brain within a few minutes to 1 hour. Patient position and interindividual variations in lumbosacral CSF volume affect xenobiotic distribution as does baricity, which is the ratio of the specific gravity of the xenobiotic to the specific gravity of CSF at 98.6°F (37°C). Hyperbaric xenobiotics typically distribute in accordance with gravitational forces. However, in overdose or administration of xenobiotics unintended for intrathecal administration, distribution, reabsorption, and clinical effects are unpredictable. The inadvertent administration of the wrong medication into the CSF is potentially fatal. This error usually occurs with misidentification or mislabeling of medications during pharmacy preparation or at the bedside. For patients with indwelling devices, medications intended for intravenous delivery are occasionally connected inadvertently to the intrathecal catheter.

Several factors affect the clinical toxicity of intrathecal medications. Ionized xenobiotics are likely to disrupt neurotransmission, as do hyperosmolar or lipophilic xenobiotics. Patients administered the wrong xenobiotic into a subcutaneous CSF reservoir often suffer immediate alterations in mental status. Patients often present with exaggerated symptoms and findings typically associated with the xenobiotic. For example, patients with intrathecal morphine overdose present with symptoms of opioid toxicity. Other manifestations of intrathecal errors, regardless of the xenobiotic, include pain and paresthesias, often ascending in nature, and autonomic instability, especially with extremes of blood pressure and hyperreflexic myoclonic spasms similar to those that occur in patients with tetanus. Seizures or a depressed level of consciousness also occur. The time of onset of these life-threatening symptoms is determined by the dose and characteristics of the xenobiotic.

## XENOBIOTIC RECOVERY FROM CEREBROSPINAL FLUID

Once a medication delivery error is identified, rapid intervention is mandatory. In cases in which outcome is uncertain or not previously described, the exposure should be treated as potentially fatal. Any existing access to the CSF, ideally in the lumbosacral area, should be maintained. Immediate withdrawal of CSF, in volumes as high as 75 mL in adults, is indicated. This can be replaced with isotonic solutions: lactated Ringer, 0.9% normal sodium chloride, or Plasma-Lyte. Some authors recommend the initial volume removal of 100 mL be performed in 20- to 30-mL aliquots. This is a reasonable initial intervention for potentially fatal intrathecal exposures. For children, multiple aliquots of 5 to 10 mL can be removed and replaced with isotonic fluid. If the patient can tolerate an upright position, this has the potential to limit cephalad movement of xenobiotics. A neurosurgical consultation should be obtained to consider the placement of cerebral ventricular access for the performance of continuous CSF lavage. This procedure, also known as ventriculolumbar perfusion, involves continuous instillation (as great as 150 mL/h) of an isotonic solution into the cerebral ventricular system with CSF drainage through a lumbar site. Another intervention involves placement of an epidural catheter into a higher intrathecal space above the lumbar drainage site so that an isotonic solution can be perfused through the catheter and drained caudally. This serves as a readily available, rapid intervention for patients awaiting placement of an emergent ventriculostomy. Extreme caution should be undertaken to avoid delivery of antidotes directly into the CSF, unless specific data support their use.

## SPECIFIC EXPOSURES

Fatalities have resulted from inadvertant intrathecal administration of aminophylline, bortezomib, cytarabine, leucovorin, methotrexate, methylene blue, potassium chloride, tramadol, tranexamic acid, and vincristine. A comprehensive list of all intrathecal errors and their outcomes can be found in the 11th edition of *Goldfranks Toxicologic Emergencies.*

## PUMP MALFUNCTIONS AND ERRORS

Pump malfunctions cause a sudden decrease or increase in the amount of drug delivered to the intrathecal space. Insufficient drug delivery will result in clinical manifestations of withdrawal especially in pumps containing opioids, baclofen, or clonidine. Catheters infrequently kink, migrate, or become obstructed by an inflammatory mass. Patients on chronic therapy are at highest risk of severe withdrawal signs and symptoms. Patients will require intensive oral and intravenous therapy until intrathecal delivery can be re-established.

Pump failures also result in overinfusion. Intrathecal pump overdoses occur with pump errors and errors in refilling pumps that are otherwise intact. Some pumps also contain two access sites, one of which is contiguous with the intrathecal space and allows for CSF withdrawal or injection of nonionic contrast media for imaging. Errors occur when a concentrated bolus is inadvertently injected into this port instead of the reservoir, resulting in a massive, sometimes fatal, overdose.

When intrathecal overdose is suspected from either a refill error or pump malfunction, the clinical service that placed and manages the pump should be consulted. The consultant can assist in device interrogation and gaining CSF access. Either re-accessing the CSF port immediately or placing a spinal needle into the intrathecal space at another site is critical for the withdrawal of CSF. Large-volume drainage (> 100 mL in adults in 20–30-mL aliquots) with isotonic fluid replacement as required, as well as other supportive measures such as intravenous naloxone if opioid intoxication is present. Some of these patients will require care in an intensive care unit. If the consultant is not readily available, emptying the depot port will automatically cause the pump motor to stop.

## ERROR PREVENTION

All intrathecal medication errors are preventable. Mechanisms for prevention include trained pharmacists, nurses, and administering physicians, specialized packaging and handling, use of minibags for intrathecal medications whenever feasible, preadministration of any intravenous medications, removal of all syringes and other medications from the area, and a checklist and time out, with two persons reviewing all labels. Non-locking systems are being adopted to limit connection errors.

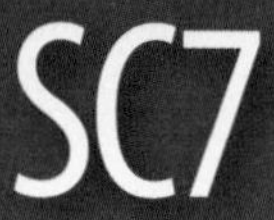

Special Considerations

# EXTRAVASATION OF VESICANT XENOBIOTICS

Extravasation injuries are among the most consequential local toxic events. When the vesicant chemotherapeutics leak into the perivascular space, significant necrosis of skin, muscles, and tendons occurs, with resultant loss of function, infection, and deformity. Early findings are often difficult to distinguish from other forms of local drug toxicity, such as irritation and hypersensitivity, which are self-limiting and typified by an immediate onset of a burning sensation, pruritus, erythema, and a flare reaction of the vein receiving the infusion. The extravasation of monoclonal antibodies causes minimal discomfort and inflammation.

Extravasations are more frequent with inexperienced clinicians, and peripheral intravenous lines that involve poor vessel integrity and blood flow, such as in patients with numerous venipuncture attempts; limited venous and lymphatic drainage caused by either obstruction or surgical resection; and the use of venous access overlying a joint. Extravasation injuries from implanted ports in central veins typically occurs from inadequate placement of the needle, needle dislodgment, fibrin sheath formation around the catheter, perforation of the superior vena cava, and fracture of the catheter.

The factors associated with a poor outcome from extravasation injuries are areas of the body with little subcutaneous tissue; increased concentrations of extravasate; increased volume and duration of contact with tissue; and the type of chemotherapeutic. Vesicants, such as doxorubicin, daunorubicin, dactinomycin, epirubicin, idarubicin, mechlorethamine, mitomycin, and the vinca alkaloids, produce more significant local tissue destruction than other types of chemotherapeutics, such as irritants. The extravasation injuries from taxanes appear similar to the vesicants but are less severe in response and more delayed in presentation.

## MANAGEMENT

Management recommendations derived from the literature and their theoretical foundations are given in Table SC7–1. Once extravasation is suspected, the infusion should be immediately halted. The venous access should be maintained to permit aspiration of as much of the infusate as possible and administration of an antidote, if indicated. We recommend early surgical irrigation (with a dermotomy or fasciotomy as indicated) of the extravasation site for an extravasation containing more than 5 mL of a vesicant. Hyaluronidase enhances absorption of an extravasation with a vinca alkaloid or etoposide. Hyaluronidase is also used in the treatment of extravasations with a hyperosmotic infusate (eg, total parenteral nutrition, calcium, potassium, 10%–50% dextrose, and nafcillin). Human recombinant hyaluronidase is available as 150 units/mL, and recommendations are to administer it as five separate and equally spaced subcutaneous injections of 0.2 mL (30 units) using a 25-gauge or smaller needle at the leading edge of the infiltrate. Wounds that are either cancerous or infected should not be treated with hyaluronidase.

**TABLE SC7–1 Management of Extravasation Injuries**

| | *Therapy* | *Purpose/Mechanism* |
|---|---|---|
| **General** | Stop infusion and maintain intravenous cannula at the site | Decreases further extravasation |
| | Aspirate extravasate from the site by accessing the original intravenous cannula | Minimizes amount of chemotherapeutic localized at the site |
| | Apply dry cool compresses for 1 hour, every 8 hours for 3 days (except for vinca alkaloids see below) | Localizes area of involvement and diminishes cellular uptake of the chemotherapeutic |
| | Elevate extremity and administer analgesia | Promotes drainage, prevents dependent edema, and provides comfort |
| **Chemotherapeutic Specific** | | |
| Anthracyclines | Dexrazoxane 1,000 mg/m$^2$, administered daily by IV (max. 2,000 mg per day), on days 1 and 2, and 500 mg/m$^2$ on day 3 (max. 1,000 mg); dose is decreased for patients with kidney disease | Limits free radical formation |
| Mechlorethamine | Add 1.6 mL of 25% sodium thiosulfate to 8.4 mL of sterile water for injection to make a 4% solution | Prevents tissue alkylation |
| | Infiltrate the site of extravasation with 2 mL of 4% sodium thiosulfate per milligram of mechlorethamine at the site | |
| Mitomycin | Dimethyl sulfoxide (DMSO): 55%–99% (w/v) applied topically and allowed to air dry | Free radical scavenger |
| Vinca alkaloids and epipodophyllotoxins | Apply dry warm compresses for 1 hour, every 8 hours for 3 days | Promotes systemic absorption of the chemotherapeutic |
| | Hyaluronidase: Inject subcutaneously 150 units/mL into the site as 5 separate and equally spaced injections of 0.2 mL using a 25-gauge or smaller needle at the leading edge of the infiltrate | Degrades hyaluronic acid to enhance systemic absorption of the chemotherapeutic |

Patients treated with hyaluronidase require monitoring for allergic reactions, such as anaphylaxis, although the newer human recombinant form is less allergenic than animal-derived hyaluronidase.

The wound should be observed closely for the first 7 days, and a surgeon consulted if either pain persists or evidence of ulceration appears. In patients with severe extravasations for which there is a high likelihood of necrosis (doxorubicin), and an area where there may be significant potential for long-term morbidity such as over joints, early surgical consultation is recommended. If tissue ulceration occurs, initial management is often restricted to sterile dressings to prevent secondary infections. Once the area of necrotic skin is clearly delineated, surgical debridement is reasonable. Some patients require surgical reconstruction or skin grafts depending on the extent of the injury.

## ANTIDOTES

Sodium thiosulfate is recommended for mechlorethamine extravasation and is believed to inactivate the xenobiotic by reacting with the active ethylenimmonium ring. For anthracycline extravasations, dexrazoxane is recommended. Dexrazoxane limits free radical cellular damage by chelating iron and directly acting as an antioxidant. Patients need to be monitored with complete blood counts and serum aminotransferase concentrations because dexrazoxane can cause reversible bone marrow suppression and can result in hepatotoxicity.

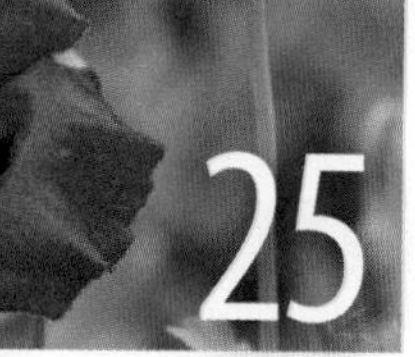

# 25 ANTIMIGRAINE MEDICATIONS

## PATHOPHYSIOLOGY OF MIGRAINE HEADACHES

A migraine headache is a neurovascular disorder often initiated by a trigger and characterized by a headache, which is preceded by an aura 20% of the time. The headache lasts 4 to 72 hours in adults and 1 to 48 hours in children and is typically a unilateral, pulsatile headache of moderate to severe intensity with associated nausea, photophobia, and/or phonophobia and is typically worsened by routine physical activity.

The treatment of migraines encompasses a wide variety of xenobiotics that can be broadly classified either as prophylactic or abortive therapies (Table 25–1). Triptans are considered the drugs of choice for abortive migraine therapy following acetaminophen and nonsteroidal antiinflammatory drugs (NSAIDs).

**TABLE 25–1 Xenobiotics Used in Migraine Treatment[a]**

| *Prophylactic* | *Abortive* |
|---|---|
| β-Adrenergic antagonists | Acetaminophen |
| ACE inhibitors | Antiemetics: Metoclopramide, prochlorperazine |
| Acetazolamide | Aspirin |
| Angiotension II receptor antagonist | Butalbital |
| Antiepileptics: Carbamazepine, gabapentin, levetiracetam, topiramate, valproic acid, zonisamide | Butyrophenones: Droperidol, haloperidol |
| Antipsychotics: Aripiprazole, olanzapine, quetiapine | Caffeine |
| Benzodiazepines | Calcitonin gene-related peptide antagonists |
| Butterbur root | Corticosteroids |
| Calcium channel blockers | Ergots |
| Coenzyme Q10 | Lasmiditan |
| Cyclic antidepressants | Lidocaine (intranasal) |
| Cyproheptadine | Magnesium (intravenous) |
| Feverfew | Nonsteroidal antiinflammatory drugs |
| Flunarizine | Opioids |
| Hormonal contraceptives | Oxygen |
| Isometheptene/dichloralphenazone/acetaminophen (Midrin) | Sedative–hypnotics |
| Magnesium (oral) | Triptans |
| Monoamine oxidase inhibitors | Valproic acid |
| Melatonin | |
| Memantine | |
| Nefazodone | |
| OnabotulinumtoxinA (Botox A) | |
| Pizotifen | |
| Riboflavin | |
| Selective serotonin reuptake inhibitors | |

[a]Prophylactic xenobiotics are usually taken to prevent triggering of migraines, and abortive xenobiotics are usually taken to stop the clinical manifestations of migraines once they are triggered. However, the separation between the two groups of xenobiotics is not strict, and some xenobiotics are used in both roles. Triptans are currently considered the drug class of choice to abort moderate to severe migraine headache. ACE = angiotensin-converting enzyme.

## ERGOT ALKALOIDS

### History and Epidemiology

Ergot is the product of *Claviceps purpurea*, a fungus that contaminates rye and other grains. This fungus produces diverse substances, including ergotamine, histamine, tyramine, isomylamine, acetylcholine, and acetaldehyde. In 600 B.C., an Assyrian tablet made mention of contamination of grain believed to be by *C. purpurea*. In approximately 400 B.C., a contaminated grass that killed pregnant women was described. In the Middle Ages, epidemics causing gangrene of the extremities with mummification of limbs were depicted in the literature. The disease was called holy fire or St. Anthony's fire because of the blackened limbs resembling the charring from fire and the burning sensation expressed by its victims. Abortion and seizures were also reported with this poisoning. As early as 1582, midwives used ergot to assist in the childbirth process. In the 20th century, ergot derivatives were almost entirely limited to the treatment of vascular headaches. Ergonovine, another ergot derivative, is used in obstetric care for its stimulant effect on uterine smooth muscle. Methylergonovine is used for postpartum uterine atony and hemorrhage. Ergot derivatives have also been used as "cognition enhancers," to help manage orthostatic hypotension, and to prevent the secretion of prolactin.

### Pharmacology and Pharmacokinetics

The ergot alkaloids are divided into three groups: amino acid alkaloids, dihydrogenated amino acid alkaloids, and amine alkaloids. The pharmacokinetics of the ergot alkaloids are well defined from controlled human volunteer studies, whereas the toxicokinetics are essentially unknown (Table 25–2). The pharmacologic effects of the ergot alkaloids can be subdivided into central and peripheral effects (Table 25–3).

### Clinical Manifestations

Ergotism, a toxicologic syndrome resulting from excessive use of ergot alkaloids, is characterized by intense burning of the extremities, hemorrhagic vesiculations, pruritus, formications, nausea, vomiting, and gangrene (Table 25–3). Headache, fixed miosis, hallucinations, delirium, cerebrovascular ischemia, cerebral infarction, and convulsions are also associated with ergotism, which has been called "convulsive" ergotism. Chronic ergotism usually presents with peripheral ischemia of the lower extremities, although ischemia of cerebral, mesenteric, coronary, and renal vascular beds is well documented. Bradycardia is characteristic and believed to be a reflex baroreceptor-mediated phenomenon associated with vasoconstriction, but a reduction in sympathetic tone, direct myocardial depression, and increased vagal activity are also factors.

Chronic use of ergotamine, dihydroergotamine, methysergide, pergolide, and cabergoline causes mitral and aortic valve leaflet thickening and immobility resulting in valvular regurgitation. The mitral and aortic valves and pulmonary arteries have high concentrations of $5HT_{2B}$ receptors, which when stimulated by ergot-derived medications activate

**TABLE 25–2 Pharmacokinetics of Ergots**

| *Ergot Derivative* | *Clinical Use* | *$t_{1/2}$ (hours)* | *Duration of Action (hours)* | *Bioavailability (%)* | *Metabolism/ Elimination* | *Interactions With Serotonergic Receptors* | *Interactions With Dopaminergic Receptors* | *Interactions With α-Adrenergic Receptors* |
|---|---|---|---|---|---|---|---|---|
| Bromocriptine | Parkinsonism, amenorrhea/ prolactinemia syndrome | 60 (PO) | 1 week (suppression of prolactin) | 28 (PO) | Liver | Weak antagonist | CNS: Partial agonist/ antagonist; inhibits prolactin secretion; emetic (high) | Vasculature: Antagonist |
| Dihydroergotamine | Migraine | 2.4 | 3–4 (IM) | 100 (IM)<br>40 (Nasal)<br>< 5 (PO) | Liver metabolism<br>Bile excretion | Smooth muscles: Partial agonist/ antagonist<br>CNS: Agonist lateral geniculate nucleus | CNS: Emetic (mild)<br>Sympathetic ganglia: Antagonism | Vasculature: Partial agonist (veins); antagonist (arteries)<br>Smooth muscles: Antagonism<br>CNS/PNS: Antagonism |
| Ergonovine | Postpartum hemorrhage | 1.9 | 3 | (IV) 100 | Liver | Smooth muscles: Potent antagonist<br>Vasculature: Agonist in umbilical and placental vessels<br>CNS: Partial antagonist/agonist | CNS: Emetic (mild); inhibits prolactin (weak); partial agonist/ antagonist<br>Vasculature: Weak antagonist | Vasculature: Partial agonist |
| Ergotamine | Migraine | 2 (1.4–6.2) | 22 (IV) | 100 (IV)<br>47 (IM)<br>< 5 (PO) | Liver metabolism<br>Bile excretion | Vasculature: Partial agonist<br>Smooth muscles: Nonselective antagonist<br>CNS: Poor agonist/ antagonist | CNS: Emetic (potent) | Vasculature: Partial agonist/ antagonist<br>Smooth muscles: Partial agonist/ antagonist<br>CNS: Antagonist<br>PNS: Antagonist |
| Methylergonovine | Postpartum hemorrhage | 1.4–2 | 3 | 78 (IM)<br>60 (PO) | Liver | Smooth muscles: Potent antagonist<br>Vasculature: Agonist in umbilical and placental vessels<br>CNS: Partial antagonist/agonist | CNS: Emetic (mild); inhibits prolactin (weak); partial agonist/ antagonist<br>Vasculature: Weak antagonist | Vasculature: Partial agonist |
| Methysergide | Migraine | 1.0 (PO) | 8–24 | 13 (PO) | Liver—metabolized to methylergonovine | Vasculature: Partial agonist<br>CNS: Potent antagonist | None | None |

CNS = central nervous system; IM = intramuscular; IV = intravenous; PNS = peripheral nervous system; PO = oral.

**TABLE 25–3 Clinical Manifestations of Ergotism**

| *Central Effects* | *Peripheral Effects* |
|---|---|
| Agitation | Angina |
| Cerebrovascular ischemia | Bradycardia |
| Hallucinations | Gangrene |
| Headaches | Hemorrhagic vesiculations and skin bullae |
| Miosis (fixed) | Mesenteric infarction |
| Nausea | Myocardial infarction |
| Seizures | Renal infarction |
| Twitching (facial) | |
| Vomiting | |

cellular kinases leading to fibroblast proliferation and collagen synthesis.

### Treatment

The treatment for a patient with ergot alkaloid toxicity depends on the nature of the clinical findings. Gastric emptying should rarely be used, if at all, because vomiting is a common early occurrence and the ingestion infrequently is complicated by seizures. After an acute overdose, activated charcoal (1 g/kg) is recommended. If emesis is present, metoclopramide or a 5-$HT_3$ antagonist, such as ondansetron, is reasonable to facilitate the administration of activated charcoal. In mild cases characterized by minimal pain of the

**TABLE 25–4 Pharmacokinetics of Triptans**

| Triptan | $t_{1/2}$ (hours) | Duration of Action (hours) | Lipophilicity | Bioavailability O (%) | Metabolism/Elimination |
|---|---|---|---|---|---|
| Almotriptan | 3.0–3.7 | 24 | Unknown | 70–80 | CYP3A4, CYP2D6 MAO-A (minor) |
| Eletriptan | 3.6–6.9 | 14–16 | High | 50 | CYP3A4 |
| Frovatriptan | 25 | 24 | Low | 24–30 | CYP1A2 kidney |
| Naratriptan | 4.5–6.6 | Unknown | High | 63–74 | Kidney (major) P450 |
| Rizatriptan | 1.8–3.0 | 25 | Moderate | 40–45 | MAO-A |
| Sumatriptan | 2.0–2.5 | 4 | Low | 14; 96 (SC) | MAO-A |
| Zolmitriptan | 1.5–3.6 | 18 | Moderate | 40–49 | CYP1A2 MAO-A (minor) |

MAO = monoamine oxidase; O = oral unless otherwise stated; SC = subcutaneous.

extremities, supportive measures such as hydration and analgesia are appropriate therapy.

Immediate-release oral nifedipine is a reasonable therapy for patients with mild symptoms of vasospasm, such as dysesthesias and minimal ischemic pain of the digits. More serious cases are defined by angina, myocardial infarction, cerebral ischemia, intermittent claudication, or internal organ/mesenteric ischemia. Reasonable therapies include sodium nitroprusside, phentolamine, and intravenous calcium channel blockers, nicardipine, or clevidipine, titrated until resolution of vasoconstriction. Anticoagulation is reasonable to prevent sludging and subsequent clot formation. Benzodiazepines are recommended therapies to treat ergot- or bromocriptine-associated seizures or hallucinations.

## TRIPTANS

In 1974, investigations began on a new class of compounds that produced vasoconstrictive effects via 5-HT receptors. In 1984, sumatriptan was synthesized and its clinical success led to the rapid development of six other triptans.

### Pharmacology

Triptans are all primarily $5\text{-HT}_{1B}$ and $5\text{-HT}_{1D}$ receptor agonists and have less activity at $5\text{-HT}_{1A}$ and $5\text{-HT}_{1F}$ receptors. In the CNS, stimulation of the $5\text{-HT}_{1B}$ receptors results in cerebral vasoconstriction. Stimulation of the $5\text{-HT}_{1D}$ receptors decrease neurotransmitter release from central trigeminal nerve terminals. The triptans also inhibit dural neurogenic inflammation by preventing the release of vasoactive neuropeptides from peripheral trigeminal nerves. Other mechanisms on the second- and third-order neurons are described. All triptans are pharmacodynamically similar but pharmacokinetically different (Table 25–4).

### Clinical Manifestations

With appropriate therapeutic use, the adverse effects associated with the triptans are minimal and include nausea, vomiting, dyspepsia, flushing, and paresthesia. However, the most consequential adverse effects are chest pressure and pain, which are reported in up to 15% of sumatriptan users. Although these symptoms are usually not secondary to cardiac ischemia, myocardial ischemia and infarction are well described. Chest pain that is not cardiac in origin may result from esophageal spasm. Renal infarctions (Fig. 25–1) and ischemic colitis are also described. Other rare reports describe transient ischemic attacks and cerebral vascular hemorrhage and infarctions.

In 2006, the US Food and Drug Administration (FDA) issued an alert, warning of an increased risk of serotonin toxicity with triptans used in combination with selective serotonin reuptake inhibitors (SSRIs) or selective serotonin-norepinephrine reuptake inhibitors. Recent evidence casts doubt on the extent of this risk.

### Treatment

Treatment of patients with triptan-induced vasospasm is dependent on the route of exposure and the organ system affected. Decontamination is not feasible after subcutaneous exposures but can be effective in overdoses of oral preparations. A single dose of activated charcoal is reasonable.

Triptan-induced vasoconstriction and ischemia should be reversed with a calcium channel blocker or intravenous vasodilators, such as nitroglycerin, or by the α-adrenergic antagonist

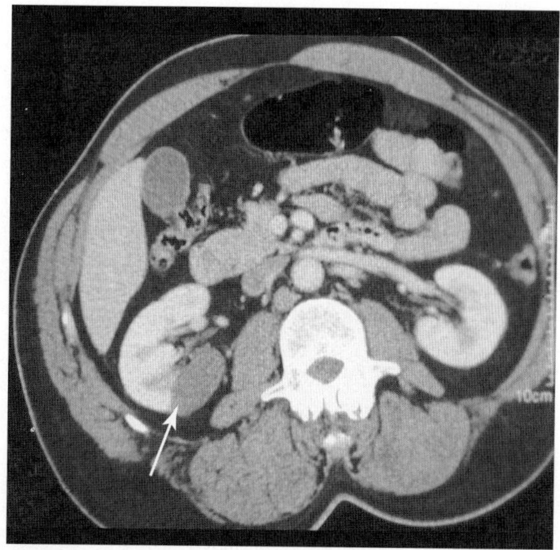


**FIGURE 25–1.** Infarction of right kidney after rizatriptan use (white arrow).

phentolamine. Many reported cases of triptan-induced vasoconstrictive compromise responded to intravenous hydration and analgesia. It is reasonable to treat triptan-associated myocardial ischemia with aspirin, heparin, and nitroglycerin.

## ISOMETHEPTENE

Isometheptene is a mild vasoconstrictor marketed as a combination preparation that includes dichloralphenazone, a muscle relaxant, and acetaminophen. It has indirect α- and β-adrenergic agonist effects, as well as minor direct α-adrenergic agonist effects on the peripheral vasculature. Cerebral vasoconstriction and myocardial infarction are reported after excessive isometheptene use. Isometheptene-associated vasoconstriction is rare, and reported treatments with calcium channel blockers or nitroglycerin are not routinely recommended.

## CALCITONIN GENE–RELATED PEPTIDE ANTAGONISTS

During migraines, calcitonin gene–related peptide (CGRP), a potent vasodilator, is among the many vasoactive peptides released from activated trigeminal nerves. Erenumab, developed for monthly subcutaneous injection, is an immunoglobulin G2 monoclonal antibody with a high affinity for the CGRP receptor and indicated for the prevention of migraines in adults. No overdoses are reported. Since the xenobiotic is a monoclonal antibody, allergic reactions are a possibility.

## 5-HT$_{1F}$ RECEPTOR AGONISTS

5-Hydroxytryptamine$_{1F}$ receptors are found on the trigeminal ganglion and the trigeminocervical complex but not on smooth muscles, coronary arteries, or cerebral vasculature. Lasmiditan is a 5-HT$_{1F}$ receptor agonist that decreases plasma protein extravasation at the trigeminal ganglion and inhibits nociceptive transmission from the trigeminocervical complex higher up to the CNS without vasoconstriction of vessels. Reported adverse effects include dizziness, fatigue, nausea, paresthesias, somnolence, vertigo, and sensation of heaviness.

# 26 THYROID AND ANTITHYROID MEDICATIONS

## HISTORY AND EPIDEMIOLOGY

Seaweed, which contains large amounts of iodine, was used to treat goiter (hypothyroidism) in Chinese medicine as early as the third century A.D. In 1863, Trousseau fortuitously discovered a treatment for Graves disease when he inadvertently prescribed a daily tincture of iodine instead of tincture of digitalis to a tachycardic, thyrotoxic young woman. In 1891, the injection of ground sheep thyroid extract was described as a treatment for myxedema. Prior to the 1950s, desiccated animal thyroid gland was commonly used to treat hypothyroidism. Two epidemics of *hamburger thyrotoxicosis* occurred in the United States (US) in the mid-1980s, secondary to consumption of ground beef contaminated with bovine thyroid gland.

Today, hypothyroidism and hyperthyroidism are relatively common endocrine disorders. Worldwide, iodine deficiency is the leading cause of hypothyroidism. According to US retail pharmaceutical statistics for prescription drugs, levothyroxine (both generic and brand combined; $T_4$) has consistently ranked in the top 5 prescriptions, with an annual average of 67 million prescriptions. Because of widespread availability of thyroid replacement therapy, many cases of intentional and unintentional overdoses with thyroid hormone are reported.

## PHARMACOLOGY

### Physiology

Thyroid function is influenced by the hypothalamus, the pituitary gland, the thyroid gland, and the target organs for the thyroid hormones (Fig. 26–1). Roughly 95% of circulating or *peripheral* thyroid hormone is $T_4$, and the remainder is $T_3$. Only 15% of the peripheral $T_3$ is secreted directly by the thyroid; the balance is a result of the peripheral conversion of $T_4$ to $T_3$. $T_3$ has approximately 3 to 4 times greater hormonal activity than $T_4$.

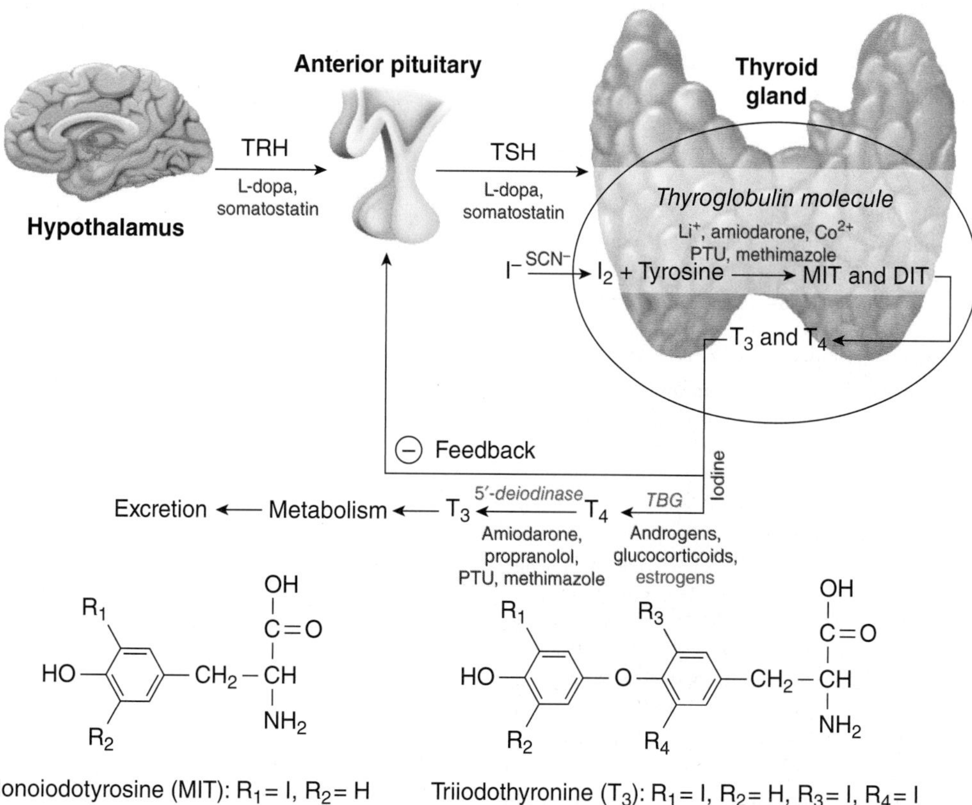


**FIGURE 26–1.** Thyroid hormone synthesis: its control, metabolism, and molecular structures. PTU = propylthiouracil; $SCN^-$ = thiocyanate; TBG = thyroxine-binding globulin; TRH = thyrotropin-releasing hormone; TSH = thyroid-stimulating hormone; $Li^+$ = lithium ion; $Co^{2+}$ = cobalt ion.

**TABLE 26–1 Pharmacokinetic Properties of Thyroid Hormones**

| *Pharmacokinetic Property* | $T_3$ | $T_4$ |
|---|---|---|
| Oral bioavailability (exogenous), % | 95 | 80 |
| Volume of distribution (L/kg) | 40 | 10 |
| Half-life (days) | 1 | 7 |
| Protein binding (normal adult), % | 99.96 | 99.6 |
| Relative potency | 3–4 | 1 |

## PHARMACOLOGY

Table 26–1 outlines some important pharmacokinetic properties of thyroid hormones. Gastrointestinal absorption of exogenous thyroid hormone occurs primarily in the duodenum and ileum and is decreased by variations in intestinal flora and binding by certain xenobiotics such as aluminum-containing antacids, calcium preparations, carbonate salts, sucralfate, iron, bile acid sequestrants (ie, cholestyramine resins, colestipol hydrochloride), and infant soy formula. In circulation, $T_3$ and $T_4$ both are highly but reversibly bound to plasma proteins, approximately 99.6% and 99.96%, respectively. Thyroxine-binding globulin binds approximately two-thirds of the circulating thyroid hormones; albumin and other proteins bind the remainder. Only 0.4% of $T_3$ and 0.04% of $T_4$ exist in the free form. Thyroid hormones undergo their ultimate metabolism peripherally, meaning outside of the thyroid gland. Xenobiotics that induce hepatic microsomal metabolism, such as rifampin, phenobarbital, phenytoin, and carbamazepine, increase the metabolic clearance of $T_3$ and $T_4$. Other xenobiotic interactions are shown in Tables 26–2 and 26–3.

## PATHOPHYSIOLOGY

Thyroid hormones are critical for optimal physiologic growth and function. Thyroid function is the most important determinant of basal metabolic rate (BMR). Additionally, the thyroid exercises a permissive effect on many hormones, notably catecholamines and insulin.

When an excess of active thyroid hormone exists, the condition is known as hyperthyroidism. Most aspects of carbohydrate and protein metabolism are increased in the presence of thyroid hormone excess. Lipid metabolism is also increased and there is an increase in cholesterol synthesis. The clinical picture consists of the manifestations of increased metabolism, along with tachycardia, tremor, anxiety, and other behavioral changes, and sometimes tachydysrhythmias such as atrial fibrillation. An increased sensitivity to catecholamines underscores the sympathomimetic effects on inotropy and chronotropy produced by thyroid hormones. $T_3$ increases the number of β-adrenergic receptors in various tissues, including cardiac cells. $T_3$ also modulates myocyte intracellular signaling mechanisms that lead to increased catecholamine effects.

Hypothyroidism, a condition characterized by decreased basal metabolic rate and decreased catecholamine effects, is a common disorder, especially in women and the elderly. Worldwide, dietary iodine deficiency remains the leading cause of hypothyroidism. Treatment of Graves disease with radioactive iodine typically results in hypothyroidism within 1 year. Thyroiditis (eg, postpartum, Hashimoto, De Quervain) is associated with either hypothyroidism or hyperthyroidism, as is exposure to certain xenobiotics such as amiodarone and lithium (Table 26–3).

**TABLE 26–2 Xenobiotic Interactions: Effects on Thyroid Hormones and Function**

| *Xenobiotic* | *Interaction* | *Effect* |
|---|---|---|
| Dopamine, levodopa, somatostatin | Inhibit TRH and TSH synthesis | No clinical hypothyroidism |
| Iodides (including amiodarone), lithium, aminoglutethimide | Inhibit thyroid hormone synthesis or release | Hypothyroidism |
| Monovalent anions ($SCN^-$, $TcO_4^-$, $ClO_4^-$) | Inhibit iodide uptake to thyroid gland | Hypothyroidism |
| Estrogens, tamoxifen, heroin, methadone, mitotane | Increase TBG | Altered thyroid hormone transport in serum ↑ Total measured thyroid hormone (vs *free* hormone) |
| Androgens, glucocorticoids | Decrease TBG | Altered thyroid hormone transport in serum ↓ Total measured thyroid hormone (vs *free* hormone) |
| Salicylates, mefenamic acid, furosemide | Displace $T_3$ or $T_4$ from TBG | Transient hyperthyroxinemia |
| Thioamides (methimazole, propylthiouracil) | Inhibit thyroid peroxidase | Decrease thyroid hormone synthesis |
| Phenytoin, carbamazepine, phenobarbital, rifampin, rifabutin | Induction of hepatic enzymes | ↓ Total thyroid hormone |
| Iopanoic acid, ipodate, amiodarone, propranolol, corticosteroids, propylthiouracil | Inhibition of 5′-deiodinase | Decrease peripheral conversion of $T_4$ (↓ $T_3$, ↑ $rT_3$) |
| Cholestyramine, colestipol, aluminum hydroxide, sucralfate, ferrous sulfate, some calcium preparations, infant soy formula | Interfere with GI absorption of $T_4$ | Decreased oral bioavailability of $T_4$ |
| Interleukin-α, interleukin-2 | Induction of autoimmune thyroid disease | Hyperthyroidism or hypothyroidism |

GI = gastrointestinal; TBG = thyroid-binding globulin; TRH = thyroid-releasing hormone; TSH = thyroid-stimulating hormone. Thiocyanate ($SCN^-$), pertechnetate ($TcO_4^-$), and perchlorate ($ClO_4^-$).

## CLINICAL MANIFESTATIONS

Signs and symptoms of toxicity from exogenous thyroid hormone resemble those of catecholamine excess, such as tachycardia, tachydysrhythmias (usually atrial fibrillation or flutter), thromboembolism, and cardiac failure. Hyperthermia occurs either secondary to the thermogenic effects of thyroid hormones or from psychomotor agitation.

### Acute Toxicity

Acute overdoses with thyroid hormone preparations most commonly occur with oral levothyroxine. Significant ingestions of levothyroxine usually do not manifest clinically until

**TABLE 26–3 Common Xenobiotics That Alter Thyroid Function and Cause Clinically Important Effects**

| *Xenobiotic* | *Effect* | *Mechanism* |
|---|---|---|
| Lithium | Goiter (in 37% of patients)<br>Hypothyroidism (in 5%–15% of patients) | Mechanism unclear |
| Amiodarone (37% iodine by weight) | 1. Hypothyroidism (in 25% of patients)<br>2. Hyperthyroidism, type 1: in patients with preexisting goiters from low iodine intake<br>3. Hyperthyroidism, type 2: in patients with previously normal thyroid function | 1. Inhibition of 5′-deiodinase<br>2. Type 1: iodine excess stimulates thyroid hormone production<br>3. Type 2: causes thyroid inflammation |
| Propranolol | ↓ Peripheral conversion of $T_4$ to $T_3$ | Inhibition of 5′-deiodinase |
| PTU (propylthiourea) or methimazole | Decreased thyroid hormone synthesis<br>↓ Peripheral conversion of $T_4$ to $T_3$ | Inhibition of thyroid peroxidase<br>Inhibition of 5′-deiodinase |
| Corticosteroids | ↓ Peripheral conversion of $T_4$ to $T_3$ | Inhibition of 5′-deiodinase |
| Iodine | 1. Low dose: transient or no effect<br>2. High doses (> 10 mg/day): ↓ thyroid hormone secretion<br>3. Transient thyrotoxicosis (ie, Jod-Basedow effect) with rapid correction of hypothyroidism from iodine deficiency<br>4. Delirium<br>5. Caustic injury [from topical iodine] | 1. Transiently stimulates thyroid hormone secretion<br>2. Inhibition of thyroid hormone synthesis<br>3. Increases thyroid hormone synthesis<br>4. Mechanism unclear<br>5. Direct cytotoxic injury to cells |
| Iodinated contrast material | 1. Rapid ↓ peripheral conversion of $T_4$ to $T_3$ (adjunctive treatment in thyroid storm)<br>2. Prolonged suppression of $T_4$ to $T_3$<br>3. Causes thyrotoxicosis and thyroid storm<br>4. Iodide "mumps" (parotitis) | 1. Inhibition of 5′-deiodinase<br>2. Mechanism unclear<br>3. Mechanism unclear<br>4. Idiopathic, toxic accumulation of iodide |
| Radioactive iodine | Treatment of hyperthyroidism, causes hypothyroidism | Uptake into thyroid follicles causes local destruction |
| Anion inhibitors[a] | ↓ Iodine uptake into thyroid follicle, used in iodide-induced hyperthyroidism | Blocks uptake of iodide into the thyroid gland by competitive inhibition |

[a]Thiocyanate ($SCN^-$), pertechnetate ($TcO_4^-$), and perchlorate ($ClO_4^-$).

7 to 10 days after the exposure but are (rarely) reported to manifest as early as 1 to 3 days after ingestion. Slow peripheral conversion of $T_4$ to $T_3$ and the time to nuclear receptor activation and protein synthesis account for this latency. In contrast, acute overdoses involving preparations containing $T_3$ can manifest in the first 12 to 24 hours after exposure.

In children, acute thyroxine overdoses are almost universally benign owing to their typically unintentional nature and lower doses ingested. Most remain asymptomatic or only develop mild symptoms. Ingestions in adults have a wide range of toxicity. Symptoms can resemble thyrotoxicosis, and in extreme cases, thyroid storm. Hyperthermia, dysrhythmias, and severe agitation are well described. Hemiparesis, muscle weakness, coma, respiratory failure, sudden death, myocardial infarction, cardiac failure, focal myocarditis, rhabdomyolysis with muscle necrosis, delayed palmar desquamation (more than 2 weeks after ingestion), and hematuria are also described.

### Chronic Toxicity

Following chronic excessive thyroid hormone ingestions, patients present with thyrotoxicosis or a have a more subtle and insidious presentation. Classically, the chronic ingestion of excess thyroid hormone occurs in patients with hypothyroidism, psychiatric disorders, and eating disorders. Significant weight loss, anxiety, and accelerated osteoporosis can develop. More severe manifestations, as described above, can also occur.

## DIAGNOSTIC TESTING

Traditionally, thyroid testing was undertaken using combinations of measurements of total $T_4$ and some measurement of hormone binding ($T_3$ uptake). Assessment of the pituitary production of TSH has greatly improved in recent years. Supersensitive assays for TSH are now the primary tests used for screening. Suppressed or elevated concentrations of TSH can be reflexively followed up with a free $T_4$ assay and, if necessary, a total $T_3$ assay and other tests (Table 26–4).

The clinical manifestations of thyrotoxicosis and thyroid storm are well known to occur at normal, low, moderate, and high concentrations of $T_3$ and $T_4$. This lack of correlation between symptoms and serum concentrations is also true for exogenous thyroid hormone ingestion. Routine analysis of laboratory thyroid function tests in the setting of acute thyroid hormone overdose is unlikely to affect management and therefore not routinely recommended.

## MANAGEMENT

### General

Based on the existing literature, conservative management is adequate in most cases of acute, unintentional thyroxine ingestions in both adults and children. Most children with acute overdose are managed with home observation and follow-up appointments. Gastrointestinal decontamination is rarely necessary. Activated charcoal administration is recommended for ingestions greater than 5,000 μg of thyroxine when no contraindications exist. Orogastric lavage is reasonable in early presentations with massive intentional thyroxine ingestions (> 10,000–50,000 μg) in suicidal adults or ingestions of preparations containing large amounts of $T_3$. These patients should be admitted in anticipation of severe symptoms.

Treatment should be based on the development of symptoms and should include rehydration, airway protection, and control of sympathomimetic symptoms, mental status alterations, and hyperthermia. Empiric treatment with β-adrenergic antagonists is not recommended.

**TABLE 26–4 Diagnostic Tests for Thyroid Hormone and Thyroid Function**

| *Diagnostic Test* | *Normal Values*[a] | *Comments* |
|---|---|---|
| TSH | 0.5–4.7 IU/mL | Available assays with respective detection limits:<br>First-generation 1.0 IU/L<br>Second-generation 0.1 IU/L<br>Third-generation 0.01 IU/L |
| Total $T_4$ by RIA | 4.5–12.5 mg/dL (58–161 nmol/L) | ↑ In pregnancy, estrogens, oral contraceptives |
| Total $T_3$ by RIA | 80–200 ng/dL (0.9–2.8 nmol/L) | ↑ In pregnancy, estrogens, oral contraceptives |
| Free $T_4$ | 8–18 pg/mL (10–23 pmol/L) | ↑ In hyperthyroidism, exogenous thyroxine ingestion |
| Free $T_3$ | 2.3–4.2 pg/mL (3.5–6.5 pmol/L) | ↑ In hyperthyroidism, exogenous thyroid hormone ($T_3$ or $T_4$) |

[a]Interlaboratory and interassay variations occur.
RIA = radioimmunoassay; TSH = thyroid-stimulating hormone.

### Agitation

When sedation is required, parenteral benzodiazepines and barbiturates are recommended. Sedation with antipsychotics such as haloperidol and droperidol should be avoided because their significant anticholinergic properties can exacerbate thyrotoxic symptoms. In addition, these drugs may prolong the QT interval and predispose to malignant dysrhythmias.

### Catecholaminelike Excess and Cardiovascular Symptoms

β-Adrenergic antagonists are recommended for significant tachycardia, dysrhythmias, and other symptoms of catecholamine excess. The principal mechanism of action of β-adrenergic antagonists in hyperthyroidism is antagonism of β-receptor–mediated effects. In addition to their sympatholytic effects, β-adrenergic antagonists inhibit 5-deiodinase, thereby decreasing peripheral conversion of $T_4$ to $T_3$. Propranolol is the most frequently used β-adrenergic antagonist in thyrotoxic patients. Starting doses of 1 to 2 mg of propranolol IV every 10 to 15 minutes are recommended. Very high doses may be required. Oral propranolol can be used for symptoms in patients who are both hemodynamically and medically stable. Oral doses, in the range of 20 to 120 mg every 6 hours, are recommended. When β-adrenergic antagonists are contraindicated, such as in patients with asthma or severe congestive heart failure, calcium channel blockers are recommended. Continuous electrocardiographic and hemodynamic monitoring is indicated when parenteral β-adrenergic antagonists are used or when patients require hospitalization.

When nonselective β-adrenergic antagonists are contraindicated, as in patients with asthma or severe congestive heart failure, $β_1$-adrenergic receptor selective antagonists (such as atenolol or metoprolol) or calcium channel blockers are recommended. Among calcium channel blockers, diltiazem is the most studied.

### Hyperthermia

Antipyretics are recommended for hyperthermia, and acetaminophen is the drug of choice. Aspirin, particularly high doses (1.5–3 g/day), should be avoided as it carries a theoretical risk of increased thyrotoxicity from displacement of $T_3$ and $T_4$ from thyroxine-binding globulin. It is important to note, however, that hyperthermia, especially extreme hyperthermia (> 106°F [41°C]), is most likely secondary to psychomotor agitation and excess heat production from the hypermetabolic, catecholaminergic, thyrotoxic state. Extreme hyperthermia should be rapidly and aggressively treated with active external cooling with ice baths as well as β-adrenergic antagonism, sedation with benzodiazepines and/or barbiturates, and intubation with paralysis if necessary.

### Other Therapies

Bile acid sequestrants, such as cholestyramine and colestipol, and aluminum hydroxide (antacids) and sucralfate bind to exogenous $T_4$ and decrease GI absorption (Table 26–2). However, because the evidence supporting their effectiveness is poor, they are not routinely recommended for thyroid hormone overdose. Although use of antithyroid drugs such as propylthiouracil (PTU), corticosteroids, and iodine contrast media in thyroxine overdose has theoretical benefits, these xenobiotics are not validated, potentially harmful, and unlikely to offer additional benefit, or be superior to conventional therapy with activated charcoal, β-adrenergic antagonism, and sedation. These treatments are not recommended as adjunctive therapies for treatment of exogenous thyroxine overdose.

### Extracorporeal Drug Removal

The use of extracorporeal drug removal procedures, such as plasma exchange or plasmapheresis, exchange transfusion (in children), and charcoal hemoperfusion, is reported in extreme cases of thyroid hormone overdose and thyroid storm. In one series, plasmapheresis was found to be more effective than hemoperfusion in the extraction of thyroxine. It is only reasonable to perform early plasmapheresis in the exceptional situation of a known massive ingestion of thyroid hormone or for a critically ill patient following thyroid hormone ingestion. The outcomes from most ingestions of thyroid hormone will be favorable with good supportive care, sedation, and β-adrenergic antagonism.

## XENOBIOTICS WITH ANTITHYROID EFFECTS

### Thioamides

Methimazole and PTU are the two principal thioamides used in the treatment of hyperthyroidism in the US. Carbimazole, which is bioactivated methimazole, is available in Europe and China. Methimazole and PTU both inhibit the activity of thyroid peroxidase in the thyroid gland. PTU has the added effect of inactivation of 5-deiodinase, which decreases the peripheral conversion of $T_4$ to the metabolically more active $T_3$.

Adverse effects occur in 3% to 12% of patients taking thioamides. The most common adverse effect is a maculopapular pruritic rash. Methimazole, PTU, and to a lesser extent carbimazole can cause immune-mediated, dose-, and age-related agranulocytosis and neutrophil dyscrasias and liver function test abnormalities. This potentially life-threatening adverse effect is treated with granulocyte colony-stimulating factor. Premature withdrawal of thioamides can lead to rebound symptoms and thyrotoxic states.

Very little data exist regarding overdose with thioamides. A 12-year-old girl with a previous thyroidectomy, who was estimated to have ingested 5,000 to 13,000 mg of PTU, developed only a transient decreased $T_3$ and elevated alkaline phosphatase. No other serious sequelae have been associated with acute overdose of thioamides.

## Iodides

Prior to the development of thioamides, iodide salts were the principal treatment for hyperthyroidism. Iodides decrease thyroid hormone concentrations by inhibiting formation and release. In thyroid storm, high-dose iodides (> 2 g/day) decrease thyroid hormone release and produce substantial improvements by 2 to 7 days.

The adverse reaction to excessive amounts of iodide salts, termed iodism, is characterized by cutaneous rash, laryngitis, bronchitis, esophagitis, conjunctivitis, drug fever, metallic taste, salivation, headache, and bleeding diathesis. Immune-mediated hypersensitivity symptoms consisting of urticaria, angioedema, eosinophilia, vasculitis, arthralgia, or lymphadenitis, and, rarely, anaphylactoid reactions are reported. Chronic iodide therapy has also produced goiters, hypothyroidism, and, rarely, hyperthyroidism. Iodide mumps is a well-described but rare disorder that is characterized by severe sialadenitis (or parotitis), allergic vasculitis, and/or conjunctivitis following administration of ionic and nonionic iodine-containing contrast media and oral iodide salts. Symptoms tend to occur within 12 hours and resolve spontaneously within 48 to 72 hours. As much as 10 g of sodium iodide has been administered IV without development of signs or symptoms of toxicity.

Potassium iodide (KI) is used prophylactically after exposure to large amounts of nuclear fallout to prevent uptake of radioactive iodine into the thyroid gland (Antidotes in Brief: A44).

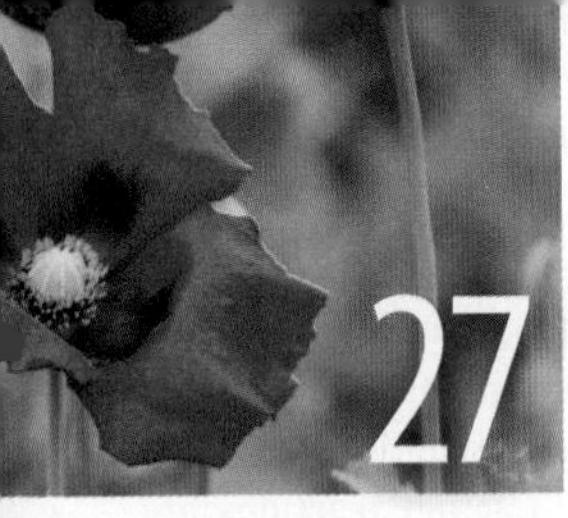



# 27 ANTIBACTERIALS, ANTIFUNGALS, AND ANTIVIRALS

## HISTORY AND EPIDEMIOLOGY

The introduction of penicillin in the 1940s revolutionized the care of patients with infectious diseases. Antimicrobials, including all categories of antibacterials, antifungals, and antivirals, significantly improve the clinical care and outcome of infected patients. Since early in their introduction, the development of antimicrobial-resistant strains of these pathogens has driven an increase in the number of antimicrobials necessary to combat infections. This, in turn, continues to increase the overall potential for toxicity after use. Fortunately, with most antimicrobials, toxicity due to acute overdose is limited and chronic therapeutic doses are safe.

However, antimicrobials are more commonly associated with allergic reactions than are other pharmaceuticals. The reason is hypothesized to be either a result of their high frequency of use, repeated intermittent prescriptions, or environmental contamination. A complete allergy history is essential to minimize these adverse drug reactions in patients being considered for antimicrobial therapy. Also, many adverse drug reactions attributed to antimicrobials are difficult to predict even when given patient- and population-specific parameters.

## PHARMACOLOGY AND TOXICOLOGY

Antimicrobial pharmacology is aimed at the destruction of microorganisms through the inhibition of cell cycle reproduction or the altering of a critical function within a microorganism. Table 27–1 lists antimicrobials and their associated

**TABLE 27–1 Antimicrobial Pharmacology and Adverse Effects**

| *Antimicrobial* | *Antimicrobial Mechanism of Action* | *Acute Overdose* | *Chronic Administration* |
|---|---|---|---|
| **Antibacterial** | | | |
| Aminoglycosides | Inhibit 30s ribosomal subunit | Neuromuscular blockade—inhibit the release of acetylcholine from presynaptic nerve terminals and act as an antagonist at acetylcholine receptors | Nephrotoxicity/ototoxicity—form an iron complex that inhibits mitochondrial respiration and causes lipid peroxidation |
| Penicillins, cephalosporins, and other β-lactams | Inhibit cell wall mucopeptide synthesis | Seizures—agonist at picrotoxin-binding site, causing GABA antagonism | Hypersensitivity—immune |
| Chloramphenicol | Inhibits 50s ribosomal subunit and inhibits protein synthesis in rapidly dividing cells | Cardiovascular collapse | "Gray baby syndrome"<br>Same as mechanism of action |
| Fluoroquinolones | Inhibit DNA topoisomerase and DNA gyrase; bind to cations ($Mg^{2+}$) | Seizures, acute kidney injury | Not entirely known; bind to cations ($Mg^{2+}$), tendon rupture, hyperglycemia, or hypoglycemia |
| Linezolid | Inhibits bacterial protein synthesis through inhibition of *N*-formylmethionyl-tRNA | None clinically relevant | MAOI activity: vasopressor response to tyramine; serotonin toxicity with SSRI and possibly meperidine |
| Macrolides, lincosamides, and ketolides | Inhibit 50s ribosomal subunit in multiplying cells | Prolong QT interval: blocks delayed rectifier potassium channel, torsade de pointes | Not entirely known; cytotoxic effect; exacerbation of myasthenia gravis |
| Nitrofurantoin | Bacterial enzymatic inhibitor | Gastritis | Dermatologic, hematologic, pancreatitis, parotitis, hepatitis, crystalluria, pulmonary fibrosis |
| Sulfonamides | Inhibit paraaminobenzoic acid and/or paraaminoglutamic acid in the synthesis of folic acid | None clinically relevant | Hypersensitivity—metabolite acts as hapten, leading to hemolysis/methemoglobinemia; exposure to UVB causes free radical formation |
| Tetracyclines | Inhibit 30s and 50s ribosomal subunits; bind to aminoacyl transfer RNA | None clinically relevant | Photosensitivity reaction<br>Pregnancy: Discoloration of teeth of offspring |
| Vancomycin | Inhibits glycopeptidase polymerase in cell wall synthesis | "Red man syndrome"—anaphylactoid | Nephrotoxicity |
| **Antifungal** | | | |
| Amphotericin B | Binds with ergosterol on cytoplasmic membrane to create pores to facilitate organelle leak | Dysrhythmias and cardiac arrest | Nephrotoxicity—vehicle deoxycholate may be involved; nephrocalcinosis |
| Triazoles and imidazoles | Increase permeability of cell membranes | None clinically relevant | None clinically relevant |

GABA = γ-aminobutyric acid; MAOI = monoamine oxidase inhibitor; SSRI = selective serotonin reuptake inhibitor; UVB = ultraviolet B light.

mechanisms of activity, toxicologic effects, and related toxicologic mechanisms. Often the mechanisms for toxicologic effects following acute overdose differ from their therapeutic mechanisms.

## ANTIBACTERIALS

### Aminoglycosides

Aminoglycosides that are in current use in the United States (US) and their toxicities are shown in Table 27–2. Overdoses, almost exclusively the result of dosing errors, are rarely life threatening, and most patients can be safely managed with minimal intervention. At therapeutic doses, aminoglycosides exacerbate concomitant neuromuscular blockade by inhibiting presynaptic calcium channels, thereby inhibiting the release of acetylcholine from presynaptic nerve terminals. Patients at risk for enhanced neuromuscular blockade include those with abnormal neuromuscular junction function, such as occurs with myasthenia gravis or botulism.

*Adverse Drug Reactions Associated With Therapeutic Use.* Adverse drug reactions correlate more closely with elevated trough serum concentrations than with elevated peak concentrations. When aminoglycosides are administered at high doses or during once-daily dosing, sepsislike chills and malaise occur, which are likely due to excipients delivered during the infusion.

*Nephrotoxicity.* The mechanism of nephrotoxicity and ototoxicity is incompletely understood but involves the formation of reactive oxygen species in the presence of iron. Both the inhibition of mitochondrial respiration resulting in lipid peroxidation and the stimulation of glutamate activated *N*-methyl-D-aspartate (NMDA) receptors are hypothesized to play a role. The incidence of nephrotoxicity with aminoglycoside therapy is estimated at 10% to 25%. Renal tubular toxicity occurs through reabsorption. In addition to tubular toxicity, renal injury also occurs through effects on the glomerulus and vascular system. Acute kidney injury does not generally occur before 7 to 10 days of standard-dose therapy and the diagnosis is often delayed because injury occurs days prior to elevations in serum creatinine concentration. Laboratory abnormalities include granular casts, proteinuria, elevated urinary sodium, and increased fractional excretion of sodium. Usually acute kidney injury (AKI) is reversible. Risk factors for the development of nephrotoxicity include increasing age, chronic kidney disease (CKD), female sex, previous aminoglycoside therapy, liver dysfunction, large total dose, long duration of therapy, frequent doses, high trough concentrations, the presence of other nephrotoxic xenobiotics, and shock. Because the uptake of aminoglycosides into organs is saturable, once-daily high-dose regimens are less problematic than several lesser doses given in a single day.

**TABLE 27–2 Predominant Manifestations of Aminoglycoside Toxicity**

| *Cochlear* | *Cochlear and Vestibular* | *Vestibular* | *Renal* |
|---|---|---|---|
| Kanamycin | Amikacin | Streptomycin | Amikacin |
| Neomycin | Gentamicin | | Gentamicin |
| | Tobramycin | | Kanamycin |
| | | | Neomycin |
| | | | Streptomycin |
| | | | Tobramycin |

*Ototoxicity.* Both cochlear and vestibular dysfunction occur after acute or prolonged exposure to aminoglycosides. Vestibular toxicity occurs in 0.4% to 10% of patients. Symptoms include vertigo or tinnitus. Full-tone audiometric testing first shows high-frequency hearing loss, which subsequently progresses in select cases. Given the inability of cochlear hair cells to regenerate, all hearing loss that develops is permanent. After early diagnosis of vestibular dysfunction, select patients improve after discontinuation of the xenobiotic. Withdrawal of the offending xenobiotic is indicated in patients with either nephrotoxicity or ototoxicity caused by an aminoglycoside antibiotic. Supportive care is the mainstay of therapy.

### Penicillins

Penicillin is derived from the fungus *Penicillium* and many semisynthetic derivatives have found clinical utility. Acute oral overdoses of the various penicillins are usually not life threatening. The most frequent complaints following acute overdose are nausea, vomiting, and diarrhea. Seizures can occur in persons given large intravenous or cerebral intraventricular doses of penicillins. More than 50 million units administered intravenously in less than 8 hours are generally required to produce seizures in adults. Penicillin-induced seizures are mediated through binding to the picrotoxin-binding site on the neuronal chloride channel near the γ-aminobutyric acid (GABA)–binding site. The treatment of patients who develop penicillin-induced seizures should emphasize benzodiazepines followed by other GABA agonists, if necessary. There are rare reports of hyperkalemia resulting in electrocardiographic abnormalities after the rapid intravenous infusion of potassium penicillin G to patients with CKD.

*Adverse Drug Reactions Associated With Therapeutic Use.* Penicillins are associated with a myriad of adverse drug reactions after therapeutic use, the most common of which are allergic in nature.

*Acute Allergy.* Penicillins are the pharmaceuticals most commonly implicated in the development of acute anaphylactic reactions. The incidence of penicillin hypersensitivity occurs in 5% of patients, with 1% of penicillin reactions manifesting as anaphylaxis. Anaphylactic reactions are severe, life-threatening, immunoglobulin E (IgE)–mediated immune reactions involving multiple organ systems that typically occur immediately after exposure. Table 27–3 lists the classifications of anaphylactic reactions. Life-threatening clinical manifestations include angioedema, tongue and airway edema, bronchospasm, bronchorrhea, dysrhythmias, cardiovascular collapse, and cardiac arrest.

Treatment is supportive with careful attention to airway, breathing, and circulation. Specific therapy for anaphylaxis is epinephrine 0.01 mg/kg in children (up to the adult dose of 0.3–0.5 mg) given as 1:1,000 (1 mg/mL) dilution intramuscularly (IM) every 5 to 15 minutes. Oxygen, intravenous

**TABLE 27–3 Classification of Anaphylactic Reactions**

| Grade | Description |
|---|---|
| I | Large local contiguous reaction (> 15 cm) |
| II | Pruritus (urticaria), generalized |
| III | Asthma, angioedema, nausea, vomiting |
| IV | Airway (asthma, lingual edema, dysphagia, respiratory distress, laryngeal edema) |
| | Cardiovascular (hypotension, cardiovascular collapse) |

use of epinephrine (1 μg/min), intravenous crystalloid, and inhaled $\beta_2$-adrenergic agonists are warranted in severe cases, as are corticosteroids. Refractory cases of hypotension may respond to glucagon and methylene blue administration (Antidotes in Brief: A20 and A43).

***Amoxicillin-Clavulanic Acid and Drug-Induced Liver Injury (DILI).*** The predominant distribution of penicillin-induced hepatotoxicity is cholestatic hepatitis, which typically occurs 1 to 8 weeks after initiation of therapy. The mechanism of hepatotoxicity is not clear, but it is hypothesized to be immunoallergic and related to clavulanate, a β-lactamase inhibitor, or one of its metabolites. Treatment is supportive and clinical findings typically resolve after the discontinuation of therapy.

***Hoigne Syndrome and Jarisch–Herxheimer Reaction.*** The most common adverse drug reactions occurring after administration of large intramuscular or intravenous doses of procaine penicillin G are the Hoigne syndrome and the Jarisch–Herxheimer reaction. The Hoigne syndrome is characterized by extreme apprehension and fear, illusions or hallucinations (both visual and auditory), tachycardia, systolic hypertension, and, occasionally, seizures that begin within minutes of injection. Procaine is implicated as the etiology because of the similarity to events that occur after the administration of other local anesthetics known as the so-called caine reaction.

The Jarisch–Herxheimer reaction is a self-limited reaction that develops within a few hours of antibiotic therapy for the treatment of spirochetal diseases (eg, syphyilis or Lyme disease), leptospirosis, and in Q fever. Myalgias, chills, headache, rash, and fever spontaneously resolve within 18 to 24 hours, even with continued antibiotic therapy. The pathogenesis of this reaction is likely either endotoxin induced from the lysed spirochete or cytokine elevation.

### Cephalosporins

Cephalosporins are semisynthetic derivatives of cephalosporin C produced by the fungus *Acremonium,* previously called *Cephalosporium.* Cephalosporins have a ring structure similar to that of penicillins and are generally divided into first, second, third, fourth, and fifth generations based on their antimicrobial spectrum. Effects occurring after acute overdose of cephalosporins resemble those occurring with penicillins. Some cephalosporins also have epileptogenic potential similar to penicillin. Case reports demonstrate seizures after inadvertent intraventricular administration. Management of patients with cephalosporin overdose is similar to those with penicillin overdose.

***Adverse Drug Reactions Associated With Therapeutic Use.*** Cephalosporins rarely cause an immune-mediated acute hemolytic crisis. Also like penicillins, first-generation cephalosporins are associated with chronic toxicity, including interstitial nephritis and hepatitis.

***Cross-Hypersensitivity.*** The extent of cross-reactivity between penicillins and cephalosporins in an individual patient is largely determined by the type of penicillin allergic response experienced by the patient and the structural similarity of the β-lactam side determinants. The incidence of anaphylaxis to cephalosporins is between 0.0001% and 0.1%, with a threefold increase in patients with previous penicillin allergy. The overall cross-reactivity rate is approximately 1% between penicillin and a first- or second-generation cephalosporin. Cross-reactivity between penicillin and third-, fourth-, or fifth-generation cephalosporins is likely to be negligible because of a dissimilar antigenic side chain.

***N-Methylthiotetrazole Side-Chain Effects.*** Cefazolin and cefotetan are the only available cephalosporins containing an *N*-methylthiotetrazole (nMTT) side chain. As these cephalosporins undergo metabolism, they release free nMTT, which inhibits the enzyme aldehyde dehydrogenase. In conjunction with ethanol consumption, use of these medications can cause a disulfiramlike reaction (Chaps. 49 and 51). The nMTT side chain is also associated with hypoprothrombinemia. Treatment of patients suspected of hypoprothrombinemia caused by these cephalosporins consists of clotting factor replacement, if bleeding is evident, and vitamin $K_1$ in doses required to reactivate vitamin K cofactors (Chap. 31 and Antidotes in Brief: A17).

### Other β-Lactam Antimicrobials

Included in this group are monobactams such as aztreonam and carbapenems such as doripenem, ertapenem, imipenem/cilastatin, and meropenem. Effects occurring after acute overdose and the management of other β-lactam antimicrobials resemble those occurring after penicillin exposure. Imipenem has epileptogenic potential in both overdose and therapeutic dosing and at a higher risk than other carbapenems.

***Adverse Drug Reactions Associated With Therapeutic Use.*** The risk factors for developing imipenem-related seizures include central nervous system disease, prior seizure disorder, and abnormal kidney function.

***Cross-Hypersensitivity.*** Aztreonam is a monobactam that does not contain the antigenic components required for cross-allergy with penicillins, and generalized cross-allergenicity is not expected.

### Trimethoprim–Sulfamethoxazole

Trimethoprim and sulfamethoxazole work in tandem as antibacterials effectively preventing tetrahydrofolic acid synthesis in bacterial cells. Significant toxicity after acute overdose is not expected. Hyperkalemia can occur as a result of the ability of trimethoprim to competitively inhibit sodium channels in the distal nephron, causing impairment in renal potassium excretion. Clinically significant hyperkalemia is reported in patients concurrently on other xenobiotics that increase potassium and among those with CKD. Other effects commonly reported after use of trimethoprim–sulfamethoxazole combinations include cutaneous allergic reactions, hematologic disorders, methemoglobinemia, hypoglycemia, rhabdomyolysis, neonatal kernicterus, and psychosis. Trimethoprim also inhibits the renal tubular secretion of creatinine, resulting in an increase in serum creatinine measurement. The rise in creatinine is independent of glomerular filtration rate and resolves on drug discontinuation.

## Chloramphenicol

Chloramphenicol was originally derived from *Streptomyces venezuelae* and is now synthetically produced. Chloramphenicol inhibits protein synthesis in rapidly proliferating cells. Metabolic acidosis occurs as a result of the inhibition of mitochondrial enzymes, oxidative phosphorylation, and mitochondrial biogenesis. Acute overdose of chloramphenicol commonly causes nausea and vomiting. Infrequently, sudden cardiovascular collapse can occur 5 to 12 hours after acute overdoses. Cardiovascular compromise is more frequent in patients with serum concentrations higher than 50 μg/mL. Orogastric lavage should be used after recent ingestions when the patient has not vomited, and oral or nasogastric activated charcoal 1 g/kg should also be given.

Extracorporeal means of eliminating chloramphenicol should be employed in patients presenting early after a life-threatening history of ingestion, particularly if they have severe hepatic or renal dysfunction.

***Adverse Drug Reactions Associated With Therapeutic Use.*** The classic description of chronic chloramphenicol toxicity is the "gray baby syndrome." Children with this syndrome exhibit vomiting, anorexia, respiratory distress, abdominal distension, green stools, lethargy, cyanosis, ashen color, metabolic acidosis, hypotension, and cardiovascular collapse.

Approximately 90% of chloramphenicol is metabolized via glucuronyl transferase, forming a glucuronide conjugate. The remainder is excreted renally unchanged. Infants, in particular, are predisposed to the gray baby syndrome because they have a limited capacity to form a glucuronide conjugate of chloramphenicol and, concomitantly, a limited ability to excrete chloramphenicol in the urine.

There are two types of bone marrow suppression that occur after use of chloramphenicol. The most common type is dose dependent and occurs with high serum concentrations of chloramphenicol. Clinical manifestations usually occur within several weeks of therapy and include anemia, thrombocytopenia, leukopenia, and, very rarely, aplastic anemia. A second type occurs through inhibition of protein synthesis in the mitochondria of marrow cell lines. This type causes the development of aplastic anemia, which is not dose related, generally occurs in susceptible patients within 5 months of treatment, and has an approximately 50% mortality rate.

## Fluoroquinolones

The fluoroquinolones are a structurally similar, synthetically derived group of antimicrobials that have diverse antimicrobial activities. Like other antimicrobials, the fluoroquinolones rarely produce life-threatening effects following acute overdose, and most patients can be safely managed with minimal intervention. Rarely, acute overdose of a fluoroquinolone results in AKI or seizures. Treatment for AKI includes discontinuation of the fluoroquinolone and supportive care. Improvement in kidney function usually occurs within several days. Seizures are reported with ciprofloxacin and likely result from the inhibition of GABA or from elevation of neuronal glutamate. Treatment is supportive, using benzodiazepines and, if necessary, barbiturates to increase inhibitory tone.

***Adverse Drug Reactions Associated With Therapeutic Use.*** Several fluoroquinolones are substrates and/or inhibitors of CYP isoenzymes. Serious adverse drug reactions related to fluoroquinolone use consist of central nervous system toxicity, cardiovascular toxicity, hepatotoxicity, and notable musculoskeletal toxicity.

Fluoroquinolones prolong the QT interval and are reported to result in torsade de pointes. Prolongation is due to the ability of fluoroquinolones to block the rapid component of the delayed rectifier potassium current ($I_{Kr}$). Treatment of patients presenting with QT interval prolongation includes immediate discontinuation of the offending drug and supportive care. Fluoroquinolones also rarely result in potentially fatal hepatotoxicity. This adverse effect was most notable with trovafloxacin, which was withdrawn from the US market.

Fluoroquinolones should be used with caution in children and pregnant women because of their potential adverse drug reactions on developing cartilage and bone. A US Food and Drug Administration review concluded that because of these risks, these drugs should be reserved for when there is no alternative available.

## Macrolides and Ketolides

The macrolide antimicrobials include various forms of erythromycin (base, ethylsuccinate, gluceptate, lactobionate, stearate), azithromycin, clarithromycin, and fidaxomicin. Ketolides are similar in pharmacology to macrolides; telithromycin is the only available xenobiotic at this time. Acute oral overdoses of macrolide antimicrobials are not life threatening, and symptoms, which are generally confined to the gastrointestinal tract, include nausea, vomiting, and diarrhea. Intravenous overdoses can cause dysrhythmias.

Intravenous and oral therapeutic use of macrolides causes QT interval prolongation and dysrhythmias. The QT interval prolongation occurs as a result of blockade of delayed rectifier potassium currents $I_{Kr}$.

***Adverse Events Associated With Interactions With Xenobiotics.*** Erythromycin and most other macrolides are potent inhibitors of CYP3A4. Azithromycin is the exception. Clinically significant interactions occur with a variety of therapeutics. In addition, macrolides interact with the absorption and renal excretion of xenobiotics that are substrates for P-glycoprotein, and they also interfere with the normal gut flora responsible for metabolism.

***End-Organ Effects.*** The most common toxic effect of macrolides after chronic use is hepatitis, which is hypothesized to be immune mediated. Erythromycin estolate is the macrolide most frequently implicated in causing cholestatic hepatitis. Large doses (> 4 g/day) of macrolides are associated with high-frequency sensorineural hearing loss that typically resolves following discontinuation of therapy. Telithromycin contains a carbamate side chain that is hypothesized to interfere with the normal function of neuronal cholinesterase. It should be used cautiously in patients with myasthenia gravis, particularly patients receiving pyridostigmine, because of the risk of cholinergic crisis.

Clindamycin has a structure and clinical effects similar to macrolides. Neuromuscular blockade is reported after intravenous dosing errors.

### Sulfonamides

Sulfonamides antagonize *para*-aminobenzoic acid or *para*-aminobenzyl glutamic acid, which are required for the biosynthesis of folic acid. Acute oral overdoses of sulfonamides are usually not life threatening, and symptoms are generally confined to nausea, although allergy and methemoglobinemia occur rarely. Treatment is similar to acute oral penicillin overdoses.

***Adverse Drug Reactions Associated With Therapeutic Use.*** The most common adverse drug reactions associated with sulfonamide therapy are nausea and cutaneous hypersensitivity reactions. The incidence of adverse reactions to sulfonamides, including allergy, is increased in HIV-positive patients and is positively correlated to the number of previous opportunistic infections experienced by the patient. This is caused by a reduction in the mechanisms available for detoxification of free radical formation, as cysteine and glutathione concentrations are low in these patients. Methemoglobinemia and hemolysis also occur rarely. Bone marrow suppression is rare, but the incidence is increased in patients with folic acid or vitamin $B_{12}$ deficiency, and in children, pregnant women, patients with alcoholism, dialysis patients, and immunocompromised patients, as well as in patients who are receiving other folate antagonists. Other adverse drug reactions include hypersensitivity pneumonitis, Stevens–Johnson syndrome, toxic epidermal necrolysis, stomatitis, aseptic meningitis, hepatotoxicity, renal injury, and central nervous system toxicity.

### Tetracyclines

Currently available tetracyclines include demeclocycline, doxycycline, minocycline, and tetracycline. Significant toxicity after acute overdose of tetracyclines is unlikely. Gastrointestinal effects consisting of nausea, vomiting, and epigastric pain are reported.

***Adverse Drug Reactions Associated With Therapeutic Use.*** Tetracycline should be avoided in children during the first 6 to 8 years of life or by pregnant women after the 12th week of gestation because of the risk for secondary tooth discoloration in children or fetuses. Other effects associated with tetracyclines include nephrotoxicity, hepatotoxicity, skin hyperpigmentation in sun-exposed areas, and hypersensitivity reactions. More severe hypersensitivity reactions, vertigo, xenobiotic-induced lupus, and pneumonitis are reported after minocycline use, as are cases of necrotizing vasculitis of the skin and uterine cervix, and lymphadenopathy with eosinophilia. Demeclocycline rarely causes nephrogenic diabetes insipidus.

### Vancomycin

Vancomycin is obtained from cultures of *Nocardia orientalis*. Acute oral overdoses of vancomycin rarely cause significant toxicity, and most cases can be treated with supportive care alone. After large, iatrogenic, rapidly infused intravenous overdoses, AKI can occur in patients with preexisting kidney disease because of sustained high serum concentrations. In these patients, multiple doses of activated charcoal and hemodialysis are effective in enhancing clearance.

***Adverse Drug Reactions Associated With Therapeutic Use.*** After rapid infusions of intravenous vancomycin, result in the development of the "red man syndrome," which occurs through an anaphylactoid (non–IgE-mediated) mechanism. Symptoms include chest pain, dyspnea, pruritus, urticaria, flushing, and angioedema. Spontaneous resolution occurs typically within 15 minutes. Other symptoms attributable to red man syndrome include hypotension, cardiovascular collapse, and seizures. The incidence of red man syndrome is approximately 14% when 1 g is given over 10 minutes and falls dramatically to only 3.4% when given over 1 hour.

Chronic use of vancomycin results in reversible nephrotoxicity, particularly in patients with prolonged excessive steady-state serum concentrations. Concomitant administration of aminoglycoside antimicrobials increases the risk of nephrotoxicity. Vancomycin also causes, though rarely, thrombocytopenia and neutropenia.

## ANTIFUNGALS

Numerous antifungals are available. Toxicity related to the use of antifungals is variable and is based generally on their mechanism of action.

### Amphotericin B

Amphotericin B is a potent antifungal derived from *Streptomyces nodosus.* Development of lipid and colloidal formulations of amphotericin B attenuates the adverse drug reactions associated with amphotericin B. Significant findings in amphotericin B overdose include hypokalemia, increased aspartate aminotransferase concentrations, and cardiac complications. Dysrhythmias and cardiac arrest have occurred following doses of 5 to 15 mg/kg of amphotericin B. Care should be used in the doses of amphotericin B administered according to specific formulation design, as these are not interchangeable. For example, intravenous therapy for fungal infections includes a usual dose of 0.25 to 1 mg/kg/day of amphotericin B or 3 to 4 mg/kg/day of amphotericin B cholesteryl. The potential for significant dosage errors and their sequelae is readily apparent in this comparison.

***Adverse Drug Reactions Associated With Therapeutic Use.*** Infusion of amphotericin B results in fever, rigors, headache, nausea, vomiting, hypotension, tachycardia, and dyspnea. Slower rates of infusion and lower total daily doses mitigate symptoms of early infusion–related reactions as does pretreatment with diphenhydramine. In addition, acetaminophen, ibuprofen, and hydrocortisone are helpful in alleviating febrile effects.

Eighty percent of patients exposed to amphotericin B will sustain some degree of kidney dysfunction. Initial distal renal tubule damage causes renal artery vasoconstriction, ultimately resulting in azotemia. Potassium and magnesium wasting, proteinuria, decreased renal concentrating ability, renal tubular acidosis, and hematuria can also occur. Strategies to reduce renal toxicity after amphotericin B include intravenous saline or magnesium and potassium supplementation. Other adverse drug reactions reported after treatment with amphotericin B include normochromic, normocytic anemia secondary to decreased erythropoietin release; respiratory insufficiency with infiltrates; and, rarely, dysrhythmias, tinnitus, thrombocytopenia, peripheral neuropathy, and leukopenia. Exchange transfusion should be used in neonates and infants after large intravenous overdoses.

### Azole Antifungals: Triazole and Imidazoles

Triazole antifungals include fluconazole, isavuconazonium, itraconazole, posaconazole, terconazole, and voriconazole. Common imidazoles include butoconazole, clotrimazole, econazole, ketoconazole, miconazole, and tioconazole. Severe toxicity is not expected in the overdose setting. Hepatotoxicity, thrombocytopenia, and neutropenia are uncommon. Rare case reports implicate voriconazole in the development of toxic epidermal necrolysis. Most of the toxic effects noted after the use of these xenobiotics result from their xenobiotic interactions. Fluconazole, itraconazole, ketoconazole, and miconazole competitively inhibit CYP3A4, which is responsible for the metabolism of many xenobiotics. Table 27–4 lists other organ system manifestations associated with antifungals and other antimicrobials.

## ANTIPARASITICS

Antiparasitics such as mebendazole, albendazole, ivermectin, praziquantel, and pyrantel pamoate generally have limited toxicity in overdoses, although significant toxicity can be found after the use of antimalarials for the treatment of malaria or following overdose (Chap. 28). Common symptoms after therapeutic use are gastrointestinal in nature and include abdominal pain, nausea, vomiting, and diarrhea. A single case of ivermectin-associated hepatic failure has been reported 1 month after a single dose.

## ANTIVIRALS

Acyclovir, famciclovir, and valacyclovir are generally well tolerated in therapeutic doses and overdoses. Neurotoxicity and, less commonly, AKI are reported after therapeutic use, and similar findings are expected after overdose. The most common neurotoxic complaints include lethargy, confusion, and ataxia. Acute kidney injury occurs as the result of precipitation of acyclovir crystals within the renal tubules with resultant obstructive effects. A single case report describes a patient with AKI with crystalluria after ingestion of 30 g of valacyclovir.

**TABLE 27–4 Major Organ System Manifestations Associated With Antimicrobial Toxicity**

| *Antimicrobial* | *System* | *Signs/Symptoms/ Laboratory Findings* |
|---|---|---|
| **Antibacterials** | | |
| Bacitracin | Immune | Hypersensitivity reactions |
| Clindamycin | Immune | Hypersensitivity reactions |
| | Gastrointestinal | Nausea, vomiting, diarrhea |
| | Neurologic | Dizziness, headache, vertigo |
| Colistimethate (colistin sulfate) | Renal | Decreased function, acute tubular necrosis |
| | Neurologic | Peripheral paresthesias, confusion, coma, seizures, neuromuscular blockade |
| Metronidazole | Neurologic | Peripheral neuropathy, seizures |
| | Gastrointestinal | Nausea, vomiting |
| | Other | Disulfiram like reactions |
| Nitrofurantoin | Gastrointestinal | Nausea, vomiting, diarrhea |
| | Hepatic | Jaundice |
| | Immune | Rash, acute and chronic pulmonary hypersensitivity |
| | Neurologic | Peripheral neuropathy |
| Polymyxin B sulfate | Neurologic | Muscle weakness, seizures |
| | Renal | Azotemia, proteinuria |
| Selenium sulfide | Cutaneous | Contact dermatitis, alopecia (rare) |
| Silver sulfadiazine | Cutaneous | Contact dermatitis |
| | Hematologic | Anemia, aplastic anemia |
| **Antifungals** | | |
| Carbol-fuchsin solution (phenol/resorcinol/fuchsin) | Gastrointestinal | Nausea, vomiting, diarrhea |
| Gentian violet | Gastrointestinal | Nausea, vomiting, diarrhea |
| | Immune | Rash (rare) |
| Griseofulvin | Renal | Proteinuria |
| | Hepatic | Increased enzymes |
| | Gastrointestinal | Nausea, vomiting, diarrhea |
| | Immune | Neutropenia |
| | Other | Disulfiram like reactions, increased porphyrins |
| Nystatin | Gastrointestinal | Nausea, vomiting, diarrhea |
| Salicylic acid | Gastrointestinal and dermal | Higher concentrations are caustic |
| Undecylenic acid and undecylenate salt | Gastrointestinal | Nausea, vomiting, diarrhea |

## ANTIMICROBIALS SPECIFIC TO THE TREATMENT OF HIV AND RELATED INFECTIONS

The evaluation and management of patients infected with HIV continues to evolve. Medications used to manage this disorder have increased life expectancy as new, more powerful antivirals and xenobiotic combinations become available. Therapeutics for HIV commonly consist of a combination of xenobiotics from different classes. The current recommendations include highly active antiretroviral therapy

(HAART), which involves the use of two nucleoside reverse transcriptase inhibitors (NRTI) along with a third antiretroviral. Options include an integrase strand transfer inhibitor (INSTI), a nonnucleoside reverse transcriptase inhibitor (NNRTI), a protease inhibitor (PI) with a pharmacokinetic enhancer (cobicistat or ritonavir), or a C-C chemokine receptor type 5 (CCR5) antagonist. The unique mechanisms that each xenobiotic offers aid in inhibiting viral replication and in minimizing xenobiotic resistance. Drug and dosage errors, particularly in infants, are of significant concern and have resulted in iatrogenic overdose. These drugs also have success in the antiviral treatment of hepatitis C infection. This section focuses on overdoses and major toxic effects from HIV-directed antiviral therapy, as well as from xenobiotics that are specifically used in the management of opportunistic infections.

Several drug interactions are also possible because these xenobiotics are substrates for both inducers and inhibitors of several CYP isoenzymes and P-glycoprotein–associated metabolic systems. Table 27–5 lists the common antimicrobials used to treat HIV-related opportunistic infections and their common adverse effects.

## Specific Antiretroviral Classes

***Nucleoside Analog Reverse Transcriptase Inhibitors.*** The nucleoside analog reverse transcriptase inhibitors inhibit transcription

**TABLE 27–5 Antimicrobials Used to Treat Common Opportunistic Infections, Overdose Effects, and Common Adverse Drug Effects**

| *Antimicrobial* | *Opportunistic Infection* | *Overdose Effects* | *Common Adverse Drug Effects* |
|---|---|---|---|
| Albendazole | Microsporidiosis | No reported cases | Increased AST/ALT, nausea, vomiting, and diarrhea; hematologic (rare), encephalopathy, AKI, rash |
| Amphotericin B | Aspergillosis<br>Candidiasis<br>Coccidioidomycosis<br>Cryptococcosis<br>Histoplasmosis<br>Leishmaniasis<br>Paracoccidioidomycosis<br>Penicilliosis | Hypokalemia, hypomagnesemia, increased AST, dysrhythmias and cardiac arrest | Infusion-related fever, rigors, headache, nausea, vomiting, hypotension, tachycardia, and dyspnea. Phlebitis, AKI, potassium and magnesium wasting, proteinuria, decreased renal concentrating ability, renal tubular acidosis, hematuria, anemia, dysrhythmias, tinnitus, thrombocytopenia, peripheral neuropathy, leukopenia |
| Antimony (pentavalent) | Leishmaniasis | AKI | AKI, multiorgan system failure |
| Atovaquone | *Pneumocystis jiroveci* (formerly *carinii*) pneumonia (PCP) | No clinical effects | Rashes, anemia, leukopenia, increased AST/ALT |
| Azithromycin | *Mycobacterium avium* complex | Nausea, vomiting, diarrhea. Intravenous; dysrhythmias | QT interval prolongation, nausea, vomiting, diarrhea |
| Clarithromycin | *Mycobacterium avium* complex | Nausea, vomiting, diarrhea | QT interval prolongation, nausea, vomiting, diarrhea |
| Caspofungin | Aspergillosis | No reported cases | Phlebitis, headache, hypokalemia, increased AST/ALT, fever |
| Clindamycin | *Pneumocystis jiroveci* (formerly *carinii*) pneumonia (PCP)<br>*Toxoplasma gondii* | Intravenous; neuromuscular blockade | Esophageal ulcers, diarrhea, and *Clostridium difficile* enterocolitis |
| Dapsone | *Pneumocystis jiroveci* (formerly *carinii*) pneumonia (PCP) | Nausea, vomiting, diarrhea, methemoglobinemia, hemolysis | Bone marrow suppression, hepatitis, rash |
| Ethambutol | *Mycobacterium avium* complex | Severe toxicity not expected | Optic neuropathy |
| Fluconazole | Coccidioidomycosis<br>Histoplasmosis | Severe toxicity not expected | Hepatotoxicity, thrombocytopenia, and neutropenia |
| Flucytosine | Cryptococcosis | No reported cases | Bone marrow suppression, hepatotoxicity, nausea, vomiting, diarrhea, rash |
| Foscarnet | Cytomegalovirus | No reported cases | Azotemia, hypocalcemia, and kidney failure (common); anemia, leukopenia, thrombocytopenia, fever, headache, seizures, genital and oral ulcers, fixed-drug eruptions, nausea, vomiting, diarrhea, headaches, seizures, coma, diabetes insipidus, hypophosphatemia, hypokalemia, hypomagnesemia |
| Fumagillin | Microsporidiosis | No reported cases | Neutropenia, thrombocytopenia |
| Ganciclovir | Cytomegalovirus | Severe toxicity not expected | Leukopenia, worsening of kidney function; can also cause nausea, vomiting, diarrhea, increased AST/ALT, anemia, thrombocytopenia, headache, dizziness, confusion, seizures |

(*Continued*)

**TABLE 27–5 Antimicrobials Used to Treat Common Opportunistic Infections, Overdose Effects, and Common Adverse Drug Effects (*Continued*)**

| *Antimicrobial* | *Opportunistic Infection* | *Overdose Effects* | *Common Adverse Drug Effects* |
|---|---|---|---|
| Itraconazole | Histoplasmosis | No reported cases | Hepatotoxicity, thrombocytopenia, and neutropenia |
| Nitazoxanide | Cryptosporidiosis<br>Microsporidiosis | No reported cases | Hypotension, headache, abdominal pain, nausea, vomiting; may cause green-yellow urine discoloration |
| Paromomycin | Cryptosporidiosis | No reported cases | Ototoxicity, nephrotoxicity, pancreatitis |
| Pentamidine | *Pneumocystis jiroveci* (formerly *carinii*) pneumonia (PCP) | 40 times dosing error in a 17-month-old child resulted in cardiac arrest | Hypoglycemia (early) followed by hyperglycemia, azotemia; can cause hypotension, torsade de pointes, phlebitis, rash, Stevens–Johnson syndrome, hypocalcemia, hypokalemia, anorexia, nausea, vomiting, metallic taste, leukopenia, thrombocytopenia |
| Primaquine | *Pneumocystis jiroveci* (formerly *carinii*) pneumonia (PCP) | No reported cases | Neutropenia, hemolytic anemia, methemoglobinemia, leukocytosis; hypertension |
| Pyrimethamine | *Toxoplasma gondii* | No reported cases | Agranulocytosis, aplastic anemia, thrombocytopenia, leukopenia |
| Rifabutin | *Mycobacterium avium* complex | High doses (> 1 g daily): arthralgia/arthritis | Nausea, vomiting, diarrhea; can cause hepatotoxicity, neutropenia, thrombocytopenia, hypersensitivity reactions |
| Sulfadiazine | *Toxoplasma gondii* | AKI and hypoglycemia | Rash, Stevens–Johnson syndrome, toxic epidermal necrolysis, erythema multiforme; headaches, depression, hallucinations, ataxia, tremor, crystalluria, hematuria, proteinuria, and nephrolithiasis |
| Trimethoprim–sulfamethoxazole | *Pneumocystis jiroveci* (formerly *carinii*) pneumonia (PCP)<br>*Toxoplasma gondii*<br>Isosporiasis | Severe toxicity not expected | Hyperkalemia, allergy, hematologic disorders, methemoglobinemia, hypoglycemia, rhabdomyolysis, neonatal kernicterus, psychosis |
| Trimetrexate | *Pneumocystis jiroveci* (formerly *carinii*) pneumonia (PCP) | Severe toxicity not expected; treat similarly to methotrexate (Chap. 24) | Myelosuppression, nausea, vomiting, histaminergic reactions |
| Valganciclovir | Cytomegalovirus | Severe toxicity not expected; expect to be similar to ganciclovir | Anemia, neutropenia, thrombocytopenia; nausea, vomiting, headache, peripheral neuropathy |
| Voriconazole | Aspergillosis | Severe toxicity not expected | Hepatotoxicity, thrombocytopenia, neutropenia, toxic epidermal necrolysis |

AKI = acute kidney injury; ALT = alanine aminotransferase; AST = aspartate aminotransferase.

of viral RNA into its subsequent DNA. Currently available xenobiotics include abacavir, didanosine (ddI), emtricitabine, lamivudine, stavudine, and zidovudine.

Overdose Effects: Many intentional overdoses of reverse transcriptase inhibitors occur without major toxicologic effects. The most serious adverse effect is the development of a metabolic acidosis with elevated lactate concentration. After the incorporation of the nucleoside analog into mitochondrial DNA by viral RNA reverse transcriptase enzymes, the faulty DNA results in impaired polymerase-$\gamma$ activity. This results in decreased production of mitochondrial DNA electron transport proteins, which ultimately inhibits oxidative phosphorylation. Organ system toxicity follows in addition to the development of acidemia. The reported mortality in patients with NRTI-associated metabolic acidosis associated with elevated lactate is 33% to 57%. Patients with NRTI-associated acidemia are reported to recover more quickly after the use of cofactors such as thiamine, riboflavin, L-carnitine, vitamin C, and antioxidants. The indications for the use of these xenobiotics are unclear at this time; however, because of the relative lack of toxicity, administration is reasonable.

Chronic Effects: Development of acidemia is more commonly associated with therapeutic use of reverse transcriptase inhibitors than with acute overdose. The mechanism is likely identical to that described above. Other drug-specific adverse reactions include hematologic toxicity after zidovudine, pancreatitis with didanosine, hypersensitivity after abacavir, and sensory peripheral neuropathy after stavudine and didanosine.

***Nonnucleoside Reverse Transcriptase Inhibitors.*** The nonnucleoside reverse transcriptase inhibitors bind directly to reverse transcriptase enzymes enabling allosteric inhibition of enzymatic function. Delavirdine, efavirenz, etravirine, nevirapine, and rilpivirine comprise the currently available xenobiotics. There is a paucity of acute overdose data on these xenobiotics, although they generally appear to have limited toxicity. An infant received 40 times the therapeutic dose of nevirapine with mild neutropenia and a metabolic acidosis with elevated lactate concentration. Treatment is entirely supportive until more information is available. The nonnucleoside reverse transcriptase inhibitors are also limited in toxicity after chronic use.

*Protease Inhibitors.* Protease inhibitors inhibit viral replication. Currently available xenobiotics include atazanavir, darunavir, fosamprenavir, indinavir, nelfinavir, ritonavir, saquinavir, and tipranavir. Data after protease inhibitor overdose are limited. A literature review found diarrhea and hyperlipidemia to be common findings after therapeutic use. Less common were hepatitis, rash, hyperbilirubinemia, paresthesias, and nephrolithiasis. Drug interactions can occur due to almost uniform inhibition of CYP3A and effects on P-glycoprotein as well as additional effects and/or substrates for other CYP isoenzymes. A unique finding is an altered fat distribution pattern that, over time, results in central obesity, "buffalo hump," breast enlargement, cushingoid appearance, and peripheral wasting.

*Fusion Inhibitors.* This class of xenobiotics interferes with the binding or entry of the HIV virion into the cell. No acute overdose data are available for this class, but after chronic use, hypersensitivity, gastrointestinal complaints, hepatotoxicity, and infusion reactions seem to be of greatest concern. The currently available drug is enfuvirtide.

*Cellular Chemokine Receptor (CCR5) Antagonist.* These drugs bind to chemokine coreceptors found on CD4 cells, which then ultimately prevents the entry of the HIV virion into the cell. The currently available drug is maraviroc. There are no overdose or adverse events reported; however, maraviroc has a boxed warning due to another CCR5 inhibitor, which was halted in development because of substantial hepatotoxicity.

*Integrase Inhibitor.* This class of xenobiotics prevents the activity of the enzyme responsible for the incorporation of the virus into DNA. The currently available xenobiotics are dolutegravir, elvitegravir, and raltegravir. No information is currently available regarding its toxicity after acute overdose.

# 28 ANTIMALARIALS

The malaria parasite has caused untold grief throughout human history. The name originated from Italian *mal aria* (bad air) because the ancient Romans believed the disease was caused by the decay in marshes and swamps and was carried by the malodorous "foul" air emanating from these areas. Today, nearly half of the world's population lives in areas where malaria is endemic. In 2015, there were 212 million estimated malaria cases, leading to 429,000 deaths. Despite using prophylactic medications, an estimated 30,000 world travelers will acquire malaria annually.

## MALARIA OVERVIEW

Malaria is an infection of protozoan parasites in the *Plasmodium* genus with a unique life cycle involving the *Anopheles* mosquito as vector (Fig. 28–1). Six *Plasmodium* spp cause malaria in humans (Table 28–1). The majority of cases worldwide are caused by *P. falciparum* and *P. vivax*, with *P. falciparum* responsible for the overwhelming majority of deaths.

## ANTIMALARIAL HISTORY

The bark of the cinchona tree, the first effective remedy for malaria, was introduced to Europeans more than 350 years ago. The toxicity of its active ingredient, quinine, was noted from the inception of its use. Pharmaceutical advances occurred, funded largely by the United States (US) military during World War II, yielding 4-aminoquinolines, 8-aminoquinolines, and novel antifolates. To combat emerging strains of drug-resistant *P. falciparum* that developed during the Vietnam conflict, alternate quinine derivatives (amino

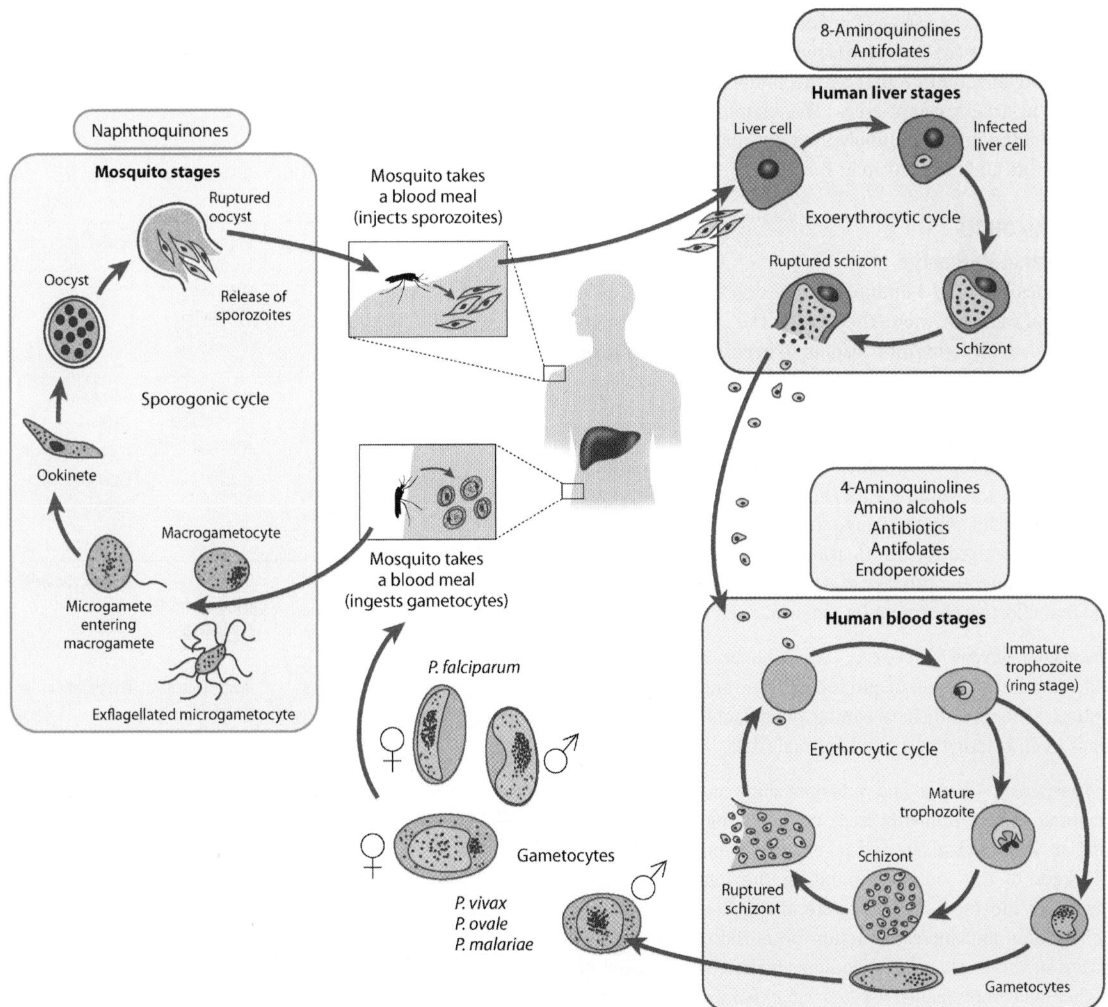


**FIGURE 28–1.** Life cycle stages during which antimalarials exert their effects.

**TABLE 28–1** *Plasmodium* spp Affecting Humans

| *Species* | *Distribution* | *Fever Cycle (days)* | *RBC Preference* | *Parasitemia* | *Comments* |
|---|---|---|---|---|---|
| *P. falciparum* | Widespread throughout tropics | 2 or less (sub-tertian) | All ages | Can be high | Most fatalities |
| *P. knowlesi* | Malaysia and neighboring countries | 1 | All ages | Can be high | Zoonosis (primary host Macaque monkey), severe disease in humans |
| *P. malariae* | Worldwide | 3–4 (quartan) | Old | Low | Chronic infections, late recrudescence |
| *P. ovale curtisi* | Africa | 2–3 (tertian) | Young | Low | Relapses/hepatic hypnozoites |
| *P. ovale wallikeri* | Africa | 2–3 (tertian) | Young | Low | Relapses/hepatic hypnozoites<br>More severe symptoms, increased parasitemia compared to *P. ovale curtis* |
| *P. vivax* | Predominantly Asia | 2–3 (tertian) | Young | Low | Relapses/hepatic hypnozoites |

alcohols) were developed. Other drugs used to treat malaria include the folate inhibitors, selected antibiotics, the sulfonamide sulfadoxine, the tetracyclines, and the macrolides (Chap. 27). With the introduction of each new drug, resistance developed. In the past 2 decades, the search for active xenobiotics has returned to a natural product, the Chinese herb qinghaosu, which contains dihydroartemisinin. These drugs are primarily used as part of artemisinin-based combination therapy (ACT), which is recommended by the World Health Organization (WHO) as the preferred treatment of malaria in drug-resistant areas. This chapter highlights the toxicity of the most commonly used antimalarials classified by structure and mechanism in Table 28–2.

## AMINO ALCOHOLS

### Antimalarial Mechanism

Amino alcohols and 4-aminoquinolines concentrate in parasite food vacuoles, where they inhibit the ability of the parasite to detoxify hemozoin, leading to accumulation of toxic heme by-products and parasite death.

### Quinine

The therapeutic benefits of the bark of the cinchona tree have been known for centuries. As early as 1633, cinchona bark was used for its antipyretic and analgesic effects, and in the 1800s, it was used for the treatment of "rebellious palpitations." Quinine, the primary alkaloid in cinchona bark, was the first effective treatment for malaria.

***Pharmacokinetics and Toxicokinetics.*** See Table 28–3 for the pharmacokinetic properties of quinine. Quinine and quinidine are optical isomers and share similar pharmacologic effects as class IA antidysrhythmics and antimalarials.

***Pathophysiology.*** Quinine and quinidine share anti- and prodysrhythmic effects primarily from an inhibiting effect on the cardiac sodium channels and potassium channels (Chap. 30). Blockade of the sodium channel in the inactivated state decreases inotropy, slows the rate of depolarization, slows conduction, and increases action potential duration. Inhibition of this rapid inward sodium current is increased at higher heart rates (called *use-dependent blockade*), leading to

**TABLE 28–2** Antimalarial Classification and Mechanisms

| *Class* | *Examples* | *Antimalarial Mechanism* | *Life Cycle Stage Effect* |
|---|---|---|---|
| Amino alcohols | Halofantrine<br>Lumefantrine<br>Mefloquine<br>Quinine | Inhibit heme digestion | Erythrocytic cycle[a] |
| 4-Aminoquinolines | Amodiaquine<br>Chloroquine<br>Hydroxychloroquine<br>Piperaquine | Inhibit heme digestion | Erythrocytic cycle[a] |
| 8-Aminoquinolines | Diethylprimaquine<br>Primaquine | Oxidant stress | Liver stages<br>Hypnozoiticidal |
| Endoperoxides | Artemether<br>Artesunate<br>Artemisinin<br>Artemisone<br>Dihydroartemisinin | Unknown but oxidant stress likely contributes | Erythrocytic cycle[a] |
| Antifolates | Cycloguanil<br>Chlorproguanil<br>Dapsone<br>Proguanil<br>Pyrimethamine<br>Trimethoprim | Inhibit dihydrofolate reductase | (All growing stages)<br>Erythrocytic cycle[a]<br>Exoerythrocytic cycle[b] |
| Antibiotics | Sulfonamides<br>Sulfadoxine | Inhibit dihydropteroate synthetase | Erythrocytic cycle[a] |
| | Cyclines<br>Doxycycline<br>Tetracycline | Inhibit protein synthesis | Erythrocytic cycle[a] |
| | Macrolides<br>Azithromycin<br>Clindamycin | Apicoplast disruption | Erythrocytic cycle[a] |
| Naphthoquinones | Atovaquone | Inhibit mitochondrial respiration | Mosquito sporogonic cycle[c] |

[a]Blood schizonticidal and blood gametocidal. [b]Liver schizonticidal but not effective against hypnozoites. [c]Altered oocyst development.

**TABLE 28–3 Pharmacokinetic Properties of Antimalarials**

| *Antimalarial* | *Bioavailability (%)* | *Time to Peak (hours) (oral)* | *Protein Bound (%)* | *Volume of Distribution (L/kg)* | *Half-Life* | *Urinary Excretion (%)* | *Metabolism* | *Comments* |
|---|---|---|---|---|---|---|---|---|
| Artemisinin | Limited | — | Large | — | 2–5 h | — | CYP2B6, CYP3A4 | Autoinduction of its own first-pass effect<br>CYP2B6 inducer<br>CYP2C19 inducer |
| Atovaquone | Varies | 5–6 | 99 | 4.7–13 | 2–3 d | < 1 | Primarily excreted unchanged in the feces | Increased bioavailability with fatty foods<br>Enterohepatic cycling |
| Dihydroartemisinin | 30 | 1–2 | — | 1–35 | 1–2.3 h | — | — | — |
| Chloroquine | 80–89 | 1.5–3 | 50–65 | 32–262 | 5–12 d | 55 | CYP2C8<br>CYP3A4 | CYP2D6 inhibitor |
| Dapsone | 90 | 2–8 | 70–80 | 0.5–2 | 21–30 h | 20 | CYP2C19 | Enterohepatic circulation<br>Genetic polymorphisms |
| Halofantrine | Low, varies | 4–7 | — | > 100 | 1–6 d | — | CYP3A4 | Active metabolite |
| Lumefantrine | Varies | 2–66 | 99 | 0.4–8.9 | 3 d | — | CYP3A4 | Active metabolite<br>CYP2D6 inhibitor |
| Mefloquine | > 85 | 6–24 | 98 | 15–40 | 15–27 d | < 1 | CYP3A4 | Stereospecific activity<br>Inactive metabolite |
| Piperaquine | Low, varies with diet | 3–6 | 99 | 529–877 | 13–28 d | — | CYP3A4 | |
| Primaquine | 75 | 1–3 | 75 | 3–8 | 4–9 h | 4 | CYP2C19<br>CYP2D6<br>CYP3A4 | Active metabolites primarily responsible for therapeutic and toxic effects<br>Genetic polymorphisms |
| Proguanil | 60 | 4–5 | 75 | 13–23 | 12–21 h | 40–60 | CYP2C19<br>CYP3A4 | Active metabolite |
| Pyrimethamine | > 95 | 2–6 | 87 | 2–7 | 3–4 d | 16–32 | Hepatic | — |
| Quinine | 76 | 1–3 | 70–90 | 1.8–4.6 | 9–15 h | 20 | CYP3A4<br>CYP2D6<br>CYP2C9<br>CYP1A2 | Protein binding increased in alkaline environments<br>CYP2D6 inhibitor |

— = poorly studied or unknown.

a rate-dependent widening of the QRS complex. Inhibition of the potassium channels suppresses the repolarizing delayed rectifier potassium current, particularly the rapidly activating component, leading to prolongation of the QT interval. The resultant increase in the effective refractory period is also rate dependent, causing greater repolarization delay at slower heart rates and predisposing to torsade de pointes. As a result, syncope and sudden dysrhythmogenic death occur. An additional α-adrenergic antagonist effect contributes to the syncope and hypotension occurring in quinine toxicity. Quinidine possesses antimuscarinic activity in therapeutic dosing.

Inhibition of the adenosine triphosphate (ATP)–sensitive potassium channels of pancreatic β cells results in the release of insulin, similar to the action of sulfonylureas (Chap. 20). Patients at increased risk of quinine-induced hyperinsulinemia include those patients receiving high-dose intravenous (IV) quinine, patients with intentional overdose, and patients with other metabolic stresses (eg, concurrent malaria, pregnancy, malnutrition, and ethanol consumption).

The mechanism of quinine-induced ototoxicity appears to be multifactorial. Microstructural lengthening of the outer hair cells of the cochlea and organ of Corti occurs. Additionally, vasoconstriction and local prostaglandin inhibition within the organ of Corti contribute to decreased hearing. Inhibition of the potassium channel also impairs hearing and produces vertigo.

Although older theories suggested that quinine caused retinal ischemia, the preponderance of evidence points to a direct toxic effect on the retina and possibly the optic nerve fibers. Quinine also antagonizes cholinergic neurotransmission in the inner synaptic layer. Quinine has direct irritant effects on the gastrointestinal (GI) tract and stimulates the brain stem center responsible for nausea and emesis.

***Clinical Manifestations.*** Patients receiving even therapeutic doses often experience a syndrome known as "cinchonism," which typically includes GI complaints, headache, vasodilation, tinnitus, and decreased auditory acuity. Vertigo, syncope, dystonia, tachycardia, diarrhea, and abdominal pain are also described. Acute quinine overdose typically leads to GI complaints, tinnitus, and visual symptoms within hours, but the time course varies. Significant overdose is heralded by cardiovascular and central nervous system (CNS) toxicity. Death can occur within hours to days, usually from a combination of shock, ventricular dysrhythmias, respiratory arrest, or acute kidney injury (AKI). The average oral lethal dose of quinine is 8 g, although a dose as small as 1.5 g is reported to cause death.

Cardiovascular manifestations include prolongation of the PR interval, prolongation of the QRS complex, prolongation of the QT interval, and ST depression with or without T wave inversion. Dysrhythmias and complete heart block are reported. Quinine toxicity can also result in significant hypotension.

Although not commonly reported, mild hyperinsulinemia and resultant hypoglycemia occur in cases of oral quinine overdose. Eighth cranial nerve dysfunction results in tinnitus and deafness. These findings usually resolve within 48 to 72 hours, and permanent hearing impairment is unlikely. Ophthalmic presentations include blurred vision, visual field constriction, diplopia, altered color perception, mydriasis, photophobia, scotomata, and sometimes complete blindness. The onset of blindness is invariably delayed and usually follows the onset of other manifestations by at least 6 hours. Improvement in vision is usually slow, occurring over a period of months following severe toxicity.

Hypokalemia likely results from an intracellular shift of potassium rather than a true potassium deficit. Hemolysis also occurs in patients with glucose-6-phosphate dehydrogenase (G6PD) deficiency.

***Diagnostic Testing.*** Quinine toxicity is somewhat correlated with total serum concentrations. In general, serum concentrations greater than 5 μg/mL cause cinchonism, greater than 10 μg/mL visual impairment, greater than 15 μg/mL cardiac dysrhythmias, and greater than 22 μg/mL death.

Unfortunately, quantitative serum testing is not rapidly or widely available.

***Management.*** Patients frequently vomit spontaneously. Orogastric lavage is not routinely recommended except for patients with recent, substantial (potentially life-threatening) ingestions with no spontaneous emesis. Activated charcoal effectively adsorbs quinine and additionally decreases serum concentrations by altering enteroenteric circulation but should only be administered in patients with a low risk of aspiration or protected airways.

Expectant treatment should be initiated, including oxygen, cardiac and hemodynamic monitoring, IV fluid resuscitation, and frequent ECG and blood glucose measurements. In general, patients should be monitored until vital signs normalize, mental status improves, and laboratory values stabilize. Asymptomatic patients with suspected overdose should be monitored for 6 to 12 hours depending on variables as above, before medical clearance.

**Cardiac.** In patients with a QRS complex of more than 100 milliseconds (ms), we recommend treating with sodium bicarbonate alkalinization to achieve a serum pH of 7.45 to 7.55, as would be done in patients with cardiotoxicity associated with cyclic antidepressant overdoses (Antidotes in Brief: A5). Since hypertonic sodium bicarbonate will worsen existing hypokalemia, potentially exacerbating the effect of potassium channel blockade, potassium monitoring and supplementation are recommended for significant hypokalemia (< 3.0 mmol/L).

The QT interval should be carefully monitored for prolongation. If necessary, interventions for torsade de pointes, including magnesium administration, potassium supplementation, and overdrive pacing, should be initiated (Antidotes in Brief: A16).

Hypotension refractory to IV crystalloid boluses should be treated with vasopressors. Extracorporeal life support is reasonable in cases of refractory shock.

**Hypoglycemia.** A low serum glucose concentration should be supported with an adequate infusion of dextrose. Octreotide should be used for cases of refractory hypoglycemia at a dose of 50 μg (1 μg/kg in children) subcutaneously every 6 hours (Antidotes in Brief: A9).

**Ophthalmic.** There is no specific, effective treatment for quinine retinal toxicity.

***Enhanced Elimination.*** Multiple-dose activated charcoal (MDAC) decreases the half-life of quinine from approximately 8 hours to about 4.5 hours and increases clearance by 56%. Direct evidence of clinical benefit is lacking. Nevertheless, MDAC is recommended unless contraindications exist (Antidotes in Brief: A1). Because quinine has a relatively large volume of distribution and is highly protein bound, hemoperfusion, hemodialysis, and exchange transfusion have only a limited effect on drug removal and are not routinely recommended.

## Mefloquine

***Pharmacokinetics and Toxicodynamics.*** See Table 28–3 for the pharmacokinetic properties of mefloquine.

***Clinical Manifestations.*** Common side effects with prophylactic and therapeutic dosing include nausea, vomiting, and diarrhea. These side effects are noted particularly in the extremes of age and with high therapeutic dosing. Similar findings should be expected in acute overdose. Bradycardia is commonly reported. With prophylactic use, neither the PR interval nor the QRS complex is prolonged, but QT interval prolongation is reported. Reports of torsade de pointes and other ventricular dysrhyhtmias are rare, but the increase in QT interval and risk of torsade de pointes are increased when mefloquine is used concurrently with quinine, chloroquine, or most particularly, with halofantrine.

Mefloquine is commonly associated with neuropsychiatric side effects. During prophylactic use, 10% to 40% of patients experience insomnia and bizarre or vivid dreams and complain of dizziness, headache, fatigue, mood alteration, and vertigo. The risk of serious neuropsychiatric adverse effects (seizures, altered mental status, inability to ambulate due to vertigo, ataxia, or psychosis) during prophylaxis is estimated to be one in 10,600 but is reported to be as high as one in 200 with therapeutic dosing.

The effect of mefloquine on the pancreatic potassium channel is much less than that of quinine, resulting in only a mild increase in insulin secretion. Symptomatic hypoglycemia has not been reported as an effect of mefloquine alone in healthy individuals but has occurred with concomitant use of ethanol and in a severely malnourished patient with acquired immunodeficiency syndrome (AIDS). In overdose, particularly when accompanied by ethanol use or starvation, hypoglycemia can be severe.

*Management.* In overdose, treatment is primarily supportive with monitoring for potential adverse effects. Decontamination with activated charcoal is indicated if the patient presents soon after the ingestion. Specific monitoring for ECG abnormalities, hypoglycemia, and liver injury should be provided. Central nervous system effects usually resolve within a few days, but persistent, permanent, and delayed-onset CNS effects are reported, such that observation for full resolution of CNS effects would not be practical.

### Halofantrine

Because of erratic absorption, the potential for lethal cardiotoxicity, and concern for cross-resistance with mefloquine, halofantrine is not presently recommended for malaria prophylaxis by the US Centers for Disease Control and Prevention.

*Pharmacokinetics and Toxicodynamics.* See Table 28–3 for the pharmacokinetic properties of halofantrine.

*Clinical Manifestations.* The primary toxicity from therapeutic and supratherapeutic doses is prolongation of the QT interval and the risk of torsade de pointes and ventricular fibrillation. Palpitations, hypotension, and syncope occur. First-degree atrioventricular (AV) block is common, but bradycardia is rare. Dysrhythmias are also likely in the context of combined overdose or combined or serial therapeutic use with other xenobiotics that cause QT interval prolongation, particularly mefloquine. Other side effects, including nausea, vomiting, diarrhea, abdominal cramps, headache, and lightheadedness, which frequently occur in therapeutic use, are also expected in overdose. Less frequently described side effects include pruritus, myalgias, and rigors. Seizures, minimal liver enzyme abnormalities, and hemolysis are described.

*Management.* Management of patients with halofantrine overdose should focus on decontamination, supportive care, monitoring for QT interval prolongation, and treatment of any associated dysrhythmias. Based on rare case reports, nonoverdose evidence, and known erratic absorption, observation of asymptomatic overdose patients for 24 hours before medical clearance would be a reasonable approach.

### Lumefantrine

Lumefantrine is structurally similar to halofantrine. It is primarily used as a partner drug in the artemisinin-based combination therapy (ACT) artemether plus lumefantrine.

Little toxicity of lumefantrine alone or in combination is reported. Studies do not show QT interval prolongation or evidence of cardiac toxicity related to lumefantrine.

## 4-AMINOQUINOLINES

The structurally related compounds chloroquine and amodiaquine were once used extensively for malaria prophylaxis. However, with the development of resistance, they are now used in fewer geographic regions. Hydroxychloroquine is similar to chloroquine in therapeutic, pharmacokinetic, and toxicologic properties. The side effect profiles of the two are slightly different, favoring chloroquine use for malarial prophylaxis and hydroxychloroquine use as an antiinflammatory in rheumatic diseases such as rheumatoid arthritis and lupus erythematosus. Piperaquine is structurally similar to chloroquine but is primarily used in conjunction with artemisinin compounds as a component of an ACT.

### Antimalarial Mechanism

The 4-aminoquinolines interfere with the digestion of heme and hemozoin formation in a manner similar to that of the amino alcohols.

### Chloroquine and Hydroxychloroquine

*Pharmacokinetics and Toxicodynamics.* See Table 28–3 for the pharmacokinetic properties of chloroquine. Chloroquine is slowly distributed from the blood compartment to the larger central compartment, leading to transiently high whole blood concentrations shortly after ingestion that are thought to be responsible for the rapid development of profound cardiorespiratory collapse typical of chloroquine toxicity.

*Pathophysiology.* The pathophysiologic mechanisms of chloroquine and hydroxychloroquine are similar to quinine. Most notably, sodium and potassium channel blockade are the likely primary mechanisms of cardiovascular toxicity. Although less common in quinine toxicity, hypokalemia is extremely common in chloroquine overdose. The mechanism appears to be a shift of potassium from the extracellular to the intracellular space and not a true potassium deficit.

*Clinical Manifestations.* Severe chloroquine poisoning is usually associated with ingestions of 5 g or more in adults, systolic blood pressure less than 80 mm Hg, QRS complex duration of more than 120 ms, ventricular fibrillation, hypokalemia, and serum chloroquine concentrations exceeding 25 μmol/L (8 μg/mL). Symptoms usually occur within 1 to 3 hours of ingestion. Neurologic manifestations include CNS depression, dizziness, headache, and seizures. Ophthalmic manifestations are infrequent in acute chloroquine toxicity and transient in nature. Acute hydroxychloroquine toxicity is similar to chloroquine toxicity.

*Management.* Aggressive supportive care is recommended, including oxygen, cardiac and hemodynamic monitoring, large-bore IV access, and serial blood glucose concentrations. Orogastric lavage is recommended for life-threatening ingestions presenting early, but there is little evidence of efficacy. Activated charcoal adsorbs chloroquine well and is also recommended. The frequent development of precipitous cardiovascular and CNS toxicity should be anticipated before initiating any type of GI decontamination.

Early aggressive management of severe chloroquine toxicity decreases the mortality rate. This includes early endotracheal intubation and mechanical ventilation. High doses of epinephrine, 0.25 μg/kg/min, increasing by 0.25 μg/kg/min until an adequate systolic blood pressure (> 90 mm Hg) is achieved, is recommended based on experimental and clinical evidence. Clinicians should be mindful that high doses of epinephrine could exacerbate preexisting hypokalemia.

The use of diazepam to augment the treatment of dysrhythmias and hypotension is a unique use of this drug. When early mechanical ventilation was combined with the administration of high-dose diazepam and epinephrine in patients severely poisoned by chloroquine, a dramatic improvement in survival compared with historical control participants (91% vs 9% survival) occurred. Although the definitive study has yet to be done, high-dose diazepam therapy (2 mg/kg IV over 30 minutes followed by 1–2 mg/kg/day for 2–4 days) is recommended for serious toxicity (Antidotes in Brief: A26). Diazepam or an equivalent benzodiazepine should also be used to treat seizures and for sedation.

The use of sodium bicarbonate for correction of QRS complex prolongation is also controversial. Although alkalinization would be expected to counteract the effects of sodium channel blockade, it could also exacerbate preexisting hypokalemia. In the setting of normal potassium, sodium bicarbonate is a reasonable intervention to counteract QRS complex prolongation.

Hypokalemia in the setting of chloroquine overdose correlates with the severity of the toxicity. Potassium replacement in this setting is, again, controversial because it has not been shown that potassium supplementation will improve cardiac toxicity. In fact, several reports suggest a possible protective effect of hypokalemia in acute chloroquine toxicity. This should be balanced against the fact that severe hypokalemia can itself result in lethal dysrhythmias. Based on the available evidence, potassium replacement for severe hypokalemia would be a reasonable intervention, but it is essential to anticipate rebound hyperkalemia as chloroquine toxicity resolves and redistribution of intracellular potassium occurs.

Because chloroquine and hydroxychloroquine have high volumes of distribution and significant protein binding, enhanced elimination procedures are not beneficial.

### Piperaquine

See Table 28–3 for the pharmacokinetic properties of piperaquine. Cardiovascular toxicity with piperaquine requires cumulative doses 5 times higher than that of chloroquine. Hepatotoxicity occurs after chronic exposure in animals. Patients with overdose should be managed with supportive measures and expectant observation, including cardiovascular and CNS monitoring.

### Amodiaquine

Amodiaquine has pharmacologic properties similar to others in the 4-aminoquinolone family. Amodiaquine fell out of favor as a prophylactic treatment as a result of serious and sometimes fatal liver and bone marrow toxicity. Reports of amodiaquine toxicity suggest that involuntary movements, muscle stiffness, dysarthria, syncope, and seizures can occur. There is no overdose experience reported. Aggressive symptomatic and supportive care and expectant observation, including cardiovascular and CNS monitoring, should be provided for possible poisoning.

## 8-AMINOQUINOLINES

### Primaquine

Primaquine and its related compounds are licensed by the US Food and Drug Administration (FDA) for the prevention of *P. ovale* and *P. vivax* relapse caused by hepatic hypnozoites (Fig. 28–1).

***Antimalarial Mechanism.*** The antimalarial action of primaquine is poorly understood but thought to be related to increasing the oxidative stress of erythrocytes, obstructing proper parasitic development.

***Pharmacokinetics and Toxicodynamics.*** See Table 28–3 for the pharmacokinetic properties of primaquine.

***Pathophysiology.*** Although primaquine blocks sodium channels both in vitro and in animal models, significant cardiovascular toxicity has not been reported, but experience with primaquine overdose is limited primarily to case reports. The predominant clinical toxicity of primaquine relates to its ability to cause red blood cell (RBC) oxidant stress.

***Clinical Manifestations.*** Gastrointestinal irritation is common, and dose related. The extent of hemolysis in G6PD-deficient individuals depends on the extent of enzyme activity; those with greater enzyme activity have less severe hemolysis than those with less enzyme activity. Overdose with primaquine is rarely reported, and unintentional overdoses have led to methemoglobinemia requiring IV methylene blue (Chap. 97).

***Management.*** Therapy should be directed at minimizing absorption with appropriate decontamination and diagnosing then treating significant methemoglobinemia or hemolysis. Activated charcoal is a reasonable early intervention (Antidotes in Brief: A1). Methylene blue (Antidotes in Brief: A43) is recommended for patients who are symptomatic with methemoglobinemia. Treatment of hemolysis necessitates avoiding further exposure to primaquine and possibly exchange transfusion in severe cases.

## ENDOPEROXIDES

### Artemisinin and Derivatives

The medicinal value of natural artemisinin, the active ingredient of *Artemisia annua* (sweet wormwood or qinghao), has been known for thousands of years. Its antimalarial properties were first recognized by Chinese herbalists in A.D. 340, but the primary active component of qinghaosu, now known as artemisinin, was not isolated until 1974. Artemisinin and its semisynthetic derivatives, artesunate, artemether, arteether, and dihydroartemisinin, are the most potent and rapidly acting of all antimalarials. Because of their extremely short half-lives, the artemisinins are now used in combination with drugs with longer half-lives to delay or prevent the emergence of resistance. Artemisinin-based combination therapies are currently recommended by the WHO for the treatment of uncomplicated malaria, but only one has been licensed for use in the US: artemether and lumefantrine. The others are artemether plus lumefantrine, artesunate plus mefloquine, artesunate plus pyrimethamine–sulfadoxine, artesunate plus amodiaquine, and dihydroartemisinin and piperaquine.

***Antimalarial Mechanism.*** The artemisinins have a unique structure containing a 1,2,4-trioxane ring. The endoperoxide linkage within this ring is cleaved when it comes into contact with ferrous iron, releasing free radicals that destroy the parasite.

***Pharmacokinetics and Toxicodynamics.*** See Table 28–3 for the pharmacokinetic properties of artemisinin.

***Clinical Manifestations.*** These drugs have a very low incidence of side effects. Uncommon side effects include nausea, vomiting, abdominal pain, diarrhea, and dizziness. Rare reports of adverse CNS effects during therapeutic use suggest the possibility of CNS depression, seizures, or cerebellar symptoms after intentional self-poisoning. When serial ECGs were obtained, a small but statistically significant decrease in heart rate was noted coincident with peak drug concentrations. In one therapeutic trial, 7% of adult patients receiving artemether had an asymptomatic QT interval prolongation of at least 25%. Changes in the QRS complex are not reported.

## NAPHTHOQUINONES

### Atovaquone

Atovaquone is a structural analog of ubiquinone, or coenzyme Q, a mitochondrial protein involved in electron transport. Atovaquone disrupts the protozoal mitochondrial membrane potential, leading to inhibition of several parasite-specific enzymes, ultimately leading to the inhibition of pyrimidine synthesis, which is necessary for protozoal survival and replication. Atovaquone alone, primarily used to treat *Pneumocystis jiroveci* and babesiosis, is relatively well tolerated. Side effects include maculopapular rash, erythema multiforme (rarely), GI complaints, and mild aminotransferase elevations. Three cases of 3- to 42-fold overdose or excess dosing have been reported. No symptoms occurred in one case (at 3 times therapeutic serum concentration). Rash occurred in another, and in the third case, methemoglobinemia was attributed to a simultaneous overdose of dapsone.

Atovaquone is reported to have extensive enterohepatic cycling, with 94% of the drug eliminated in the feces. Although there is no evidence, MDAC is a reasonable intervention in severe overdose patients.

## ANTIFOLATES AND ANTIBIOTICS

### Antimalarial Mechanism

Proguanil, pyrimethamine, and the antibiotic trimethoprim interfere with malarial folate metabolism by inhibiting dihydrofolate reductase at concentrations far lower than that required to produce comparable inhibition of mammalian enzymes. Dapsone and sulfonamide antibiotics also disrupt malarial folate metabolism, but by inhibiting a different enzymatic reaction—dihydropteroate synthase.

### Pharmacokinetics and Toxicodynamics

See Table 28–3 for the pharmacokinetic properties of pyrimethamine, proguanil, and dapsone.

Dapsone is chiefly metabolized by CYP2C19 to dapsone hydroxylamine. This hydroxylamine metabolite has a long half-life, partially because of enterohepatic recirculation, and concentrate in erythrocytes leading to oxidant stress resulting in methemoglobinemia and hemolysis.

### Clinical Manifestations

The side effects of proguanil during prophylaxis include nausea, diarrhea, and mouth ulcers. Because of the interference with folate metabolism, megaloblastic anemia is a rare but potential complication. Megaloblastic bone marrow toxicity is reported in patients with chronic kidney disease. Rarely, neutropenia, thrombocytopenia, rash, and alopecia are also noted. In a single case report, hypersensitivity hepatitis was described.

Overdose of pyrimethamine alone is rare. In children, it results in nausea, vomiting, a rapid onset of seizures, fever, and tachycardia. Blindness, deafness, and developmental delay have followed. Chronic high-dose use is associated with a megaloblastic anemia and bone marrow suppression, requiring folate replacement.

The sulfonamides, including the sulfone dapsone, have a long history of causing idiosyncratic reactions, including neutropenia, thrombocytopenia, eosinophilic pneumonia, aplastic anemia, neuropathy, and hepatitis. Rare occurrence of life-threatening erythema multiforme major and toxic epidermal necrolysis, associated with pyrimethamine–sulfadoxine prophylaxis, has limited the use of this combination.

Acute ingestion of dapsone results in nausea, vomiting, and abdominal pain. After overdose, dapsone produces RBC oxidant stress, leading to methemoglobinemia and, to a much lesser extent, sulfhemoglobinemia through formation of an active metabolite (Chap. 97). Hemolysis may be either immediate or delayed. Dapsone, in particular, is known for its tendency to cause prolonged methemoglobinemia.

### Management

Folinic acid (leucovorin) is a reasonable intervention after an overdose of proguanil or pyrimethamine (Antidotes in Brief: A12). Other efforts should include supportive care.

After dapsone ingestion, clinically significant methemoglobinemia should be treated with methylene blue (Antidotes in Brief: A43). The long half-life of dapsone and its metabolites often makes repetitive doses of methylene blue necessary. Multiple-dose activated charcoal is recommended for patients with a dapsone overdose and no contraindications. Cimetidine inhibits the production of the hydroxylamine metabolite, decreasing methemoglobin levels during therapeutic dapsone dosing. Cimetidine administration is a reasonable intervention after dapsone overdose.

## NEW DIRECTIONS

The development of drug resistance and search for treatments with improved efficacy, compliance, and side-effect profiles fuels an ongoing pursuit for better antimalarials. Tafenoquinone is an 8-aminoquinoline with greater activity against liver-stage parasites than primaquine. It appears to have fewer side effects than primaquine, less hemolytic toxicity, and a longer half-life, enabling less frequent dosing that could increase compliance. At the time of this writing, tafenoquine was recently approved by the US FDA for malaria prophylaxis and radical cure in patients over 16 years old with *P. vivax*. A number of new ACTs are being studied in different countries but are not yet recommended by the WHO because of insufficient evidence. These new ACTs include combinations of artesunate and pyronaridine, arterolane and piperaquine, artemisinin and piperaquine base, and artemisinin and napthoquine.

The complicated structure and life cycle of malaria protozoa has made the development of an effective malaria vaccine an elusive undertaking. Despite these difficulties, the Malaria Vaccine Technology Roadmap has focused strategic efforts since 2006. The most advanced vaccine in development, RTS,S/AS01, provides modest protection (26%–50%) against *P. falciparum*. Funding for a large-scale implementation pilot using this vaccine is established. Vaccinations in several sub-Saharan African countries began in 2018.

# 29 ANTITUBERCULOUS MEDICATIONS

## HISTORY AND EPIDEMIOLOGY

Approximately one-third of the total population of the world, or 2 billion people, are infected with *Mycobacterium tuberculosis.* An estimated 10.4 million new cases of disease are diagnosed annually. Isoniazid (INH) was introduced into clinical practice in 1952. In 2006, 20% of *M. tuberculosis* isolates were resistant to at least isoniazid and rifampin, called multidrug-resistant tuberculosis (MDR-TB), and 2% were identified as highly resistant or extensively drug-resistant tuberculosis (XDR-TB), with resistance to many additional drugs—defined as all fluoroquinolones and at least one of three injectable drugs (capreomycin, kanamycin, and amikacin).

At present, populations that remain at risk for tuberculosis (TB) include HIV-positive patients, people who are undomiciled, people with alcoholism, injection drug users, healthcare workers, prisoners, prison workers, and Native Americans. In addition, the TB rate in foreign-born persons is nearly 10 times higher than in United States (US)-born persons. In the US population, countries of birth generating the highest number of TB cases are Mexico, the Philippines, India, and Vietnam. The use of multiple drugs in regimens against MDR-TB and XDR-TB results in significant adverse drug effects in approximately 40% of patients, and this increases to approximately 70% in treatment against coinfection with human immunodeficiency virus (HIV).

## ISONIAZID

### Pharmacology

Isoniazid (INH, or isonicotinic hydrazide) is structurally related to nicotinic acid (niacin, or vitamin $B_3$), nicotinamide adenosine dinucleotide (NAD), and pyridoxine (vitamin $B_6$). It is a prodrug that undergoes metabolic activation by KatG, a catalase peroxidase in *M. tuberculosis* that produces a highly reactive intermediate, which in turn interacts with InhA. InhA is a mycobacterial enzyme that is required for the synthesis of important components of mycobacterial cell walls.

### Pharmacokinetics

Orally, INH is rapidly absorbed, reaching peak serum concentrations typically within 2 hours. Isoniazid diffuses into all body fluids with a volume of distribution of approximately 0.6 L/kg and has negligible binding to serum proteins. The metabolism of INH is shown in Figure 29–1.

Pharmacogenetic differences in the acetylation steps affect efficacy and toxicity. Based on the activity of NAT2, patients are described as homozygous fast acetylators (FF), heterozygous fast acetylators (FS), and homozygous slow acetylators (SS) and are distinguishable phenotypically as fast, intermediate, and slow acetylators. Slow acetylators have less presystemic clearance, or first-pass effect, than do fast acetylators. Fast acetylators metabolize INH 5 to 6 times faster than slow acetylators, resulting in serum INH concentrations that are 30% to 50% lower in fast acetylators than in slow acetylators. Slow acetylators are at increased risk of peripheral neuropathy, and dose adjustments mitigate this risk. There is no significant association between either genetic aceytlation polymorphisms or CYP activity and hepatotoxicity.

### Pathophysiology

*Mechanism of Toxicity.* Isoniazid induces a functional pyridoxine deficiency via two main mechanisms (Fig. 29–2). This results in refractory seizures because of a relative lack of γ-aminobutyric acid (GABA), the primary inhibitory neurotransmitter in the central nervous system (CNS), and an excess of glutamate, the primary stimulatory neurotransmitter in the CNS. As shown, pyridoxine is converted in vivo to an active form, pyridoxal-5′-phosphate, which serves as an important cofactor in the synthesis of GABA. Isoniazid metabolites inhibit the enzyme pyridoxine phosphokinase, which converts pyridoxine (vitamin $B_6$) to its active form, pyridoxal-5′-phosphate. Glutamic acid decarboxylase (GAD) is unable to catalyze GABA synthesis from glutamate, and GABA aminotransferase degrades the inhibitory neurotransmitter. Pyridoxine depletion is further compounded when INH directly reacts with pyridoxal phosphate to produce an inactive hydrazone complex that is renally excreted and thereby increases loss of this required cofactor.

### Interactions With Other Drugs and Foods

Drug–drug interactions associated with INH are mediated through alteration of hepatic metabolism of several CYP enzymes. The majority of these interactions are inhibitory, with decreased CYP-mediated transformations, particularly demethylation, oxidation, and hydroxylation. Table 29–1 summarizes additional INH drug and food interactions.

### Pregnancy

Isoniazid is listed as a US Food and Drug Administration (FDA) class C drug. A weekly regimen is preferred, and coadministration of pyridoxine is strongly recommended. Although INH readily and rapidly enters breast milk, breastfeeding during therapy is acceptable.

### Clinical Manifestations of Isoniazid Toxicity

*Acute Toxicity.* Isoniazid produces the triad of seizures refractory to conventional therapy, severe metabolic acidosis, and coma. These clinical manifestations appear as soon as 30 minutes after ingestion. The case fatality rate of a single acute ingestion classically is as high as 20%. Vomiting, slurred speech, dizziness, and tachycardia typically represent early manifestations of toxicity, although seizures are uncommonly the initial sign of acute overdose. Seizures characteristically occur after the ingestion of greater than 20 mg/kg of INH and invariably occur with ingestions greater than 35 to 40 mg/kg. Because GABA, the primary inhibitory neurotransmitter, is

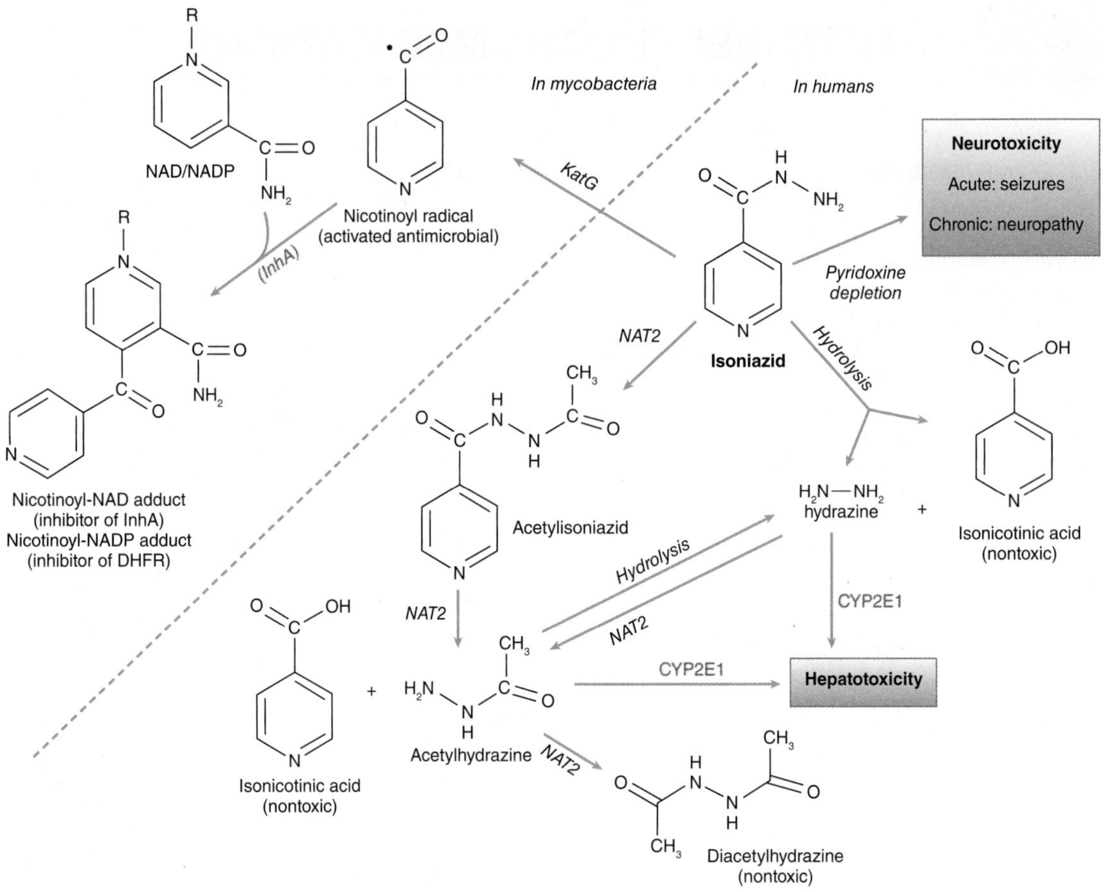

**FIGURE 29–1.** Metabolism of isoniazid (INH). INH metabolism occurs via the enzyme *N*-acetyltransferase type 2 (NAT2), hydrolysis, and further oxidation via CYP2E1 into both nontoxic and hepatotoxic metabolites. Hepatotoxicity is multifractional and occurs directly via hepatotoxic metabolites and indirectly via induced apoptosis and steatosis. DHFR = dihydrofolate reductase; InhA = mycobacterial enoyl-acyl carrier protein reductase; KatG = mycobacterial catalase peroxidase.

depleted in acute INH toxicity, seizure activity is often refractory to typical antiepileptic therapy, persisting until GABA concentrations are restored therapeutically.

Acute INH toxicity is often associated with an anion gap metabolic acidosis associated with a high serum lactate concentration. Typically, arterial pH ranges between 6.80 and 7.30, although survival in the setting of an arterial pH of 6.49 was reported. Paralyzed animals poisoned with INH do not develop elevated lactate concentrations, a finding that suggests the lactate arises from intense muscular activity associated with seizures. In acute severe INH toxicity, coma as long as 24 to 36 hours is reported, persisting beyond both the termination of seizures and the resolution of acidemia. Additional sequelae from acute INH toxicity include rhabdomyolysis, acute kidney injury, hyperglycemia, glycosuria, ketonuria, hypotension, and hyperthermia.

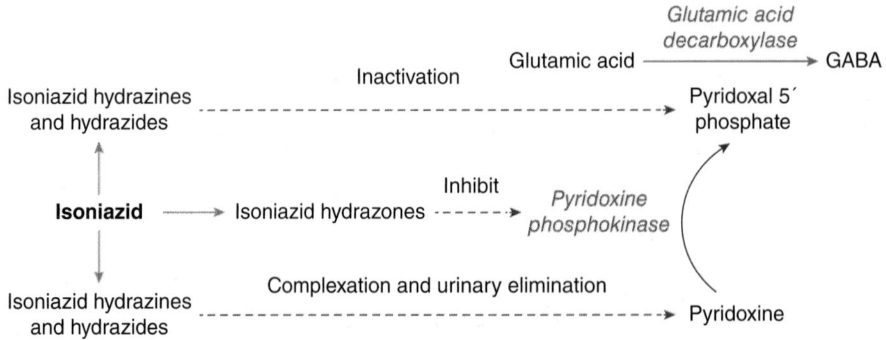


**FIGURE 29–2.** The effect of isoniazid on γ-aminobutyric acid (GABA) synthesis.

**TABLE 29–1 Adverse Reactions and Drug Interactions of Antituberculous Drugs**

| *Drug* | *Major Adverse Reactions* | *Drug Interactions: Clinical Effect* | *Monitoring* | *Comments* |
|---|---|---|---|---|
| Isoniazid (INH) | *Acute:* seizures, acidosis, coma, hyperthermia, oliguria, anuria<br>*Chronic:* elevation of aminotransferases, autoimmune hepatitis, arthritis, anemia, hemolysis, eosinophilia, peripheral neuropathy, optic neuritis, vitamin $B_6$ deficiency (pellagra) | Rifampin, PZA, ethanol: hepatic necrosis<br>Warfarin: increased INR<br>Theophylline: tachycardia, vomiting, seizures, acidosis<br>Phenytoin: increased phenytoin concentrations<br>Carbamazepine: altered mental status<br>Lactose: decreased INH absorption<br>Antacids: decreased INH absorption<br>Red wine/soft cheese: tyramine reaction<br>Fish (scombroid): flushing, pruritus | Hepatic aminotransferases, ANA, CBC | HIV enteropathy may decrease absorption |
| Rifampin | *Acute:* diarrhea, periorbital edema<br>*Chronic:* elevation of aminotransferases, reddish discoloration of body fluids | Protease inhibitors: decreased serum concentration of protease inhibitor<br>Delavirdine: increased HIV resistance<br>Cyclosporine: graft rejection<br>Warfarin: decreased INR<br>Oral contraceptives: ineffective contraception<br>Methadone: opioid withdrawal<br>Phenytoin: higher frequency of seizures<br>Theophylline: decreased theophylline concentrations<br>Verapamil: decreased cardiovascular effect | If administered with HIV antiretrovirals, viral titers should be followed. Hepatic aminotransferases; monitor serum concentrations of drugs (ie, phenytoin, cyclosporine) or clinical markers of efficacy (ie, INR) | Interactions of rifampin with several HIV medications are very poorly described; changes in dosing or dosing interval for both rifampin and antiretroviral drugs are commonly required; teratogenic |
| Ethambutol | *Chronic:* optic neuritis, loss of red–green discrimination, loss of peripheral vision | | Visual acuity, color discrimination | Contraindicated in children too young for formal ophthalmologic examination |
| Pyrazinamide (PZA) | *Chronic:* elevation of aminotransferases, decreased urate excretion | INH: increased rates of hepatotoxicity (when extended courses or high-dose PZA used) | Hepatic aminotransferases | Courses of therapy of ≤ 2 months are recommended |
| Cycloserine | *Chronic:* depression, paranoia, seizures, megaloblastic anemia | INH: increased frequency of seizures | CBC, psychiatric monitoring | |
| Ethionamide | *Chronic:* orthostatic hypotension, depression | Cycloserine: increases CNS effects | Blood pressure, pulse, orthostasis | |
| *para*-Aminosalicylic acid | *Chronic:* malaise, GI upset, elevation of aminotransferases, hypersensitivity reactions, thrombocytopenia | | Hepatic aminotransferases, CBC | |
| Capreomycin | *Chronic:* hearing loss, tinnitus, proteinuria, sterile abscess at IM injection sites | | Audiometry, kidney function tests | |

ANA = antinuclear antibodies; CBC = complete blood count; CNS = central nervous system; HIV = human immunodeficiency virus; INR = international normalized ratio.

***Chronic Toxicity.*** Chronic therapeutic INH use is associated with a variety of adverse effects. Overall incidence of adverse reactions to INH is estimated to be 5.4%, the most serious of which is hepatocellular necrosis. Although asymptomatic elevation of aminotransferases is common in the first several months of treatment, the onset of hepatitis uncommonly presents up to 1 year after starting INH therapy. Hepatotoxicity is associated with chronic overdose, increasing age, comorbid conditions such as malnutrition, and combinations of antituberculous drugs. Overt hepatic failure typically occurs when INH therapy is continued after the onset of hepatocellular injury in both adults and children. Isoniazid-induced hepatitis arises via two pathways. The first involves an immunologic mechanism resulting in hepatic injury that is thought to be idiopathic. The second, more common, mechanism involves direct hepatic injury by INH or its metabolites. The metabolites believed responsible are acetylhydrazine and hydrazine (Fig. 29–1).

Peripheral neuropathy and optic neuritis are other known adverse drug effects of chronic INH use. The exact pathophysiology of INH-induced neurotoxicity is not known but is believed to be caused by pyridoxine deficiency aggravated by the formation of pyridoxine-INH hydrazones. Peripheral neuropathy, the most common complication of INH therapy, presents in a stocking-glove distribution that progresses proximally. Although primarily sensory in nature, myalgias and weakness are also reported. Peripheral neuropathy is generally observed in severely malnourished, alcoholic, uremic, or diabetic patients; it is also associated with slow acetylator status, an effect that leads to increased

INH concentrations and, consequently, increased pyridoxine depletion.

### Diagnostic Testing

Acute INH toxicity is a clinical diagnosis that is inferred by history and confirmed by measuring serum INH concentrations. Because serum INH concentrations are not widely available, clinicians cannot rely on serum concentrations to confirm the diagnosis or initiate therapy. Because of the risk of hepatitis associated with chronic INH use, hepatic aminotransferases should be regularly monitored after therapy is started. In critically ill patients, serum should be assessed for acidemia, kidney function, creatine phosphokinase (CPK), and urine myoglobin, indicating rhabdomyolysis and possible acute kidney injury.

### Management

*Acute Toxicity.* The antidote for INH-induced neurologic dysfunction is pyridoxine (Antidotes in Brief: A15). We recommend a pyridoxine dose in grams that should equal the amount of INH ingested in grams, with a first dose of up to 5 g intravenously in adults. Unknown quantities of ingested INH warrant initial empiric treatment with a pyridoxine dose of no more than 5 g (pediatric dose: 70 mg/kg to a maximum of 5 g). When patients have seizures that persist beyond administration of the initial dose, an additional similar dose of pyridoxine is recommended.

Benzodiazepines such as lorazepam, midazolam, or diazepam, which should be used to potentiate the antidotal efficacy of pyridoxine, are often ineffective as the sole treatment of acute severe INH poisoning because of their reliance on GABA to exert their activity. Phenytoin has no intrinsic GABAergic effect and is not recommended. Barbiturates have potent direct and indirect GABA agonist activity and are expected to be as effective or more effective than the benzodiazepines. The efficacy of propofol in terminating INH-induced seizures is unstudied in humans but is reasonable in cases of refractory status epilepticus.

It is recommended that asymptomatic patients who present to the emergency department within 2 hours of ingestion of toxic amounts of INH receive prophylactic administration of 5 g of oral or IV pyridoxine. Asymptomatic patients should be observed for a 6-hour period for signs of toxicity. Acute toxicity is unlikely to manifest more than 6 hours beyond ingestion.

It is reasonable to perform early gastrointestinal (GI) decontamination by administering activated charcoal enterally by mouth to patients who are awake and able to comply with therapy or via nasogastric tube in intubated patients if there are no contraindications. Orogastric lavage is not routinely recommended but is reasonable shortly after a large INH ingestion.

Hemodialysis has clearance rates reported as high as 120 mL/min, but is rarely if ever indicated for initial management of INH toxicity. However, hemodialysis is reasonable following massive ingestion, when adequate supplies of pyridoxine are not available.

*Chronic Toxicity.* Hepatitis (defined as aminotransferase concentrations more than 2–3 times baseline) resulting from therapeutic INH administration mandates termination of therapy. Pyridoxine does not reverse hepatic injury; consequently, surveillance for and recognition of hepatocellular injury remain essential. Cases of hepatitis refractory to medical therapy, requiring liver transplantation, are reported.

Neurotoxicity is commonly treated with as much as 50 mg/day of oral pyridoxine, although doses as low as 6 mg/day are reportedly effective.

## RIFAMYCINS

### Pharmacology

Rifamycins are a class of macrocyclic antibiotics derived from the actinomycete *Amycolatopsis mediterranei.* Xenobiotics in this class include rifampin (a semisynthetic derivative), rifabutin, and rifapentine. Rifampin inhibits the initial steps in RNA chain polymerization. Disruption of RNA synthesis interrupts transcription and therefore inhibits protein synthesis, leading to cell death.

### Pharmacokinetics and Toxicokinetics

Oral rifampin reaches peak serum concentrations in 0.25 to 4 hours. Rifampin is secreted into the bile and undergoes enterohepatic recirculation. The half-life of rifampin, which is normally 1.5 to 5 hours, increases in the setting of hepatic dysfunction. Additionally, rifampin autoinduces its metabolism to shorten its half-life by approximately 40%. Rifampin is distributed widely into body compartments. Rifampin and rifapentine are US FDA pregnancy class C, whereas rifabutin is class B.

### Drug–Drug Interactions

Rifamycins are potent inducers of CYP enzymes, which result in numerous drug interactions. Additionally, the ability of rifampin to induce CYP3A4 is strongly correlated with P-glycoprotein (P-gp) concentrations. P-glycoprotein is a transmembrane protein that functions as a cellular efflux pump of endogenous and exogenous xenobiotics; variations in expression of P-gp significantly affect the bioavailability of many xenobiotics and subsequent drug–drug interactions. Concurrent administration of rifampin thus affects the metabolism of a wide array of drugs (Table 29–1).

### Clinical Manifestations

*Acute Toxicity.* Isolated rifamycin overdose infrequently produces serious acute effects. The most common side effects of acute rifampin overdose are GI in nature, consisting of epigastric pain, nausea, vomiting, and diarrhea. Other common effects include an anaphylactoid reaction manifested by flushing, urticarial rash, angioedema, and facial and periorbital edema. This occurs in both adults and children. Central nervous system effects of overdose include fatigue, drowsiness, headache, dizziness, ataxia, confusion, and obtundation.

*Chronic Toxicity.* Hepatitis occurs more frequently in patients taking combination therapy with INH than in those taking INH alone and results from the ability of rifampin to induce cytochromes responsible for INH hepatotoxicity. Liver injury, when attributable to rifampin alone, is predominantly cholestatic, suggesting that clinical surveillance for hepatic injury is important, along with regular biochemical monitoring.

A hypersensitivity reaction that is associated with rifampin therapy presents with an influenzalike syndrome. The antituberculous drug-induced hypersensitivity syndrome, formerly called DRESS syndrome (drug rash with eosinophilia and systemic symptoms), occurs in up to 20% of patients receiving high doses or intermittent (less than twice weekly) dosing and includes fever, chills, myalgias, eosinophilia, hemolytic anemia, thrombocytopenia, or interstitial nephritis.

### Diagnostic Testing and Management

Management of patients with acute rifampin overdose is primarily observational and supportive. Stabilization of vital signs is usually adequate, although clinicians should remain vigilant for toxicity from coingestants. Activated charcoal is reasonable but not routinely recommended.

## ETHAMBUTOL

### Pharmacology

Ethambutol is bacteriostatic against *Corynebacterium, Mycobacterium*, and *Nocardium* (CMN group) bacteria. Ethambutol inhibits arabinosyl transferases, interfering with biosynthesis of arabinogalactan and liparabinomannan, thus inhibiting polymerization of arabinose subunits within the arabinoglycan layer of mycobacterial cell walls.

### Pharmacokinetics

Only the D(+) isomer is used therapeutically because the L(−) isomer is the major contributor to optic neuritis, but both enantiomers are bactericidal. About 80% of an oral dose is absorbed. Maximum serum concentrations are reached within 4 hours of oral administration. Ethambutol is approximately 20% to 30% protein bound and has a half-life of 4 to 6 hours. Three-fourths of a standard dose is excreted unchanged in the urine by a combination of glomerular filtration and tubular secretion.

Ethambutol is US FDA pregnancy class C. Although ethambutol is excreted into breast milk in approximately a 1:1 ratio with serum, it is considered to be compatible with breastfeeding.

### Clinical Manifestations and Management

Acute overdose of ethambutol is generally well tolerated, although at least one death has been reported. More commonly, nausea, abdominal pain, confusion, visual hallucinations, and optic neuropathy occur after acute ingestions of greater than 10 g. Stabilization of vital signs is recommended, and although GI decontamination with activated charcoal was a hallmark of therapy, it is not routinely recommended.

The most significant effect of the therapeutic use of ethambutol is unilateral or bilateral ocular toxicity presenting typically as painless blurring of vision, cecocentral scotomas (at and around the blind spot in the central field), and less commonly decreased perception of color and loss of peripheral vision. Patients develop ocular toxicity as soon as 2 days after starting ethambutol or as delayed as 2 years after starting therapy. Management of chronic toxicity from ethambutol involves cessation of therapy.

### Diagnostic Testing and Management

All patients should receive neuroophthalmic testing before ethambutol therapy. The use of visual evoked potentials is especially useful in identifying subclinical optic nerve disease. Furthermore, patients should receive regular visual acuity examinations, and clinicians should encourage patients to report any subjective visual symptoms.

## PYRAZINAMIDE

### Pharmacology and Pharmacokinetics

Pyrazinamide (PZA) is a structural analog of nicotinamide with a mechanism of action similar to that of INH. Similar to INH, PZA is a prodrug. Pyrazinamide kills the bacteria by disruption of mycolic acid biosynthesis. Pyrazinamide is also active at neutral pH under certain conditions of decreased metabolism such as reduced temperature, which will facilitate drug susceptibility testing. After oral administration, PZA is rapidly absorbed, with maximum concentrations occurring within 1 to 2 hours of administration and a half-life of approximately 9 hours. Hepatic metabolism to pyrazinoic acid and 5-hydroxypyrazinoic acid occurs with the metabolites subsequently renally excreted. Drug clearance of PZA increases with continuing therapy, causing decreased serum PZA concentration within 1 to 2 months.

Pyrazinamide is US FDA pregnancy class C but is rarely used in pregnancy because the risk of poorly defined birth defects. Pyrazinamide is minimally excreted into breast milk and is presumed safe for breastfeeding.

### Diagnostic Testing and Treatment

Proper dosing of PZA and short courses of therapy are the two most important factors in preventing toxicity. Treatment for hepatotoxicity involves cessation of PZA therapy in conjunction with supportive care.

## CYCLOSERINE

Cycloserine, previously avoided because of its adverse effects, is being used increasingly as second-line treatment with other tuberculostatic medications when treatment with primary antituberculous medications (INH, rifampin, ethambutol, and streptomycin) fails or as initial therapy when drug susceptibility testing indicates either MDR-TB or XDR-TB. Cycloserine is a structural analog of alanine and demonstrates inhibition of D-alanine racemase and D-alanine ligase, which are involved in peptidoglycan cell wall synthesis. After oral doses, 70% to 90% of the drug is absorbed, and peak concentrations are reached in 3 to 8 hours. Less than 35% of the cycloserine is metabolized, and the remaining xenobiotic is excreted unchanged in the urine.

Toxicity is dose dependent and occurs in as many as 50% of patients taking cycloserine. Cycloserine is a partial agonist at the NMDA/glycine receptor, which contributes to neurologic effects such as somnolence, headache, tremor, dysarthria, vertigo, confusion, irritability, and seizures. Psychiatric manifestations include paranoid reactions, depression, and suicidal ideation. Reversible hypersomnolence and asterixis are reported with cycloserine, suggesting reversible thalamic neurotoxicity, which is corroborated by magnetic resonance imaging. Whenever this drug is used, monitoring serum concentrations is recommended. Optimal peak treatment concentrations are between 20 and 35 μg/L, and adverse effects are more common with peak concentrations above 35 mg/L. Toxicity usually appears within the first 2 weeks of therapy and ceases upon discontinuation. Cycloserine is US FDA pregnancy class C. Cycloserine acceptable in women who are breastfeeding only if no safer therapy is available for the mother.

Reports of cycloserine overdose are scarce; however, use of peritoneal dialysis was reported in one case of intentional cycloserine ingestion in a woman who had previously undergone a unilateral nephrectomy, with observation of improvement in CNS effects and effective decrease in serum concentrations of cycloserine. In patients with evidence of CNS toxicity from cycloserine overdose and impaired kidney function, it is reasonable to consider extracorporeal drug removal.

## ETHIONAMIDE

Ethionamide is a congener of INH that is thought to have a similar mechanism of action as INH, causing cell death from disruption of mycolic acid biosynthesis. Ethionamide is rapidly absorbed, widely distributed, and crosses the blood–brain barrier. Oral doses yield peak serum concentrations within approximately 3 hours of administration. The half-life is approximately 2 hours. The most common adverse symptoms associated with ethionamide are GI irritation and anorexia. Toxic effects such as orthostatic hypotension, depression, and drowsiness are common. Rash, purpura, and gynecomastia are observed, as are tremor, paresthesias, and olfactory disturbances.

Ethionamide is US FDA pregnancy class C. Data regarding the incidence and safety of breastfeeding while receiving ethionamide also are lacking. Reports of ethionamide overdose are absent from the literature.

## *para*-AMINOSALICYLIC ACID

*para*-Aminosalicylic acid (PAS) is incorporated into the folate pathway to generate a toxic antimetabolite analog, which then inhibits dihydrofolate reductase (DHFR). *para*-Aminosalicylic acid is readily absorbed from the gut and is rapidly distributed in all tissues, especially the pleural fluid and caseous material. A population-based determination of volume of distribution was 79 L in a study of adult volunteers. *para*-Aminosalicylic acid has a half-life of approximately 1 hour and is renally excreted. Adverse effects of PAS occur in 10% to 30% of patients and include anorexia, nausea, vomiting, diarrhea, sore throat, and malaise. Between 5% and 10% of patients receiving PAS develop hypersensitivity reactions characterized by high fever, rash, and arthralgias. Hematologic abnormalities including agranulocytosis, leukopenia, eosinophilia, thrombocytopenia, and acute hemolytic anemia are reported. *para*-Aminosalicylic acid was removed by hemodialysis in patients with kidney failure in small amounts but is of uncertain clinical use. Data regarding the safety of PAS in pregnancy and breastfeeding are lacking. Reports of PAS overdose are absent from the literature.

### Capreomycin

Capreomycin is a cyclic polypeptide currently used more frequently because of its antibacterial activity against MDR-TB and intracellular TB bacilli. Capreomycin interferes with ribosomes and inhibits protein translation but also appears to act by other mechanisms such as alterations in topoisomerase or the glyoxylate shunt pathway. Because of poor absorption after oral dosing, capreomycin must be administered intramuscularly. Toxicity associated with capreomycin use includes tinnitus, hearing loss, proteinuria, and electrolyte disturbances, although severe acute kidney injury is rare. Risk of toxicity is increased in patients with chronic kidney disease and the elderly. Eosinophilia, leukocytosis, and rashes are described. Pain and sterile abscesses at the site of capreomycin injection are reported. Capreomycin is US FDA pregnancy class C. Data are lacking regarding the safety of capreomycin in pregnancy and breastfeeding. Capreomycin overdose is not described.

## BEDAQUILINE

### Pharmacology and Pharmacokinetics

Bedaquiline is a diarylquinoline that received conditional approval in 2012 by the US FDA for the treatment of MDR-TB. It exerts its antituberculous effects via inhibition of mycobacterial ATP synthase. Bedaquiline is relatively slowly absorbed after oral administration, with peak plasma concentrations achieved at 4 to 6 hours. Bedaquiline is more than 99% protein bound and has an estimated volume of distribution of 164 L in adults. Bedaquiline is metabolized primarily by CYP3A4 and is primarily excreted in the feces. The terminal half-life for bedaquiline and *N*-desmethyl bedaquiline is estimated to be 5.5 months. Bedaquiline overdose has not been described. Bedaquiline is US FDA pregnancy class B.

### Adverse Effects

The most frequently reported adverse effects included nausea, vomiting, headache, and arthralgias; additional adverse effects include dizziness, elevated aminotransferases, myalgias, diarrhea, and QT interval prolongation.

### Drug–Drug Interactions

Concomitant administration with rifamycins increases clearance of bedaquiline 5-fold and significantly decreases serum concentration of bedaquiline; this practice should be avoided pending further evaluation of the safety profile of bedaquiline. Bedaquiline should be used with caution in patients who are also taking medications that inhibit CYP3A4, as these are expected to lead to higher serum concentration of bedaquiline and potential resultant toxicity; there are currently no data regarding appropriate dose adjustments in these situations.

### Monitoring

Monitoring of serum potassium, magnesium, and calcium concentrations, as well as aspartate aminotransferase and alanine aminotransferase, is recommended at baseline and then monthly thereafter while taking bedaquiline. Because of the dysrhythmogenic effects due to QT interval prolongation, an ECG should be obtained prior to initiation of treatment with bedaquiline and at weeks 2, 4, 8, 12, and 24 after starting treatment. Monthly ECGs are recommended in patients taking bedaquiline concurrently with other QT interval–prolonging xenobiotics. Reports of overdose are lacking from the medical literature.

## DELAMANID

Delamanid, is a newer antituberculous medication that received conditional approval in 2014 from the European Medicines Agency and the Japanese drug regulatory authority; it is not currently approved by the US FDA. Delamanid exerts its effects by inhibiting synthesis of methoxymycolic and ketomycolic acids, resulting in destabilization of the mycobacterial cell wall; in contrast with INH, it does not inhibit α-mycolic acid synthesis. The pharmacologic profile of delamanid has yet to be satisfactorily determined. Adverse effects reported with delamanid therapy include nausea, vomiting, tinnitus, headache, palpitations, and QT interval prolongation. Because of its potential dysrhythmogenic effects due to QT interval prolongation, an ECG should be obtained before initiation of treatment with delamanid, and at weeks 2, 4, 8, 12, and 24 after starting treatment. Monthly ECGs are recommended in patients taking delamanid concurrently with other QT interval–prolonging xenobiotics. Delamanid overdose is not described in the literature.

# A15 PYRIDOXINE

## INTRODUCTION

Pyridoxine (vitamin $B_6$), a water-soluble vitamin, is administered as an antidote for isonicotinic acid hydrazide (isoniazid, INH), *Gyromitra esculenta* mushrooms, hydrazines, and ethylene glycol overdoses.

## HISTORY

Pyridoxine deficiency is rare in healthy patients consuming a modern diet but is most common in patients with malnutrition, alcohol use disorder, and autoimmune, liver, kidney, and digestive diseases. The classic findings including seborrheic dermatitis, cheilosis, stomatitis, and glossitis, and peripheral neuropathy was first characterized in the early 20th century. A rare genetic abnormality that produces pyridoxine-responsive seizures in newborns was described in 1954.

## PHARMACOLOGY

### Chemistry

Pyridoxine hydrochloride was chosen as the commercial preparation because of its stability. The active form of pyridoxine is the phosphate ester of pyridoxal (pyridoxal-5′-phosphate, PLP).

### Mechanism of Action

Pyridoxal-5′-phosphate is an important cofactor in more than 100 enzymatic reactions, including decarboxylation and transamination of amino acids, and the metabolism of tryptophan to 5-hydroxytryptamine and methionine to cysteine. Iatrogenic pyridoxine deficiency in animals produces seizures associated with reduced brain concentrations of PLP, glutamic acid decarboxylase, and γ-aminobutyric acid (GABA).

Isoniazid and methylated hydrazines such as monomethyl hydrazine produce a syndrome resembling vitamin $B_6$ deficiency by inhibiting the enzyme pyridoxine phosphokinase that converts pyridoxine to PLP (Fig. 29–2). In addition, they directly combine with both pyridoxine and PLP, causing inactivation and rapid excretion by the kidney. Pyridoxal-5′-phosphate is a coenzyme for L-glutamic acid decarboxylase, which facilitates the synthesis of GABA from L-glutamic acid.

Decreased GABA reduces cerebral inhibition and increased glutamate enhances cerebral excitation, resulting in seizures. The administration of large doses of pyridoxine overcomes the deficiency.

### Pharmacokinetics

Pyridoxine is not protein bound, has a volume of distribution of 0.6 L/kg, and easily crosses cell membranes; in contrast, PLP is nearly entirely plasma protein bound. After intravenous infusion of 100 mg of pyridoxine over 6 hours, the PLP concentration increases rapidly in plasma and in erythrocytes. Oral pyridoxine in doses of 600 mg is 50% absorbed within 20 minutes of ingestion by a first-order process with rapid achievement of peak plasma concentrations of pyridoxine, PLP, and pyridoxal.

## ROLE IN HYDRAZIDE- AND HYDRAZINE-INDUCED SEIZURES

### Animal Studies

In a dog model of INH-induced toxicity, pyridoxine reduced the severity of seizures and the time to seizure and prevented the mortality of a previously lethal dose of INH in a dose-dependent fashion. As single antiepileptics, phenobarbital, pentobarbital, phenytoin, ethanol, and diazepam were ineffective in controlling seizures and mortality, but when combined with pyridoxine, each protected the animals from seizures and death.

### Human Data

Clinical experience with INH overdose in humans demonstrates rapid seizure control following pyridoxine administration. In addition to controlling seizures, the administration of pyridoxine also appears to restore consciousness. Similar experiences are reported for monomethylhydrazine (MMH) poisoning and ingestions of *G. esculenta*.

## ROLE IN ETHYLENE GLYCOL POISONING

Pyridoxal-5′-phosphate is a cofactor in the conversion of glycolic acid to nonoxalate compounds (Fig. 79–2). Patients poisoned with ethylene glycol should receive pyridoxine IV in an attempt to shunt metabolism preferentially away from the production of oxalic acid.

## ADVERSE EFFECTS AND SAFETY ISSUES

Pyridoxine is neurotoxic to animals and humans when administered chronically in supraphysiologic doses. Delayed peripheral neurotoxicity occurred in patients taking daily doses of 200 mg to 6 g of pyridoxine for 1 month. Healthy volunteers administered 1 or 3 g/day developed a distal sensory axonopathy after 1.5 months on the high-dose and 4.5 months on the low-dose regimens. Pyridoxine also induces a sensory neuropathy when massive doses are administered either as a single dose or over several days. Acute dosing in excess of 375 mg/kg carries a similar risk potential.

## PREGNANCY AND LACTATION

Pyridoxine is Food and Drug Administration pregnancy category A. Although there has never been a controlled trial in pregnant women of gram doses of pyridoxine, the benefit of using pyridoxine for INH-induced seizures would clearly exceed the theoretical risk to the fetus. Pyridoxine enters breast milk and is considered compatible with breastfeeding when 10- to 25-mg doses are ingested. However, concentrations of pyridoxine in breast milk after maternal gram doses of pyridoxine are not known, and it is reasonable to be concerned for the infant and temporarily avoid breastfeeding after gram amounts of pyridoxine are given.

## DOSING AND ADMINISTRATION

A safe and effective pyridoxine regimen for INH overdoses in adults is 1 g of pyridoxine for each gram of INH ingested, to a maximum of 5 g or 70 mg/kg. Initial doses of pyridoxine in children probably should not exceed 70 mg/kg. These doses are sufficient in the majority of patients but can be repeated if necessary. For patients who are actively seizing, it is reasonable to give pyridoxine as a slow IV infusion at approximately 0.5 g/min until the seizures stop or the maximum dose has been reached. When the seizures stop, the remainder of the dose should be infused over 4 to 6 hours to maintain pyridoxine availability while the INH is being eliminated. In the event of inadequate availability of IV pyridoxine, oral pyridoxine should be administered.

Using the INH dosage regimen is reasonable for poisoning from monomethyl hydrazine or *Gyromitra* spp but has never been formally studied in humans. Pyridoxine should not be the sole agent used for INH or monomethyl hydrazine poisoning. Benzodiazepine and barbiturates should be used with pyridoxine in an attempt to achieve synergistic control of seizures. If the seizures do not respond to the initial therapeutic interventions, they can be repeated, followed by intravenous propofol, and if necessary neuromuscular blockade and general anesthesia with video electroencephalogram monitoring.

We recommend that patients poisoned with ethylene glycol receive 100 mg/day of pyridoxine IV in an attempt to shunt metabolism preferentially away from the production of oxalic acid.

## FORMULATION

Pyridoxine HCl is available parenterally at a concentration of 100 mg/mL in 1-mL ampules. An IV dose of 5 g of pyridoxine requires 50 (1 mL) ampules containing 100 mg/mL. This is an exception to the rule that appropriate doses of medications rarely require multiple dosages of this magnitude. This also emphasizes the necessity of keeping an adequate supply available in the emergency department as well as in the pharmacy. Oral pyridoxine is available in many tablet strengths from 10 to 500 mg from various manufacturers.

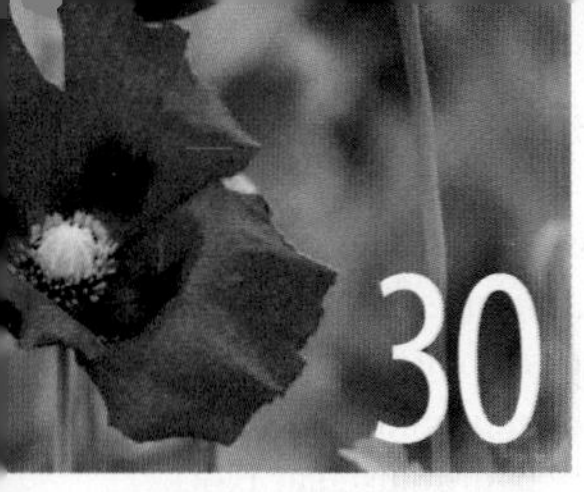

# 30 ANTIDYSRHYTHMICS

## HISTORY AND EPIDEMIOLOGY

The term *dysrhythmia* encompasses an array of abnormal cardiac rhythms that range in clinical significance from merely annoying to instantly life threatening. The word *arrhythmia* can be defined as a lack of rhythm. Some references state they are synonyms for irregular heartbeat, and others define arrhythmia as irregular heartbeat and dysrhythmia as a disturbance to an otherwise normal rhythm. Throughout the text, we have chosen the term *dysrhythmia*. Antidysrhythmics include all medications that are used to treat any of these various dysrhythmias.

For many years, antidysrhythmics were considered among the most rational of the available cardiac medications. However, this belief changed dramatically following publication of the Cardiac Arrhythmia Suppression Trials (CAST and CAST II), which highlighted lethal prodysrhythmic events.

This chapter focuses on the medications that serve primarily as antidysrhythmics and, with the exception of lidocaine (found in Chap. 37), have few other medicinal indications. In addition, the toxicities from β-adrenergic antagonists and $Ca^{2+}$ channel blockers, which have indications in addition to dysrhythmia control, are discussed separately in Chaps. 32 and 33. The toxicology of cardioactive steroids such as digoxin is discussed in Chap. 35.

## CLASSIFICATION OF ANTIDYSRHYTHMICS

Antidysrhythmics modify impulse generation and conduction by interacting with various membrane $Na^+$, $K^+$, and $Ca^{2+}$ channels. Generally, antidysrhythmics manifest electrophysiologic effects either through alteration of the channel pore or, more commonly, by modification of its gating mechanism (Fig. 30–1). The Vaughan-Williams classification of antidysrhythmics by electrophysiologic properties emphasizes the connection between the basic electrophysiologic actions and the antidysrhythmic effects. Although initially proposed as a descriptive model for electrophysiologic actions and not for clinical effects, the Vaughan-Williams classification is commonly invoked as a user-friendly guide to clinical therapy. A more rational classification would match the electrophysiologic effects of the antidysrhythmics with their molecular interactions on different regions of the various ion channels, such as channel gating and pore conductance. This discussion of antidysrhythmics uses the Vaughan-Williams classification, recognizing its shortcomings. The pharmacokinetic properties of the various medications are summarized in Table 30–1.

## CLASS I ANTIDYSRHYTHMICS

All antidysrhythmics in Vaughan-Williams class I (A, B, and C) alter $Na^+$ conductance through cardiac voltage-gated, fast inward $Na^+$ channels (Fig. 30–1). Blockade of these $Na^+$ channels slows the rise of phase 0 of the cellular action potential, which correlates with a reduction in the rate of depolarization of the myocardial cell (or $V_{max}$). Similarly, conduction through the myocardium is slowed, producing a measurable prolongation of the QRS complex on the surface electrocardiogram (ECG). Correspondingly, slowed intramyocardial conduction is associated with reduced contractility, manifesting as negative inotropy.

The differences among class I antidysrhythmics are directly related to their pharmacologic relationships with the $Na^+$ channel. Type IB antidysrhythmics have their highest affinity for inactivated $Na^+$ channels. Inactivation occurs at the end of depolarization, during early repolarization, and during periods of myocardial ischemia. These xenobiotics also have rapid "on–off" binding kinetics and are thus bound only briefly, during late electrical systole, and are completely unbound during diastole. The degree of binding increases as the heart rate accelerates because the duration of diastole decreases, and the relative proportion of time spent in systole increases; this is termed *use dependence*. Because all IB antidysrhythmics do not bind to activated $Na^+$ channels, in therapeutic doses they do not affect the rate of rise of phase 0 of the action potential, or Vmax, and have no effect on the ECG.

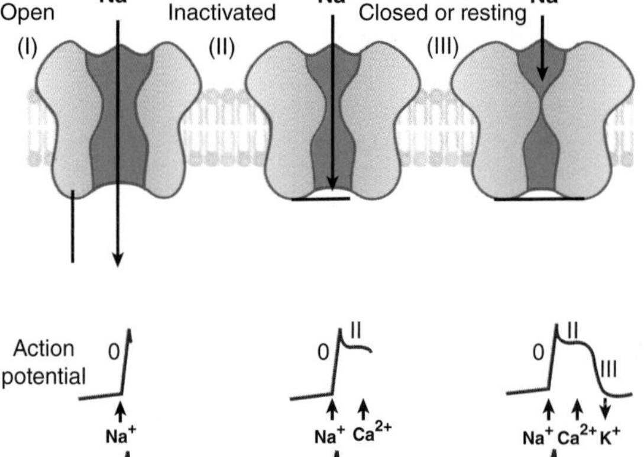


**FIGURE 30–1.** Sodium channel blockade. On appropriate signal, $Na^+$ channel activation occurs, at which time the $Na^+$ channel converts from the resting (III) state to the open state (I). This allows $Na^+$ influx to initiate phase 0 of the action potential, or cellular depolarization. The $Na^+$ channels subsequently assume the inactivated state by closure of an inactivation gate; this is a voltage-dependent phenomena and occurs concomitantly with, although more slowly than, channel activation. Cellular depolarization is maintained for a period of time by other ion channels that form the plateau of the action potential. Before reactivating, $Na^+$ channels must convert back to the resting state, which also occurs in a voltage-gated fashion. Many antidysrhythmics stabilize the inactivated state of the channel and, by slowing conversion to the resting state, prevent its reopening, reducing the excitability of the cell. Because this is a population phenomenon, there are dose-dependent effects on channel blockade; thus, more xenobiotics interfere with more channels. Interestingly, certain xenobiotics, such as aconitine, stabilize the open state of the $Na^+$ channel and produce persistent depolarization. ECG = electrocardiogram.

**TABLE 30–1 Antidysrhythmics: Pharmacology, Pharmacokinetics, and Adverse Effects**

| *Antidysrhythmic* | *Route* | *Primary Route of Elimination* | *Elimination Half-Life* | *Channel Blockade* | *Volume of Distribution L/kg* | *Protein Binding (%)* | *Adverse Effects and Complicating Factors* | *Other* |
|---|---|---|---|---|---|---|---|---|
| *Class IA* | | | | | | | | |
| Disopyramide | PO | Liver, kidney | Variable | $Na^+$ ($\tau = 9$ s), $K^+$, $Ca^{2+}$ | $0.59 \pm 0.15$ | 35–95 depending on plasma concentration | CHF, negative inotropic effects, anticholinergic, torsade de pointes, heart block, hypoglycemia QRS and QT prolonged | |
| Procainamide | IV, PO | 50%–60% unchanged in kidney; active hepatic metabolite (NAPA) | PA: 3-4 h ↑ CKD NAPA: 6–10 h ↑ CKD | $Na^+$($\tau = 1.8$ s), $K^+$ | $1.9 \pm 0.3$ | $16 \pm 9$ | Hypotension (ganglionic blockade), QRS and QT prolonged, fever, SLE-like syndrome, torsade de pointes | NAPA: active metabolite, renally eliminated, $K^+$ channel blocker; half-life, 6–10 h A sustained-release PA preparation is available |
| Quinidine | PO | Liver, kidney, 10%–20% unchanged | 6–8 h ↑ liver disease (to > 50 h) and CKD (to 9–12 h) | $Na^+$($\tau = 3$ s), $K^+$, $Ca^{2+}$ | $2.7 \pm 1.2$ | $87 \pm 3$ | Heart block, sinus node dysfunction, QRS and QT prolonged, hypotension, hypoglycemia, torsade de pointes, thrombocytopenia, ↑ digoxin concentration | |
| *Class IB* | | | | | | | | |
| Lidocaine | SC, IV, PO (30% BA) | Liver, active metabolite (MEGX CYP3A4) | Distribution 8 min after bolus Terminal elimination, 2 h | $Na^+$($\tau = 0.1$ s) | $1.1 \pm 0.4$ | $70 \pm 5$ | Fatigue, agitation, paresthesias, seizures, hallucinations, rarely bundle branch block | Metabolites: GX and MEGX are less potent as $Na^+$ channel blockers than lidocaine |
| Mexiletine | IV, PO | Liver (CYP 2D6) | 10–24 h | $Na^+$($\tau = 0.3$ s) | $4.9 \pm 0.5$ | $63 \pm 3$ | See lidocaine | |
| Phenytoin | IV, PO | Liver | | $Na^+$($\tau = 0.2$ s) | $0.64 \pm 0.04$ | $89 \pm 23$ | Hypotension and asystole related to IV propylene glycol infusion, nystagmus, ataxia | |
| Tocainide | IV, PO | Kidney, liver | 9–14 h | $Na^+$($\tau = 0.4$ s) | $3.0 \pm 0.2$ | $10 \pm 15$ | See lidocaine; aplastic anemia, interstitial pneumonia | |
| *Class IC* | | | | | | | | |
| Flecainide | IV, PO | Liver (CYP2D6), 75%; kidney, 25% | 20 h | $Na^+$($\tau = 11$ s), $Ca^{2+}$, $K^+$ | $4.9 \pm 0.4$ | $61 \pm 10$ | Negative inotropic effects, bradycardia, heart block, ventricular fibrillation, ventricular tachycardia, neutropenia, QT prolonged | Two major metabolites, one with minor activity, meta-*O*-dealkylated flecainide; and inactive meta-*O*-dealkylated lactam of flecainide |

(*Continued*)

**TABLE 30–1 Antidysrhythmics: Pharmacology, Pharmacokinetics, and Adverse Effects (*Continued*)**

| *Antidysrhythmic* | *Route* | *Primary Route of Elimination* | *Elimination Half-Life* | *Channel Blockade* | *Volume of Distribution L/kg* | *Protein Binding (%)* | *Adverse Effects and Complicating Factors* | *Other* |
|---|---|---|---|---|---|---|---|---|
| Moricizine | PO | Liver | 2–4 h | $Na^+$($\tau$ = 10 s) | ? | 95 | ↑ Mortality after myocardial infarction, bradycardia, CHF, ventricular fibrillation, ventricular tachycardia | |
| Propafenone | IV, PO | Liver (CYP2D6) extensive first pass | 2–10 h | $Na^+$($\tau$ = 1 s), $K^+$ | 3.6 ± 2.1 | 85 ± 95 | Asthma, congestive heart failure, hypoglycemia, AV block, QRS and QT prolonged, bradycardia, ventricular fibrillation, ventricular tachycardia | Active metabolite 5-OH-propafenone |
| ***Class II*** | | | | | | | | |
| β-Adrenergic antagonists | IV, PO | Variable | Variable | β-Adrenergic receptor | Variable | Variable | CHF, asthma, hypoglycemia, Raynaud disease | See Chap. 32 |
| ***Class III*** | | | | | | | | |
| Amiodarone | IV, PO | Liver (100%) (CYP3A4) | 2 mo | $Na^+$, $K^+$, $Ca^{2+}$ | 66 ± 44 | 99.98 ± 0.01 | Negative inotropic effects, pulmonary fibrosis, corneal microdeposits, thyroid function abnormalities, hepatitis photosensitivity, ↑ concentrations of; diltiazem, quinidine, procainamide, flecainide, and digoxin, QT prolonged | Desethylamiodarone; has comparable activity to the parent compound |
| Dofetilide | IV, PO | Kidney | 7.5 h | $K^+$ | 3.6 ± 0.8 | 64 | Torsade de pointes, QT prolonged | |
| Dronedarone | PO | Liver (CYP3A4) | 13–19 h | $Na^+$, $K^+$, $Ca^{2+}$ | 20 | > 98 | Contraindicated in decompensated heart failure, atrial fibrillation that cannot be converted; liver, thyroid, and pulmonary toxicity, QT prolonged | Active *N*-debutyl metabolite (10%–33% potency) |
| Ibutilide | IV | Kidney | 2–12 h; average, 6 h | $K^+$, $Na^+$ opener | 11 | 40 | Torsade de pointes, heart block, QT prolonged | |
| ***Class IV*** | | | | | | | | |
| $Ca^{2+}$ channel blockers | IV, PO | Variable | Variable | $Ca^{2+}$ | Variable | Variable | Asystole (if used IV with IV β-adrenergic antagonists), AV block, hypotension, CHF, constipation, ↑ digoxin concentration | See Chap. 33 |

(*Continued*)

**TABLE 30–1 Antidysrhythmics: Pharmacology, Pharmacokinetics, and Adverse Effects (*Continued*)**

| *Antidysrhythmic* | *Route* | *Primary Route of Elimination* | *Elimination Half-Life* | *Channel Blockade* | *Volume of Distribution L/kg* | *Protein Binding (%)* | *Adverse Effects and Complicating Factors* | *Other* |
|---|---|---|---|---|---|---|---|---|
| ***Unclassified*** | | | | | | | | |
| Adenosine | IV | All cells (intracellular adenosine deaminase) | Seconds | Nucleoside-specific G protein–coupled adenosine receptors, ↑ $Ca^{2+}$ currents activate ACh-sensitive $K^+$ current | | | Transient asystole < 5 s, chest pain, dyspnea, atrial fibrillation, ↓ BP, effects potentiated by dipyridamole and in heart transplant patients, ↑ dose needed with methylxanthine use | |
| Digoxin | IV, PO | (Chap. 35) | | | | | | |
| Magnesium Sulfate | (Antidotes in Brief: A16) | | | | | | | |

$\tau_{recovery}$ describes the time it takes for the $Na^+$ channel to recover from blockade.
ACh = acetylcholine; AV = atrioventricular; BA = bioavailable; BP = blood pressure; CHF = congestive heart failure; CKD = chronic kidney disease; GX = glycine xylidide; IV = intravenous; NAPA = *N*-acetylprocainamide; MEGX = monoethylglycylxylidide; PA = procainamide; PO = oral; SC = subcutaneous; SLE = systemic lupus erythematosus.

Alternatively, the class IC antidysrhythmics either act preferentially on activated $Na^+$ channels or they release from the $Na^+$ channels very slowly and thus are still bound during the next cardiac cycle. This prolonged channel blockade and reduced channel reactivation results in both greater pharmacologic effects and toxicity, even at slow heart rates. Class IA antidysrhythmics fall between the other two subclasses.

Many class I antidysrhythmics also have effects on cardiac $K^+$ channels. Slowing of $K^+$ efflux prolongs the duration of the action potential and accounts for the persistence of refractoriness, and produces QT interval prolongation. Because class IB antidysrhythmics have no effect on myocardial $K^+$ channels, they do not alter refractoriness or the QT interval.

## Class IA Antidysrhythmics: Procainamide, Quinidine, and Disopyramide

***Procainamide.*** Procainamide is used to suppress either atrial or ventricular tachydysrhythmias. Importantly, procainamide undergoes hepatic biotransformation by acetylation to *N*-acetylprocainamide (NAPA), the rate of which is genetically determined, and rapid acetylators are prone to developing toxicity. Although NAPA lacks the $Na^+$ channel–blocking activity of procainamide, it prolongs the action potential duration through blockade of the $K^+$ rectifier currents and is independently responsible for the production of cardiac dysrhythmias.

Both procainamide and NAPA are renally eliminated and accumulate in patients with chronic kidney disease (CKD). Although the chronic use of procainamide is commonly accompanied by the development of antinuclear antibodies and infrequently progresses to drug-induced systemic lupus erythematosis, this syndrome is not associated with acute poisoning. Other reported adverse effects include seizures and antimuscarinic effects with acute overdose and myopathic pain, hepatitis, thrombocytopenia, and agranulocytosis after long-term use.

Serum procainamide concentrations should be determined as part of therapeutic drug monitoring (therapeutic: 4–12 μg/mL); NAPA concentrations should also be monitored in patients with CKD (therapeutic: 10–20 μg/mL). In patients with procainamide overdose, both procainamide and NAPA concentrations should be obtained, although a direct prognostic role is not defined.

***Quinidine.*** Quinidine was once widely used for the management of atrial or ventricular dysrhythmias but has largely fallen out of favor because of its adverse effects. Quinidine has substantial cardiotoxicity that includes intraventricular conduction abnormalities and a prolonged QT interval. "Quinidine syncope," in which patients on therapeutic doses of quinidine experience paroxysmal, transient loss of consciousness, is almost exclusively a result of torsade de pointes.

Because quinidine shares many pharmacologic properties with quinine (Chap. 28), patients occasionally have cinchonism after either chronic or acute quinidine overdose. This syndrome includes abdominal symptoms, tinnitus, and altered mental status. Quinidine-induced blockade of $K^+$ channels in pancreatic islet cells causes uncontrolled insulin release, leading to hypoglycemia. The antimuscarinic effects can produce classical anticholinergic findings such as dry mouth and flushed skin, and alpha-adrenergic antagonism contributes to hypotension.

Serum quinidine concentrations greater than 14 μg/mL are associated with cardiotoxicity, as evidenced by a 50% increase in the duration of either the QRS complex or QT interval. These concentrations have limited utility in clinical management.

***Disopyramide.*** Disopyramide is more likely than other class IA antidysrhythmics to produce negative inotropy and congestive heart failure. This effect is related to the blockade of myocardial $Ca^{2+}$ channels. The mono-*N*-dealkylated metabolite of disopyramide produces the most pronounced antimuscarinic effects of the class. Lethargy, confusion, and hallucinations are prominent in overdose. Disopyramide causes hyperinsulinemic hypoglycemia through its antagonism of $K^+$ channels in the pancreatic islet cells.

***Management of Class IA Antidysrhythmic Toxicity.*** Management concentrates on assessment and correction of cardiovascular dysfunction. After airway evaluation and IV line placement, an ECG and continuous ECG monitoring are of paramount importance. Activated charcoal is recommended for early-presenting patients with a protected airway and an ingestion of a potentially toxic amount of medication. Gastric lavage is reasonable for patients with life-threatening ingestions who present within several hours depending on the severity and probability of retained ingestant.

For patients who have widening of the QRS complex duration, bolus administration of IV hypertonic sodium bicarbonate is recommended (Antidotes in Brief: A5). Hypotension in the setting of QRS complex prolongation responds favorably to hypertonic sodium bicarbonate, which enhances inotropy by both accelerating depolarization and raising intravascular volume. In addition to hypertonic sodium bicarbonate, rapid infusion of 0.9% NaCl to expand intravascular volume and to simultaneously increase myocardial contractility by enhancing the Starling force is reasonable. In refractory cases, dobutamine or a catecholamine such as epinephrine or norepinephrine is recommended based on the assessment of the hemodynamic requirements for inotropy versus pressor effect. Extracorporeal life support is reasonable in refractory cases. Because disopyramide also blocks $Ca^{2+}$ channels, $Ca^{2+}$ administration is reportedly beneficial and is reasonable to administer in appropriate doses.

We recommend treating patients with stable ventricular dysrhythmias occurring in the setting of class IA antidysrhythmic poisoning with hypertonic sodium bicarbonate or lidocaine. Because lidocaine has rapid on–off receptor kinetics, it displaces the "slower" class IA antidysrhythmic from the binding site on the $Na^+$ channel, effectively reducing channel blockade. Magnesium sulfate and overdrive pacing can prevent recurrent torsade de pointes after initial spontaneous resolution or defibrillation. Hemodialysis and hemoperfusion are reasonable means to remove NAPA, but there is not sufficient evidence to support their use of for quinidine or disopyramide poisoning.

### Class IB Antidysrhythmics: Lidocaine, Tocainide, Mexiletine, and Moricizine

***Lidocaine.*** Lidocaine is a synthetic derivative of cocaine. Its predominant clinical uses are as a local anesthetic and, for mechanistically similar reasons, to control ventricular dysrhythmias. Lidocaine prevents myocardial reentry and subsequent dysrhythmias by preferentially suppressing conduction in compromised tissue. After an IV bolus, lidocaine rapidly enters the central nervous system (CNS) but quickly redistributes into the peripheral tissue with a distribution half-life of approximately 8 minutes. Lidocaine is metabolized to an active metabolite, monoethylglycylxylidide (MEGX), that bioaccumulates because of its substantially longer half-life.

Patients with massive lidocaine exposures develop both CNS and cardiovascular effects, generally in that order. Because of its rapid entry into the CNS, acute lidocaine poisoning typically produces CNS dysfunction, with paresthesias or seizures, as the initial manifestation. Concomitant respiratory arrest generally occurs. Shortly after the CNS effects, depression in the intrinsic cardiac pacemakers leads to sinus arrest, atrioventricular (AV) block, intraventricular conduction delay, hypotension, or cardiac arrest. If the patient is supported through this period, the xenobiotic rapidly distributes away from the heart, and spontaneous cardiac function returns.

Chronic lidocaine toxicity most commonly occurs as a result of therapeutic misadventure in patients on lidocaine infusions. Toxicity after appropriate dosing is most likely to occur in patients with reduced hepatic blood flow as occurs with congestive heart failure, liver disease, or concomitant therapy with CYP3A4 and CYP1A2 inhibitors.

***Mexiletine.*** Mexiletine is currently available in oral form for the management of ventricular dysrhythmias and chronic neuropathic pain. Its metabolism, predominantly through CYP2D6, is accelerated by concomitant use of phenobarbital, rifampin, and phenytoin.

Adverse effects with therapeutic dosing are primarily neurologic and are similar to those that occur with lidocaine. The few reported cases of mexiletine overdose describe prominent cardiovascular effects such as complete heart block, torsade de pointes, and asystole. Neurotoxicity resulting from overdose includes self-limited seizures, generally in the setting of cardiotoxicity.

***Moricizine.*** Moricizine possesses the general qualities of class I antidysrhythmics but is difficult to specifically subclassify because it has properties that place it in both classes IB and IC. Clinical experience with overdose is limited but is expected to be similar to that of other class I antidysrhythmics.

***Management of Class IB Antidysrhythmic Toxicity.*** The focus of the initial management for IV lidocaine-induced cardiac arrest is continuous cardiopulmonary resuscitation to allow lidocaine to redistribute away from the heart. Catecholamine administration is recommended for the management of resistant hypotension, and if refractory toxicity persists, extracorporeal life support is reasonable. When bradydysrhythmias do not respond to atropine, a chronotrope such as norepinephrine or isoproterenol is recommended. Lidocaine-induced seizures, and those related to lidocaine analogs, are generally brief in nature and do not require specific therapy. For patients requiring treatment, an IV benzodiazepine is recommended; rarely, a barbiturate is required. Similarly, although IV lipid emulsion is often described as useful for the resuscitation of patients with life-threatening local anesthetic overdose (local anesthetic systemic toxicity), its use for lidocaine-poisoned patients is limited to case reports and likely unnecessary given the rapid time course of recovery. As such, lipid emulsion is not recommended for lidocaine poisoning except in cases of severe and prolonged toxicity that are refractory to other therapies (Antidotes in Brief: A23). Enhanced elimination techniques are limited after IV poisoning because of the rapid time course of poisoning. There is no role for extracorporeal drug removal.

### Class IC Antidysrhythmics: Flecainide and Propafenone

***Flecainide.*** Flecainide, a derivative of procainamide, is orally administered to maintain sinus rhythm in patients with structurally normal hearts who have atrial fibrillation or supraventricular tachycardia. Kidney disease, medication interactions, and congestive heart failure all decrease the clearance of flecainide and its active metabolite. Therapeutic doses produce left ventricular dysfunction with worsening congestive heart failure presumably from antagonistic effects on $Ca^{2+}$ channels.

Flecainide toxicity is associated with an increase in QRS complex duration, prolongation of the PR interval, and prolongation of the QT interval. The duration of the QRS complex has significant prognostic value: a QRS duration of 200 ms or greater is predictive of the need for mechanical circulatory support. The combination of marked QRS complex and PR interval changes, associated with minimal QT interval prolongation, is characteristic of flecainide toxicity and contrasts with those described with other antidysrhythmics.

***Propafenone.*** Propafenone blocks fast inward $Na^+$ channels, is a weak β-adrenergic antagonist, and is an L-type $Ca^{2+}$ channel blocker. Propafenone overdose produces sinus bradycardia, ventricular dysrhythmias, and negative inotropy. The ECG often shows a right bundle branch block pattern, first-degree AV block, and prolongation of the QT interval. Generalized seizures have occurred.

***Management of Class IC Antidysrhythmic Toxicity.*** Management concentrates on assessment and correction of cardiovascular dysfunction. After airway evaluation and IV line placement, an ECG and continuous ECG monitoring are of paramount importance. Activated charcoal is recommended for early-presenting patients with a protected airway and an ingestion of a potentially toxic amount of medication. Gastric lavage is reasonable for patients with life-threatening ingestions who present within several hours depending on the severity and probability of retained ingestant.

Standard management strategies should be instituted for hypotension, such as fluid resuscitation, and for seizures, with benzodiazepines as well as careful attention to maintaining the airway as indicated. Additionally, therapy for hypotension and the ECG manifestations of class IC poisoning include IV hypertonic sodium bicarbonate to overcome the $Na^+$ channel blockade. As with β-adrenergic antagonists, an animal model and human case reports suggest that hyperinsulinemic euglycemic therapy is beneficial after propafenone poisoning. In patients with refractory bradycardia, pacing should be attempted with the caveat that the efficacy of an external or internal pacemaker may be limited because of the xenobiotic-induced increased electrical pacing threshold of the ventricle. Successful therapy with extracorporeal life support is reported and is recommended in patients with severe toxicity when available. Intravenous lipid emulsion therapy is reasonable for those who are seriously ill, deteriorating, and refractory to conventional therapy (Antidotes in Brief: A23). Extracorporeal removal is not recommended at this time.

## CLASS III ANTIDYSRHYTHMICS

### Amiodarone, Dofetilide, Dronedarone, and Ibutilide

The class III antidysrhythmics prevent and terminate reentrant dysrhythmias by prolonging the action potential duration and effective refractory period without slowing conduction velocity during phase 0 or 1 of the action potential. This effect on the action potential is generally caused by blockade of the rapidly activating component of the delayed rectifier $K^+$ current, which is responsible for repolarization. Thus, common ECG effects at therapeutic doses include prolongation of the PR and QT intervals and abnormal T and U waves.

***Amiodarone and Dronedarone.*** Amiodarone is structurally similar to both thyroxine and procainamide and 40% of its molecular weight is iodine. Dronedarone is an analog of amiodarone that does not contain iodine. Both medications are used primarily to terminate or prevent atrial fibrillation, and although dronedarone is less effective, it is not associated with many of the potentially severe adverse effects of amiodarone. In addition to their class III antidysrhythmic effects, amiodarone and dronedarone also have weak α- and β-adrenergic antagonist activity and can block both L-type $Ca^{2+}$ channels and inactivated $Na^+$ channels. The ability of amiodarone to compete for P-glycoprotein is responsible for several drug interactions, including elevated digoxin and cyclosporin concentrations and enhanced anticoagulation effectiveness of warfarin.

Ventricular dysrhythmias and sinus bradycardia are the most serious cardiac complications of therapeutic doses of amiodarone. Other complications associated with long-term amiodarone therapy do not occur after short-term IV use and include pulmonary, thyroid, corneal, hepatic, and cutaneous toxicity. Dronedarone rarely causes hepatic or pulmonary toxicity. Pneumonitis, the most consequential extracardiac adverse effect, occurs in up to 5% of patients taking the xenobiotic therapeutically. Amiodarone pneumonitis typically occurs only after years of therapy. Its occurrence appears to be dose related: a daily dose of greater than 400 mg is a risk factor, and pneumonitis is rare in those taking less than 200 mg daily. Manifestations of pneumonitis include dyspnea, cough, hemoptysis, crackles, hypoxia, and radiographic changes.

Thyroid dysfunction, either amiodarone-induced thyrotoxicosis (AIT) or amiodarone-induced hypothyroidism (AIH), occurs in approximately 4% of patients. Amiodarone-induced hypothyroidism is more common than AIT when iodine intake is sufficient. Amiodarone-induced hypothyroidism is likely caused by an exaggerated Wolff-Chaikoff effect, in which iodine inhibits the organification and release of thyroid hormone. Amiodarone-induced thyrotoxicosis appears to exist in two distinct forms: type I AIT, which occurs in patients with abnormal thyroid glands and iodine-induced excessive thyroid hormone synthesis and release, and type II AIT, in which destructive thyroiditis leads to release of thyroid hormone from the damaged follicular cells. The diagnosis is confirmed with standard thyroid function testing (thyroid-stimulating hormone, total triiodothyronine and free thyroxine) (Chap. 26).

Corneal microdeposits are extremely common during chronic therapy and lead to vision loss. Abnormal elevation of hepatic enzymes occurs in more than 30% of those on long-term therapy, and the hepatotoxicity progresses to cirrhosis. Periodic monitoring of aminotransferases is recommended. Slate-gray or bluish discoloration of the skin is common, particularly in sun-exposed portions of the body.

***Dofetilide.*** Dofetilide is approved for conversion of atrial fibrillation or atrial flutter to a normal sinus rhythm. Dofetilide increases the effective refractory period more substantially in atrial tissue than in ventricular fibers, accounting for this clinical indication. Dofetilide prolongs the QT interval but does not change either the PR interval or QRS complex in humans.

Although limited data are available, the expected and reported adverse cardiac events include ventricular tachycardia, particularly torsade de pointes. The approximate incidence of torsade de pointes in patients receiving high therapeutic doses of the medication is 3%. Few cases of overdose are reported but include cases of nonfatal ventricular tachycardia and fatal ventricular fibrillation.

***Ibutilide.*** Ibutilide is an antidysrhythmic with predominant class III activity used for the rapid conversion of atrial fibrillation and flutter to normal sinus rhythm. Because of its extensive first-pass metabolism, ibutilide can only be administered parenterally. In addition to its effects on the delayed rectifier current, ibutilide activates a slow inward $Na^+$ current. Ibutilide prolongs the QT interval and causes torsade de pointes, especially in patients with congenital long-QT syndrome and in women.

Acute kidney injury, including biopsy-identified crystals, is reported in association with ibutilide cardioversion, but a causal relationship is not yet definitive. Acute overdose information, only available in limited form (four patients) through the manufacturer, suggests that ventricular dysrhythmias and high-degree AV conduction abnormalities should be expected.

### Management of Class III Antidysrhythmic Toxicity

Treatment experience with class III antidysrhythmic overdose is limited. Isoproterenol, magnesium sulfate, and overdrive pacing can prevent recurrent torsade de pointes after initial spontaneous resolution or defibrillation.

Oral activated charcoal is recommended if patients present shortly after overdose. Extracorporeal drug removal is not expected to be beneficial in general, either because of extensive protein binding or because of large volumes of distribution. It is reasonable to implement extracorporeal life support for refractory shock. It is reasonable to administer intravenous lipid emulsion in patients with severe amiodarone poisoning refractory to standard resuscitative efforts.

## ANTIDYSRHYTHMICS–UNCLASSIFIED

Adenosine is administered as a rapid IV bolus to terminate reentrant supraventricular tachycardia. The effects of adenosine are mediated by its interaction with adenosine ($A_1$) receptors that activate acetylcholine-sensitive outward $K^+$ current in the atrium, sinus nodes, and AV nodes. The resultant hyperpolarization reduces the rate of cellular firing. Adverse effects of adenosine administration are very common and include transient asystole, dyspnea, chest tightness, flushing, hypotension, and atrial fibrillation. Fortunately, most of the adverse effects of adenosine are transient because of its rapid metabolism to inosine by both extracellular and intracellular deaminases. The clinical effects are potentiated by dipyridamole, an adenosine uptake inhibitor, and by denervation hypersensitivity in cardiac transplant recipients. Methylxanthines block adenosine receptors (Chap. 36). In this setting, larger-than-usual doses of adenosine are required to produce an antidysrhythmic effect. Overdose of adenosine is not reported. Treatment is supportive because of the rapid elimination of the medication.

Digoxin, a cardioactive steroid, is often considered a member of this class. A complete discussion of digoxin can be found in Chap. 35.

Magnesium ion is occasionally included in this class as well because of its ability to prevent the development of recurrent torsade de pointes. A complete discussion of magnesium sulfate can be found in Antidotes in Brief: A16.

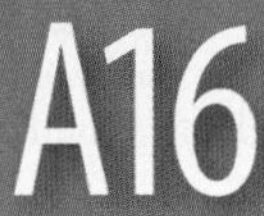


# MAGNESIUM

## INTRODUCTION

Magnesium is an essential cofactor in more than 350 enzyme reactions in cardiac, neurologic, neuromuscular, and endocrine processes, as well as in basic energy, structural, nucleic acid, and signal transduction pathways. Magnesium as chloride, citrate, hydroxide, oxide, or sulfate is used to treat xenobiotic-associated hypomagnesemia and as an adjunctive treatment for cardiovascular toxins, fluoride toxicity, and in patients with alcohol use disorder.

## HISTORY

In 1695, magnesium sulfate ($MgSO_4$) was determined to be the main component of Epsom salts. $MgSO_4$ was used to treat tetanus in 1906 and seizures in 1923. $MgSO_4$ was used to suppress paroxysmal tachycardia in the 1930s and 1940s. $MgSO_4$ continues in use as a uterine tocolytic, a bronchodilator, a migraine therapy, and a nutritional adjunct to prevent hypomagnesemia in hyperalimentation.

## PHARMACOLOGY

### Chemistry and Preparation

Magnesium has the atomic number 12, with a molecular weight of 24.3 Da. Despite having a smaller atomic radius than calcium, magnesium binds water tighter, with two hydration shells, leading to a radius 400 times larger than its dehydrated form. This property underlies its calcium antagonism. Despite similar chemical reactivity and charge, magnesium does not lose its hydration shell as easily as calcium and remains too large to fit into calcium channels to which it is otherwise attracted.

### Related Agents

The use of magnesium as an oral saline cathartic (eg, magnesium citrate, magnesium hydroxide, and $MgSO_4$) is discussed in Antidotes in Brief: A2.

### Pharmacokinetics

Adults contain approximately 1 mole (21–28 g) of magnesium; homeostasis balances intestinal absorption and renal excretion. A normal serum magnesium concentration is 1.5 to 2.0 mEq/L (1.7–2.4 mg/dL; 0.7–1 mmol/L). Magnesium is approximately 30% to 40% protein bound. Extracellular magnesium represents only 1% of the body's total stores, with the remaining magnesium found in bone (~60%), muscle (~20%), and soft tissues (~19%). After being absorbed, magnesium is eliminated by the kidney at a rate proportional to the plasma concentration and glomerular filtration.

After a 4-g IV loading dose followed by a 1-g/h continuous maintenance infusion of $MgSO_4$, serum magnesium concentrations approximately double from 0.74 to 0.85 mmol/L to 1.48 to 1.70 mmol/L at 30 minutes and remain constant for at least 24 hours. After intramuscular administration, the magnesium concentration does not peak until 90 to 120 minutes and is followed by a slow decline back to baseline concentrations over 4 to 8 hours. Oral bioavailability ranges between 19% and 30% depending on the salt form, and peak concentrations are achieved at about 4 hours after administration.

### Pharmacodynamics and Mechanisms of Action

Selected key magnesium actions provide the physiologic basis for antidotal strategies. Magnesium acts as a calcium channel blocker. In the heart, this produces negative inotropy in isolated preparations. However, it results in positive inotropy in healthy human volunteers, presumably because of decreased systemic and pulmonary arterial vascular resistance. Additionally, limiting calcium outflow from the sarcoplasmic reticulum and restricting outward potassium movement appear to underlie the role of magnesium in the reduction of sinus node rate firing, increased atrioventricular (AV) node refractoriness, and suppression of ectopy. In the pulmonary system, the inhibitory actions of magnesium on smooth muscle lead to a weak bronchodilating effect. In the nervous system, the glutamate *N*-methyl-D-aspartate (NMDA) receptor mediates excitatory neurotransmission that is blocked by magnesium. Magnesium similarly blocks N- (and L-) type calcium channels to inhibit catecholamine release from adrenergic nerves.

## ROLE IN XENOBIOTIC-INDUCED HYPOMAGNESEMIA

The choice of oral or IV repletion should depend on the degree of hypomagnesemia and the clinical scenario, with IV treatment used for severe cases.

## ROLE IN POISONING BY CARDIAC TOXINS

Digoxin inhibits the action of magnesium-dependent sodium-potassium adenosine triphosphatase ($Na^+,K^+$-ATPase). In controlled animal studies, hypomagnesemia enhanced the lethality of cardioactive steroid toxicity. In another animal experiment, $MgSO_4$ reversed cardioactive steroid-induced inhibition of $Na^+,K^+$-ATPase. In humans, $MgSO_4$ suppresses digoxin-associated extrasystoles and reduces digoxin-associated tachydysrhythmias. Magnesium also stabilized refractory digoxin-associated ventricular dysrhythmias when digoxin-specific antibody fragments were unavailable. On the basis of these data, it is reasonable to administer magnesium to patients with tachydysrhythmias and evidence of digoxin poisoning, even in the setting of normal digoxin concentrations.

Magnesium sulfate has been used sporadically to treat patients with other specific cardiovascular poisonings such as amitriptyline and aconite, and to limit the adverse effects of ibutilide. It is also used routinely in the treatment of patients with drug-induced torsade de pointes. Based on the limited available data, it is reasonable to ensure eumagnesemia in patients with a prolonged QT interval and to administer magnesium in patients with progressive QT interval prolongation due to poisoning. After an episode of torsade de pointes, it is recommended to administer IV $MgSO_4$.

## ROLE IN ETHANOL DISORDERS AND THIAMINE DEFICIENCY

Chronic alcohol use is associated with hypomagnesemia. Magnesium is an essential cofactor of the thiamine-dependent enzymes transketolase and pyruvate dehydrogenase, and magnesium increases the activity of a third critical thiamine-dependent enzyme α-ketoglutarate dehydrogenase. Magnesium deficiency results in a loss of thiamine from tissues and limits the response to exogenous thiamine. In a controlled trial of patients with chronic alcohol use disorder, those given $MgSO_4$ in addition to thiamine demonstrated significantly greater transketolase activity.

Separately, magnesium was evaluated for its role in mitigating the consequences of alcohol withdrawal and neuronal hyperactivity. In a double-blind, placebo-controlled trial of patients with alcohol withdrawal, four doses of IM $MgSO_4$ (2 g every 6 hours) did not alter chlordiazepoxide use or the incidence of diaphoresis, tremor, vomiting, hallucinations, or withdrawal severity. This is in contrast to the findings of a retrospective review of 781 patients with alcoholism being treated for detoxification, which documented a lower seizure incidence in the patients treated with magnesium. Given the significant prevalence of magnesium and thiamine deficiency in individuals with alcoholism and the critical role of magnesium in thiamine efficacy, it is reasonable to actively screen for magnesium deficiency and administer magnesium to patients with documented hypomagnesemia, those with moderate to severe alcohol withdrawal, and those at risk for Wernicke encephalopathy.

## ROLE IN PESTICIDE POISONING

Because magnesium diminishes calcium channel–mediated synaptic acetylcholine release, it was hypothesized that $MgSO_4$ might ameliorate organic phosphorus (OP) effects at the neuromuscular junction and elsewhere. In a small controlled trial of patients given 4 g/day of IV $MgSO_4$, the requirement for atropine and oximes did not differ compared to control patients receiving standard care, but the duration of hospitalization decreased, and the mortality rate decreased from 15% to 0%. A larger double-blind, randomized clinical trial of patients with OP poisoning found that 4 g of $MgSO_4$ IV reduced atropine requirements over 30 minutes and reduced the need for intubation and intensive care unit stay but did not alter the mortality rate. Currently, the use of $MgSO_4$ is not routinely recommended in patients with organic phosphorus poisoning.

## ROLE IN HYDROFLUORIC ACID AND FLUORIDE-RELEASING XENOBIOTICS

Calcium administration (Antidotes in Brief: 32) remains a mainstay of treatment for patients with hydrofluoric acid (HF) burns. Relatively small skin surface area burns with concentrated HF can lead to profound hypomagnesemia, which, if left unaddressed, can contribute to death. Survival and mitigation of lethal dysrhythmias in HF or sodium fluoride ingestion both typically require large amounts of magnesium and calcium. It is reasonable to administer magnesium in cases of systemic toxicity from fluoride-releasing xenobiotics.

## ADVERSE EFFECTS AND SAFETY ISSUES

The side effects of excessive $MgSO_4$ administration include bradycardia, hypotension, and cardiac arrest; respiratory depression; gastrointestinal complaints of nausea, vomiting, and thirst; and neurologic sequelae of restlessness, confusion, a sense of impending doom, central nervous system depression, weakness, areflexia, and paralysis. In the event of hypermagnesemia or hypocalcemia leading to significant symptoms (eg, respiratory muscle paralysis, hypotension, or dysrhythmia), IV calcium (Antidotes in Brief: 32) is used to counteract the effects.

## PREGNANCY AND LACTATION

In 2013, the status of magnesium was changed from pregnancy class A to D (positive evidence of human fetal risk, but the potential benefits are acceptable in certain situations despite its risks). Magnesium distributes into breast milk during parenteral magnesium administration. Although caution should be exercised when $MgSO_4$ is administered to a nursing mother, the American Academy of Pediatrics considers $MgSO_4$ to be compatible with breastfeeding.

## DOSING AND ADMINISTRATION

Magnesium dosing varies significantly. In the setting of magnesium deficiency, several grams of $MgSO_4$ provided over the first day in divided doses of 1 to 2 g are often required for repletion, with frequent serum determinations to guide therapy. For torsade de pointes in adults, 2 g (25–50 mg/kg in children up to 2 g) of $MgSO_4$ intravenously is recommended. By comparison, 4 to 6 g of IV $MgSO_4$ is recommended to initiate therapy for severe preeclampsia or eclampsia with maintenance doses typically of 1 to 2 g/h. Both normal magnesium and potassium concentrations should be ensured in patients with a prolonged QT interval, and given the lack of consensus, it would be reasonable to administer magnesium in patients with progressive QT interval prolongation from poisoning. The recommended dose mirrors that for torsade de pointes: 2 g of $MgSO_4$ in adults followed by infusion or intermittent doses of 0.5 to 1 g/h with endpoints guided by the specific clinical circumstances. The rate of administration depends on the clinical scenario. For example, in a seizing patient with eclampsia, a dose of 4 g $MgSO_4$ is rapidly provided over 5 minutes. In nonemergent scenarios, $MgSO_4$ is administered at a rate not to exceed 150 mg/min. Magnesium requirements in fluoride poisoning are guided by serum magnesium and clinical assessment. Magnesium sulfate should be diluted to a less than or equal to 20% concentration for IV administration.

## FORMULATION AND ACQUISITION

A variety of $MgSO_4$ formulations are available for parenteral administration: 4% (40 mg/mL) or 8% (80 mg/mL) in sterile water volumes ranging from 100 mL to 1 L. Magnesium sulfate injection, 50% in water (500 mg/mL), is typically supplied as 2 or 10 mL.

# 31 ANTITHROMBOTICS

## HISTORY AND EPIDEMIOLOGY

Antithrombotics have numerous clinical applications, including the treatment of coronary artery disease, cerebrovascular events, hypercoagulable states, deep vein thrombosis (DVT), and pulmonary embolism (PE). The discovery of modern-day oral anticoagulants originated after investigations of a hemorrhagic disorder in Wisconsin cattle in the early 20th century that resulted from the ingestion of spoiled sweet clover silage. The hemorrhagic agent, eventually identified as bishydroxycoumarin, would be the precursor to its synthetic congener warfarin (named after the *W*isconsin *A*lumni *R*esearch *F*oundation).

During the period from 2011 to 2015, the American Association of Poison Control Centers listed anticoagulants in the top 25 xenobiotic categories associated with the largest number of fatalities. The total number of cases of reported antithrombotic exposures to the American Association of Poison Control Centers was 96,498 with 130 deaths during that 5-year period. In 2011, dabigatran and warfarin led the United States (US) Food and Drug Administration (FDA) Safety Information and Adverse Event Reporting Program's list of adverse drug events, with 3,781 reports of serious adverse events associated with dabigatran, including 542 patient deaths.

## PHYSIOLOGY

### Balance Between Coagulation and Anticoagulation

This section summarizes the critical steps of the coagulation cascade. Coagulation consists of a series of events that prevent blood loss and assist in the restoration of blood vessel integrity. Within the cascade, coagulation factors exist as inert precursors and are transformed into enzymes when activated. Activation of the cascade occurs through one of two distinct pathways, the *intrinsic* and *extrinsic* systems (Fig. 31–1). The *intrinsic* and *extrinsic* pathways are linked at factor X. After being activated, these enzymes catalyze a series of reactions that ultimately converge to generate thrombin (IIa) with the subsequent formation of a fibrin clot. Platelets interact with proteins of the coagulation cascade through surface receptors for factors V, VIII, IX, and X. As a final step, factor XIII assists in the cross-linking of fibrin to form a stable thrombus. The stimulus to form clot is balanced by antithrombin (AT), and proteins C, S, and Z, which serve as inhibitors. Additionally, endogenous thrombolysis serves to assure the fluidity of the blood.

## DEVELOPMENT OF COAGULOPATHY

Impaired coagulation results from decreased production or enhanced consumption of coagulation factors, the presence of inhibitors of coagulation, activation of the fibrinolytic system, or abnormalities in platelet number or function. Decreased production of coagulation factors results from congenital and acquired etiologies. Although congenital disorders of factor VIII (hemophilia A), factor IX (Christmas factor Hemophilia B), factor XI, and factor XII (Hageman factor) are all reported, their overall incidence is still quite low. Clinical conditions that result in acquired factor deficiencies are much more common and result from either a decrease in synthesis or activation. Factors II, V, VII, and X are entirely synthesized in the liver, making hepatic dysfunction a common cause of acquired coagulopathy. In addition, factors II, VII, IX, and X also require postsynthetic modification by an enzyme that uses vitamin K as a cofactor, such that vitamin K deficiency (from malnutrition, changes in gut flora secondary to xenobiotics, or malabsorption) and inhibition of vitamin K cycling (from warfarin) are capable of impairing coagulation.

Excessive consumption of coagulation factors usually results from massive activation of the coagulation cascade. Massive activation occurs during severe bleeding or disseminated intravascular coagulation (DIC). Inhibitors of the coagulation cascade (circulating anticoagulants) are of two types: immunoglobulins to coagulation factors or antibodies to phospholipid membrane surfaces. Immunoglobulins develop without obvious cause, are part of a systemic autoimmune disorder, or result from repeated transfusions with exogenous factors (as occurs in patients with hemophilia). Antibodies to factors V, VII to XI, and XIII are described. The clinical syndromes associated with antibody inhibitors are similar to those associated with deficiencies of the particular coagulation factors involved.

## GENERAL MANAGEMENT

In general, a single dose of activated charcoal (AC) decreases absorption of oral anthrombotics and should be given unless contraindicated. In addition to general supportive measures, the patient should be placed in a supervised medical and psychiatric environment that offers protection against external or self-induced trauma and permits observation for the onset of coagulopathy. Blood transfusion is required for any patient with a history of blood loss or active bleeding who is hemodynamically unstable, has impaired oxygen transport, or is expected to become unstable. Although a transfusion of packed red blood cells (PRBCs) is ideal for replacing lost blood, it cannot correct a coagulopathy, so patients will continue to bleed. Massive transfusion protocols (MTPs) aim to correct coagulopathy with an array of blood products, electrolytes, and antifibrinolytics. If available, it is reasonable to use an MTP for unstable patients. If an MTP is not available, whole blood is reasonable in severe cases because it contains many components, including platelets, white blood cells, and non–vitamin K–dependent factors.

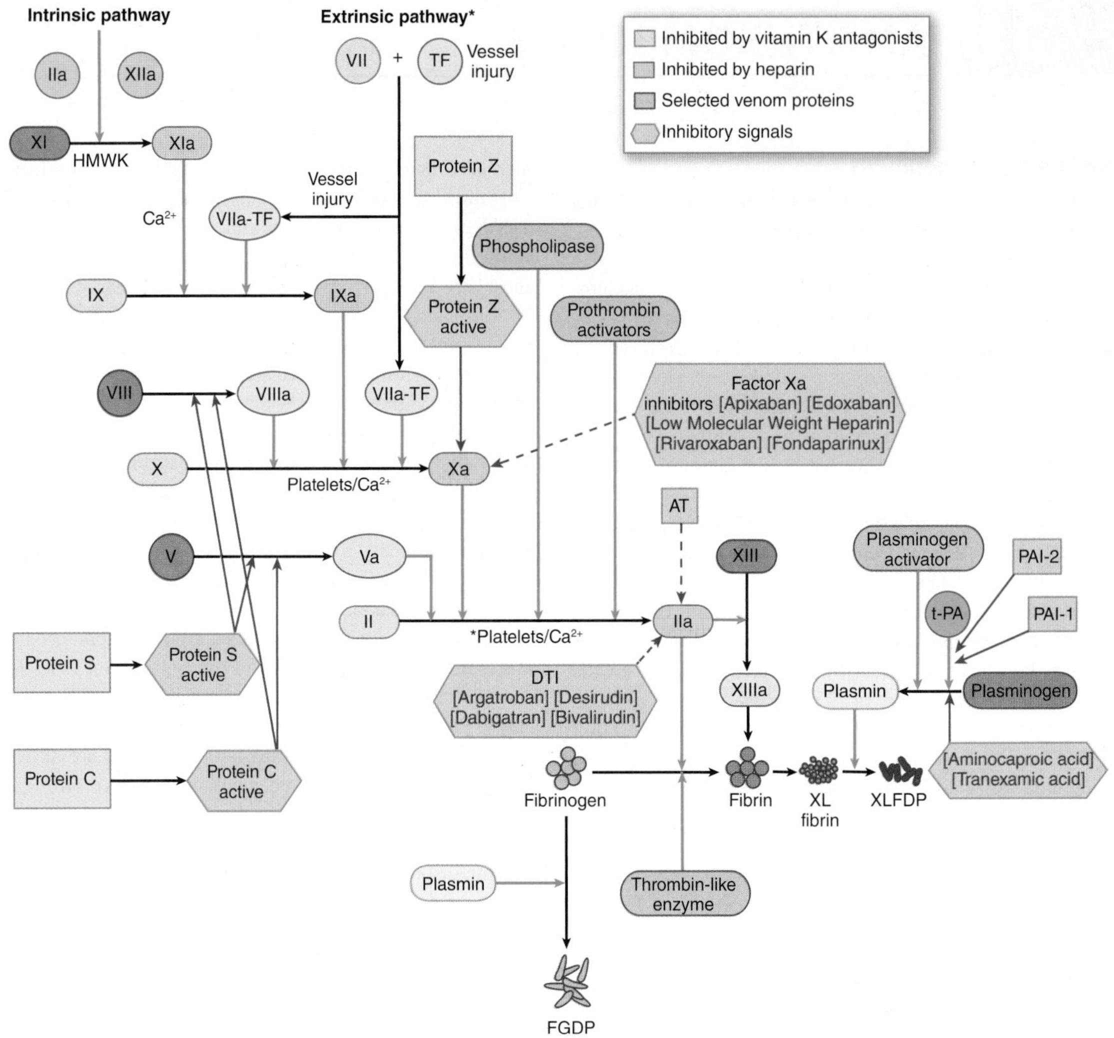


**FIGURE 31–1.** A schematic overview of the coagulation, platelet activation, and fibrinolytic pathways indicating where phospholipids on the platelet surface interact with the coagulation pathway intermediates. Arrows are not shown from platelets to phospholipids involved in the tissue factor VIIa and the factor IX to VIIIa interactions to avoid confusion. Interactions of selected venom proteins are indicated in the purple boxes. The diagram is not complete with reference to the multiple sites of interaction of the serine protease inhibitors (SERPINs) to avoid overcrowding. Solid red lines indicate inhibition of a reaction effect. Black arrows refer to chemical conversion of coagulation factors. Green arrows represent activation of the chemical conversion pathway. Dashed red lines indicate inhibition of a specific clotting factor. *Refer to **Figs. 31–4** and **31–5** for the platelet activation pathway. DTI = direct thrombin inhibitor; FDP = fibrin degradation products; FGDP = fibrinogen degradation product; HMWK = high-molecular-weight kininogen; TF = tissue factor; t-PA = tissue plasminogen activator; XL = cross-linked.

## VITAMIN K ANTAGONISTS

### Warfarin and "Warfarinlike" Anticoagulants

The vitamin K antagonist (VKA) anticoagulants inhibit the vitamin K cycle (Fig. 31–2). The vitamin K–sensitive enzymatic step that occurs in the liver involves the γ-carboxylation of residues on the amino terminal end of the precursor proteins to form a unique amino acid γ-carboxyglutamate, which allows them to chelate calcium to facilitate binding to phospholipid membranes during activation of the coagulation cascade.

Vitamin K is inactive until it is reduced from its quinone form to a quinol (or hydroquinone) form in hepatic microsomes. This reduction of vitamin K must precede the carboxylation of the precursor factors. The carboxylation activity is coupled to an epoxidase activity for vitamin K, whereby vitamin K is oxidized simultaneously to vitamin K 2,3-epoxide. This inactive form of the vitamin is converted back to the active form by two successive reductions. All VKAs interfere with this conversion (Fig. 31–2).

### Pharmacology of Vitamin K Antagonists

Oral warfarin is well absorbed, and peak serum concentrations occur approximately 3 hours after administration. Because only the free warfarin is therapeutically active, concurrent administration of xenobiotics that alter the concentration of free warfarin, either by competing for binding to albumin or by inhibiting warfarin metabolism, markedly influences the anticoagulant effect. Although vitamin K

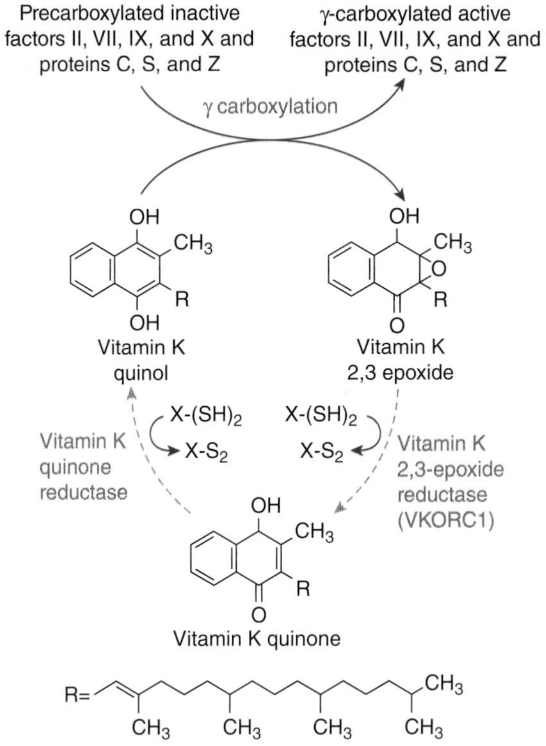

**FIGURE 31–2.** The vitamin K cycle. Dotted lines represent pathways that can be blocked with warfarin and warfarinlike anticoagulants. The aliphatic side chain (R) of vitamin K is shown below the metabolic pathway. VKORC1 = vitamin K reductase complex 1.

regeneration is altered almost immediately, the anticoagulant effect of VKAs is delayed until the existing stores of vitamin K are depleted and the active coagulation factors are removed from circulation. Thus, most patients require at least 15 hours before the effect is evident on the international normalized ratio (INR).

Some VKAs, known as *superwarfarins* or long-acting VKAs, were designed to be effective rodenticides in warfarin-resistant rodents. Their mechanism of action is identical to that of other VKAs, but they are highly lipid soluble and saturate hepatic enzymes at very low concentrations. These factors make them about 100 times more potent than warfarin and give them a longer duration of action.

## Clinical Manifestations

Although intentional ingestions of warfarin-containing products are uncommon, adverse drug events resulting in excessive anticoagulation and bleeding frequently occur. The most serious complication of excessive therapeutic anticoagulation is intracranial bleeding, which is reported to occur in as many as 2% of patients on long-term therapy, which is an 8- to 10-fold increase in risk compared with patients who are not anticoagulated.

Many cases of intentional overdose of long-acting VKAs are reported. The clinical courses of these patients are characterized by a severe coagulopathy that last weeks to months, often accompanied by consequential blood loss. Most patients do not seek medical care until bruising or bleeding is evident, which often occurs many days after ingestion. The most common sites of bleeding are the gastrointestinal (GI) and genitourinary tracts.

Patients with unintentional ingestions must be distinguished from those with intentional ingestions because the former demonstrate a low likelihood of developing a coagulopathy and have rare morbidity or mortality. Single small unintentional ingestions of warfarin or warfarin-containing rodenticides pose a minimal threat to normal patients. Prolongation of the INR is unlikely with a single small ingestion of a long-acting VKA rodenticide. Clinically significant anticoagulation is even rarer, but can result, however, after small repeated ingestions.

## Laboratory Assessment

Table 31–1 summarizes appropriate laboratory testing. We recommend a single INR at a minimum of 2 days after the exposure for children with one-time ingestions of a long-acting VKA. No testing in necessary for single unintentional ingestions of warfarin. A baseline INR is usually unnecessary but is reasonable if there is a suspicion of an antecedent ingestion or chronic exposure is suspected. For patients with an acute and significant long-acting VKA overdose, daily INR evaluations for 2 days are adequate to identify most patients at risk for coagulopathy. When blood loss is evident, serial determinations of hemoglobin concentration are indicated.

## Treatment of Vitamin K Antagonist–Induced Coagulopathy

Life-threatening bleeding secondary to VKA toxicity should be immediately reversed with factor replacement followed by vitamin $K_1$ (Table 31–1). We recommend factor replacement with four-factor prothrombin complex concentrate (PCC) as a first-line treatment for major bleeding in the setting of VKA-induced coagulopathy. The typical doses range between 25 and 50 units/kg with the largest dose based on a maximum weight of 100 kg. Some PCCs contain heparin and are contraindicated in patients with a history of heparin-induced thrombocytopenia (HIT) and heparin-induced thrombocytopenia and thrombosis syndrome (HITT). In those cases, factor eight inhibitor bypassing activity (FEIBA), an activated prothrombin complex concentrate (aPCC), is recommended. If PCCs are unavailable, fresh frozen plasma (FFP) at a dose of 15 mL/kg should be adequate to reverse VKA-induced coagulopathy.

Activated recombinant factor VII (rFVIIa) is approved for patients with hemophilia or various factor inhibitors and has successfully reversed warfarin toxicity. However, adverse outcomes, such as arterial thrombotic events, occur at higher than acceptable rates. We do not recommend routine use of rFVIIa for reversing VKA-associated coagulopathy. If FFP, PCC, and FEIBA are not available, then it is reasonable that rFVIIa be given only in life-threatening situations.

Treatment with vitamin $K_1$ takes several hours to activate enough factors to reverse a patient's coagulopathy, and this delay is potentially fatal. Repetitive, large doses of vitamin $K_1$ (on the order of 60 mg/day or greater) are reported in some patients with massive ingestions. If complete reversal of INR prolongation occurs or is desirable (as in most cases of life-threatening bleeding) and the underlying

**TABLE 31–1 Antithrombotics: Laboratory Testing, Antidotes, and Treatment Strategies**

| | *Laboratory Testing Results (Expected)* | *Antidotes and Treatment Strategies* |
|---|---|---|
| ***Antiplatelet Agents***<br>Cyclooxygenase inhibitors<br>Phosphodiesterase inhibitors<br>Adenosine reuptake inhibitors<br>Adenosine diphosphate receptor inhibitors<br>Glycoprotein IIb/IIIa inhibitors | Bleeding time prolonged; platelet function assays abnormal | Desmopressin 0.3 μg/kg IV over 15–30 min for life-threatening bleeding; platelet administration is controversial but is recommended in life-threatening situations |
| ***Antithrombin Agonists*** | | |
| Unfractionated heparin | PTT prolonged; TT abnormal; ACT elevated; fibrinogen normal, anti–factor Xa activity increased | 1 mg of protamine per 100 units of heparin[a]. In overdose, if unknown quantity of heparin administered, treat based on ACT:[b]<br>ACT < 150 s: no protamine needed<br>ACT 200–300 s: 0.6 mg/kg protamine<br>ACT 300–400 s: 1.2 mg/kg protamine<br>Alternatively, empiric treatment with 25–50 mg of protamine<br>Ciraparantag (in clinical trials) |
| Low-molecular-weight heparin (eg, enoxaparin, dalteparin) | Anti–factor Xa activity increased; PTT is insensitive | 1 mg of protamine per 100 anti–factor Xa units (or 1 mg of enoxaparin) given in the previous 8 h. Administer an additional 0.5 mg protamine per 100 anti–factor Xa units if bleeding continues. Protamine does not completely neutralize LMWHs. |
| ***Direct Thrombin Inhibitors*** | PTT prolonged; TT prolonged; ECT prolonged; anti–factor Xa activity elevated (at low concentrations, PT and PTT may be normal); dTT prolonged | |
| Dabigatran | | Activated charcoal in overdose<br>Idarucizumab 5 g IV<br>If idarucizumab is unavailable:<br>4F-PCC administration with up to 100 units/kg in repeated 50 unit/kg doses as needed. If bleeding continues 30 min after PCC, give FEIBA.<br>Hemodialysis<br>FFP 15 mL/kg |
| Bivalirudin<br>Argatroban | | Stop the infusion |
| ***Direct Factor Xa Inhibitors***<br>Rivaroxaban<br>Apixaban<br>Edoxaban | PT and PTT can be normal or prolonged (varies with reagents); anti–factor Xa activity elevated with specific modified chromogenic antifactor Xa assay[d] | AC in overdose<br>PCC[c] administration with up to 50 units/kg in repeated 25 unit/kg doses as needed<br>Andexanet alfa[e]<br>Low dose: 400 mg IV<br>High dose: 800 mg IV<br>Ciraparantag (in clinical trials) |
| ***Fibrinolytics*** | PT and PTT prolonged; TT abnormal; fibrinogen abnormal | Cryoprecipitate (adults, 1 unit/5 kg body weight; children 5-10 mL/kg)<br>Factor replacement with 15 mL/kg of FFP or 50 units/kg of PCC[c]<br>For life-threatening hemorrhage, give tranexamic acid at 1 g intravenously over 10 minutes followed by 1 g over 8 h. If tranexamic acid is unavailable, IV aminocaproic acid is recommended as a loading dose of 5 g over 1 h followed by an infusion at 1 g/h for 23 h. Stop infusion if bleeding ceases. |
| ***Pentasaccharide*** | | |
| Fondaparinux | Fondaparinux-specific anti-Xa assay<br>PTT does not reflect degree of anticoagulation | PCC administration with up to 50 units/kg in repeated 25 unit/kg doses as needed to maximum of 100 units/kg |
| ***Vitamin K Antagonist*** | | |
| Warfarin | *Early* (PT (INR) prolonged; PTT normal)<br>*Late* (PT (INR) and PTT prolonged; TT and fibrinogen normal) | Vitamin K (**Table 31–2**)<br>Factor replacement with 4F-PCC[c] or if not available FFP (15 mL/kg) for major or life-threatening hemorrhage |

[a]May need to repeat in 2–8 h because of potential heparin rebound. [b]Use of activated clotting time (ACT) is only validated in the operative setting after cardiopulmonary bypass. [c]In patients with a history of heparin-induced thrombocytopenia, avoid prothrombin complex concentrate (PCC) (except Profilnine) and use factor eight inhibitor bypassing activity (FEIBA) or recombinant factor VII (rFVIIa). [d]No readily available method to assess extent of anticoagulation at this time. [e]FDA approved for rivaroxaban and apixaban (but should also be effective for edoxaban), and low dose vs high dose is based on timing and amount of last dose of anti-Xa inhbitor.

AC = activated charcoal; ECT = ecarin clotting time; dTT= dilute thrombin time; FFP = fresh-frozen plasma; 4F-PCC = four-factor prothrombin complex concentrate; INR = international normalized ratio; LMWH = low-molecular-weight heparin; PCC = prothrombin complex concentrate; PT = prothrombin time; PTT = partial thromboplastin time; TT = thrombin time.

medical condition of the patient still requires some degree of anticoagulation, the patient can then receive anticoagulation with heparin after the bleeding is controlled and clinical stability restored.

Vitamin $K_1$ is preferable over the other forms of vitamin K; the other forms are ineffective, potentially toxic, and are unavailable in the US. Parenteral administration of vitamin $K_1$ (phytonadione) is traditionally preferred as initial therapy by many authors, but success can also be achieved with early oral therapy, especially when the coagulopathy is not severe. In most cases, the patient can be switched to oral vitamin $K_1$ for long-term care (Antidotes in Brief: A18).

For patients with non–life-threatening bleeding, the clinician must evaluate whether anticoagulation is required for long-term care. In patients not requiring chronic anticoagulation, we recommend treating even small elevations of the INR with vitamin $K_1$ alone to prevent deterioration in coagulation status and reduce the risk of bleeding. For patients requiring chronic anticoagulation, we agree with the American College of Chest Physicians (ACCP) guidelines for the management of patients with elevated INRs (Table 31–2).

### Treatment of Long-Acting Vitamin K Antagonist Overdoses

In patients with unintentional, small ingestions of long-acting VKAs, the risk of coagulopathy is low. However, it takes days to develop coagulopathy. Administration of AC is recommended to prevent absorption in acute ingestions if no contraindication exists. In contrast to ingestions of warfarin, we recommend not to give prophylactic vitamin $K_1$ to asymptomatic patients with unintentional ingestions of long-acting VKAs because (1) if the patient develops a coagulopathy, it will last for weeks, and the one or two doses of vitamin $K_1$ given will not prevent complications; (2) a gradual decline in coagulation factors occurs over the first day of anticoagulation, so an individual would not be expected to develop a life-threatening coagulopathy in 1 or 2 days; and (3) after vitamin $K_1$ is administered, the onset of an INR abnormality will be delayed, which could impair the ability of the clinician to recognize a coagulation abnormality, possibly requiring the patient to undergo an unnecessarily prolonged observation period.

**TABLE 31–2 Recommendations for Management of Elevated International Normalized Ratio or Bleeding in Patients Receiving Vitamin K Antagonists**

| *International Normalized Ratio* | *Recommendation*[a] |
|---|---|
| < 4.5; no significant bleeding | Lower or omit the next dose of warfarin. |
| ≥ 4.5–10; no significant bleeding | Omit warfarin for the next one or two doses. |
| > 10; no evidence of bleeding | Give oral vitamin $K_1$ (1–2.5 mg). If more rapid reversal is necessary, give oral vitamin $K_1$ (≤ 5 mg) and wait 24 h. Give additional vitamin $K_1$ orally (1–2 mg) as needed. |
| Serious bleeding at any INR value or life-threatening bleeding | Hold warfarin therapy and give 4F-PCC supplemented with vitamin $K_1$ (5–10 mg by slow IV[a] infusion). Vitamin $K_1$ administration often needs to be repeated every 12 h. |

[a]Intravenous (IV) infusion of vitamin $K_1$ rarely may cause severe anaphylactoid reactions

4F-PCC = four-factor prothrombin complex concentrate; INR = international normalized ratio.

Treatment of a patient with a coagulopathy resulting from a long-acting VKA overdose is essentially the same as the treatment of oral anticoagulant toxicity, with certain exceptions. Although initial parenteral vitamin $K_1$ doses as high as 400 mg have been required for reversal, daily oral vitamin $K_1$ requirements are often in the range of 50 to 200 mg (Antidotes in Brief: A18).

Patients with long-acting VKA overdose should be followed until their coagulation studies remain normal without treatment for several days. This usually requires daily or even twice-daily INR measurements until the INR is at the lower limit of the therapeutic range. Periodic coagulation factor analysis (particularly factor VII), however, provides an early marker of toxicity resolution.

### Nonbleeding Complications of Vitamin K Antagonists

Warfarin therapy is associated with four nonhemorrhagic lesions of the skin: urticaria, purple toe syndrome, warfarin skin necrosis, and warfarin-related nephropathy. Evidence suggests a link between warfarin skin necrosis and protein C deficiency. Protein C synthesis is also dependent on vitamin K. Because the half-life of protein C is shorter than that of many of the vitamin K–dependent coagulation factors, protein C concentrations fall rapidly during the first hours of warfarin therapy. This results in an imbalance that actually favors coagulation, and skin necrosis results because of microvascular thrombosis in dermal vessels. This disorder is also described in patients with protein S and AT deficiencies as well as idiosyncratically. If necrosis occurs, warfarin should be discontinued, and heparin should be initiated to decrease thrombosis of postcapillary venules. Some patients also require surgical debridement. The purple toe syndrome, in contrast to warfarin-induced skin necrosis, is presumed to result from small atheroemboli that are no longer adherent to their plaques by clot.

Warfarin-related nephropathy (WRN) is a form of nonhemorrhagic warfarin toxicity. In patients with chronic kidney disease (CKD), an acute increase in the INR above 3 is associated with an increase in serum creatinine and accelerated reduction in kidney function. The etiology of the WRN is attributed to acute tubular injury and glomerular bleeding.

## ANTITHROMBIN AGONISTS

### Heparin

Conventional heparin, also known as unfractionated (UFH), is a heterogeneous group of molecules within the class of glycosaminoglycans. Heparin inhibits thrombosis by accelerating the binding of AT to thrombin (activated factor II) and other serine proteases involved in coagulation. Thus, factors IX to XII, kallikrein, and thrombin are inhibited. The therapeutic effect of heparin is usually measured through the activated PTT. The activated clotting time (ACT) is more useful for monitoring large therapeutic doses or in the overdose situation. Low-molecular-weight heparins (LMWHs) are 4,000- to 6,000-Da fractions obtained from conventional heparin. As such, they share many of the pharmacologic and toxicologic properties of conventional heparin. The major differences between LMWHs and conventional heparin are greater bioavailability, longer half-life, more predictable anticoagulation with fixed dosing, targeted activity against activated factor X, and less targeted activity against thrombin. As a result of this targeted factor X activity, LMWHs have minimal effect on the activated PTT, thereby eliminating either the need for or the usefulness of monitoring. However, in certain instances (eg, patients with CKD, pregnancy), monitoring of anti–factor Xa activity is performed to assess adequacy of anticoagulation and to prevent the risk of bleeding.

Heparin is unable to cross cellular membranes and heparin must be administered parenterally. After parenteral administration, heparin remains in the intravascular compartment, in part bound to globulins, fibrinogen, and low-density lipoproteins, resulting in a volume of distribution of 0.06 L/kg. Because of its rapid metabolism in the liver by a heparinase, heparin has a short duration of effect. The duration of anticoagulant effect is usually reported as 1 to 3 hours. Low-molecular-weight heparins are nearly 90% bioavailable after SC administration and have an elimination half-life of 3 to 6 hours. Anti–factor Xa activity peaks between 3 and 5 hours after dosing.

### Clinical Manifestations

Intentional overdoses with heparin are rare. Most overdose cases involve iatrogenic administration of large amounts of heparin as a medication error. However, intentional overdoses of LMWHs are reported, although none of them were fatal. Similar adverse effects to UFH are also reported with LMWHs and include epidural or spinal hematoma, intrahepatic bleeding, abdominal wall hematomas, psoas hematoma after lumbar plexus block, and intracranial bleeding in patients with central nervous system (CNS) malignancy.

### Diagnostic Testing

For therapeutic anticoagulation, the effect of heparin is usually monitored with activated partial thromboplastin time (aPTT). For patients undergoing cardiovascular procedures, the ACT is used to monitor them because they require higher dose heparin. More recently, an anti-Xa assay specific for heparin was US FDA approved. Heparin dosing is titrated based on the anti-Xa assay results, with therapeutic ranges higher than prophylactic ranges. Low-molecular-weight heparins are usually administered at fixed doses for venous thromboembolism (VTE) prophylaxis or at weight-based doses for VTE treatment. Laboratory monitoring is not done unless patients are pregnant, have CKD, or are obese. In these cases, anti-Xa activity is measured, with target ranges varying based on agent and dosing regimen.

### Treatment

After stabilization of the airway and breathing, significant blood loss should be replaced and the coagulopathy reversed, if indicated. Because of the relatively short duration of action of heparin, observation alone is indicated if significant bleeding has not occurred. For a patient requiring anticoagulation, serial aPTT determinations will indicate when it is safe to resume therapy. If significant bleeding occurs, either removal of the heparin or reversal of its anticoagulant effect is indicated. Because heparin has a very small volume of distribution, it can be effectively removed by exchange transfusion. Although this technique has been used successfully in neonates, protamine has also safely been given to neonates without a history of fish allergy or previous exposure to protamine or protamine-containing insulin.

When severe bleeding occurs, protamine sulfate partially neutralizes UFH (Table 31–1). One milligram of protamine sulfate injected intravenously neutralizes 100 units of UFH. The dose of protamine should be calculated from the dose of heparin administered if known and assuming the approximate half-life of heparin to be 60 to 90 minutes; the amount of protamine should not exceed the amount of heparin expected to be found intravascularly at the time of infusion (Antidotes in Brief: A19).

If life-threatening bleeding occurs after LMWH administration, we also recommend treating patients with protamine. Approximately 1 mg protamine will neutralize 100 anti–factor Xa units of enoxaparin for up to 8 hours after LMWH administration. A second dose of 0.5 mg protamine per 100 anti–factor Xa units is reasonable if bleeding continues. If more than 8 hours has elapsed, a smaller dose of protamine should be administered. The maximum dose of 50 mg should not be exceeded.

## NONBLEEDING COMPLICATIONS

Postoperative thrombocytopenia that occurs in the first 1 or 2 days after surgery usually results from platelet consumption. This early fall in platelet count tends to cause concern for drug-induced thrombocytopenia called HIT because postoperative VTE prophylaxis with heparin is usually started simultaneously. However, postoperative thrombocytopenia usually improves by the third postoperative day, distinguishing itself from HIT, which typically occurs between days 5 and 10 after heparin initiation. In patients who were previously treated with heparin, HIT-related events sometimes occur within 24 hours after reexposure.

Heparin-induced thrombocytopenia affects up to 5% of patients receiving heparin and results from antibody formation to platelet factor 4 (PF4), causing platelet aggregation. A more severe form of thrombocytopenia, HITT (formerly known as HIT-2 or the white clot syndrome) occurs in up to 55% of patients with untreated HIT. The antibodies against the heparin–PF4 complex activate platelets, which leads to platelet–fibrin thrombotic events.

Patients present with either hemorrhagic or thromboembolic complications. Treatment of patients with HIT includes discontinuation of heparin or LMWH and immediate use of alternative anticoagulant such as lepirudin, argatroban, or danaparoid.

In addition to HIT and HITT, necrotizing skin lesions and hyperkalemia from aldosterone suppression also rarely occur in patients receiving heparin therapy. Osteoporosis is also reported in patients on long-term therapy with UFH.

## DIRECT THROMBIN INHIBITORS

Hirudin and its congeners (lepirudin and desirudin) are used in patients with acute coronary syndromes, for the prevention of thromboembolic disease, and in patients with HITT. Unfortunately, all of these direct thrombin inhibitors (DTIs) are short acting and require parenteral administration.

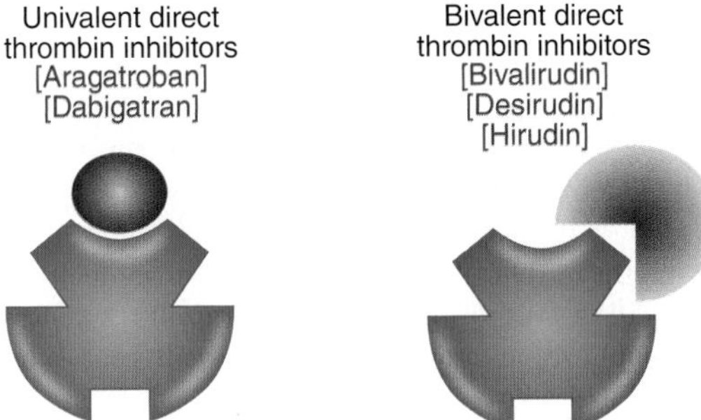


**FIGURE 31–3.** Thrombin has four separate binding sites. Each site is specific for substrate, inhibitor, or cofactors. Bivalent direct thrombin inhibitors, such as hirudin and bivalirudin, bind the active site and one of two exosites. Univalent direct thrombin inhibitors, such as dabigatran, bind only the active site.

Because of the potential therapeutic limitations of warfarin (eg, dosing, risk of bleeding, narrow therapeutic window), direct oral anticoagulants were developed with directed activity against specific clotting factors. Dabigatran was approved for systemic anticoagulation in patients with nonvalvular atrial fibrillation in the US and many other countries. Later it was approved for the treatment and prophylaxis of VTE.

## Pharmacology

Thrombin has four separate binding sites, each of which is specific for substrate, inhibitor, or cofactors. Whereas bivalent DTIs, such as hirudin and bivalirudin, bind the active site and one of two exosites (binding sites outside of the active site), univalent DTIs, such as dabigatran, bind just the active site (Fig. 31–3). By directly inhibiting thrombin, anticoagulation is possible without the need for AT. Unlike heparin, DTIs are able to enter clots and inhibit clot-bound thrombin because of their small size, offering the distinct advantage of restricting further thrombus formation.

Desirudin, bivalirudin, and argatroban are all administered parenterally. Dabigatran is orally administered as dabigatran etexilate. This prodrug has no anticoagulant properties, and serum esterase coverts it to dabigatran, the active drug. At therapeutic doses, peak concentrations occur in 2 hours (Table 31–3). Approximately 35% of dabigatran is protein bound; 85% is eliminated renally, with 78% of it eliminated within the first 24 hours. Its mean terminal half-life is approximately 8 to 12 hours. The manufacturer recommends either dose adjustment or avoidance of concomitant administration of P-glycoprotein inhibitors in patients with renal insufficiency.

## Clinical Manifestations

Intentional overdoses with the DTIs are rare events. Although there are reports of patients who develop significant coagulopathy after unintentional ingestion of excess dabigatran, the more common scenario is that patients become overanticoagulated because of improper dosing in patients with CKD or failure to adjust dosing in patients who develop acute kidney injury (AKI). There are numerous published case reports of patients bleeding while anticoagulated with dabigatran, including intracranial bleeding, GI bleeding, hematuria, and hemoptysis.

## Laboratory Assessment

Monitoring the anticoagulant effect in the setting of DTI use is complex. For bivalirudin and argatroban, serial aPTT measurements are commonly used to estimate the degree of anticoagulation. Admittedly, the aPTT is not a good test because the degree of anticoagulation does not follow a linear relationship. This is particularly emphasized with dabigatran, the most recently developed DTI. The aPTT increases at higher dabigatran concentrations, but the relationship is nonlinear, with the aPTT plateauing at dabigatran concentrations greater than 200 ng/mL. Furthermore, the PT and INR are usually elevated, but they do not correlate with the anticoagulant

**TABLE 31–3 Pharmacology of Oral Antithrombotics[a]**

| | *Warfarin* | *Dabigatran* | *Rivaroxaban* | *Apixaban* | *Edoxaban* |
|---|---|---|---|---|---|
| $T_{max}$ (h) | 3 | 2 | 3 | 1–3 | 1–2 |
| $t_{1/2}$ (h)[a] | 35 | 8–12 | 5–13 | 8–15 | 10–15 |
| Protein binding (%) | 97 | 35 | > 90 | 87 | 55 |
| Metabolism and elimination | Hepatic metabolites (primarily CYP1A2, CYP3A4, and CYP2C9) excreted via renal and biliary systems | 80%–85% renal; 15%–20% biliary | 33% renal (unchanged); 33% renal metabolite; 33% hepatic metabolite | 25% renal; 55% fecal; 15% hepatic metabolite | 35% renal; 49% fecal; 16% hepatic metabolism |
| Drug interactions | Many interactions | P-gp inducers; rifampin | Combined P-gp and strong CYP3A4 inhibitors and inducers | Strong dual inhibitors of CYP3A4 and P-gp<br>Combined CYP3A4 and P-gp inducers | Rifampin |

[a]Antithrombotic metabolism and plasma half-life ($t_{1/2}$) may be altered by a number of factors such as diet, genetic polymorphisms, and kidney disease.

P-gp = P-glycoprotein; $T_{max}$ = time to maximum blood concentration.

effect of dabigatran. Dilute thrombin time (dTT) and ecarin clotting time (ECT) are proposed as more accurate reflections of the anticoagulation effect. Although some hospitals are able to obtain a thrombin time (TT) in a clinically relevant time, the dTT and the ECT are usually unavailable.

### Treatment of Direct Thrombin Inhibitor–Induced Coagulopathy

In the event of an acute ingestion of dabigatran, AC is indicated based on data from an in vitro model. An overdose of argatroban was successfully treated with FFP. With widespread dabigatran use, the absence of a reversal agent became a potentially deadly complication. The manufacturer fast-tracked the development of idarucizumab, a monoclonal antibody targeting dabigatran. In a prospective study containing 90 patients who received 5 g of IV idarucizumab for urgent reversal of dabigatran-induced coagulopathy, reversal of coagulopathy occurred in 100% of patients despite 18 deaths in the study population. Study investigators noted that hemostasis in bleeding patients was restored at a median of 11.4 hours after administration of idarucizumab. The standard dose of idarucizumab, 5 g, will be insufficient in reversing coagulopathy in patients with these extremely high dabigatran concentrations.

Before the US FDA approval of idarucizumab in 2015, the manufacturer suggested several strategies to treat patients with significant bleeding while anticoagulated with dabigatran. Transfusion of RBCs and FFP in addition to supportive care were the mainstays of treatment (Table 31–1). Recombinant factor FVIIa, PCCs, and hemodialysis were also used, but these interventions are incompletely studied.

Hemodialysis for dabigatran removal remains a controversial intervention. A single study showed that after a subtherapeutic dose of dabigatran in patients with stage 5 CKD, the extraction ratios were up to 68% at 4 hours after the initiation of hemodialysis. Although this suggests that dabigatran is effectively removed from the serum, the greater implication of this finding is unknown. Although the safety and efficacy of these adjunctive therapies are unknown, they are reasonable in patients with serious bleeding if idarucizumab is not available or if a patient continues to have life-threatening hemorrhage despite idarucizumab administration. Repletion of blood volume and coagulation factors with PCC is reasonable. If maximal efforts at repletion of blood volume and coagulation factors are ineffective, then hemodialysis followed by continuous venovenous hemodialysis is reasonable if the patient can tolerate the procedure hemodynamically.

## FACTOR Xa INHIBITORS

Rivaroxaban was the first orally active direct factor Xa inhibitor approved for VTE and stroke prophylaxis and treatment. Compared with warfarin, rivaroxaban prevented more strokes or systemic thromboembolic events and significantly reduced the number of intracranial hemorrhages in patients with nonvalvular atrial fibrillation. Apixaban is another oral factor Xa inhibitor that is approved by the US FDA for VTE prophylaxis in patients with atrial fibrillation. Numerous studies showed benefit of apixaban in preventing VTE in specific populations while simultaneously lowering mortality or specific types of bleeding, such as intracranial hemorrhage. However clinical trials of both Xa inhibitors in patients with recent acute coronary syndromes showed poor results. Edoxaban and betrixaban are the newest of the approved factor Xa inhibitors based on studies for VTE prophylaxis in patients with atrial fibrillation and for the treatment of VTE disease.

### Pharmacology

The factor Xa inhibitors are ideal anticoagulants because their site of action is the intersection of the intrinsic and extrinsic pathways, preventing thrombin activation. These drugs reversibly inhibit factor Xa without any cofactor requirements. Rivaroxaban and apixaban selectively bind free and clot-bound factor Xa without inhibiting related serine proteases, including thrombin, trypsin, plasmin, or other activated clotting factors. In addition, rivaroxaban and apixaban inhibit tissue factor or collagen-induced thrombin formation.

Rivaroxaban has an oral bioavailability of approximately 80%. Inhibition of factor Xa peaks approximately 3 hours after administration of the rivaroxaban. This inhibition lasts for approximately 12 hours. However, kidney or liver disease lengthens its duration of action (Table 31–3). Concomitant use of CYP3A4 inhibitors or P-glycoprotein inhibitors is contraindicated because of increased risk of drug accumulation of up to 160%.

The oral bioavailability of apixaban is approximately 66%. Apixaban is primarily distributed to the blood compartment and is approximately 87% protein bound. Peak serum concentrations occur between 1 and 3 hours postingestion. There are multiple elimination pathways, suggesting that patients with either renal or hepatic impairment should be able to tolerate apixaban safely.

Edoxaban is orally administered and has a bioavailability of 61.8%. P-glycoprotein appears to be the key factor as a transporter of edoxaban. Edoxaban metabolism is minor, and the compound is largely excreted in the urine and feces. Approximately 35% of an oral dose is eliminated renally, and 49% of the oral dose is excreted in the feces. Peak edoxaban concentrations occur 1 to 2 hours after ingestion, and the terminal half-life is 10 to 14 hours.

### Clinical Manifestations

Hemorrhage is the most concerning consequence of the factor Xa inhibitors, even at therapeutic doses, and hemorrhage does not necessarily occur in overdose. Although many reports confirm prolonged INRs after acute overdoses of both rivaroxaban and apixaban, at the time of this writing, there are no reports of hemorrhage.

### Diagnostic Testing

Studies in healthy volunteers show that rivaroxaban inhibits factor Xa activity and prolongs PT and aPTT. Unfortunately, PT and aPTT are not reliable measures of the anticoagulant effect of rivaroxaban because results vary widely depending on the reagent used. Chromogenic anti–factor Xa activity reliably measures rivaroxaban effect over a large range of concentrations.

### Treatment of Factor Xa Inhibitor–Induced Coagulopathy

A study in healthy volunteers demonstrated that rivaroxaban absorption is decreased after AC administration up to 8 hours after a single oral dose of rivaroxaban. Another study showed that AC at 2 hours and 6 hours after single-dose apixaban ingestion also reduced apixaban absorption. The administration of AC after an acute overdose is therefore recommended (Table 31–1). A single human study evaluated the use of four-factor PCC in reversing patients given rivaroxaban 20 mg twice daily for 2.5 days. The PT and endogenous thrombin time rapidly normalized after administration of 50 units/kg of PCC. Because of its high protein binding, hemodialysis is unlikely to be an effective adjunct method to accelerate rivaroxaban removal.

Although the half-lives of the factor Xa inhibitors are substantially shorter than that of warfarin, normalization of hemostasis often requires more than 24 hours without intervention. During this time, supportive measures such as restoration of intravascular volume are helpful but do not correct the xenobiotic-induced coagulopathy. Prothrombin complex concentrates at a starting dose of 25 units/kg improves laboratory parameters immediately after infusion, but their effect on hemostasis is unknown. In severe cases, repeat doses may need to be administered.

Andexanet alfa is a recombinant protein recently US FDA approved for reversal of anticoagulation caused by factor Xa inhibitors. Studies in healthy volunteers demonstrated that andexanet alfa administration given to patients who had achieved a steady-state concentration of either apixaban or rivaroxaban resulted in rapid reduction in plasma-free inhibitor concentrations and increased thrombin formation. In an open-label single-group study, andexanet alfa was given to patients who had ingested a factor Xa inhibitor within 18 hours of acute major bleeding onset. After infusion of andexanet alfa, 79% of patients achieved hemostasis and antifactor Xa activity decreased 12 hours after andexanet alfa infusion. Thrombotic events occurred in 6% of patients within 3 days of andexanet alfa infusion, and 15% of the patients died (Antidotes in Brief: A17).

## PENTASACCHARIDES

Pentasaccharides are synthetic anticoagulants that possess activity against factor Xa and are used for the prevention and treatment of VTE. Fondaparinux is the only pentasaccharide currently available for clinical use. The pentasaccharide binds to AT with an affinity higher than that of heparin facilitating the formation of the AT–factor Xa complex. Routine measurements of coagulation are not generally performed. When the degree of anticoagulation needs to be assessed, the fondaparinux-specific anti-Xa assay is the most helpful. The pentasaccharides have long half-lives and have no reliable reversal agent if bleeding occurs; they do not bind to protamine. If a patient develops significant bleeding from fondaparinux, it is reasonable to administer 25 to 50 units/kg of PCC in addition to standard supportive measures.

## FIBRINOLYTICS

The fibrinolytic system is designed to remove unwanted clots while leaving those clots protecting sites of vascular injury intact. Plasminogen exists as a proenzyme that is converted to the active form, plasmin, by plasminogen activators. The actions of plasmin are nonspecific in that it degrades fibrin clots and some plasma proteins and coagulation factors. Inhibition of plasmin occurs through $\alpha_2$-antiplasmin. Tissue plasminogen activator is released from the endothelium and is under the inhibitory control of two inactivators known as tissue plasminogen activator inhibitors 1 and 2 (t-PAI-1 and t-PAI-2). Under physiological conditions, endogenous t-PA does not induce a fibrinolytic state because there is no fibrin to initiate the conversion of plasminogen to plasmin.

Although all fibrinolytics enhance fibrinolysis, they differ in their specific sites of action and duration of effect. Tissue plasminogen is clot specific (ie, it does not increase fibrinolysis in the absence of a thrombus). Newer thrombolytics such as reteplase and tenecteplase possess longer half-lives that facilitate administration via bolus dosing rather than infusion. On the other hand, streptokinase, urokinase, and anistreplase are not clot specific. Tissue plasminogen activator has the shortest half-life and duration of effect (5 minutes and 2 hours, respectively) and anistreplase the longest (90 minutes and 18 hours, respectively). Streptokinase has the additional risk of potential severe allergic reaction on rechallenge, limiting its use to once in a lifetime.

### Clinical Manifestations

Although the incidence of bleeding requiring transfusion is as high as 7.7% after high-dose (150 mg) t-PA and 4.4% after low-dose t-PA, the incidence of intracranial hemorrhage with t-PA appears to be similar to the newer fibrinolytics (monteplase, tenecteplase, reteplase, and lanoteplase). Reviews of multiple trials suggest that life-threatening events such as intracranial hemorrhage occur in 0.30% to 0.58% of patients receiving anistreplase, 0.42% to 0.73% of patients receiving alteplase, and 0.08% to 0.30% of patients receiving streptokinase. Regardless of the thrombolytic used, the frequency of bleeding events is similar, with the exception that lanoteplase has a decreased incidence of significant hemorrhage.

### Treatment

Patients with minor hemorrhagic complications caused by the fibrinolytics should receive supportive care as necessary, with focus on volume replacement and attempts to control the bleeding if possible. However, for patients with significant bleeding such as intracranial hemorrhage, it is reasonable to administer fibrinogen and coagulation factor replacement with cryoprecipitate, FFP, or PCC. When studied, postfibrinolytic patients with expanding intracranial hematomas

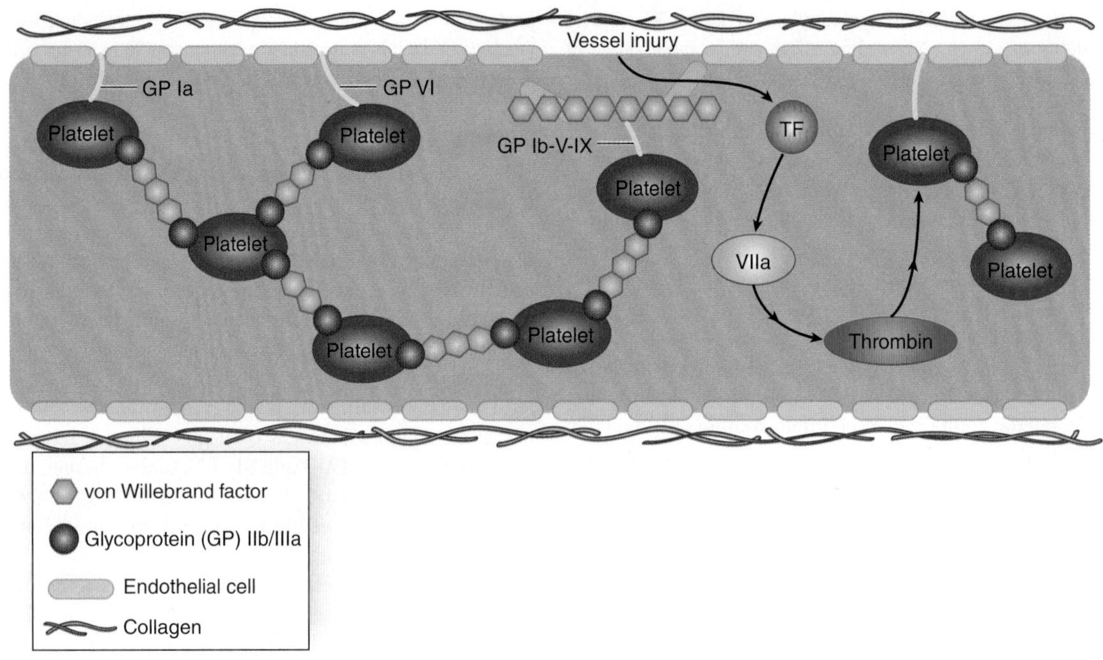


**FIGURE 31–4.** A schematic diagram of platelet aggregation. An injury to the endothelium results in initial platelet tethering by means of von Willebrand factor (vWF) and glycoprotein (GP) Ib-V-IX. Platelet GP VI and Ia tether the platelets to exposed collagen. GP IIb-IIIa is expressed on the surface of the platelets and allows platelet cross-linking with vWF bridging. TF = tissue factor.

tended to have severe hypofibrinogenemia, highlighting the need for cryoprecipitate repletion. If fibrinogen and factor replacement are ineffective, then antifibrinolytics such as aminocaproic acid and tranexamic acid are recommended (Table 31–1). These antifibrinolytics prevent activation of plasmin by competing with fibrin to bind to plasminogen and plasmin.

Aminocaproic acid is administered orally or intravenously. When administered intravenously, a loading dose of 4 to 5 g over 1 hour is followed by an infusion of 1 to 1.25 g/h with a maximum of 30 g given in 24 hours. The infusion should be stopped before 24 hours if the bleeding has ceased. Aminocaproic acid should not be given to patients with hematuria. These patients are at risk for developing obstructive AKI from ureteral clots that cannot be lysed.

Tranexamic acid is dosed as a 1-g infusion over 10 minutes, followed by 1 g over 8 hours. In the Japanese Observational Study for Coagulation and Thrombolysis in Early Trauma (J-OCTET) study, early administration of tranexamic acid resulted in lower rates of mortality, including in the subset of patients with primary brain injury. Unfortunately, aminocaproic acid and tranexamic acid are associated with generalized tonic-clonic seizures in up to 7.6% of patients. The precise mechanism of seizures is not known. In murine studies, competitive antagonism of glycine receptors is suggested.

## ANTIPLATELET DRUGS

Under normal conditions, vascular endothelium provides thromboregulators that prevent thrombus formation. When the endothelium becomes compromised, exposed collagen triggers two cascades of events to promote platelet aggregation. First, a tissue factor–mediated pathway indirectly activates platelets. Tissue factor, either from the damaged vessel wall or carried in the blood, complexes with factor VIIa and activates factor IX and the extrinsic pathway of the coagulation cascade. Thrombin then directly stimulates further platelet adhesion. Second, when von Willebrand factor (vWF) adheres to the exposed endothelium, platelet glycoprotein (GP) Ib-V-IX binds to the vWF and anchors platelets to the site of vascular injury. In addition, platelet GP VI and Ia tether the platelets to exposed collagen (Fig. 31–4).

After platelet adhesion, modulators such as ADP and thromboxane $A_2$ ($TXA_2$) maintain platelet activation. Intracellular signaling results in the release of arachidonic acid (AA) via phospholipase $A_2$. Next, AA is converted into prostacyclin via cyclooxygenase-1 (COX-1) or cyclooxygenase-2 (COX-2). This stimulates the production of $TXA_2$, which further propagates platelet activation and aggregation.

These mediators recruit more platelets to the area of vessel injury. Glycoprotein IIb/IIIa is expressed on the surface of the platelets and allows platelet cross-linking via this receptor with vWF acting as a bridge. Thrombus formation perpetuates platelet aggregation and adhesion to the vessel wall. Platelet GP IIb/IIIa activation results in further thrombus formation by binding fibrinogen and vWF, essential to the linking of platelets.

Antiplatelet therapies aim to decrease platelet activation or aggregation by inhibiting one of the steps in the many pathways, leading to GP IIb/IIIa activation of platelets (Fig. 31–5).

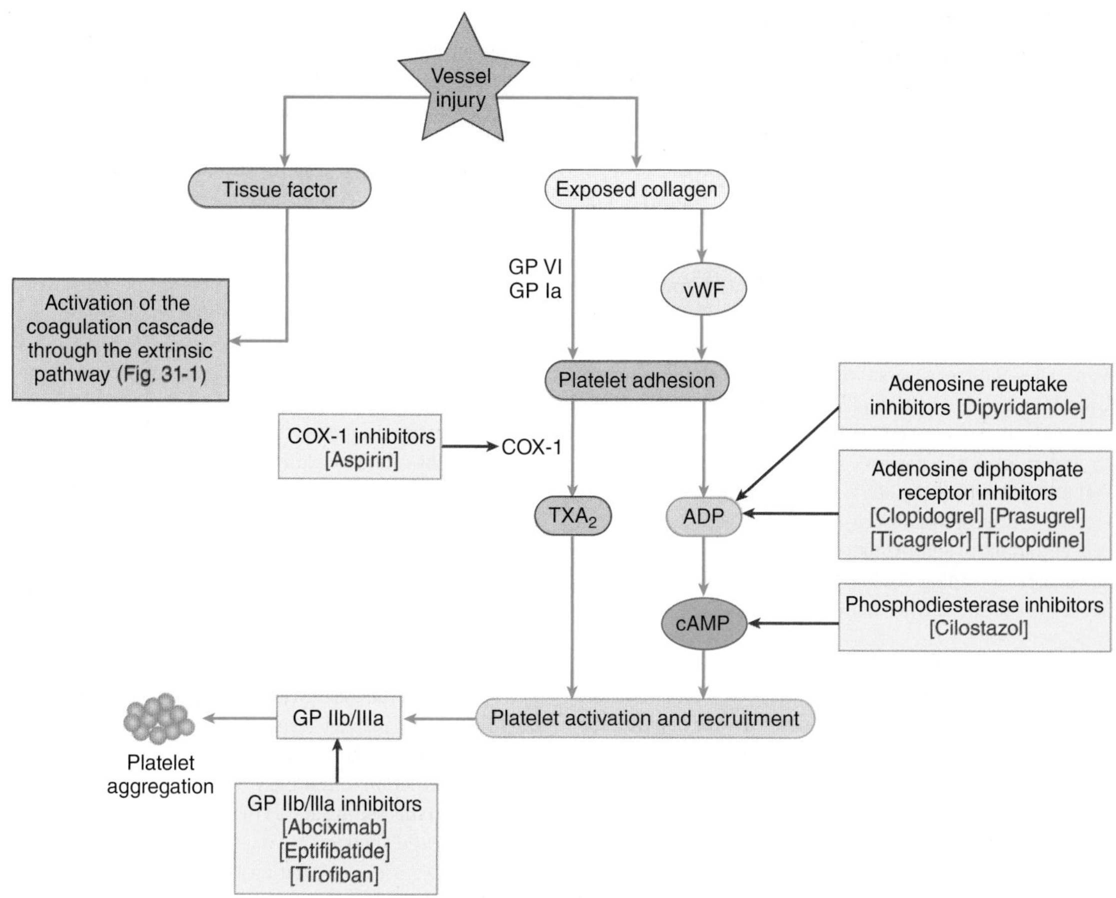


**FIGURE 31–5.** The antiplatelet drugs act in various stages of platelet aggregation. ADP = adenosine diphosphate; cAMP = cyclic adenosine monophosphate; COX-1 = cyclooxygenase 1; GP = glycoprotein; $TXA_2$ = thromboxane $A_2$; vWF = von Willebrand factor.

## CYCLOOXYGENASE INHIBITORS

Aspirin acetylates the COX-1 enzyme, prevents substrate binding to the enzyme, and results in irreversible inhibition of $TXA_2$ generation. Aspirin dosed between 75 and 150 mg offers the best odds reduction in secondary prevention of MI and stroke compared with other doses. Although effective in preventing vascular events, the risks of bleeding and GI irritation are consequential.

## CYCLIC ADENOSINE MONOPHOSPHATE MODULATORS

### Phosphodiesterase Inhibitors

Cilostazol is a phosphodiesterase inhibitor marketed for the treatment of intermittent claudication secondary to peripheral vascular disease (PVD). By increasing cyclic adenosine monophosphate (cAMP), vasodilation is achieved by inhibiting smooth muscle contraction. Additionally, cAMP inhibits platelet aggregation.

### Adenosine Reuptake Inhibitors

Dipyridamole has antiplatelet properties, although its mechanism of action is not completely known. Evidence suggests that by inhibiting degradation of cAMP and by blocking adenosine reuptake, intracellular cAMP accumulates and inhibits platelet aggregation. Compared with clopidogrel, dipyridamole and aspirin offer no improvement in stroke prevention and an increase in the risk of major bleeding.

## ADENOSINE DIPHOSPHATE RECEPTOR INHIBITORS

Platelets require stimulation of P2Y1 and P2Y12, ADP receptors, to inhibit adenylate cyclase. Cyclic AMP formation decreases as a result of the inhibition of adenylate cyclase, and the platelet loses its ability to activate. Clopidogrel, prasugrel, ticagrelor, cangrelor, and ticlopidine are ADP receptor inhibitors. By increasing cAMP concentrations through inhibition of the P2Y12 receptor, these xenobiotics are able to inhibit platelet activation.

Ticlopidine is typically taken orally at 250 mg twice daily. Despite its rapid absorption with peak plasma concentrations between 1 and 3 hours, peak platelet inhibition occurs 1 week after initiation. The relatively high risk of neutropenia; the risks of agranulocytosis, thrombocytopenia, and thrombotic thrombocytopenic purpura–hemolytic uremic syndrome; and the development of newer generation ADP receptor inhibitors have rendered the use of ticlopidine obsolete.

Clopidogrel irreversibly binds and inhibits ADP receptors. Maximal platelet inhibition is achieved between day 4 and 7 after initiation of maintenance doses but occurs 2 to 4 hours after a 600-mg loading dose. Clopidogrel requires conversion via CYP2C19 to form its active metabolite, but the lack of CYP2C19 efficacy leaves up to one-third of patients resistant to clopidogrel. Clopidogrel is dosed at 75 mg/day. The risk of bleeding remains a major concern associated with the use of clopidogrel, particularly in dual antiplatelet regimens. Prasugrel also requires conversion to an active metabolite, which occurs within 30 minutes of dosing. CYP2C19 inhibition or concomitant proton pump inhibitor administration does not alter efficacy. Cangrelor is another ADP receptor inhibitor with rapid onset of action. It has a short half-life, between 2.6 and 3.3 minutes. Rates of adverse events such as severe bleeding are favorable compared with clopidogrel when used during percutaneous coronary intervention.

Ticagrelor is the newest of the ADP receptor inhibitors that exerts its effects by allosterically and reversibly inhibiting the ADP receptor. Absorption is rapid with peak plasma concentrations in approximately 2.5 hours. Dosing of ticagrelor includes a loading dose of 180 mg followed by a maintenance dose of 90 mg twice daily.

## GLYCOPROTEIN IIb/IIIa INHIBITORS

Abciximab is a monoclonal Fab antibody that binds the GP IIb/IIIa receptor. When administered with heparin and aspirin in patients undergoing coronary artery intervention, stent thrombosis, MI, and mortality all decrease. Abciximab is administered as an IV bolus followed by an infusion because its half-life is short. However platelet function is inhibited for up to 24 hours. Eptifibatide is a synthetic GP IIb/IIIa based on snake venom disintegrin. An IV loading dose is followed by an infusion. Tirofiban also inhibits the GP IIb/IIIa receptor and has similar clinical efficacy compared with eptifibatide. Up to 10% of patients treated with GP IIb/IIIa inhibitors have major bleeding events. Thrombocytopenia can also occur as a result of antigenic recognition of the xenobiotic-bound platelets.

### Laboratory Assessment

Bleeding time is traditionally the most useful and widely available test used to assess platelet function. However, its popularity has decreased because of its insensitivity, invasiveness, scarring, and high degree of variability. A variety of platelet function assays exist, but few are widely available.

### Management

When managing bleeding in patients taking antiplatelet xenobiotics, blood transfusion should be used in patients with significant blood loss. However, transfusion of PRBCs will not increase platelet adhesion or aggregation. Unfortunately, the published literature that assesses interventions on bleeding patients maintained on antiplatelet xenobiotics is conflicting, and there is no clear consensus on appropriate reversal strategies and agents. The most widely evaluated intervention is platelet transfusion. Many studies show that platelet transfusion is potentially harmful and independently predicts increased mortality and bleeding (Table 31–1). Although transfusing platelets is associated with worse outcomes, it is important to notice that these studies only demonstrate association and not causation. Therefore, blood transfusion to replace lost volume and coagulation factors is reasonable. It is also reasonable to administer platelets to patients in extremis, such as those requiring massive transfusion caused by extensive blood loss.

Desmopressin is approved for the treatment of inherited defects of hemostasis and potentiates thrombosis by releasing vWF and factor VIII from the endothelium into the plasma. In these patients, complications such as arterial thrombosis and MI are reported after desmopressin administration. A single study evaluated the administration of desmopressin on platelet aggregation and platelet activity in healthy volunteers given a single dose of clopidogrel. They found that platelet reactivity and platelet aggregation increased after desmopressin administration. There is not enough information to routinely recommend the use of desmopressin in this setting at this time.

In the case of abciximab, cessation of the infusion results in a rapid decrease in circulating antibodies. If severe bleeding occurs, platelet transfusion after discontinuation of the infusion is effective in restoring platelet activation and aggregation. Although not formally studied, case reports of patients with protracted platelet inhibition in the setting of eptifibatide use and end-stage CKD suggest that hemodialysis restores platelet aggregation capacity. However, there are insufficient data at this time to routinely recommend this intervention, especially because initiating hemodialysis typically takes several hours, during which time platelet function typically improves. Unlike abciximab platelet toxicity, transfusion of platelets to patients receiving eptifibatide is believed to be ineffective in restoring platelet function.

## SNAKE VENOMS

A detailed discussion of snake envenomations is found in **Chap. 92** and **Special Considerations: SC9**.

Antidotes in Brief

# A17 PROTHROMBIN COMPLEX CONCENTRATES AND DIRECT ORAL ANTICOAGULANT ANTIDOTES

## INTRODUCTION

Prothrombin complex concentrate (PCC) is a lyophilized powder that primarily contains coagulation factors II, VII, IX, and X that is used to correct coagulopathy from vitamin K antagonists while avoiding the volume complications of plasma. Although some direct oral anticoagulants (DOACs) now have a reversal agent, PCCs are still used to attempt rapid reversal of DOAC-induced coagulopathy because of cost and availability issues. The manufacturer of dabigatran developed idarucizumab, a monoclonal antibody to treat bleeding complications associated with that drug. Similarly, andexanet alfa was recently approved to treat bleeding associated with Xa inhibitors.

## PROTHROMBIN COMPLEX CONCENTRATES

### History

Prothrombin complex concentrates were initially used for the treatment of patients with hemophilia A. That iteration of PCC is referred to as 3F-PCC because it contains a lower concentration of factor VII compared with 4F-PCC in an attempt to limit thrombogenic complications. The use of 4F-PCC became routine when consensus guidelines recommended their use to reverse warfarin-associated coagulopathy.

### Pharmacology

Different prothrombin complex concentrates contain variable amounts of factors II, VII, IX, and X. They also include proteins C and S (Table A17–1).

### Mechanism of Action

Vitamin K antagonists impair the synthesis of γ-carboxylated factors II, VII, IX, and X in the coagulation cascade. Prothrombin complex concentrates correct warfarin-associated coagulopathy by direct replacement of factors whose synthesis was inhibited.

### Pharmacokinetics and Pharmacodynamics

In a study of 15 healthy volunteers receiving 4F-PCC, maximal concentration of factors and proteins C and S occurred at the earliest sampling point, at 5 minutes postinfusion, and remained stable for the first hour. Terminal half-lives are shown in Table A17–2. In one prospective study treating patients with warfarin-induced coagulopathy, normalization of INR was achieved within 30 minutes after completion of 4F-PCC infusion and remained stable for 48 hours. In another randomized controlled trial, the INR was normalized in 62% of participants 30 minutes after 4F-PCC infusion.

### Adverse Effects and Safety Issues

Because some forms of PCC contain small amounts of heparin, they are contraindicated in patients with a history of heparin-induced thrombocytopenia (HIT) and heparin-induced thrombocytopenia and thrombosis syndrome (HITT). Since PCCs are made from human blood, they can theoretically transmit infectious diseases, although the risk is exceedingly low because of safeguards in the manufacturing process. Fatal and nonfatal thrombotic events are reported with 4F-PCC use including myocardial infarction (MI), arterial thrombosis, venous thrombosis, pulmonary embolism (PE), cerebrovascular accident, and disseminated intravascular coagulation. Data from one publication cited a less than 1% rate of thrombosis. Hypersensitivity to 4F-PCC is reported to have an incidence of 3%. Other side effects include headache, gastrointestinal disturbances, arthralgias, and hypotension.

### Pregnancy and Lactation

There are no studies or data available to elucidate the risks of PCC use in pregnancy or breastfeeding. If a pregnant woman is anticoagulated with warfarin and requires emergent reversal, fresh-frozen plasma (FFP) should be used. If the volume associated with FFP is a concern because of the risk of volume overload, providers can use PCCs but with the caveat that the effects on the pregnancy and fetus are unknown.

### Dosing and Administration

Most countries use 4F-PCC for the reversal of vitamin K antagonist (VKA)-induced anticoagulation along with vitamin K. The only brand of 4F-PCC currently approved for VKA reversal in the United States (US) is Kcentra. Dosing of Kcentra is based on the international normalized ratio (INR) and actual body weight, with a maximum weight of 100 kg (Table A17–3). All US studies evaluating the safety and efficacy of 4F-PCC have enrolled adults. However, PCCs have been increasingly used in children.

**TABLE A17–1 Content of Prothrombin Complex Concentrates Available in the United States***

| | *Factors II, IX, X Present* | *Factor VII Present* | *Proteins S and C Present* | *Heparin Present* |
|---|---|---|---|---|
| Four-factor prothrombin complex concentrate (Kcentra) | Yes (not activated) | Yes (not activated) | Yes | Yes |
| Three-factor prothrombin complex concentrate (Profilnine) | Yes (not activated) | Little to none (not activated) | Yes | No |
| Factor VIII Inhibitor Bypassing Activity (FEIBA) | Yes (not activated) | Yes (mostly activated) | Yes | No |

* = Outside of the United States other 4-factor PCCs such as Octaplex and Cofact Proplex are marketed.

**TABLE A17–2 Coagulation Factor and Protein Pharmacokinetics After Four-Factor Prothrombin Complex Concentrate in Healthy Volunteers**

| | *Factor II* | *Factor VII* | *Factor IX* | *Factor X* | *Protein C* | *Protein S* |
|---|---|---|---|---|---|---|
| Terminal half-life (h) | 59.7 (45.5–65.9) | 4.2 (3.9–6.6) | 16.7 (14.2–67.7) | 30.7 (23.7–41.1) | 47.2 (28.4–65.1) | 49.1 (39–59.7) |
| Volume of distribution (mL/kg) | 71 (61.2–78.9) | 41.8 (39.3–52.5) | 92.4 (76.2–182.2) | 56.1 (52.9–60.1) | 62.9 (50.1–65) | 76.6 (69.8–85.8) |

### Four-Factor Versus Three-Factor Prothrombin Complex Concentrates

Numerous studies have evaluated the efficacy and safety of 4F-PCC versus 3F-PCC. Several retrospective studies indicate faster reversal, higher rates of reversal, and lower mortality rates in patients receiving 4F-PCC compared with 3F-PCC. However, in several retrospective studies, the efficacy was about equal regardless of which formulation of PCC was used, and although the rates of thromboembolic complications were similar, thrombotic complications were higher if 4F-PCC was given.

### Four-Factor Prothrombin Complex Concentrates Versus FFP

Although several studies conclude that PCC leads to more rapid correction of INR compared with FFP, they are biased toward PCC by giving unequal doses of factor replacement. Typically, the patients in the PCC groups received a dose of 25 to 50 IU/kg (replacement 50%–100%), but patients in the FFP group received 10 to 15 mL/kg (replacement 20%–30%). Theoretical advantages of PCCs over FFP include a smaller volume of infusion, bypassing blood type matching, avoidance of delay for thawing of plasma, and predictable dosing of factors. Despite its significantly increased cost, PCC possesses a lower risk of infection transmission compared with FFP.

### Other Uses for Prothrombin Complex Concentrates

***Prothrombin Complex Concentrates for Direct Oral Anticoagulants.*** Prothrombin complex concentrates can be used to treat coagulopathy from the DOACs. Some evidence suggests limited efficacy in dabigatran-induced coagulopathy. Similarly, PCC was used to partially reverse the anticoagulant activity of rivaroxaban in healthy volunteers. For patients requiring emergent reversal of dabigatran-induced anticoagulation, PCC is a reasonable second-line agent for achieving reversal of anticoagulation if idarucizumab is unavailable. For patients requiring emergent reversal of factor Xa inhibitor–induced anticoagulation, PCC is also a reasonable second-line therapy if andexanet alfa is unavailable.

***Prothrombin Complex Concentrates in Liver Disease.*** There are studies evaluating the use of PCC to reverse coagulopathy associated with liver disease. Unfortunately, the rate of INR reversal in patients with liver disease treated with 4F-PCC seems to be significantly less than rates for elevated INRs for other reasons such as warfarin-associated coagulopathy. One study compared the use of FFP versus PCC versus rFVIIa to facilitate procedures in critically ill patients with liver disease. Patients receiving PCC and rFVIIa experienced expedited procedures and required fewer blood products compared with those receiving FFP. At this time, there is currently insufficient information to routinely recommend PCC administration to patients with liver disease for the sole purpose of INR correction. For patients with the collective criteria of liver disease, elevated INR, and life-threatening hemorrhage, it would be reasonable to give PCC.

***Prothrombin Complex Concentrates in Trauma.*** There is not enough evidence to recommend routine use of PCC to correct coagulopathy from trauma at this time.

**TABLE A17–3 Kcentra Dosing Recommendations**

| Pretreatment INR | 2–< 4 | 4–6 | > 6 |
|---|---|---|---|
| Dose of Kcentra: units of factor IX/kg body weight | 25 | 35 | 50 |
| Maximum dose (units of factor IX) | Not to exceed 2,500 IU | Not to exceed 3,500 IU | Not to exceed 5,000 IU |

INR = international normalized ratio.

Table from manufacturer's prescribing insert.

### Availability

The only brand of 4F-PCC currently available in the US is Kcentra. Another brand of 4F-PCC, Octaplex, is being evaluated for US Food and Drug Administration (FDA) approval. 3F-PCC is available as Profilnine.

### Activated Prothrombin Complex Concentrates (aPCCs)

Similar to 4F-PCCs, aPCCs contain factors II, VII IX, and X. However, the difference between the two PCCs is that aPCCs contain activated factor VII instead of nonactivated factor VII. The only aPCC product currently available in the US is factor eight inhibitor bypassing activity (FEIBA) used for patients with hemophilia A and B who have developed inhibitors. Because FEIBA does not contain heparin, it is the recommended therapy to reverse warfarin-associated coagulopathy in critically ill patients with HIT or HITT. Unfortunately, this indication is not extensively studied. In one study comparing the aPCC FEIBA versus FFP for reversing warfarin-associated coagulopathy, aPCC was superior to FFP in time to reversal of anticoagulation. However, it should be noted that patients in the aPCC group received more overall factor replacement than the patients in the FFP group.

There is no standard dose of aPCC for coagulopathy reversal. Providers should weigh the risks and benefits of aPCC use in anticoagulated patients. Typical doses for treating bleeding or for perioperative management range between 50 and 100 units/kg with the units measuring the amount of factor VIII inhibitor bypass activity. One study evaluated fixed doses of aPCC in adult patients because lower doses resulted in cessation of bleeding in 93% of patients. In this study, patients with an INR of less than 5 received 500 units of aPCC. Patients with INR of greater than 5 received 1,000 units of aPCC; 87% of patients survived to discharge, and no thrombotic complications were noted. Given the thrombogenic potential of FEIBA, this lower dose recommendation is reasonable if FFP is unavailable in warfarin-anticoagulated patients. In patients requiring reversal of direct factor Xa–induced anticoagulation, there are very little data on ideal dosing. If andexanet alpha or another antidote is unavailable, it is reasonable to administer aPCC to patients with a contraindication to nonactivated PCC in aliquots of 25 units/kg up to a maximum of 100 units/kg. This therapy should be reserved for critically ill patients who need emergent reversal of their anticoagulation.

### Recombinant Factor VIIa

Recombinant factor VIIa is approved for patients with hemophilia or various factor inhibitors and has been successfully used to reverse VKA toxicity. Off-label use of rFVIIa to reverse VKA coagulopathy is not recommended because of a high frequency of thrombotic events. However, if FFP and PCC (activated or nonactivated) cannot be administered or are unavailable, then it is reasonable to administer only rFVIIa in life-threatening situations.

## IDARUCIZUMAB

### History

Idarucizumab received accelerated approval by the FDA in 2015 because there were no other definitive antidotes or means of reversal for dabigatran.

### Pharmacology and Chemistry

Idarucizumab is a humanized monoclonal antibody fragment to dabigatran.

### Mechanism of Action

Idarucizumab binds directly to dabigatran at an affinity of approximately 350 times higher than the affinity of dabigatran to thrombin. When dabigatran is bound to idarucizumab, its anticoagulant effect is deactivated.

### Pharmacokinetics and Pharmacodynamics

The binding of idarucizumab to dabigatran is irreversible given its high affinity for dabigatran. Peak plasma concentrations occur immediately after infusion. The volume of distribution of idarucizumab is approximately 0.06 L/kg. Because idarucizumab is primarily located in plasma, it is able to bind plasma dabigatran. Extravascular dabigatran likely moves back into the vascular space to reequilibrate. If there is excess or unbound intravascular idarucizumab available, it will be able to bind any newly arriving dabigatran to further neutralize dabigatran and its anticoagulant effects. After peak concentrations are reached, the initial half-life of idarucizumab is approximately 45 minutes. Four hours after administration, only 4% of the peak idarucizumab concentration is detectable in plasma. At that point, the half-life ranges between 4.5 and 8.1 hours.

In human studies, idarucizumab administration results in normalization of a battery of functional clotting assays, such as clotting time, aPTT, and thrombin time. In a prospective study of patients taking dabigatran who required rapid reversal of anticoagulation for either life-threatening hemorrhage or for emergent surgery or procedures, patients who received 5 g of intravenous (IV) idarucizumab had a reversal rate of 100%, but no clear clinical advantage. In patients undergoing an emergent procedure, normal intraoperative hemostasis was noted in 85% of cases. Some of these cases may have had partial responses to other blood products administered. Despite the apparent rapid reversal of anticoagulation by idarucizumab in most cases, some patients experience a recurrent coagulopathy between 12 and 24 hours after receiving idarucizumab, perhaps caused by dabigatran redistribution as noted above.

### Adverse Effects and Safety Issues

In premarketing studies, idarucizumab was tested in over 200 volunteers and well tolerated in doses up to 8 g. No hypersensitivity reactions or severe antibody reactions were reported in any of the volunteers. Thrombotic events such as DVT, PE, MI, or ischemic stroke are reported after idarucizumab use in 6% to 7% of treated patients. Patients with hereditary fructose intolerance are at risk for serious adverse effects because the medication contains sorbitol, which is converted to fructose upon digestion.

### Other Uses of Idarucizumab

Several reports describe the use of idarucizumab to reverse the anticoagulant effect of dabigatran before thrombolytic therapy in patients with acute ischemic strokes. Because quality clinical studies that assess the safety and efficacy of this practice are lacking, we cannot currently recommend this practice.

### Pregnancy and Lactation

There are no studies or data available to elucidate the risks of idarucizumab use in pregnancy or while breastfeeding. There are also no available data regarding excretion of idarucizumab in breast milk.

### Dosing and Administration

Idarucizumab is dosed at 5 g either as two consecutive infusions of 2.5 g or by syringe bolus. There is no evidence that one approach is better than the other. In a small subset of patients, coagulopathy recurs between 12 and 24 hours after receiving idarucizumab. If these patients have clinically significant bleeding or need for a procedure, it is reasonable to administer a second dose of idarucizumab at 5 g.

### Availability

Idarucizumab is available as a parenteral solution with each vial containing 2.5 g of idarucizumab in 50 mL of fluid for injection.

## ANDEXANET ALFA

### History

Given the increasing use of oral factor Xa inhibitors, there was motivation to find a safe and efficacious reversal agent. Andexanet alfa is a recombinant protein that reverses anticoagulation caused by factor Xa inhibitors.

### Pharmacology and Mechanism of Action

Andexanet alfa binds factor Xa inhibitors and inhibits the catalytic activation of thrombin. It also blocks the factor Va binding site on factor X, which is necessary for anticoagulation.

### Pharmacokinetics and Pharmacodynamics

A study in healthy elderly volunteers demonstrated that andexanet alfa administration given to participants with a steady-state concentration of either apixaban or rivaroxaban resulted in rapid reduction in plasma free inhibitor concentrations and increased thrombin formation. Immediately after andexanet alfa infusion, antifactor Xa activity decreased by more than 90%. However, within 1 to 2 hours, concentrations were comparable to those of the placebo group.

### Adverse Effects and Safety Issues

In healthy volunteers, there were no serious or thrombotic complications in any of the participants. However, thrombotic complications occurred in 18% of clinically anticoagulated patients reversed with andexanet alfa during the 30-day follow-up period. One-third of these events occurred in the first 72 hours after infusion. Only 27% of patients were restarted on their anticoagulation during the 30-day follow-up period and 15% of patients died. There are no reports of anaphylaxis in human or animal studies.

### Pregnancy and Lactation

There are no data available to elucidate the risks of andexanet alfa use in pregnancy or while breastfeeding.

### Dosing and Administration

Andexanet alfa is administered intravenously in a low-dose or high-dose protocol based on the timing and amount of the last dose of rivaroxaban and apixaban. All patients are administered a loading dose over 15 to 30 minutes. A 2-hour infusion dose is then given immediately after the loading dose. For patients who received a factor Xa inhibitor more than 7 hours before andexanet alfa administration, the loading dose is 400 mg, and the infusion dose is 480 mg. For patients who received a factor Xa inhibitor within 7 hours of andexanet alfa administration, the loading dose is 800 mg, and the infusion dose is 960 mg.

### Availability

Andexanet alfa received US FDA approval in 2018 for the reversal of rivaroxaban and apixiban-associated hemorrhage. It is available as a lyophylized powder in single-use vials of 100 mg of recombinant coagulation factor X.

# A18 VITAMIN $K_1$

Vitamin $K_1$ (phytonadione) is indicated for the reversal of elevated prothrombin times and international normalized ratios (INRs) in patients with xenobiotic-induced vitamin K deficiency. Acquired vitamin K deficiency most commonly results from therapeutic administration of warfarin or following the ingestion of the long-acting anticoagulant rodenticides (LAARs) such as brodifacoum.

## HISTORY

It was noted in 1929 that chickens fed a poor diet developed spontaneous bleeding. In 1935, Dam and coworkers discovered that incorporating a fat-soluble substance, defined as a "koagulation factor," into the diet could correct the bleeding, leading to the name vitamin K.

## PHARMACOLOGY

### Chemistry

Vitamin K, an essential fat-soluble vitamin, is actually a broad term that encompasses at least two distinct natural forms. Vitamin $K_1$ (phytonadione, phylloquinone) is the only form synthesized by plants and algae. Most of the vitamin K ingested in the diet is vitamin $K_1$. Vitamin $K_2$ (menaquinones) is actually a series of compounds synthesized by bacteria.

### Related Vitamin K Compounds

Vitamin $K_1$ (phytonadione) is the only vitamin K preparation that should be used to reverse anticoagulant-induced vitamin K deficiency or to treat infants or pregnant women. Vitamins $K_3$ (menadione) and $K_4$ (menadiol sodium diphosphate) are no longer approved by the United States (US) Food and Drug Administration (FDA) because they produce hemolysis, hyperbilirubinemia, and kernicterus in neonates, as well as hemolysis in G6PD-deficient patients.

### Mechanism of Action

A postsynthetic modification of coagulation factors II, VII, IX, and X and proteins S, C, and Z requires γ-carboxylation of the glutamate residues in a vitamin K–dependent process. Only the reduced ($K_1H_2$, hydroquinone) form of vitamin K is biologically active. During the carboxylation step, the active reduced vitamin $K_1$ is converted to an epoxide. This 2,3-epoxide is reduced and recycled to the active $K_1H_2$ in a process that is inhibited by warfarin (Fig. 31–2). Vitamin $K_1$ is activated to vitamin $K_1H_2$ enzymes that use both NADH and NADPH in a pathway that is relatively insensitive to warfarin. Exogenous phytonadione allows γ-carboxylation of clotting factors that are present and does not rely on recycling.

### Daily Requirement

The human daily requirement for vitamin K is small; the US Food and Nutrition Board set the recommended daily allowance at 1 μg/kg/day of phylloquinone for adults.

## PHARMACOKINETICS OF DIETARY VITAMIN K

Dietary vitamin K in the form of phylloquinone and menaquinones is solubilized with the bile salts, free fatty acids, and monoglycerides to enhance absorption. Vitamin K, bound to chylomicrons, enters the circulation via the lymphatic system and then is taken up by the liver. In the plasma, vitamin K is primarily in the phylloquinone form, whereas liver stores are menaquinones and 10% phylloquinone.

### Pharmacokinetics of Oral and Parenterally Administered Vitamin $K_1$

The pharmacokinetics of oral and intramuscular (IM) vitamin $K_1$ were compared in healthy volunteers. Baseline serum vitamin $K_1$ concentrations were 0.23 ng/mL. After the oral administration of 5 mg of vitamin $K_1$, peak serum concentrations of 90 ng/mL were achieved between 4 and 6 hours. These concentrations dropped to a steady state of 3.8 ng/mL and exhibited a half-life of about 4 hours. Intramuscular administration of 5 mg of vitamin $K_1$ resulted in peak serum concentrations of only 50 ng/mL, with delays from 2 to 30 hours after administration and with the maintenance of a plateau for about 30 hours. Consequently, IM administration is not recommended.

### Pharmacodynamics of Administered Vitamin $K_1$

The time necessary for the INR to return to a safe or normal range is variable and dependent on the rate of absorption of vitamin $K_1$, the serum concentration achieved, and the time necessary for the synthesis of activated clotting factors. A decrease in the INR often occurs within several hours, although it often takes 8 to 24 hours to reach target values. While the onset of action for the IV route is faster, this is not clinically meaningful as all routes of administration act too slowly to control serious bleeding. However, in a retrospective analysis of 64 patients requiring vitamin K for nonurgent reversal of anticoagulation before a procedure, the IV route corrected more patients to an INR less than 4 at 4 hours than the oral route (66.6% vs 25.0%).

### Vitamin K Deficiency and Monitoring

Vitamin K deficiency can result from inadequate intake, malabsorption, or interference with the vitamin K cycle. Determination of vitamin K deficiency is usually established on the basis of a prolonged prothrombin time (PT), which is a surrogate marker of specific coagulation factors. Measurement of the vitamin K–dependent factors, II, VII, IX, and X, is an effective way to determine the adequacy of vitamin $K_1$ dosing.

## ROLE IN XENOBIOTIC-INDUCED VITAMIN K DEFICIENCY

Warfarin and LAARs are strong irreversible inhibitors of the vitamin K 2,3-epoxide reductase, which regenerates vitamin K into its active ($K_1H_2$, hydroquinone) form.

Under ideal nutritional circumstances in a healthy individual, vitamin K is recycled, and only 1 μg/kg/day is required in adults to maintain adequate coagulation. In the presence of warfarin or superwarfarins, additional vitamin $K_1$ must be administered over many days to supply this active cofactor for each and every carboxylation step because it can no longer be recycled.

## ADVERSE EFFECTS AND SAFETY ISSUES

Although vitamin $K_1$ can be administered orally, subcutaneously, intramuscularly, or intravenously, the oral route is preferred for maintenance therapy because this route is virtually free of adverse effects. The preparations available for IV administration are rarely (0.03%) associated with nonimmune hypersensitivity reactions when dilute administrations are given over 1 hour.

## PREGNANCY AND LACTATION

Vitamin $K_1$ is listed as US FDA pregnancy Category C. Vitamin $K_1$ is the treatment of choice for vitamin K deficiency during pregnancy and for prevention of hemorrhagic disease in newborns and is compatible with breastfeeding.

## DOSING AND ADMINISTRATION

The management of patients with elevated INRs secondary to excessive warfarin is described in Table 31–2. Reported cases of LAAR poisoning have required as much as 50 to 250 mg of vitamin $K_1$ daily for weeks to months. A recommended starting approach for a patient who has overdosed on LAAR is 25 to 50 mg of vitamin $K_1$ orally three to four times a day for 1 to 2 days. For unusually large oral vitamin K doses, the IV formulation can be given orally. The INR should be monitored, and the vitamin $K_1$ dose adjusted accordingly. When the INR is less than 2, a downward titration in the dose of vitamin $K_1$ should be made on the basis of factor VII analysis.

Intravenous administration of vitamin $K_1$ should be reserved for serious or life-threatening hemorrhage at any elevation of INR. Under these circumstances, supplementation with prothrombin complex concentrate (PCC) and fresh-frozen plasma (FFP) is recommended. A starting dose of 10 mg of vitamin $K_1$ is recommended. To minimize the risk of nonimmune hypersensitivity reactions, the preparation should be diluted with preservative-free 5% dextrose, 0.9% sodium chloride, or 5% dextrose in 0.9% sodium chloride and administered slowly, using an infusion pump, over a minimum of 1 hour. Subcutaneous administration is not generally recommended because of less predictable absorption.

## FORMULATION AND ACQUISITION

Vitamin $K_1$ is available for IV and as phytonadione injection emulsion in 2 mg/mL and 10 mg/mL ampules. Oral vitamin $K_1$ is available in 5-mg tablets.

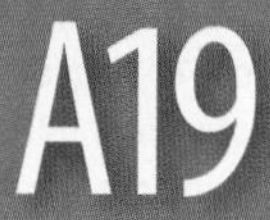

# A19 PROTAMINE

Protamine is a rapidly acting antidote used for reversing the anticoagulant effects of unfractionated heparin (UFH) and for some of the effects of low-molecular-weight heparins (LMWH).

## HISTORY

In 1868, Friedric Miescher discovered and named the basic protein that resides in the sperm of salmon as protamine. The antidotal properties of protamine were recognized in the late 1930s, leading to its approval as an antidote for heparin overdose in 1968. However, the largest body of literature pertaining to protamine originates from its use in neutralizing heparin after cardiopulmonary bypass and dialysis procedures.

## PHARMACOLOGY

### Chemistry

Heparin is a large electronegative substance that is rapidly complexed by the electropositive protamine, forming an inactive salt. Commercially available protamine sulfate is derived from the sperm of mature testes of salmon and related species.

### Related Protamine Variants

In animal studies, synthetic protamine variants, not yet available for clinical use, were effective in reversing the anticoagulant effects of LMWH and are reported to be less toxic than protamine.

### Mechanism of Action

Heparin is an indirect anticoagulant, requiring a cofactor antithrombin III (AT). Since the binding of heparin to protamine is stronger than the binding of heparin to AT, protamine rapidly inactivates heparin and reverses its anticoagulant effects. Low-molecular-weight heparins have a reduced ability to inactivate thrombin because of lesser AT binding, but preferentially inactivate factor Xa compared to UFH, allowing equal efficacy. However, the ability of protamine to bind to LMWH is limited by the smaller chain length and molecular weight and the lesser sulfate charge density.

## PHARMACOKINETICS AND PHARMACODYNAMICS

Protamine has a very rapid onset of action and can neutralize the effects of heparin within 5 minutes. Its half-life is short, typically less than 10 minutes.

## ROLE IN REVERSING HEPARIN

Protamine is indicated to reverse anticoagulant effects of heparin. Multiple controlled human trials substantiate the effectiveness of protamine in terminating the effects of heparin. Protamine should be used in patients with consequential bleeding from excessive heparin.

## ROLE IN REVERSING LOW-MOLECULAR-WEIGHT HEPARIN

In contrast to heparin, there is no proven method for completely neutralizing LMWH. Protamine neutralizes the anti-IIa activity and a variable portion of the anti-Xa activity of LMWH. No human studies offer strong evidence for or against a beneficial effect of protamine as treatment for hemorrhage after LMWH use. Protamine is reasonable therapy for LMWH excess associated with hemorrhage, but complete reversal should not be expected, and caution should limit the protamine dose.

## ADVERSE EFFECTS, RISK FACTORS, AND SAFETY ISSUES

Although millions of patients have been exposed to protamine during cardiopulmonary bypass surgery, only approximately 100 deaths are associated with the use of protamine. Adverse effects associated with protamine include both rate-related and non–rate-related hypotension, anaphylactic and anaphylactoid reactions, bradycardia, thrombocytopenia, leukopenia, decreased oxygen consumption, acute respiratory distress syndrome, pulmonary hypertension, and anticoagulant effects.

The strong net-positive charge of protamine is likely responsible for some of the adverse effects. Additionally, the protamine-heparin complex activates the arachidonic acid pathway, and the production of thromboxane is at least partly responsible for some of the hemodynamic changes, including pulmonary hypertension. Multiple other mechanisms have been proposed.

Risk factors for protamine-induced adverse reactions include prior exposure to protamine in insulin, exposure during previous surgery with protamine reversal, vasectomy, fish allergy, or a rapid protamine infusion rate. A prospective study reported a 0.06% incidence of anaphylactic reactions to protamine in all patients undergoing coronary artery bypass, but a 2% incidence in patients with diabetes using NPH (neutral protamine Hagedorn) insulin.

## RISK FOR ADVERSE DRUG REACTIONS

There are limited options to replace protamine for the reversal of heparin in patients who have previously experienced anaphylaxis after protamine therapy or in patients who are suspected of being at high risk. Pretreatment with antihistamines and corticosteroids is often sufficient for immune-mediated mechanisms but will probably not be beneficial for pulmonary vasoconstriction and non–immune-mediated hypersensitiity reactions.

## PREGNANCY AND LACTATION

Protamine is United States Food and Drug Administration Pregnancy Category C. Protamine is reasonable to reverse or partially reverse the bleeding in a pregnant woman considered secondary to UFH or LMWH, respectively. Protamine excretion in breast milk is unknown.

## DOSING AND ADMINISTRATION

### Dosing in Cardiopulmonary Bypass

Protamine is most frequently used at the end of cardiopulmonary bypass operations to reverse the effects of heparin, and many regimens are used. We recommend using a ratio of 0.3 to 1 mg of protamine to 100 units of heparin and subsequently titrating based on normalization of the activating clotting time (ACT) point-of-care testing.

### Heparin Rebound

A heparin anticoagulant rebound effect is noted after cardiopulmonary bypass and is attributed to the presence of detectable circulating heparin several hours after apparently adequate heparin neutralization with protamine. The incidence of heparin rebound and the need for additional protamine range from 4% to 42%, depending on the neutralization protocol.

### Dosing for Heparin and Low-Molecular-Weight Heparins

One milligram of protamine will neutralize approximately 100 units (1 mg) of UFH. Because excessive protamine can act as an anticoagulant, the dose chosen should always be an underestimation of that which is needed. In the case of unintentional overdose, the half-life of heparin should be considered, because half of the administered dose of heparin is eliminated within 60 to 90 minutes if kidney function is normal. This means that if bleeding occurs 2 hours after a single dose, only half of that initial dose will require reversal with protamine. In the case of an overdose without bleeding, the short half-life of heparin and the potential risks of protamine administration usually argue for a conservative approach of patient observation, rather than protamine reversal of anticoagulation. If protamine use is necessary to treat active bleeding, a dose of no greater than 50 mg must be administered intravenously over 15 minutes to limit rate-related hypotension, which results from nitric oxide-mediated vascular dilation.

Most studies demonstrate incomplete protamine neutralization of the LMWHs enoxaparin, dalteparin, and tinzaparin. We recommend administering 1 mg of protamine per 100 anti–factor Xa units, in which 1 mg of enoxaparin equals 100 anti–factor Xa units if administered within 8 hours of the LMWH. A second dose of 0.5 of mg protamine should be administered per 100 anti–factor Xa units if bleeding continues. If more than 8 hours has elapsed, then a smaller fractional dose of protamine should be administered based on the actual time from the initiation of therapy.

The dosing of protamine in children for the reversal of heparin is similar to that of adults if the dose of heparin was given within 30 minutes and is 1 mg of protamine/100 units heparin received. However if the dose of heparin has been 30 to 60 minutes earlier, then the dose of protamine should be 0.5 to 0.75 mg/100 units of heparin received. For 60 to 120 minutes after the heparin dose, the protamine dose is 0.375 to 0.5 mg/100 units heparin received, and for longer than 120 minutes, the protamine dose is 0.25 mg to 0.375 mg/100 units of heparin received. The maximum dose in each of these circumstances is 50 mg.

## DOSING IN THE UNKNOWN OVERDOSE SETTING

When faced with a patient believed to have received an overdose of an unknown quantity of heparin, the decision to use protamine should be determined by the presence of a prolonged activated partial thromboplastin time (aPTT) and whether persistent bleeding is present. In each circumstance, the potential risks of protamine use (especially in those who have had a prior life-threatening reaction to protamine, as well as in a patients with diabetes receiving NPH insulin) and the risks of continued heparin anticoagulation should be evaluated. Because of the routine nature of heparin reversal following cardiopulmonary bypass, consultation with members of the bypass team may be helpful.

An empiric dose of protamine is determined by the baseline ACT: (1) an ACT of less than 200 seconds necessitates no protamine, (2) an ACT of 200 to 300 seconds necessitates 0.6 mg/kg, and (3) an ACT of 300 to 400 seconds necessitates 1.2 mg/kg. These doses should be given up to a single maximum dose of 50 mg. The dose can be repeated if dictated by persistent bleeding and an elevated aPTT, thrombin time, and ACT. The ACT should be repeated 5 to 15 minutes after protamine administration and in 2 to 8 hours to evaluate for potential heparin rebound. Further dosing should be based on these values and the patient's clinical condition. When an ACT is unavailable, protamine 25 mg to a maximum of 50 mg should be administered to an adult and adjusted accordingly.

## AVAILABILITY

Protamine is available either as a parenteral solution ready for injection or as a powder to be reconstituted with 5 mL of sterile or bacteriostatic water for injection. When the vials containing 50 mg of protamine are used, they should be shaken vigorously after the water is added.

# 32 β-ADRENERGIC ANTAGONISTS

## HISTORY

In 1948, Raymond Alquist postulated that the ability of epinephrine's to produce hypertension and tachycardia were best explained by the existence of two distinct sets of receptors that he generically named α and β receptors. British pharmacist Sir James Black was influenced by Alquist's work and recognized the potential clinical benefit of a β-adrenergic antagonist. In 1958, Black synthesized the first β-adrenergic antagonist, pronethalol. Pronethalol was briefly marketed but was discontinued because it produced thymic tumors in mice. Propranolol was soon developed and marketed in the United Kingdom in 1964 and in the United States (US) in 1973. New medications soon followed, and by 1979, there were 10 β-adrenergic antagonists available in the US. There are currently 20 US Food and Drug Administration–approved β-adrenergic antagonists with additional β-adrenergic antagonists available worldwide (Table 32–1). They are commonly used in the treatment of cardiovascular disease, tremor, thyroid disease, migraines, panic attack, and glaucoma.

## EPIDEMIOLOGY

Intentional β-adrenergic antagonist overdose, although relatively uncommon, continues to account for a number of deaths annually. Compared with the other β-adrenergic antagonists, propranolol accounts for a disproportionate number of reported cases of self-poisoning and deaths. This may be explained by the fact that propranolol is frequently prescribed to patients with diagnoses such as anxiety, stress, and migraine who may be more prone to suicide attempts.

## PHARMACOLOGY

### The Cardiac Cycle

Under normal conditions, heart rate is determined by the rate of spontaneous discharge of specialized pacemaker cells that comprise the sinoatrial (SA) node (Fig. 32–1). Depolarization of cells in the SA node spreads to surrounding atrial cells, where it triggers the opening of fast sodium channels. This initiates an electric current that spreads from cell to cell along specialized pathways to depolarize the entire heart. This depolarization, referred to as cardiac excitation, is linked to mechanical activity of the heart by the process of electrical–mechanical coupling.

***Myocyte Calcium Flow and Contractility.*** During systole, voltage-gated slow $Ca^{2+}$ channels (L-type channels) on the myocyte membrane open in response to cell depolarization, allowing $Ca^{2+}$ to flow down its concentration gradient into the myocyte (Fig. 32–2). During diastole, several ion pumps actively remove calcium from the cytoplasm.

***β-Adrenergic Receptors and the Heart.*** β-Adrenergic receptors are divided into $\beta_1$, $\beta_2$, and $\beta_3$ subtypes. In the healthy heart, approximately 80% of human cardiac β-adrenergic receptors are $\beta_1$, and 20% are $\beta_2$. Human hearts also contain a small number of $\beta_3$-adrenergic receptors. The relative density of cardiac $\beta_2$-adrenergic receptors increases with heart failure. $\beta_1$-Adrenergic receptors mediate increased inotropy by a well-described pathway involving cAMP, which acts as a second messenger to activate protein kinases (Fig. 32–3).

Cardiac $\beta_2$-adrenergic receptors are dually linked to both excitatory Gs proteins and inhibitory Gi proteins. Under normal conditions, the Gs pathway predominates in human cardiac $\beta_2$-adrenergic receptors, and $\beta_2$-adrenergic stimulation increases contractility, relaxation, and chronotropy through the protein kinase pathway described earlier. However, in a failing heart, the inhibitory Gi protein pathway becomes dominant, and $\beta_2$-adrenergic stimulation inhibits cardiac function. The $\beta_3$-adrenergic receptors are best understood as metabolic regulators in adipose tissue. The role of cardiac $\beta_3$-adrenergic receptors is poorly understood, but evidence suggests that they prevent the maladaptive myocardial remodeling that occurs with chronic sympathetic overstimulation.

### Noncardiac Effects of β-Adrenergic Receptor Activation

β-Adrenergic receptors mediate smooth muscle relaxation in several organs. Relaxation of arteriolar smooth muscle, predominately by $\beta_2$-adrenergic stimulation, reduces peripheral vascular resistance and decreases blood pressure. This counteracts α-adrenergic–mediated arteriolar constriction. In the lungs, $\beta_2$-adrenergic receptors mediate bronchodilation. Third trimester uterine tone and contractions are inhibited by $\beta_2$-adrenergic agonists, and gut motility is decreased by both $\beta_1$- and $\beta_2$-adrenergic stimulation.

β-Adrenergic receptors play a role in the immune system. Mast cell degranulation is inhibited by $\beta_2$-adrenergic stimulation, explaining the role of epinephrine in aborting and treating anaphylaxis. Also, insulin secretion is increased by $\beta_2$-adrenergic receptor stimulation. Despite increased insulin concentrations, the net effect of $\beta_2$-adrenergic receptor stimulation is to increase glucose because of increased skeletal muscle and hepatic glycogenolysis, and hepatic gluconeogenesis. $\beta_2$-Adrenergic receptors cause glucagon secretion from pancreas and act at fat cells to cause lipolysis and thermogenesis. Skeletal muscle potassium uptake is increased by $\beta_2$-adrenergic stimulation. Finally, renin secretion is increased by $\beta_1$-adrenergic stimulation, resulting in increased blood pressure.

### Action of β-Adrenergic Antagonists

β-Adrenergic antagonists competitively antagonize the effects of catecholamines at β-adrenergic receptors and blunt the chronotropic and inotropic response to catecholamines. Severe bradycardia and hypotension often result in patients who take additional medications that impair cardiac conduction or contractility or in those with underlying cardiac or medical conditions that make them reliant on sympathetic stimulation. In addition to slowing the rate of SA node discharge, β-adrenergic antagonists inhibit ectopic pacemakers and slow conduction through atrial and atrioventricular (AV) nodal tissue.

**TABLE 32–1 Pharmacologic Properties of the β-Adrenergic Antagonists**

| | *Adrenergic Blocking Activity* | *Partial Agonist Activity (ISA)* | *Membrane-Stabilizing Activity* | *Vasodilating Property* | *Log D*[a] | *Protein Binding (%)* | *Oral Bioavailability (%)* | *Half-Life (h)* | *Metabolism* | *Volume of Distribution (L/kg)* |
|---|---|---|---|---|---|---|---|---|---|---|
| Acebutolol | $\beta_1$ | Yes | Yes | No | 0.52 | 25 | 40 | 2–4 | Hepatic or renal | 1.2 |
| Atenolol | $\beta_1$ | No | No | No | −2.03 | < 5 | 40–50 | 5–9 | Renal | 1 |
| Betaxolol (tablets and ophthalmic) | $\beta_1$ | No | Yes | Yes (calcium channel blockade) | 0.56 | 50 | 80–90 | 14–22 | Hepatic or renal | 4.9–8.8 |
| Bisoprolol | $\beta_1$ | No | No | No | 0.11 | 30 | 80 | 9–12 | Hepatic or renal | 3.2 |
| Bucindolol | $\beta_1$, $\beta_2$ | $\beta_2$ | NA | Yes ($\beta_2$ agonism and $\alpha_1$ blockade) | NA | NA | 30 | 8 +/− 4.5 | Hepatic | NA |
| Carteolol (ophthalmic) | $\beta_1$, $\beta_2$ | Yes | No | Yes ($\beta_2$ agonism and nitric oxide mediated) | −0.42 | 30 | 85 | 5–6 | Renal | NA |
| Carvedilol (long-acting form available) | $\alpha_1$, $\beta_1$, $\beta_2$ | No | Yes | Yes ($\alpha_1$ blockade, calcium channel blockade) | 3.16 | ~98 | 25–35 | 6–10 | Hepatic | 2 |
| Celiprolol | $\alpha_2$, $\beta_1$ | $\beta_2$ | NA | Yes ($\beta_2$ agonism, nitric oxide mediated) | NA | 22–24 | 30–70 | 5 | Hepatic | NA |
| Esmolol | $\beta_1$ | No | No | No | −0.22 | 50 | NA | ~8 min | RBC esterases | 2 |
| Labetalol | $\alpha_1$, $\beta_1$, $\beta_2$ | $\beta_2$ | Low | Yes ($\alpha_1$ blockade, $\beta_2$ agonism) | 0.99 | 50 | 20–33 | 4–8 | Hepatic | 9 |
| Levobunolol (ophthalmic) | $\beta_1$, $\beta_2$ | No | No | No | 0.56 | NA | NA | 6 | NA | NA |
| Metipranolol (ophthalmic) | $\beta_1$, $\beta_2$ | No | No | No | 0.53 | NA | NA | 3–4 | NA | NA |
| Metoprolol (long-acting form available) | $\beta_1$ | No | Low | No | −0.34 | 10 | 40–50 | 3–4 | Hepatic | 4 |
| Nadolol | $\beta_1$, $\beta_2$ | No | No | No | −0.84 | 20–30 | 30–35 | 10–24 | Renal | 2 |
| Nebivolol | $\beta_1$ | No | NA | Yes (nitric oxide mediated) | NA | 98 | 12–96 | 8–32 | Hepatic | 10–40 |
| Oxprenolol | $\beta_1$, $\beta_2$ | Yes | Yes | No | NA | 80 | 20%–70% | 1–3 | Hepatic | 1.3 |
| Penbutolol | $\beta_1$, $\beta_2$ | Yes | No | No | 2.05 | 90 | ~100 | 5 | Hepatic or renal | NA |
| Pindolol | $\beta_1$, $\beta_2$ | Yes | Low | No | −0.19 | 50 | 75–90 | 3–4 | Hepatic or renal | 2 |
| Propranolol (long-acting form available) | $\beta_1$, $\beta_2$ | No | Yes | No | 0.99 | 90 | 30–70 | 3–5 | Hepatic | 4 |
| Sotalol | $\beta_1$, $\beta_2$ | No | No | No | −1.82 | 0 | 90 | 9–12 | Renal | 2 |
| Timolol (tablets and ophthalmic) | $\beta_1$, $\beta_2$ | No | No | No | −1.99 | 60 | 75 | 3–5 | Hepatic or renal | 2 |

[a]Log D is the octanol/water partition coefficient at a pH of 7.

ISA = intrinsic sympathomimetic activity; NA = information not available; RBC = red blood cell.

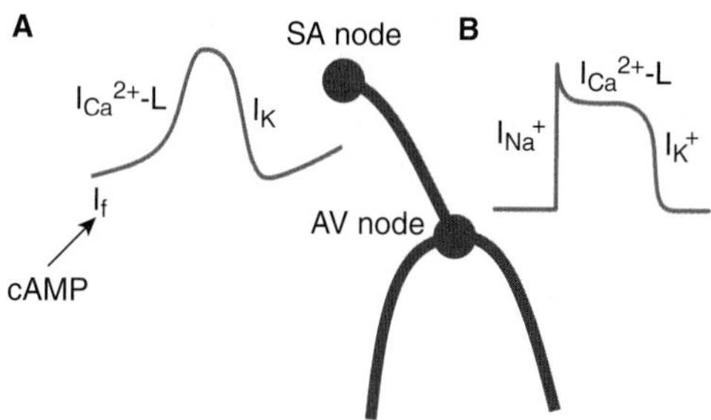


**FIGURE 32–1.** The cardiac conduction system. (**A**) The cardiac cycle begins when pacemaker cells in the sinoatrial (SA) node depolarize spontaneously. Traditionally, this depolarization was attributed to inward "pacemaker" currents ($I_f$). There is now evidence that pacemaker cell depolarization may also be driven by cyclical calcium release from a "calcium clock" in the sarcoplasmic reticulum (SR). β-Adrenergic stimulation increases both the frequency of the "calcium clock" by a protein kinase A (PKA)-mediated effect and the magnitude of the pacemaker current secondary to a direct effect of cyclic adenosine monophosphate (cAMP). These effects both increase the heart rate. Cholinergic stimulation has the opposite effects and results in bradycardia. Pacemaker cells lack fast $Na^+$ channels. Pacemaker cell depolarization triggers the opening of voltage-gated type calcium channels ($I_{Ca^{2+}}$-L), and the impulse is transmitted to surrounding cells. (**B**) Coordinated SA nodal depolarization generates an impulse sufficient to open fast $Na^+$ channels in surrounding atrial tissue, and the impulse spreads along specialized pathways to depolarize the atria and ventricles. AV = atrioventricular.

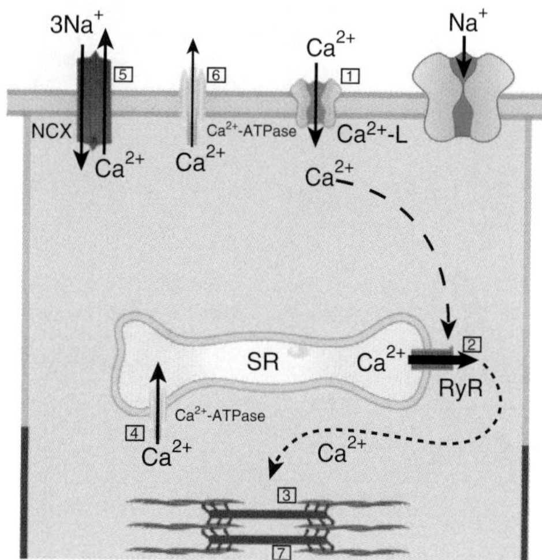


**FIGURE 32–2.** Fluctuations in $Ca^{2+}$ concentrations couple myocyte depolarization with contraction and myocyte repolarization with relaxation. (1) Depolarization, driven by $Na^+$ influx through $Na^+$ channels, causes voltage-gated $Ca^{2+}$ channels to open and calcium to flow down its concentration gradient into the myocyte. (2) This $Ca^{2+}$ current triggers the opening of $Ca^{2+}$ release channels in the sarcoplasmic reticulum (SR), and calcium pours out of the SR. The amount of $Ca^{2+}$ released from the SR is proportional to the initial inward $Ca^{2+}$ current and to the amount of calcium stored in the SR. (3) At rest, actin-myosin interaction is prevented by troponin. When $Ca^{2+}$ binds to troponin, this inhibition is removed, actin and myosin slide relative to each other, and the cell contracts.

After contraction, calcium is actively removed from the myocyte to allow relaxation. (4) Most $Ca^{2+}$ is actively pumped into the SR, where it is bound to calsequestrin. Calcium stored in the SR is thus available for release during subsequent depolarizations. The sarcoplasmic $Ca^{2+}$ ATPase is inhibited by phospholamban (**Fig. 32–3**). (5) NCX, the $Ca^{2+}$, $Na^+$ antiporter, couples the flow of three molecules of $Na^+$ in one direction to that of a single molecule of $Ca^{2+}$ in the opposite direction. This transporter is passively driven by electrochemical gradients, which usually favor the inward flow of sodium coupled to the extrusion of calcium. Extrusion of $Ca^{2+}$ is inhibited by high intracellular sodium or extracellular $Ca^{2+}$ concentrations and by cell depolarization. Under these conditions, the pump may "run in reverse."(6) Some calcium is actively pumped from the cell by a $Ca^{2+}$ ATPase. (7) As myocyte $Ca^{2+}$ concentrations fall, $Ca^{2+}$ is released from troponin, and the myocyte relaxes.

β-Adrenergic antagonists limit the detrimental effects of chronic adrenergic overstimulation and have become standard of care for patients with all stages of compensated chronic heart failure. The antihypertensive effect of β-adrenergic antagonists is counteracted by a reflex increase in peripheral vascular resistance. This effect is augmented by the $\beta_2$-adrenergic antagonism of nonselective β-adrenergic antagonists.

Some patients with reactive airways disease experience severe bronchospasm after using β-adrenergic antagonists because of loss of $\beta_2$-adrenergic–mediated bronchodilation. $\beta_2$-Adrenergic antagonists also impair the ability to recover from hypoglycemia and sometimes mask the sympathetic discharge that serves to warn of hypoglycemia. β-Adrenergic antagonism inhibits catecholamine-mediated potassium uptake at skeletal muscle. This causes slight elevations in serum potassium concentration. Although $\beta_2$-adrenergic stimulation augments insulin release, β-adrenergic antagonists seldom lower insulin concentrations. In fact, they occasionally cause hypoglycemia, especially in children, by interference with glycogenolysis and gluconeogenesis.

## PHARMACOKINETICS

The pharmacokinetic properties of the β-adrenergic antagonists are shown in Table 32–1 and depend in large part on their lipophilicity. Propranolol is the most lipid soluble, and atenolol is the most water soluble. The highly lipid-soluble β-adrenergic antagonists cross lipid membranes rapidly and concentrate in adipose tissue. These properties allow rapid entry into the central nervous system (CNS) and typically result in large volumes of distribution. In contrast, highly water-soluble medications cross lipid membranes slowly, distribute in total body water, and tend to have less CNS toxicity. The highly lipid-soluble β-adrenergic antagonists are highly protein bound and poorly excreted by the kidneys. They require hepatic biotransformation before they can be eliminated and accumulate in patients with liver failure. In contrast, the water-soluble β-adrenergic antagonists tend to be slowly absorbed, poorly protein bound, and renally eliminated. They accumulate in patients with kidney failure.

### $\beta_1$ Selectivity (Acebutolol, Atenolol, Betaxolol, Bisoprolol, Celiprolol, Esmolol, Metoprolol, and Nebivolol)

$\beta_1$-Selective antagonists avoid some of the adverse effects of the nonselective antagonists. These medications are safer for patients with asthma, diabetes mellitus, or peripheral vascular disease. Their $\beta_1$-adrenergic selectivity, however, is incomplete, and adverse reactions secondary to $\beta_2$-adrenergic antagonism occur with therapeutic dosage as well as in overdose.

### Membrane-Stabilizing Effects (Acebutolol, Betaxolol, Carvedilol, Oxprenolol, and Propranolol)

β-Adrenergic antagonists that inhibit fast sodium channels (also known as type I antidysrhythmic activity) are said to possess "membrane-stabilizing activity." No significant

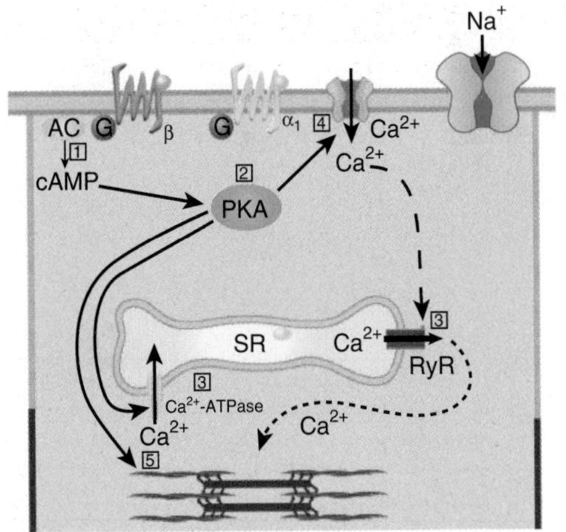


**FIGURE 32–3.** $\beta_1$-Adrenergic agonists are positive inotropes by virtue of their ability to activate protein kinase A (PKA). (1) $\beta_1$-Adrenergic receptors are coupled to $G_s$ proteins, which activate adenylate cyclase when catecholamines bind to the receptor. This causes increased formation of cyclic adenosine monophosphate (cAMP) from adenosine triphosphate (ATP). (2) Increased cAMP concentrations activate PKA, which mediates the ultimate effects of β-adrenergic receptor stimulation by phosphorylating key intracellular proteins. (3) Phosphorylation of phospholamban disinhibits the sarcoplasmic reticulum (SR) $Ca^{2+}$ ATPase, resulting in increased SR calcium stores available for release during subsequent depolarizations, and phosphorylation of SR calcium release channels enhances $Ca^{2+}$ release from SR stores during contraction. (4) Phosphorylation of voltage-gated $Ca^{2+}$ channels increases $Ca^{2+}$ influx through these channels during systole. (5) Troponin phosphorylation improves cardiac performance by facilitating $Ca^{2+}$ unbinding during diastole. $\beta_2$-Adrenergic receptors are also coupled to $G_s$ proteins and mediate positive inotropy through a cAMP mechanism. Increased cAMP directly increases heart rate (**Fig. 32–1A**).

membrane stabilization occurs with therapeutic use of β-adrenergic antagonists, but this property contributes to toxicity in overdose by impairing cardiac conduction.

### Intrinsic Sympathomimetic Activity (Acebutolol, Carteolol, Oxprenolol, Penbutolol, and Pindolol)

These xenobiotics are partial agonists at β-adrenergic receptors and are said to have intrinsic sympathomimetic activity (ISA), and thus theoretically avoid the dramatic decrease in resting heart rate that occurs with β-adrenergic antagonism. Their clinical advantage over classic β-adrenergic antagonists is not demonstrated in controlled trials.

### Potassium Channel Blockade (Acebutolol and Sotalol)

Sotalol is unique because of its ability to block the delayed rectifier potassium current responsible for repolarization. This prolongs the action potential duration and is manifested on the electrocardiogram by a prolonged QT interval. The prolonged QT interval predisposes to torsade de pointes and ventricular dysrhythmias, which rarely complicate the therapeutic use of sotalol. Acebutolol also prolongs the QT interval presumably secondary to blockade of outward potassium channels.

### Vasodilation (Betaxolol, Bucindolol, Carteolol, Carvedilol, Celiprolol, Labetalol, and Nebivolol)

Labetalol and some newer β-adrenergic antagonists (betaxolol, bucindolol, carteolol, carvedilol, celiprolol, nebivolol) are also vasodilators. Labetalol and carvedilol are nonselective β-adrenergic antagonists that also possess α-adrenergic antagonist activity. Nebivolol is a selective $\beta_1$-adrenergic antagonist that causes vasodilation by release of nitric oxide. Bucindolol, carteolol, and celiprolol vasodilate because they are agonists at $\beta_2$-adrenergic receptors. Celiprolol and carteolol also vasodilate because of nitric oxide–mediated effects. Despite theoretical advantages, β-adrenergic antagonists with vasodilating properties have not been proven to be more beneficial than other β-adrenergic antagonists for patients with congestive heart failure. These β-adrenergic antagonists should not be given without appropriate α-adrenergic blockade in situations of catecholamine excess such as pheochromocytoma. In these conditions, $\beta_2$-adrenergic–mediated vasodilation is essential to counteract α-adrenergic–mediated vasoconstriction, and β-adrenergic antagonists result in unopposed α-adrenergic effect, causing dangerous increases in vascular resistance. Even xenobiotics with combined α- and β-adrenergic antagonist properties, such as labetalol, can cause this problem. Labetalol is more potent as a β-adrenergic antagonist than as an α-adrenergic antagonist depending on whether is it given orally (3:1 ratio) or intravenously (7:1 ratio).

### Other Preparations (Ophthalmic Preparations and Combined Products)

Therapeutic use of ophthalmic solutions containing β-adrenergic antagonists rarely causes systemic adverse effects such as bradycardia, high-grade AV block, heart failure, and bronchospasm. Several combination tablets containing both β-adrenergic antagonists and thiazide diuretics are available to treat hypertension in the US. Internationally, products containing β-adrenergic antagonists in combination with calcium channel antagonists are available.

## PATHOPHYSIOLOGY

Most of the toxicity of β-adrenergic antagonists is due to their ability to competitively antagonize the action of catecholamines at cardiac β-adrenergic receptors. The peripheral vascular effects of β-adrenergic antagonism are less prominent in overdose. β-Adrenergic antagonists also appear to have toxic effects independent of their action at catecholamine receptors, possibly because of interference with calcium handling at the level of the SR.

β-Adrenergic antagonists also interfere with calcium uptake into intracellular organelles. Interference with cytosolic calcium handling stimulates calcium-sensitive outward potassium channels, resulting in myocyte hyperpolarization and subsequent refractory bradycardia. In experiments with isolated rat hearts, calcium improved the function of rat hearts poisoned with β-adrenergic antagonists. Although cardiovascular effects are most prominent in overdose, β-adrenergic antagonists also cause respiratory depression. This effect is centrally mediated and is an important cause of death in spontaneously breathing animal models of β-adrenergic antagonist toxicity.

## CLINICAL MANIFESTATIONS

Isolated β-adrenergic antagonist overdose in healthy people is often benign. This is partially explained by the fact that β-adrenergic antagonism is often well tolerated in healthy persons who do not rely on sympathetic stimulation to maintain cardiac output. In particular, unintentional ingestions in children rarely result in significant toxicity. β-Adrenergic antagonists severely impair the ability of the heart to respond to peripheral vasodilation, bradycardia, or decreased contractility caused by other xenobiotics. Therefore, even relatively benign vasoactive xenobiotics cause catastrophic toxicity when coingested with β-adrenergic antagonists. The most important predictor of toxicity in healthy patients with β-adrenergic antagonist overdose is likely the presence of a cardioactive coingestant. Nevertheless, severe toxicity and death occur in healthy persons who have ingested β-adrenergic antagonists alone.

The clinical findings of toxicity generally occur within hours after β-adrenergic antagonist overdose. Propranolol overdose, in particular, is often complicated by the rapid development of hypoglycemia, seizures, coma, and dysrhythmias. Most patients who ingest immediate-release products develop symptoms within 6 hours of ingestion. These observations do not apply to sotalol, which is well known to cause delayed toxicity in overdose, or to sustained-release preparations.

Patients with symptomatic β-adrenergic antagonist overdose are most often hypotensive and bradycardic. Decreased SA node function results in sinus bradycardia, sinus pauses, or sinus arrest. Impaired AV conduction manifested as prolonged PR interval or high-grade AV block occurs rarely. Prolonged QRS complex duration and QT interval duration occur, and severe poisoning results in asystole. Congestive heart failure often complicates β-adrenergic antagonist overdose. Delirium, coma, and seizures occur most commonly in the setting of severe hypotension but also occur with normal blood pressure, especially with exposure to the more lipophilic medications such as propranolol. Respiratory depression and apnea may have an additional role in toxicity. Hypoglycemia often complicates β-adrenergic antagonist poisoning in children but is uncommon in acutely poisoned adults. Clinical use of β-adrenergic antagonists slightly increases serum potassium concentration, but significant hyperkalemia is rare.

### $\beta_1$ Selectivity (Acebutolol, Atenolol, Betaxolol, Bisoprolol, Esmolol, Metoprolol, and Nebivolol)

In overdose, cardioselectivity is largely lost, and deaths caused by $\beta_1$-adrenergic selective antagonists are reported.

### Membrane-Stabilizing Effects (Acebutolol, Betaxolol, Carvedilol, Oxprenolol, and Propranolol)

Propranolol possesses the most membrane-stabilizing activity of this class. Impaired AV conduction and QRS complex prolongation are reported. Hypotension is often out of proportion to bradycardia, from propranolol overdose.

### Lipid Solubility

In overdose, the more lipophilic β-adrenergic antagonists more often cause delirium, coma, and seizures even in the absence of hypotension.

### Intrinsic Sympathomimetic Activity (Acebutolol, Carteolol, Oxprenolol, Penbutolol, and Pindolol)

There is little experience with overdose of these xenobiotics, but ISA would theoretically make these xenobiotics safer than the other β-adrenergic antagonists. However, deaths due to acute toxicity from many of these xenobiotics are reported.

### Potassium Channel Blockade (Acebutolol and Sotalol)

In patients with sotalol overdose, large increases in QT interval and ventricular dysrhythmias, including multifocal ventricular extrasystoles, torsade de pointes, ventricular tachycardia, and ventricular fibrillation, are well documented. Sotalol overdose often causes delayed and prolonged toxicity, although changes on the electrocardiogram (ECG) appear to occur early. The greatest QT interval prolongation occurrs up to 15 hours after ingestion, and the risk of ventricular dysrhythmias is greatest between 4 and 20 hours.

### Vasodilation (Betaxolol, Bucindolol, Carteolol, Carvedilol, Celiprolol, Labetalol, and Nebivolol)

Overdose with labetalol appears to be similar to that of other β-adrenergic antagonists with hypotension and bradycardia as prominent features. Similar to conventional β-adrenergic antagonists, carvedilol overdose causes hypotension and bradycardia. Experience with overdose of the newer vasodilating β-adrenergic antagonists is limited.

### Other Preparations (Ophthalmic Preparations, Sustained Release, and Combined Products)

There is very little published experience with overdoses of the sustained-release β-adrenergic antagonists, but it is reasonable to expect that overdose with these xenobiotics will result in both a delayed onset and prolonged duration of toxicity. Acute overdose of ophthalmic β-adrenergic antagonists has not been reported. Patients who take mixed overdoses with calcium channel blockers and β-adrenergic antagonists are difficult to manage because of synergistic toxicity. Overdoses with combined β-adrenergic antagonist and calcium channel blocker preparations such as felodipine and metoprolol or atenolol and nifedipine have not been well reported, but these combinations would be expected to be quite dangerous in overdose.

## DIAGNOSTIC TESTING

All patients with an intentional overdose of a β-adrenergic antagonist require an ECG and continuous cardiac monitoring. Serum glucose should be measured regardless of mental status. A chest radiograph and assessment of oxygen saturation should be obtained if the patient is at risk for or has symptoms of congestive heart failure. Patients with bradycardia of uncertain etiology should have thyroid function, potassium, kidney function, and cardiac enzymes measured. Serum concentrations of β-adrenergic antagonists are not readily available for routine clinical use but may prove helpful in making a retrospective diagnosis in selected cases.

## MANAGEMENT

Airway and ventilation should be maintained with endotracheal intubation if necessary. Because laryngoscopy sometimes induces a vagal response, it is reasonable to give atropine before intubation of patients with bradycardia. The initial treatment of patients with bradycardia and hypotension consists of atropine and an intravenous (IV) fluid bolus.

These measures will likely be insufficient in patients with severe toxicity requiring administration of vaospressors or antidotes.

Gastrointestinal (GI) decontamination is warranted for all persons who have ingested significant amounts of a β-adrenergic antagonist. Orogastric lavage is recommended for patients with significant toxic effects such as seizures, hypotension, or bradycardia only if the patient presents in a time frame when the medication is still expected to be in the stomach. Orogastric lavage is also recommended for patients who present shortly after massive ingestion of large (gram amount), of propranolol, or one of the other more toxic β-adrenergic antagonists (ie, acebutolol, betaxolol, metoprolol, oxprenolol, sotalol). Orogastric lavage causes vagal stimulation and carries the risk of worsening bradycardia, so it is reasonable to pretreat patients with standard doses of atropine or, at a minimum, be prepared to treat if it develops. Orogastric lavage should be followed with activated charcoal. Activated charcoal alone is recommended for persons with minor effects after an overdose with one of the more water-soluble β-adrenergic antagonists who present within several hours after ingestion (Antidotes in Brief: A1). Whole-bowel irrigation with polyethylene glycol is reasonable in addition to activated charcoal for patients who have ingested sustained-release preparations (Antidotes in Brief: A2).

Seizures or coma associated with cardiovascular collapse is treated by attempting to restore circulation. Seizures in the patient with relatively normal vital signs should be treated with an adequate trial of benzodiazepines followed by barbiturates or propofol if benzodiazepines fail. Refractory seizures are rare in patients with isolated β-adrenergic antagonist overdose.

## Specific Management

Patients who fail to respond to atropine and fluids require management with the inotropes discussed later (Fig. 32–4). When time permits, it is preferable to introduce new medications sequentially so that the effects of each may be assessed. We recommend glucagon followed by calcium and high-dose insulin euglycemia therapy. In critically ill patients, there may not be enough time for this stepwise approach, and multiple treatments may be started simultaneously. If these therapies fail, we suggest starting a catecholamine pressor. Mechanical life support with intraaortic balloon pump (IABP) or extracorporeal circulation is recommended when medical management fails.

## Glucagon

Cardiac glucagon receptors, like β-adrenergic receptors, is coupled to Gs proteins. Glucagon binding increases adenylate cyclase activity independent of β-adrenergic receptor binding. The inotropic effect of glucagon is enhanced by its ability to inhibit phosphodiesterase and thereby prevent cAMP breakdown.

Glucagon successfully reversed bradydysrhythmias and hypotension in patients unresponsive to isoproterenol therapies and was formerly routinely recommended for administration early in the management of patients with severe toxicity. Case reports, case series, and reviews document

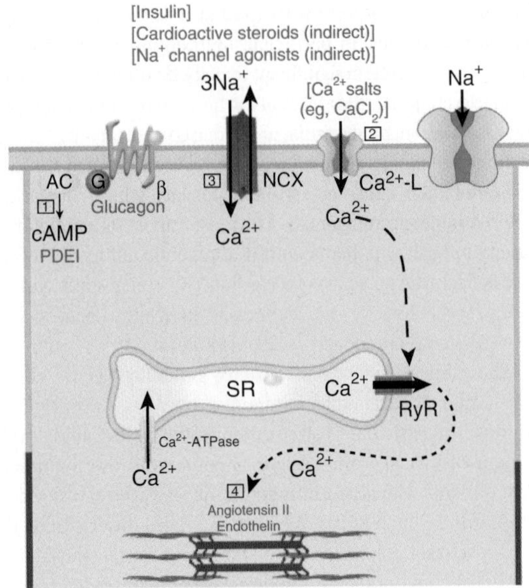


**FIGURE 32–4.** Positive inotropes improve cardiac function by a number of mechanisms, which usually result in increased intracellular $Ca^{2+}$. (1) Xenobiotics that increase cyclic adenosine monophosphate (cAMP). Glucagon receptors and β-adrenergic receptors are coupled to $G_s$ proteins so that receptor binding increases cAMP by activation of adenylate cyclase. Phosphodiesterase inhibitors increase cAMP by inhibiting its breakdown. (2) Xenobiotics that increase calcium influx. Calcium salts increase calcium influx through L-type $Ca^{2+}$ channels by a direct mass effect. (3) Xenobiotics that inhibit extrusion of calcium via the $Na^+$ $Ca^{2+}$ exchange pump: Xenobiotics that increase intracellular sodium such as digoxin and $Na^+$ channel agonists (eg, aconitine) and those such as 4-aminopyridine that prolong the action potential duration alter the electrochemical gradients in a way that hinders the extrusion of calcium. (4) Xenobiotics that increase the sensitivity of the contractile elements to calcium. Angiotensin II and endothelin do this by inducing an intracellular alkalosis. The calcium sensitizers levosimendan and pimobendan are used to treat heart failure in some countries. NCX = the calcium-sodium antiporter.

full or partial beneficial hemodynamic response to glucagon administration in β-adrenergic antagonist toxicity, although often, it is unsuccessful.

Because the management of β-adrenergic antagonist toxicity is often complicated, many other therapies, including atropine, epinephrine, norepinephrine, dopamine, dobutamine, and various combinations, are used with variable success. High-dose insulin (HDI) (Antidotes in Brief: A21) and lipid emulsion (Antidotes in Brief: A23) are also used. In canine studies, HDI therapy has a more sustained effect on hemodynamic parameters and an improved survival rate compared with glucagon. We recommend HDI early in the resuscitation of severe β-adrenergic antagonist overdoses with myocardial depression. We do not routinely recommend glucagon for patients with undifferentiated hypotension and bradycardia.

Glucagon sometimes causes vomiting with risk of aspiration, and it is reasonable to pretreat with an antiemetic but to remain cognizant of the fact that many antiemetics cause QT interval prolongation (Antidotes in Brief: A20).

## Calcium

Calcium chloride successfully reverses hypotension in patients with β-adrenergic antagonist overdose. The adult starting dose of calcium gluconate is 3 g of the 10% solution given intravenously. For patients with persistent hypotension, we recommend repeating this same dose of calcium gluconate every 10 to 20 minutes up to a total of 9 g. The initial dose of calcium gluconate in children is 60 mg/kg up to 3 g followed by repeat boluses every 10 to 20 minutes, as needed for persistent hypotension, up to a total of 180 mg/kg (Antidotes in Brief: A32).

### Insulin and Glucose

High-dose insulin combined with sufficient glucose to maintain euglycemia is beneficial in β-adrenergic antagonist poisoning. High-dose insulin is simple to use and safe (with appropriate monitoring of glucose and potassium) and does not require invasive monitoring. For these reasons, we recommend using HDI and glucose infusions for patients with β-adrenergic antagonist toxicity who have not responded to fluids, atropine, and glucagon. Although the dose of insulin is not definitively established, therapy typically begins with a bolus of 1 unit/kg of regular human insulin along with 0.5 g/kg of dextrose. If blood glucose is greater than 300 mg/dL (16.7 mmol/L), the dextrose bolus is not necessary. A concentrated infusion of regular insulin (10 units/mL) should follow the bolus starting at 1 unit/kg/h. A continuous dextrose infusion, beginning at 0.5 g/kg/h, may be needed. Glucose should be monitored every 15 to 30 minutes until stable and then every 1 to 2 hours and titrated to maintain the blood glucose between 100 and 250 mg/dL. Cardiac function should also be reassessed every 10 to 15 minutes, and if it remains depressed, the insulin infusion should be increased up to 10 units/kg/h as required (rarely higher). It is important to continue monitoring glucose and electrolytes for several hours after insulin is discontinued (Antidotes in Brief: A21).

### Catecholamines

Patients who do not respond to the preceding therapies usually require a catecholamine infusion. The choice of catecholamine is somewhat controversial. Epinephrine seems to be more effective than isoproterenol. Experience is limited with dobutamine, which is not always effective in patients with β-adrenergic antagonist overdose. In the setting of β-adrenergic antagonism, catecholamines with substantial α-adrenergic agonist properties can increase peripheral vascular resistance without improving contractility, resulting in acute cardiac failure. Because of this uncertainty, we recommend that catecholamine use be guided by hemodynamic monitoring either using noninvasive techniques such as bioimpedance or echocardiographic monitoring or by direct invasive measures of determining cardiac performance. If advanced monitoring is unavailable and the diagnosis of β-adrenergic antagonist overdose is fairly certain, it is reasonable to begin epinephrine. The infusion should be stopped immediately if the patient becomes more hypotensive or develops congestive heart failure.

### Lipid Emulsion

Intravenous administration of lipid emulsion has a potential role in selected cases of severe β-adrenergic antagonist overdose. Human experience with the use of lipid emulsion in β-adrenergic antagonist overdose is limited largely to case reports, but both dramatic recoveries and immediate cardiac arrest are reported. Another concern with using lipid emulsion in severely poisoned patients is that it may cause mechanical problems with the equipment used in extracorporeal membrane oxygenation (ECMO). Given these concerns and limited evidence supporting its efficacy in β-adrenergic antagonist overdose, lipid emulsion should not be used routinely in patients poisoned with β-adrenergic antagonists. It is reasonable to administer lipid emulsion in patients poisoned with a lipid-soluble β-adrenergic antagonist who have cardiac arrest or circulatory failure that does not respond to usual therapy, especially if mechanical life support is not promptly available. A typical dose is a bolus of 1.5 mL/kg of 20% lipid emulsion followed by an infusion of 0.25 mL/kg/min (Antidotes in Brief: A23).

### Phosphodiesterase Inhibitors

The phosphodiesterase inhibitors amrinone, milrinone, and enoximone are theoretically beneficial in β-adrenergic antagonist overdose because they inhibit the breakdown of cAMP by phosphodiesterase and hence increase cAMP independently of β-adrenergic receptor stimulation. Phosphodiesterase inhibitors have been used clinically to treat β-adrenergic antagonist–poisoned patients, but experience is limited. Therapy with phosphodiesterase inhibitors is often limited by hypotension secondary to peripheral vasodilation. Furthermore, these xenobiotics are difficult to titrate because of relatively long half-lives. For these reasons, they are not routinely recommended in β-adrenergic antagonist–poisoned patients, especially in patients without arterial and pulmonary artery pressure monitoring.

### Ventricular Pacing

Ventricular pacing is not a particularly useful intervention in patients with β-adrenergic antagonist toxicity, but it will increase the heart rate in some patients. Unfortunately, in many cases there will be failure to capture, while in others, pacing increases the heart rate with no increase in cardiac output or blood pressure. Occasionally, ventricular pacing even decreases blood pressure perhaps secondary to loss of organized atrial contraction or because of impaired ventricular relaxation. For these reasons, transvenous ventricular pacing is not recommended for management of β-adrenergic antagonist toxicity except for heart rate control in patients with an IABP. A trial of transcutaneous pacing is always reasonable in patients with symptomatic bradycardia.

### Extracorporeal Removal

Extracorporeal removal is not routinely recommended in patients with β-adrenergic antagonist overdose. It is unlikely to be effective for most β-adrenergic antagonists because of their large volumes of distribution or high protein binding. Although extracorporeal removal is a reasonable consideration in patients with severe toxicity from a water-soluble β-adrenergic antagonist (such as atenolol), it is often technically limited because of the patient's hemodynamics. Extracorporeal removal could potentially be used in combination with ECMO for an appropriate drug.

### Mechanical Life Support

It is important to remember that a patient with circulatory failure from an acute overdose will typically recover without sequelae if ventilation and circulation are maintained until the xenobiotic is eliminated. When the preceding medical treatment fails, it is recommended to use extracorporeal life support (ECLS). Extracorporeal life support includes venoarterial extracorporeal membrane oxygenation (VA-ECMO), emergency cardiac bypass, IABP, or left ventricular assist devices. Consistent with several recent reviews of ECLS in poisoned patients, we recommend that ECLS be used, in centers where it is available, in β-adrenergic antagonist–poisoned patients with persistent cardiac arrest or circulatory failure unresponsive to standard therapy. Given the high risk of complications, including severe bleeding, stroke, and intracranial hemorrhage, ECLS should be reserved for severely poisoned patients who are failing medical therapy.

### Special Circumstances

The preceding discussion applies to the generic management of patients with β-adrenergic antagonists. Certain β-adrenergic antagonists have unique properties that modify their toxicity. The management considerations for these unique agents are discussed next.

***Sotalol.*** In addition to bradycardia and hypotension, sotalol toxicity results in a prolonged QT interval and ventricular dysrhythmias, including torsade de pointes. Sotalol-induced bradycardia and hypotension should be managed as with other β-adrenergic antagonists. Specific management of patients with sotalol overdose includes correction of hypokalemia and hypomagnesemia. Overdrive pacing and magnesium infusions are recommended for prevention of recurrent episodes in patients who have developed sotalol-induced torsade de pointes.

***Peripheral Vasodilation (Betaxolol, Bucindolol, Carteolol, Carvedilol, Celiprolol, Labetalol, and Nebivolol).*** Treatment of patients who have overdosed with one of the vasodilating β-adrenergic antagonists is similar to that for patients who ingest other β-adrenergic antagonists.

***Membrane-Stabilizing Effects (Acebutolol, Betaxolol, Carvedilol, Oxprenolol, and Propranolol).*** It might be expected that hypertonic sodium bicarbonate would be beneficial in treating the ventricular dysrhythmias that occur with these xenobiotics. Unfortunately, there is limited experience with the use of sodium bicarbonate in this situation, and the experimental data are mixed. Because sodium bicarbonate is a relatively safe and simple intervention, we recommend that it be used in addition to standard therapy for β-adrenergic antagonist–poisoned patients with QRS complex prolongation or ventricular dysrhythmias. Sodium bicarbonate would not be expected to be beneficial in sotalol-induced ventricular dysrhythmias and, by causing hypokalemia, may actually increase the risk of torsade de pointes. The usual dose of hypertonic sodium bicarbonate is 1 to 2 mEq/kg given as an IV bolus (Antidotes in Brief: A5).

### Observation

All patients who have bradycardia, hypotension, abnormal ECGs, or CNS toxicity after β-adrenergic antagonist overdose should be observed in a critical care setting until these findings resolve. Toxicity from regular-release β-adrenergic antagonist poisoning other than sotalol usually occurs within the first 6 hours. Therefore, patients without any findings of toxicity after an overdose of a regular-release β-adrenergic antagonist other than sotalol can safely be discharged from medical care after an observation time of 6 to 8 hours if they remain asymptomatic with normal vital signs and a normal ECG and have had GI decontamination with activated charcoal. Because ingestion of extended-release preparations is associated with delayed toxicity, these patients should be observed for 24 hours in an intensive care unit. We recommend that all patients with sotalol overdose be monitored for at least 12 hours. Patients who remain stable without QT interval prolongation can then be discharged from a monitored setting.

# A20 GLUCAGON

## INTRODUCTION

The traditional role of glucagon was to reverse life-threatening hypoglycemia in patients with diabetes mellitus unable to receive dextrose in the outpatient setting. However, in clinical toxicology, glucagon is used early in the management of β-adrenergic antagonist and calcium channel blocker toxicity to improve hemodynamics while bridging to other therapies. Clinical use is hampered by its relative high cost, rapid tachyphylaxis, complex administration regimen, and propensity to induce emesis.

## HISTORY

Glucagon was discovered in 1922, the year after the discovery of insulin. Originally viewed as a mere contaminant in insulin products, glucagon was eventually attributed to pancreatic α-cells and sequenced in 1957. The positive inotropic and chronotropic effects of glucagon were recognized in the 1960s. Clinical use in human poisonings began in 1971. Despite decades of use, glucagon has never been subjected to a controlled trial, and systematic reviews fail to demonstrate a clear benefit over traditional inotropes and vasopressors.

## PHARMACOLOGY

### Chemistry and Preparation

Glucagon is a single-chain polypeptide counterregulatory hormone with a molecular weight of 3,500 Da that is secreted by the α-cells of the pancreas. The current product is synthesized by recombinant DNA technology.

### Mechanism of Action

Glucagon receptors are found in the heart, brain, and pancreas. Binding of glucagon to cardiac receptors is closely correlated with activation of cardiac adenylate cyclase. Binding of glucagon to its receptor results in coupling of Gs protein that stimulates adenylate cyclase to convert adenosine triphosphate (ATP) to cAMP. Evidence suggests an additional mechanism of action of a glucagon metabolite (mini-glucagon) that stimulates phospholipase $A_2$, releasing arachidonic acid. Arachidonic acid increases cardiac contractility through an effect on calcium.

### Cardiovascular Effects

The inotropic action of glucagon is related to an increase in cardiac cAMP concentrations. Glucagon increases cAMP to augment the sarcoplasmic reticulum calcium pool. Glucagon improves chronotropy at both the sinus node and the atrioventricular (AV) junctional region, even in the presence of escape rhythms. Both the positive inotropic and chronotropic actions of glucagon are very similar to those of the β-adrenergic agonists, except that they are not blocked by β-adrenergic antagonists.

### Pharmacokinetics and Pharmacodynamics

The volume of distribution of glucagon is 0.25 L/kg. The plasma, liver, and kidney extensively metabolize glucagon with an elimination half-life of 8 to 18 minutes. In human volunteers, after a single IV bolus, the cardiac effects of glucagon begin within 1 to 3 minutes, are maximal within 5 to 7 minutes, and persist for 10 to 15 minutes. The onset of action after intramuscular and subcutaneous administration occurs in about 10 minutes, with a peak at about 30 minutes. Tachyphylaxis (desensitization of receptors) may occur with repetitive dosing.

### Volunteer Studies

In 21 patients with heart failure, 3- to 5-mg intravenous (IV) boluses of glucagon increased the force of contraction, heart rate, cardiac index, blood pressure, and stroke work. There were no changes in systemic vascular resistance, left ventricular end-diastolic pressure, or stroke index. In nine patients who received glucagon (50 μg/kg), coronary blood flow increased by 30%. Patients who received 1 mg via IV bolus also had an increase in cardiac index, but systemic vascular resistance fell, probably secondary to vascular smooth muscle relaxation. Patients who received an infusion of 2 to 3 mg/min for 10 to 15-minutes responded similarly to those who received the 3- to 5-mg IV boluses, but patients receiving boluses experienced significant dose-limiting nausea and vomiting.

## ROLE IN THE MANAGEMENT OF β-ADRENERGIC ANTAGONIST TOXICITY

One early management strategy for patients with β-adrenergic antagonist toxicity included provision of large doses of competitive β-agonists such as isoproterenol. Glucagon successfully reversed bradydysrhythmias and hypotension in patients unresponsive to the aforementioned therapy and was routinely recommended for administration early in the management of patients with severe toxicity. Case reports, case series, and reviews document full or partial beneficial hemodynamic response to glucagon administration in β-adrenergic antagonist toxicity, although at times, it is unsuccessful.

Because the management of β-adrenergic antagonist toxicity is often complicated, many other therapies, including atropine, epinephrine, norepinephrine, dopamine, dobutamine, and various combinations are used with variable success. High-dose insulin (HDI) (Antidotes in Brief: A21) and lipid emulsion (Antidotes in Brief: A23) are also used. In canine studies, HDI therapy has a more sustained effect on hemodynamic parameters and an improved survival rate compared with glucagon. We recommend HDI early in the resuscitation of severe β-adrenergic antagonist overdoses with myocardial depression. We recommend glucagon use in refractory anaphylaxis in patients taking β-adrenergic antagonists. We do not routinely recommend glucagon for patients with undifferentiated hypotension and bradycardia.

### Combined Effects with Phosphodiesterase Inhibitors and Calcium

Previous strategies for enhancing the effects of glucagon have involved combining it with a $PDE_3$ inhibitor such as amrinone. In a canine model of propranolol toxicity, both amrinone and milrinone alone were comparable to glucagon, but the combination of amrinone and glucagon resulted in a decrease in mean arterial pressure. Although the evidence for the effectiveness of combining glucagon with a PDE inhibitor was demonstrated in animal models and human case reports, we recommend against the use of this approach.

The relationship between calcium and the chronotropic effects of glucagon was demonstrated in rats. Maximal chronotropic effects of glucagon are dependent on a normal circulating ionized calcium. Both hypocalcemia and hypercalcemia blunt the maximal chronotropic response.

## ROLE IN CALCIUM CHANNEL BLOCKER TOXICITY

Animal studies demonstrate the ability of glucagon to improve heart rate and AV conduction and reverse the myocardial depression produced by nifedipine, diltiazem, and verapamil without a demonstrable survival benefit. A canine model of verapamil toxicity comparing glucagon to HDI, only revealed a survival benefit for HDI. While human case reports demonstrate improved hemodynamics, including in cases refractory to other standard measures, many other reports document no improvement. Therefore, it is reasonable to try glucagon therapy if easily available while preparing for HDI administration.

## ROLE IN REVERSAL OF HYPOGLYCEMIA

Glucagon was once proposed as part of the initial treatment for all comatose patients because it stimulates glycogenolysis in the liver. The theoretical rationale for this approach is only partially sound in that glucagon requires time to act and will often be ineffective in a patient with depleted glycogen stores, such as in patients with prolonged fasting, severe liver disease, alcoholism, starvation, adrenal insufficiency, or chronic hypoglycemia. Because IV administration of 0.5 to 1.0 g/kg of dextrose rapidly reverses hypoglycemia and does not rely on glycogen stores for its effect, it is preferred over glucagon (Antidotes in Brief: A8). Glucagon is reasonable as a temporizing measure, until medical help can be obtained, in the home where IV dextrose is not an option, or when IV access is not rapidly available.

## ADVERSE EFFECTS AND SAFETY ISSUES

Side effects associated with glucagon include dose-dependent nausea, vomiting, hyperglycemia, hypoglycemia, and hypokalemia; relaxation of the smooth muscle of the stomach, duodenum, small bowel, and colon; and, rarely, urticaria, respiratory distress, and hypotension. Glucagon increased the release of catecholamines in a patient with a pheochromocytoma, resulting in a hypertensive crisis, which was treated with phentolamine.

## PREGNANCY AND LACTATION

Glucagon is United States Food and Drug Administration Pregnancy Category B. There are no reports of glucagon use during lactation.

## DOSAGE AND ADMINSTRATION

The dosing regimen for glucagon in toxicologic emergencies has never been formally studied. Intravenous infusion of an initial dose of 50 μg/kg (3–5 mg in a 70-kg adult) over 3 to 10 minutes is recommended and likely minimizes nausea and vomiting. If the initial dose is ineffectual, a higher dose (up to 10 mg) is reasonable. If the higher dose appears beneficial, then either repeat doses of 3 to 5 mg as needed or a continuous infusion of 2 to 5 mg/h (titrated to a maximum of 10 mg/h) in 5% dextrose in water may serve as a temporizing measure while waiting for HDI to become effective.

## FORMULATION AND ACQUISITION

Glucagon (rDNA origin) is available as a sterile, lyophilized white powder in a vial alone or accompanied by sterile water for reconstitution. The glucagon powder should be reconstituted with 1 mL of sterile water for injection, after which the vial should be shaken gently until the powder completely dissolves.

# 33 CALCIUM CHANNEL BLOCKERS

## HISTORY AND EPIDEMIOLOGY

In 1964, Fleckenstein described an inhibitory action of verapamil and prenylamine on excitation–contraction coupling that was similar to calcium depletion. By the late 1970s, the clinical use of calcium channel blockers (CCBs) was widely accepted for a variety of cardiovascular indications, including hypertension, dysrhythmias, and angina. The cardiovascular drug class is one of the leading causes drug-associated poisoning fatality. Within this class, CCBs were the most common cardiovascular drugs involved in poisoning fatalities.

## PHARMACOLOGY

Calcium ($Ca^{2+}$) ion channels exist as either voltage-dependent or ligand-gated channels. There are many types of voltage-gated $Ca^{2+}$ channels, including P-, N-, R-, T-, Q-, and L-type channels (Table 33–1). The primary action of all CCBs available in the United States is antagonism of the L-type or "long-acting" voltage-gated $Ca^{2+}$ channels. Calcium channel blockers are often classified into three groups based on their chemical structure (Table 33–2). It is often more logical to classify them as nondihydropyridine versus dihydropyridine CCBs. Verapamil and diltiazem have inhibitory effects on both the sinoatrial (SA) and atrioventricular (AV) nodal tissue and thus are commonly used for the treatment of hypertension, to reduce myocardial oxygen demand, and to achieve rate control in a variety of tachydysrhythmias. In contrast, the dihydropyridines have very little direct effect on the myocardium at therapeutic doses and act primarily as peripheral vasodilators. They are therefore commonly used for conditions with increased vascular tone such as hypertensive emergencies, aortic dissection, and post subarachnoid hemorrhage vasospasm. Experimental studies suggest that dihydropyridine CCBs also release nitric oxide in a dose-dependent fashion.

## PHARMACOKINETICS AND TOXICOKINETICS

All CCBs are well absorbed orally, but many have low bioavailability because of extensive hepatic first-pass metabolism. When the CCBs reach the liver, they undergo hepatic oxidative metabolism predominantly via CYP3A4 enzymes. All CCBs are highly protein bound even in supratherapeutic concentrations, which restricts the role of extracorporeal removal. Volumes of distribution are generally large and listed in Table 33–2. The CCBs undergo a significant, but variable, amount of renal excretion after metabolism with a small percentage eliminated in the urine unchanged.

One interesting aspect of the pharmacology of CCBs is their potential for drug–drug interactions; CYP3A4, which metabolizes most CCBs, is also responsible for the initial oxidation of numerous other xenobiotics. Verapamil and diltiazem specifically compete for CYP3A4 and can decrease the clearance of many xenobiotics. Verapamil and diltiazem also inhibit P-glycoprotein–mediated drug transport into peripheral tissues that results in elevated serum concentrations of xenobiotics. Unlike diltiazem and verapamil, the dihydropyridines do not affect the clearance of other xenobiotics via CYP3A4 or P-glycoprotein–mediated transport.

## PHYSIOLOGY AND PATHOPHYSIOLOGY

Calcium plays an essential role in many cellular processes throughout the body, and many types of cells depend on the maintenance of a $Ca^{2+}$ concentration gradient across cell membranes in order to function. The extracellular $Ca^{2+}$ concentration is approximately 10,000 times greater than the intracellular concentration. This concentration gradient is important for contraction and relaxation of muscle cells. In myocardial cells, $Ca^{2+}$ influx is slower relative to the initial $Na^+$ influx that initiates cellular depolarization and

**TABLE 33–1 Voltage-Gated Calcium Channel Subtypes**

| *Type* | *Distribution* | *Function* | *Blocked By* |
|---|---|---|---|
| T (transient) | Polysynaptic nerve terminals and cardiac nodal tissue | Pacemaker activity | Mibefradil |
| R | Neural tissue | Neurotransmitter release | Cadmium |
| Q | Presynaptic nerve terminals | Neurotransmitter release | Agatoxin |
| P (Purkinje) | Cerebellar Purkinje neurons | Neurotransmitter release | Agatoxin |
| N (neuronal) | Presynaptic nerve terminals | Catecholamine release | ω-Conotoxin |
| L (long-acting) | Myocardium and smooth muscle | Muscular contraction | Verapamil, diltiazem, dihydropyridines |

**TABLE 33–2 Classification of Calcium Channel Blockers Available in the United States**

| *Class* | *Specific Compounds* | *Volume of Distribution (L/kg)* | *Time to Peak[a] Concentrations (h)* |
|---|---|---|---|
| Phenylalkylamine | Verapamil | 3–5 | 1–2 |
| Benzothiazepine | Diltiazem | 5.3 | 2–4 |
| Dihydropyridines | Amlodipine | 21 | 6–12 |
| | Clevidipine | 0.17 | <1 |
| | Felodipine | 10 | 2.5–5 |
| | Isradipine | 3 | 1–2 |
| | Nicardipine | 8.3 | 1–4 |
| | Nifedipine | 0.75 | 2.5–5 |
| | Nimodipine | 2 | 1–2 |
| | Nisoldipine | 1.6 | >6 |

[a]All values are for ingestion of a therapeutic dose of an immediate-release formulation.

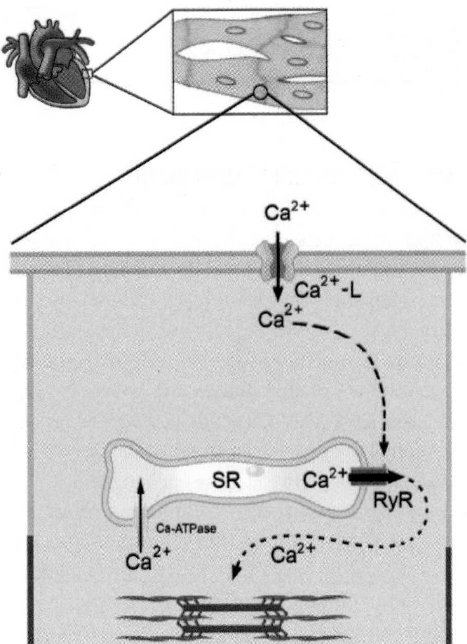


**FIGURE 33–1.** Normal contraction of myocardial cells. The L-type voltage-gated $Ca^{2+}$ channels ($Ca^{2+}$-L) open to allow $Ca^{2+}$ ion influx during myocyte depolarization. This causes the concentration-dependent release of more $Ca^{2+}$ ions from the ryanodine receptor (RyR) of the sarcoplasmic reticulum (SR).

prolongs this depolarization, creating the plateau phase (phase 2) of the action potential. The $Ca^{2+}$ subsequently stimulates a receptor-operated $Ca^{2+}$ channel on the sarcoplasmic reticulum (SR), known as the ryanodine receptor, releasing $Ca^{2+}$ from the vast stores of the SR into the cytosol. This is often termed *$Ca^{2+}$-induced $Ca^{2+}$ release.* Calcium then binds troponin C, which causes a conformational change that displaces troponin and tropomyosin from actin, allowing actin and myosin to bind, resulting in a contraction (Fig. 33–1).

At therapeutic doses, the dihydropyridine CCBs such as nifedipine have little effect at the myocardium and have most of their effect at the peripheral vascular tissue; thus, they have more potent vasodilatory effects compared with the nondihydropyridine CCBs. Dihydropyridines bind the $Ca^{2+}$ channel best at less-negative membrane potentials. Because the resting potential for myocardial muscle (−90 mV) is lower than that of vascular smooth muscle (−70 mV), dihydropyridines bind preferentially in the peripheral vascular tissue.

The toxicity of CCBs is largely an extension of their therapeutic effects within the cardiovascular system. Calcium channel blocker poisoning also results in blockade of L-type $Ca^{2+}$ channels located in the pancreas. This results in decreased insulin release and hyperglycemia.

## CLINICAL MANIFESTATIONS

The hallmarks of patients with CCB poisoning are hypotension and bradycardia, which result from depression of myocardial contraction and peripheral vasodilation. Myocardial conduction is impaired, producing AV conduction abnormalities, idioventricular rhythms, and complete heart block, most commonly with nondihydropyridine poisoning. Junctional escape rhythms occur in patients with significant poisonings. The negative inotropic effects are often so profound, particularly with verapamil, that ventricular contraction is completely ablated.

Hypotension is the most common and life-threatening finding in acute CCB poisoning, caused by a combination of decreased inotropy, bradycardia, and peripheral vasodilation. Patients can present asymptomatically early after ingestion and subsequently deteriorate rapidly to severe cardiogenic shock. The associated clinical findings reflect the degree of cardiovascular compromise and hypoperfusion, particularly to the central nervous system. Early symptoms include fatigue, dizziness, and lightheadedness. Alteration in mentation in the absence of hypotension should prompt the clinician to evaluate for other causes. Severely poisoned patients manifest syncope, altered mental status, coma, and sudden death. Acute respiratory distress syndrome (ARDS) is also described with severe CCB poisoning. This is due to precapillary vasodilation with a subsequent increase in transcapillary pressure. The elevated pressure gradient results in increased capillary transudates and possible interstitial edema.

In mild to moderate overdose of dihydropyridine CCBs, the predominantly peripheral effect induces a reflex tachycardia. However, severe poisoning with any CCBs usually results in loss of receptor selectivity, resulting in bradycardia.

## DIAGNOSTIC TESTING

All patients with suspected CCB poisoning should be considered at risk for cardiovascular collapse and be evaluated with an electrocardiogram (ECG) followed by continuous cardiac and hemodynamic monitoring. A chest radiograph, pulse oximetry, end-tidal carbon dioxide ($EtCO_2$), and serum chemistry should also be obtained if any degree of hypoperfusion is suspected. Assessment of electrolytes, including magnesium, and a serum digoxin concentration in a bradycardic patient with unknown exposure history are indicated, although a careful history, if possible, may narrow down the etiology. Assays for CCB serum concentrations are not routinely available and therefore have no role in the management of patients poisoned with CCBs. Hyperglycemia is considered a poor prognostic sign in cases of severe CCB poisoning. In a retrospective study, the initial mean serum glucose concentration was 188 mg/dL (10.4 mmol/L) in patients who met a composite endpoint of requiring vasopressors, a pacemaker, or death versus 122 mg/dL (6.8 mmol/L) in those not requiring intervention.

## MANAGEMENT

### Overview

All patients with suspected CCB poisoning should undergo prompt evaluation even when the initial vital signs are normal. This urgency is due to the potential to initiate early gastrointestinal (GI) decontamination and pharmacologic therapies before patients manifest severe poisoning. Intravenous (IV) access should be obtained, and initial treatment should be directed toward GI decontamination of patients with large recent ingestions. All patients who become

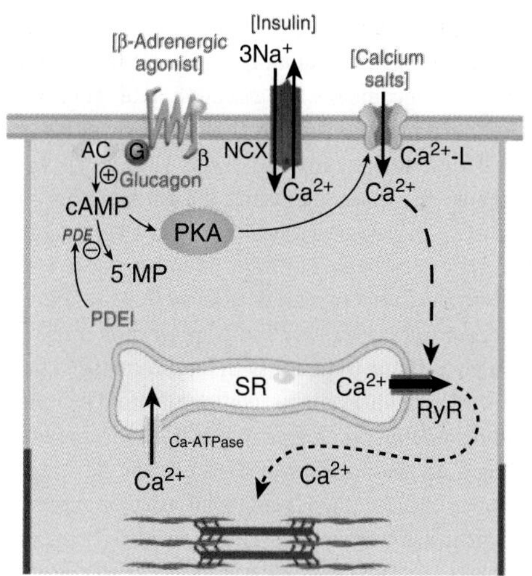


**FIGURE 33–2.** Myocardial toxicity of calcium channel blockers (CCBs) and use of antidotal therapies. Calcium channel blockers reduce calcium ion influx through the L-type $Ca^{2+}$ channel ($Ca^{2+}$-L) and thus reduce contractility. The entry of calcium via voltage-gated channels ($Ca^{2+}$-L) initiates a cascade of events that result in actin-myosin coupling and contractions. Mechanisms to increase intracellular $Ca^{2+}$ include recruitment of new or dormant $Ca^{2+}$ channels by increasing cyclic adenosine monophosphate (cAMP) by stimulating its formation by adenylate cyclase (AC) with glucagon (see text). The use of calcium salts may increase the [$Ca^{2+}$] gradient across the cellular membrane to further its influx and improve contractility. The mechanism by which insulin therapy enhances inotropy is not fully known. 5′MP = 5′-monophosphate; NCX = $Ca^{2+}$, $Na^+$ antiporter; PDEI = phosphodiesterase inhibitor; PKA = protein kinase A; RyR = ryanodine receptor; SR = sarcoplasmic reticulum.

hypotensive should initially receive a fluid bolus of 10 to 20 mL/kg of crystalloid. Caution is required because excessive fluid resuscitation should not be given to patients with congestive heart failure, evidence of ARDS, or chronic kidney disease. Pharmacotherapy should focus on maintenance or improvement of both cardiac output and peripheral vascular tone (Fig. 33–2).

## Gastrointestinal Decontamination

Because CCB poisoning is a leading cause of poisoning fatality, attempts to prevent absorption from the GI tract are recommended, assuming there are no contraindications. This is particularly important if sustained-release CCBs are ingested. Patients who present early with minimal or no symptoms can have delayed cardiovascular toxicity, which can be profound and refractory to conventional treatment, making early GI decontamination a cornerstone in CCB management.

We recommend that all patients with CCB ingestions should receive 1 g/kg of activated charcoal (AC) orally or via nasogastric tube as long as the airway is stable or protected and the patient is not vomiting. Multiple-dose activated charcoal (MDAC) (0.5 g/kg every 4–6 hours) without a cathartic is reasonable for nearly all patients with either sustained-release pill ingestions or signs of continuing absorption (Antidotes in Brief: A1).

Orogastric lavage is reasonable in the uncommon scenario when patients present early (1–2 hours postingestion) after large ingestions and for those who are critically ill and require immediate endotracheal intubation, although the effects of orogastric lavage after overdose of a sustained-release CCB are not specifically studied. If the pill or tablet size is known to be too large to fit through the pores in the orogastric tube, lavage is not recommended. When performing orogastric lavage in a CCB-poisoned patient, it is important to remember that lavage increases vagal tone and potentially exacerbates any bradydysrhythmias; we routinely pretreat with atropine. Whole-bowel irrigation (WBI) with polyethylene glycol solution (1–2 L/h orally or via nasogastric tube in adults, up to 500 mL/h in children) is reasonable for patients who ingest sustained-release products and for whom there are no contraindications (Antidotes in Brief: A2).

## Atropine

Atropine is often first-line therapy for patients with symptomatic bradycardia from xenobiotic poisoning. Unfortunately, reports of patients with severe CCB poisoning demonstrate atropine to be largely ineffective. However, given its availability, familiarity, efficacy in mild poisonings, and safety profile, atropine is recommended as initial therapy in patients with symptomatic bradycardia.

***Dose.*** The dosing of atropine for xenobiotic-induced bradycardia is similar to the dose used for Advanced Cardiac Life Support. Dosing should begin with 0.5 to 1.0 mg (minimum of 0.1 mg in children > 5 kg; 0.02 mg/kg in children) intravenously every 2 or 3 minutes up to a maximum dose of 3 mg in all patients with symptomatic bradycardia.

## Calcium

Calcium is another treatment often used for CCB poisoning to increase extracellular $Ca^{2+}$ concentration with an increase in transmembrane concentration gradient. Pretreatment with IV $Ca^{2+}$ prevents hypotension without diminishing the antidysrhythmic efficacy with therapeutic verapamil use in patients with reentrant supraventricular tachydysrhythmias. This also is observed with CCB poisoned patients for whom $Ca^{2+}$ tends to improve blood pressure more than heart rate. Unfortunately, this effect is often limited and short lived.

***Dose.*** For poisoned adults, an initial IV infusion of approximately 13 to 25 mEq of $Ca^{2+}$ (10–20 mL of 10% $CaCl_2$ or 30–60 mL of 10% $Ca^{2+}$ gluconate) is given over 10 minutes followed by repeat doses every 10 minutes up to two doses then every 20 to 60 minutes as needed. It is important to monitor $Ca^{2+}$ concentration every 30 to 60 minutes (Antidotes in Brief: A32).

## Glucagon

There are reports of both successes and failures of glucagon in CCB-poisoned patients who failed to respond to fluids, $Ca^{2+}$, or dopamine and dobutamine. We do not routinely recommend glucagon for patients with undifferentiated hypotension and bradycardia, and only use it as a temporizing measure in the critically ill while other therapies are being optimized.

***Dose.*** Dosing for glucagon is not well established. An initial dose of 3 to 5 mg IV, slowly over 3 to 5 minutes is reasonable. If there is no hemodynamic improvement within 5 minutes, retreatment with a dose of 4 to 10 mg is reasonable. The initial pediatric dose is 50 μg/kg. Because of the short half-life of glucagon, repeat doses are often required. A maintenance infusion can be initiated only if a desired effect is achieved (Antidotes in Brief: A20).

### High-Dose Insulin Therapy

High-dose insulin (HDI) therapy is the treatment of choice for patients who are severely poisoned by CCBs (Antidotes in Brief: A21). Many CCB-poisoned patients have been successfully treated with HDI therapy as demonstrated by improved hemodynamic function, mainly resulting from improved contractility, with little effect on heart rate.

***Dose.*** We recommend beginning with a bolus of 1 unit/kg of regular human insulin along with 0.5 g/kg of dextrose. If blood glucose is greater than 300 mg/dL (17 mmol/L), the dextrose bolus is unnecessary. A concentrated infusion of regular insulin (10 units/mL) should follow the bolus starting at 1 unit/kg/h titrated up to 2 units/kg/h if there is no improvement after 30 minutes. Even higher doses (10 units/kg/h) of insulin have been successfully reported, and we recommend escalating to this dose if 1 to 2 units/kg/h is not successful. A continuous dextrose infusion, beginning at 0.5 g/kg/h, should also be started. It is essential to note that the development of hypoglycemia is an indication to increase glucose delivery rather than decrease the insulin infusion rate.

### Intravenous Lipid Emulsion

The use of intravenous lipid emulsion (ILE) as an antidote is best studied for the treatment of local anesthetic systemic toxicity with expanded use for the treatment of nonlocal anesthetic overdose such as with CCBs (Antidotes in Brief: A23).

There is controversy regarding whether ILE is a valuable treatment for CCB poisoning because of inconsistently reported outcomes and the possibility that ILE enhances intestinal absorption of ingested xenobiotics. Intravenous lipid emulsion also has the potential for interfering with the circuitry of extracorporeal membrane oxygenation (ECMO) and reducing the efficacy of resuscitation medications. The Lipid Emulsion Workgroup's evidence-based recommendation on the use of ILE in CCB poisoning state that in the setting of life-threatening and non–life-threatening CCB poisoning, ILE should not be used as first-line therapy. The use of ILE is reasonable for CCB-induced severe cardiovascular toxicity that persists despite maximal treatment with standard resuscitative measures (including GI decontamination) and when ECMO and other ECLS are not available.

### Adjunctive Pharmacologic Treatment

Other pharmacotherapies are studied in the setting of CCB poisoning but have limited data and therefore we do not recommend routine use. These therapies include digoxin, levosimendan, and methylene blue (Antidotes in Brief: A43).

### Inotropes and Vasopressors

Catecholamines are often administered after first-line therapy, such as when atropine, $Ca^{2+}$, glucagon, and isotonic fluids, fail. There are numerous cases that describe either success or failure with various inotropes and vasopressors, including epinephrine, norepinephrine, dopamine, isoproterenol, dobutamine, and vasopressin. Based on experimental and clinical data, no single inotrope or vasopressor is consistently effective. Experimental data show that all vasopressors are generally inferior to HDI with significantly more adverse effects such as tissue ischemia with long-term use. That being said, they are readily available, commonly used by most clinicians, and sometimes effective. While it is reasonable to start inotropes and vasopressors in the critically ill, the authors recommend against their prolonged use in patients with poor myocardial contractility. This is most likely to occur in patients who have taken nondihydropyridine calcium channel blockers. High-dose insulin is recommended for patients with impaired perfusion that is refractory to large doses of vasopressors even when there is no associated poor contractility.

### Adjunctive Hemodynamic Support

The most severely CCB-poisoned patients will not respond to any pharmacologic intervention. Transthoracic or IV cardiac pacing is reasonable in an attempt to improve heart rate, but failure to achieve electrical capture and increases in the heart rate with no effect on blood pressure are well reported. Intraaortic balloon pump (IABP) is another invasive supportive option that is reasonable to attempt in CCB poisoning refractory to pharmacologic therapy. Because IABPs are ECG gated, in patients with very low heart rates, IABP often fails to increase cardiac output. Severely CCB-poisoned patients have also been supported for days and subsequently recovered fully with much more invasive technology such as extracorporeal membrane oxygenation (ECMO) and emergent open and percutaneous cardiopulmonary bypass. The advantage of ECMO over IABP is that it is independent of cardiac electrical and mechanical activity.

## DISPOSITION

Patients who manifest signs or symptoms of toxicity should be admitted to an intensive care setting. Because of the potential for delayed toxicity, patients who ingest sustained-release products should be admitted for 24 hours to a monitored setting even if they are asymptomatic. Criteria for safe discharge or medical stability apply only to patients with a reliable history of an ingestion of an "immediate-release" preparation who have received adequate GI decontamination, who are asymptomatic and have had serial ECGs over 6 to 8 hours that have remained unchanged.

# A21 HIGH-DOSE INSULIN

## HISTORY

Insulin was discovered and named in 1922, but it took 30 years before its first clinical use. In the past 2 decades, insulin has gained increased attention and importance in the management of a spectrum of critical illnesses, including sepsis, heart failure, and cardiovascular drug toxicity. The benefits of insulin go well beyond simple glucose control. In xenobiotic-induced myocardial depression, the use of high-dose insulin (HDI) can mitigate toxicity.

## PHARMACOLOGY

### Chemistry and Physiology

The hallmarks of severe β-adrenergic antagonist (BAA) and calcium channel blocker (CCB) toxicity are bradycardia and decreased inotropy that compromise cardiac output and produce cardiogenic shock. In some cases, peripheral vasodilation also occurs, especially in the context of dihydropyridine CCB ingestions. Associated metabolic derangements resemble diabetes with hyperglycemia, insulin deficiency, insulin resistance, and acidemia. The nonstressed heart primarily catabolize's free fatty acids for its energy needs. However, the stressed myocardium switches its preferred energy substrate to carbohydrates. The greater the degree of shock, the greater the carbohydrate demand. The liver responds to stress by making more glucose available via glycogenolysis but this is a limited process. As a result, blood glucose concentrations increase temporarily. Hyperglycemia is noted both in animal models and in human cases of some cardiac drug overdoses, and the degree of hyperglycemia correlates directly with the severity of shock resulting from verapamil and diltiazem. Calcium channel blockers directly inhibit pancreatic calcium channels to inhibit insulin release. They also create a state of insulin resistance by interfering with glucose transporter 1 (GLUT-1) and phosphatidylinositol 3-kinase (PI3K) glucose transport. As a result of diminished circulating insulin and inhibited enzymatic glucose uptake, glucose movement into cells becomes concentration dependent and insufficient to support myocardial demand in CCB poisoning.

### Mechanism of Action

High-dose insulin therapy supports the metabolic demands associated with cardiogenic shock and augments calcium processing, thereby increasing myocardial contractility and improving tissue perfusion. Insulin-mediated improved contractility appears to be a critical factor leading to survival from cardiogenic shock. Insulin improves drug-induced cardiac function and work efficiency. Interestingly, in BAA and CCB studies using HDI, survival occurs without dramatic improvement in hypotension or bradycardia, which may be due to the vasodilatory properties of insulin. These vasodilatory effects occur in the systemic, coronary, and pulmonary vasculature. The mechanism is likely due to activation of the PI3K pathway enhancing endothelial nitric oxide synthase (eNOS) activity. Vasodilation in concert with improved cardiac contractility allows for improved tissue perfusion. There is also evidence that insulin exerts an effect beyond enhanced carbohydrate usage via direct effects on calcium and, to a lesser extent, potassium and sodium ion homeostasis. Insulin increases available intracellular calcium by enhancing reverse mode sodium–calcium exchange, with a resultant increase in the sarcoplasmic reticulum (SR) calcium load, thus causing increased contractility.

### Pharmacokinetics and Pharmacodynamics

Regular insulin administered as HDI therapy is given intravenously, so gastrointestinal absorption is not an issue. The peak plasma concentration is essentially immediate. The onset and peak of the cardiovascular effect of insulin is roughly 15 to 40 minutes. Insulin is slightly soluble in water, has a volume of distribution of roughly 21 L in an adult human, and demonstrates protein binding of roughly 5%, which can increase in a patient with diabetes with insulin antibodies. More than half of insulin metabolism occurs in the liver, but there is also a sizable degree that occurs in adipose tissue, muscle, and the kidneys. The elimination half-life of conventional doses of intravenously administered insulin is roughly 5 to 10 minutes, and it is partially eliminated in both the kidneys and the bile.

## ROLE IN DRUG-INDUCED CARDIOVASCULAR TOXICITY

Based on the experimental studies and aggregate human cases, HDI will most likely benefit patients with cardiac drug-induced myocardial depression. High-dose insulin is recommended for patients with impaired perfusion that is refractory to large doses of vasopressors even when there is no associated poor contractility. Myocardial function should be measured or estimated. Options include cardiac ultrasonography or through machine-estimated cardiac output using pulse contour analysis attached to a standard arterial catheter. Myocardial function can also be measured more invasively via placement of a pulmonary artery catheter.

The predominant clinical effect of insulin is increased cardiac contractility with subsequent improvement in perfusion, often without initial increase in blood pressure. Contractility typically increases within 15 to 40 minutes after initiating insulin and often allows for a decrease in concurrent vasopressor use, sparing the toxicity of these xenobiotics.

## ADVERSE EVENTS AND SAFETY ISSUES

The major anticipated adverse event associated with the use of high doses of insulin is hypoglycemia. Although hypoglycemia is a potential consequence of HDI therapy, clinically significant hypoglycemia is rare. A combination of rigorous glucose monitoring and dextrose administration can prevent hypoglycemia and avoid unnecessary cessation of insulin treatment. Patients typically received empiric supplemental dextrose based on frequent glucose monitoring. There is likely a ceiling requirement for dextrose as glucose transport is saturable. A typical dextrose dose is 25 g/h, which is often necessary beyond cessation of insulin for most cases.

Another anticipated consequence of insulin treatment is hypokalemia. Although serum potassium concentrations often decrease below normal laboratory ranges, HDI does not typically cause profound hypokalemia. The observed decrease reflects a shifting of potassium from the extracellular to intracellular space that occurs as a result of the action of insulin. Patients maintain normal total body potassium stores and do not experience true deficiency unless they have other reasons for potassium loss. There is a theoretical risk of excessive potassium replacement in the instance of lowered serum potassium but normal total body stores. Other observed ion changes during insulin therapy include hypomagnesemia and hypophosphatemia.

## PREGNANCY AND LACTATION

Regular insulin is United States Food and Drug Administration Pregnancy Category B and is compatible with breastfeeding.

## DOSING AND ADMINISTRATION

Based on experimental and clinical experience, we recommend using HDI early in the resuscitation of severe BAA- and CCB-induced myocardial depression. This recommendation is supported by multidisciplinary consensus guidelines. It is also reasonable to use HDI for other xenobiotic-induced cardiogenic shock that is failing resuscitation with inotropes and vasopressors. When myocardial function is decreased, insulin therapy is initiated by first administering a 1-unit/kg bolus of regular human insulin along with 0.5-g/kg bolus of dextrose; if blood glucose is greater than 300 mg/dL (16.7 mmol/L), the dextrose bolus is not necessary. An infusion of regular insulin should immediately follow the bolus starting at 1 unit/kg/h. Ideally, this insulin infusion should be concentrated to prevent fluid overload that would occur with large doses. We typically concentrate the infusion at 10 unit/mL compared with the typical insulin infusion concentration of 1 unit/mL used for diabetic ketoacidosis. This unusual pharmacy formulation requires close collaboration with hospital pharmacists. Concentrated insulin solutions are stable for 14 days. A continuous dextrose infusion, beginning at 0.5 g/kg/h, is concurrently recommended when necessary. Dextrose can be started as $D_{10}W$, especially without central venous access and while determining the dextrose need, but it is ultimately best delivered as $D_{25}W$ and $D_{50}W$ via central venous access, also with the intent to lessen large fluid volumes that would otherwise be necessary with administration of more dilute dextrose solutions.

If possible, cardiac function should be reassessed every 10 to 15 minutes after starting HDI therapy. If cardiac function remains depressed, then the insulin dose should be increased. Although we typically recommend increasing the dose of insulin to a maximum of 10 units/kg/h, doses up to 22 units/kg/h have been used, and the maximum dose is not established. The blood glucose should be monitored every 15 to 30 minutes until stable and then every 1 to 2 hours. The dextrose infusion should be increased to maintain blood glucose concentrations of 100 to 180 mg/dL (5.5–10 mmol/L) rather than reducing the insulin.

The serum potassium concentration should be measured during HDI therapy. If it is low, especially when potassium loss is suspected, then supplementation is indicated to maintain the concentration in the "mildly hypokalemic" range (2.8–3.2 mEq/L). A reasonable time frame is to evaluate serum potassium hourly while actively titrating the insulin infusion and every 6 hours after the infusion rate is stabilized. Magnesium and phosphorus should also be measured and supplemented as indicated.

The ultimate goal of HDI is improvement in organ perfusion as demonstrated by increased cardiac output, improved mental status, adequate urine output, and reversal of metabolic abnormalities, as indicated by improved serum lactate, bicarbonate, pH, and base excess. This improvement is often, but not always, accompanied by an improvement in mean arterial blood pressure. Because insulin improves both cardiac function and perfusion while slightly vasodilating, treatment goals should focus more on organ perfusion and outcome as opposed to simply the numerical blood pressure.

The typical duration of therapy is 1 to 2 days, although HDI has been used for up to 4 days. We recommend reducing the insulin infusion rate by 1 unit/kg/h after the patient has stabilized and reassessing hourly for additional infusion reduction while maintaining adequate perfusion. In many patients, the dextrose infusion will continue to be necessary after the insulin is reduced and ultimately eliminated. The reduction of insulin and dextrose will cause potassium shifting, which should also be monitored.

# 34 OTHER ANTIHYPERTENSIVES

As our understanding of the medical complications of chronic hypertension has grown, an increasing number of antihypertensive drugs have become available (Table 34–1). Most of the adverse effects and toxicity in overdose are exaggerated pharmacologic effects.

## CLONIDINE AND OTHER CENTRALLY ACTING ANTIHYPERTENSIVES

Clonidine is an imidazoline compound that has potent $\alpha_2$-adrenergic agonist effects. Clonidine is the best understood and the most commonly used of all the centrally acting antihypertensives, a group that includes methyldopa, guanfacine, and guanabenz. Although these drugs differ chemically and structurally, they all decrease blood pressure in a similar manner—by reducing the sympathetic outflow from the central nervous system (CNS). Although the use of clonidine as an antihypertensive has decreased, it has found a wide variety of new applications including in attention deficit hyperactivity disorder (ADHD), peripheral nerve and spinal anesthesia, and the management of substance withdrawal.

**TABLE 34–1 Antihypertensives and Pharmacologically Related Xenobiotics**

| |
|---|
| β-Adrenergic antagonists (Chap. 32) |
| Calcium channel blockers (Chap. 33) |
| Sympatholytics (antagonize α-adrenergic vasoconstriction) |
| Central $\alpha_2$-adrenergic agonists |
| Clonidine, dexmedetomidine, guanabenz,[a] guanfacine,[a] methyldopa,[a] tizanidine |
| Central imidazoline agonists |
| Moxonidine, rilmenidine |
| Ganglionic blockers |
| Trimethaphan[a] |
| Peripheral adrenergic neuron antagonists |
| Guanadrel,[a] metyrosine,[a] reserpine[a] |
| Peripheral $\alpha_1$-adrenergic antagonists |
| Doxazosin, prazosin, silodosin, terazosin |
| Diuretics |
| Thiazides |
| Bendroflumethiazide,[a] chlorthalidone,[a] chlorothiazide, hydrochlorothiazide, hydroflumethiazide,[a] indapamide, methyclothiazide,[a] metolazone, polythiazide,[a] trichlormethiazide[a] |
| Loop diuretics |
| Bumetanide, ethacrynic acid, furosemide, torsemide |
| Potassium-sparing diuretics |
| Amiloride, eplerenone, spironolactone, triamterene |
| Vasodilators |
| Diazoxide,[a] hydralazine, minoxidil,[a] nitroprusside |
| Angiotensin-converting enzyme inhibitor |
| Benazepril, captopril, enalapril, fosinopril, lisinopril, moexipril, perindopril, quinapril, ramipril, spirapril, trandolapril |
| Angiotensin II receptor blockers |
| Azilsartan, candesartan, eprosartan, irbesartan, losartan, olmesartan, telmisartan, valsartan |
| Direct renin inhibitors |
| Aliskiren |

[a]Included for historical reference; use as an antihypertensive is limited in the United States.

### Pharmacology

Clonidine and the other centrally acting antihypertensives exert their hypotensive effects primarily by stimulating two sets of receptors: presynaptic $\alpha_2$-adrenergic receptors and imidazoline receptors. Central $\alpha_2$-adrenergic receptor agonism enhances the activity of inhibitory neurons in the vasoregulatory regions of the CNS, including the locus ceruleus, resulting in decreased norepinephrine release. Central agonism by imidazolines results in decreased sympathetic outflow to the periphery and reduces the heart rate, vascular tone, and, ultimately, arterial blood pressure. Imidazolines also have profound effects at imidazoline receptors, one of their primary sites of action. There are three recognized classes of imidazoline receptors. Imidazoline-1 ($I_1$) receptors mediate hypotensive effects of imidazolines by functioning upstream from presynaptic $\alpha_2$-adrenergic receptors, likely in addition to other physiologic effects. Imidazoline-2 ($I_2$) receptors are involved in pain perception modulation and interact with monoamine oxidases A and B. Imidazoline-3 ($I_3$) receptors have effects on glucose homeostasis within pancreatic β-islet cells. Clonidine also has opioidlike effects that are mediated through $I_2$ receptors and through the release of β-endorphin, which directly stimulates opioid receptors.

### Pharmacokinetics

Clonidine is well absorbed from the GI tract (approximately 75%) with an onset of action within 30 to 60 minutes. The plasma concentration peaks at 2 to 3 hours and lasts as long as 8 hours.

Clonidine has 20% to 40% protein binding (primarily to albumin) and an apparent volume of distribution of 3.2 to 5.6 L/kg. Nearly half of clonidine is eliminated unchanged via the kidneys. The remained is hydroxylated by multiple hepatic enzymes.

The patch formulation of clonidine allows slow, continuous delivery of drug over a prolonged period of time, typically 1 week. Each patch contains significantly more drug than is delivered during the prescribed duration of use, and much of the drug remains in the patch after discontinuing its use. Both of these issues raise concern for overdose.

Guanabenz and guanfacine are structurally and pharmacologically very similar. They are well absorbed orally, achieving peak concentrations within 3 to 5 hours, and both have large volumes of distribution (4–6 L/kg for guanfacine and 7–17 L/kg for guanabenz). Guanabenz is metabolized predominantly in the liver and undergoes extensive first-pass effect, whereas guanfacine is eliminated equally by the liver and kidney. Neither drug has significant active metabolites.

Methyldopa is a prodrug that requires conversion to α-methylnorepinephrine for activity. Approximately 50% of an oral dose of methyldopa is absorbed and peak serum concentrations are achieved in 2 to 3 hours. Methyldopa has a small volume of distribution (0.24 L/kg) and little protein binding (15%). It is eliminated in the urine, both as parent compound and after hepatic sulfation.

### Pathophysiology

In therapeutic oral dosing, clonidine and the other centrally acting antihypertensives have little effect on the peripheral $\alpha_2$ receptors or the peripheral sympathetic nervous system. However, when serum concentrations increase as in overdose, peripheral postsynaptic $\alpha_2$-adrenergic stimulation occurs, producing temporary vasoconstriction and hypertension. Shortly afterward, however, potent centrally mediated sympathetic inhibition becomes the predominant effect, and bradycardia with hypotension ensues.

### Clinical Manifestations

Although the majority of the published cases involve clonidine, the signs and symptoms of poisoning with any centrally acting antihypertensive are similar. The CNS and cardiovascular toxicity reflect an exaggeration of their pharmacologic action. Common signs include CNS depression, bradycardia, hypotension, and occasionally hypothermia. Most patients who ingest clonidine and the other similarly acting drugs will manifest symptoms rapidly, usually within 30 to 90 minutes. The exception may be methyldopa, which requires metabolism to be activated, possibly delaying the onset of toxicity beyond 2 hours.

Central nervous system depression is the most frequent clinical finding and can vary from mild lethargy to coma. Respirations are often slow and shallow with intermittent deep sighing breaths. The CNS and respiratory depression typically resolves over 12 to 36 hours. Other manifestations of this CNS depression include hypotonia, hyporeflexia, and irritability.

Sinus bradycardia, usually associated with hypotension, is common following overdose. Other conduction abnormalities including first-degree heart block, Wenckebach block, 2:1 atrioventricular block, and complete heart block are described both in overdose and after therapeutic dosing.

Paradoxically, severe hypertension may occur early in dosing, particularly during intravenous administration, or in massive overdoses. Typically, this hypertensive effect is short-lived, as the central sympatholytic effects become predominant and hypotension ensues. However, in patients with massive ingestions, protracted hypertension requires pharmacologic intervention.

Hypothermia is associated with overdoses involving centrally acting antihypertensives, likely a result of $\alpha$-adrenergic effects within the thermoregulatory center. Fatalities are rare. This may be because these drugs effectively block all sympathetic outflow from the CNS and this physiologic effect is not essential for life. The CNS depression resulting in hypoventilation, hypoxia, and poor airway protection may be more pronounced in fatalities.

### Diagnostic Testing

Because clonidine and other centrally acting antihypertensives are not routinely included in serum or urine toxicologic assays, management decisions should be based on clinical parameters. No electrolyte or hematologic abnormalities are associated with this exposure. Because of the potential for bradydysrhythmias and hypoventilation, an electrocardiogram (ECG) and continuous cardiac and pulse oximetry monitoring are recommended during the assessment.

### Management

Appropriate therapy begins with particular focus on the patient's respiratory and hemodynamic status. Administration of activated charcoal (AC) is the primary mode of GI decontamination in most cases of ingestion; however, altered mental status and severe respiratory depression typically limit the ability to administer AC. Patients often present following the onset of symptoms rather than immediately after ingestion, and patients respond well to supportive care. In cases involving clonidine patch ingestions, whole-bowel irrigation (WBI) is a reasonable intervention.

All patients with CNS depression should be evaluated for hypoxia and hypoglycemia. Respiratory compromise, including apnea, often responds well to simple auditory or tactile stimulation. Significant arousal during preparation for intubation often precludes the need for mechanical ventilation. Endotracheal intubation should be performed in patients who fail to arouse to stimuli or those with evidence of airway compromise. Patients with isolated hypotension should initially be treated with IV boluses of crystalloid. Bradycardia is typically mild and well tolerated, but if symptomatic bradycardia occurs, atropine is recommended and is usually effective.

Clonidine-poisoned patients, particularly children, often show increased arousal, respiratory effort, heart rate, and blood pressure after naloxone administration. Because of the short duration of effects of naloxone (20–60 minutes), redosing or continuous infusions are often required. As with some synthetic opioids, clinical improvement sometimes occurs only after high doses (4–10 mg) of naloxone, and some patients have no response regardless of dose used.

Early-onset hypertension in imidazoline toxicity is typically self-limited, and therapy should be cautiously undertaken. If hypertension is severe or prolonged, treatment with a short-acting and titratable antihypertensive such as IV nicardipine is reasonable.

### Withdrawal

Abrupt cessation of central antihypertensive therapy results in withdrawal, which is characterized by excessive sympathetic activity. Symptoms include agitation, insomnia, tremor, palpitations, and hypertension that begin between 16 and 48 hours after cessation of therapy. Ventricular tachycardia, myocardial stunning, and myocardial infarction are reported. Although this phenomenon is associated with all centrally acting $\alpha_2$-agonists, it appears to be most prominent in the shorter acting clonidine and guanabenz. Reasonable treatment strategies include administering oral clonidine, followed by a closely monitored tapering of the dosing over several weeks, or use of benzodiazepines.

## CENTRAL IMIDAZOLINE AGONISTS

Moxonidine and related rilmenidine are second-generation centrally acting oral antihypertensives. They selectively attach at $I_1$ imidazoline binding sites with much less affinity for the $\alpha_2$-adrenergic receptor. Therapeutically, moxonidine is used both as monotherapy or in combination with other antihypertensives. Case reports of seizures (resolving with benzodiazepines) without development of hypotension suggest the possibility of peripheral effects similar to clonidine in overdose. Dexmedetomidine is a centrally acting imidazoline agonist used for sedation in intensive care settings. In contrast to moxonidine and rilmenidine, dexmedetomidine is highly selective for the $\alpha_2$-adrenergic receptor and has profound sedating, analgesic-sparing, and sympatholytic effects. Side effects include bradycardia and hypotension. Tachycardia, agitation, and hypertension are reported following dexmedetomidine withdrawal and can be treated with either oral clonidine or resumption of dexmedetomidine based on the patient's clinical status.

## OTHER SYMPATHOLYTIC ANTIHYPERTENSIVES

Several other antihypertensives decrease the effects of the sympathetic nervous system. Often termed *sympatholytics*, they can be classified as ganglionic blockers, presynaptic adrenergic neuron antagonists, or $\alpha_1$-adrenergic antagonists, depending on their mechanism of action. These drugs are rarely used clinically and little is known about their effects in overdose.

### Presynaptic Adrenergic Neuron Antagonists

These drugs exert their sympatholytic action by decreasing norepinephrine release from presynaptic nerve terminals. In overdose, an extension of their pharmacologic effects is expected. Severe orthostatic hypotension should be anticipated and treated with intravenous crystalloid boluses and a direct-acting vasopressor. If reserpine is involved, significant CNS depression should also be anticipated.

### Peripheral $\alpha_1$-Adrenergic Antagonists

The selective $\alpha_1$-adrenergic antagonists include prazosin, terazosin, and doxazosin. The $\alpha_1$-receptor is a postsynaptic receptor primarily located on vascular smooth muscle, although it is also found in the eye and in the gastrointestinal (GI) and genitourinary tracts. In overdose, hypotension and CNS depression ranging from lethargy to coma are reported. Treatment of peripheral $\alpha_1$-adrenergic agonist overdose includes supportive care, IV crystalloid boluses, and a vasopressor, with phenylephrine being a logical initial choice.

## DIRECT VASODILATORS

### Hydralazine, Minoxidil, and Diazoxide

These drugs produce vascular smooth muscle relaxation independent of innervation or known pharmacologic receptors that is attributed to stimulation of nitric oxide release from vascular endothelial cells. As vasodilation occurs, the baroreceptor reflexes, which remain intact, produce an increased sympathetic outflow to the myocardium, resulting in an increase in heart rate and contractile force. Hydralazine, minoxidil, and diazoxide are effective orally. Minoxidil is also used topically in a 2% solution to promote hair growth, and ingestion can cause significant poisoning. Diazoxide, although previously used to rapidly reduce blood pressure in hypertensive emergencies, is rarely used.

Adverse effects associated with daily hydralazine use include several immunologic phenomena such as hemolytic anemia, vasculitis, acute glomerulonephritis, and most notably a lupus-like syndrome. The common toxic manifestations of these xenobiotics in overdose are an extension of their pharmacologic action. Symptoms include lightheadedness, syncope, palpitations, and nausea. Signs include tachycardia alone or with flushing or alterations in mental status, typically related to the degree of hypotension.

In the case of hydralazine, minoxidil, or diazoxide overdose, GI decontamination with AC is reasonable followed by routine supportive care, with special consideration to maintaining adequate mean arterial pressure. If intravenous crystalloid boluses are insufficient, then a peripherally acting $\alpha$-adrenergic agonist, such as norepinephrine or phenylephrine, is reasonable as the next therapy. Dopamine and epinephrine should be avoided to prevent an exaggerated myocardial response and tachycardia from $\beta$-adrenergic stimulation.

### Nitroprusside

Sodium nitroprusside is effectively a prodrug, exerting its vasodilatory effects only after its breakdown and the release of nitric oxide. The nitroprusside molecule also contains five cyanide radicals that, although gradually released, occasionally produce cyanide or thiocyanate toxicity. This cyanide detoxification process in healthy adults is not usually exceeded at a sodium nitroprusside infusion rate of 2 μg/kg/min. A variety of factors including poor nutrition, critical illness, surgery, diuretic use, and young age place patients at risk for developing cyanide toxicity. Therefore, depending on the balance of cyanide release and the rate of cyanide detoxification, cyanide toxicity can develop within hours. Infusion rates greater than 4 μg/kg/min of nitroprusside for longer than 12 hours are expected to overwhelm the capacity for detoxifying cyanide. Signs and symptoms of cyanide toxicity include alteration in mental status; anion gap metabolic acidosis; elevated lactate concentration; and in late stages, hemodynamic instability. If cyanide poisoning does occur, hydroxycobalamin is the current treatment of choice (Chap. 96).

One method of preventing cyanide toxicity from sodium nitroprusside is to expand the thiosulfate pool available for detoxification by the concomitant administration of sodium thiosulfate. Dosing of 1 g of sodium thiosulfate for every 100 mg of nitroprusside is typically sufficient to prevent cyanide accumulation. Thiocyanate thus formed is either renally eliminated or accumulates in patients with chronic kidney disease (CKD) or acute kidney injury (AKI), and produces thiocyanate toxicity. The signs and symptoms of thiocyanate toxicity begin to appear at serum concentrations of 60 μg/mL (1 mmol/L) and are very nonspecific, ranging from nausea, vomiting, fatigue, and dizziness to confusion, delirium, and seizures. Severe thiocyanate toxicity causes life-threatening effects, such as hypotension with intracranial pressure elevation, when serum concentrations are above 200 μg/mL. Hemodialysis clears thiocyanate from the serum; patients with significant clinical manifestations of thiocyanate toxicity benefit from hemodialysis.

Another therapy used to prevent cyanide toxicity from sodium nitroprusside is a simultaneous infusion of hydroxocobalamin. Dosing of 25 mg/h has successfully reduced cyanide toxicity in humans. As with thiosulfate, simultaneous infusion of hydroxocobalamin does not interfere with the vasodilatory effects of sodium nitroprusside. Because of the relative higher cost of hydroxocobalamin as well its interactions with some laboratory tests, thiosulfate should remain the mainstay of prophylaxis against sodium nitroprusside–induced cyanide toxicity (Antidotes in Brief: A41 and A42).

## DIURETICS

Diuretics are divided into three main groups: (1) the thiazides and related compounds, including hydrochlorothiazide and chlorthalidone; (2) the loop diuretics, including furosemide, bumetanide, and ethacrynic acid; and (3) the potassium-sparing diuretics, including amiloride, triamterene, and spironolactone. Two other groups of diuretics, the carbonic anhydrase inhibitors, such as acetazolamide, and osmotic diuretics, such as mannitol, are not used as antihypertensive therapy.

The thiazides produce their diuretic effect by inhibition of sodium and chloride reabsorption in the distal convoluted tubule. Loop diuretics, in contrast, inhibit the coupled transport of sodium, potassium, and chloride in the thick ascending limb of the loop of Henle.

The most common toxicity associated with diuretics is metabolic alkalosis and occurs during chronic therapy or overuse. Hyponatremia (< 120 mEq/L) presents as headache, nausea, vomiting, confusion, seizures, or coma. Other electrolyte abnormalities include hypokalemia and hypomagnesemia, which may precipitate ventricular dysrhythmias and sudden death.

Despite the widespread use of these drugs, acute overdoses are distinctly rare. Major signs and symptoms include GI distress, brisk diuresis, possible hypovolemia and electrolyte abnormalities, and altered mental status. Assessment focuses on fluid and electrolyte status, which should be corrected as needed.

## ANGIOTENSIN-CONVERTING ENZYME INHIBITORS

Angiotensin-converting enzyme (ACE) inhibitors (ACEIs) are among the most widely prescribed antihypertensives. In general, these drugs are well absorbed from the GI tract, reaching peak serum concentrations within 1 to 4 hours. Enalapril and ramipril are prodrugs and require hepatic metabolism to produce their active forms. These drugs are primarily eliminated via the kidneys.

All ACEIs bind directly to the active site of angiotensin-converting enzyme, which is found in the lung and vascular endothelium, preventing the conversion of angiotensin I to angiotensin II. Because angiotensin II is a potent vasoconstrictor and stimulant of aldosterone secretion, vasodilation, decreased peripheral vascular resistance, decreased blood pressure, increased cardiac output, and a relative increase in renal, cerebral, and coronary blood flow occur.

### Management

The toxicity of ACEIs in overdose appears to be limited. Hypotension occurs in select patients but deaths are rarely reported in isolated ACEI ingestions. Treatment is supportive and symptomatic. Activated charcoal alone is sufficient in most cases and should be given as long as no contraindications exist. Intravenous crystalloid boluses are often effective in correcting hypotension, although in rare cases, catecholamines are required. Although the role of naloxone in the setting of ACEI overdose remains unclear, a trial of naloxone is reasonable in opioid-naïve patients. Case reports suggest success with IV angiotensin II in patients with refractory hypotension.

## ANGIOTENSIN-CONVERTING ENZYME INHIBITOR–INDUCED ANGIOEDEMA

The pathogenesis of acquired angioedema involves multiple vasoactive substances, including histamine, prostaglandin $D_2$, leukotrienes, and bradykinin. Because ACE also inactivates bradykinin and substance P, ACE inhibition results in elevations in bradykinin concentrations that appear to be the primary cause of both ACEI angioedema and cough (Fig. 34–1). Unlike anaphylaxis, there is no evidence that the ACEI angioedema phenomenon is immunoglobulin E (IgE) mediated, although these two entities can be difficult to differentiate clinically. The overall incidence is only approximately 0.1%, and one-third of these reactions occur within hours of the first dose, and another third occurs within the first week. Women, African Americans, and patients with a history of idiopathic angioedema appear to be at greater risk.

Treatment varies depending on the severity and rapidity of the swelling. Because of its propensity to involve the tongue, face, and oropharynx, the airway must remain the primary focus of management. A nasopharyngeal airway is often helpful. If there is any potential for or suggestion of airway compromise, then early endotracheal intubation should be performed. Fiberoptic intubation or other rescue

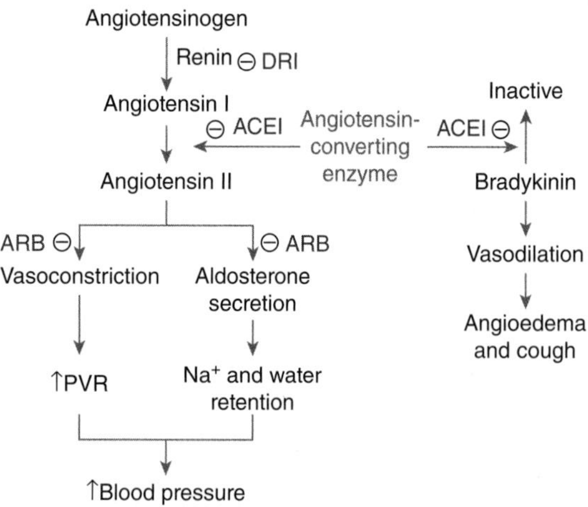


**FIGURE 34–1.** An overview of the normal function of the renin-angiotensin-aldosterone system (RAAS) and the mechanisms of action of angiotensin-converting enzyme inhibitors (ACEIs), angiotensin II receptor blockers (ARBs), and direct renin inhibitors (DRIs) on that system. PVR = peripheral vascular resistance.

techniques are often required because of tongue swelling. Because ACEI angioedema is not an IgE-mediated phenomenon, pharmacologic therapy targeting an allergic cascade such as epinephrine, diphenhydramine, and corticosteroids should not be expected to be effective. However, when the history is unclear, these medications should not be withheld to ensure providing life-saving therapy to someone having a severe IgE-mediated allergic reaction.

Newer potential treatment modalities target various points along the cascade of events associated with hereditary angioedema such as the bradykinin receptor antagonist icatibant. Fresh-frozen plasma (FFP) is also described to reverse or slow the progression of both hereditary and ACEI angioedema because it contains kinase II, which acts as an ACE and thus leads to the degradation of accumulated bradykinin. Doses range from 1 to 5 units of FFP (200–250 mL/unit) with most using an infusion of 2 units of FFP as initial, and typically definitive, treatment. All patients with mild or rapidly resolving angioedema should be observed for several hours to ensure that the swelling does not progress or return. If FFP is unavailable or contraindicated success is reported with tranexamic acid (1-2g IV) is reasonable. Patients developing angioedema from ACEI therapy should be instructed to discontinue them permanently and to consult their primary care physicians about other antihypertensive options. Because this is a mechanistic and not allergic adverse effect, the use of any other ACEIs is contraindicated.

## ANGIOTENSIN II RECEPTOR BLOCKERS

These drugs are rapidly absorbed from the GI tract, reaching peak serum concentrations in 1 to 4 hours, and they are either eliminated unchanged in the feces, or, after undergoing hepatic metabolism via CYP3A4 and CYP2C9, are eliminated in the bile. The ARBs block whereas the ACEIs decrease the formation of angiotensin II, they act by antagonizing angiotensin II at the type 1 angiotensin (AT-1) receptor (Fig. 34–1). Despite the mechanistic evidence that ARBs do not affect bradykinin, rare serious cases of angioedema associated with ARB therapy are reported.

There are few published reports of isolated overdoses involving ARBs. Adverse signs and symptoms reflect orthostatic or absolute hypotension and include palpitations, diaphoresis, dizziness, lethargy, or confusion. Hypotension should be treated with crystalloid boluses and catecholamine therapy. One theoretical treatment for hypotension produced by ARBs and ACEIs is methylene blue (Antidotes in Brief: A43). A reasonable starting dose of methylene blue, when used as a vasopressor, is 2 mg/kg with subsequent intermittent boluses or possibly continuous infusions starting at 0.5 mg/kg/h with a maximum daily dose of 7 mg/kg.

## DIRECT RENIN INHIBITORS

Direct renin inhibitors such as aliskiren exert their antihypertensive effects by inhibiting circulating renin in the renin–angiotensin–aldosterone system (RAAS). Aliskiren is well tolerated and is an effective antihypertensive both as monotherapy and in combination with other antihypertensives, including hydrochlorothiazide, CCBs, and β-adrenergic antagonists. However, aliskiren is contraindicated in patients receiving ARBs or ACEIs because of an increase in adverse vascular events. There are no reported overdoses; however, hypotension should be anticipated and treatment that includes supportive care, including IV crystalloid and catecholamines, seems reasonable.

# 35 CARDIOACTIVE STEROIDS

## HISTORY AND EPIDEMIOLOGY

In 1785, William Withering wrote the first systematic account about the effects of the foxglove plant. Foxglove, the most common source of plant cardioactive steroids (CASs) was initially used as a diuretic and for the treatment of "dropsy" (edema) and Withering eloquently described its "power over the motion of the heart, to a degree yet unobserved in any other medicine." In the past, CASs were the primary treatment for congestive heart failure and control of ventricular response rate in atrial tachydysrhythmias. Because of their narrow therapeutic index, acute and chronic toxicities remain important problems.

Most cases of pharmaceutically induced CAS toxicity encountered in the United States result from digoxin; other internationally available but much less commonly used preparations are digitoxin, ouabain, lanatoside C, deslanoside, and gitalin. Cardioactive steroid toxicity also results from exposure to certain plants or animals, including oleander (*Nerium oleander*); yellow oleander (*Thevetia peruviana*), which is implicated in the suicidal deaths of thousands of patients in Southeast Asia; foxglove (*Digitalis* spp); lily of the valley (*Convallaria majalis*); common milkweed (*Asclepias syriaca*); sea mango (*Cerbera manghas*); dogbane (*Apocynum cannabinum*); and red squill (*Urginea maritima*). Toxicity has resulted from ingestion of the dried secretion of toads from the *Bufo* species, which contains a bufadienolide-class CAS. Although there have been no reported human exposures, fireflies of the *Photinus* species (*P. ignitus*, *P. marginellu*, and *P. pyralis)* contain the CAS lucibufagin, which is structurally a bufadienolide.

## CHEMISTRY

Cardioactive steroids contain an aglycone or "genin" nucleus structure with a steroid core and an unsaturated lactone ring attached at C-17. Cardioactive glycosides contain additional sugar groups attached to C-3. The sugar residues confer increased water solubility and enhance the ability of the molecule to enter cells. Cardenolides are primarily plant-derived aglycones with a five-membered unsaturated lactone ring. The bufadienolide and lucibufagin groups of CAS molecules are mainly animal derived and contain a six-membered unsaturated lactone ring. Thus, when the aglycone digoxigenin is linked to one or more hydrophilic sugar (digitoxoses) moieties at C-3, it forms digoxin, a cardiac glycoside (Fig. 35–1).

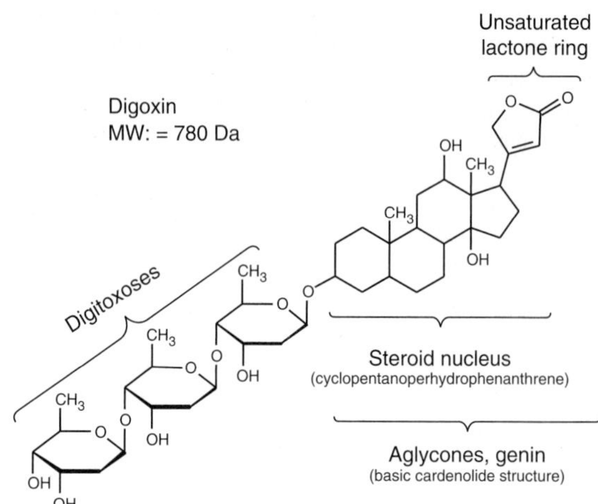


**FIGURE 35–1.** The chemical composition of cardioactive steroids.

## PHARMACOKINETICS

The correlation between clinical effects and serum concentrations is based on steady-state concentrations, which are dependent on absorption, distribution, and elimination (Table 35–1). Physiologic changes in CAS kinetics occur with functional decline of the liver, kidney, and heart and dynamics with electrolyte abnormalities, including hypomagnesemia, hypercalcemia, hypernatremia, and commonly hypokalemia. Therefore, serum concentrations of CAS should be monitored to avoid inadvertent toxicity. Drug interactions between digoxin and other pharmaceuticals commonly result from changes in organ perfusion or P-glycoprotein inhibition. Also, a significant amount of digoxin is inactivated in the gastrointestinal (GI) tract by enteric bacteria, primarily *Eggerthella lenta*. Inhibition of this inactivation by the alteration of the GI flora by many antibiotics, particularly

**TABLE 35–1 Pharmacology of Selected Cardioactive Steroids**

| *Pharmacology* | *Digoxin* | *Digitoxin* |
|---|---|---|
| Onset of action | | |
| PO | 1.5–6 h | 3–6 h |
| IV | 5–30 min | 30 min–2 h |
| Maximal effect (h) | | |
| PO | 4–6 | 6–12 |
| IV | 1.5–3 | 4–8 |
| Intestinal absorption (%) | 40–90 (mean, 75) | > 95 |
| Plasma protein binding (%) | 25 | 97 |
| Volume of distribution (L/kg) | 5–7 (adults)<br>16 (infants)<br>10 (neonates)<br>4–5 (adults with kidney failure) | 0.6 (adults) |
| Elimination half-life (days) | 1.6 | 6–7 |
| Route of elimination (%) | Renal (60%–80%), with limited hepatic metabolism | Hepatic metabolism (80%) |
| Enterohepatic circulation (%) | 7 | 26 |

IV = intravenous; PO = oral.

macrolides, results in increased bioavailability and increased serum CAS concentrations.

## MECHANISMS OF ACTION AND PATHOPHYSIOLOGY

### Electrophysiologic Effects on Inotropy

Cardioactive steroids increase the force of contraction of the heart (positive inotropic effect) by increasing cytosolic $Ca^{2+}$ during systole (Fig. 35–2).

### Effects on Cardiac Electrophysiology

At supratherapeutic serum concentrations, CASs increase automaticity and shorten the repolarization intervals of the atria and ventricles (Table 35–2). There is a concurrent decrease in the rate of depolarization and conduction

**TABLE 35–2 Electrophysiologic Effects of Cardioactive Steroids on the Myocardium**

| | *Atria and Ventricles* | *AV Node* | *Electrocardiography Findings* |
|---|---|---|---|
| Excitability | ↑ | — | Extrasystoles, tachydysrhythmias |
| Automaticity | ↑ | — | Extrasystoles, tachydysrhythmias |
| Conduction velocity | ↓ | ↓ | ↑ PR interval, AV block |
| Refractoriness | ↓ | ↑ | ↑ PR interval, AV block, decreased QT interval |

AV = atrioventricular.

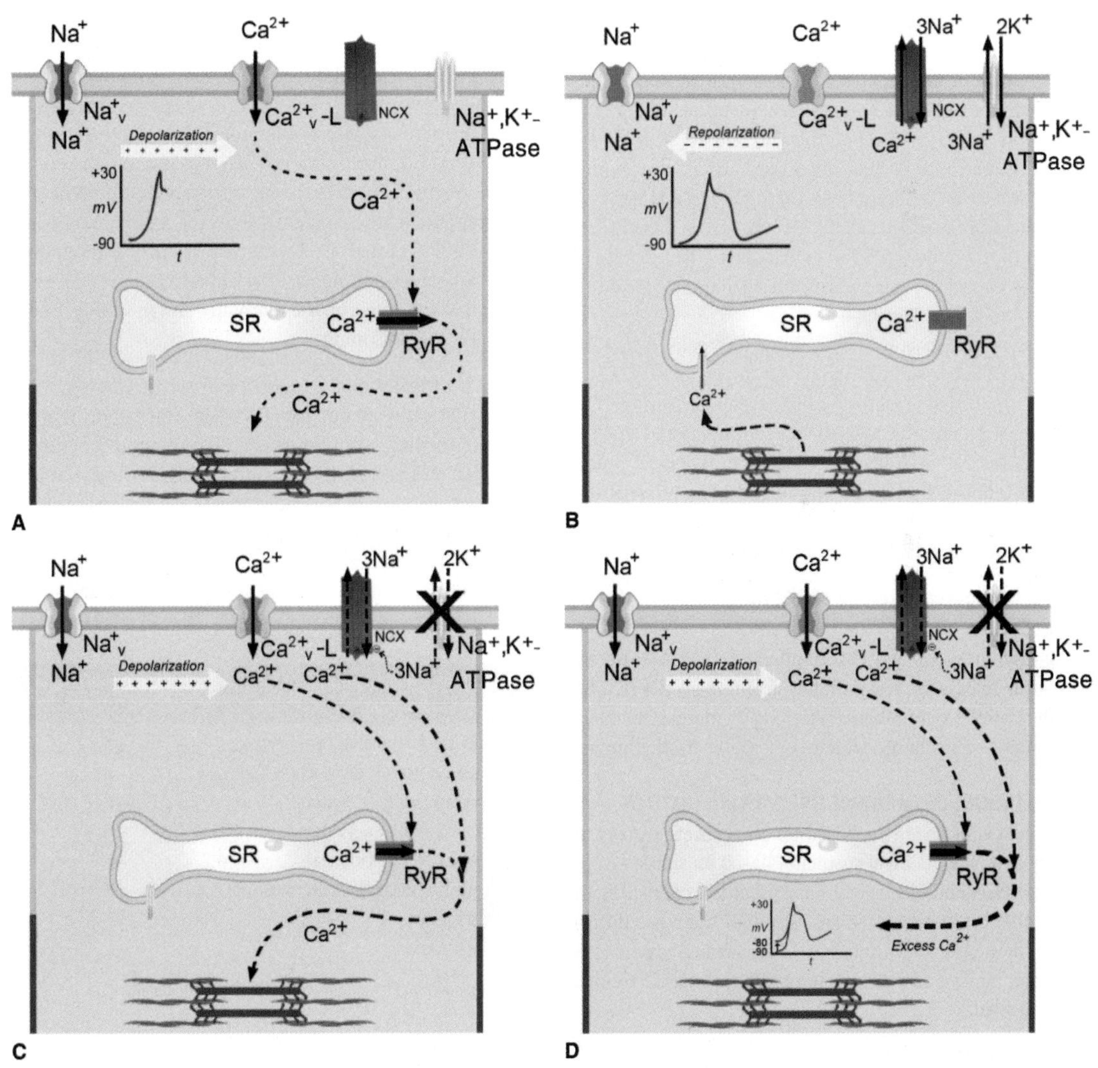


**FIGURE 35–2.** Pharmacology and toxicology of the cardioactive steroids (CASs). (**A**) Normal depolarization. Depolarization occurs after the opening of fast $Na^+$ channels; the increase in intracellular potential opens voltage-dependent $Ca^{2+}$ channels, and the influx of $Ca^{2+}$ induces the massive release of $Ca^{2+}$ from the sarcoplasmic reticulum (SR), producing contraction. (**B**) Normal repolarization. Repolarization begins with active expulsion of $3Na^+$ ions in exchange for $2K^+$ ions using an ATPase. This electrogenic ($3Na^+$ for $2K^+$) pump creates a $Na^+$ gradient used to expel $Ca^{2+}$ via an antiporter (NCX). The SR sequesters its $Ca^{2+}$ load via a separate ATPase. (**C**) Pharmacologic CAS. Digitalis inhibition of the $Na^+$, $K^+$-ATPase raises the intracellular $Na^+$ content, preventing the antiporter from expelling $1Ca^{2+}$ in exchange for $3Na^+$. The net result is an elevated intracellular $Ca^{2+}$, resulting in enhanced inotropy through enhanced SR calcium release. (**D**) Toxicologic CAS. Excessive elevation of the intracellular $Ca^{2+}$ elevates the resting potential, producing myocardial sensitization and predisposing to dysrhythmias. RyR = ryanodine receptor.

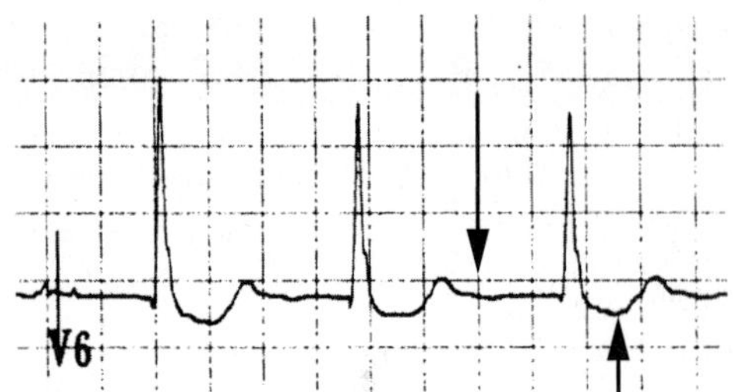


**FIGURE 35–3.** Digitalis effect noted in the lateral precordial lead, V6. Note the prolonged PR interval (long arrow) and the repolarization abnormality (scooping of the ST segment) (short arrow).

through the sinoatrial (SA) and atrioventricular (AV) nodes, respectively. This is mediated directly by depression of myocardial tissue and indirectly via an enhancement in vagally mediated parasympathetic tone. These changes in nodal conduction are reflected on the electrocardiogram (ECG) by a decrease in ventricular response rate to suprajunctional rhythms and by PR interval prolongation. The effects of CASs on ventricular repolarization are related to the elevated intracellular resting potential caused by accumulated cytosolic $Ca^{2+}$ that manifests on the ECG as QT interval shortening and ST-segment and T-wave forces opposite in direction to the major QRS forces. The last effect results in the characteristic scooping of the ST segments (referred to as the *digitalis effect*; Fig. 35–3).

Excessive increases in intracellular $Ca^{2+}$ caused by CAS toxicity result in delayed afterdepolarizations (DADs). Occasionally, DADs initiate a cellular depolarization that manifests as a premature ventricular contraction. Hypokalemia reduces $Na^+,K^+$-ATPase activity and enhances pump inhibition induced by CASs. Hypomagnesemia reduces the $Na^+,K^+$-ATPase exchange activity, enhancing the inhibitory effects and increasing the sensitivity to CASs.

### Effects of Cardioactive Steroids on the Autonomic Nervous System

The parasympathetic system is affected by CASs by an increase in release of acetylcholine from vagal fibers. The CAS effect on the sympathetic system is an increase in efferent sympathetic discharge, which exacerbates dysrhythmias.

## MANIFESTATIONS OF CARDIOACTIVE STEROID TOXICITY

Detection of CAS toxicity is based on an accurate history of CAS exposure, high clinical suspicion based on subtle symptoms, and ECG and electrolyte abnormalities, coupled with a detectable CAS concentration. Although there are differences in the signs and symptoms of acute versus chronic CAS poisoning, adults and children have similar manifestations when poisoned.

### Noncardiac Manifestations

***Acute Toxicity.*** An asymptomatic period of several minutes to several hours often follows a single administered toxic dose of CAS. The first clinical effects are typically nausea, vomiting, or abdominal pain. Central nervous system effects of acute toxicity include lethargy, confusion, and weakness that are not caused by hemodynamic changes. The absence of nausea and vomiting within several hours after exposure makes severe acute CAS poisoning unlikely.

***Chronic Toxicity.*** Chronic toxicity is often difficult to diagnose as a result of its insidious development and protean manifestations. Gastrointestinal findings include anorexia, nausea, vomiting, abdominal pain, and weight loss. Neuropsychiatric disorders include delirium, confusion, drowsiness, headache, hallucinations, and, rarely, seizures. Visual disturbances rarely include transient amblyopia, photophobia, blurring, scotomata, photopsia, decreased visual activity, and aberrations of color vision (chromatopsia) such as yellow halos (xanthopsia) around lights.

***Electrolyte Abnormalities.*** Elevated serum potassium concentrations frequently occur in patients with acute CAS poisoning. Hyperkalemia has important prognostic implications because the serum potassium concentration is a better predictor of lethality than either the initial ECG changes or the serum CAS concentration. In one study conducted before digoxin-specific Fab (DSFab) was available, approximately 50% of the patients with serum potassium concentrations of 5.0 to 5.5 mEq/L died. Although a serum potassium concentration less than 5.0 mEq/L was associated with no deaths, all 10 patients with serum potassium concentrations greater than 5.5 mEq/L died. However, correction of the hyperkalemia alone does not increase patient survival; it is a marker for, but not the cause of, the morbidity and mortality associated with CAS poisoning.

### Cardiac Manifestations

***General.*** With therapeutic use, CASs slow tachydysrhythmias without causing hypotension. With poisoning, alterations in cardiac rate and rhythm result in nearly any dysrhythmia with the exception of a rapidly conducted supraventricular tachydysrhythmia because of the prominent AV nodal depressive effect of CASs (Table 35–3). Although no single dysrhythmia is pathognomonic of CAS toxicity, toxicity should be

| TABLE 35–3 Cardiac Dysrhythmias Associated With Cardioactive Steroid Poisoning |
|---|
| ***Myocardial Irritability Causing Dysrhythmias*** |
| Atrial flutter and atrial fibrillation with AV block |
| Bidirectional ventricular tachycardia |
| Nonparoxysmal atrial tachydysrhythmias with AV block |
| Nonsustained ventricular tachycardia |
| Premature and sustained ventricular contractions |
| Ventricular bigeminy |
| Ventricular fibrillation |
| ***Primary Conduction System Dysfunction Causing Dysrhythmias*** |
| Junctional tachycardia |
| AV dissociation |
| High-degree AV block |
| Sinus bradycardia |
| Exit blocks |
| His-Purkinje dysfunction |
| SA nodal arrest |

AV = atrioventricular; SA = sinoatrial.

suspected when there is increased automaticity with impaired conduction through the SA and AV nodes. Bidirectional ventricular tachycardia is nearly diagnostic, although it may also occur with poisoning by aconitine and other uncommon xenobiotics. Dysrhythmias, including atrial tachycardia with high-degree AV block, result from the complex electrophysiologic influences on both the myocardium and conduction system of the heart that stem from direct, vagotonic, and other autonomic actions of the CASs.

## DIAGNOSTIC TESTING

Properly obtained and interpreted serum digoxin concentrations aid significantly in the management of patients with suspected digoxin toxicity, as well as in the management of patients poisoned by other CASs. Although most institutions report a therapeutic range for serum digoxin concentration from 0.5 to 2.0 ng/mL (SI units, 1.0–2.6 nmol/mL), current understanding suggests an upper limit of 1.0 ng/mL is preferable to maintain benefit while decreasing the risk of toxicity. Care must be taken to interpret the concentration as a correlate with other factors—the clinical condition of the patient; the interval between the last dose and the time the blood sample was taken; the presence of other metabolic abnormalities; and the use of other xenobiotics.

Cardioactive steroid poisoning is multifactorial, and using the upper limit of the therapeutic range of digoxin as the sole indicator of toxicity is misleading because there is an overlap in serum digoxin concentrations between toxic and nontoxic patients. Asymptomatic patients with CAS concentrations obtained before completion of distribution that are above the therapeutic range are less often toxic but require close observation and retesting. Patients with mean serum concentrations above 2 ng/mL for digoxin and above 40 ng/mL for digitoxin measured 6 hours after the last dose often are clinically toxic.

Digoxin assays frequently, but unpredictably, cross-react with other plant- or animal-derived CASs. Although a monoclonal digoxin immunoassay accurately only quantifies the serum digoxin concentration, an elevated digoxin concentration in the correct clinical setting will qualitatively assist in establishing a presumptive diagnosis of nonpharmaceutical CAS exposure (Chaps. 16 and 91).

## ENDOGENOUS DIGOXINLIKE IMMUNOREACTIVE SUBSTANCES

Some patients have a positive digoxin assay resulting from an endogenous digoxinlike immunoreactive substances (EDLIS) that are structurally and functionally similar to prescribed CASs. These substances are found in patients with increased inotropic need or reduced renal clearance, including neonates; patients with end-stage kidney disease, liver disease, subarachnoid hemorrhage, congestive heart failure, insulin-dependent diabetes, stress, or hypothermia; after strenuous exercise; and in pregnancy. Clinical observations indicate that the serum digoxin concentration contributed by EDLIS is usually less than 2 ng/mL.

Other endogenous substances that can cross-react with the digoxin assay to produce a false-positive result include bilirubin and spironolactone.

## THERAPY

### Acute Management Overview

Initial treatment of a patient with acute CAS poisoning includes providing general care (eg, GI decontamination, monitoring for dysrhythmias, measuring electrolyte and digoxin concentrations) and administering DSFab. Secondary care includes treating complications such as dysrhythmias and electrolyte abnormalities.

### Gastrointestinal Decontamination

Lavage is rarely recommended because efficacy is limited because of rapid absorption from the gut and due to the emetic effects of the drug itself. Because many CASs, such as digitoxin and digoxin, are recirculated enterohepatically, both late and repeated activated charcoal (AC) administration (1 g/kg of body weight every 2–4 hours for up to four doses) are beneficial in reducing serum concentrations. Activated charcoal is recommended in CAS-toxic patients if definitive therapy with digoxin-specific Fab is not immediately available or when kidney function is impaired.

### Advanced Management

***Digoxin-Specific Antibody Fragments.*** Definitive therapy for patients with life-threatening dysrhythmias from CAS toxicity is to administer DSFab. Table 35–4 lists the indications for administering digoxin-specific Fab. Extensive discussion is found in Antidotes in Brief: A22.

***Other Cardiac Therapeutics.*** Secondary treatments used in patients with symptomatic CAS poisoning include the use of atropine for supraventricular bradydysrhythmias or high degrees of AV block (Antidotes in Brief: A35). Phenytoin and lidocaine were used to manage CAS-induced ventricular tachydysrhythmias and ventricular irritability with some success prior to the introduction of DSFab. When used, phenytoin should be slowly IV infused (~50 mg/min) or administered in increments of 100 mg repeated every 5 minutes until control of the dysrhythmias is achieved or a maximum of 1,000 mg has been given in adults or 15 to 20 mg/kg in children. Fosphenytoin has not been evaluated in this setting. Lidocaine is given as a 1 to 1.5 mg/kg IV bolus followed by a continuous infusion at 1 to 4 mg/min in adults or as a 1 to 1.5 mg/kg IV bolus followed by 30 to 50 μg/kg/min in children

| TABLE 35–4 Indications for Administration of Digoxin-Specific Antibody Fragments |
|---|
| Any digoxin-related life-threatening dysrhythmias, regardless of SDC<br>—Includes ventricular tachycardia or ventricular fibrillation or progressive bradydysrhythmias such as atropine-resistant symptomatic sinus bradycardia or second- or third-degree heart block |
| Potassium concentration > 5 mEq/L in the setting of acute digoxin poisoning |
| Chronic elevation of SDC associated with dysrhythmias, significant GI symptoms, or altered mental status |
| SDC ≥ 15 ng/mL at any time or ≥ 10 ng/mL 6 h postingestion, regardless of clinical effects |
| Acute ingestion of 10 mg of digoxin in an adult |
| Acute ingestion of 4 mg of digoxin in a child |
| Poisoning with a nondigoxin cardioactive steroid |

GI = gastrointestinal; SDC = serum digoxin concentration.

as required to control the rhythm disturbance (Chap. 30). Current indications for the use of phenytoin and lidocaine in the setting of CAS toxicity are rare.

### Pacemakers and Cardioversion

External or transvenous pacemakers have had limited indications in the management of patients with CAS poisoning. In one retrospective study, patients who received internal pacemakers had worse outcomes. It is reasonable to attempt transthoracic pacing for atropine-unresponsive bradydysrhythmias in settings when definitive care (DSFab) is delayed or unavailable. In CAS-poisoned patients with unstable rhythms, such as unstable ventricular tachycardia or ventricular fibrillation, cardioversion and defibrillation, respectively, are indicated.

### Electrolyte Therapy

***Potassium.*** Hypokalemia and hyperkalemia exacerbate CAS cardiotoxicity even at "therapeutic" digoxin concentrations. When hypokalemia is noted in conjunction with tachydysrhythmias or bradydysrhythmias, potassium replacement should be administered with serial monitoring of the serum potassium concentration. In non-life-threatening cases, digoxin-specific Fab administration generally should be withheld until the hypokalemia is corrected because the life-threatening manifestations of CAS cardiotoxicity often resolve when the potassium is normalized. In hyperkalemic patients, reduction in potassium concentrations should be initiated with care to avoid hypokalemia prior to administering DSFab, because the serum potassium will decrease rapidly after DSFab treatment.

Although calcium is beneficial in most hyperkalemic patients, in the setting of CAS poisoning, administration of calcium salts is considered to be potentially dangerous.

Although rate of administration of $Ca^{2+}$ may play a role in exaggerating CAS cardiac toxicity, calcium administration should be avoided because better, safer, alternative treatments, such as DSFab, insulin, and sodium bicarbonate, are available for CAS-induced hyperkalemia.

***Magnesium.*** Hypomagnesemia also occurs in CAS-poisoned patients secondary to the contributory factors mentioned with hypokalemia, such as long-term diuretic use to treat congestive heart failure. Hypomagnesemia increases myocardial digoxin uptake and decreases cellular $Na^+$,$K^+$-ATPase activity. Cardioactive steroid–toxic patients found to be hypomagnesemic should have magnesium repleted (Antidotes in Brief: A16).

### Extracorporeal Removal of Cardioactive Steroids

All extracorporeal techniques are ineffective in enhancing the elimination of digoxin because of its large volume of distribution, which makes it relatively inaccessible to these techniques.

Antidotes in Brief

# A22 DIGOXIN-SPECIFIC ANTIBODY FRAGMENTS

## INTRODUCTION

Digoxin-specific antibody fragments (DSFab) are indicated for the management of patients with digoxin and digitoxin toxicity, as well as toxicity from other pharmaceutical, plant, and animal cardioactive steroids (CASs; eg, ouabain, dogbane, oleander, squill, and *Bufo* and *Birgus* species).

## HISTORY

The production of antibody fragments to treat patients poisoned with digoxin followed the development of digoxin antibodies for measuring serum digoxin concentrations by radioimmunoassay (RIA). This RIA technique permitted the correlation between serum digoxin concentrations and clinical digoxin toxicity. In 1967, Butler and Chen suggested that purified antidigoxin antibodies with a high affinity and specificity should be developed to treat digoxin toxicity in humans.

Intact IgG antidigoxin antibodies reversed digoxin toxicity in dogs. Unfortunately, the urinary excretion of digoxin was delayed, free digoxin was released, and there was significant concern with regard to the development of hypersensitivity reactions. To make antibodies that were both safer and effective in humans, whole IgG antidigoxin antibodies were cleaved yielding two antigen-binding fragments (Fab) and one Fc fragment. Because the Fc fragment does not bind antigen and increases the potential for hypersensitivity reactions, it was eliminated. In 1976, Digibind was used with clinical success, and it became commercially available in 1986, before being discontinued in 2011. Another commercial product, DigiFab, approved by the United States (US) Food and Drug Administration (FDA) in 2001, is currently available.

## PHARMACOLOGY

### Chemistry and Preparation

DigiFab is prepared from the blood of healthy sheep that were immunized with a digoxin derivative, digoxin-dicarboxymethoxylamine. Papain digestion yields digoxin-specific Fab fragments, each of which has a molecular weight of approximately 46,200 Da.

### Mechanism of Action

Immediately after intravenous (IV) administration, the antigen-binding fragments bind intravascular free digoxin (or digitoxin). Uncomplexed antibody fragments then diffuse into the interstitial space, where they bind free digoxin. This causes digoxin to dissociate from the external surface of $Na^+$,$K^+$-adenosine triphosphatase (ATPase) enzyme and restore its function.

### Pharmacokinetics

The pharmacokinetics of Digibind and DigiFab (previously named DigiTAb) were compared in human volunteers. At 30 minutes after infusion of either DSFab, the serum free digoxin concentration was below the level of detection and remained so for several hours. A few patients in both groups had free digoxin concentrations rebound to 0.5 ng/mL at approximately 18 hours. The elimination half-life of total digoxin averaged 18 hours for DigiFab. In another study, the elimination half-life of the DSFab-glycoside complex was 20 to 30 hours, with free digoxin concentrations rising between 8 and 12 hours. The volume of distribution was 0.3 L/kg for DigiFab. Similar findings were described after the first clinical use of Digibind.

When a bolus dose strategy was compared to a loading dose followed by a continuous infusion, the second strategy increased the ratio of digoxin bound to uncomplexed DSFab in the serum from 50% to 70% presumably because when the entire dose is given as a bolus some elimination of DSFab occurs before optimally binding.

Pharmacokinetic studies in patients with kidney failure demonstrate that the half-life of DSFab is prolonged 10-fold, with no change in the apparent DSFab $V_d$. In this situation, serum DSFab concentrations can remain detectable for 2 to 3 weeks or more. Case reports and series demonstrate that free digoxin concentrations can persist and reappear up to 10 days after administration of DSFab to patients with end-stage kidney disease compared with 12 to 24 hours in patients with normal kidney function.

In an attempt to hasten digoxin elimination with and without DSFab treatment, various extracorporeal modalities were explored, with predictably disappointing results given the large $V_d$ of digoxin and the size of the digoxin–antibody complex. A multispecialty working group, which reviewed the available literature, recommended against performing extracorporeal treatments in patients with severe digoxin poisoning when DSFab is administered.

### Pharmacodynamics

At the tissue level, in ex vivo isolated human ventricular myocardium with a 1.5-fold higher than equimolar DSFab dosing, digoxin toxicity was reversed within 30 minutes. The maximal rate of digoxin removal from $Na^+$,$K^+$-ATPase was limited by the dissociation rate of digoxin from $Na^+$,$K^+$-ATPase, with a half-life for this decay ranging from 46 to 54 minutes. In six toxic patients in whom free digoxin or digitoxin concentrations were measured, free serum concentrations decreased to zero or near zero within 1 to 2 minutes after administration of DSFab. In 36 patients with chronic digoxin poisoning, free digoxin concentrations decreased to almost zero after administration.

In a multicenter study of 150 patients, the mean time to initial response from the completion of the Digibind infusion was 19 minutes, and the mean time to complete response was 88 minutes. In another study of 63 patients, therapeutic response generally occurred by 30 minutes, and complete response sometimes took hours. Life-threatening dysrhythmia reversal occurred within a mean of 3.2 hours in 34 patients.

## ROLE IN DIGOXIN TOXICITY

A large study evaluating adult and pediatric patients with acute and chronic digoxin toxicity established the efficacy of Digibind. Of the 148 patients evaluated for cardiovascular manifestations of toxicity before treatment, 79 patients (55%) had high-grade atrioventricular (AV) block, 68 (46%) had refractory ventricular tachycardia, 49 (33%) had ventricular fibrillation, and 56 (37%) had hyperkalemia. Complete resolution of all signs and symptoms of digoxin toxicity occurred in 80% of cases. Partial response was observed in 10% of patients, and of the 15 patients who did not respond, 14 were moribund before initiation of therapy or later found to not be digoxin toxic. The success of Digibind was further demonstrated when 54% of patients who had cardiac arrest survived to discharge compared with 100% mortality before the availability of DSFab. In a postmarketing surveillance study of 717 patients, 50% of patients had a complete response to treatment, 24% had a partial response, and 12% had no response. In the 89 patients with no response, digoxin was deemed contributory in only 14 patients. Other studies show similarly impressive results. Newborns, infants, and children have all been successfully treated with DSFab.

## ROLE OF DIGOXIN-SPECIFIC ANTIBODY FRAGMENTS WITH OTHER CARDIOACTIVE STEROIDS

Digoxin-specific antibody fragments were designed to have high-affinity binding for digoxin and digitoxin. There are structural similarities, however, among the CASs. In fact, detectable "digoxin concentrations" using immunoassays were reported with some, but not all, nondigoxin CASs. Since this interference suggests a potential for cross-reactivity between DSFab and other CASs, DSFab has variable efficacy for multiple natural CAS poisonings, including those unique CASs in common and yellow oleander (*Nerium oleander* and *Thevetia peruviana*), dogbane (*Apocynum cannabinum*), lily of the valley (*Convallaria majalis*), the ordeal bean (*Tanghinia venenifera*), (red) squill (sea onion, *Urginea maritima*), sea mango (*Cerbera manghas*), *Bufo* toad species, and coconut crab (*Birgus latro L.*).

Larger doses of DSFab may be required in cases of poisoning by other CASs because of the lower affinity binding of DSFab for these toxins with doses as high as 20 vials (800 mg) given. We recommend that treatment decisions be based on clinical and diagnostic findings such as electrocardiogram (ECG) or electrolyte abnormalities (eg, life-threatening dysrhythmias, shock or hemodynamic instability, potassium concentrations > 5 mEq/L, and those provided in Table 35–4), with initial therapy consisting of 10 to 20 vials in cases of nonpharmaceutical cardioactive steroid poisonings. Subsequent doses should be based on clinical response. Gastrointestinal decontamination is recommended because of the potential ongoing absorption of ingested products.

## INDICATIONS FOR DIGOXIN-SPECIFIC ANTIBODY FRAGMENTS

Life-threatening, or potentially life-threatening, toxicity from any CAS should prompt DSFab treatment. Patients with known or suggestive CAS exposure with progressive bradydysrhythmias, including symptomatic sinus bradycardia or second- or third-degree heart block unresponsive to atropine, and patients with severe ventricular dysrhythmias, such as ventricular tachycardia or ventricular fibrillation, should also be treated with DSFab. Ventricular tachycardia with a fascicular block is likely to be a digoxin toxic rhythm. We recommend treating with DSFab patients with a potassium concentration exceeding 5 mEq/L that is attributable to a CAS in the presence of other manifestations of acute or chronic digoxin toxicity. Digoxin-specific antibody fragments are recommended for acute ingestions greater than 4 mg in a healthy child (or > 0.1 mg/kg) or 10 mg in a healthy adult, with a lower threshold in compromised patients. Serum concentrations of greater than or equal to 10 ng/mL soon after an acute ingestion may predict the need for treatment with DSFab. Because older adults are at greatest risk of lethality with digoxin poisoning, the treatment threshold for patients older than 60 years of age is recommended to be lower. Before the advent of DSFab, the mortality rate in patients older than 60 years of age was 58% compared with 8% in patients younger than 40 years of age. A rapid progression of clinical signs and symptoms, such as cardiac and gastrointestinal toxicity and an elevated or rising potassium concentration, in the presence of an acute overdose, suggests a potentially life-threatening exposure necessitating DSFab.

Cardioactive steroid toxicity causes an increase in intracellular calcium, and the administration of exogenous calcium may further exacerbate conduction abnormalities and potentially result in cardiac arrest, unresponsive to further resuscitation. Thus, in a patient with an unknown exposure who is clinically ill with characteristics suggestive of poisoning by a CAS, DSFab should be administered early in the management and always before administration of calcium gluconate or chloride. The CAS effects can be reversed, obviating the risk associated with the administration of calcium. It also can be difficult to distinguish clinically between digoxin poisoning and intrinsic cardiac disease, which the administration of DSFab can resolve.

A computer-based simulation model concluded that treatment with DSFab could decrease length of hospitalization by 1.5 days, a major cost containment benefit.

## ADVERSE EFFECTS AND SAFETY ISSUES

Digoxin-specific antibody fragments are generally safe and effective. Uncommon reported adverse effects include hypokalemia as a consequence of reactivation of the $Na^+,K^+$-ATPase; withdrawal of the inotropic or AV nodal blocking effects of digoxin, leading to congestive heart failure or a rapid ventricular rate in patients with atrial fibrillation; and, rarely, allergic reactions.

Patients with allergies to papain, chymopapain, or other papaya extracts or the pineapple enzyme bromelain may be at risk for allergic reactions because trace residues of papaya may remain in the DSFab. Patients with an allergy to sheep

**TABLE A22–1 Sample Calculation Based on History of Acute Digoxin Ingestion**

| *Adult* | *Child* |
|---|---|
| Weight: 70 kg | Weight: 10 kg |
| Ingestion: 50 (0.25 mg) digoxin tablets | Ingestion: 50 (0.25 mg) digoxin tablets |
| Calculation:<br>0.25 mg × 50 = 12.5 mg ingested dose<br>12.5 mg × 0.80 (assume 80% bioavailability) = 10 mg (absorbed dose)<br>$\frac{10\text{ mg}}{0.5\text{ mg/vial}} = 20\text{ vials}$ | Calculation: Same as for adult. Child will require 20 vials. |

protein or those who have previously received ovine antibodies or ovine Fab may also be at risk for allergic reactions, although this is not reported. In life-threatening cases, DSFab is still reasonable as long as the clinician is prepared to treat these allergic reactions.

## PREGNANCY AND LACTATION

Digoxin-specific antibody fragments are US FDA Pregnancy Category C. Digoxin-specific antibody fragment use should not be withheld in maternal poisoning because of pregnancy. It is unknown whether DSFab is excreted into breast milk, but it is considered compatible with breastfeeding.

## DOSING AND ADMINISTRATION

The dose of DSFab depends on the total body load (TBL) of digoxin. Estimates of digoxin TBL can be made in three ways: (1) estimate the quantity of digoxin acutely ingested and assume 80% bioavailability (milligrams ingested × 0.8 equals TBL), which is on the higher end of the value incorporated into successful treatment regimens; (2) obtain a serum digoxin concentration and, using a pharmacokinetic formula, incorporate the apparent $V_d$ of digoxin and the patient's body weight (in kilograms); or (3) use an empiric dose based on the average requirements for an acute or chronic overdose in an adult or child. Each of these methods of estimating the dose of DSFab has limitations. Sample calculations for each of these methods are shown in Tables A22–1 to A22–3. The number of vials is rounded up to the next whole vial, which provides some margin against the limitations of the calculations. The clinician should always be prepared to increase or repeat the dose if symptoms fail to resolve.

**TABLE A22–3 Empiric Dosing Recommendations**

| *Acute Ingestion* | *Chronic Toxicity* |
|---|---|
| Adult: 10–20 vials | Adult: 3–6 vials |
| Child:[a] 10–20 vials | Child:[b] 1–2 vials |

[a]Monitor for volume overload in very small children. [b]The prescribing information contains a table for infants and children, with corresponding serum concentrations.

Because of the increasing cost of DSFab and availability concerns, several authors have suggested partial or "semi-molar" neutralization in various scenarios, particularly in cases of chronic toxicity in which full reversal might exacerbate the underlying tachydysrhythmias for which digoxin was originally prescribed. Many chronically poisoned patients have been safely treated with partial neutralization. It is reasonable to follow this approach with close clinical monitoring. However, recurrent dysrhythmias attributed to persistent digoxin toxicity are reported in acutely overdosed patients who receive partial neutralizing doses. Pending direct comparative trials and when resources are available, we recommend full equimolar dosing in patients with acute toxicity.

Each 40-mg vial of DigiFab (which binds 0.5 mg of digoxin) should be reconstituted with 4 mL of sterile water for IV injection and gently mixed to provide a solution containing 10 mg/mL of DSFab. DigiFab should be administered slowly as an IV infusion over at least 30 minutes unless the patient is critically ill, in which case the DigiFab can be given by IV bolus. For infants and small children, the manufacturer recommends diluting the 40-mg vial with 4 mL of sterile water for IV injection and administering the dose undiluted using a tuberculin syringe.

**TABLE A22–2 Sample Calculations Based on the Serum Digoxin Concentration[a]**

| *Adult* | *Child* | *Quick Estimation (for Adults and Children)* |
|---|---|---|
| Weight: 70 kg<br>SDC: 10 ng/mL<br>$V_d$: 5-7 L/kg<br>Calculation:[b]<br>$\text{No. of vials}^c = \frac{\text{Total body load (mg)}}{0.5\text{ mg/vial}}$<br>$= \frac{\text{SDC} \times V_d \times \text{Patient wt (kg)}}{1{,}000 \times 0.5\text{ mg/vial}}$<br>$\text{No. of vials}^c = \frac{10\text{ ng/mL} \times 5\text{ L/kg} \times 70\text{ kg}}{1{,}000 \times 0.5\text{ mg/vial}}$<br>No. of vials = 7 | Weight: 10 kg<br>SDC: 10 ng/mL<br>$V_d$: 5 L/kg<br>Calculation:[b]<br>$\text{No. of vials}^c = \frac{10\text{ ng/mL} \times 5\text{ L/kg} \times 10\text{ kg}}{1{,}000 \times 0.5\text{ mg/vial}}$<br>No. of vials = 1 | $\text{No. of vials}^c = \frac{\text{SDC (ng/mL)} \times \text{Patient wt (kg)}}{100}$ |

[a]If the serum digoxin concentration (SDC) is provided in units of nmol/L, a factor of 0.78 is used to convert to ng/mL. [b]1,000 is a conversion factor to change ng/mL to mg/L.
[c]Round up to the nearest whole vial to determine the number of vials indicated.
$V_d$ = volume of distribution.

## MEASUREMENT OF SERUM DIGOXIN CONCENTRATION AFTER DIGOXIN-SPECIFIC ANTIBODY FRAGMENT ADMINISTRATION

Most laboratories are not equipped to determine free serum digoxin concentrations within a clinically reasonable timeframe. This is relevant because after DSFab administration, total serum digoxin concentrations are clinically meaningless because they represent both free and bound digoxin and may rise up to 10- to 20-fold compared with pretreatment values or provide falsely low serum concentrations, depending on the test. Newer commercial methods, using ultrafiltration or immunoassays, make free digoxin concentration measurements easier to perform and therefore more clinically useful, but they remain associated with errors in the underestimation or overestimation of the free digoxin concentration. Free digoxin concentrations are particularly useful in patients with end-stage kidney disease.

Additional pitfalls in the measurement and utility of serum digoxin concentrations include endogenous and exogenous factors. Spironolactone, eplerenone, canrenone, and the prodrug of canrenone potassium canrenoate can positively or negatively interfere with serum digoxin measurements, depending on the analytical method. Endogenous digitalis-like substances are described in infants, women in the third trimester of pregnancy, high altitude exposure, hypothermia, acute respiratory distress syndrome, essential hypertension, congestive heart failure, right ventricular dysfunction, hypertrophic cardiomyopathy, kidney and liver failure, kidney and liver transplant recipients, and critically ill patients without liver or kidney disease.

## FORMULATION AND ACQUISITION

Digoxin-specific antibody fragments are available in the US as DigiFab. Vials contain 40 mg of purified lyophilized digoxin-immune ovine immunoglobulin fragments, approximately 75 mg of mannitol USP, and approximately 2 mg of sodium acetate USP as a buffer.

# 36 METHYLXANTHINES AND SELECTIVE $\beta_2$-ADRENERGIC AGONISTS

| Therapeutic concentrations | |
|---|---|
| Theophylline | 5–15 µg/mL (28–83 µmol/L) |
| Caffeine | 1–10 µg/mL |

## HISTORY AND EPIDEMIOLOGY

The methylxanthines including caffeine, theobromine, and theophylline are used ubiquitously throughout the world, most commonly in beverages imbibed for their stimulant, mood-elevating, and fatigue-abating effects. Methylxanthines are the active ingredients in coffee (caffeine), tea (caffeine), and chocolate (theobromine), while the primary pharmaceutical is theophylline. Selective $\beta_2$-adrenergic agonists were developed for the treatment of bronchoconstriction while avoiding the adverse effects of epinephrine and isoproterenol.

The overwhelming preponderance of caffeine consumed is in beverages; a lesser portion is consumed in foods and tablets or capsules (Table 36–1). Guarana, a plant with very high caffeine content, is used for weight loss and athletic performance enhancement. Medicinally, caffeine is used to treat neonatal apnea and bradycardia syndrome; as an analgesic adjuvant; and as an adjuvant treatment for migraine headaches and postlumbar puncture headaches.

Theophylline, or its water-soluble salt aminophylline, is used to treat asthma and chronic obstructive pulmonary diseases. Theophylline was once the mainstay of therapy for such diseases, but more selective $\beta_2$-adrenergic agonists are now more commonly used. In neonates, theophylline and aminophylline are used similarly to caffeine to treat neonatal apnea and bradycardia syndrome.

### Spectrum of Toxicity

Methylxanthine toxicity is classified as acute, acute on chronic, or chronic. Acute methylxanthine toxicity can be intentional, unintentional, or iatrogenic. Chronic theophylline toxicity results largely from altered metabolism. In contrast, acute on chronic theophylline toxicity represents acute overdose in patients normally maintained on theophylline. Chronic toxicity from caffeine most typically results from frequent self-administration of excessive caffeine. *Caffeinism* is a syndrome associated with chronic caffeine use, consisting of headache, palpitations, tachycardia, insomnia, and delirium. Theobromine poisoning is reported in veterinary literature and typically results from dogs or other small animals ingesting cocoa or chocolate. Because of its greater thermogenic and ergogenic activity relative to caffeine, theobromine is now an ingredient of numerous energy and sports drinks used for stimulation and athletic enhancement, but human toxicity is unreported. Use of selective $\beta_2$-adrenergic agonists is widespread. Adverse effects are associated with both therapeutic dosing and overdose. Clenbuterol, a long-acting $\beta_2$-adrenergic agonist used for treating bronchoconstriction in countries outside the United States, emerged as an abused anabolic xenobiotic. Food poisoning by consumption of animal meat from livestock treated with clenbuterol occurs in Europe.

## PHARMACOLOGY

### Methylxanthines

Methylxanthines cause the release of endogenous catecholamines, resulting in stimulation of $\beta_1$- and $\beta_2$-adrenergic receptors. Concentrations of endogenous catecholamines are extremely elevated in patients with acute methylxanthine poisoning. Methylxanthines are also adenosine antagonists, and, at supratherapeutic doses, phosphodiesterase inhibitors. Because phosphodiesterase is responsible for degradation of intracellular cyclic adenosine monophosphate (cAMP), and cAMP is the postsynaptic second messenger

**TABLE 36–1 Caffeine and Stimulant Content of Commonly Used Products**

| *Product* | *Caffeine Content in Typical Single Serving (mg)* | *Volume of Typical Single Serving (mL)* | *Other Relevant Beverage Ingredients* | *Category* |
|---|---|---|---|---|
| Arizona AZ RX Energy Shot | 110 | 240 | Niacin, vitamin $B_{12}$ | Dietary supplement |
| Caffeine pill (Vivarin, No-Doz) | 200 | — | — | Medication |
| Chocolate (Hershey Kiss) | 1 | — | — | Food |
| Chocolate milk | 10–15 | 240 | Theobromine | Beverage |
| Coffee (regular) | 115–175 | 330 | | Beverage |
| Cola | 30 | 330 | | Beverage |
| Espresso | 55 | 30 | | Beverage |
| Five-Hour Energy | 207 | 60 | Niacin, taurine, vitamin $B_6$, vitamin $B_{12}$ | Dietary supplement |
| Hot chocolate | 8 | 240 | Theobromine | Beverage |
| Red Bull | 110 | 250 | Taurine | Beverage |
| Tea (black) | 40–100 | 240 | Theobromine, theophylline | Beverage |

system of β-adrenergic stimulation, clinical effects are similar to adrenergic stimulation.

### Selective $\beta_2$-Adrenergic Agonists

Selective $\beta_2$-adrenergic agonists act specifically at $\beta_2$-adrenergic receptors, resulting in an increase in intracellular cAMP, which leads to relaxation of vascular, bronchial, and uterine smooth muscle; glycogenolysis in skeletal muscle; and hepatic glycogenolysis and gluconeogenesis.

## PHARMACOKINETICS AND TOXICOKINETICS

### Caffeine Pharmacokinetics

Caffeine is bioavailable by oral, intravenous, subcutaneous, intramuscular, and rectal routes of administration. Oral bioavailability approaches 100%. Caffeine rapidly diffuses into the total-body water and readily crosses the blood–brain barrier and the placenta. The volume of distribution is 0.6 L/kg, and 36% is protein bound. Caffeine is metabolized primarily by the isoenzyme CYP1A2. Neonates demethylate caffeine, producing theophylline, and also possess the unique ability to convert theophylline to caffeine. The elimination half-life is 4.5 hours in healthy, adult, nonsmoking patients.

### Caffeine Toxicokinetics

Therapeutic dosing in adults is 100 to 200 mg orally every 4 hours; a typical loading dose in neonates is 20 mg/kg, with daily maintenance dosing of 5 mg/kg. Based on case reports and series, lethal dosing in adults is estimated at 150 to 200 mg/kg, and death is associated with serum concentrations greater than 80 μg/mL.

### Theophylline Pharmacokinetics

Theophylline is approximately 100% bioavailable by the oral route. Many of the available oral preparations are sustained release, designed to provide stable serum concentrations over a prolonged period of time with less frequent dosing. Peak absorption generally occurs 6 to 10 hours after ingestion of therapeutic doses of sustained-release theophylline pharmaceuticals. However, following overdose, the time to peak absorption may be doubled. Similar to caffeine, theophylline rapidly diffuses into the total-body water with a volume of distribution of 0.45 L/kg and 56% protein binding. Theophylline is metabolized primarily by CYP1A2. In healthy, adult, nonsmoking patients, the half-life is 4.5 hours. Infants and the elderly, as well as patients with CYP1A2 inhibition, pregnant patients, and patients with cirrhosis, have longer half-lives than healthy children and adult nonsmoking patients.

### Theophylline Toxicokinetics

As in the case of caffeine, theophylline exhibits Michaelis-Menten kinetics, presumably when greater than a single therapeutic dose is taken. Therapeutic serum concentrations of theophylline are 5 to 15 μg/mL. Life-threatening toxicity, including seizures, ventricular dysrhythmias, and death, are associated with serum concentrations of 80 to 100 μg/mL in acute overdoses, and serum concentrations of 40 to 60 μg/mL in chronic toxicity.

### Theobromine Pharmacokinetics and Toxicokinetics

Theobromine is well absorbed from the gut and is 77% bioavailable. Theobromine has 21% protein binding, a volume of distribution of 0.62 L/kg, and a plasma half-life of 6 to 10 hours. Theobromine undergoes hepatic metabolism by CYP1A2 and CYP2E1.

### Selective $\beta_2$-Adrenergic Agonist Pharmacokinetics

The $\beta_2$-adrenergic agonists are bioavailable by both inhalation and ingestion. Absorption, distribution, and elimination are quite variable. The half-life of albuterol is approximately 4 hours, and less than 5% crosses the blood–brain barrier. Terbutaline is partially metabolized in the liver, mainly to inactive conjugates. With parenteral administration, 60% of a given dose is excreted in the urine unchanged. Clenbuterol has a half-life of approximately 22 hours and a prolonged duration of action. It is more potent than other $\beta_2$-adrenergic agonists, with a typical therapeutic dose of 20 to 40 μg, as opposed to milligram doses for other $\beta_2$-adrenergic agonists.

### Selective $\beta_2$-Adrenergic Agonist Toxicokinetics

Overdose of albuterol, which happens predominantly in young children, uncommonly causes significant effects. For oral albuterol poisoning, 1 mg/kg appears to be the dose threshold for developing clinically significant toxicity.

## METHYLXANTHINE AND $\beta_2$-ADRENERGIC AGONIST TOXICITY

Caffeine, theobromine, and theophylline all affect the same organ systems and cause qualitatively similar effects, although their potencies differ.

### Gastrointestinal

In overdose, methylxanthines cause nausea. Most significant acute overdoses result in severe and protracted emesis. Direct effects on the medullary vomiting center and local effects on gastric acidity contribute to gastrointestinal symptoms. This emesis is often difficult to control despite the use of potent antiemetics.

### Cardiovascular

Methylxanthines are cardiac stimulants and result in positive inotropy and chronotropy. Tachydysrhythmias, especially supraventricular tachycardias (SVTs), are common in methylxanthine toxicity. Adenosine antagonism, catecholamine excess, and electrolyte disturbances, particularly hypokalemia, contribute to the development of dysrhythmias. Dysrhythmias occur more commonly and at lower serum concentrations in cases of chronic poisoning. At elevated serum concentrations, methylxanthines result in peripheral vasodilation causing a characteristic widened pulse pressure.

### Pulmonary

Methylxanthines stimulate the central nervous system (CNS) respiratory center, causing tachypnea and hyperpnea. Respiratory alkalosis, respiratory failure, respiratory arrest, and acute respiratory distress syndrome all occur.

### Neuropsychiatric

The stimulant and psychoactive properties of methylxanthines, particularly caffeine, elevate mood and improve performance of manual tasks. Headache, anxiety, agitation, insomnia, tremor, irritability, hallucinations, and seizures occur from caffeine or theophylline poisoning. Seizures are a major complication of methylxanthine poisoning and tend to be severe and recurrent and refractory to conventional treatment. Antagonism of adenosine, the endogenous neurotransmitter responsible for halting seizures, contributes to the seizures associated with methylxanthine overdose.

### Musculoskeletal

Methylxanthines increase intracellular calcium content and increase striated muscle contractility, secondarily decreasing muscle fatigue. They also increase muscle oxygen consumption and increase the basal metabolic rate. Tremor is common, and other manifestations of excitation include fasciculations, hypertonicity, myoclonus, and rhabdomyolysis.

### Metabolic

Numerous metabolic derangements result from acute methylxanthine toxicity. All result from excess adrenergic stimulation and subsequent increased metabolism. Severe hypokalemia, hypomagnesemia, and hypophosphatemia are accompanied by hyperglycemia and a metabolic acidosis with increased serum lactate concentration.

## CHRONIC METHYLXANTHINE TOXICITY

Patients chronically receiving theophylline or caffeine have higher total body stores of these xenobiotics and often underlying medical disorders and thus develop toxicity with a smaller amount of additional theophylline or caffeine. Signs and symptoms of chronic toxicity are usually more subtle or nonspecific, such as anorexia, nausea, palpitations, or emesis, but chronic toxicity also presents as seizures or dysrhythmias. In the absence of protracted emesis or seizures, the initial electrolytes other than potassium and blood gases are expected to be normal in patients with chronic methylxanthine toxicity.

## CHRONIC METHYLXANTHINE USE

Data on the effect of caffeine on many chronic health issues are mixed and highly contradictory. Hypokalemia secondary to excessive consumption of caffeine-containing beverages is reported.

## CAFFEINE WITHDRAWAL

Caffeine induces tolerance and a withdrawal syndrome; headache, yawning, nausea, drowsiness, rhinorrhea, lethargy, irritability, nervousness, a disinclination to work, and depression. Withdrawal begins 12 to 24 hours after cessation and lasts up to 1 week.

## REPRODUCTION

Massive doses of methylxanthines are teratogenic, but the doses of typical use are not associated with birth defects. Human studies of fertility, fetal loss, and fetal outcome produce divergent results, and the effects of methylxanthine use during gestation are unclear.

## DIAGNOSTIC TESTING

An electrocardiogram (ECG), serum electrolytes, and a serum caffeine or theophylline concentration are indicated in cases of methylxanthine toxicity. Because toxicity is dose related in acute overdose, serum concentrations of caffeine and theophylline correlate with toxicity. Overdose of caffeine causes a spuriously elevated serum theophylline concentration. Serial theophylline concentrations, and to a lesser extent caffeine concentrations, are used to guide response to decontamination and extracorporeal drug-removal techniques. As such, concentrations should be obtained immediately and repeated every 1 to 2 hours until a downward trend is evident. Likewise, serum electrolytes, particularly potassium, should be monitored serially as long as the patient remains symptomatic. Cardiac monitoring should continue until the patient is free of dysrhythmias other than sinus tachycardia, has a decreasing serum methylxanthine concentration, and is stable.

## MANAGEMENT

### General Principles and Gastrointestinal Decontamination

After ensuring adequacy of airway, breathing, and circulation, supportive care, and maintenance of vital signs, decisions regarding gastrointestinal (GI) decontamination can be made. Activated charcoal (AC) is the only GI decontamination that should be routinely considered for methylxanthine ingestion.

### Orogastric Lavage

Orogastric lavage is an acceptable option for patients with methylxanthine ingestions capable of causing severe toxicity or fatality given an appropriate time frame (Chap. 3) and who are not already experiencing spontaneous emesis. If orogastric lavage can be performed safely, an approximated dose of ingestion of 50 mg/kg of theophylline tablets is a reasonable threshold. Most patients with caffeine ingestion are unlikely to be appropriate for orogastric lavage because concentrated caffeine is most commonly in powder, liquid, or rapidly disintegrating tablets, and caffeine is very rapidly absorbed from the stomach. Therefore, we recommend orogastric lavage for caffeine tablet ingestions of 50 mg/kg or greater that have occurred 60 minutes or less from the time orogastric lavage can be started. At the completion of orogastric lavage, the lavage tube should be used to deliver an appropriate dose of AC. If a nasogastric tube is used, it may be left in place for delivery of multiple-dose activated charcoal (MDAC).

### Activated Charcoal

Activated charcoal adsorbs methylxanthines and selective $\beta_2$-adrenergic agonists present in the GI tract and limits their absorption. Multiple-dose activated charcoal enhances the elimination of methylxanthines and is recommended for any significant ingestion. Multiple-dose activated charcoal enhances elimination of theophylline, and probably caffeine and theobromine, by "gut dialysis" (Antidotes in Brief: A1). For $\beta_2$-adrenergic agonist ingestions, only a single dose of AC is recommended.

### Whole-Bowel Irrigation

A brief period of initial whole-bowel irrigation (WBI) is reasonable for patients with ingestion of sustained-release theophylline tablets (Antidotes in Brief: A2). Polyethylene glycol electrolyte lavage solution used for WBI can displace theophylline already bound to AC. This is a concern in patients who have taken several doses of AC before WBI, in which desorption of methylxanthine from AC will result in some additional methylxanthine available for GI absorption.

## Specific Treatment

***Gastrointestinal Toxicity.*** Methylxanthine-induced vomiting is usually severe and prolonged. Use of a highly effective antiemetic, such as ondansetron or granisetron, sometimes in large doses is reasonable. However, most antiemetics are capable of resulting in QT interval prolongation, particularly in the setting of likely hypokalemia and hypomagnesemia, both common with methylxanthine toxicity. We recommend confirmation of a normal QT interval before antiemteic use. Phenothiazine antiemetics are contraindicated in methylxanthine poisoning because they are typically ineffective, and they lower the seizure threshold. Less effective antiemetics such as metoclopramide are reasonable if ondansetron or granisetron is unavailable or if the maximal ondansetron or granisetron dose has been reached or if the QT interval is already prolonged. Histamine ($H_2$) blockers and proton pump inhibitors are reasonable in any patient with hematemesis.

***Cardiovascular Toxicity.*** Hypotension should initially be treated by administration of isotonic intravenous fluid, such as 0.9% sodium chloride or lactated Ringer solution, in bolus volumes of 20 mL/kg. If an acceptable blood pressure cannot be maintained despite several fluid boluses, vasopressors should be administered. A pure α-adrenergic agonist, such as phenylephrine, is recommended, although norepinephrine is also acceptable. When hypotension is refractory to vasopressor therapy, cautious administration of a β-adrenergic antagonist such as esmolol is reasonable. Any β-adrenergic antagonist therapy should ideally be preceded and accompanied by repeated assessment of cardiac output and vascular resistance to help guide therapy.

Administration of adenosine should not be expected to convert a methylxanthine-induced SVT. Primary treatment for SVT includes administration of benzodiazepines, which work to abate CNS stimulation and concomitant release of catecholamines. More focused pharmacologic therapy to treat SVT includes the administration of a β-adrenergic antagonist or calcium channel blocker. In the nonasthmatic patient, a β-adrenergic antagonist is recommended. However, because of the risk of provoking bronchospasm, calcium channel blockers are preferred in patients with reactive airways disease. Correction of hypokalemia and hypomagnesemia is important when ventricular dysrhythmias are present.

***Central Nervous System Toxicity.*** Administration of a benzodiazepine is recommended for anxiety, agitation, or seizures. Unfortunately, the seizures associated with methylxanthine toxicity are severe and often refractory to treatment. In patients with seizures not controlled with one or two therapeutic doses of a benzodiazepine, a barbiturate or propofol is recommended. No delay should occur before administering such medications as permanent CNS injury seems more common with methylxanthine-associated seizures than with many other causes. It is important to note that phenytoin and fosphenytoin are of no benefit in controlling methylxanthine-induced seizures.

***Metabolic Abnormalities.*** Methylxanthines and $\beta_2$-adrenergic agonists shift potassium intracellularly and hypokalemia resolves on recovery. Thus, aggressive attempts to correct hypokalemia result in hyperkalemia after the β-adrenergic agonist effects abate. Hypokalemia is generally well tolerated and does not require potassium supplementation unless patients are symptomatic or have ECG changes of abnormal T waves or QT interval prolongation. Correction of hypokalemia is crucial in methylxanthine poisoning associated with ventricular dysrhythmias. Hyperglycemia does not usually necessitate treatment since it is a transient effect.

***Musculoskeletal Toxicity.*** The use of benzodiazepines is a reasonable treatment for fasciculations, hypertonicity, myoclonus, and rhabdomyolysis. Rhabdomyolysis necessitates therapy with IV fluid and sodium bicarbonate (Antidotes in Brief: A5).

## Enhanced Elimination

Methylxanthine toxicity lends itself well to several methods of enhanced elimination. Multiple-dose activated charcoal is extremely effective at enhancing elimination of theophylline. The pharmacologic similarity of the methylxanthines suggests that MDAC is probably effective in caffeine or theobromine poisoning. The efficacy of MDAC combined with the safety and ease with which this therapy can be administered makes MDAC the mainstay of enhanced elimination in methylxanthine toxicity as long as emesis can be controlled (Antidotes in Brief: A1).

Although intermittent hemodialysis has a long record of efficacy in treating methylxanthine toxicity, in some settings when hemodialysis is not an option, continuous kidney replacement therapy (CKRT) is an alternative treatment. Particularly in infants, MDAC, CKRT, and exchange blood transfusion are effective methods of enhanced elimination, and these may be used concurrently, particularly if hemodialysis is not feasible.

Consensus guidelines give specific indications for extracorporeal removal of theophylline, which are also reasonably applied to caffeine poisoning (Table 36–2). Extracorporeal treatment should be continued until clinical improvement is apparent or the concentration is less than 15 mg/L (83 μmol/L). Intermittent hemodialysis is the preferred method of extracorporeal removal, but hemoperfusion or CKRT is reasonable if hemodialysis is not feasible. Exchange transfusion is an adequate alternative to hemodialysis in neonates. Multiple-dose activated charcoal should be continued during extracorporeal treatment.

**TABLE 36–2 Methylxanthine Poisoning: Indications for Hemodialysis or Charcoal Hemoperfusion**

1. Extracorporeal xenobiotic removal is recommended if:
   a. Serum theophylline or caffeine concentration > 100 mg/L (555 mmol/L).
   b. Seizures are present.
   c. Life-threatening dysrhythmias are present.
   d. Shock is present.
   e. Theophylline or caffeine concentration is rising despite optimal treatment.
   f. Clinical deterioration occurs despite optimal therapy.
2. Extracorporeal xenobiotic removal is suggested if:
   a. Theophylline or caffeine > 60 mg/L (333 mmol/L) in chronic exposure.
   b. The patient is < 6 months or > 60 years of age and the theophylline or caffeine > 50 mg/mL (278 mmol/L) in chronic exposure.
   c. Gastrointestinal decontamination cannot be performed.

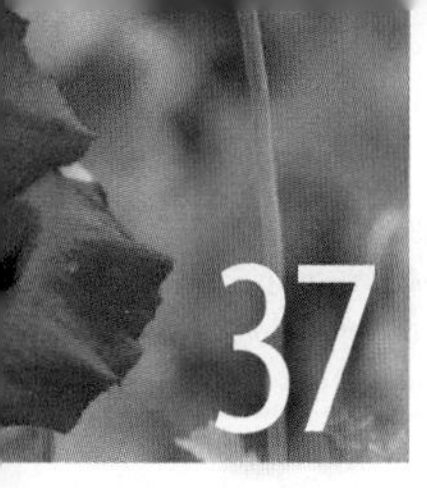



# 37 LOCAL ANESTHETICS

## HISTORY AND EPIDEMIOLOGY

Until the 1880s, the only available analgesics were centrally acting depressants such as alcohol and opioids, which blunted the perception of pain rather than addressing the underlying cause. In 1860, Albert Niemann extracted cocaine (Chap. 48) from the leaves of *Erythroxylon coca.* In 1884, Koller performed glaucoma surgery with only topical cocaine anesthesia. Although the clinical benefits of cocaine anesthesia were significant, so were its toxic and addictive potential. In 1904, Einhorn synthesized procaine, but its short duration of action limited its clinical utility. The potent, long-acting local anesthetics dibucaine and tetracaine were synthesized in the 1920s, but unfortunately, these anesthetics were not safe for regional anesthetic techniques because of systemic toxicity. Lidocaine was synthesized in 1943 and several other anesthetics followed. Considering the frequency of local anesthetic use, both within and outside healthcare facilities, clinically significant toxic reactions are relatively uncommon. Among them, poisoning from nonprescription topical benzocaine is the most common. Benzocaine spray is the most important cause of severe acquired methemoglobinemia in the hospital setting (Chap. 97).

## PHARMACOLOGY

Local anesthetics fall into one of two chemically distinct groups: amino esters and amino amides. The basic structure of all local anesthetics has three major components. A lipophilic, aromatic ring is connected by an ester or amide linkage to a short alkyl, intermediate chain that is bound to a hydrophilic tertiary (or, less commonly, secondary) amine.

All local anesthetics function by reversibly binding to specific receptor proteins within the membrane-bound sodium channels of conducting tissues. These receptors are reached only via the cytoplasmic (intracellular) side of the cell membrane. Blockade of ion conductance through the sodium channel eventually leads to failure to form and propagate action potentials. The analgesic effect results from inhibiting axonal transmission of the nerve impulse in small-diameter myelinated and unmyelinated nerve fibers that carry pain and temperature sensation. Local anesthetic blockade is much stronger for channels that are activated (open) or inactivated than for channels that are resting. Analogous to the use-dependent kinetics of class I antidysrhythmics, pain fibers have a higher firing rate and longer action potential (ie, more time with the sodium channel open or inactivated) than other fiber types and therefore are more susceptible to local anesthetic action.

These effects also occur in other conductive tissues reliant on a sodium current in the heart and brain and are the primary mechanism of toxicity. However, local anesthetics may interact with other cellular systems at clinically relevant concentrations. There is growing evidence that local anesthetics can directly affect many other organ systems and functions, such as the coagulation, immune, and respiratory systems, at concentrations much lower than those required to achieve sodium channel blockade.

The primary determinant of the onset of action of a local anesthetic is its $pK_a$ as it affects the drugs lipophilicity (Table 37–1). At physiologic pH (7.4), xenobiotics with a lower $pK_a$ have relatively more uncharged molecules free to cross the nerve cell membrane, producing a faster onset of action than xenobiotics with a higher $pK_a$. Onset of action is also influenced by the total dose of local anesthetic administered as it affects concentration for diffusion. Potency is highly correlated with lipid solubility, and protein binding is correlated with the duration of action.

**TABLE 37–1 Pharmacologic Properties of Local Anesthetics**

| | $pK_a$ | Protein Binding (%) | Log D[a] | Relative Potency | Duration of Action | Approximate Maximum Allowable Subcutaneous Dose (mg/kg) |
|---|---|---|---|---|---|---|
| **Esters** | | | | | | |
| Chloroprocaine | 9.3 | Unknown | 1.17 | Intermediate | Short | 10 |
| Cocaine | 8.7 | 92 | 1.14 | Low | Medium | 3 |
| Procaine | 9.1 | 5 | 0.72 | Low | Short | 10 |
| Tetracaine | 8.4 | 76 | 2.23 | High | Long | 3 |
| **Amides** | | | | | | |
| Bupivacaine | 8.1 | 95 | 2.45 | High | Long | 2 |
| Etidocaine | 7.9 | 95 | 3.16[b] | High | Long | 4 |
| Lidocaine | 7.8 | 70 | 2.36 | Low | Medium | 4.5 |
| Mepivacaine | 7.9 | 75 | 0.93 | Intermediate | Medium | 4.5 |
| Prilocaine | 8.0 | 40 | 0.75 | Intermediate | Medium | 8 |
| Ropivacaine | 8.2 | 95 | 1.92 | Intermediate | Long | 2–3 |

[a]Log D is the octanol/water partition coefficient at a pH of 7. [b]Log D for etidocaine is at a pH of 7.4.

## PHARMACOKINETICS

A distinction must be made between local disposition (distribution and elimination) and systemic disposition. Local distribution is influenced by several factors, including spread of the local anesthetic by bulk flow, diffusion, transport via local blood vessels, and binding to local tissues. Local elimination occurs through systemic absorption and transfer into the general circulation and by local hydrolysis of amino ester anesthetics. Systemic absorption is dependent on the avidity of binding of local anesthetics to tissues near the site of injection and on local perfusion.

All local anesthetics, except cocaine, cause peripheral vasodilation by direct relaxation of vascular smooth muscle, which enhances the vascular absorption. The addition of epinephrine (5 μg/mL) decreases the rate of vascular absorption, thereby improving the depth and prolonging the duration of local action.

The two classes of local anesthetics undergo metabolism by different routes. The amino esters are rapidly metabolized by plasma cholinesterase to the major metabolite para-aminobenzoic acid (PABA). The amino amides are metabolized more slowly in the liver to a variety of metabolites unrelated to PABA. Patients with atypical or low concentrations of plasma cholinesterase are at increased risk for systemic toxicity from amino ester local anesthetics. Factors that decrease hepatic blood flow or that impair hepatic function increase the risk of toxic reactions to the amino amides and make management of serious reactions more difficult.

## CLINICAL MANIFESTATIONS OF TOXICITY

Although the most common adverse reactions to local anesthetics are vasopressor syncopal events associated with injection, the following sections focus on their local and systemic toxicity.

### Toxic Reactions

***Regional Side Effects and Tissue Toxicity.*** At a sufficient concentration, all local anesthetics are directly cytotoxic to nerve cells. However, in clinically relevant doses, they rarely produce localized nerve damage. However, significant direct neurotoxicity results from intrathecal injection or infusion of local anesthetics for spinal anesthesia. When nerve damage occurs, it is often attributed to the use of excessively concentrated solutions, hyperbaric solutions, the preservative sodium bisulfite, or inappropriate formulation (eg, extreme pH).

### Systemic Side Effects

***Allergic Reactions.*** Allergic reactions to local anesthetics are extremely rare. Less than 1% of all adverse drug reactions caused by local anesthetics are caused by true IgE-mediated allergic reactions. The amino esters are responsible for the majority of true allergic reactions. When hydrolyzed, the amino ester local anesthetics produce PABA, a known allergen. Cross-sensitivity among the amino ester anesthetics is common. If a history of prior allergic reaction to a particular anesthetic is obtained from a patient requiring a local anesthetic, a preservative free drug from the opposite class can be chosen as there is no cross-reactivity between the amides and esters.

**TABLE 37–2** Toxic Intravenous (IV) Doses of Local Anesthetics

| *Local Anesthetic* | *Minimum IV Toxic Dose of Local Anesthetic in Humans (mg/kg)* |
|---|---|
| Bupivacaine | 1.6 |
| Chloroprocaine | 22.8 |
| Etidocaine | 3.4 |
| Lidocaine | 6.4 |
| Mepivacaine | 9.8 |
| Procaine | 19.2 |
| Tetracaine | 2.5 |

***Methemoglobinemia.*** Methemoglobinemia is frequently reported as an adverse effect of topical and oropharyngeal benzocaine use and is also reported with use of lidocaine, tetracaine, or prilocaine. Most reports of methemoglobinemia associated with local anesthetics are the result of an excessive dose. When clinically indicated, we recommend treating patients with symptomatic methemoglobinemia with intravenous methylene blue (Chap. 97 and Antidotes in Brief: A43).

***Systemic Toxicity.*** Systemic toxicity for all local anesthetics correlates with serum concentrations. Factors that determine the concentration include dose; rate of administration; site of injection; the presence or absence of a vasoconstrictor; and the degree of tissue–protein binding, fat solubility, and $pK_a$ of the local anesthetic. The brain and heart are the primary target organs for systemic toxicity. Toxicity is also related to the metabolism of a given local anesthetic. The rapidity of elimination from the plasma influences the total dose delivered to the central nervous system (CNS) or heart. The amino esters are rapidly hydrolyzed in the plasma and eliminated, explaining their relatively low potential for systemic toxicity. Although these factors make it difficult to establish safe doses of local anesthetics, Table 37–2 summarizes the estimates of minimal toxic IV doses of various local anesthetics.

***Central Nervous System Toxicity.*** Systemic toxicity in humans usually presents initially with CNS abnormalities. The rapidity with which a particular serum concentration is achieved influences anesthetic toxicity. Volunteers tolerated a higher serum concentration of etidocaine when it was infused slowly. Both metabolic and respiratory acidoses increase local anesthetic–induced CNS toxicity. Acidemia decreases plasma protein binding, increasing the amount of free drug available for CNS diffusion despite promoting the charged form of the amine group. A gradually increasing blood concentration of lidocaine produces a common pattern of symptoms and signs (Fig. 37–1). In contrast, bupivacaine toxicity often presents with cardiotoxicity.

***Cardiovascular Toxicity.*** Cardiovascular (CV) side effects are the most significant manifestations of local anesthetic toxicity. Shock and CV collapse are related to effects on vascular tone, inotropy, and dysrhythmias related to

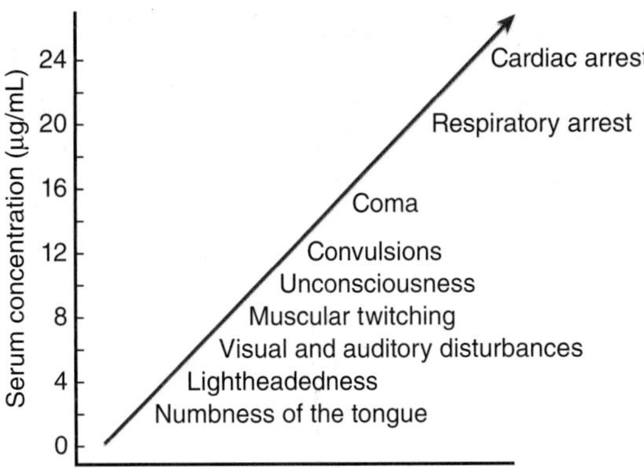


**FIGURE 37–1.** Relationship of signs and symptoms of toxicity to serum lidocaine concentrations.

indirect CNS and direct cardiac and vascular effects of the local anesthetic. For most local anesthetics (except bupivicaine), CNS toxicity develops at a lower plasma concentration than is needed to produce cardiac toxicity; that is, they have a high CV/CNS toxicity ratio.

All local anesthetics directly produce a dose-dependent decrease in cardiac contractility, with the effects roughly proportional to their peripheral anesthetic effect. Impaired conduction results from blockade of the fast sodium channels of cardiac myocytes, which slows impulse conduction in the sinoatrial and atrioventricular (AV) nodes, the His-Purkinje system, and atrial and ventricular muscles. These changes are reflected on the electrocardiogram (ECG) by increases in PR interval and QRS complex duration. At progressively higher anesthetic concentrations, hypotension, sinus arrest with a junctional escape rhythm, and eventually cardiac arrest occur. Cardiovascular toxicity of local anesthetics usually occurs after a sudden increase in serum concentration, as in unintentional intravascular injection. Cardiovascular toxicity is rare in other circumstances because high serum concentrations are necessary to produce this effect and because CNS toxicity precedes CV events, providing a warning. Bupivacaine is significantly more cardiotoxic than most other local anesthetics in common use and likely results from effects on intracellular energy dynamics. Inadvertent intravascular injection produces near simultaneous signs of CNS and cardiovascular toxicity. Table 37–3 outlines the spectrum of acute local anesthetic reactions.

**TABLE 37–3 Types of Local Anesthetic Reactions**

| *Cause* | *Major Clinical Features* |
|---|---|
| Local anesthetic toxicity (intravascular injection) | Immediate seizure or dysrhythmias |
| Reaction to adjuvant epinephrine | Tachycardia, hypertension, headache |
| Vasodepressor syncope | Bradycardia, hypotension, pallor, loss of consciousness, rapid onset and recovery consciousness |
| Allergic reaction | Anaphylaxis |
| High spinal or epidural block | Bradycardia, hypotension, respiratory distress, respiratory arrest |

## DIAGNOSTIC TESTING

The patient should be attached to continuous cardiac monitoring, and an ECG should be obtained to detect dysrhythmias and conduction disturbances. Serum electrolytes, blood urea nitrogen, creatinine, and a blood gas analysis should be obtained to help assess the cause of cardiac dysrhythmias. Cooximetry should be obtained in patients in whom methemoglobinemia is suspected clinically. Rapid, sensitive assays are available for measuring concentrations of lidocaine and its monoethylglycinexylidide (MEGX) metabolite. Assays for determining serum concentrations of other local anesthetics are not routinely available. Treatment should never be delayed while waiting for results of xenobiotic concentration determinations.

## TREATMENT

If toxicity results from ingestion of liquid medications, it is reasonable to give oral activated charcoal within 1 to 2 hours of ingestion, provided airway protective reflexes are intact. Contaminated mucous membranes should be washed off. Neither hemodialysis nor hemoperfusion has proven utility.

### Treatment of Local Anesthetic Central Nervous System Toxicity

At the first sign of possible CNS toxicity, administration of the drug must be discontinued. One hundred percent oxygen should be supplied immediately, and ventilation should be supported if necessary. Although most seizures caused by local anesthetics are self-limited, they should be treated quickly because the hypoxia and acidemia exacerbate toxicity. Benzodiazepines are recommended for initial treatment of local anesthetic–induced seizures, followed by barbiturates and propofol if necessary. When severe systemic toxicity occurs, the CV system must be monitored closely because CV depression often goes unnoticed while seizures are being treated. Since local anesthetic–induced myocardial depression occurs even with preserved blood pressure, it is important to be aware of early signs of cardiac toxicity, including ECG changes.

### Treatment of Local Anesthetic Cardiovascular Toxicity

Treatment of CV toxicity is complicated by the complex effects of local anesthetics on the heart. Initial therapy should focus on correcting the physiologic derangements that potentiate the cardiac toxicity of local anesthetics, including hypoxemia, acidemia, and hyperkalemia. If a potentially massive intravascular local anesthetic injection is suspected, maximizing oxygenation of the patient before CV collapse occurs is critical.

Advanced Cardiac Life Support (ACLS) protocols should be followed when dealing with most local anesthetic cardiac toxicity. Atropine supplemented with electrical pacing is reasonable to treat bradycardia. Use of sodium bicarbonate early in resuscitation to prevent acidemia-mediated potentiation of cardiac toxicity is reasonable. Bupivacaine-induced dysrhythmias often are refractory to cardioversion, defibrillation, and pharmacologic treatment. With toxicity from bupivacaine and etidocaine, if the patient does not respond promptly to therapy, cardiopulmonary resuscitation is expected to be difficult and prolonged (1–2 hours) before depression of the cardiac conduction system spontaneously reverses as a result of redistribution and metabolism of the drugs. Cardiopulmonary bypass has been used in some cases but increasingly, extracorporeal life support using venoarterial extracorporeal membrane oxygenation (VA-ECMO) is being used.

### Intravenous Lipid Emulsion (ILE)

Numerous case reports describe successful use of ILE to treat patients in cardiac arrest from local anesthetics. After initiating ACLS protocols, including ensuring adequate oxygenation and ventilation, we recommend that ILE be given as soon as possible after signs of significant local anesthetic toxicity become manifest. The suggested dosing for a patient in cardiac arrest is a 1.5-mL/kg bolus of 20% ILE over 1 minute while continuing chest compressions followed by continuous infusion of 0.25 mL/kg/min. More details on ILE therapy are provided in Antidotes in Brief: A23.

### Prevention of Systemic Toxicity of Local Anesthetics

The keys to prevention are to use the lowest possible anesthetic concentration and volume consistent with effective anesthesia and to avoid a significant intravascular injection. Extravascular placement is demonstrated by ultrasonographic guidance and by careful, slow aspiration before injection of a small test dose of anesthetic mixed with epinephrine. The epinephrine helps assess intravascular injection by observing for a CV response. Vigilance for early signs of CNS and cardiac toxicity is essential.

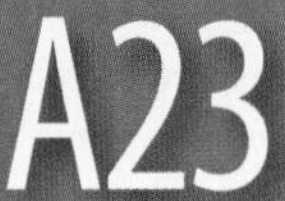

# LIPID EMULSION

## INTRODUCTION

The use of intravenous lipid emulsion (ILE) is best studied for the treatment of local anesthetic systemic toxicity. However, it is also used for the treatment of overdose from other lipophilic xenobiotics.

## HISTORY

Lipid emulsion has been used as one component of parenteral nutrition for more than 40 years and is also used as a diluent for intravenous (IV) drug delivery of highly lipophilic xenobiotics such as amphotericin and propofol. Bupivacaine toxicity is uncommon and sometimes refractory to Advanced Cardiac Life Support (ACLS) measures (Chap. 37). Intravenous lipid emulsion showed evidence of efficacy in animal models of bupivacaine toxicity. Because of this success and the limitations of other therapies, ILE was attempted in humans with local anesthetic toxicity. It was subsequently recommended by several anesthesia and medical toxicology specialty societies for the treatment of patients with local anesthetic toxicity, especially bupivacaine. In 2008, the first case of nonlocal anesthetic toxicity treated with ILE was published. Subsequently, ILE was used in many human and animal poisonings with varied results.

## PHARMACOLOGY

### Chemistry and Preparation

Lipid emulsion is composed of two types of lipids, triglycerides and phospholipids. Triglycerides (primarily linoleic, linolenic, oleic, palmitic, and stearic acids) are hydrophobic molecules that are formed when three fatty acids are linked to one glycerol. Phospholipids contain two fatty acids bound to glycerol and a phosphoric acid moiety. Phospholipids are amphipathic; the nonpolar fatty acids are hydrophobic, and the polar phosphate head is hydrophilic. This allows it to solubilize nonpolar xenobiotics in aqueous serum.

The lipids are dispersed in the serum by forming an emulsion of small lipid droplets, in which the phospholipids form a layer around a triglyceride core. The hydrophobic fatty acid component of the phospholipid molecule is directed toward the triglycerides while the hydrophilic glycerol component is directed outward away from the triglyceride core. The presence of small amounts of glycerol, which is hydrophilic, allows the lipid droplets to be suspended as an emulsion in water and serum. The lipid emulsion is a white, milky liquid that is sterile, nonpyrogenic, isosmotic, and has an average pH of 8 (range, 6–9). Lipid emulsions are easily delivered through a peripheral or central vein and intraosseously. After IV administration, lipid emulsions are found in the serum as lipid droplets that resemble chylomicrons and turn the serum turbid or milky for several hours.

### Related Lipid Formulations

Most supporting literature for the treatment of local anesthetic toxicity with ILE uses branded Intralipid™ or standard long-chain triglyceride mixtures. Other lipid emulsions, which contain mixtures of long-chain and medium-chain triglycerides, are also reportedly successful in clinical cases of poisoning. However, formulations containing oleic acid are theoretically problematic at high doses because IV sodium oleate induces acute respiratory distress syndrome (ARDS) in animals and ingestion of sodium oleate was reported to produce severe respiratory distress.

### Mechanism of Action

The mechanisms of action of parenteral lipid emulsion in toxicology are not clearly proven. The three proposed mechanisms of action of ILE are modulation of intracellular metabolism; a lipid sink, sponge, or conduit mechanism; and activation of ion channels.

***Modulation of Intracellular Metabolism.*** Bupivacaine blocks carnitine-dependent mitochondrial lipid transport and inhibits adenosine triphosphatase (ATPase) synthetase in the electron transport chain. Verapamil inhibits intracellular processing of fatty acids, but it also inhibits insulin release and produces insulin resistance. This reduces the consumption of free fatty acid (FFA) during shock, perhaps caused by the high oxygen demand required of fatty acid oxidation. The cyclic antidepressant amitriptyline depresses human myocardial contraction independent of an effect on conduction and inhibits medium- and short-chain fatty acid metabolism. Propranolol changes intracellular energy from primarily fatty acid to carbohydrate-dependent metabolism.

Theoretically, the administration of large amounts of fatty acids could overcome blocked or inhibited enzymes by mass action, providing energy to an energy "starved" heart, reversing toxicity. In a canine model, the positive effects of ILE on myocardial contraction after ischemia were mediated by improved mitochondrial metabolism. Other models did not report a similar benefit on mitochondrial energy shifts with ILE administration, raising the question as to whether or not an exogenous source of FFAs such as provided by lipid emulsion, is actually useful in a xenobiotic-induced shock state.

***Lipid Sink, Sponge, or Conduit Mechanism.*** This mechanism theorizes that lipid emulsion "soaks up" lipid-soluble xenobiotic, removing it from the site of toxicity. In a variation of this proposed mechanism, ILE sequesters the xenobiotic out of the aqueous plasma, which bathes the tissue, and within a nonaqueous part of the plasma that is not in contact with the site of toxicity. Intravenous lipid emulsion is also thought to alter the distribution of lipid-soluble xenobiotics and redistribute them away from the site of toxicity into an area with high lipid content (ie, create a "lipid conduit").

In animal experiments lipid emulsion decreased the distribution of bupivacaine, clomipramine, amiodarone, amitriptyline, bupropion, and verapamil into peripheral compartments. These findings in experimental models and case reports are used to support the lipid sink or sponge model, in which ILE removes a xenobiotic from the compartment of toxicity into the plasma, thereby raising the plasma concentration. Alternatively, the increased concentrations are also explained by an increased perfusion of tissues and release of the drug. Additional indirect evidence supports the lipid sink or sponge and a nonmetabolic mechanism as illustrated by differences in central nervous system (CNS) and myocardial metabolism. Although the myocardium can utilize fatty acids for metabolism, the CNS does not use fatty acids to a substantial degree, implying that the reversal of sedation reported with ILE administration results from xenobiotic removal from the CNS in the lipid phase as opposed to an altered metabolism.

The degree of lipid solubility of a xenobiotic is measured using the partition coefficients log P or log D. The editors of this text consider the log D at pH of 7 as the best evaluation of lipid solubility in normal plasma. Physiologic conditions that vary lipid solubility alter the amount of xenobiotic partitioning into the serum lipid and the likely success of ILE. In an in vitro model, the distribution of bupivacaine and ropivacaine in lipid emulsion decreased at lower pH.

***Activation of Ion Channels.*** Lipid emulsion is hypothesized to activate either or both $Ca^{2+}$ and $Na^{+}$ channels. In experimental models of isolated animal cells expressing grafted $Ca^{2+}$ and $Na^{+}$ channels, linolenic and stearic acids decreased bupivacaine-induced $Na^{+}$ channel blockade; fatty acids directly activated myocardial $Ca^{2+}$ channels; and oleic, linoleic, and linolenic acids directly increased $Ca^{2+}$ current with an increase in dysrhythmias. Unfortunately, these data are not representative of the clinical scenario of administration of ILE in humans or animals, and the amount of ILE used in this setting cannot be converted to a meaningful dosing regimen.

***Mechanism of Action: Conclusion.*** Despite the lack of definitive studies on mechanisms of action, the lipid sink, conduit, and sponge model is the most compelling because beneficial effects from ILE are most frequently noted for lipid-soluble xenobiotics independent of their mechanisms of toxicity.

### Pharmacokinetics

Lipid droplets are primarily hydrolyzed by lipoprotein lipase on the capillary endothelium of adipose and hepatic tissue. The half-life of intravenously administered lipid emulsion is 30 to 60 minutes and can vary substantially depending on the patient's clinical status, lipid emulsion dose, and droplet size. More than 2.5 g of lipid/kg/day (12.5 mL/kg of 20% ILE or 875 mL in a 70-kg person) overwhelms lipoprotein lipase activity, resulting in marked decreased clearance. Mean droplet sizes vary across lipid emulsion formulations, and larger droplet sizes have slower clearances and are removed by reticuloendothelial phagocytosis.

### Pharmacodynamics

For use as energy, triglycerides are transported into the mitochondria by carnitine palmitoyltransferase, where they undergo β-oxidation sequentially releasing acetylcoenzyme A (acetyl-CoA). Acetyl-CoA enters the citric acid cycle, ultimately generating adenosine triphosphate (ATP). Although glucose, lactate, and fatty acid metabolism all produce acetyl-CoA, fatty acid metabolism produces the largest amount of energy; 1 mole of glucose produces 36 moles of ATP, and 1 mole of stearic acid produces 146 moles of ATP.

## ROLE IN LOCAL ANESTHETIC TOXICITY

Based on the experimental evidence in bupivacaine toxicity, ILE was successfully used in several reported human cases of cardiovascular collapse from local anesthetic overdose. The first human case occurred after the inadvertent IV administration of bupivacaine and mepivacaine during an interscalene block. The patient developed cardiac arrest and was treated with cardiopulmonary resuscitation (CPR) and ACLS for 20 minutes but only had return of spontaneous circulation after administration of the first dose of ILE (100 mL of 20% ILE followed by 0.5 mL/kg/min for 2 hours). In a review of 76 human case reports of ILE use for resuscitation for local anesthetic toxicity, the majority reported some improvement. The absence of a control group and publication bias inherent to case reporting hamper interpretation of these data. A randomized trial that gave healthy volunteers local anesthetics to the point of early neurotoxicity was unable to demonstrate a benefit of ILE. Similarly, a pretreatment model showed no difference in electroencephalographic patterns in patients given lidocaine after ILE versus control.

We recommend administering ILE when there is rapid progression of bupivacaine toxicity affecting the CNS (agitation, confusion, seizures) or cardiovascular system (hypertension, tachycardia, ventricular dysrhythmias, hypotension, conduction blocks). The use of ILE for the same indications in other local anesthetics is reasonable. In the setting of cardiovascular collapse, ILE is recommended with CPR and standard ACLS. Lipid emulsion should be stored for easy and rapid access in operating rooms or in areas where local anesthetics are frequently used.

## ROLE IN NON–LOCAL ANESTHETIC TOXICITY

After the experience with bupivacaine toxicity, ILE was evaluated for toxicity of calcium channel blockers, cyclic antidepressant, β-adrenergic antagonists, organic phosphorus compounds, amiodarone, cocaine, and many other xenobiotics, with conflicting results.

To date, the latest and most exhaustive systematic review found more than 159 case reports, 137 of which are in humans, three low-quality randomized control trials, and one observational study of ILE for resuscitation in non–local anesthetic toxicity. All three randomized controlled trials failed to demonstrate a meaningful advantage for ILE. Despite successful reports, data on the efficacy of ILE are severely limited by reporting biases, therapeutic effects resulting from additional coadministered therapies, and coingestant xenobiotic toxicity. A study on fatality cases of the United States (US) National Poison Database system from 2006 to 2016 reported more than 450 cases of unsuccessful use of ILE for various overdoses, attesting to the fact that this therapy requires controlled studies to determine its effectiveness and adverse effect profile when used for poisonings.

The Lipid Emulsion Workgroup, composed of representatives of all major toxicology associations, published evidence-based recommendations in which ILE was recommended for cardiac arrest from bupivacaine toxicity and after failure of other modalities in patients with amitriptyline and bupropion toxicity and toxicity from other local anesthetics. The workgroup could not find evidence to recommend ILE in other situations because of a lack of data or balance between risks and possible benefits. However, given the lack of data, which yield overall neutral opinions from the Lipid Emulsion Workgroup, the authors of this textbook provide the following recommendation pending new available evidence. Lipid emulsion can be administered for patients with hemodynamic instability refractory to standard resuscitation measures when the risk-to-benefit ratio of interaction with other pharmacological or specific antidotal therapies or extracorporeal life support (ECLS) measures such as extracorporeal membrane oxygenation (ECMO) is carefully evaluated. Thus it is reasonable that lipid emulsion be used in the setting of severe toxicity (prolonged cardiovascular instability with nonperfusion or poor perfusion caused by hypotension, or dysrhythmias or seizures) resulting from a lipid-soluble xenobiotic(s) despite maximal treatment with standard resuscitation measures even if the current available evidence for the efficacy of this therapy is of very low grade. Standard antidotal therapy and resuscitative measures are shown to be superior or equivalent to lipid emulsion and should not be abandoned in a rush to administer ILE.

## ADVERSE EFFECTS AND SAFETY ISSUES

Potential complications of ILE include acute kidney injury, cardiac arrest, ventilation-perfusion mismatch, ARDS, venous thromboembolism, hypersensitivity, fat embolism, fat overload syndrome, pancreatitis, extracorporeal circulation machine circuit obstruction, allergic reaction, and increased susceptibility to infection. Intravenous lipid emulsion causes pulmonary toxicity by at least two mechanisms: occlusion of the pulmonary vasculature with microscopic fat emboli, or metabolism of linoleic acid to arachidonic acid and then into vasoactive prostaglandins. In patients with ARDS, ILE administration increases pulmonary artery pressures, pulmonary shunting, and pulmonary vascular resistance, and decreases partial pressures of oxygen in the alveoli/fraction of inspired oxygen ratio ($Pao_2/Fio_2$). The pulmonary effect of ILE in ARDS may be related to infusion rate. In patients with ARDS, 500 mL of 20% ILE infused over 5 hours resulted in an increase in pulmonary pressures, but a slower infusion over 10 hours left pulmonary pressures unchanged.

Large doses or rapid infusions of ILE have the potential to induce a fat overload syndrome, characterized by hyperlipemia, fever, fat infiltration, hepatomegaly, jaundice, splenomegaly, anemia, leukopenia, thrombocytopenia, coagulation disturbances, seizures, and coma. Particularly when administered early in the clinical course of an oral overdose, ILE has the potential to increase gastrointestinal absorption or facilitate distribution of lipid-soluble xenobiotics, resulting in increased toxicity. In orogastric models of amitriptyline and verapamil overdose, ILE increased concentrations and increased systemic toxicity. Intravenous lipid emulsion also has the potential to interact with other essential antidotes and especially epinephrine and vasopressin. If an antidote is lipid soluble, it may be incorporated by the ILE and result in decreased effectiveness.

Hyperlipidemia after using ILE interferes with many laboratory studies, making them uninterpretable. This interference lasts for several hours and is dependent in part on the type of laboratory system used. In vitro testing of ILE demonstrated that colorimetric methods were more prone to the effects of ILE than potentiometric methods. Troponin-I, sodium, potassium, chloride, calcium, bicarbonate, and urea assays had the least interference. Albumin and magnesium assays demonstrated significant interference. Amylase, lipase, phosphate, creatinine, total protein, alanine aminotransferase, creatine kinase, and bilirubin became unmeasurable.

## DOSING AND ADMINISTRATION

Dosing was initially arbitrarily defined for local anesthetic toxicity, specifically bupivacaine, with generalization of this dosing regimen to poisoning by other local anesthetics and other xenobiotics. The American Society of Regional Anesthesia and Pain Management, the Association of Anesthetists of Great Britain and Ireland, and the American Heart Association accepted similar guidelines and recommendations on the use of ILE in local anesthetic toxicity. These societies recommend a dose of 1.5 mL/kg bolus of 20% ILE followed by 0.25 mL/kg/min or 15 mL/kg/h to run for 30 to 60 minutes. They suggest repeating this bolus several times for persistent dysrhythmias and that the infusion rate can be increased if blood pressure decreases. The precise dose of ILE for non–local anesthetics has not been studied, and it is not known if boluses or infusion are more effective. The reasonable safe total dose is also unknown but would depend on the degree of toxicity and response to previous doses of ILE. The most common route of administration is IV either peripherally or via central catheters. The intraosseous route was also utilized, although it was seldomly reported as successful. The American College of Medical Toxicology published interim guidance on the use of ILE in lipophilic xenobiotic toxicity. They recommend a bolus dose of 1.5 mL/kg of 20% ILE, followed by repeat boluses of ILE for persistent severe symptoms and that the bolus "may" be followed by an infusion for 30 to 60 minutes of 0.25 mL/kg/min or to a maximum total dose of 10 mL/kg. To date, no experimental, animal, or human clinical studies exist to inform on what benefit, if any, could be expected from any infusion of ILE. The adverse effects described previously were mostly reported with ILE infusions, which provide 10 to 20 times the bolus amount in 60 minutes. We agree on a maximum total dose of 10 mL/kg.

### Pregnancy and Lactation

Intravenous lipid emulsion is a Pregnancy Category C pharmaceutical. It is not known whether ILE can cause fetal harm when administered to gravid patients. Few cases of ILE resuscitation have been published in pregnant patients. Potentially, large doses can result in elevated triglyceride concentrations, and lipid globules may occlude placental vasculature. The risk of potential toxicity should be weighed against potential benefit to the pregnant woman and fetus. There is no reported risk of ILE on breastfeeding infants.

## FORMULATION AND ACQUISITION

Lipid emulsion is available in parenteral formulation of 5%, 10%, 20%, and 30% solutions. The 20% solution is the formulation we recommend and the one used most often in the literature.

# 38 INHALATIONAL ANESTHETICS

## HISTORY AND EPIDEMIOLOGY

Paracelsus, a Swiss physician and alchemist, is credited with the earliest use of ether as an inhalational anesthetic in animals. Modern anesthetic practice began in 1846 at the Massachusetts General Hospital, when the dentist William Morton gave the first public demonstration of the ability of inhaled ether vapor to alleviate the pain of surgery. Observations on circulatory and respiratory physiology eventually led to an understanding of the effects of inhalation gases and vapors. In the last decade of the 18th century, centers for the "pneumatic treatment" of disease were established in Birmingham and Bristol, England. Experiments with ether that was inhaled via a funnel and with nitrous oxide were conducted at these institutions.

In Great Britain in 1847, James Simpson, an obstetrician, first used ether to relieve the pain of labor. He subsequently adopted chloroform for this purpose because of its more pleasant odor and more rapid induction and emergence. Over the next century, several "volatile" anesthetics were introduced, including ethyl chloride in 1848, divinyl ether in 1933, trichloroethylene in 1934, and ethyl vinyl ether in 1947. All of these inhalational anesthetics had significant safety problems associated with their use, including combustibility and direct organ toxicity.

Advances in fluorine chemistry led to the cost-effective incorporation of fluorine into molecules used in the development of modern anesthetics.

## PHARMACOLOGY

Because a wide range of chemically distinct xenobiotics can produce anesthesia, it is unlikely that a unique receptor exists for inhaled anesthetics; it is more likely that the volatile anesthetics probably cause general anesthesia by modulating synaptic function from within cell membranes. The most likely targets for the inhalational anesthetics are the ion channels that control the ion flow across the cytoplasmic membrane. Many of the side effects of the inhalational anesthetics result directly from ion channel effects in nonneural tissue, primarily cardiac cell membranes.

Reversible changes in neurologic function cause loss of perception and reaction to pain, unawareness of immediate events, and loss of memory of those events. The common pharmacologic mechanisms for general anesthesia include the physical–chemical behavior of volatile hydrocarbons with lipids and proteins within the hydrophobic regions of biologic membrane.

General anesthesia works through the physicochemical behavior of volatile hydrocarbons within the hydrophobic regions of biologic membrane lipids and proteins. The potency of the various inhaled anesthetics correlates with their lipid solubility in the lipid portion of cell membranes. This mechanism is known as the *Meyer-Overton lipid-solubility theory*.

## PHARMACOKINETICS

Because the inhaled anesthetics enter the body through the lungs, the factors that influence their absorption by blood and distribution to other tissues include the solubility in blood, blood flow through the lungs, blood flow distribution to the various organs, solubility in tissue, and the mass of the tissue. The goal of inhalation anesthesia is to develop and maintain a satisfactory partial pressure of anesthetic in the brain, the primary site of action. For the inhaled anesthetics, potency is commonly referred to as the minimum alveolar concentration (MAC) of the anesthetic. This is the alveolar concentration at 1 atm that prevents movement in response to a painful stimulus in 50% of subjects. The MAC is used when comparing the effects of equipotent doses of anesthetics on various organ functions.

## NITROUS OXIDE

Nitrous oxide is the most commonly used inhalational anesthetic in the world. Its advantages include a mild odor, absence of airway irritation, rapid induction and emergence, potent analgesia, and minimal respiratory and circulatory effects. When administered using current standards of monitoring to prevent unintentional hypoxia, it is remarkably safe. Unfortunately, nitrous oxide also has a potential for abuse, particularly among hospital and dental personnel. Death and permanent brain damage are reported, but are indirect toxic effects, secondary to hypoxia.

Deaths may rarely occur when patients receive commercially prepared nitrous oxide from tanks contaminated with impurities such as nitric oxide or nitrogen dioxide. Injury can also result from the physical properties. Because nitrous oxide is 35 times more soluble in blood than is nitrogen, any compliant air-containing space, such as bowel, will increase in size, whereas noncompliant spaces, such as the eustachian tubes, will exhibit an increase in pressure. These effects occur because nitrous oxide diffuses along the concentration gradient from the blood into a closed space much more rapidly than nitrogen can be transferred in the opposite direction. Clinical consequences include bowel distension, tympanic membrane rupture, or, more importantly, rapid progression of a pneumothorax to tension pneumothorax.

### Hematologic Effects

Bone marrow depression includes leukopenia with hypoplastic bone marrow and megaloblastic erythropoiesis, which typically develops 3 to 5 days after initial exposure and is followed by thrombocytopenia. Recovery usually occurs within 4 days after discontinuation. The hematologic effects of exposure to nitrous oxide strongly resemble the biochemical characteristics of pernicious anemia, which results from a deficiency of vitamin $B_{12}$, or cyanocobalamin. The cobalt moiety in the enzyme functions as a methyl carrier in its transfer from 5-methyltetrahydrofolate to homocysteine to form

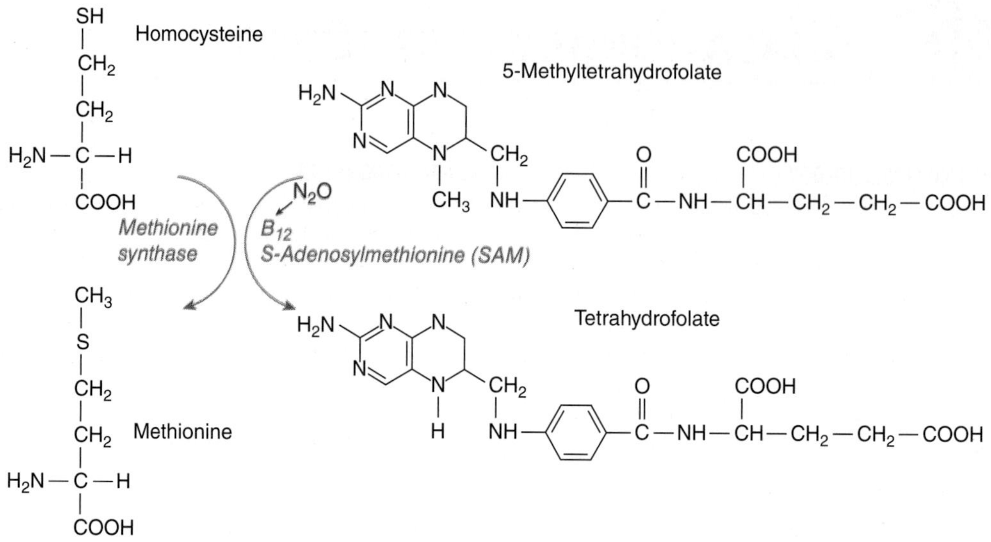

**FIGURE 38–1.** Hematologic effects of exposure to nitrous oxide ($N_2O$) resemble those characteristic of pernicious anemia and are related to oxidation and inactivation of vitamin $B_{12}$. The irreversible blockade of methionine synthase impairs DNA synthesis and myelin production.

methionine (Fig. 38–1). Nitrous oxide oxidizes the cobalt ion, converting vitamin $B_{12}$ from the active monovalent form ($Co^+$) to the inactive divalent form ($Co^{2+}$), which irreversibly inhibits methionine synthase. The metabolic consequences of this inhibition are significant because methionine and tetrahydrofolate are required for both DNA synthesis and myelin production. This interference is responsible for the development of bone marrow depression and polyneuropathy resembling the characteristic findings that occur in pernicious anemia.

### Neurologic Effects

Disabling polyneuropathy in healthcare workers who habitually used nitrous oxide was first described in 1978. The neurologic disorder improved slowly when the patients abstained from further nitrous oxide use. This neuropathy is clinically indistinguishable from subacute combined degeneration of the spinal cord associated with pernicious anemia, which is characterized by sensorimotor polyneuropathy and often combined with signs of posterior and lateral spinal cord involvement. Signs and symptoms include numbness and paresthesias in the extremities, weakness, and truncal ataxia. Neurologic changes develop only after several months of frequent exposure to nitrous oxide.

### Immunologic Effects

Nitrous oxide is associated with decreased proliferation of human peripheral blood mononuclear cells and decreased neutrophil chemotaxis. The clinical implications of this have yet to be determined.

### Cardiovascular Effects

Nitrous oxide increases postoperative homocysteine concentrations and impairs endothelial function by inhibiting an enzyme that converts homocysteine to methionine. Chronic homocysteinemia is associated with cardiovascular disease. Once again it is unclear if this has any clinical implications.

### Treatment

***General.*** Removal of the affected person from the toxic environment should be the initial intervention.

***Specific.*** Acute overdose of nitrous oxide can lead to life-threatening hypoxia. Patients admitted with respiratory compromise should be administered supplemental oxygen and monitored for 24 hours. Supportive treatment such as intensive care unit (ICU) care and mechanical ventilation is warranted in the presence of severe respiratory failure.

The treatment regimen for the neurologic sequelae of vitamin $B_{12}$ deficiency from nitrous oxide toxicity includes parenteral vitamin $B_{12}$ and oral methionine. Vitamin $B_{12}$ is recommended by either (1) intramuscular injection of 1,000 μg vitamin $B_{12}$ daily for 1 to 2 weeks followed by weekly injection of 1,000 μg for 4 to 9 weeks and then monthly injection of 1,000 μg until clinical resolution or (2) daily oral administration of 1,000 to 2,000 μg of vitamin $B_{12}$ until clinical resolution. Methionine was also successfully used when vitamin $B_{12}$ treatment alone failed to improve neurologic effects. There is no guideline for dosing methionine for patients with nitrous oxide toxicity, although case reports have used a 3-g daily oral regimen. The bone marrow abnormalities associated with nitrous oxide toxicity should be treated with a single 30-mg intravenous (IV) dose of folinic acid (Antidotes in Brief: A12).

## HALOGENATED HYDROCARBONS

The inhaled anesthetics were initially considered to be biochemically inert. Early reports of toxicity following their administration were poorly explained and attributed to direct effects on susceptible organs. It is now clear that the inhalational anesthetics are not inert but are metabolized in vivo, and that their metabolites are responsible for acute and chronic toxicity.

### Halothane Hepatitis

Two distinct types of hepatotoxicity are associated with the use of halothane. The first is a mild dysfunction that develops in approximately 20% of exposed patients. Patients exhibit modest elevations of serum aminotransferase concentrations within a few days of anesthetic exposure. Recovery is complete. In contrast, a life-threatening hepatitis occurs in approximately 1 in 10,000 exposed patients and produces fatal massive hepatic necrosis in 1 of 35,000 patients. Factors that increase the risk of developing hepatotoxicity from halothane include multiple exposures, obesity, female gender, age, and ethnic origin.

### Mechanism of Toxicity

Halothane is the most extensively metabolized inhalational anesthetic. Volatile metabolites are free radicals, which directly produce acute hepatic toxicity by irreversibly binding to and destroying hepatocellular structures. Alternatively, by acting as haptens, they trigger an immune-mediated hypersensitivity response. The high percentage of patients with halothane hepatitis who had recent reexposure is most consistent with the latter mechanism.

The use of halothane for inhalational anesthesia has markedly decreased in North America with the widespread availability of newer, safer halogenated anesthetics. Halothane is still widely used in some countries because it is inexpensive and provides a smooth induction of anesthesia.

Isoflurane and desflurane are pungent gases that can be airway irritants. Isoflurane, desflurane, and sevoflurane all appear to have low hepatotoxic potential. Cross-sensitivity may exist, such that prior exposure to one anesthetic triggers hepatotoxicity upon subsequent exposure to a different anesthetic.

### Nephrotoxicity

Methoxyflurane causes a vasopressin-resistant polyuric kidney insufficiency (nephrogenic diabetes insipidus) that lasts from 10 to 20 days in most patients, but occasionally longer. Toxicity is a result of inorganic fluoride ($F^-$) released during biotransformation of methoxyflurane. In the kidney, $F^-$ inhibits adenylate cyclase, thereby interfering with the normal action of antidiuretic hormone on the distal convoluted tubules. Methoxyflurane is no longer used, although sevoflurane may produce transient decreases in urine concentrating ability. However, clinically evident kidney impairment almost never occurs with the use of either enflurane or sevoflurane.

## INHALATIONAL ANESTHETIC–RELATED CARBON MONOXIDE POISONING

### Pharmacology

Desflurane, enflurane, and isoflurane contain a difluoromethoxy moiety that can be degraded to carbon monoxide (CO). This occasionally results in patient exposure to toxic CO concentrations, and in rare instances, to severe CO poisoning. The true incidence of CO exposure during clinical anesthesia is unknown, and no adequate passive means to routinely detect intraoperative exposure exists.

Carbon monoxide production is inversely proportional to the water content of $CO_2$ absorbents. Soda lime and Baralyme, the two most frequently used $CO_2$ absorbents, are sold wet (13%–15% water by weight), but wet absorbents dry with high gas-inflow rates. Higher concentrations of CO are most apt to be present during the first case following a weekend because of drying of the $CO_2$ absorbent from a continuous inflow of dry oxygen over the weekend. If an anesthetic machine is found with the fresh-gas flow on at the beginning of the day, it is reasonable to replace the absorbent. Changing from the use of Baralyme to soda lime should also be considered as a protective measure. Clinical monitors in routine use in the operating room cannot detect CO, although more advanced monitors may do so either directly or indirectly.

## LONG-TERM USE OF HALOGENATED ANESTHETICS IN INTENSIVE CARE UNITS

Halogenated anesthetics have been used since the 1990s in ICUs for long-term sedation of patients receiving mechanical ventilation and more recently as part of the treatment for patients with refractory status epilepticus. Use is limited by concerns regarding atmospheric pollution, but also ambient ICU air, and high costs (because of a lack of rebreathing systems in the ICU). Potential advantages include more rapid awakening and shorter times to extubation with minimal risk of toxicity.

Isoflurane is being used as a first choice for long-term sedation during mechanical ventilation in some ICUs. Reversible psychomotor dysfunction was reported in 3.6% of patients who received isoflurane for more than 12 hours as a primary sedative during mechanical ventilation and was more common in children. Reversible magnetic resonance imaging (MRI) abnormalities developed in two patients who received inhaled isoflurane for a prolonged time (35 and 85 days).

## CHRONIC EXPOSURE TO WASTE ANESTHETIC GASES

Exposure to waste anesthetic gas produces short- and long-term effects. Common short-term effects are lethargy and fatigue in staff members who are exposed to significant quantities of waste anesthetic gas. Chronic long-term effects correlate with the concentration of gas and duration of exposure. Epidemiologic studies suggest increased risks of hepatic, kidney, and neurologic disease, higher spontaneous abortion rates, reduced fertility, and a higher rate of congenital abnormalities in the offspring of dentists and dental assistants chronically exposed to nitrous oxide.

## ABUSE OF HALOGENATED VOLATILE ANESTHETICS

Fatal or life-threatening complications occur when halogenated inhalational anesthetics are used for nonanesthetic purposes (suicide attempts, mood elevation, topical treatment of herpes simplex labialis). When ingested, halothane usually produces a gastroenteritis with vomiting, followed by depression of consciousness, hypotension, shallow breathing, bradycardia with extrasystoles, and respiratory failure. Coma usually resolves within 72 hours. The diagnosis should be suspected when these features occur in a patient with the odor (sweet/fruity) of halothane on his or her breath. Supportive care, including endotracheal intubation and nasogastric lavage, should be provided with protection for potentially exposed staff. Full recovery can occur without permanent organ injury.

Intravenous injections of halothane may occur as a suicide attempt or unintentionally during induction of anesthesia. Following IV injection, coma, hypotension, and acute respiratory distress syndrome should be expected. Transient coma and apnea probably are secondary to a halothane bolus reaching the brain on its first pass through the bloodstream. Redistribution then occurs, explaining the rapid awakening. The ARDS that develops after injection of halothane most likely results from a direct toxic effect of high concentrations of the hydrocarbon on the pulmonary vasculature. Most reported cases of halothane misuse by inhalation involve hospital personnel. Inhalation of halothane produces a pleasurable sensation similar to that described with glue sniffing. Death may result from upper airway obstruction following loss of consciousness or from dysrhythmias.

# 39 NEUROMUSCULAR BLOCKERS

## HISTORY AND EPIDEMIOLOGY

Curare is the generic term for the resinous arrowhead poisons used to paralyze hunted animals. The curare alkaloids are derived from the bark of the *Strychnos* vine, and the most potent alkaloids, the toxiferines, are derived from *Strychnos toxifera*. Curare (d-tubocurarine) was introduced into clinical anesthesia in 1943, and its use spanned almost 40 years until it was replaced by superior nondepolarizing neuromuscular blockers that caused less histamine release and hypotension. Around the same time in the 1950s that curare gained popularity in the operating room, succinylcholine also came to clinical use to facilitate orotracheal intubation. Understanding the pharmacokinetics and pharmacodynamics of the depolarizing and nondepolarizing neuromuscular blockers (NDNMBs) is critical to maximizing benefit while minimizing toxicity.

## MECHANISM OF NEUROMUSCULAR TRANSMISSION AND BLOCK

The purpose of neuromuscular blockers (NMBs) is to reversibly inhibit transmission at the skeletal neuromuscular junction (NMJ). All NMBs have at least one positively charged quaternary ammonium moiety that binds to the postsynaptic nicotinic acetylcholine (nACh) receptor at the NMJ, inhibiting its normal activation by acetylcholine (ACh). Activation of this receptor opens a sodium channel that leads to myocyte depolarization. Skeletal muscle paralysis can occur by several mechanisms. Figure 39–1 reviews the function of the NMJ and illustrates the mechanisms by which different xenobiotics can cause paralysis.

Modulation of postsynaptic ACh receptor activity at the neuromuscular junction can produce paralysis by one of two mechanisms: depolarizing (phase I block) and nondepolarizing (phase II block). Succinylcholine is the only depolarizing NMB (DNMB) in current clinical use; the other drugs discussed are all NDNMBs. The NDNMBs cause skeletal muscle paralysis by competitively inhibiting the effects of ACh and thus preventing muscle depolarization.

## PHARMACOKINETICS

The NMBs are highly water soluble and relatively insoluble in lipids and thus cross the blood–brain barrier (BBB) poorly. Table 39–1 presents their relevant pharmacology.

## COMPLICATIONS OF NEUROMUSCULAR BLOCKERS

Complications associated with the use of NMBs include (1) problems associated with the care of a patient who is therapeutically paralyzed (eg, undetected hypoventilation caused by ventilator or airway problems, impaired ability to monitor neurologic function, unintentional patient awareness, peripheral nerve injury, deep vein thrombosis, and skin breakdown); (2) immediate side effects; and (3) effects occurring following prolonged drug exposure.

### Consciousness

The NMBs do not affect consciousness, and therefore, a sedative must be coadministered in conscious patients. The pupillary light reflex, an important indicator of midbrain function, is preserved in healthy subjects who have received

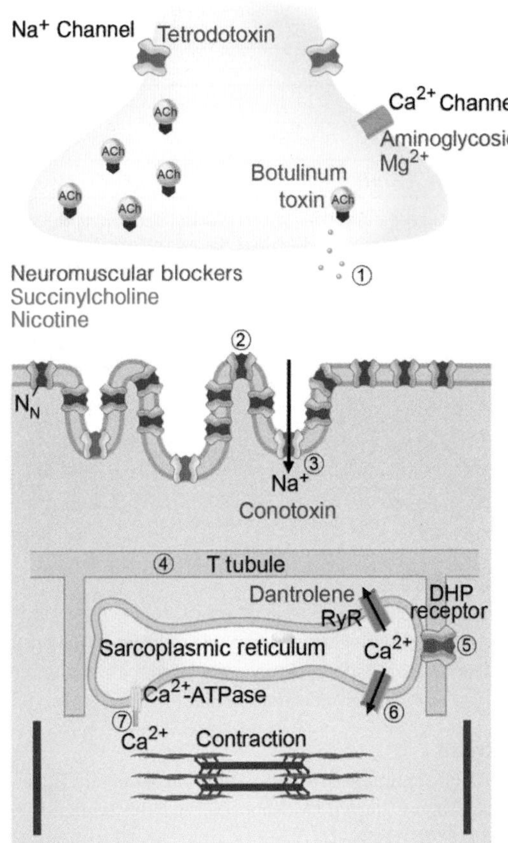


**FIGURE 39–1.** Excitation–contraction coupling in skeletal muscle. At the neuromuscular junction, acetylcholine (1) released from the presynaptic nerve terminal crosses the 50-nm synaptic cleft to reach the nicotinic acetylcholine (nACh) receptor (2). When an agonist simultaneously occupies both receptor sites, this ion channel opens, becoming nonselectively permeable to monovalent cations, resulting in an influx of $Na^+$ and an efflux of $K^+$. This produces local membrane depolarization (endplate potential), which in turn opens voltage-gated $Na^+$ channels (3). A depolarization of sufficient amplitude generates a propagated muscle action potential (MAP), which is conducted along the muscle membrane and down the transverse (T) tubules (4). In the T tubule, the MAP triggers a voltage-gated calcium channel (7) and the dihydropyridine receptor (5), which then activates the skeletal muscle ryanodine receptor/channel (6). To allow the fastest activation of mammalian skeletal muscle, calcium diffusion is not necessary for activation of the type 1 ryanodine receptor (RyR-1); instead, there is a direct electrical (protein) linkage between the dihydropyridine (DHP) receptor and the ryanodine receptor. Active ATPase-driven calcium reuptake terminates muscle contraction. Many factors influence the activity of the RyR-1 channel, including $Ca^{2+}$, $Mg^{2+}$, and xenobiotics such as inhalational anesthetics that accelerate $Ca^{2+}$ release in persons susceptible to malignant hyperthermia. Antagonists such as conotoxin are red and agonists such as nicotine are green.

**TABLE 39–1 Pharmacology of Selected Neuromuscular Blockers**

| *Generic Name* | *Class* | *Duration* | *Initial Dose (mg/kg)*[a,b] | *Onset (min)*[c] | *Clinical Duration (min)*[d] |
|---|---|---|---|---|---|
| Succinylcholine | Depolarizer | Ultrashort | 0.6–1 | 1–1.5 | 3–7 |
| Atracurium | Nondepolarizer, benzylisoquinolinium | Intermediate | 0.4 | 2–4 | 20–40 |
| Cisatracurium | | Intermediate | 0.1 | 2–4 | 20–40 |
| Pancuronium | Nondepolarizer, aminosteroid | Long | 0.1 | 3–6 | 60–90 |
| Rocuronium | | Intermediate | 0.6 | 1.5–3 | 30–40 |
| Vecuronium | | Intermediate | 0.1 | 2–4 | 20–40 |
| | *Renal Excretion (%)*[e] | *Biliary Excretion (%)*[f] | *Metabolite* | *Histamine Release* | *Effect on Heart Rate* |
| Succinylcholine | < 10 | Minimal | Succinic acid | Minimal | Bradycardia (rare) |
| Atracurium | 5–10 | Minimal | Laudanosine | Minimal | No |
| Cisatracurium | 10–20 | Minimal | Laudanosine | No | No |
| Pancuronium | 40–60 | 10–20 | 3-Desacetyl-pancuronium[g] | No | Tachycardia |
| Rocuronium | 10–20 | 50–70 | No | No | Tachycardia at high dose |
| Vecuronium | 15–25 | 40–70 | 3-Desacetyl-vecuronium | No | No |

[a]Cisatracurium is labeled as milligram of base per milliliter. Other drugs are labeled and packaged as milligram of salt per milliliter. [b]Typical initial dose is approximately $2 \times ED_{95}$ (mg/kg). [c]Onset is time from bolus to 100% block. [d]Clinical duration is time from drug injection until 25% recovery of single twitch height. [e]Percent renal excretion in the first 24 h of unchanged drug; if high, associated with prolongation of clinical effect. [f]Percent biliary excretion in first 24 h of unchanged drug; if high, associated with prolongation of clinical effect. [g]Active metabolite.

Data from Donati F. Neuromuscular blocking drugs for the new millennium: current practice, future trends—comparative pharmacology of neuromuscular blocking drugs. *Anesth Analg*. 2000;90(suppl):S2-S6; McManus MC. Neuromuscular blockers in surgery and intensive care, part 1. *Am J Health Syst Pharm*. 2001;58:2287-2299; and Murray MJ, et al. Clinical practice guidelines for sustained neuromuscular blockade in the adult critically ill patient. *Crit Care Med*. 2002:30:142-156.

NDNMBs because pupillary function is mediated by muscarinic cholinergic receptors, for which the NMBs have no affinity.

### Histamine Release

Neuromuscular blockers may elicit dose- and injection rate–related nonimmunologic histamine release from tissue mast cells. The NMBs most commonly associated with histamine release are atracurium and succinylcholine.

### Anaphylaxis

Anaphylactic reactions are rare, with rocuronium and succinylcholine being the two NMBs most often cited as offenders.

### Control of Respiration

At subparalyzing doses, NDNMBs blunt the hypoxic ventilatory response (HVR) but not the ventilatory response to hypercapnia. At paralyzing doses, they prevent the mechanics of ventilation.

### Autonomic Side Effects

The neuronal nACh receptors found in autonomic ganglia are less susceptible to block by NMBs. Notably, tubocurarine also blocks nACh receptors at the parasympathetic ganglia, causing tachycardia, and at the sympathetic ganglia, blunting the sympathetic response.

Dysrhythmias, including bradycardia, junctional rhythms, ventricular dysrhythmias, and cardiac arrest, occur rarely after succinylcholine. This most likely results from stimulation of the cardiac muscarinic receptors and can be prevented by pretreatment with atropine.

## INTERACTIONS OF MUSCLE RELAXANTS WITH OTHER DRUGS AND PATHOLOGIC CONDITIONS

There are significant interactions of NMBs with many medications and coexisting medical conditions (Table 39–2).

## PHARMACOLOGY OF SUCCINYLCHOLINE

Succinylcholine is hydrolyzed mostly by plasma (pseudo-) cholinesterase (ChE) and to a slight extent by alkaline hydrolysis. At an induction dose of 1 mg/kg IV, succinylcholine theoretically increases cerebral blood flow, cortical electrical activity, intracranial pressure (ICP), and intraocular pressure, but the clinical implications of these effects are unclear.

## TOXICITY OF SUCCINYLCHOLINE

The important adverse drug reactions associated with succinylcholine include anaphylaxis, prolonged drug effect, hyperkalemia, acute rhabdomyolysis in patients with muscular dystrophy, malignant hyperthermia (MH) in susceptible patients, masseter spasms or trismus in patients with congenital myopathies, and cardiac dysrhythmias. This is especially relevant for children who present with undiagnosed or a clincally subtle myopathy.

### Prolonged Effect

The effects of succinylcholine can last for several hours if metabolism is slowed because of decreased or abnormal plasma ChE.

### Hyperkalemia

Succinylcholine typically causes a transient serum $K^+$ concentration increase of approximately 0.5 mEq/L within minutes

**TABLE 39–2 Effect of Prior Administration of Xenobiotics on Subsequent Response to Succinylcholine or Nondepolarizing Neuromuscular Blockers**

| *Xenobiotic* | *Response to Succinylcholine* | *Response to Nondepolarizer* | *Comments* |
|---|---|---|---|
| Aminoglycosides (eg, amikacin, gentamicin) | Potentiates | Potentiates | Dose-related decrease in presynaptic ACh release. Decrease postjunctional response to ACh. Partially reversible with calcium administration. The ability of neostigmine to reverse this effect is unpredictable. |
| Anticholinesterase, peripherally acting: neostigmine, edrophonium | Prolongs succinylcholine (except edrophonium) | No effect | Neostigmine, pyridostigmine, and physostigmine inhibit plasma AChE and prolong succinylcholine block. Edrophonium does not inhibit plasma cholinesterase. |
| Anticholinesterase, centrally acting: donepezil | Potentiates | No effect | Inhibits AChE (junctional >> plasma); long half-life (70 h). |
| β-Adrenergic antagonist: propranolol | Potentiates in cats, effects in humans uncertain | Potentiates | When given alone, unmasks myasthenic syndrome. Blocks ACh binding at postsynaptic membrane. Reversal of block with neostigmine causes severe bradycardia. |
| β-Adrenergic antagonist: esmolol | ? Mild prolongation | Slows onset of rocuronium | Competes for PChE or red blood cell cholinesterase. |
| Botulinum toxin | ? | Early potentiation, delayed resistance | Subclinical systemic denervation leads to hypersensitivity. |
| Calcium channel blockers | Potentiates | Potentiates | Causes calcium channel block pre- and postjunctionally. Verapamil has local cholinesterase inhibitor effect on nerve. Inhibits block reversal of NDNMBs by cholinesterase inhibitors. |
| Carbamazepine | ? | Inhibits, shortened duration | Chronic therapy causes resistance to NDNMB, except for atracurium. |
| Cardioactive steroids | More prone to cardiac dysrhythmias | Pancuronium increases catecholamines and causes dysrhythmias | |
| Dantrolene | ? | Potentiates | Blocks excitation–contraction coupling by blocking ryanodine receptor channel in sarcoplasmic reticulum of skeletal muscle. |
| Furosemide | Potentiates or inhibits | Potentiates or inhibits | Biphasic dose response in cats; protein kinase inhibition at low doses and phosphodiesterase inhibition at high doses. Diuretic-related hypokalemia potentiates pancuronium in cats. |
| Glucocorticoids | ? | Inhibits | Chronic steroid use induces resistance to pancuronium and decreases plasma cholinesterase activity by 50%. Steroids ± NDNMB associated with myopathies. |
| Inhalational anesthetics: isoflurane | Potentiates | Potentiates | Decreases CNS activity and potentiates NMB in anesthetic doses-dependent fashion (postsynaptic and muscle effects). Halothane causes less muscle relaxation than isoflurane. |
| Lidocaine | Potentiates | Low dose potentiates block; high dose inhibits nerve terminals and blocks ACh binding site at postsynaptic membrane | The fast $Na^+$ channel blockers decrease action potential propagation, ACh release, postsynaptic membrane sensitivity, and muscle excitability. Weak inhibitor of PChE. This potentially is observed with all local anesthetics, but practically lidocaine is the only one that is intravenously administered. |
| Lithium | Prolongs onset and duration | Prolongs effect of pancuronium | Inhibits synthesis and release of ACh. Lithium alone causes myasthenic reaction. |
| Magnesium | Potentiates; blocks fasciculations | Potentiates or prolongs blocks | Decreases prejunctional ACh release, postjunctional membrane sensitivity, and muscle excitability. |
| NDNMB: pancuronium, vecuronium, rocuronium | "Precurarization" with NDNMB shortens the onset and decreases side effects of succinylcholine; pancuronium increases block duration | Chronic NDNMB induces resistance to their effect; mixing different NDNMBs causes greater than additive effects, especially combining pancuronium with tubocurarine or metocurine | Prior NDNMB inhibits plasma PChE and prolongs mivacurium and succinylcholine block. Rank order: pancuronium > vecuronium > atracurium. Heterozygotes for atypical PChE develop phase II block when given succinylcholine and pancuronium. |
| Organic phosphorus compounds | Potentiates | ? | Irreversible PChE inhibitor that totally blocks enzyme activity. |
| Phenelzine (MAOI) | Prolongs | ? | Decreases PChE activity. |

(*Continued*)

**TABLE 39–2 Effect of Prior Administration of Xenobiotics on Subsequent Response to Succinylcholine or Nondepolarizing Neuromuscular Blockers (*Continued*)**

| *Xenobiotic* | *Response to Succinylcholine* | *Response to Nondepolarizer* | *Comments* |
|---|---|---|---|
| Phenytoin | ? | Resistant, shortened duration | Acutely, potentiates NDNMB paralysis. With chronic use (except for atracurium), phenytoin induces resistance to NDNMB and increases metabolism. This increases the initial dose and decreases the repeat dosing interval. |
| Polypeptide antibiotics: polymyxin | Potentiates | Potentiates | Causes severe weakness and induces postsynaptic neuromuscular block. Neostigmine increases block. |
| Succinylcholine | Small initial doses of succinylcholine are used to limit muscular fasciculations | Pancuronium and vecuronium are slightly prolonged by prior succinylcholine | |
| Theophylline | | Inhibits | The combination of pancuronium and theophylline increases cardiac dysrhythmias. |
| Cyclic antidepressants (CA) | | | The combination of pancuronium and CA causes cardiac dysrhythmias due to sympathetic effects. |

ACh = acetylcholine; AChE = acetylcholinesterase; CNS = central nervous system; MAOI = monoamine oxidase inhibitor; NDNMB = nondepolarizing neuromuscular blocker; NMB = neuromuscular blocker; NMJ = neuromuscular junction; PChE = plasma cholinesterase.

Data from Crowe S, Collins L. Suxamethonium and donepezil: a cause of prolonged paralysis. *Anesthesiology*. 2003;98:574-575; Flacchino F, et al. Sensitivity to vecuronium after botulinum toxin administration. *J Neurosurg Anesthesiol*. 1997;9:1491153; Fleming NW, et al. Neuromuscular blocking action of suxamethonium after antagonism of vecuronium by edrophonium, pyridostigmine or neostigmine. *Br J Anaesth*. 1996;77:492-495; Kaeser HE. Drug-induced myasthenic syndromes. *Acta Neurol Scand Suppl*. 1984;100:39-47; Kato M, et al. Inhibition of human plasma cholinesterase and erythrocyte acetylcholinesterase by nondepolarizing neuromuscular blocking agents. *J Anesth*. 2000;14:30-34; Ostergaard D, et al. Adverse reactions and interactions of the neuromuscular blocking drugs. *Med Toxicol Adverse Drug Exp*. 1989; 4:351-368; and Viby-Mogensen J. Interaction of other drugs with muscle relaxants. In: Katz RL, ed. *Muscle Relaxants: Basic and Clinical Aspects*. New York, NY: Grune & Stratton; 1985:233-256.

both in normal individuals and in persons with kidney failure. The acute hyperkalemic response to succinylcholine is greatly exaggerated with coexisting myopathy or proliferation of extrajunctional muscle ACh receptors. Conditions that are associated with proliferation of ACh receptors include head or spinal cord injury, stroke, neuropathy, prolonged use of NDNMBs because of muscle pathology, direct trauma, crush or compartment syndrome, or muscular dystrophy; critical illness due to hemorrhagic shock, neuropathy, myopathy, or prolonged immobility; thermal burn or cold injury; and sepsis lasting several days. After a neurologic injury, susceptibility to hyperkalemia begins within 4 to 7 days and persists for an extended period of time. Severe hyperkalemia can be mitigated, but not prevented, by a small dose of an NDNMB.

### Rhabdomyolysis

Severe hyperkalemia rarely occurs in the absence of a clinical history that readily discloses an obvious risk factor, with one important exception. An acute or delayed onset of rhabdomyolysis, hyperkalemia, ventricular dysrhythmias, cardiac arrest, and death are reported in apparently healthy children who were subsequently found to have a myopathy. If there is coexisting fever, muscle rigidity, hyperlactatemia, or metabolic and respiratory acidosis, the presumptive diagnosis of MH should also prompt immediate therapy with dantrolene.

### Malignant Hyperthermia

Malignant hyperthermia, a syndrome characterized by extreme skeletal muscle hypermetabolism, is inherited as an autosomal dominant trait with variable penetrance. Mutations of the RYR1 receptor are detected in 50% to 70% of patients with MH (Fig. 39–1). Triggering xenobiotics that can precipitate an attack of MH include succinylcholine and volatile inhalational anesthetics (the prototypical xenobiotic is halothane). Rarely, MH is triggered by severe exercise in a hot climate, IV potassium (which depolarizes the muscle membrane), antipsychotics, or infection.

In the operating room, MH most often presents abruptly soon after initial exposure to a triggering anesthetic, although the onset of MH may be delayed several hours during the anesthesia or occur as long as 12 hours after surgery. The immediate systemic manifestations of MH result from extreme skeletal muscle hypermetabolism. The uncontrolled release of calcium from the terminal cisternae of the sarcoplasmic reticulum causes skeletal muscle contraction. Although generalized muscular rigidity is a specific sign of MH, it is only observed in 40%; masseter spasm is a finding observed in 27% of MH patients. Futile calcium cycling by sarcoplasmic $Ca^{2+}$-ATPase rapidly depletes intracellular adenosine triphosphate and leads to anaerobic metabolism. Clinically, MH presents as hypermetabolism with an increase in cardiac output and sinus tachycardia; increased $CO_2$ production causes hypercapnia; increased $O_2$ consumption can cause mixed venous $O_2$ desaturation, arterial hypoxemia, anaerobic metabolism, metabolic acidosis, elevated lactate concentration, cyanosis, and skin mottling; and excess heat production that leads to a rapid increase in core temperature with hyperthermia. The antidote for MH is dantrolene (Antidotes in Brief: A24), and the other essential aspects of therapy are rapid initial diagnosis, discontinuation of triggering anesthetics, and active cooling (Table 39–3).

### Muscle Spasms

When administered to persons genetically predisposed to myotonia, succinylcholine precipitates tonic muscular contractions, ranging from trismus (which prevents orotracheal

**TABLE 39–3 Therapy for Malignant Hyperthermia (MH)[a]**

***Acute Phase Treatment of MH***

1. Call for help. Immediately summon experienced help when MH is suspected. Call MH hotline, 800-644-9737.
2. Discontinue triggers: volatile inhalational anesthetics and succinylcholine.
3. Hyperventilate with 100% $O_2$ with flow ≥ 10 L/min and monitor end-tidal $CO_2$.
4. Halt procedure as soon as possible and continue sedation and analgesia with nontriggering agents: opioids and benzodiazepines.
5. Administer dantrolene, initial IV bolus of 2.5 mg/kg followed by additional boluses (every 15 minutes), until signs of MH are controlled (tachycardia, rigidity, increased end-tidal $CO_2$, hyperthermia). Typically, a total dose of 10 mg/kg IV controls symptoms, but occasionally 30 mg/kg is required.
   - Dantrium/Revonto:[b] Each 20-mg vial is reconstituted by adding 60 mL of sterile water.
   - Ryanodex: Each 250-mg vial is reconstituted by adding 5 mL of sterile water.
6. Monitor core temperature closely (tympanic membrane, nasopharynx, esophagus, rectal, or pulmonary artery) and actively cool the patient with core temperature > 39°C (immersion in ice-water slurry is preferred; cooling by peritoneal or gastric lavage, or surface cooling techniques is also reasonable).
7. Hyperkalemia is common and should be treated with hyperventilation, IV calcium gluconate (30 mg/kg up to 3 g) or chloride (10 mg/kg up to 1 g), sodium bicarbonate, IV dextrose, and insulin. Hypokalemia should be treated with caution because of the potential for rhabdomyolysis induced hyperkalemia.[c]
8. Sodium bicarbonate. 1.2 mEq/kg is reasonable if blood gas values have not yet been obtained or if clinically indicated.
9. Monitor continuously: ECG, pulse oximetry, end-tidal $CO_2$, core temperature, CVP, urine output; and serially measure: arterial and mixed venous blood gases, metabolic profile (especially potassium), calcium, CBC, coagulation indices, and creatine kinase.
10. Dysrhythmias usually respond to dantrolene, cooling, and correction of acidemia and hyperkalemia. If dysrhythmias persist or are life threatening, standard antidysrhythmics are indicated, including amiodarone, magnesium, and procainamide.
    - Calcium channel blockers (verapamil or diltiazem) should not be used to treat dysrhythmias because they may cause hyperkalemia and cardiac arrest.
11. Ensure adequate urine output by restoration of intravascular volume followed by administration of mannitol or furosemide. Insert a urinary bladder catheter and consider central venous or pulmonary artery catheterization.
12. For emergency consultation, refer to the MHAUS at http://www.mhaus.org/. Call the MH Emergency Hotline:
    - Inside the United States or Canada, call 800-MH-HYPER (800-644-9737).
    - Outside the United States and Canada, call 001 315-464-7079.

***Postacute Phase Treatment of MH***

1. Observe the patient in an ICU setting for at least 24 h because recrudescence of MH occurs in 25% of cases, particularly after a fulminant case resistant to treatment. Observe for pulmonary edema, kidney failure, and compartment syndrome.
2. Administer dantrolene 1 mg/kg IV q4–6h or 0.25 mg/kg/h by infusion for at least 24 h after the episode.
3. Serially monitor arterial blood gases, metabolic profile, CBC, creatine kinase, calcium, phosphorus, coagulation indices, urine and serum myoglobin, and core body temperature until they return to normal values.
4. Counsel the patient and family regarding MH and further precautions.
   - For nonemergency patient referrals, contact the MHAUS at 800-644-9737, 1 North Main Street, PO Box 1069, Sherburne, NY 13460.
   - Report patients who have had an acute MH episode to the North American MH Registry of MHAUS at 888-274-7899.
   - Alert family members to the possible dangers of MH and anesthesia.
5. Recommend an MH medical identification tag or bracelet for the patient, which should be worn at all times.

[a]The guidelines may not apply to every patient and of necessity must be altered according to specific patient needs. [b]There are two formulations of dantrolene, Dantrium/Revonto and Ryanodex. [c]Sudden unexpected cardiac arrest in children: Children younger than about 10 years of age who experience sudden cardiac arrest after succinylcholine administration in the absence of hypoxemia and anesthetic overdose should be treated for acute hyperkalemia first. In this situation, calcium chloride should be administered along with means to reduce serum potassium. They should be presumed to have subclinical muscular dystrophy, and a pediatric neurologist should be consulted.

CBC = complete blood count; CVP = central venous pressure; ECG = electrocardiogram; ICU = intensive care unit; IV = intravenous; MHAUS = Malignant Hyperthermia Association of the United States.

Modified from Malignant Hyperthermia Association of the United States (mhaus.org).

intubation) to severe generalized myoclonus and chest wall rigidity (which prevent ventilation). Because the myotonic contractions are independent of neural activity, they cannot be aborted by an NDNMB. Usually the contractions are self-limited, but occasionally they will be life threatening if an airway cannot be established and hypoxemia ensues.

## PHARMACOLOGY OF NONDEPOLARIZING NEUROMUSCULAR BLOCKERS

Table 39–1 details the pharmacology and toxicity of these drugs.

## TOXICITY OF NONDEPOLARIZING NEUROMUSCULAR BLOCKERS

The most important toxic effects of the NDNMBs are accumulation of laudanosine and persistent weakness.

### Laudanosine

Metabolism of atracurium and cisatracurium generates laudanosine, which crosses the blood–brain and placental barriers but lacks any neuromuscular blocking activity. Laudanosine is excreted primarily in the bile, and its elimination is prolonged in patients with liver disease, biliary obstruction, and kidney disease. In the CNS, laudanosine has an inhibitory effect at the γ-aminobutyric acid, nACh, and opioid receptors. At high serum concentrations in experimental animals, laudanosine causes dose-related neuroexcitation, myoclonic activity (> 14 μg/mL), and generalized seizures (> 17 μg/mL), but in humans, seizures directly attributable to atracurium are not reported.

### Persistent Weakness Associated with Nondepolarizing Neuromuscular Blockers

Short-term blockade with an NDNMB usually resolves promptly upon discontinuation. When an NDNMB is administered for more than 48 hours, there is a risk that weakness will persist longer than anticipated based on the kinetics of drug elimination. In addition, critical illness is associated with dysfunction of the peripheral nerve, NMJ, and muscle (Table 39–4).

**TABLE 39–4 Acute Neuromuscular Pathology Associated With Critical Illness or Nondepolarizing Neuromuscular Blockers**

| | *Critical Illness Polyneuropathy* | *Residual Neuromuscular Block* | *Disuse (Cachectic) Myopathy* | *Critical Illness Myopathy* |
|---|---|---|---|---|
| Sensory | Moderate to severe, distal > proximal | Normal | Normal | Normal |
| Motor | Symmetric weakness, lower > upper extremity, proximal > distal or diffuse, respiratory failure | Diffuse symmetric weakness, respiratory failure | Diffuse weakness, proximal > distal | Symmetric weakness, proximal > distal or diffuse, respiratory failure |
| Creatine phosphokinase | Normal | Normal | Normal | Elevated in ≤ 50% |
| Electrodiagnostic studies (EMG, NCV) | Axonal degeneration of motor > sensory, reduced sensory and motor compound action potentials, normal NCV | Fatigue at NMJ assessed by fade on repetitive nerve stimulation | Normal EMG and NCV | Myopathic changes, muscle membrane inexcitability, normal NCV |
| Muscle biopsy | Denervation atrophy | Normal | Atrophy of type 2 fibers, no myosin loss, no necrosis | Atrophy of type 2 fibers, myosin loss, mild myonecrosis, no inflammatory infiltration |

EMG = electromyography; NCV = nerve conduction velocity; NMJ = neuromuscular junction.

Data from Bolton CF. Critical illness polyneuropathy and myopathy. *Crit Care Med*. 2001;29:2388-2390; Lacomis D. Critical illness myopathy. *Curr Rheumatol Rep*. 2002;4:403-408; Lacomis D, Campellone JV. Critical illness neuromyopathies. *Adv Neurol*. 2002;88:325-335; and Leijten FSS, de Weerd AW. Critical illness polyneuropathy: a review the literature, definition and pathophysiology. *Clin Neurol Neurosurg*. 1994;96:10-19.

## PHARMACOLOGY OF REVERSAL DRUGS

### Acetylcholinesterase Inhibitors

Termination of NMB effect initially results from drug redistribution and later from drug elimination, metabolism, or chemical antagonism. Partial pharmacologic antagonism of a NDNMB is achieved by giving a reversal agent that inhibits junctional AChE and thereby increases ACh, which can overcome the competitive inhibition caused by residual NDNMB (Table 39–5). The most common and troublesome clinical side effect of ChE inhibition is bradycardia, which usually is prevented by coadministration of an antimuscarinic such as atropine.

### Sugammadex

Sugammadex reverses the effect of steroidal NMBs (roccuronium and vecuronium) by directly binding them in a 1:1 ratio to form a complex that does not bind to the nicotinic receptors. Administration of IV sugammadex results in rapid removal of NMB from plasma, which facilitates the movement of NMBs from the NMJ into plasma through a concentration gradient effect, where they bind to any free remaining sugammadex.

The doses of sugammadex based on actual body weight are:

- 2 mg/kg for shallow blockade: if spontaneous recovery has been reached up to the reappearance of the second twitch to train-of-four stimulation after rocuronium and vecuronium blockage
- 4 mg/kg for profound blockage: if one or two posttetanic counts and response to train-of-four stimulation after rocuronium and vecuronium blockade
- 16 mg/kg for immediate reversal: 3 minutes after administration of 1.2 mg/kg of rocuronium. Immediate reversal of vecuronium is unstudied.

**TABLE 39–5 Pharmacology of Intravenous Neuromuscular Blockade Reversal Drugs and Coadministered Antimuscarinics**

| | *Anticholinesterases* | | |
|---|---|---|---|
| | *Neostigmine* | *Pyridostigmine* | *Edrophonium* |
| Initial dose (mg/kg) | 0.04–0.08 | 0.2–0.4 | 0.5–1.0 |
| Onset (min) | 7–11 | 10–16 | 1–2 |
| Duration (min) | 60–120 | 60–120 | 60–120 |
| Recommended antimuscarinic | Glycopyrrolate | Glycopyrrolate | Atropine (preferred because the time of onset is better paired with edrophonium) |

| | *Antimuscarinics* | |
|---|---|---|
| | *Glycopyrrolate* | *Atropine* |
| Structure | Quaternary ammonium | Tertiary amine |
| Initial dose (mg/kg) | 0.01–0.02 | 0.02–0.03 |
| Onset (min) | 2–3 | 1 |
| Duration (min) | 30–60 | 30–60 |
| Elimination | Renal | Renal |
| Crosses blood–brain barrier | No | Yes |

## CHOICE OF REVERSAL

Choice of reversal between sugammadex versus acetylcholinesterase inhibitor is complex. Sugammadex offers two major advantages: rapid reversal and lack of cholinergic side effects. Its disadvantages include a lack of affinity for nonsteroidal NDNMB and a variable affinity for steroidal NMB (rocuronium > vecuronium >> pancuronium).

## DIAGNOSTIC TESTING

Quantitative methods employing high-performance liquid chromatography and mass spectrometry are available for analysis of blood and tissue NMB (both NDNMB and succinylcholine) and metabolite concentrations.

# A24 DANTROLENE SODIUM

## INTRODUCTION

Dantrolene relaxes skeletal muscle without causing paralysis. It is the only therapy proven to be effective for both treatment and prophylaxis of malignant hyperthermia (MH). Malignant hyperthermia is a rare life-threatening condition of skeletal muscle that overwhelms the ability of the body to supply oxygen, remove carbon dioxide, and regulate body temperature and can quickly lead to circulatory collapse if untreated.

## HISTORY

Dantrolene was first synthesized in 1967 in a study of hydantoin derivatives as potential muscle relaxants. Four years later, it was used in oral form to treat skeletal muscle spasticity secondary to neurologic disorders. The ability of intravenous (IV) dantrolene to rapidly reverse MH was first reported in humans in 1982.

## PHARMACOLOGY

Dantrolene is highly lipophilic, and widespread use had to wait until there was a suitable IV preparation. Oral dantrolene exhibits variable absorption by the small intestine, bioavailability is up to 70%, and peak blood concentrations are achieved 3 to 6 hours after ingestion. Dantrolene is metabolized in the liver to 5-hydroxydantrolene, an active metabolite that is excreted in the urine. Elimination half-lives are 6 to 9 hours for dantrolene and 15.5 hours for the 5-hydroxydantrolene metabolite. In one study of children ages 2 to 7 years, the dantrolene elimination half-life was 10 hours, and that for 5-hydroxydantrolene was 9 hours. At therapeutic concentrations, dantrolene inhibits binding of [$^{3}$H]ryanodine to the ryanodine receptor type 1 (RYR-1) on the sarcoplasmic reticulum membrane of skeletal muscle, causing a dose-dependent inhibition of both the steady and peak components of calcium release. This reduces the free myoplasmic calcium concentration and thereby directly inhibits excitation–contraction coupling. Dantrolene does not bind to the cardiac ryanodine receptor (RYR-2) and thus does not have any direct cardiac effects.

## ROLE IN MALIGNANT HYPERTHERMIA AND OTHER HYPERTHERMIAS

Dantrolene is indicated for treatment of the fulminant skeletal muscle hypermetabolism characteristic of MH and for treatment following an acute episode of MH to prevent recrudescence. It is reasonable to administer dantrolene for patients with severe hyperthermia, when the diagnosis of MH cannot be excluded with certainty, especially in the presence of a known trigger such as succinylcholine.

Dantrolene use is reported in hyperthermic syndromes other than MH, including neuroleptic malignant syndrome, heat stroke, serotonin toxicity, monoamine oxidase inhibitor interaction or overdose, methylenedioxymethamphetamine ("ecstasy") overdose, intrathecal baclofen withdrawal, and thyroid storm. Given the lack of evidence-based support for these conditions, dantrolene therapy is not routinely recommended for indications other than MH. However, given that (1) the differential diagnosis of a hyperthermic syndrome does not necessarily exclude (and often includes) that of MH, (2) the definitive diagnosis of a hyperthermic syndrome may be subtle or delayed, and (3) MH may occur simultaneously with another hyperthermic syndrome, it is reasonable to give dantrolene when MH cannot be specifically excluded because its use may be lifesaving and response to standard cooling measure is not rapidly effective. It bears emphasis that dantrolene provided for hyperthermia does not substitute for rapid cooling and resuscitation.

## ADVERSE EFFECTS AND SAFETY ISSUES

Because extravasation can cause tissue necrosis, dantrolene should only be given through a central vein or a large peripheral vein. In healthy volunteers, dantrolene 2.5 mg/kg does not reduce respiratory rate, vital capacity, or peak expiratory flow rate. Dantrolene and verapamil should not be used in combination because of the risk of hyperkalemia and hypotension. Intravenous calcium salts are safe to administer with dantrolene if needed, such as for the treatment of cardiac dysrhythmias or hyperkalemia (during an episode of MH).

## PREGNANCY AND LACTATION

Dantrolene carries a Pregnancy Category C designation. Dosing during pregnancy is based on total body weight. Dantrolene rapidly crosses the placenta and is slowly excreted in breast milk. At the concentrations achieved in serum or breast milk, there are no reports of significant adverse neonatal effects; however, it is suggested that breastfeeding be withheld until 48 hours after the last dose of dantrolene.

## FORMULATION

Of the two formulations of dantrolene currently available (Dantrium or Revonto, and Ryanodex), Ryanodex offers significant advantages over the older formulations. Dantrium and Revonto are supplied as a sterile lyophilized powder in a 70-mL vial that contains 20 mg of dantrolene sodium and 3,000 mg of mannitol. After addition of 60 mL of sterile water to each vial, each vial is shaken for approximately 20 seconds and until the solution becomes clear. Ryanodex is supplied as a sterile nanocrystalline powder suspension containing 250 mg of dantrolene sodium (or 12.5 times more dantrolene per vial than the older formulations) and 125 mg of mannitol. Each vial of Ryanodex is reconstituted with 5 mL of preservative-free sterile water. The reconstituted vial is shaken for 10 seconds until a uniform orange color suspension forms and administered by IV bolus into a free running infusion line of either 0.9% sodium chloride or 5% dextrose solution.

A single vial of Ryanodex is sufficient to provide a loading dose for a patient weighing up to 100 kg, and it can be mixed and administered in less than 1 minute. For the older dantrolene formulations, a 100-kg patient would require 12.5 vials to be prepared in a much larger volume of sterile water, a process that could take 15 to 20 minutes and involve multiple providers to mix and administer.

## DOSING

The initial dose of dantrolene for treatment of acute MH is a 2.5 mg/kg IV bolus; it is repeated every 15 minutes until the signs of hypermetabolism are reversed, or until a total dose of about 10 mg/kg has been administered. Occasionally higher doses are required. Following initial treatment, at least 1 to 2 mg/kg IV should be given every 6 hours for 1 to 3 days to prevent recrudescence of the syndrome. The key point is that the total dose of dantrolene is determined by titration to a metabolic end point—resolution of skeletal muscle hypermetabolism. When an effective dose of dantrolene is given, signs of muscle hypermetabolism start to normalize within 30 minutes.

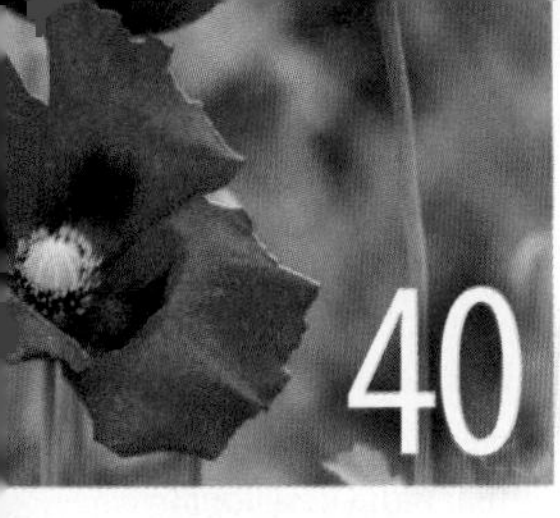




# 40 ANTIPSYCHOTICS

## HISTORY AND EPIDEMIOLOGY

The development of antipsychotic drugs dramatically altered the practice of psychiatry. Before the introduction of chlorpromazine in 1950, patients with schizophrenia were treated with nonspecific sedatives such as barbiturates or chloral hydrate. Agitated patients were housed in large "mental institutions" and often placed in physical restraints, and thousands underwent surgical disruption of the connections between the frontal cortices and other areas of the brain (leucotomy). By 1955, approximately 500,000 patients with mental health disorders were institutionalized in the United States (US). The advent of antipsychotic drugs in the 1950s revolutionized the care of these patients. These drugs, originally termed *major tranquilizers* and subsequently *neuroleptics,* dramatically reduced the characteristic hallucinations, delusions, thought disorders, and paranoia—the "positive" symptoms of schizophrenia. Clozapine, which came into clinical use in the 1970s, marked a major advance in pharmacotherapy in that it not only was associated with a low risk of movement disorders but it also improved the "negative" symptoms of schizophrenia. These "negative symptoms," such as avolition, alogia, and social withdrawal, although often less outwardly apparent than the positive symptoms, result in significant disability. Reports of life-threatening agranulocytosis led to the withdrawal of clozapine from the US market in 1974, although it was reintroduced in 1990 with stringent monitoring requirements. However, the unique therapeutic and pharmacologic properties of clozapine led to its characterization as an *atypical* antipsychotic, the forerunner and prototype of many other second-generation antipsychotics that have now largely supplanted the earlier drugs in clinical practice.

The true incidences of antipsychotic overdose and adverse effects are not known with certainty. Some patients never seek medical attention, and others are misdiagnosed. Even among those who seek medical attention and are correctly diagnosed, notification of poison centers or other adverse event reporting systems is discretionary and incomplete. With these limitations in mind, a few observations can be made. The vast majority of poison center calls involving antipsychotics pertain to intentional overdoses and are associated with a large percentage of fatalities.

## PHARMACOLOGY

### Classification

Antipsychotics are classified in several ways, according to their chemical structures, their receptor binding profiles, or as *typical* or *atypical* antipsychotics. Table 40–1 outlines the taxonomy of some of the more commonly used antipsychotics. Classification by chemical structure was most useful before the 1970s, when phenothiazines and butyrophenones constituted most of the antipsychotics in clinical use. Of greater clinical utility is the classification of antipsychotics according to their binding affinities for various receptors (Table 40–2).

However, by far the most widely used classification system categorizes antipsychotics as either *typical* or *atypical.* Typical (also called *traditional*; *conventional*; or, *first-generation*) antipsychotics dominated the first 40 years of antipsychotic therapy. They were subcategorized according to their affinity for the $D_2$ receptor as either low potency (exemplified by thioridazine and chlorpromazine) or high potency (exemplified by haloperidol). The concept of atypicality connotes different features to pharmacologists and clinicians. From a clinical perspective, atypical (*second-generation*) antipsychotics treat both the positive and negative symptoms of schizophrenia, are less likely than traditional drugs to produce extrapyramidal symptoms (EPS), and cause little or no elevation of the serum prolactin concentration. From a pharmacologic perspective, many atypical antipsychotics also inhibit the activity of serotonin at the $5\text{-HT}_{2A}$ receptor. Some antipsychotics are classified as third generation, reflecting the property of antagonism (or partial antagonism) of $D_2$ receptors with agonism at $5\text{-HT}_{1A}$ receptors.

### Mechanisms of Antipsychotic Action

Of the many contemporary theories of schizophrenia, the most enduring has been the *dopamine hypothesis.* This theory posits that the "positive symptoms" of schizophrenia result from excessive dopaminergic signaling in the mesolimbic and mesocortical pathways. There are at least five subtypes of dopamine receptors ($D_1$ through $D_5$), but schizophrenia principally involves excess signaling at the $D_2$ subtype, and antagonism of $D_2$ neurotransmission is the *sine qua non* of antipsychotic activity.

Antipsychotics interfere with signaling at other receptors to varying degrees, including muscarinic receptors, $H_1$ histamine receptors, and α-adrenergic receptors. The extent to which these receptors are blocked at therapeutic doses can be used to predict the adverse effect of each antipsychotic profile (Table 40–2). Several antipsychotics also block voltage-gated fast sodium channels ($I_{Na}$). Although this effect is of little consequence during therapy, in the setting of overdose, this can slow cardiac conduction (phase 0 depolarization) and impair myocardial contractility. This effect, most notable with the phenothiazines, is both rate and voltage dependent and is therefore more pronounced at faster heart rates and less negative transmembrane potentials. Blockade of the delayed rectifier potassium current ($I_{Kr}$) can produce prolongation of the QT interval, creating a substrate for development of ventricular dysrhythmias including torsade de pointes.

**TABLE 40–1 Classification of Commonly Used Antipsychotics**

| Classification | Antipsychotic | Usual Daily Adult Dose (mg) | Volume of Distribution (L/kg) | Half-Life (Range, h) | Protein Binding (%) | Active Metabolite |
|---|---|---|---|---|---|---|
| *Typicals* | | | | | | |
| Butyrophenones | Droperidol | 1.25–30 | 2–3 | 2–10 | 85–90 | N |
| | Haloperidol | 1–20 | 18–30 | 14–41 | 90 | Y |
| Diphenylbutylpiperidines | Pimozide | 1–20 | 11–62 | 28–214 | 99 | Y |
| **Phenothiazines** | | | | | | |
| Aliphatic | Chlorpromazine | 100–800 | 10–35 | 18–30 | 98 | Y |
| | Methotrimeprazine | 2–50 | 23–42 | 17–78 | NR | Y |
| | Promazine | 50–1,000 | 30–40 | 8–12 | 98 | N |
| | Promethazine | 25–150 | 9–25 | 9–16 | 93 | Y |
| Piperazine | Fluphenazine | 0.5–20 | 220 | 13–58[b] | 99 | NR |
| | Perphenazine | 8–64 | 10–35 | 8–12 | > 90 | NR |
| | Prochlorperazine | 10–150 | 13–32 | 17–27 | > 90 | NR |
| | Trifluoperazine | 4–50 | NR | 7–18 | > 90 | Y |
| Piperidine | Mesoridazine | 100–400 | 3–6 | 2–9 | 98 | Y |
| | Thioridazine | 200–800 | 18 | 26–36 | 96 | Y |
| | Pipotiazine | 25–250 (monthly IM depot) | 7.5 | 3–11 | NR | N |
| **Thioxanthenes** | Chlorprothixene | 30–300 | 11–23 | 8–12 | NR | NR |
| | Flupentixol | 3–6 | 7–8 | 7–36 | NR | NR |
| | Thiothixene | 5–30 | NR | 12–36 | > 90 | NR |
| | Zuclopenthixol | 20–100 | 10 | 20 | NR | NR |
| *Atypicals* | | | | | | |
| Benzamides | Amisulpride | 50–1,200 | 5.8 | 12 | 16 | N |
| | Raclopride | 3–6 | 1.5 | 12–24 | NR | N |
| | Remoxipride | 150–600 | 0.7 | 3–7 | 80 | Y |
| | Sulpiride | 200–1,200 | 0.6–2.7 | 4–11 | 14–40 | N |
| Benzepines | | | | | | |
| Dibenzodiazepine | Clozapine | 50–900 | 15–30 | 6–17 | 95 | Y |
| Dibenzoxazepine | Loxapine[a] | 20–250 | NR | 2–8 | 90–99 | Y |
| Thienobenzodiazepine | Olanzapine | 5–20 | 10–20 | 21–54 | 93 | N |
| Dibenzothiazepine | Quetiapine | 150–750 | 10 | 3–9 | 83 | N |
| **Indoles** | | | | | | |
| Benzisoxazole | Risperidone | 2–16 | 0.7–2.1 | 3–20 | 90 | Y |
| | Paliperidone | 1–12 mg (IM 25–150 monthly) | 7 | 23 | 74 | N |
| | Iloperidone | 12–14 | 30–36 | 18–33 | 96 | Y |
| Imidazolidinone | Sertindole | 12–24 | 20–40 | 24–200 | 99 | Y |
| Benzisothiazole | Ziprasidone | 40–160 | 2 | 4–10 | 99 | N |
| | Lurasidone | 20–160 | 80–90 | 29–37 | 99 | Y |
| Dibenzo-oxepino pyrroles | Asenapine | 5–20 | 20–25 | 13–39 | 95 | N |
| Quinolinones | Aripiprazole | 10–30 | 5 | 47–68 | 99 | Y |

[a]Loxapine's atypical profile is lost at doses > 50 mg/day; it is sometimes therefore categorized as a typical antipsychotic. [b]For hydrochloride salt; enanthate and decanoate have ranges of 3–4 days and 5–12 days, respectively.

IM = intramuscular; N = no; NR = not reported; Y = yes.

Several antipsychotics exhibit a relatively high degree of antagonism at the 5-$HT_{2A}$ receptor, which imparts two important therapeutic properties: (1) greater effectiveness for the treatment of the negative symptoms of schizophrenia and (2) a significantly lower incidence of EPS. A more detailed description of the pharmacology of the most commonly used second-generation antipsychotics is warranted in light of their increasing role in therapy.

Clozapine binds to dopamine receptors ($D_1$–$D_5$) and serotonin receptors (5-$HT_{1A/1C}$, 5-$HT_{2A/2C}$, 5-$HT_3$, and 5-$HT_6$) with moderate to high affinity. It also antagonizes $\alpha_1$-adrenergic, $\alpha_2$-adrenergic, and $H_1$ histamine receptors. It has the highest binding affinity of any atypical antipsychotic at $M_1$ muscarinic receptors. Despite this feature, clozapine paradoxically activates the $M_4$ muscarinic receptor and frequently produces sialorrhea during therapy.

**TABLE 40–2 Clinical and Toxicologic Manifestations of Selected Antipsychotics**

| | *$\alpha_1$-Adrenergic Antagonism* | *Muscarinic Antagonism* | *Fast Sodium Channel ($I_{Na}$) Blockade* | *Delayed Rectifier ($I_{Kr}$) Blockade* |
|---|---|---|---|---|
| Clinical effect | Hypotension | Central and peripheral anticholinergic effects | QRS complex widening; myocardial depression | QT interval prolongation; torsade de pointes |
| ***Typical*** | | | | |
| Chlorpromazine | +++ | ++ | ++ | ++ |
| Fluphenazine | – | – | + | + |
| Haloperidol | – | – | + | ++ |
| Loxapine | +++ | ++ | ++ | + |
| Mesoridazine | +++ | +++ | +++ | ++ |
| Perphenazine | + | – | + | ++ |
| Pimozide | + | – | + | ++ |
| Thioridazine | +++ | +++ | +++ | +++ |
| Trifluoperazine | + | – | + | ++ |
| ***Atypical*** | | | | |
| Amisulpride | – | – | – | ++ |
| Asenapine | ++ | – | – | – |
| Aripiprazole | ++ | – | – | – |
| Clozapine | +++ | +++ | – | + |
| Iloperidone | +++ | – | – | ++ |
| Lurasidone | – | – | – | – |
| Olanzapine | ++ | +++ | – | – |
| Paliperidone | ++ | – | – | + |
| Quetiapine | +++ | +++ | + | – to + |
| Remoxipride | – | – | – | – |
| Risperidone | ++ | – | – | – |
| Sertindole | + | – | – | ++ |
| Ziprasidone | ++ | – | – | +++ |

+ to ++ = effect present in increasing degree; – = effect is absent; – to + = presence of effect minimal or absent.

Olanzapine binds with high affinity to serotonin (5-$HT_{2A/2C}$, 5-$HT_3$, and 5-$HT_6$) and dopamine receptors ($D_1$, $D_2$, and $D_4$), although its potency at $D_2$ receptors is lower than that of most traditional antipsychotics. It is an exceptionally potent $H_1$ antagonist and also has a high affinity for $M_1$ receptors and is a relatively weak $\alpha_1$-adrenergic antagonist.

Risperidone has high affinity for serotonin receptors (5-$HT_{2A/2C}$), $D_2$ receptors, and $\alpha_1$-adrenergic receptors and $H_1$ receptors. Paliperidone is the major active metabolite of risperidone and is available orally and as a long-acting parenteral preparation that exhibits a similar receptor binding profile.

Quetiapine is a weak antagonist at $D_2$, $M_1$, and 5-$HT_{1A}$ receptors, but it is a potent antagonist of $\alpha_1$-adrenergic and $H_1$ receptors.

Ziprasidone is an antagonist at $D_2$ and several serotonin (5-$HT_{2A/2C}$, 5-$HT_{1D}$, and 5-$HT_7$) receptors, but it also displays agonist activity at 5-$HT_{1A}$ receptors. Its $\alpha_1$-adrenergic antagonist activity is particularly strong. In addition, it is a strong inhibitor of the delayed rectifier channel ($I_{Kr}$) and can significantly prolong cardiac repolarization. Lurasidone is an active metabolite of risperidone. It exhibits high affinity for $D_2$ and 5-$HT_{2A}$ receptors, as well as for 5-$HT_{1A}$ and 5-$HT_7$, but low affinity for $\alpha_1$-adrenergic receptors and no appreciable affinity for muscarinic or $H_1$ receptors.

Aripiprazole is a novel antipsychotic that binds avidly to $D_2$ and $D_3$ receptors as well as 5-$HT_{1A}$, 5-$HT_{2A}$, and 5-$HT_{2B}$ receptors. Aripiprazole acts as a partial agonist at 5-$HT_{1A}$ receptors but is an antagonist at 5-$HT_{2A}$ receptors. Like aripiprazole, bifeprunox is a partial agonist at $D_2$ and 5-$HT_{1A}$ receptors. It is characterized as a third-generation antipsychotic and has no appreciable affinity for serotonin 5-$HT_{2A}$ and 5-$HT_{2C}$, muscarinic, or $H_1$ receptors.

Amisulpride preferentially blocks dopamine receptors in limbic rather than striatal structures. At low doses, it blocks presynaptic $D_2$ and $D_3$ receptors with high affinity, thereby accentuating dopamine release, and at high doses, it blocks postsynaptic $D_2$ and $D_3$ receptors. It has no appreciable affinity for serotonergic, histaminergic, adrenergic, and cholinergic receptors.

Sertindole is a second-generation antipsychotic recently reintroduced into the US market after being voluntarily withdrawn in 1998 over concerns about its effects on the QT interval. It binds to striatal $D_2$ receptors, and antagonizes 5-$HT_{2A}$ and $\alpha_1$-adrenergic receptors. Between 3.1% and 7.8% of patients receiving sertindole develop QT intervals greater than 500 ms.

Asenapine is a second-generation antipsychotic administered sublingually because of its high first-pass metabolism. It acts as an antagonist at multiple dopamine, 5-HT, histamine, and $\alpha$-adrenergic receptors but has no appreciable activity at muscarinic receptors or on the QT interval.

## PHARMACOKINETICS AND TOXICOKINETICS

With a few exceptions, the antipsychotics have similar pharmacokinetic characteristics regardless of their chemical classification (Table 40–1). Most are lipophilic; have a large volume of distribution; and with the exception of asenapine, are generally well absorbed. Plasma concentrations generally peak within 2 to 3 hours after a therapeutic dose but can be delayed after overdose.

Most antipsychotics are substrates for one or more isoforms of the hepatic cytochrome (CYP) enzyme system. For example, haloperidol, perphenazine, thioridazine, sertindole, and risperidone are extensively metabolized by the CYP2D6 system. Drugs that inhibit CYP2D6 (eg, paroxetine, fluoxetine, and bupropion) can increase concentrations of these antipsychotics, increasing the risk of adverse effects. In contrast, metabolism of clozapine and asenapine is primarily mediated by CYP1A2, and increased clozapine concentrations follow exposure to CYP1A2 inhibitors such as fluvoxamine, macrolide, or fluoroquinolone antibiotics or upon smoking cessation.

## PATHOPHYSIOLOGY AND CLINICAL MANIFESTATIONS

Table 40–3 lists the adverse effects of antipsychotics. Some of these effects develop primarily following overdose, but others occur during the course of therapeutic use.

**TABLE 40–3 Adverse Effects of Antipsychotics**

| | | |
|---|---|---|
| Central nervous system | | Somnolence, progressing to coma |
| | | Respiratory depression with loss of airway reflexes |
| | | Hyperthermia |
| | | Seizures |
| | | Extrapyramidal syndromes |
| | | Central anticholinergic syndrome |
| Cardiovascular | | |
| | Clinical | Tachycardia |
| | | Hypotension (orthostatic or resting) |
| | | Myocardial depression |
| | | Myocarditis (clozapine) |
| | Electrocardiographic | QRS complex prolongation |
| | | Right deviation of terminal 40 ms of frontal plane axis |
| | | QT interval prolongation |
| | | Torsade de pointes |
| | | Ventricular dysrhythmias |
| | | Nonspecific repolarization changes |
| Endocrine | | Amenorrhea, oligomenorrhea, or metrorrhagia |
| | | Breast tenderness and galactorrhea |
| | | Glucose dysregulation |
| Gastrointestinal | | Impaired peristalsis |
| | | Dry mouth[a] |
| Genitourinary | | Urinary retention |
| | | Ejaculatory dysfunction |
| | | Priapism |
| Ophthalmic | | Mydriasis or miosis; visual blurring |
| Dermatologic | | Impaired sweat production |
| | | Cutaneous vasodilation |

[a]An exception is clozapine, which can cause sialorrhea.

## ADVERSE EFFECTS DURING THERAPEUTIC USE

### The Extrapyramidal Syndromes

The EPSs (Table 40–4) are a group of disorders that share the common feature of abnormal muscular activity. Among the typical antipsychotics, the incidence of EPS is highest with the more potent antipsychotics such as haloperidol and lower with less potent antipsychotics such as chlorpromazine. Atypical antipsychotics are associated with an even lower incidence of EPS. However, it is important to note that EPS occur during treatment with any antipsychotic, regardless of typicality or potency.

### Acute Dystonia

Acute dystonia is a movement disorder characterized by sustained involuntary muscle contractions, often involving the muscles of the head and neck, including the extraocular muscles and the tongue, but occasionally involving the extremities. Spasmodic torticollis, facial grimacing, protrusion of the tongue, and oculogyric crisis are among the more common manifestations. Laryngeal dystonia is a rare but potentially life-threatening variant that is easily misdiagnosed because it presents with throat pain, dyspnea, stridor, and dysphonia rather than the more characteristic features of dystonia. Acute dystonia typically develops within a few hours of starting of treatment but may be delayed in onset for several days. Left untreated, dystonia resolves slowly over several days after the offending antipsychotic is withdrawn. Risk factors for acute dystonia include male gender, young age (children are particularly susceptible), a previous episode of acute dystonia, and recent cocaine use.

***Treatment of Acute Dystonia.*** The response to parenteral anticholinergics is generally rapid and dramatic, and benztropine is recommended as the first-line treatment (2 mg intravenously or intramuscularly in adults or 0.05 mg/kg in children). Diphenhydramine is often more readily available, and it is also reasonable to use (50 mg intravenously or intramuscularly in adults, or 1 mg/kg in children). It is important to recognize that additional doses of anticholinergics are often necessary because the duration of action of most antipsychotics exceeds that of either benztropine or diphenhydramine. We recommend that patients in whom acute dystonia jeopardizes respiration be observed for at least 12 to 24 hours after initial resolution.

### Akathisia

Akathisia (from the Greek phrase "not to sit") is characterized by a feeling of restlessness, anxiety, or sense of unease, often in conjunction with the objective finding of an inability to remain still. Patients with akathisia frequently appear uncomfortable or fidgety. They typically rock back and forth while standing or repeatedly cross and uncross their legs while seated. Akathisia is sometimes misinterpreted as a manifestation of the underlying psychiatric disorder rather than an adverse effect of drug therapy. Like acute dystonia, akathisia tends to occur relatively early in the course of treatment and coincides with peak antipsychotic concentrations in plasma. The incidence appears highest with typical, high-potency antipsychotics and lowest with atypical

**TABLE 40–4 The Extrapyramidal Syndromes**

| *Disorder* | *Time of Maximal Risk* | *Features* | *Postulated Mechanism* | *Suggested Treatments* |
|---|---|---|---|---|
| Akathisia | Hours to days | Restlessness and general unease; inability to sit still | Mesocortical $D_2$ antagonism | Dose reduction, trial of alternate drug, propranolol, benzodiazepines, anticholinergics |
| Dystonia | Hours to days | Sustained, involuntary muscle contraction, including torticollis, blepharospasm, oculogyric crisis | Imbalance of dopaminergic or cholinergic transmission | Anticholinergics, benzodiazepines |
| Neuroleptic malignant syndrome | 2–10 days | Many (Table 40–5): altered mental status, rigidity, hyperthermia, autonomic instability, catatonia, mutism | $D_2$ antagonism in striatum, hypothalamus, and mesocortex | Cooling, benzodiazepines, supportive care, bromocriptine, amantadine, or other direct-acting dopamine agonist |
| Parkinsonism | Weeks | Bradykinesia, rigidity, shuffling gait, masklike facies, resting tremor | Postsynaptic striatal $D_2$ antagonism | Dose reduction, anticholinergics, dopamine agonists |
| Tardive dyskinesia | 3 months to years | Late-onset involuntary choreiform movements, orobuccal lingual masticatory movements | Excess dopaminergic activity | Recognize early and stop offending drug; addition of other antipsychotics; cholinergics; valbenazine |

antipsychotics. Most cases develop within days to weeks after initiation of treatment or an increase in dose.

*Treatment of Akathisia.* Akathisia can be difficult to treat. A reduction in the antipsychotic dose is a reasonable initial intervention. If this fails or is impractical, substitution of another (generally atypical) antipsychotic drug or treatment with lipophilic β-adrenergic antagonists such as propranolol lessens akathisia. Benzodiazepines produce short-term relief, and anticholinergics such as benztropine lessen akathisia in some patients but are more likely to be effective for akathisia induced by antipsychotics with little or no intrinsic anticholinergic activity.

## Parkinsonism

Antipsychotics occasionally produce a parkinsonian syndrome characterized by rigidity, akinesia or bradykinesia, and postural instability. It is similar to idiopathic Parkinson disease, although the classic "pill-rolling" tremor is often less pronounced. The syndrome typically develops during the first few months of therapy, particularly with high-potency antipsychotics. It is more common among older women, and in some patients, it represents iatrogenic unmasking of latent Parkinson disease. Parkinsonism results from antagonism of postsynaptic $D_2$ receptors in the striatum.

*Treatment of Drug-Induced Parkinsonism.* The addition of an anticholinergic often attenuates symptoms at the expense of additional side effects. A dopamine agonist such as amantadine is sometimes added, particularly in older patients who may be less tolerant of anticholinergics, but this may aggravate the underlying psychiatric disturbance and is not generally recommended.

## Tardive Dyskinesias

The adjective *tardive*, meaning delayed, is used to distinguish these movement disorders from the Parkinsonian movements described earlier. Potential risk factors for tardive dyskinesia include older age, alcohol use, affective disorder, prior electroconvulsive therapy, and diabetes mellitus. Several distinct tardive syndromes are recognized, including the classic orobuccal lingual masticatory stereotypy, chorea, dystonia, myoclonus, blepharospasm, and tics. It is generally accepted that the atypical antipsychotics are associated with a lower incidence of tardive dyskinesia and other drug-related movement disorders.

*Treatment of Tardive Dyskinesia.* Tardive dyskinesia is highly resistant to the usual pharmacologic treatments for movement disorders. Despite the absence of good data, proposed strategies for management of tardive dyskinesia begin with primary prevention (avoidance of antipsychotic therapy when possible and use of the lowest effective dose). Tetrabenazine, an inhibitor of vesicular monoamine transporter type 2 ($VMAT_2$), was suggested as the first-line treatment, although it is expensive and may cause somnolence, depression, or parkinsonism. Valbenazine, a more recently approved $VMAT_2$ inhibitor with a longer half-life, appears to be better tolerated than tetrabenazine. For focal tardive dyskinesia (cervical or oromandibular, for example), botulinum toxin injections are sometimes used.

## Neuroleptic Malignant Syndrome

Neuroleptic malignant syndrome (NMS) is a potentially life-threatening emergency. The reported incidence of NMS ranges from 0.2% to 1.4% of patients receiving antipsychotics, but less severe episodes may go undiagnosed or unreported. Most cases of NMS are diagnosed in young adulthood, with the frequency of diagnosis diminishing gradually thereafter. The pathophysiology of NMS is incompletely understood but involves abrupt reductions in central dopaminergic neurotransmission in the striatum and hypothalamus, altering the core temperature "set point" and leading to impaired thermoregulation and other manifestations of autonomic dysfunction. Although NMS most often occurs during treatment with a $D_2$ receptor antagonist, withdrawal of dopamine agonists sometimes produces an indistinguishable syndrome.

The vast majority of NMS cases occur in the context of therapeutic use of antipsychotics rather than after overdose. Postulated risk factors for the development of NMS include young age, male gender, extracellular fluid volume contraction, use of high-potency antipsychotics, depot preparations, cotreatment with lithium, multiple drugs in combination, and rapid dose escalation. The mortality rate of NMS associated with first-generation antipsychotics is estimated at approximately 16%, and the rate associated with second-generation antipsychotics is estimated at 3%.

The manifestations of NMS include the tetrad of altered mental status, muscular rigidity (classically described as "lead pipe"), hyperthermia, and autonomic dysfunction. These findings appear in any sequence, although a review of 340 NMS cases found that mental status changes and rigidity usually preceded the development hyperthermia and autonomic instability. Signs typically evolve over a period of several days, with the majority occurring within 2 weeks of antipsychotic initiation. However, it is important to recognize that NMS occurs even after prolonged use of an antipsychotic, particularly after a dose increase, the addition of another antipsychotic, or the development of intercurrent illness.

There are no universally accepted criteria for the diagnosis of NMS, and more than a dozen sets of criteria have been proposed. An international group published the results of a Delphi consensus panel regarding the diagnosis of NMS (Table 40–5). A validation exercise suggested that an aggregate cutoff score of 74 (of a possible 100) was associated with the highest degree of agreement between expert-generated criteria and *Diagnostic and Statistical Manual of Mental Disorders,* criteria (sensitivity, 69.6%; specificity, 90.7%). It may be difficult to distinguish NMS from other xenobiotic-induced hyperthermia syndromes, such as those associated with anticholinergics (antimuscarinics) (Chap. 22) and the serotonergics (Chap. 42), all of which share common features of elevated temperature, altered mental status, and neuromuscular abnormalities. The most important differentiating feature is the medication history.

**TABLE 40–5 Suggested Diagnostic Criteria for the Neuroleptic Malignant Syndrome**

| *Criterion* | *Priority Score* |
|---|---|
| Exposure to a dopamine antagonist or withdrawal of a dopamine agonist in previous 72 hours | 20 |
| Hyperthermia (> 100.4°F or 38.0°C on at least two occasions, measured orally) | 18 |
| Rigidity | 17 |
| Mental status alteration (reduced or fluctuating level of consciousness) | 13 |
| Creatine kinase elevation (at least four times the upper limit of normal) | 10 |
| Sympathetic nervous system lability, defined as at least two of:<br>Blood pressure elevation (SBP or DBP ≥ 25% above baseline)<br>Blood pressure fluctuation (≥ 20% DBP change or ≥ 25% SBP change in 24 hours)<br>Diaphoresis<br>Urinary incontinence | 10 |
| Hypermetabolic state (defined as heart rate increase ≥ 25% above baseline and respiratory rate increase ≥ 50% above baseline) | 5 |
| Negative workup for other toxic, metabolic, infectious, or neurologic causes | 7 |

DBP = diastolic blood pressure; SBP = systolic blood pressure.

***Treatment of Neuroleptic Malignant Syndrome: General Measures.*** The provision of good supportive care is the cornerstone for treatment of NMS. It is essential to recognize the condition as an emergency and to withdraw the offending xenobiotic immediately. When NMS ensues after abrupt discontinuation of a dopamine agonist such as levodopa, the drug should be reinstituted promptly. Most patients with suspected NMS should be admitted to an intensive care unit. Supplemental oxygen should be administered, and assisted ventilation is necessary in cases of respiratory failure, which results from one or more of central hypoventilation, loss of protective airway reflexes, rigidity of the chest wall muscles, or oversedation.

The hyperthermia associated with NMS is multifactorial in origin and, when present, warrants rapid treatment. Antipyretics are not effective. Immersion of patients with severe drug-induced hyperthermia (> 106°F) in an ice-water bath has been shown to rapidly lower body temperature (Chap. 48). Other strategies are inferior to ice water immersion and are not recommended unless immersion is impractical or unsafe.

Hypotension should be treated initially with isotonic crystalloid followed by vasopressors if necessary. Maintenance of intravascular volume and adequate renal perfusion are recommended to reduce the incidence of myoglobinuric acute kidney injury in patients with high creatine kinase concentrations. Venous thromboembolism is a major cause of morbidity and mortality in patients with NMS, and prophylactic doses of low-molecular-weight heparin are reasonable in patients who likely will be immobilized for more than 12 to 24 hours.

***Pharmacologic Treatment of Neuroleptic Malignant Syndrome.*** Benzodiazepines are the most widely used pharmacologic adjuncts for treatment of NMS and are recommended as first line-therapy. Dantrolene and bromocriptine are not well studied, and their incremental benefit over good supportive care is debated. The primary disadvantage of benzodiazepines is that they will cloud the assessment of the patient's mental status. Although dantrolene is not recommended as a routine treatment in patients with NMS, it is reasonable in those with prominent muscular rigidity or rhabdomyolysis, despite sedation. Bromocriptine is a centrally acting dopamine agonist given orally or by nasogastric tube at dosages of 2.5 to 10 mg three or four times daily. The rationale for its use rests in the belief that reversal of antipsychotic-related striatal $D_2$ antagonism will ameliorate the manifestations of NMS. While it is recommended in patients with moderate to severe NMS, dopaminergics are associated with exacerbation of underlying psychiatric illness.

***Electroconvulsive Therapy.*** Electroconvulsive therapy (ECT) is reported to dramatically improve the manifestations of NMS, presumably by enhancing central dopaminergic transmission. As with drug therapies for NMS, the effectiveness of ECT remains unproven, but its use seems reasonable in patients with severe, persistent, or treatment-resistant NMS as well as those with residual catatonia or psychosis after resolution of other manifestations.

## ACUTE OVERDOSE

Antipsychotic overdose produces a spectrum of toxic manifestations involving multiple organ systems, but the most serious toxicity involves the CNS and cardiovascular system. Some of these manifestations are present to a minor degree during therapeutic use, although they tend to be most pronounced during the early period of therapy and dissipate with continued use.

Depressed level of consciousness is a common and dose-dependent feature of antipsychotic overdose, ranging from somnolence to coma. It may be associated with impaired airway reflexes, but significant respiratory depression is uncommon in the absence of other factors. Many antipsychotics, including several of the atypical antipsychotics, are potent muscarinic antagonists and produce anticholinergic features in overdose.

Mild elevations in body temperature are common and reflect impaired heat dissipation. Tachycardia is a common finding in patients with antipsychotic overdose and reflects reduced vagal tone and, with some antipsychotics, a compensatory response to hypotension. Hypotension is a common feature of antipsychotic overdose and is generally caused by peripheral $\alpha_1$-adrenergic blockade and, particularly with the phenothiazines, reduced myocardial contractility.

The electrocardiographic (ECG) manifestations of antipsychotic overdoses vary, sometimes exhibiting similarities to those of cyclic antidepressant toxicity (Chap. 41). These include prolongation of the QRS complex and a rightward deflection of the terminal 40 milliseconds of the QRS complex, typically manifesting as a tall, broad terminal positive deflection of the QRS complex in lead aVR. These changes reflect blockade of the inward sodium current ($I_{Na}$). Prolongation of the QT interval results from blockade of the delayed rectifier potassium current ($I_{Kr}$), creating a substrate for development of torsade de pointes and other ventricular dysrhythmias.

## DIAGNOSTIC TESTS

The diagnosis of antipsychotic poisoning is supported by the clinical history, the physical examination, and a limited number of adjunctive tests. Both the clinical and ECG findings are nonspecific and shared by other drug classes. Moreover, the absence of typical ECG changes does not exclude a significant antipsychotic ingestion, particularly early after overdose, and at least one additional ECG is recommended in the following 2 to 3 hours. Plasma concentrations of antipsychotics are not widely available, do not correlate well with clinical signs and symptoms, and do not help guide therapy. Urine immunoassays for tricyclic antidepressants occasionally produce a false-positive result in the presence of phenothiazines.

## MANAGEMENT

The care of a patient with an antipsychotic overdose should proceed with the recognition that other drugs, particularly other psychotropics, may have been coingested and can confound both the clinical presentation and management. Regularly encountered coingestants include antidepressants, sedative–hypnotics, opioids, anticholinergics, valproic acid, and lithium, as well as ethanol and nonprescription analgesics such as acetaminophen and aspirin.

Supportive care is the cornerstone of treatment for patients with antipsychotic overdose. Supplemental oxygen should be administered if hypoxia is present. Intubation and ventilation are rarely required for patients with single xenobiotic ingestions but may be necessary for patients with very large overdoses of antipsychotics or coingestion of other CNS depressants. Patients with altered mental status should receive thiamine, as well as parenteral dextrose if hypoglycemia is present. Naloxone is recommended based on clinical grounds (Antidotes in Brief: A4). All symptomatic patients should undergo continuous cardiac monitoring. An ECG should be recorded upon presentation and reliable venous access obtained. Asymptomatic patients with a normal ECG 6 hours after overdose are at exceedingly low risk of complications and generally do not require ongoing cardiac monitoring. Symptomatic patients and those with an abnormal ECG should have continuous monitoring for a minimum of 24 hours.

### Gastrointestinal Decontamination

Gastrointestinal decontamination with activated charcoal (1 g/kg by mouth or nasogastric tube) is recommended for patients who present within a few hours of a large or multidrug overdose and have no contraindications. Orogastric lavage and whole-bowel irrigation likely will not improve clinical outcomes and should be used rarely if ever in the management of patients with isolated antipsychotic overdose.

### Treatment of Cardiovascular Complications

Hypotension should be treated initially with appropriate titration of 0.9% sodium chloride. If vasopressors are required, direct-acting agonists such as norepinephrine or phenylephrine are recommended. Progressive prolongation of the QRS complex is usually associated with reduced cardiac output and malignant ventricular dysrhythmias. Sodium bicarbonate (1–2 mEq/kg IV) is the first-line therapy for ventricular dysrhythmias and is recommended for patients with dysrhythmias or QRS complex greater than 0.12 seconds (Antidotes in Brief: A5). Either repeated boluses of hypertonic sodium bicarbonate or a continuous infusion is recommended to achieve a target blood pH of no greater than 7.55. When administering sodium bicarbonate to patients with antipsychotic overdose, caution must be taken to avoid hypokalemia because many of these antipsychotics block cardiac potassium channels, thereby prolonging the QT interval. If significant conduction abnormalities or ventricular dysrhythmias persist despite the use of sodium bicarbonate, lidocaine (Class IB) (1–2 mg/kg, followed by continuous infusion) is a reasonable second-line antidysrhythmic. Class IA antidysrhythmics, class IC antidysrhythmics, and class III antidysrhythmics can aggravate cardiotoxicity and are contraindicated.

Prolongation of the QT interval requires no specific treatment other than monitoring and correction of potential contributing causes such as hypokalemia and hypomagnesemia. After torsade de pointes has resolved spontaneously or after cardioversion, intravenous magnesium sulfate is recommended to lessen the likelihood of recurrence, taking care to prevent hypotension, which is dose and rate dependent. Overdrive pacing with isoproterenol or transcutaneous or transvenous pacing is recommended if the patient does not respond to magnesium; however, magnesium is preferred because pacing may worsen rate-dependent sodium channel blockade.

Most antipsychotics exhibit a high degree of lipophilicity in addition to significant cardiovascular toxicity. Considerable enthusiasm has emerged for the use of intravenous lipid emulsion (ILE) therapy for patients with significant cardiac toxicity from lipophilic drugs (Antidotes in Brief: A23). However, published evidence-based recommendations on the use of ILE in acute poisoning note the very low quality of evidence supporting the intervention for most poisonings. As a result, it is reasonable to give ILE only in cases of not rapidly treatable cardiovascular collapse after antipsychotic overdose. Dosing for ILE is not well established, but a reasonable protocol begins with 20% lipid emulsion given as a bolus of 1.5 mL/kg (Antidotes in Brief: A23). Extracorporeal circulatory support is reasonable in critically ill patients unresponsive to other therapies.

### Treatment of Seizures

Seizures associated with antipsychotic overdose are generally short-lived and often require no pharmacologic treatment. Multiple or refractory seizures should prompt a search for other causes, including hypoglycemia and ingestion of other proconvulsant xenobiotics. When treatment is necessary, benzodiazepines such as lorazepam, midazolam, or diazepam generally suffice, although phenobarbital is a reasonable second-line therapy. Patients with refractory seizures should respond to propofol infusion or general anesthesia. Finally, seizures abruptly lower serum pH and thereby increase the cardiotoxicity of antipsychotics by enhancing binding to the sodium channel; therefore, an ECG should be obtained after resolution of seizure activity.

### Treatment of the Central Antimuscarinic Syndrome

Many of the older and newer generation antipsychotics have pronounced anticholinergic properties. Case reports and observational studies suggest that physostigmine (Antidotes in Brief: A11) can safely and effectively ameliorate the agitated delirium associated with the central antimuscarinic (anticholinergic) syndrome. It should not be used in patients with ventricular dysrhythmias, any degree of heart block, or prolongation of the QRS complex. If physostigmine is used, it is recommended to be given in 0.5-mg increments every 3 to 5 minutes, with close observation.

### Enhanced Elimination

No pharmacologic rationale supports the use of multiple-dose charcoal or manipulation of urinary pH to increase the clearance of antipsychotics. Because most antipsychotics have large volumes of distribution and extensive protein binding, extracorporeal removal is unwarranted and should be performed only if the patient has coingested other xenobiotics amenable to extracorporeal removal.

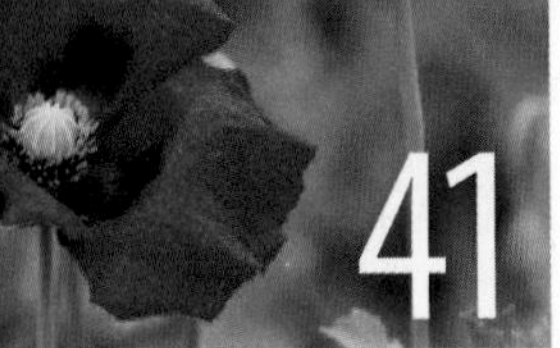

# 41 CYCLIC ANTIDEPRESSANTS

## HISTORY AND EPIDEMIOLOGY

The term *cyclic antidepressant* (CA) refers to a group of pharmacologically related xenobiotics used for treatment of depression, neuralgic pain, migraines, enuresis, and attention deficit hyperactivity disorder (ADHD). This class includes the traditional tricyclic antidepressants (TCAs), such as imipramine, desipramine, amitriptyline, nortriptyline, doxepin, trimipramine, protriptyline, and clomipramine, as well as other cyclic antidepressants such as the tetracyclic, maprotiline, and the dibenzoxapine amoxapine. Imipramine was the first TCA used for treatment of depression in the late 1950s. From the 1960s until the late 1980s, the TCAs were the major pharmacologic treatment for depression in the United States. However, by the early 1960s, cardiovascular and central nervous system (CNS) toxicities were recognized as major complications in patients with TCA overdoses. Although with the advent of selective serotonin reuptake inhibitors (SSRIs) the use of CAs for depression has decreased, other medical indications, including chronic pain, sleep disorders, obsessive-compulsive disorder, and, particularly in children, enuresis and ADHD, have emerged, resulting in their continued use.

## PHARMACOLOGY

The TCAs are classified into tertiary and secondary amines based on the presence of a methyl group on the propylamine side chain (Table 41–1). The tertiary amines amitriptyline and imipramine are metabolized to the secondary amines nortriptyline and desipramine, respectively, which themselves are marketed as antidepressants. At therapeutic doses, CAs inhibit presynaptic reuptake of norepinephrine and serotonin, functionally increasing the amount of these neurotransmitters at CNS receptors. Additional pharmacologic mechanisms of CAs are responsible for their side effects with therapeutic dosing and clinical effects after overdose. All of the CAs are competitive antagonists of the muscarinic acetylcholine receptors, although they have different affinities. The CAs also antagonize peripheral $\alpha_1$-adrenergic receptors. The most prominent effects of CA overdose result from binding to the cardiac sodium channels, which is also described as a membrane-stabilizing effect (Fig. 41–1). The TCAs are potent inhibitors of both peripheral and central postsynaptic histamine receptors. Finally, the CAs interfere with chloride conductance by binding to the picrotoxin site on the γ-aminobutyric acid (GABA)–chloride complex.

## PHARMACOKINETICS AND TOXICOKINETICS

In therapeutic dosing, the CAs are rapidly and almost completely absorbed from the gastrointestinal (GI) tract, with peak concentrations occurring between 2 and 8 hours. In overdose, the decreased GI motility delays CA absorption. Because of extensive first-pass metabolism by the liver, the oral bioavailability of CAs is low and variable, although metabolism saturates in overdose, increasing bioavailability.

**TABLE 41–1 Cyclic Antidepressants—Classification by Chemical Structure**

| | |
|---|---|
| ***Tertiary Amines*** | |
| Amitriptyline<br>Clomipramine<br>Doxepin<br>Imipramine<br>Trimipramine | Imipramine $CH_2CH_2CH_2N(CH_3)_2$ |
| ***Secondary Amines*** | |
| Desipramine<br>Nortriptyline<br>Protriptyline | Nortriptyline $CHCH_2CH_2N(CH_3)H$ |
| **Amoxapine** | N, N, N=, O, Cl |
| **Maprotiline** | $CH_2CH_2CH_2N(CH_3)H$ |

The CAs are highly lipophilic and have large and variable volumes of distribution (15–40 L/kg). Less than 2% of the ingested dose is present in blood several hours after overdose, and serum CA concentrations decline biexponentially. The CAs are extensively bound to $\alpha_1$-acid glycoprotein (AAG) in the plasma. Changes in AAG concentration or pH alter the percentage of free or unbound drug. Specifically, a low blood pH increases the amount of free drug. Elimination half-lives for therapeutic doses of CAs vary from 7 to 92 hours. The apparent half-lives are also prolonged following overdose as a result of ongoing absorption and saturable metabolism. A small fraction (15%–30%) of CA elimination occurs through biliary and gastric secretion. The metabolites are then reabsorbed in the systemic circulation. Less than 5% of CAs are excreted unchanged by the kidney.

## PATHOPHYSIOLOGY

The CAs slow phase 0 depolarization of the action potential in the distal His-Purkinje system and the ventricular myocardium (Fig. 41–1). Impaired depolarization within the ventricular conduction system slows the propagation of ventricular depolarization, which manifests as prolongation of the QRS

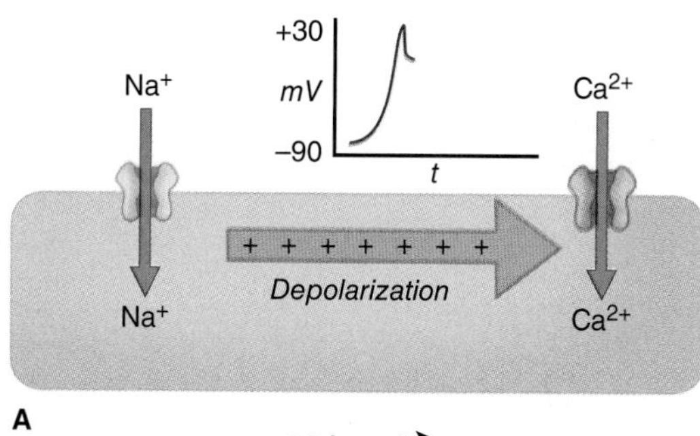


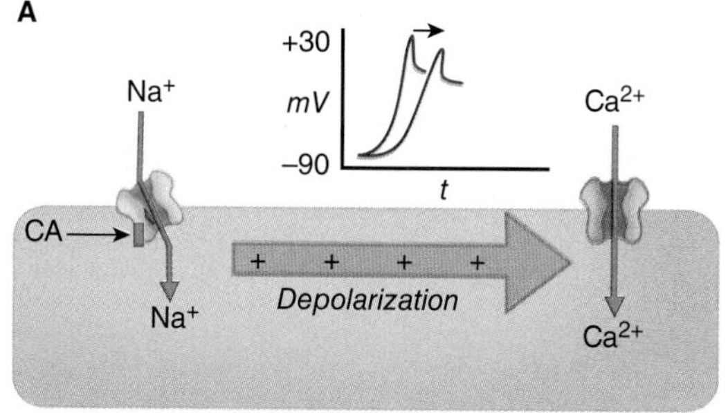


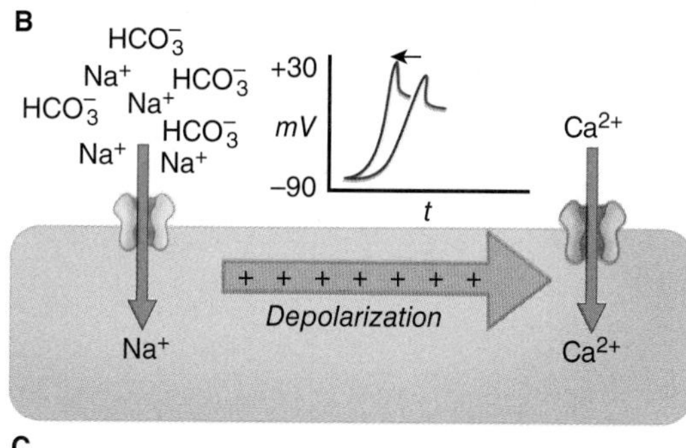


**FIGURE 41–1.** Effects of cyclic antidepressants (CAs) on the fast sodium channel. (**A**) Sodium depolarizes the cell, which both propagates conduction, allowing complete cardiac depolarization, and opens voltage-dependent $Ca^{2+}$ channels, producing contraction. (**B**) CAs and other sodium channel blockers alter the conformation of the sodium channel, slowing the rate of rise of the action potential, which produces both negative dromotropic and inotropic effects. (**C**) Raising the $Na^+$ gradient across the affected sodium channel speeds the rate of rise of the action potential, counteracting the drug-induced effects. Raising the pH removes the CA from the binding site on the $Na^+$ channel. See **Fig. 41–3** for the effects noted on the electrocardiograph.

complex on the electrocardiogram (ECG) (Figs. 41–2 and 41–3). The right bundle branch has a relatively longer refractory period, and it is affected disproportionately by xenobiotics that slow intraventricular conduction. This slowing of depolarization results in a rightward shift of the terminal 40 milliseconds (T40-ms) of the QRS complex axis and the right bundle branch block pattern that is noted on the ECG of patients who are exposed to or overdose on a CA. Because CAs are weakly basic, they are increasingly ionized as the ambient pH falls and less ionized as the pH rises. Changing the ambient pH therefore alters their binding to the sodium channel. Because 90% of the binding of CA to the sodium channel occurs in the ionized state, alkalinizing the blood facilitates the movement of the CA away from the hydrophilic sodium channel and into the lipid membrane (Antidotes in Brief: A5).

Sinus tachycardia is caused by the antimuscarinic, vasodilatory (reflex tachycardia), and sympathomimetic effects of the CAs. Wide-complex tachycardia most commonly represents aberrantly conducted sinus tachycardia rather than ventricular tachycardia. However, by prolonging anterograde conduction, nonuniform ventricular conduction can result, leading to reentrant ventricular dysrhythmias. Prolongation of the QT interval results primarily from slowed depolarization (ie, QRS complex prolongation) rather than altered repolarization. Although QT interval prolongation predisposes to the development of torsade de pointes, this dysrhythmia is uncommon in patients with CA poisoning in whom tachycardia is prominent.

Hypotension is caused by direct myocardial depression secondary to altered sodium channel function, which disrupts the subsequent excitation-contraction coupling of myocytes and impairs cardiac contractility. Peripheral vasodilation from α-adrenergic blockade also contributes prominently to postural hypotension.

Agitation, delirium, and depressed sensorium are primarily caused by central anticholinergic and antihistaminic effects. Cyclic antidepressant–induced seizures may result from a combination of an increased concentration of monoamines (particularly norepinephrine), muscarinic antagonism, neuronal sodium channel alteration, and GABA inhibition.

## CLINICAL MANIFESTATIONS

The progression of clinical toxicity is unpredictable and often rapid. Patients commonly present with minimal apparent clinical abnormalities, only to develop life-threatening cardiovascular and CNS toxicity within hours. Acute ingestion of 10 to 20 mg/kg of most CAs causes significant cardiovascular and CNS manifestations (therapeutic dose, 2–4 mg/kg/day). Thus, in adults, ingestions of more than 1 g of a CA are usually associated with life-threatening effects.

### Acute Toxicity

Most of the reported toxicity from CAs derives from patients with acute ingestions, especially in patients who are chronically taking the medication. Clinical manifestations of these two cohorts do not appear to be different, and most studies do not distinguish between them.

### Acute Cardiovascular Toxicity

Cardiovascular toxicity is primarily responsible for the morbidity and mortality attributed to CAs. Refractory hypotension caused by myocardial depression is the most common cause of death from CA overdose. Hypoxia, acidosis, volume depletion, seizures, or concomitant ingestion of other cardiodepressant or vasodilating drugs exacerbate hypotension and predispose to ventricular dysrhythmia. The most common dysrhythmia observed after CA overdose is sinus tachycardia. The ECG typically demonstrates a rightward shift of the T40-ms QRS complex axis and a prolongation of the QRS complex duration. Prolongation of the PR interval, QRS complex, and QT interval can occur in the setting of both therapeutic and toxic amounts of TCAs. Wide-complex tachycardia is the characteristic potentially life-threatening dysrhythmia observed in patients with severe toxicity (Fig. 41–2).

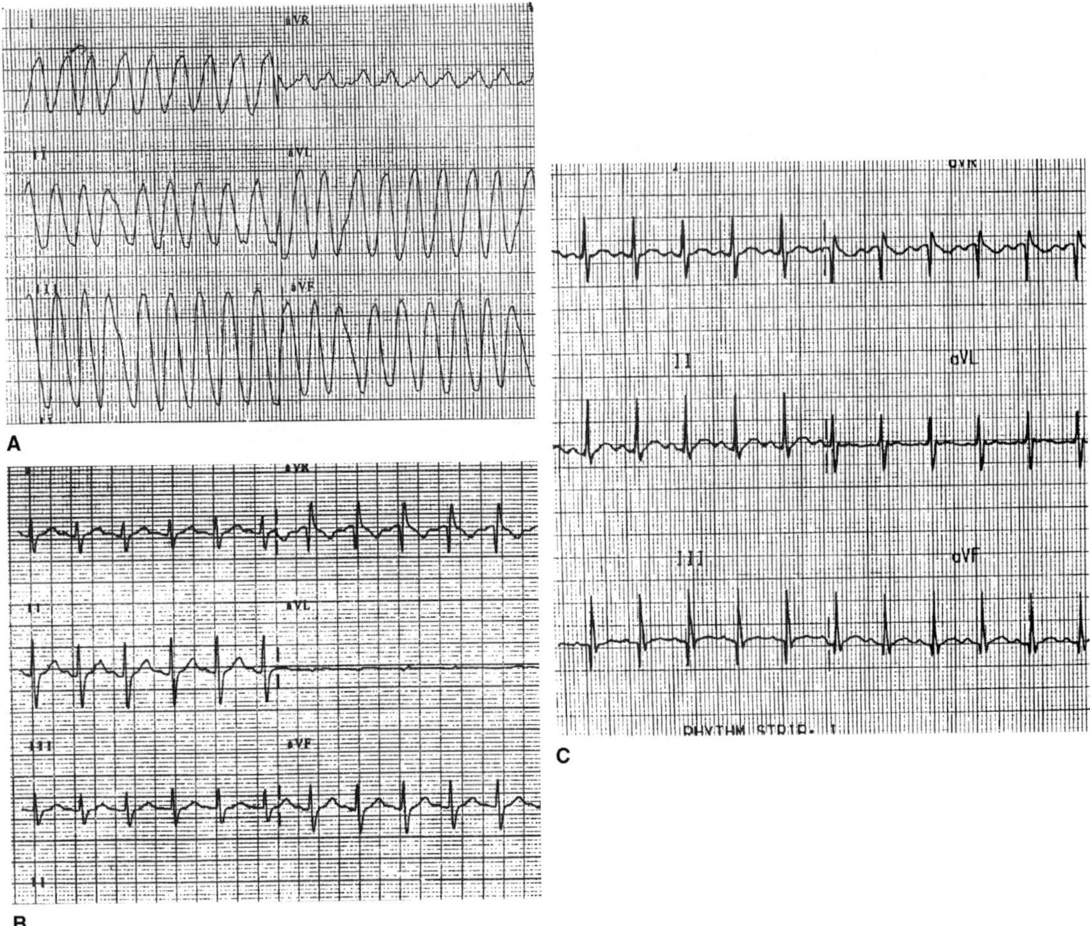

**FIGURE 41–2.** (**A**) Electrocardiograph (ECG) shows a wide-complex tachycardia with a variable QRS complex duration (minimum, 220 ms). (**B**) ECG 30 minutes after presentation following sodium bicarbonate administration shows narrowing of the QRS complex duration to 140 ms and an amplitude of the R in $aV_R$ of 6.0 mm. (**C**) ECG 9 hours after presentation shows further narrowing of the QRS complex to 80 ms and decrease in the amplitude of the R in $aV_R$ to 4.5 mm. *(Reproduced with permission from Liebelt EL. Targeted management strategies for cardiovascular toxicity from tricyclic antidepressant overdose: the pivotal role for alkalinization and sodium loading. Pediatr Emerg Care. 1998 Aug;14(4):293-298.)*

### Acute Central Nervous System Toxicity

Delirium, agitation, and psychotic behavior with hallucinations most likely result from antagonism of muscarinic and histaminergic receptors. These alterations in consciousness usually are followed by lethargy, which is followed by rapid progression to coma. Seizures usually are generalized and brief, most often occurring within 1 to 2 hours of ingestion. Status epilepticus is uncommon. Abrupt deterioration in hemodynamic status, namely hypotension and ventricular dysrhythmias, often develops during or within minutes after a seizure and likely results from seizure-induced acidemia exacerbating cardiovascular toxicity.

### Other Clinical Effects

Anticholinergic effects can occur early or late in the course of CA toxicity. Pupils are dilated and poorly reactive to light. Other anticholinergic effects include dry mouth, dry flushed skin, urinary retention, and ileus. Although prominent, these findings are typically inconsequential. Pulmonary complications include acute respiratory distress syndrome, aspiration pneumonitis, and multisystem organ failure.

### Chronic Toxicity

Chronic CA toxicity usually manifests as exaggerated side effects, such as sedation and sinus tachycardia, or is identified by supratherapeutic drug concentrations in the blood in the absence of an acute overdose. Chronic CA toxicity does not appear to cause life-threatening effects.

### Unique Toxicity from "Atypical" Cyclic Antidepressants

Although the incidence of serious cardiovascular toxicity is lower in patients with amoxapine overdoses, the incidence of seizures is significantly greater than with the traditional CAs. Moreover, seizures are more frequent, or status epilepticus occurs. Similarly, the incidences of seizures and cardiac dysrhythmias and duration of coma are greater with maprotiline toxicity compared with the CAs.

## DIAGNOSTIC TESTING

Diagnostic testing for patients with CA poisoning primarily relies on indirect bedside tests (ECG) and other qualitative laboratory analyses. Quantification of CA concentration provides little help in the acute management of patients with CA

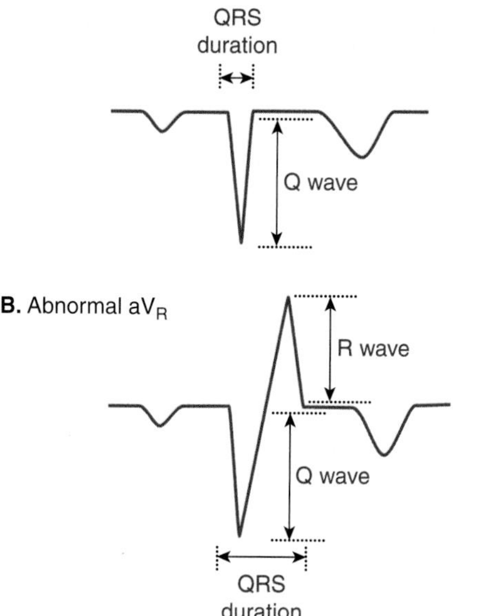


**FIGURE 41–3.** (**A**) Normal QRS complex in lead aVR. (**B**) Abnormal QRS complex in a patient with cyclic antidepressant (CA) poisoning. The R wave in lead $aV_R$ is measured as the maximal height in millimeters of the terminal upward deflection in the QRS complex. In this example, the QRS complex duration is prolonged, indicating significant CA poisoning.

overdose but provides adjunctive information to support the diagnosis.

### Electrocardiography

A rightward T40-ms axis shift is a sensitive indicator of drug presence. An abnormal terminal rightward axis is easily estimated by observing a negative deflection (terminal S wave) in leads I and aVL and a positive deflection (terminal R wave) in lead aVR (Fig. 41–3). The maximal limb lead QRS complex duration is an easily measured ECG parameter that is a sensitive indicator of toxicity. A landmark investigation reported that 33% of patients with a limb lead QRS complex duration greater than or equal to 100 ms developed seizures, and 14% developed ventricular dysrhythmias. No seizures or dysrhythmias occurred in those patients whose QRS complex duration remained less than 100 ms. There was a 50% incidence of ventricular dysrhythmias among patients with a QRS complex duration greater than or equal to 160 ms. No ventricular dysrhythmias occurred in patients with a QRS complex duration less than 160 ms. Evaluation of lead aVR on a routine ECG is also reported to predict toxicity (Figs. 41–2 and 41–3). Some patients also develop a type 1 Brugada pattern.

### Laboratory Tests

Determination of serum CA concentrations has limited utility in the immediate evaluation and management of patients with acute overdoses. Although CA concentrations greater than 1,000 ng/mL usually are associated with significant clinical toxicity such as coma, seizures, and dysrhythmias, life-threatening toxicity occurs in patients with serum concentrations of less than 1,000 ng/mL. The duration of the QRS complex is more predictive of adverse events than the CA concentration.

## MANAGEMENT

Any person with a suspected or known ingestion of a CA requires immediate evaluation and treatment. The patient should be attached to a cardiac monitor, an ECG should be obtained, and intravenous access should be secured. Early intubation is recommended for patients with CNS depression or hemodynamic instability because of the potential for rapid clinical deterioration. An ECG should be obtained for all patients. Laboratory tests, including concentrations of glucose and electrolytes, should be performed for all patients with altered mental status, as well as blood gas analysis to both assess the degree of acidemia and guide alkalinization therapy. Interventions for maintenance of blood pressure and peripheral perfusion must be performed early to avoid irreversible damage.

### Gastrointestinal Decontamination

Anticholinergic actions of some CAs decrease spontaneous gastric emptying, allowing unabsorbed drug to remain in the stomach for several hours. However, because of the potential for rapid deterioration of mental status and seizures, orogastric lavage should not be performed on patients without a protected airway. As such, this procedure should be limited to patients presenting shortly after ingestion (within 2 hours) who have already undergone endotracheal intubation for depressed mental status or other clinical toxicity. Endotracheal intubation should not routinely be performed for the sole purpose of GI decontamination. Activated charcoal (AC) is recommended in all patients presenting within 2 hours of ingestion with a normal mental status, and in patients with altered mental status and a protected airway. Irrespective of age, an additional dose of AC several hours later is reasonable in a seriously poisoned patient in whom unabsorbed drug may still be present in the GI tract or in the case of desorption of CAs from AC.

### Wide-Complex Dysrhythmias, Conduction Delays, and Hypotension

The mainstay of therapy for treating wide-complex dysrhythmias and for reversing conduction delays and hypotension is the combination of serum alkalinization and sodium loading. Increasing the extracellular concentration of sodium overwhelms the effective blockade of sodium channels, presumably through gradient effects (Fig. 41–1). Hypertonic sodium bicarbonate effectively reduces QRS complex prolongation, increases blood pressure, and reverses or suppresses ventricular dysrhythmias caused by CAs (Antidotes in Brief: A5). Indications include conduction delays (QRS complex > 100 ms) and hypotension. No evidence supports prophylactic alkalinization in the absence of cardiovascular toxicity (eg, QRS complex duration < 100 ms). In addition, alkalinization inevitably decreases potassium and ionized calcium, which results in QT interval prolongation.

A bolus, or rapid infusion over several minutes, of hypertonic sodium bicarbonate (1–2 mEq/kg) is recommended initially. Additional boluses every 3 to 5 minutes are recommended until the QRS complex duration narrows and the hypotension improves (Fig. 41–2). Blood pH should be carefully monitored after several bicarbonate boluses, aiming for a target pH of no greater than 7.50 or 7.55. Because CAs redistribute from the tissues into the blood over several hours, it is reasonable to begin a continuous sodium bicarbonate infusion to maintain the pH in this range. It is reasonable to administer hypertonic saline or sodium acetate in situations in which alkalinization with sodium bicarbonate is not possible. Hyperventilation of an intubated patient is a more rapid and easily titratable method of serum alkalinization but is not as effective as sodium bicarbonate in reversing cardiotoxicity. Alkalinization should be continued for at least 12 to 24 hours after the ECG has normalized because of the redistribution of the drug from the tissue.

### Antidysrhythmic Therapy

Lidocaine should be used for ventricular dysrhythmias not responsive to sodium bicarbonate therapy. Because phenytoin exacerbates ventricular dysrhythmias in animals and fails to protect against seizures, its use is not recommended. The use of class IA and class IC antidysrhythmics is absolutely contraindicated because they have similar pharmacologic actions to CAs and thus will worsen the sodium channel inhibition and exacerbate cardiotoxicity.

### Hypotension

Standard initial treatment for hypotension should include volume expansion with isotonic saline or sodium bicarbonate. Hypotension unresponsive to these therapeutic interventions necessitates the use of inotropic or vasopressor support and possibly extracorporeal cardiovascular support. Based on the available data, pharmacologic effects, theoretical concerns, and experience, norepinephrine (0.1–0.2 μg/kg/min) is recommended for hypotension that is unresponsive to volume expansion and hypertonic sodium bicarbonate therapy. If these measures fail to correct hypotension, extracorporeal life support measures are reasonable, if available.

### Additional Therapies

There is no evidence to support intravenous lipid emulsion use for non–life-threatening toxicity. Intravenous lipid emulsion is reasonable for cardiac arrest after CA poisoning and for refractory hypotension or cardiac dysrhythmias if other interventions fail but should not be used as a first-line therapy and should not delay serum alkalinization in patients with cardiovascular toxicity (Antidotes in Brief: A23).

### Central Nervous System Toxicity

Seizures caused by CAs usually are brief and often stop before treatment can be initiated. Recurrent seizures, prolonged seizures (> 2 minutes), and status epilepticus require prompt treatment to prevent worsening acidemia, hypoxia, and development of hyperthermia and rhabdomyolysis. Benzodiazepines are effective as first-line therapy for seizures. If this therapy fails, either a barbiturate or propofol is recommended. Propofol controls refractory seizures resulting from amoxapine toxicity. Failure to respond to barbiturates or propofol should prompt the use of neuromuscular paralysis and general anesthesia with continuous electroencephalographic monitoring. Phenytoin is contraindicated for seizures because data not only demonstrate a failure to terminate seizures but also suggest enhanced cardiovascular toxicity.

Use of flumazenil in a patient with known or suspected CA ingestion is contraindicated (Antidotes in Brief: A25). Physostigmine was used in the past to reverse the acute CNS toxicity (Antidotes in Brief: A11). However, physostigmine is contraindicated because it precipitates bradycardia and asystole.

### Enhanced Elimination

No specific treatment modalities have demonstrated clinically significant efficacy in enhancing the elimination of CAs. Hemodialysis and hemoperfusion are ineffective and should not be performed.

### Hospital Admission Criteria

All patients who present with known or suspected CA ingestion should undergo continuous cardiac monitoring and serial ECGs for a minimum of 6 hours. The following algorithm is reasonable: if the patient is asymptomatic at presentation, undergoes GI decontamination, has normal ECGs, or has sinus tachycardia (with normal QRS complexes) that resolves and the patient remains asymptomatic in the healthcare facility for a minimum of 6 hours without any treatment interventions, the patient may be medically cleared for psychiatric evaluation or discharged home, as appropriate. The disposition of patients with persistent isolated sinus tachycardia, prolonged QT interval with no concomitant altered mental status, or blood pressure changes is not clearly defined. In one study of isolated CA overdose, patients with a heart rate greater than 120 beats/min and a QT interval greater than 480 ms had an increased likelihood of major toxicity. These patients are candidates for observation with continuous ECG monitoring and serial ECGs for 24 hours.

### Inpatient Cardiac Monitoring

Patients admitted to the hospital for significant poisoning should be monitored for 24 hours after termination of alkalinization, antidysrhythmics, and inotrope or vasopressors. They should have returned to baseline mental status prior to discharge.

# 42 SEROTONIN REUPTAKE INHIBITORS AND ATYPICAL ANTIDEPRESSANTS

## INTRODUCTION

In the United States (US), major depressive disorder is a leading cause of disability and affects almost 7% of all adults. The exact etiology of depression and the mechanism by which increased serotonergic and norepinephrine neurotransmission modulates mood remain unclear. Although termed *selective serotonin reuptake inhibitors* (SSRIs), these antidepressants have complex pharmacologic effects and interact with a number of other receptors and neurotransmitters.

## HISTORY AND EPIDEMIOLOGY

Serotonin (5-hydroxytryptamine) got its name after its initial discovery as a vasoconstrictor. The SSRIs were initially marketed in the US in the early 1980s and are today considered one of the first-line therapies for treatment of major depressive disorders. The SSRIs are as effective as the cyclic antidepressants (CAs) and monoamine oxidase inhibitors (MAOIs) for the treatment of major depression, have fewer significant adverse events associated with therapeutic use, and are less problematic in overdose (Chaps. 41 and 44).

## PATHOPHYSIOLOGY

The SSRIs selectively inhibit serotonin reuptake via the serotonin transporter (SERT). Serotonergic neurons are located almost exclusively in the median raphe nucleus of the brainstem, where they extend into and are in close proximity to norepinephrine neurons that are located primarily in the locus ceruleus (Fig. 42–1). The interplay between norepinephrine and serotonin likely explains the effectiveness of antidepressants that do not directly modulate serotonin neurotransmission.

## PHARMACOKINETICS AND TOXICOKINETICS

Table 42–1 lists the pharmacology, therapeutic doses, and metabolism of the available SSRIs and atypical antidepressants. Important pharmacokinetic and pharmacodynamic drug interactions are reported with therapeutic dosing (see Serotonin Toxicity). The SSRIs and their active metabolites are substrates for and potent inhibitors of CYP2D6 and other cytochrome P450 metabolizing enzymes (CYPs).

## PATHOPHYSIOLOGY

The causes of depression and the mechanisms by which antidepressants ameliorate depressive symptoms are not well understood. The current postulated causes of depression include a disruption in function in the signal transduction cascade or subsequent events that influence the regulation of neuronal ion channels, receptor modulation, neurotransmitter release, synaptic potentiation, and neuronal survival. Multiple neurotransmitters are likely involved, including

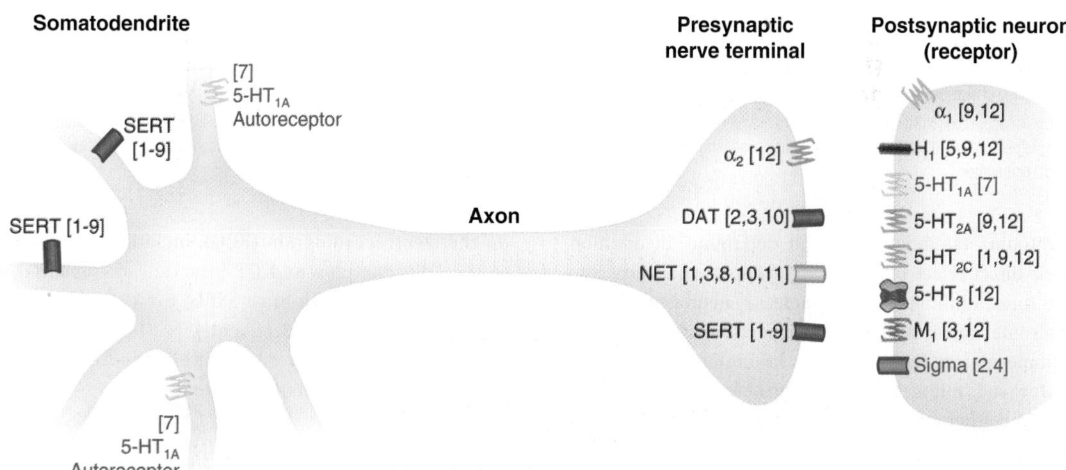


**FIGURE 42–1.** Sites of action of select serotonin and noradrenergic antidepressants. Xenobiotics in green numbers are agonists, and those in red numbers are antagonists. (**A**) All of the following inhibit the serotonin transporter (SERT) and affect other receptors: (1) fluoxetine blocks norepinephrine reuptake transporter (NET) (weak) and 5-$HT_{2C}$; (2) sertraline blocks the dopamine reuptake transporter (DAT) (weak) and binds to the sigma receptor; (3) paroxetine blocks NET (weak) and the muscarinic receptor ($M_1$) and inhibits nitric oxide synthase (NOS); (4) fluvoxamine binds to the sigma receptor; (5) citalopram has mild histamine receptor ($H_1$) receptor inhibition and increases QTc prolongation at high doses; (6) escitalopram is a pure selective serotonin reuptake inhibitor (SSRI); (7) serotonin reuptake inhibitors/partial receptor agonists (SPARIs) include the partial 5-$HT_{1A}$ agonist vilazodone (also for buspirone; not a SERT); (8) serotonin/norepinephrine reuptake inhibitors (SNRIs), including venlafaxine, deslafaxine, and duloxetine, indirectly increase dopamine in the prefrontal cortex); and (9) serotonin antagonist/partial agonist/reuptake inhibitors (SARIs; trazodone) block 5-$HT_{2A}$, 5-$HT_{2C}$, $H_1$, and $\alpha_1$ receptor (dose dependent). (**B**) All of the following have no SERT inhibition but exhibit other effects: (10) norepinephrine/dopamine reuptake inhibitors (NDRIs; bupropion); (11) norepinephrine reuptake inhibitors (NRIs; atomoxetine); and (12) noradrenergic and specific serotonergic antidepressants (NASSAs; mirtazapine), which block central $\alpha_2$ presynaptic receptors, 5-$HT_{2A}$, 5-$HT_{2C}$, 5-$HT_3$, $H_1$, $M_1$ (weak), and peripheral $\alpha_1$ receptor (weak). The xenobiotics listed next to the receptors affect the receptors to varying degrees of potency.

**TABLE 42–1 Drug Mechanism and Pharmacokinetic Data for Available Selective Serotonin Reuptake Inhibitors and Atypical Antidepressants[a]**

| *Drug* | *Typical Daily Dose Range (mg)* | $t_{1/2}$ *(h)* | *Major Metabolic Mechanism* | *Major Active Metabolites* | *Major Active Metabolite* $t_{1/2}$ | *Drug (d) or Metabolite (m) Inhibits CYP* |
|---|---|---|---|---|---|---|
| ***SSRIs*** | | | | | | |
| Citalopram | 20–60 | 33–37 | 2C19, 3A4, 2D6 | Monodesmethylcitalopram, didesmethylcitalopram | 59 h | None or unknown |
| Escitalopram | 10–20 | 22–32 | 2C19, 3A4, 2D6 | S(+)-Desmethylcitalopram | 59 h | None |
| Fluoxetine | 10–80 | 24–144 | 2C9, 2D6 | Norfluoxetine | 4–16 d | 2D6 (d,m), 2C19 (d,m), 2D6 (d,m), 3A4 (m) |
| Fluvoxamine | 100–300 | 15–23 | 1A2, 2D6 | None | N/A | 1A2, 2C9, 2C19, 3A4 |
| Paroxetine | 10–50 | 2.9–44 | 2D6 | None | N/A | 2D6 |
| Sertraline | 50–200 | 24 | 2C9, 2B6, 2C19, 2D6, 3A4 | Desmethylsertraline | 62–104 h | 2C19 (d,m) |
| ***SPARIs*** | | | | | | |
| Vilazodone | 10–40 | 25 | 3A4, 2C19, 2D6 | None | NA | None or unknown |
| Vortioxetine | 5–20 | 66 | 2D6, 3A4 | None | NA | None or unknown |
| ***SARIs*** | | | | | | |
| Trazodone | 50–600 | 3–9 | 2D6, 3A4 inhibitors may increase concentration | m-Chlorophenylpiperazine | ? | None or unknown |
| Nefazodone | 300–600 | 3.5 | 3A4 | Triazoledione, hydroxynefazodone | 10 hours | (m)3A4 |
| ***SNRIs*** | | | | | | |
| Desvenlafaxine | 50 | 11 | Conjugation, 2D6 | None or unknown | N/A | None or unknown |
| Duloxetine | 40–60 | 8–17 | 2D6, 1A2 | None | N/A | 2D6 |
| Levomilnacipran | 40–120 | 12 | 3A4, P-glycoprotein Minor: 2C19, 2C8 and 2D6 | None | N/A | None or unknown |
| Milnacipran | 25–200 | 6-8 | Glucuronidation | None | N/A | None |
| Venlafaxine | 75–375 | 3–4 | 2D6 | *O*-Desmethylvenlafaxine, depends on 3A4 and 2C19 for metabolism | 10 h | None or unknown |
| ***PSNR*** | | | | | | |
| Mirtazapine | 15–45 | 20–40 | 3A4 | Desmethylmirtazapine | Unknown | 3A4 induction |
| ***NDRI*** | | | | | | |
| Bupropion | 150–450 | 9.6–20.9 | 2D6 | Hydroxybupropion, erythrohydrobupropion, threohydrobupropion | 24–37 h | 2D6 |

[a]The volume of distribution for all these xenobiotics is large except for trazodone.

N/A = not applicable; NDRI = norepinephrine/dopamine reuptake inhibitor; PSNR = presynaptic serotonin and norepinephrine releaser; SARI = serotonin antagonist/partial agonist/reuptake inhibitor; SNRI = serotonin/norepinephrine reuptake inhibitor; SPARI = serotonin reuptake inhibitors/partial receptor agonists; SSRI = selective serotonin reuptake inhibitor.

serotonin, norepinephrine, and dopamine. In addition to their direct effect of increasing synaptic concentrations of serotonin, antidepressants increase neurogenesis in the prefrontal cortex and glia in oligodendrocytes and activate complementary factors such as brain-derived neurotrophic factor and mitogen-activated protein kinase. Unlike the CAs and other atypical antidepressants, the SSRIs have little direct interaction with cholinergic receptors, GABA receptors, sodium channels, or adrenergic reuptake (Table 42–2).

## CLINICAL MANIFESTATIONS

Most of the effects that occur after overdose are direct extensions of the pharmacologic activity of the SSRIs in therapeutic doses. Excess serotonergic stimulation is prominent and nonselective. Common signs and symptoms include drowsiness, tremor, nausea, and vomiting. Less commonly, central nervous system (CNS) depression and sinus tachycardia occur. Seizures and changes on the electrocardiogram (ECG), including prolongation of the QRS complex and QT interval, are reported, but they rarely occur with most SSRIs, even after large overdoses (Table 42–3). Infrequently, SSRI overdose results in life-threatening effects with fatalities often associated with coadministration of other xenobiotics.

### Citalopram

Citalopram and escitalopram cause QT interval prolongation in therapeutic doses in a linear, dose-related, and delayed manner. The development of torsade de pointes is reported in therapeutic doses but only when concurrent xenobiotics are used or when there are electrolyte abnormalities. In large case series, patients are at risk for seizures and QT interval prolongation after ingestions exceeding 600 mg of citalopram or with serum concentrations more than 40 times the expected therapeutic concentrations. Seizures were an early finding, occurring within 2 hours of ingestion, but the development of abnormalities on ECG was delayed for as long

**TABLE 42–2 Receptor Activity of Selective Serotonin Reuptake Inhibitors and Related Antidepressants**

| Drug | Mechanism | Degree of Norepinephrine Reuptake Inhibition | Degree of Serotonin Reuptake Inhibition | Degree of Dopamine Reuptake Inhibition | Degree of Peripheral α-Adrenergic Effects |
|---|---|---|---|---|---|
| ***SSRIs*** | | | | | |
| Citalopram | SSRI, antimuscarinic | 0 | ++++ | 0 | 0 |
| Escitalopram | SSRI | 0 | ++++ | 0 | 0 |
| Fluoxetine | SSRI, inhibition of 5-$HT_{2C}$ | 0 | ++++ | 0 | 0 |
| Fluvoxamine | SSRI | 0 | ++++ | 0 | 0 |
| Paroxetine | SSRI, antimuscarinic | + | ++++ | + | 0 |
| Sertraline | SSRI, weak reuptake norepinephrine and dopamine inhibitor | 0 | ++++ | + | + |
| ***Other*** | | | | | |
| Bupropion | Inhibits reuptake of biogenic amines | ++ | 0 | + | ++ |
| Duloxetine | SRI, norepinephrine reuptake inhibitor | ++ | ++++ | 0 | ++ |
| Desvenlafaxine | SRI, norepinephrine reuptake inhibitor | ++ | ++++ | 0 | ++ |
| Levomilnacipran | SRI, norepinephrine reuptake inhibitor | ++ | ++++ | 0 | 0 |
| Milnacipran | SRI, norepinephrine reuptake inhibitor | ++ | ++++ | 0 | + |
| Mirtazapine | $\alpha_2$-Adrenergic antagonism, 5-$HT_2$/5-$HT_3$ antagonism | 0 | ++++ | 0 | + |
| Nefazodone | SRI, $\alpha_1$-adrenergic antagonist | 0 | + | 0 | + |
| Trazodone | SRI, $\alpha_1$-adrenergic antagonist | 0 | + | 0 | + |
| Venlafaxine | SRI, norepinephrine reuptake inhibitor | ++ | ++++ | 0 | ++ |
| Vilazodone | SSRI, 5-$HT_{1A}$ agonist | 0 | ++++ | 0 | 0 |
| Vortioxetine | SSRI, 5-$HT_{1A}$/5-$HT_3$ agonist | 0 | ++++ | 0 | 0 |

+ = weak if any agonism; ++ = weak agonism; +++ = strong agonism; ++++ = very strong agonism; 0 = no effect; SRI = serotonin reuptake inhibitor; SSRI = selective serotonin reuptake inhibitor.

**TABLE 42–3 Predictive Analysis of the Relative Potential for Seizures and Abnormalities on Electrocardiography of Selective Serotonin Reuptake Inhibitors and Related Antidepressants**

| Drug | Seizures | QT Interval Prolongation | QRS Complex Prolongation |
|---|---|---|---|
| ***Classic SSRIs*** | | | |
| Citalopram | +++ | +++ | + |
| Escitalopram | +++ | +++ | + |
| Fluoxetine | + | 0 | 0 |
| Fluvoxamine | + | 0 | 0 |
| Paroxetine | + | 0 | 0 |
| Sertraline | + | 0 | 0 |
| ***Atypical Antidepressants*** | | | |
| Bupropion | ++++ | + | + |
| Desvenlafaxine | +++ | + | +++ |
| Duloxetine | ++++ | Unknown | Unknown |
| Levomilnacipran | Unknown | Unknown | Unknown |
| Milnacipran | Unknown | Unknown | Unknown |
| Mirtazapine | Unknown | Unknown | ++ |
| Nefazodone | 0 | 0 | 0 |
| Trazodone | + | + | 0 |
| Venlafaxine | +++ | + | +++ |
| Vilazodone | + | Unknown | Unknown |
| Vortioxetine | Unknown | Unknown | Unknown |

0 = does not cause; + = very rarely causes; ++ = rarely causes; +++ = causes; ++++ = very commonly causes; SSRI = selective serotonin reuptake inhibitor.

as 24 hours after ingestion. Although the mechanisms are unclear, experimental models suggest that the didesmethylcitalopram metabolite of citalopram prolongs the QT interval by blocking $IK_r$.

## MANAGEMENT

Adults with well-defined unintentional ingestions of up to 100 mg of citalopram and 50 mg of escitalopram can be managed safely at home with close observation. The dose at which children can be safely managed in the home is less well defined. For hospitalized patients, treatment is largely supportive. An ECG should be obtained to identify other cardiotoxic drugs, such as the CAs, to which the patient might access, and the patient should be attached to a cardiac monitor to exclude the possibility of delayed QT interval prolongation and subsequent risk for ventricular dysrhythmias. Oral activated charcoal (AC) (1 g/kg) is recommended if there are no contraindications. Lowering of blood concentrations and reduction in risk for QT interval prolongation are demonstrated when AC is given within the first 4 hours after escitalopram and citalopram ingestion. Patients who have ingested other SSRIs can be managed conservatively with a single dose of activated charcoal if not contraindicated and a short period of observation if they remain asymptomatic.

## ADVERSE EVENTS AFTER THERAPEUTIC DOSES

Adverse events commonly associated with therapeutic doses of SSRIs as well as with overdose include GI effects (anorexia, nausea, vomiting, diarrhea), sexual dysfunction, weight gain, sleep disturbance, and discontinuation syndromes. Movement disorders, most commonly akathisia, parkinsonism, myoclonus, and dystonia, also occur after SSRI use. These extrapyramidal adverse events appear to be related to the complex interplay between serotonergic and dopaminergic activity. The use of SSRIs is associated with the syndrome of inappropriate antidiuretic hormone secretion (SIADH), in which severe hyponatremia occurs rapidly. A review of the literature identified increasing age, female sex, concurrent medications known to cause hyponatremia, low body weight, a previous history of hyponatremia, and excessive fluid intake as risk factors for hyponatremia. Although reported to occur from 3 days to 4 months after initiation of therapy, SIADH occurs most frequently within the first 2 weeks of therapy.

### Serotonin Toxicity

The most common severe adverse event associated with SSRIs is the development of serotonin toxicity. This was formerly referred to in life-threatening cases as *serotonin syndrome* and *serotonin behavioral* or *hyperactivity syndrome.*

***Pathophysiology.*** The pathophysiologic mechanism of serotonin toxicity is not completely understood but likely involves excessive selective stimulation and genetic variation of serotonin 5-$HT_{2A}$ and perhaps 5-$HT_{1A}$ receptors. Serotonin toxicity occurs most frequently after use of combinations of serotonergic xenobiotics (Table 42–4) but also occurs after high therapeutic dosing or overdoses of isolated serotonergic xenobiotics.

***Manifestations.*** Signs of serotonin toxicity include altered mental status, agitation, tachycardia, myoclonus, hyperreflexia, diaphoresis, tremor, diarrhea, incoordination, muscle rigidity, and hyperthermia (Table 42–5). The neuromuscular effects are often more prominent in the lower extremities. Life-threatening effects invariably result from hyperthermia caused by excessive muscle activity.

***Diagnosis.*** Although fulminant life-threatening cases are easy to recognize, mild cases of serotonin toxicity are more difficult to distinguish from similarly appearing disorders from other causes. A modification of the Hunter Serotonin Toxicity Criteria, which included myoclonus, agitation, diaphoresis, hyperreflexia, hypertonicity, and fever, was validated in 473 patients and found to correlate best with a clinical toxicologic diagnosis of serotonin toxicity (Table 42–5). Currently, no diagnostic test capable of determining whether a patient is experiencing serotonin toxicity is available.

***Management.*** Treatment of patients with serotonin toxicity begins with supportive care and focuses on decreasing core body temperature and muscle activity. Because muscular rigidity is thought to be primarily responsible for hyperthermia and death, rapid external cooling using ice water immersion in conjunction with sedative hypnotics such as benzodiazepines is recommended to limit complications and mortality. In severe cases, neuromuscular blockade with a definitive airway is a recommended approach to achieve rapid muscle relaxation. In most patients, the manifestations of serotonin toxicity resolve within 24 hours after the offending xenobiotic is removed. However, serotonin toxicity can be prolonged when it is caused by xenobiotics with long half-lives, protracted duration of effects, or active metabolites.

Several case reports suggest success after use of 4 mg of oral cyproheptadine, an antihistamine with nonspecific serotonin antagonist effects, including 5-$HT_{1A}$ and 5-$HT_{2A}$ receptors. Patients who responded typically had no hyperthermia and only mild to moderate manifestations of serotonin toxicity.

**TABLE 42–4 Potential Causes of Serotonin Toxicity**

| |
|---|
| ***Inhibitors of Serotonin Metabolism*** |
| Linezolid |
| Methylene blue |
| Monoamine oxidase inhibitors (nonselective) |
| Phenelzine, moclobemide, clorgyline, isocarboxazid |
| Harmine and harmaline from ayahuasca preparations, psychoactive beverage used for religious purposes in the Amazon and Orinoco River basins |
| St. John's wort (*Hypericum perforatum*) |
| Syrian rue (*Peganum harmala*) |
| ***Blockers of Serotonin Reuptake*** |
| Clomipramine, imipramine |
| Cocaine |
| Dextromethorphan |
| Fentanyl |
| Meperidine |
| Pentazocine |
| SSRIs: all |
| Milnacipran |
| Tramadol |
| Trazodone, nefazodone |
| Venlafaxine |
| ***Serotonin Precursors or Agonists*** |
| L-Tryptophan |
| Lysergic acid diethylamide (LSD) |
| Triptans (sumatriptan) |
| ***Enhancers of Serotonin Release*** |
| Substituted amphetamines and analogs: phenylethylamines, especially MDMA, cathinones, aminoindanes |
| Methylone |
| Buspirone |
| Butylone |
| Cocaine |
| Lithium |
| Mirtazapine |
| ***Other*** |
| Ginseng |
| Lithium |
| Ondansetron, granisetron, and metoclopramide |
| Sibutramine |
| Ritonavir |
| Valproic acid |

MDMA = 3,4-methylenedioxymethamphetamine; SSRI = selective serotonin reuptake inhibitor.

| TABLE 42–5 Diagnostic Criteria for Serotonin Toxicity |
|---|
| ***After Introduction of a Serotonergic Xenobiotic:*** |
| Spontaneous clonus alone |
| Inducible or ocular clonus *plus* agitation *or* diaphoresis *or* hypertonicity with temperature > 38°C (100.4°F) |
| Tremor with hyperreflexia |
| ***Other Common Manifestations*** |
| Diaphoresis and shivering |
| Diarrhea |
| Hyperthermia |
| Incoordination |
| Mental status changes |
| Myoclonus |

Evidence supports the use of cyproheptadine in this patient group. We currently recommend an initial dose of 12 mg orally with subsequent doses of 2 mg repeated hourly, as needed, to achieve muscle relaxation in more severe cases.

### Differentiating Serotonin Toxicity from Neuroleptic Malignant Syndrome

Many features overlap between serotonin toxicity and the neuroleptic malignant syndrome (NMS) (Chap. 40). Although altered mental status, autonomic instability, and changes in neuromuscular tone that result in hyperthermia are common to both disorders, many differences are apparent. It is also clear that the implicated xenobiotics, time course, pathophysiology, and manifestations are distinct (Table 42–6).

## ATYPICAL ANTIDEPRESSANTS

Atypical antidepressants are defined as not belonging strictly within a specific class of antidepressants. They are not SSRIs, CAs, or MAOIs.

**TABLE 42–6 Comparison of Neuroleptic Malignant Syndrome (NMS) and Serotonin Toxicity**

| | *NMS* | *Serotonin Toxicity* |
|---|---|---|
| ***Historical Diagnostic Clue*** | | |
| Inciting drug pharmacology | Dopamine antagonist | Serotonin agonist |
| Time course of initiation of symptoms after exposure | Days to weeks | Hours |
| Duration of symptoms | Days to 2 wk | Usually 24 h |
| ***Symptoms*** | | |
| Altered mental status (depressed or confusion) | +++ | +++ |
| Altered mental status (agitation or hyperactivity) | +++ | +++ |
| Autonomic instability | +++ | +++ |
| Bradykinesia | +++ | – |
| Gastrointestinal findings (diarrhea) | – | +++ |
| Hyperthermia | +++ | +++ |
| Lead pipe rigidity | +++ | + |
| Shivering | – | +++ |
| Tremor, hyperreflexia, myoclonus | + | +++ |

– = not found; + = rare finding; +++ = common finding.

### Serotonin/Norepinephrine Reuptake Inhibitors: Venlafaxine, Desvenlafaxine, Duloxetine, Milnacipran, and Levomilnacipran

In addition to inhibiting serotonin reuptake, venlafaxine inhibits norepinephrine reuptake. Patients with acute venlafaxine overdose present with nausea, vomiting, dizziness, tachycardia, CNS depression, hypotension, hypoglycemia, hyperthermia, hepatic toxicity (including zone 3 necrosis), rhabdomyolysis, and seizures. Sodium and potassium channel blocking effects are rarely clinically apparent; however, prolongation of the QRS complex and QT interval can lead to ventricular tachycardia and death. Although no clinical data regarding efficacy are available, we recommend sodium bicarbonate to attenuate the sodium channel blocking effects that lead to QRS complex prolongation (Antidotes in Brief: A5). In addition, GI decontamination with AC with or without whole-bowel irrigation (WBI) decreases serum concentrations and decreases the incidence of seizures in select patients, particularly after the ingestion of extended-release formulations. Venlafaxine appears to be more dangerous than SSRIs and the other serotonin/norepinephrine reuptake inhibitors (SNRIs)—desvenlafaxine, duloxetine, milnacipran, and levomilnacipran—after overdose.

### Serotonin Reuptake Inhibitors/Partial Receptor Agonists: Vilazodone and Vortioxetine

Vilazodone is an SSRI with additional 5-$HT_{1A}$ receptor agonism. Little information is available about vilazodone after overdose. There has been a single report of a child with a reported ingestion of 37 mg/kg of vilazodone who developed altered mental status, signs of serotonin toxicity, and a seizure. Similarly, there is little information available regarding vortioxetine overdose, but it is anticipated to have effects similar to other SSRIs.

### Serotonin Antagonist/Partial Agonist/Reuptake Inhibitors: Trazodone and Nefazodone

Trazodone is an antagonist at 5-$HT_{2A}$ and 5-$HT_{2C}$ receptors, a partial agonist at 5-$HT_1$ receptors, and a weak serotonin reuptake inhibitor. In addition, trazodone has $\alpha$-adrenergic antagonist activity and weak $H_1$ receptor antagonism. Central nervous system depression and orthostatic hypotension are the most common complications after acute overdose of trazodone. Less common complications include seizures and cardiac conduction delays, such as QT interval prolongation and ventricular dysrhythmias, and death. Trazodone is rarely reported to cause SIADH and cholestatic hepatitis. Priapism, reported with therapeutic doses of trazodone, occurs occasionally after overdose. Treatment is supportive and includes monitoring the ECG for conduction delays and the administration of fluids and vasopressors for hypotension if necessary.

Nefazodone is an antagonist at 5-$HT_{2A}$ receptors and $\alpha$-adrenergic receptors in addition to moderate inhibition of serotonin and norepinephrine reuptake. The most common manifestations that occur after acute overdose include drowsiness, nausea, dizziness, and hypotension. Treatment is similar to trazodone overdose.

### Presynaptic Serotonin and Norepinephrine Releaser: Mirtazapine

The mechanism of action of mirtazapine is unique. It is a central presynaptic $\alpha_2$-adrenergic inhibitor that increases neuronal norepinephrine and serotonin release. Mirtazapine also blocks 5-$HT_{2A}$, 5-$HT_{2C}$, 5-$HT_3$, $H_2$, peripheral $\alpha_1$, and muscarinic acetylcholine receptors. The main effects that occur after acute mirtazapine overdoses include altered mental status, tachycardia, and hypothermia. Large overdoses cause respiratory depression and prolongation of the QT interval.

### Norepinephrine/Dopamine Reuptake Inhibitor: Bupropion

The use of bupropion, especially extended-release formulations, is common for the treatment of depression. Bupropion is also frequently used in the treatment of smoking cessation therapy, weight loss, attention deficit hyperactivity disorder, and, occasionally, in compulsive eating disorders. The pharmacologic mechanism of action of bupropion includes inhibition of reuptake of dopamine and, to a lesser extent, norepinephrine. Frequent effects that occur after overdose include tachycardia, hypertension, GI symptoms, and agitation. Large acute overdoses result in seizures (infrequently status epilepticus), QRS complex prolongation, and occasionally QT interval prolongation. In some cases, effects were delayed for up 10 hours, and seizures up to 24 hours, particularly after the ingestion of sustained-release preparations. Treatment, when required for seizures, should be supportive and includes judicious use of benzodiazepines. Cardiotoxicity and QRS complex prolongation are likely manifested through gap junctions and therefore may not be responsive to sodium bicarbonate. Evidence-based recommendations suggest the use of intravenous lipid emulsion for life-threatening bupropion overdose after other therapies fail. Intravenous lipid emulsion is not recommended in the situation of bupropion overdose without life-threatening cardiac toxicity. When a patient presents shortly after an overdose or the patient has taken a massive overdose, we recommend the use of multiple doses of AC with the addition of WBI if the airway is protected.

## DRUG DISCONTINUATION SYNDROME

The term *drug discontinuation syndrome* is used to describe the physiologic manifestations that occur after abrupt antidepressant cessation. The distinction between a withdrawal syndrome and drug discontinuation syndrome is unclear, but it likely distinguishes the manifestations occurring after therapeutic use versus misuse, such as alcohol or heroin withdrawal and SSRI discontinuation syndrome. Drug discontinuation syndromes are commonly reported after abrupt discontinuation of all antidepressants, including SSRIs and atypical antidepressants. The discontinuation syndrome usually begins within 5 days after drug discontinuation and continues up to 3 weeks. The most frequently reported symptoms include dizziness, lethargy, paresthesias, nausea, vivid dreams, irritability, and depressed mood. The syndrome is more common with SSRIs with shorter elimination half-lives (paroxetine > fluvoxamine > sertraline > fluoxetine).

Because of difficulty in distinguishing symptoms of discontinuation syndrome from underlying disease, some authors have proposed diagnostic criteria for the SSRI discontinuation syndrome. All proposed criteria include discontinuation of the SSRI associated with CNS effects, GI distress, or anxiety. The prominent CNS findings include dizziness; ataxia; vertigo; sensory abnormalities, including electric shock-like sensations and paresthesias; and behavior abnormalities, including aggression and impulsivity.

Treatment of patients should include supportive care and resumption of the discontinued drug or administration of another SSRI if the implicated drug is contraindicated. The drug then should be tapered at a rate that allows for improved patient tolerance.

Drug discontinuation syndrome is also identified to occur in neonates. It is commonly referred to as the neonatal (serotonin) abstinence syndrome (NSAS). Neonatal (serotonin) abstinence syndrome is reported to occur after in utero exposure to SSRIs and other atypical antidepressants. The incidence of NSAS was reported to be as high as 30% in a cohort of neonates whose mothers were taking SSRIs. In these cases, symptoms were generally confined to the CNS, respiratory system, and GI system and resolved over a 2-week period.

# 43 LITHIUM

Lithium concentration (serum):
Therapeutic concentration for
bipolar depression = 0.6–1.2 mEq/L (mmol/L)

## HISTORY AND EPIDEMIOLOGY

By the mid-19th century, lithium salts were used therapeutically for the treatment of gout, as well as mania and depression. The soft drink 7-Up originally contained lithium as its "active ingredient," and during the 1930s and 1940s, lithium was used as a table salt substitute for patients with congestive heart failure. In 1949, the Australian psychiatrist Cade "rediscovered" the calming effects of lithium in guinea pig experiments. In 1974, lithium was approved by the United States (US) Food and Drug Administration. Lithium is considered the most effective long-term therapy for treatment and prevention of relapse of bipolar affective disorders.

## PHARMACOLOGY

Lithium has a complex mechanism of action that remains incompletely understood after more than 50 years of clinical use and study. The therapeutic effects of lithium become evident only after chronic administration, so its mechanism of action is unlikely solely the result of acute biochemical interactions on receptors or neurotransmitter release and reuptake. Rather, a complex cascade of interactions with secondary messengers such as the β form of the multifunctional enzyme glycogen synthase kinase 3 (GSK-3β) (Fig. 43–1) and inositol monophosphatase (Fig. 43–2) is proposed.

## PHARMACOKINETICS AND TOXICOKINETICS

Lithium has a volume of distribution of between 0.6 and 0.9 L/kg. It has no discernible protein binding and distributes freely in total body water, with the exception of the cerebrospinal fluid (CSF), from which it is actively extruded. Immediate-release preparations of lithium are rapidly absorbed from the gastrointestinal (GI) tract, and peak serum concentrations are achieved within 1 to 2 hours. Sustained-release products demonstrate variable absorption, with a delay to peak of 4 to 5 hours. Although lithium is rapidly absorbed, tissue distribution is a complex phenomenon, with a significant delay to achieve steady state. Each 300-mg lithium carbonate tablet contains 8.12 mEq of lithium. Ingestion of a single 300-mg tablet is expected to increase the serum lithium concentration by approximately 0.1 to 0.3 mEq/L (assuming a volume of distribution of approximately 0.6–0.9 L/kg and a patient weight of 50–100 kg). Lithium is not metabolized and is eliminated almost entirely (95%) by the kidneys. In an adult with normal kidney function, lithium clearance varies from 10 to 40 mL/min. Lithium is handled by the kidneys much in the same way as sodium. Lithium is freely filtered, and more than 80% is reabsorbed by the proximal tubule. Any condition that makes the kidney sodium avid, such as volume depletion or salt restriction, increases lithium reabsorption in the proximal tubule.

## CLINICAL MANIFESTATIONS

Similar to other xenobiotics having prolonged redistributive phases and tissue burdens, lithium toxicity is characteristically divided into three main categories: acute, acute on chronic, and chronic. In acute lithium toxicity, the patient has no body burden of lithium present at the time of ingestion. The toxicity that develops depends on the amount ingested, along with rates of absorption, distribution, and elimination. In chronic toxicity, the patient has a stable body burden of lithium as the serum concentration is maintained in the therapeutic range, and then some factor disturbs this balance, either by enhancing absorption, or more commonly,

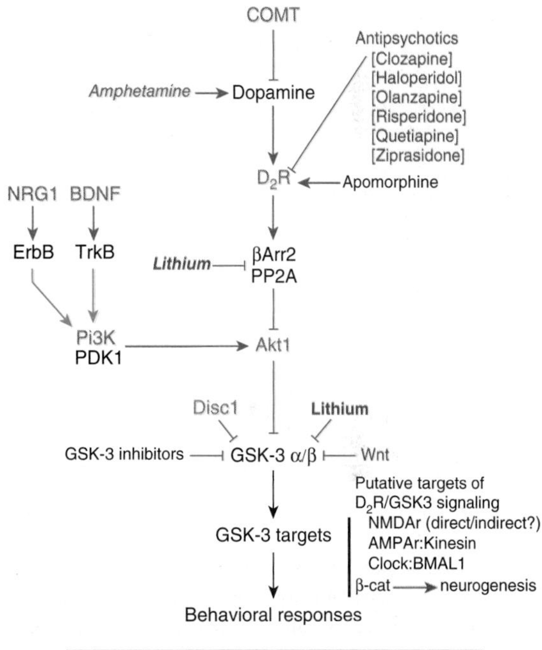


**FIGURE 43–1.** Regulation of GSK-3 (glycogen synthase kinase 3) and Akt (GSK-3β-modifying enzyme) signaling by psychoactive drugs and related network of gene products associated with mental disorders. Proteins labeled in orange are the product of genes associated with an increased risk of developing schizophrenia or bipolar disorders. Blue arrows indicate activation, and the red T arrows indicate inhibition. Black arrows indicate actions that can either activate or inhibit the function of specific substrates. Behavioral changes in dopaminergic responses have been reported in Akt1 and β-arrestin 2 knock out mice and in GSK-3β-HET mice. Growth factors, including neurotrophins, activate Akt, which phosphorylates and inhibits GSK-3, allowing activation of downstream effectors to promote cell survival. Wnt (wingless-related integration site) inhibits GSK-3, stabilizing β-catenin, which activates Wnt target genes, and promotes neurogenesis. β-cat = β-catenin; COMT = catechol-*O*-methyltransferase; $D_2R = D_2$ dopamine receptor; Disc1 = disrupted-in-schizophrenia 1; NRG1 = neuregulin 1; PDK1 = phosphatidylinositol-dependent kinase 1; Pi3K = phosphatidylinositol 3-kinase. *(Used with permission of Am Soc for Pharmacology & Experimental Therapeutics, from The physiology, signaling, and pharmacology of dopamine receptors. Beaulieu JM, Gainetdinov RR. Volume 63(1), 2011; permission conveyed through Copyright Clearance Center, Inc.)*

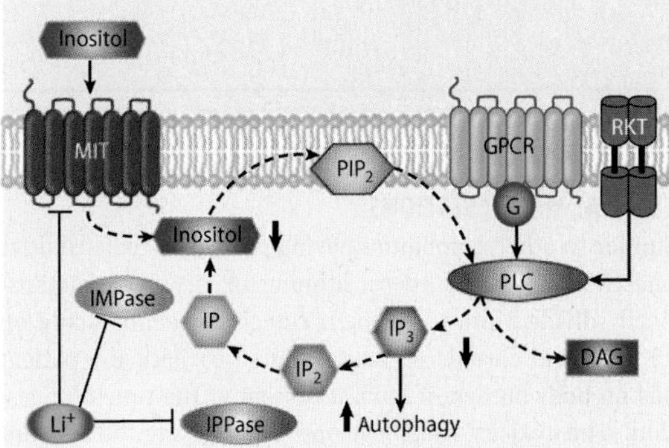


**FIGURE 43–2.** The actions of lithium on inositol depletion and autophagy induction. Extracellular signal binding to its cell surface receptor, either G protein-coupled receptor (GPCR) or RTK, activates phospholipase C (PLC), which hydrolyzes the phospholipid phosphatidyl bisphosphate ($PIP_2$) to yield second messengers inositol triphosphate ($IP_3$) and diacylglycerol (DAG). Inositol triphosphate is recycled by enzymes inositol bisphosphate phosphatase (IPPase) and inositol monophosphatase (IMPase) and converted to inositol (mainly myoinositol), which is required for $PIP_2$ resynthesis. Lithium decreases intracellular inositol concentrations by directly inhibiting IPPase, IMPase, and myoinositol transporter (MIT) that uptakes extracellular inositol. Decreased intracellular inositol concentrations are expected to subsequently reduce $PIP_2$ and prevent the formation of $IP_3$ and DAG, thus blocking transmembrane signaling and trigging the induction of autophagy. Lines with solid arrows represent stimulatory connections; lines with flattened ends represent inhibitory connections. Dashed lines represent pathways with reduced activity as a result of lithium treatment. IP = inositol monophosphate; $IP_2$ = inositol bisphosphate. *(Reproduced with permission from Chiu CT, Chuang DM. Molecular actions and therapeutic potential of lithium in preclinical and clinical studies of CNS disorders. Pharmacol Ther. 2010;128(2):281-304.)*

decreasing elimination. In acute-on-chronic toxicity, the patient ingests an increased amount of lithium (intentionally or unintentionally) in the setting of a stable body burden. With tissue saturation, any additional lithium leads to signs and symptoms of toxicity.

### Acute Toxicity

Clinical findings of acute ingestions of lithium salts begin with GI effects. Nausea, vomiting, and diarrhea are prevalent. Significant volume losses may result, leading patients to complain of lightheadedness, dizziness, and orthostasis. Neurologic manifestations occur several hours after ingestion in acute toxicity because the lithium redistributes slowly into the CNS from the serum.

### Chronic Toxicity

Lithium is primarily a neurotoxin. Approximately 27% of patients using lithium develop tremor at some point during therapeutic dosing. Other findings of chronic toxicity include fasciculations, hyperreflexia, choreoathetoid movements, clonus, dysarthria, nystagmus, and ataxia. The mental status is often altered and progresses from confusion to stupor, coma, and seizures.

The syndrome of irreversible lithium-effectuated neurotoxicity (SILENT) is a descriptive syndrome of the irreversible neurologic and neuropsychiatric sequelae of lithium toxicity that is defined as neurologic dysfunction caused by lithium in the absence of prior neurologic illness and persists for at least 2 months after cessation of the drug. Cerebellar findings predominate in patients with SILENT. One of the predictors of persistent neurologic dysfunction is the concomitant finding of hyperpyrexia, an ominous finding in patients with lithium toxicity.

### Acute-on-Chronic Toxicity

Patients undergoing chronic therapy who acutely ingest an additional amount of lithium (either intentionally or unintentionally) are at risk for signs and symptoms of both acute and chronic toxicity. These patients display prominent GI and neurologic effects, which adds some confusion to the diagnosis and management. Serum lithium concentrations in cases of acute on chronic toxicity are often difficult to interpret.

### Other Systemic Manifestations of Chronic Lithium Therapy

The most common adverse effect of chronic lithium therapy is nephrogenic diabetes insipidus (NDI), which can develop within weeks of the initiation of therapy and affects up to 40% of patients. Patients present with polyuria, thirst, and hypernatremia. Chronic lithium therapy is also associated with chronic tubulointerstitial nephropathy, as manifested by the development of acute kidney injury (AKI) and chronic kidney disease (CKD) with little or no proteinuria and biopsy findings of tubular cysts. Lithium causes a number of endocrine disorders. The most prevalent endocrine manifestation of chronic lithium therapy is hypothyroidism. The combination of hyperparathyroidism and hypercalcemia is also frequently reported in patients receiving chronic lithium therapy, most commonly in older women.

Lithium is associated with a number of electrocardiographic (ECG) abnormalities. The most commonly reported manifestation is T-wave flattening or inversion, primarily in the precordial leads, although prolongation of the QT interval is also noted.

Developmentally, in utero exposure to lithium increases the incidence of congenital heart defects (approximately 1 additional case per 100 live births), specifically right ventricular outflow obstructions (including Ebstein abnormality), in a dose-dependent fashion. Additionally, many effects similar to those that occur in patients undergoing chronic therapy are found in infants exposed in utero, including thyroid disease and neurotoxicity.

## DIAGNOSTIC TESTING

Because of the prevalence of lithium use, therapeutic drug monitoring is readily available in most settings, and serum concentrations are usually readily obtainable. A lithium concentration should be determined upon patient presentation and serial measurements obtained in most instances in which overdose or toxicity is likely, especially after ingestion of sustained-release preparations. Emphasis should be placed on the lithium concentration as a marker of exposure and response to therapy but not necessarily as a determinant of toxicity or treatment. The sample must be sent in an appropriate lithium-free tube because use of lithiated-heparin tubes will lead to false-positive results, up to an additional 4 mEq/L. Serum electrolyte concentrations and kidney function should be assessed because kidney function is important in determining the need for additional therapies, such as hemodialysis. If the patient is hypernatremic, nephrogenic diabetes insipidus should be suspected, and determinations of serum and urine osmolarity and electrolytes help confirm the diagnosis. If a deliberate ingestion has occurred, a serum acetaminophen concentration should be obtained. An ECG is also indicated.

## MANAGEMENT

The initial management and stabilization should begin with assessment and, if necessary, support of airway, breathing, and circulation. Lithium rarely, if ever, affects the patient's airway or breathing, although coingestants may. Emesis, which occurs with significant frequency after acute exposure, may lead to aspiration and respiratory compromise.

### Gastrointestinal Decontamination

For patients who present after an acute overdose or an acute-on-chronic overdose, a risk-benefit analysis of GI decontamination must be undertaken. Two factors should be considered. With an acute overdose and predominance of early GI symptoms, including emesis, self-decontamination may already have occurred. Second, immediate-release preparations are often rapidly absorbed and may not lend themselves to GI evacuation.

Gastrointestinal decontamination options are limited. Lithium salts do not bind readily to activated charcoal. Orogastric lavage has a limited role in the acute management of a patient with a lithium overdose but remains of reasonable benefit early in the clinical course after a substantial ingestion. However, immediate-release preparations are rapidly absorbed and typically produce emesis, obviating the role of lavage, and sustained-release formulations of lithium are often compounded in such a way that makes them too large to fit through even the largest pores in lavage tubes. Sodium polystyrene sulfonate (SPS) is a cationic exchange resin often used for the treatment of severe hyperkalemia. Although limited benefits are noted in animal models that are supported by a few human cases, concerns over hypokalemia, salt and water depletion, and other complications of SPS persist. We therefore recommend against the routine use of SPS in the management of acutely lithium-poisoned patients. There may be some utility in patients with chronic toxicity, especially if hemodialysis was indicated but not feasible. Newer potassium binders do not adsorb lithium.

Whole-bowel irrigation (WBI) is the only GI decontamination that has some demonstrated efficacy in eliminating lithium from volunteers. Whole-bowel irrigation is recommended for patients manifesting significant toxicity (ie, neurologic dysfunction) and who have ingested sustained-release lithium preparations and have no contraindications (eg, protected airway, no obstruction or ileus) (Antidotes in Brief: A2).

### Fluid and Electrolytes

The critical initial management of the lithium-poisoned patient should focus on restoration of intravascular volume. Many patients with lithium toxicity have volume-responsive decreases in kidney function, which we recommend managing with an infusion of 0.9% sodium chloride solution at 1.5 to 2 times the maintenance rate. This therapy increases renal perfusion, and glomerular filtration rate, which will increase lithium elimination. When the kidney is sodium avid (as in volume depletion), it will retain lithium. Urine output must be closely monitored, and any electrolyte abnormalities corrected. Caution must be used in patients with prerenal acute kidney injury, chronic kidney disease, and congestive heart failure.

Lithium-induced NDI is sometimes reversed by discontinuation of the drug and repletion of electrolytes and water, although it may be permanent. Use of amiloride, as well as acetazolamide, to mitigate lithium-induced polyuria is described, although the potential for volume contraction and stimulation of lithium reabsorption prevents recommendation of these drugs as routine adjuncts to acute care.

We recommend against any attempt to enhance elimination of lithium by forced diuresis using loop diuretics (furosemide), osmotic agents (mannitol), carbonic anhydrase inhibitors (acetazolamide), or phosphodiesterase inhibitors (aminophylline). An initial small increase in elimination may be achieved, but typically salt and water depletion subsequently develop followed by increased lithium retention. We also recommend against sodium bicarbonate administration for urinary alkalinization because it does not significantly increase elimination over volume expansion with sodium chloride and may lead to hypokalemia, alkalemia, and fluid overload.

### Extracorporeal Drug Removal

Lithium has pharmacokinetic properties that make it amenable to extracorporeal removal, and with these characteristics, it would seem to be an ideal candidate for hemodialysis. In fact, hemodialysis is often recommended for treatment of lithium toxicity. The Extracorporeal Treatments in Poisoning Workgroup (ExTRIP) consensus recommendations are adapted and shown in Table 43–1. Intermittent hemodialysis (IHD) provides clearance rates between 50 and 170 mL/min depending on blood flow. Although continuous renal replacement therapies offer lower clearance per hour than does IHD, their overall daily clearances are similar. After an initial session of IHD, a second session or more are recommended until serum lithium concentrations fall consistently below 1.0 mEq/L; clinical improvement is apparent; or as per the ExTrip consensus, after a minimum of 6 hours of therapy when a concentration is not readily available. Continuous modalities are acceptable following the initial IHD session.

**TABLE 43–1 Consensus Recommendations for Hemodialysis**[a]

| *Strength of Recommendation* | *Concentration* | *Or Clinical Features* |
|---|---|---|
| Recommended | > 4.0 mEq/L with ↓GFR | Decreased level of consciousness, seizures, or life-threatening dysrhythmias |
| Reasonable | > 5.0 mEq/L | Confusion or [$Li^+$] not expected to fall to < 1.0 mEq/L with optimal management in 36 h |

[a]↓ GFR = glomerular filtration rate < 60 mL/min.

Data from Decker BS, Goldfarb DS, Dargan PI, et al. Extracorporeal treatment for lithium poisoning: systematic review and recommendations from the EXTRIP Workgroup. *Clin J Am Soc Nephrol*. 2015;10(5):875-887.

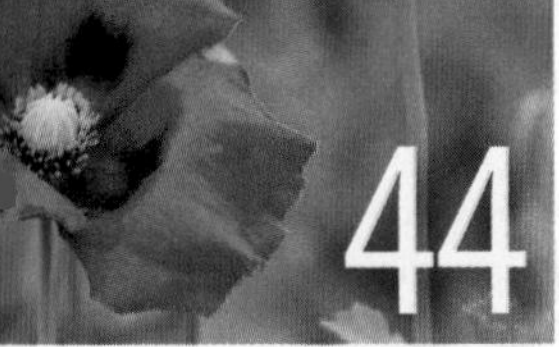

# 44 MONOAMINE OXIDASE INHIBITORS

## HISTORY AND EPIDEMIOLOGY

Monoamine oxidase (MAO) was discovered in 1928 and named when the enzyme was recognized to metabolize primary, secondary, and tertiary amines such as tyramine and norepinephrine. Subsequently, the "monoamine hypothesis" postulated depression as a condition of monoamine deficiency, and MAO inhibitors (MAOIs) targeted monoamine metabolism for therapeutic benefit. In the early 1950s, iproniazid, a drug previously used to treat tuberculosis, was found to produce favorable behavioral effects. By the mid-1950s, it was demonstrated that iproniazid inhibited MAO, and it then became the first antidepressant used clinically.

Many authors recommend the prescription of nonselective MAOIs only for resistant or atypical depression with prominent neurovegetative symptoms. However, selective and reversible MAOIs are the subject of renewed clinical applicability. Monoamine oxidase-B–selective xenobiotics, such as selegiline, are widely used for the treatment of Parkinson disease. Reversible inhibitors of MAO, such as moclobemide, are used in Europe for depression, phobias, anxiety, and other select indications.

## PHARMACOLOGY

### Chemistry

Monoamines, also known as biogenic amines, include the catecholamines (epinephrine, norepinephrine, dopamine, tyrosine), indolamines (serotonin, melatonin), and some naturally occurring amines (eg, tyramine, benzylamine). They share the presence of a single amine group and the ability to be metabolized by MAO. Deamination by MAO is one of two major routes of elimination of monoamines, with the other being extracellular degradation by catechol-*O*-methyltransferase (COMT). Serotonin and tyramine, which are not metabolized by COMT, are the exceptions to this rule.

### Monoamine Neurotransmitter Stores

Monoamine neurotransmitter synthesis, vesicle transport, vesicle storage, uptake, and degradation are described in Figure 44–1 using norepinephrine as an example. In the neuron, MAO functions as a "safety valve" to metabolize and inactivate excess monoamine neurotransmitter molecules.

### Monoamine Oxidase Isoforms

There are two MAO isoforms, each with its own substrate and inhibitor specificity (Table 44–1).

### Mechanism of Action

Monoamine oxidase inhibitors are transported into the neuron by the $Na^+$-dependent membrane norepinephrine-reuptake transporter. Inhibition of MAO prevents presynaptic degradation of monoamines, thus increasing the concentration of monoamine neurotransmitters available for synaptic storage and subsequent release (Fig. 44–1). Inhibition of MAO also results in indirect release of norepinephrine into the synapse via displacement from presynaptic vesicles in a manner like amphetamines (Chap. 46). The enzymatic inhibition produced by MAOIs precedes the clinical antidepressant effects by as long as 2 weeks. This finding, which is similar to other antidepressants, most likely relates to the relatively slow downregulation of postsynaptic central nervous system (CNS) serotonin receptors.

In overdose, MAOIs also impair norepinephrine synthesis and deplete norepinephrine stores by inhibiting dopamine-β-hydroxylase. Additionally, indirect dopamine agonism occurs via elevated synaptic concentrations of dopamine. Dopamine agonism results in β-adrenergic stimulation, peripheral vasodilation, and direct α-adrenergic stimulation at high doses.

### First-Generation Monoamine Oxidase Inhibitors: Nonselective and Irreversible

Monoamine oxidase inhibitors are a chemically heterogeneous group of xenobiotics (Fig. 44–2). First-generation MAOIs (ie, irreversible and nonselective) in clinical use worldwide include the hydrazide derivatives (phenelzine, isocarboxazid) and an amphetamine derivative (tranylcypromine). First-generation MAOIs bind covalently to MAO and irreversibly inhibit the function of the enzyme. Thus, patients taking these MAOIs are depleted of the enzyme until new MAO is synthesized, a process that typically takes up to 3 weeks. Patients taking first-generation MAOIs remain at risk for food and xenobiotic interactions during much of this period and must be placed on a restrictive diet to prevent adverse events resulting from the absorption of undigested tyramine from the gut. Many other enzyme systems are inhibited by first-generation MAOIs. The clinical implications of inhibiting these diverse enzyme systems, other than alcohol dehydrogenase and cytochrome P450 enzymes, are poorly understood.

**TABLE 44–1 Monoamine Oxidase (MAO) Isoforms: Substrate Affinities and Localization**

| | *MAO Isoforms* | |
|---|---|---|
| | *MAO-A* | *MAO-B* |
| ***Substrate Affinity*** | | |
| Dopamine | Moderate | Moderate |
| Epinephrine | Moderate | Moderate |
| Norepinephrine | High | Low |
| Serotonin | High | Low |
| Tyramine | Moderate | Moderate |
| ***Localization*** | | |
| Brain | Low | High |
| Intestine | Moderate | Low |
| Liver | Moderate | Moderate |
| Placenta | High | Absent |
| Platelets | Absent | High |

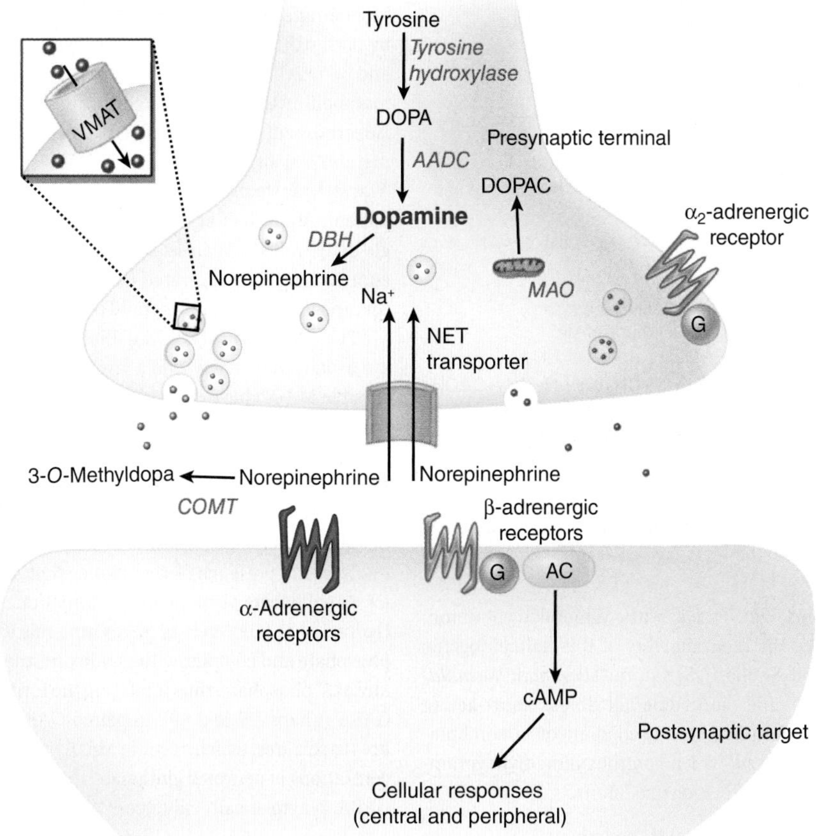


**FIGURE 44–1.** Sympathetic nerve terminal. Dopamine is synthesized in the sympathetic nerve cell and transported into vesicles, where it is converted to norepinephrine (NE) and stored in vesicles (⁘). An action potential causes the vesicles to migrate to and fuse with the presynaptic membrane. Norepinephrine diffuses across the synaptic cleft and binds with and activates postsynaptic α- and β-adrenergic receptors. Neuronal NE reuptake occurs via the monoamine transporter. Norepinephrine is transported back into vesicles by the vesicular monoamine transporter (VMAT; inset) or metabolized to 3,4-dihydroxyphenyl acetic acid (DOPAC) by mitochondrial monoamine oxidase (MAO). Norepinephrine that diffuses away from the synaptic cleft is inactivated by catechol-*O*-methyltransferase (COMT). AADC = aromatic L-amino acid decarboxylase; cAMP = cyclic adenosine monophosphate; DBH = dopamine β-hydroxylase; NET = membrane NE reuptake transporter.

### Second-Generation Monoamine Oxidase Inhibitors: Selective and Irreversible

Selective MAOIs preferentially inhibit one of the two MAO isoforms, although isoform selectivity is dose dependent.

***MAO-A Inhibitors.*** Clorgyline is an MAO-A inhibitor once thought to be useful for treatment of depression, but it has not found widespread use in psychiatry because of disappointing results from clinical trials.

***MAO-B Inhibitors.*** Selegiline and rasagiline are selective MAO-B inhibitors that are United States (US) Food and Drug Administration approved for the treatment of Parkinson disease.

### Third-Generation Monoamine Oxidase Inhibitors: Selective and Reversible

Reversible inhibitors of monoamine oxidase-A (RIMAs), such as moclobemide, selectively and reversibly inhibit MAO-A and were developed to compensate for the limitations of first- and second-generation MAOIs.

### Naturally Occurring Monoamine Oxidase Inhibitors

The extract of the plant St. John's wort (*Hypericum perforatum*) has weak MAOI activity. While it is uncertain whether this activity is responsible for its antidepressant effect, sporadic reports of hypertensive crises, cardiovascular collapse during anesthesia, and the development of serotonin toxicity are associated with use of St. John's wort. Ayahuasca, a hallucinogenic beverage used by South American natives, is an ethnobotanical mixture of dimethyltryptamine and harmala alkaloids that circumvents gastrointestinal (GI) MAO. Dimethyltryptamine, which is a potent hallucinogen, is derived from several local plant species but is not normally orally bioavailable because of its first-pass metabolism by MAO. When *Banisteriopsis caapi*, a plant containing the MAO-inhibiting

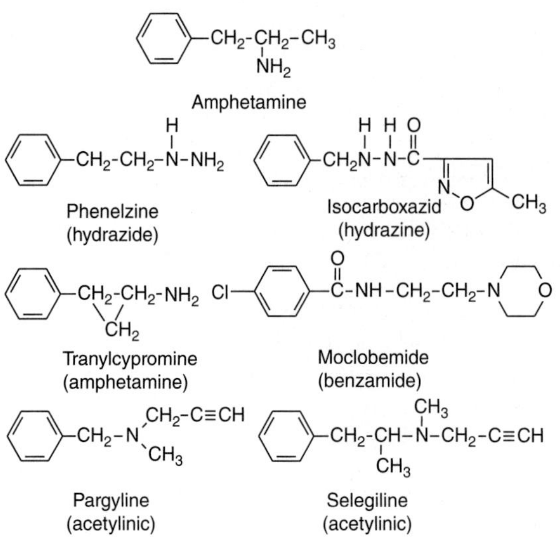

Amphetamine

Phenelzine (hydrazide)

Isocarboxazid (hydrazine)

Tranylcypromine (amphetamine)

Moclobemide (benzamide)

Pargyline (acetylinic)

Selegiline (acetylinic)

**FIGURE 44–2.** Structural similarities between amphetamine and the monoamine oxidase inhibitors (MAOIs). The words in parentheses are the chemical classes of the MAOI.

harmala alkaloids, is mixed with dimethyltryptamine-containing plants, the bioavailability of this hallucinogenic amine is increased. Similarly, Syrian rue (*Peganum harmala*) contains harmine and harmaline alkaloids, short-acting inhibitors of MAO-A. It has been used alone or in combination with *Acacia confusa*, which contains dimethyltryptamine (DMT) for similar hallucinogenic intent.

### Miscellaneous and Experimental Monoamine Oxidase Inhibitors

Other xenobiotics with nonselective MAO inhibitory properties are used for purposes unrelated to MAO inhibition. Some of these xenobiotics include furazolidone (an antiprotozoal), procarbazine (a chemotherapeutic), linezolid (an antibiotic), and azure B (a metabolite of methylene blue).

## PHARMACOKINETICS AND TOXICOKINETICS

Monoamine oxidase inhibitors are well absorbed orally, and peak plasma concentrations are reached within 2 to 3 hours. Similar to other antidepressants, these xenobiotics are lipophilic and readily cross the blood–brain barrier. Monoamine oxidase inhibitors are hepatically metabolized by both oxidation (various CYP enzymes, including CYP2D6 and CYP2C19) and acetylation (*N*-acetyltransferase), to metabolites that are excreted in the urine. Phenelzine and isocarboxazid are metabolized to hydrazides. The rate of metabolism of the hydrazide MAOIs is dependent on the *N*-acetyltransferase phenotype (ie, "acetylator status") of the patient. About half of the US population has a recessive single gene trait that causes slow acetylator status in the liver, contributing to exaggerated clinical effects despite standard therapeutic dosing or even mild overdose.

The clinical effects of MAOI inhibition occur rapidly and are usually maximal within a few days. First-generation, irreversible MAOIs have durations of effect that far surpass their pharmacologic half-lives, as discussed earlier.

## PATHOPHYSIOLOGY

MAOIs cause release of norepinephrine from sympathetic nerve terminals leading to a hyperadrenergic crises particularly in the presence of xenobiotics that serve as substrates for, or enhancers of, monoamine formation, such as tyramine. Hydrazide MAOIs such as phenelzine inactivate pyridoxal 5′ phosphate and complex with pyridoxine, the precursor of pyridoxal 5′ phosphate, thus inhibiting the formation of neuronal GABA (Chaps. 29 and 90). Impaired $GABA_A$ activity contributes to seizures, which occur in MAOI overdose. Elevated concentrations of neuronal glutamate, the excitatory precursor of GABA, synergistically enhances CNS excitation.

## ADVERSE EFFECTS

### Overdose

Toxic dose–response relationships in humans are unclear, but an overdose of 5 mg/kg of a first-generation MAOI is potentially life threatening. Patients with MAOI overdose are initially asymptomatic for several hours. Although clinical toxicity should generally be apparent within the first several hours (initially with neuromuscular and sympathetic effects), maximal toxicity is reportedly delayed up to 24 hours after overdose. Clinical manifestations of MAOI overdose are summarized in Table 44–2. Classically, the clinical course involves

**TABLE 44–2 Comparison of the Clinical Manifestations of Monoamine Oxidase Inhibitor (MAOI) Toxicity**

| *Clinical Category* | *Hyperadrenergic Crisis* | *Serotonin Toxicity* | *MAOI Overdose* |
|---|---|---|---|
| Onset | Minutes to hours | Minutes to hours | ≤ 24 h |
| Duration | Hours | Hours | Days |
| Temperature | Normal | Elevated | Elevated |
| Neurologic | Headache, hemorrhagic stroke, neuromuscular excitation | Akathisia, hyperreflexia, shivering, tremor, seizures, autonomic instability, coma<br>Myoclonus, "wet dog shakes," muscular rigidity | Neuropsychiatric effects, neuromuscular effects, headache, seizures<br>Myoclonus, muscular rigidity |
| Cardiovascular | Hypertension, dysrhythmias, myocardial injury | Hypertension, hypotension, tachycardia, palpitations, dysrhythmias | Hypertension (early), hypotension (late), tachycardia, palpitations, dysrhythmias, myocardial injury |
| Gastrointestinal | Nausea | Hyperactive bowel sounds | Nausea, vomiting, diarrhea |
| Dermatologic | Flushing, diaphoresis | Diaphoresis | Flushing, piloerection, diaphoresis |
| Ophthalmologic | Mydriasis | Mydriasis | Mydriasis, ocular clonus |

a biphasic response characterized by initial CNS excitation and peripheral sympathetic stimulation that terminates in coma and cardiovascular collapse. In addition to the effects mentioned above and listed in Table 44–2, reported complications of MAOI overdose include acute kidney injury, fetal demise, and hemolysis.

### Selegiline Overdose

Selegiline is metabolized to L-methamphetamine, which results in hypertension and tachycardia, even at therapeutic doses. Selegiline overdose produces hallucinations and convulsions and is associated with elevated urinary concentrations of L-methamphetamine and L-amphetamine.

### Moclobemide Overdose

Moclobemide overdose typically produces mild to moderate CNS depression (drowsiness, disorientation), GI effects (nausea), and cardiovascular effects (tachycardia and hypertension). Serotonin toxicity caused by the ingestion of moclobemide, alone and in combination with other serotonergics, is well described. In massive overdose, fatalities attributed solely to the toxic effects of moclobemide are reported.

### Hyperadrenergic Crisis

Hyperadrenergic crisis occurs in patients with MAO-A inhibition in the setting of exposure to other sympathomimetic drugs such as cocaine, epinephrine, or amphetamines or when tyramine-containing foods such as aged cheeses and fermented drinks are consumed (Table 44–3). Tyramine is an indirect-acting sympathomimetic amine with an amphetamine-like mechanism of action. The MAO-A present in the intestinal wall and liver extensively metabolizes dietary amines, preventing them from entering the circulation, but in the presence of irreversible MAO-A inhibition, this protective mechanism is lost, allowing tyramine and other dietary monoamines to enter the circulation.

### Serotonin Toxicity

Any xenobiotic with serotonin-potentiating activity can interact with the MAOIs to produce serotonin toxicity (Chap. 42). Serotonin toxicity most commonly occurs in patients receiving combination therapy with two or more serotonergic xenobiotics; however, it rarely occurs with usage of one serotonergic xenobiotic such as venlafaxine. Several diagnostic schemes for serotonin toxicity exist. However, the key diagnostic criterion is exposure to a serotonergic. Because no diagnostic test is yet available, the diagnosis of serotonin toxicity must be established on clinical grounds. Key clinical features of MAOI-induced serotonin toxicity are summarized in Table 44–2.

### Other Adverse Drug Reactions

Chronic use of phenelzine is also associated with an isoniazid-like peripheral neuropathy. Administration of opioids with serotonergic properties (eg, meperidine, dextromethorphan) is absolutely contraindicated because of the risk of precipitating the serotonin toxicity. Adverse drug reactions are expected with other coadministered drugs that are metabolized by cytochrome P450 enzymes because first-generation MAOIs have an extensive inhibitory effect on CYP2C9, CYP2C19, and CYP2D6. Thus, prolonged sedation and respiratory depression are reported when barbiturates (eg, phenobarbital) and benzodiazepines (eg, diazepam, lorazepam), which are both metabolized by hepatic cytochrome P450 enzymes, are coadministered. Table 44–4 summarizes analgesic safety in combination with MAOI drugs.

### Drug Discontinuation Syndrome

Monamine oxidase inhibitor drug discontinuation syndrome typically begins 24 to 72 hours after discontinuation. Classically, sudden discontinuation of MAOI produces symptoms that range from nausea, vomiting, and malaise to CNS symptoms such as agitation, psychosis, and seizures. Treatment is generally supportive and typically involves a benzodiazepine such as diazepam or lorazepam and restarting the medication if clinically indicated.

**TABLE 44–3 Dietary Restrictions for Patients Taking Monoamine Oxidase Inhibitors[a]**

| *Low Tyramine Content (0–4 mg/serving)* | *Moderate Tyramine Content (4–8 mg/serving)* | *High Tyramine Content (> 8 mg/serving)* |
|---|---|---|
| Chocolate | Avocado or guacamole | Aged, mature cheeses |
| Cottage cheese, cream cheese, yogurt, sour cream | Banana peels or stewed whole bananas | Broad beans or fava beans |
| Distilled alcohol | Meat extracts | Fermented sausage |
| Non-overripe fruit | Overripe fruit or figs | Liver |
| Soy sauce | Pasteurized light and pale beers | Red wines, selected beers |
| | | Smoked, pickled, aged, putrefying meats or fish, caviar |
| | | Yeast and meat extracts |

[a]Recommendation: Foods with high tyramine content should be avoided; those with moderate content should be consumed in restricted moderation; and those with low content can be cautiously consumed.

**TABLE 44–4 Analgesics/Anesthetics/Sedatives Safety When Combined With Monoamine Oxidase Inhibitors (MAOIs)**

| *Analgesic Class* | *Safe* | *Monitor Closely or Use Alternative if Medically Appropriate* | *Avoid Combination (Contraindicated)* |
|---|---|---|---|
| Nonprescription | Acetaminophen<br>Aspirin<br>Nonsteroidal antiinflammatory drugs | | Dextromethorphan |
| Opioids | Buprenorphine<br>Codeine<br>Morphine<br>Oxycodone | Propoxyphene | Meperidine<br>Pentazocine<br>Tramadol<br>Tapentadol |
| Nonopioids | Inhalational anesthetics<br>Nitroglycerin | Barbiturates[a]<br>Benzodiazepines[a]<br>Ketamine | |
| Local anesthetics | Lidocaine | | Cocaine |

[a]Drugs metabolized by hepatic cytochrome P450 may produce prolonged sedation and respiratory depression when combined with MAOIs.

## DIAGNOSTIC TESTING

Assessment of MAO activity is not routinely available, requires a fresh specimen (preferably jejunal biopsy), and is therefore not recommended. Evaluation of MAOI toxicity remains a clinical diagnosis. Serum concentrations of MAOIs that correlate meaningfully with clinical effects are not well established.

## MANAGEMENT

### Out of Hospital

All patients with MAOI ingestions who display suicidal intent should be referred to an emergency department (ED) for evaluation. Children with exposure to even one adult formulation MAOI tablet or selegiline patch should be referred to the ED because of the potential for late-onset significant toxicity. Patients who exhibit more than mild headache or minimal diaphoresis after an acute therapeutic error involving MAOI ingestion should be referred to an ED. Observation at home is warranted in patients who are asymptomatic and more than 24 hours have elapsed since the time of ingestion. Because of the paucity of data at this time, patients with selegiline patch ingestion should be referred to the ED for observation, even if suicidal intent is absent.

### Initial Approach in the Emergency Department

The initial evaluation must include rapid assessment and stabilization of the airway, breathing, and circulation as well as establishment of IV access, supplemental oxygen, and continuous cardiac monitoring. Hyperthermia or hemodynamic instability after MAOI ingestion is a manifestation of significant toxicity. Intravenous volume repletion should begin while focusing on stabilization of hyperthermia, seizures, and muscular rigidity. In any patient with altered mental status who will likely deteriorate, early endotracheal intubation not only protects the airway but also facilitates safe gastric decontamination measures.

### Gastrointestinal Decontamination

Orogastric lavage with a large-bore orogastric tube (36–40 Fr) is recommended if a life-threatening ingestion is suspected to have occurred within several hours before presentation. Single-dose activated charcoal is recommended orally (or via nasogastric tube) for patients who present within several hours of ingestion unless contraindications are present. The lack of early clinical findings of poisoning should not dissuade the use of GI decontamination given the potential for delayed clinical deterioration.

### Cooling Measures

Severe hyperthermia must be treated with rapid cooling. Ice baths (first choice for life-threatening hyperthermia), cold water, and fans are the mainstays of treatment. Indications for ice bath immersion to treat MAOI toxicity include a rectal temperature greater than 106°F (41.1°C), rigidity, and altered mental status. Benzodiazepines help to control muscular rigidity, seizures, and agitation and to contribute to amelioration of hyperthermia and tachycardia. Patients with refractory hyperthermia despite the above measures require nondepolarizing neuromuscular blockade in conjunction with endotracheal intubation and ventilation.

### Blood Pressure Control

Because there is characteristic fluctuation in vital signs associated with MAOI overdose, hemodynamic monitoring should be instituted even for patients who initially are stable. When supporting the patient's blood pressure, preference should be given to titratable drugs with a rapid onset and termination of action because of the potential for rapid hemodynamic changes. Use of β-adrenergic antagonists is contraindicated for control of hypertension in MAOI-related toxicity because the action of monoamines (eg, norepinephrine) at the neuronal synapse in the autonomic nervous system could result in refractory hypertension caused by unopposed α-adrenergic agonism. Patients who are normotensive at baseline and who experience MAOI-related severe hypertension can be preferably treated with phentolamine for effective control (2–5 mg IV). Alternatively, nicardipine or nitroglycerin allow for titratable blood pressure control. Tyramine-related mild hypertensive crises can theoretically be controlled with the dihydropyridine calcium channel blockers such as nifedipine and possibly the oral α-adrenergic antagonists such as terazosin but should be used with caution.

Patients who are hypotensive require support with IV fluid resuscitation and vasopressors. The direct-acting sympathetic vasopressors epinephrine and norepinephrine can be used safely in patients taking MAOIs. Rather than causing release of a stored pool of norepinephrine, they bind directly with postsynaptic α- and β-adrenergic receptors, unlike dopamine. Dopamine is contraindicated in hypotensive patients who have overdosed on MAOIs.

### Dysrhythmias

Patients with immediately life-threatening dysrhythmias require rapid cardioversion. In the presence of the nonperfusing dysrhythmias such as ventricular fibrillation, pulseless ventricular tachycardia, and torsade de pointes, unsynchronized electrical defibrillation is the treatment of choice. In patients with stable ventricular tachycardia, a trial of an antidysrhythmic such as procainamide or amiodarone is recommended. High-quality studies evaluating the use of these xenobiotics in the setting of MAOI overdose are not available.

Hemodynamically significant supraventricular tachycardia from MAOI toxicity should be corrected to prevent myocardial ischemia or infarction, ventricular dysrhythmia, and high-output heart failure. Benzodiazepines are safe and effective to treat sinus tachycardia as long as respiratory status remains monitored. Adenosine and synchronized cardioversion are unlikely to be useful in the setting of ongoing presence of the MAOI, but are reasonable in rare cases that are unresponsive to benzodiazepines.

Hemodynamically significant bradycardia from MAOI toxicity includes management of IV fluid and atropine as first-line therapy to temporize the patient with bradycardia and hypotension. Epinephrine and isoproterenol are recommended second choices while a pacemaker (transcutaneous or transvenous) is prepared.

### Management of Central Nervous System Manifestations

In any patient with acute altered mental status, hypoglycemia should be rapidly excluded. For patients with mild to moderate

CNS excitation, small incremental doses of parenteral (eg, diazepam, lorazepam, or midazolam) are recommended. Patients with seizures should be treated with benzodiazepines in standard incremental doses. Empiric administration of pyridoxine (vitamin $B_6$), intravenously at 70 mg/kg, up to 5 g in adults, is reasonable in patients with status epilepticus, particularly after massive ingestions of hydrazide-derived MAOIs such as phenelzine because of its ability to deplete endogenous pyridoxine stores (Antidotes in Brief: A15).

### Cyproheptadine

Cyproheptadine is a nonselective serotonin antagonist (with additional anticholinergic, and antihistaminic activity) that is recommended as third-line therapy (after benzodiazepine administration and cooling measures) for serotonin toxicity. It is suggested when the diagnosis of serotonin toxicity is likely, especially if incomplete response has been achieved with cooling and benzodiazepine therapy. The recommended initial dose in adults is 12 mg orally followed by 2 mg every 2 hours while symptoms continue.

### Dantrolene

Use of dantrolene in patients with serotonin toxicity is not recommended as it is neither needed nor effective (Antidotes in Brief: A24).

### Extracorporeal Elimination

Extracorporeal elimination is not recommended in the management of MAOI overdose unless other indications are present such as severe acidemia or life-threatening hyperkalemia or the need to eliminate dialyzable toxic coingestions.

### Disposition

For patients with presumed MAOI (selective or nonselective) overdose, it is reasonable to observe them with telemetry monitoring, preferably in an intensive care unit, for at least 24 hours regardless of the initial clinical findings. However, patients with MAOI–food or MAOI–xenobiotic interactions often do not require hospital admission if the interaction is mild and resolution of symptoms is complete.

# 45 SEDATIVE–HYPNOTICS

## HISTORY AND EPIDEMIOLOGY

*Sedative–hypnotics* are xenobiotics that limit excitability (sedation) or induce drowsiness and sleep (hypnosis). *Anxiolytics* (formerly known as *minor tranquilizers*) are medications prescribed for their sedative–hypnotic properties. Mythology of ancient cultures is replete with stories of xenobiotics that cause sleep or unconsciousness. Sedative–hypnotic overdoses were described in the medical literature soon after the commercial introduction of bromide preparations in 1853. Barbiturates were introduced in 1903 and quickly supplanted older xenobiotics. After their introduction in the early 1960s, benzodiazepines quickly became the most commonly used sedatives in the United States (US). Although the benzodiazepines remain the most popular prescribed anxiolytics, several benzodiazepine-receptor agonists were developed in 1989 in an attempt to circumvent some of the side effects of benzodiazepines. These drugs include zolpidem, zaleplon, zopiclone, and eszopiclone. Ramelteon and tasimelteon are newer sleep aids that function as melatonin receptor ($MT_1$ and $MT_2$) agonists.

This chapter focuses primarily on pharmaceuticals prescribed for their sedative–hypnotic effects, many of which interact with the $\gamma$-aminobutyric acid-A ($GABA_A$) receptor. Specific sedative–hypnotics such as ethanol and $\gamma$-hydroxybutyric acid (GHB) are discussed in more depth in their respective chapters (Chaps. 49 and 53).

## PHARMACODYNAMICS AND TOXICODYNAMICS

Most clinically effective sedative–hypnotics produce their physiologic effects by enhancing the function of GABA-mediated chloride channels via agonism at the $GABA_A$ receptor. These receptors are the primary mediators of inhibitory neurotransmission in the brain. The $GABA_A$ receptor is a pentameric structure composed of varying polypeptide subunits associated with a chloride on the postsynaptic membrane. Almost all sedative–hypnotics bind to $GABA_A$ receptors containing the $\alpha_1$ subunit. One exception may be etomidate, which produces sedation at the $\beta_2$ unit and anesthesia at the $\beta_3$ subunit. Benzodiazepines are effective only at $GABA_A$ receptors that also have a $\gamma_2$ subunit. The $\alpha_1$ subunit is responsible for sedation, antiepileptic activity, and amnesia, the $\alpha_2$ subunit is responsible for anxiolysis, and the $\alpha_4$ and $\alpha_6$ subunits are completely insensitive to benzodiazepines. Nonbenzodiazepine sedative–hypnotics such as zolpidem, zaleplon, and zopiclone selectively bind the $\alpha_1$ subunit and thus cause primarily sedation and not anxiolysis at therapeutic doses.

Many sedative–hypnotics also act at receptors other than the $GABA_A$ receptor. Trichloroethanol and propofol also inhibit glutamate-mediated *N*-methyl-D-aspartate (NMDA) receptors. The anxiolytic effects of clonazepam are partially explained by upregulation of serotonergic receptors. Sleep aids such as melatonin, ramelteon, and tasimelteon are agonists at melatonin receptor subtypes $MT_1$ and $MT_2$ in the suprachiasmatic nucleus of the brain. Dexmedetomidine is a central $\alpha_2$-adrenergic agonist similar to clonidine (Chap. 34).

## PHARMACOKINETICS AND TOXICOKINETICS

Most orally administered sedative–hypnotics are rapidly absorbed via the gastrointestinal (GI) tract, with the rate-limiting step consisting of dissolution and dispersion of the xenobiotic. Clinical effects are determined by their relative ability to penetrate the blood–brain barrier. Xenobiotics that are highly lipophilic penetrate most rapidly. Table 45–1 lists individual sedative–hypnotics and some of their pharmacokinetic properties. After initial distribution, many of the sedative–hypnotics undergo a redistribution phase as they are dispersed to other body tissues, specifically adipose tissue. Xenobiotics that are extensively redistributed, such as the lipophilic barbiturates, have a brief clinical effect as the early peak concentrations in the brain rapidly decline.

Many of the sedative–hypnotics are metabolized to pharmacologically active intermediates (Table 45–1). Most sedative–hypnotics are highly protein bound and therefore poorly filtered by the kidneys. Elimination occurs principally by hepatic metabolism. Chloral hydrate and meprobamate are notable exceptions.

Pharmacodynamic synergy is expected when multiple sedatives act on different receptors. Pharmacokinetic synergy occurs via alteration of metabolism. The combination of ethanol and chloral hydrate, historically known as a "Mickey Finn," has synergistic central nervous system (CNS) depressant effects. Chloral hydrate competes for alcohol and aldehyde dehydrogenases, thereby prolonging the half-life of ethanol. The metabolism of ethanol generates the reduced form of nicotinamide adenine dinucleotide (NADH), which is a cofactor for the metabolism of choral hydrate to trichloroethanol, an active metabolite. Finally, ethanol inhibits the conjugation of trichloroethanol, which in turn inhibits the oxidation of ethanol (Fig. 45–1).

## TOLERANCE AND WITHDRAWAL

*Tolerance,* defined as the progressive diminution of effect of a particular drug with repeated administrations that results in a need for greater doses to achieve the same effect, is common within this class. Tolerance occurs by multiple changes in receptors, receptor coupling, or altered metabolism. Cross-tolerance readily develops among the sedative–hypnotics. For example, chronic use of benzodiazepines decreases the binding affinity of barbiturates on the $GABA_A$ channel. Many sedative–hypnotics are also associated with drug dependence after chronic exposure. The barbiturates, benzodiazepines, and ethanol are also associated with life-threatening withdrawal syndromes.

**TABLE 45–1 Sedative–Hypnotics: Duration of Action and Active Metabolites**

| | Duration of Action[a] | Active Metabolite Important |
|---|---|---|
| ***Benzodiazepines*** | | |
| Alprazolam | S | No |
| Chlordiazepoxide | I | Yes |
| Clonazepam | L | Yes |
| Clorazepate | L | Yes |
| Diazepam | Single dose: S<br>Multiple doses: L | Yes |
| Estazolam | I | No |
| Flunitrazepam | L | Yes |
| Flurazepam | L | Yes |
| Lorazepam | I | No |
| Midazolam | S | Yes |
| Oxazepam | I | No |
| Temazepam | I | No |
| Triazolam | S | No |
| Eszopiclone | S | No |
| Zaleplon | S | No |
| Zolpidem | S | No |
| ***Barbiturates*** | | |
| Amobarbital | I | Yes |
| Butabarbital | I | Unknown |
| Mephobarbital | S | Yes |
| Methohexital | S | No |
| Pentobarbital | Single dose: S<br>Multiple doses: I | No |
| Phenobarbital | L | No |
| Primidone | I | Yes |
| Secobarbital | I | Unknown |
| ***Other*** | | |
| Chloral hydrate | I | Yes |
| Dexmedetomidine | S | No |
| Etomidate | US | Unclear |
| Propofol | US | No |
| Ramelteon | S | Yes |
| Tasimelteon | S | No |
| Suvorexant | I | No |

[a]The duration of action usually approximates the half-life (t½); some lipophilic xenobiotics have a short duration of action with a single dose because of redistribution from the central nervous system but with multiple doses become longer acting.
I = intermediate acting t½ = 6–24 h; L = long acting t½ > 24 h (a long-acting metabolite may contribute to a long duration of action); S = short acting t½ < 6 h; US = ultrashort acting t½ < 1 h.

## CLINICAL MANIFESTATIONS

Patients with sedative–hypnotic overdoses develop slurred speech, ataxia, and incoordination. Larger doses result in stupor or coma. In most instances, respiratory depression parallels CNS depression. However, not all sedative–hypnotics cause significant hypoventilation. Although the physical examination is rarely specific for a particular sedative–hypnotic, it can sometimes offer clues of exposure based on certain physical and clinical findings (Table 45–2).

Large single doses or prolonged duration of IV dosing of sedative–hypnotics can also cause toxicities due to their

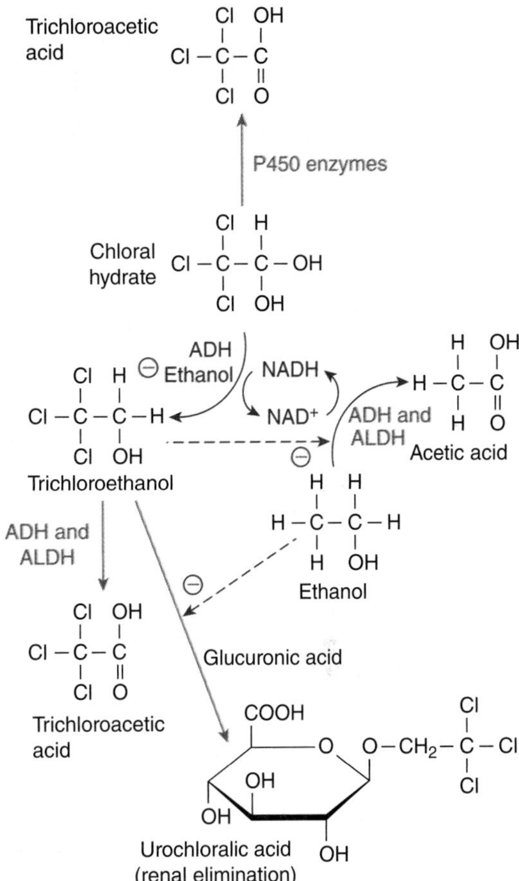


**FIGURE 45–1.** Metabolism of chloral hydrate and ethanol demonstrating the interactions between chloral hydrate and ethanol metabolism. Note the inhibitory effects (dotted lines) of ethanol on trichloroethanol metabolism and the converse. ADH = alcohol dehydrogenase; ALDH = aldehyde dehydrogenase; $NAD^+$ = nicotinamide adenine dinucleotide; NADH = nicotinamide adenine dinucleotide.

**TABLE 45–2 Clinical Findings of Sedative–Hypnotic Overdose**

| Clinical Signs | Sedative–Hypnotics |
|---|---|
| Acneiform rash | Bromides |
| Cardiotoxicity<br>Hypotension from myocardial depression<br>Dysrhythmias | <br>Meprobamate<br>Chloral hydrate |
| Coma (fluctuating) | Glutethimide, meprobamate |
| GI hemorrhage | Chloral hydrate |
| Hypothermia | Barbiturates, bromides, ethchlorvynol |
| Muscular twitching | γ-Hydroxybutyric acid, γ-butyrolactone, 1,4-butanediol, γ-valerolactone, propofol, etomidate |
| Odors (unique) | Chloral hydrate (pear), ethchlorvynol (new vinyl shower curtain) |
| Urine (discolored) | Propofol (green/pink) |

GI = gastrointestinal.

diluents. Propylene glycol accumulates with prolonged infusions of certain medications such as lorazepam. Rapid infusions of propylene glycol induce hypotension. Accumulated amounts of propylene glycol lead to metabolic acidosis and a hyperosmolar state with elevated lactate concentrations (Chap. 19).

## DIAGNOSTIC TESTING

When overdose is a primary concern in an undifferentiated comatose patient without a clear history, laboratory testing is useful to exclude comorbidities. This includes electrolytes, liver function tests, thyroid function tests, blood urea nitrogen, creatinine, glucose, venous blood gas analysis, and cerebrospinal fluid analysis as clinically indicated. With any suspected intentional overdose, a serum acetaminophen concentration should be obtained. Diagnostic imaging studies, such as neuroimaging of the head, are warranted on a case-by-case basis. Routine laboratory screening for "drugs of abuse" generally is not helpful in the management of undifferentiated comatose adult patients. Specific concentrations of xenobiotics such as ethanol or phenobarbital, although readily available at most hospitals, are rarely crucial in clinical decision making. Although immediate identification of a particular sedative–hypnotic may be helpful in predicting the duration of toxicity, it rarely affects the acute management of the patient. One exception is phenobarbital, for which urinary alkalinization and multiple-dose activated charcoal (MDAC) enhance elimination.

## MANAGEMENT

Death secondary to sedative–hypnotic overdose usually results from cardiorespiratory collapse. Careful attention should focus on monitoring and maintaining adequate airway, oxygenation, and hemodynamic support. Supplemental oxygen, respiratory support, and prevention of aspiration are the cornerstones of treatment. Hemodynamic instability should be treated initially with volume expansion. With proper supportive care and adequate airway and respiratory support as needed, patients with sedative–hypnotic overdoses should eventually recover. The cardiotoxic effects of chloral hydrate include lethal ventricular dysrhythmias caused by myocardial sensitization to catecholamines. In the setting of cardiac dysrhythmias from chloral hydrate, we recommend administering intravenous β-adrenergic antagonists.

The use of GI decontamination should be decided on a case-by-case basis. The benefits of activated charcoal (AC) must be balanced with the risks of its aspiration and subsequent potential for pulmonary toxicity. Phenobarbital overdose is one particular scenario in which MDAC increases elimination by 50% to 80%. Although the efficacy of orogastric lavage is controversial, orogastric lavage is reasonable in overdoses with xenobiotics that slow GI motility or that are known to develop concretions, specifically phenobarbital and meprobamate. Orogastric lavage in the setting of oral benzodiazepine overdoses alone is not recommended because the benefits of lavage are minimal compared with the significant risks of complications (Chap. 3).

Flumazenil, a competitive benzodiazepine antagonist, rapidly reverses the sedative effects of benzodiazepines as well as zolpidem and its congeners. However, flumazenil can precipitate life-threatening benzodiazepine withdrawal in benzodiazepine-dependent patients and should be used with caution (Antidotes in Brief: A25).

## SPECIFIC SEDATIVE–HYPNOTICS

### Barbiturates

Early deaths caused by barbiturate ingestions result from respiratory arrest and cardiovascular collapse. Delayed deaths result from acute kidney failure, pneumonia, acute respiratory distress syndrome, cerebral edema, and multiorgan system failure as a result of prolonged cardiorespiratory depression.

Oral barbiturates are preferentially absorbed in the small intestine and are eliminated by both hepatic and renal mechanisms. Shorter acting barbiturates tend to be more lipid soluble, more protein bound, have a higher pKa, and are metabolized almost completely by the liver. Longer acting barbiturates such as phenobarbital accumulate less extensively in tissues and are excreted renally as the parent drug. An example of this is phenobarbital, with a relatively low pKa (7.24). Alkalinizing the urine with sodium bicarbonate to a urinary pH of 7.5 to 8.0 can increase the elimination of phenobarbital by 5- to 10-fold. This procedure is not effective for the short-acting barbiturates because they have higher pKa values, are more protein bound, and are primarily metabolized by the liver with very little unchanged drug excreted by the kidneys (Antidotes in Brief: A5 and Chap. 4). Given the pharmacokinetic properties of barbiturates, the EXTRIP Workgroup recommends hemodialysis for cases of severe long-acting barbiturate poisoning presenting with prolonged coma, respiratory depression requiring mechanical ventilation, shock, persistent toxicity, or persistently elevated or rising serum concentrations despite MDAC. Intermittent hemodialysis and continuation of MDAC during dialysis are recommended.

### Benzodiazepines

Benzodiazepines bind to $GABA_A$ α and γ subunits. The binding of the benzodiazepine to its particular site changes the GABA receptor to "lock" into a position that promotes GABA binding to the GABA receptor. Whereas benzodiazepines that are active at the $\alpha_1$ subunit affect anxiety, sleep, and amnesia, those that are active in the $\alpha_2$ and $\alpha_3$ subunits tend to have greater anxiolytic properties. One unique property of the benzodiazepines is their relative safety even after substantial ingestion, which probably results from their GABA receptor properties. Unlike many other sedative–hypnotics, benzodiazepines do not open GABA channels independently at high concentrations.

Flumazenil is a competitive benzodiazepine receptor antagonist that is ideal for either benzodiazepine-naïve patients with a sole benzodiazepine overdose or benzodiazepine-naïve patients who develop respiratory depression after IV administration of benzodiazepines (Antidotes in Brief: A25). Caution should be exercised if flumazenil is administered to patients with an unknown overdose because seizures and dysrhythmias are reported to occur from the effects of the coingestant after the effect of the benzodiazepine has been reversed. Similarly, chronic benzodiazepine users are at risk of developing withdrawal symptoms, including seizures, after receiving flumazenil. The duration of effect of flumazenil is shorter than that of most benzodiazepines, and resedation can occur.

### Chloral Hydrate

Chloral hydrate belongs to one of the oldest classes of pharmaceutical hypnotics. Although still used sporadically in children, its use has substantially decreased. Chloral hydrate is well absorbed but is irritating to the GI tract. It has extensive tissue distribution, rapid onset of action, and rapid hepatic metabolism by alcohol and aldehyde dehydrogenases. Trichloroethanol is a lipid-soluble, active metabolite that is responsible for the hypnotic effects of chloral hydrate. It has a serum half-life of 4 to 12 hours.

Acute chloral hydrate poisoning is unique compared with that of other sedative–hypnotics because of the production of toxic metabolites. Cardiac dysrhythmias are the major cause of death. Chloral hydrate and its metabolites reduce myocardial contractility, shorten the refractory period, and increase myocardial sensitivity to catecholamines. Persistent cardiac dysrhythmias (ventricular fibrillation, ventricular tachycardia, torsade de pointes) are common terminal events. β-Adrenergic antagonists such as propranolol mitigate this myocardial sensitivity and are recommended in patients with chloral hydrate–induced dysrhythmias resistant to standard therapy.

In addition to cardiotoxicity, chloral hydrate toxicity causes vomiting, hemorrhagic gastritis, and rarely gastric and intestinal necrosis, leading to perforation and esophagitis with stricture formation. Although large ingestions of chloral hydrate are evident on abdominal radiographs because of its radiopacity, a normal radiograph should not be used to exclude chloral hydrate ingestion.

### Bromides

Bromides were used in the past as "nerve tonics," headache remedies, and anticonvulsants. Although medicinal bromides have largely disappeared from the US pharmaceutical market, bromide toxicity still occurs through the availability of bromide salts of common drugs, such as dextromethorphan hydrobromide, in large overdoses. Poisoning may also occur in immigrants and travelers from other countries where bromides are still therapeutically used.

Bromides tend to have long half-lives, and toxicity typically occurs over time as concentrations accumulate in tissue. The clinical manifestations of bromism include inappropriateness of behavior, headache, apathy, irritability, confusion, muscle weakness, anorexia, weight loss, thickened speech, psychotic behavior, tremulousness, ataxia, and eventually, coma. Delusions and hallucinations occur. Chronic use of bromides also produces dermatologic changes called bromoderma, with the hallmark characteristic of a facial acneiform rash. A spurious laboratory result of hyperchloremia with decreased or negative anion gap results from the interference of bromide with the chloride assay on some analyzers. Thus, an isolated elevated serum chloride concentration with neurologic symptoms should raise suspicion of possible bromide poisoning. Treatment with 0.9% sodium chloride (a source of chloride) and supportive care are all that is usually required, although in rare cases hemodialysis was performed.

### Carisoprodol and Meprobamate

Meprobamate was introduced in 1950 and was used for its muscle-relaxant and anxiolytic characteristics. Carisoprodol, which was introduced in 1955, is metabolized to meprobamate. Both drugs have pharmacologic effects on the $GABA_A$ receptor similar to those of the barbiturates. Similar to the barbiturates, meprobamate can directly open the GABA-mediated chloride channel and inhibits NMDA receptor currents. Of all the nonbarbiturate tranquilizers, meprobamate is most likely to produce euphoria; the exact mechanism of this is unknown. Unlike most sedative–hypnotics, meprobamate causes profound hypotension from direct myocardial depression. Adherent masses or bezoars of pills are reported in the stomach at autopsy after large meprobamate ingestions. Orogastric lavage with a large-bore tube and MDAC are reasonable for patients with a significant meprobamate ingestion while keeping in mind the risk of aspiration. Whole-bowel irrigation is also reasonable if multiple pills or small concretions are suspected. Patients can experience recurrent toxic manifestations as a result of concretion formation with delayed drug release and absorption. Careful monitoring of the clinical course is essential even after the patient shows initial improvement because recurrent and cyclical CNS depression can occur.

### Zolpidem, Zaleplon, Zopiclone, and Eszopiclone

These oral hypnotics have supplanted benzodiazepines as the most commonly prescribed sleep aid medications. Although they are structurally unrelated to the benzodiazepines, they bind preferentially to the benzodiazepine site $GABA_A$ $\alpha_1$ subunit. Therefore, they have potent hypnotic effects with less potential for dependence and antiepileptic properties.

In isolated overdoses, drowsiness and CNS depression are common. However, prolonged coma with respiratory depression is exceptionally rare. Zopiclone overdoses are rarely associated with methemoglobinemia. Flumazenil reverses the hypnotic and cognitive effects of these xenobiotics, and given the lack of antiepileptic effects of these xenobiotics, flumazenil reversal is safer than in the case of benzodiazepines (Antidotes in Brief: A25).

### Propofol

Propofol is a rapidly acting IV sedative–hypnotic that is both a postsynaptic $GABA_A$ agonist and induces presynaptic release of GABA. Propofol is also an antagonist at NMDA receptors. In addition, propofol interacts with dopamine, promotes nigral dopamine release possibly via $GABA_B$ receptors, and has partial agonist properties at dopamine ($D_2$) receptors. The onset of effect is usually less than 1 minute. The duration of action after short-term dosing is usually less than 8 minutes because of its rapid redistribution from the CNS.

Propofol use is associated with various adverse events. Acutely, propofol causes dose-related respiratory depression.

Propofol decreases systemic arterial pressure and causes myocardial depression. Prolonged propofol infusions, typically more than 48 hours at rates of 4 to 5 mg/kg/h or greater, are associated with a life-threatening propofol-infusion syndrome involving metabolic acidosis, cardiac dysrhythmias, and skeletal muscle injury. The clinical signs of propofol infusion syndrome often begin with the development of a new right bundle branch block and ST-segment convex elevations in the precordial leads of the electrocardiogram. Predisposing factors to the development include young age, severe brain injury, respiratory compromise, concurrent exogenous administration of catecholamines or glucocorticoids, inadequate carbohydrate intake, and undiagnosed mitochondrial myopathy.

Propofol disrupts mitochondrial free fatty acid utilization and metabolism, causing a syndrome of energy imbalance and myonecrosis similar to mitochondrial myopathies. Most case reports associate propofol with metabolic acidosis, elevated lactate concentration, and fatal myocardial failure in both children and young adults. However, this syndrome is also reported in older adults. Because treatment is largely supportive and outcomes are often poor, early identification and discontinuation of propofol at the first sign of toxicity are essential.

### Etomidate

Etomidate is a nonbarbiturate hypnotic primarily used for an anesthesia induction. It is active at the $GABA_A$ receptor, specifically the $\beta_2$ and $\beta_3$ subunits. The onset of action is less than 1 minute, and its duration of action is less than 5 minutes.

Etomidate is commercially available as a 2 mg/mL solution in a 35% propylene glycol solution. Propylene glycol toxicity from prolonged etomidate infusions is implicated in the development of hyperosmolar metabolic acidosis (Chap. 19). Etomidate depresses adrenal production of cortisol and aldosterone (by 11-beta-hydroxylase inhibition); therefore, it is associated with adrenocortical suppression.

### Dexmedetomidine

Dexmedetomidine is a central $\alpha_2$-adrenergic agonist that decreases central presynaptic catecholamine release, primarily in the locus ceruleus. Dexmedetomidine has minimal effect at the $GABA_A$ receptor. Unlike other sedative–hypnotics, it is not associated with significant respiratory depression. Dexmedetomidine is currently only approved for use for less than 24 hours. Extensive safety trials have not yet explored its use beyond 24 hours. The most common adverse effects from its use are nausea, dry mouth, bradycardia, and blood pressure instability (usually hypertension followed by hypotension).

### Melatonin, Ramelteon, and Tasimelteon

Melatonin and melatonin-containing products are sold as dietary supplements. Ramelteon is a synthetic melatonin-analog that is US Food and Drug Administration (FDA) approved for the treatment of chronic insomnia. Tasimelteon, the newest melatonin receptor agonist, is a US FDA-approved drug used to treat non–24-hour sleep–wake disorder that occurs in blind individuals in whom light cues do not reach the suprachiasmatic nucleus of the brain to allow for a normal sleep–wake cycle. Melatonin, ramelteon, and tasimelteon act as agonists at $MT_1$ and $MT_2$ receptors. Whereas $MT_1$ receptors are involved in sleep induction, $MT_2$ receptors are involved in regulation of the circadian sleep–wake cycle in humans.

Adverse effects of ramelteon are mild and usually include drowsiness, dizziness, fatigue, and headache. Isolated cases of bradycardia, hypotension, and seizures are reported in overdose. There are no published reports of tasimelteon toxicity from overdose.

### Suvorexant

Suvorexant is a newly approved dual orexin receptor antagonist. Orexin (also known as hypocretin) promotes wakefulness; as an orexin antagonist, suvorexant induces and maintains sleep. The most commonly reported side effect with overdose is somnolence after awakening.

# A25 FLUMAZENIL

## INTRODUCTION

Flumazenil is a competitive benzodiazepine receptor antagonist with a limited role in patients with an unknown overdose. Flumazenil also has the potential to induce benzodiazepine withdrawal symptoms, including seizures in patients who are benzodiazepine dependent. Flumazenil is the ideal antidote for patients who are both naïve to benzodiazepines and who overdose solely on a benzodiazepine such as children when there is a concern for airway protection. Flumazenil is also indicated in benzodiazepine-naïve patients whose benzodiazepines must be reversed during or after procedural sedation.

## HISTORY

Attempts to produce benzodiazepines with potent anxiolytic and antiepileptic activity and diminished sedative and muscle-relaxing properties resulted in derivatives that had high in vitro binding affinities but lacked in vivo activity. An inability to enter the central nervous system (CNS) was erroneously considered as an explanation for this discordance. However, during an experiment that attempted to demonstrate CNS penetration for these new derivatives, it was noted that when diazepam was given to incapacitate the animals, it surprisingly had a weaker than expected effect, demonstrating that these new molecules were actually receptor antagonists. Ultimately, flumazenil was developed and marketed as a benzodiazepine antagonist.

## PHARMACOLOGY

### Mechanism of Action

The benzodiazepine receptor modulates the effect of γ-aminobutyric acid (GABA) on the $GABA_A$ receptor by increasing the frequency of $Cl^-$ channel opening, leading to hyperpolarization. Agonists such as diazepam stimulate the benzodiazepine receptor to produce anxiolytic, antiepileptic, sedative–hypnotic, amnestic, and muscle relaxant effects. Flumazenil is a competitive antagonist at the $\alpha_1$ subtype of $GABA_A$ benzodiazepine receptors. Positron emission tomography investigations in adults revealed that 1.5 mg of flumazenil led to an initial receptor occupancy of 55%, and that 15 mg caused almost total blockade of benzodiazepine receptor sites.

## PHARMACOKINETICS AND PHARMACODYNAMICS

Table A25–1 summarizes the physicochemical and pharmacologic properties of flumazenil.

## ROLE IN CONSCIOUS SEDATION

When a benzodiazepine is given for conscious sedation during a procedure, flumazenil is safe and effective for reversal of prolonged sedation and partial reversal of amnesia and cognitive impairment. Most patients respond to total doses of 0.4 to 1 mg. Administering flumazenil slowly at a rate of 0.1 mg/min minimizes the symptoms associated with rapid arousal, such as confusion, agitation, and emotional lability. If recurrent sedation is to occur, it tends to appear 20 to 120 minutes after the administration of flumazenil, depending on the dose and pharmacokinetics of the previously administered benzodiazepine and the dose of flumazenil. Since flumazenil does not alter the clinical course of most patients who receive it, patients must be carefully monitored and subsequent doses of flumazenil titrated to clinical response. Because the amnestic effect of benzodiazepines and the cognitive and psychomotor effects are not fully reversed, posttreatment instructions should be reinforced in writing and given to a responsible caregiver accompanying the patient.

## ROLE IN PARADOXICAL REACTIONS

Paradoxical reactions to benzodiazepines are unpredictable and documented in as many as 10% of adults and in 3.4% of children. Common features include worsening restlessness, agitation, disorientation, irrational talking, flailing and excessive movements, hostile behavior, and dysphoria. Clinical evidence supports the efficacy of flumazenil to reverse paradoxical reactions to benzodiazepines in both adults and children.

## ROLE IN THE OVERDOSE SETTING

The use of flumazenil following overdose remains controversial. The first argument against its use is that benzodiazepines rarely cause morbidity and mortality. Proponents of flumazenil suggest that although it does not provide a mortality benefit, it reduces some complications and unnecessary

| TABLE A25–1 | Physicochemical and Pharmacologic Properties of Flumazenil |
|---|---|
| $pK_a$ | Weak base |
| LogD | 1.15 (octanol/aqueous $PO_4$ buffer) |
| Volume of distribution (SS) | 1.06 L/kg |
| Distribution half-life (min) | 4–11 |
| Metabolism | Hepatic: three inactive metabolites<br>Clearance dependent on hepatic blood flow |
| Elimination | First order |
| Protein binding (%) | 54–64 |
| Elimination half-life (min) | 54 |
| Onset of action (min) | 1–2 |
| Duration of action | Dependent on dose and elimination of benzodiazepine, time interval, dose of flumazenil, and hepatic function |

**TABLE A25–2 Indications for Flumazenil Use in the Overdose Setting**

Pure benzodiazepine overdose in a nontolerant individual who has
- CNS depression
- Normal vital signs, including $SaO_2$
- Normal ECG findings
- Otherwise normal neurologic examination

CNS = central nervous system; ECG = electrocardiogram.

diagnostic testing or endotracheal intubations in patients with predicted difficult airways or difficult weaning of mechanical ventilation. In one study, overdosed comatose patients were retrospectively assigned to either a low-risk or non–low-risk group. Low-risk patients had CNS depression with normal vital signs, no other neurologic findings, no evidence of ingestion of a tricyclic antidepressant by history or electrocardiography, no seizure history, and absence of an available history of chronic benzodiazepine use. All other patients fell into the non–low-risk category. Although flumazenil use was safe and effective in the low-risk group, the risk of seizures was substantial in the non–low-risk patients. The risks of flumazenil usually outweigh the benefits in patients with overdoses. When non–benzodiazepine-dependent patients, such as pediatric patients, ingest benzodiazepines alone in overdose with high certainty, the risks associated with flumazenil are limited. Table A25–2 summarizes some clear indications for flumazenil use in the overdose setting.

## ROLE IN NONBENZODIAZEPINE TOXICITY

### Hepatic Encephalopathy

Animal studies of hepatic encephalopathy demonstrate an increase in GABA effect, which is antagonized by flumazenil. Human studies have detected benzodiazepine binding activity in the cerebrospinal fluid and serum of patients with hepatic encephalopathy. Flumazenil somewhat improves the clinical and electrophysiologic responses in about 30% of patients with hepatic encephalopathy. Maximal improvement after flumazenil lasts approximately 1 to 2 hours and gradually dissipates within 6 hours. Existing guidelines recommend that use be reserved for patients with acute hepatic encephalopathy and a history of benzodiazepine use. There is no known survival benefit, and we do not routinely recommend flumazenil utilization for this indication.

### Ethanol Intoxication

A randomized, double-blind, crossover study was conducted in eight male volunteers given IV ethanol to achieve a constant serum ethanol concentration of 160 mg/dL. After being stabilized, the volunteers were given either placebo or 5 mg of flumazenil. Subjective and objective psychomotor tests were conducted, with no differences noted between groups. Although there are anecdotal reports of efficacy, based on mechanism of action and the study above, flumazenil likely does not have a significant effect on ethanol intoxication. Therefore, to avoid the increased risk of adverse effects, flumazenil cannot be recommended for reversal of ethanol intoxication.

**TABLE A25–3 Contraindications to Flumazenil Use**

| *History* | *Clinical* |
|---|---|
| Seizure history or current treatment of seizures | Potential ECG evidence of cyclic antidepressant use: terminal rightward 40-ms axis, QRS complex or QT interval prolongation |
| Ingestion of a xenobiotic capable of provoking seizures or cardiac dysrhythmias | Hypoxia or hypoventilation[a]<br>Hypotension<br>Head trauma |
| Long-term use of benzodiazepines | |

[a]Do not rely on flumazenil to reverse benzodiazepine-induced respiratory depression.
ECG = electrocardiogram.

### Adverse Effects and Safety Issues

Flumazenil use potentially precipitates seizures in benzodiazepine-dependent patients, the unmasking of dysrhythmias in patients with coingestion of a prodysrhythmic drug, and recurrence of sedation, which significantly limit its use. A consensus report suggested that (1) flumazenil is not a substitute for primary emergency care; (2) hypoxia and hypotension should be corrected before flumazenil is used; (3) if used, small titrated doses of flumazenil should be administered; (4) flumazenil should be avoided in patients with a history of seizures, evidence of seizures or jerking movements, or evidence of a cyclic antidepressant overdose or in unknown overdoses; and (5) flumazenil should not be used by inexperienced clinicians. We agree with those findings. Table A25–3 summarizes the contraindications and precautions essential to evaluate before flumazenil use.

## PREGNANCY AND LACTATION

Flumazenil is US FDA Pregnancy Category C. It is not known whether flumazenil is excreted in breast milk.

## DOSING AND ADMINISTRATION

Slow IV titration (0.1 mg/min) of an initial dose of 0.1 or 0.2 mg seems most reasonable in adults. Following a 1-minute or more observation period to determine an effect, it is reasonable to repeat that dose to a maximal dose of 1 mg. In pediatric patients, for the reversal of conscious sedation, the initial dose is 0.01 mg/kg (up to 0.2 mg) administered slowly as in adults. Recurrent sedation should be anticipated to occur between 20 and 120 minutes and may be sufficient to require repeated flumazenil dosing. Although not United States (US) Food and Drug Administration (FDA) approved, a continuous intravenous infusion in saline or dextrose of 0.1 to 1.0 mg/h has been employed following the loading dose.

## FORMULATION

Flumazenil is available by many manufacturers in a concentration of 0.1 mg/mL with parabens in 5- and 10-mL vials.

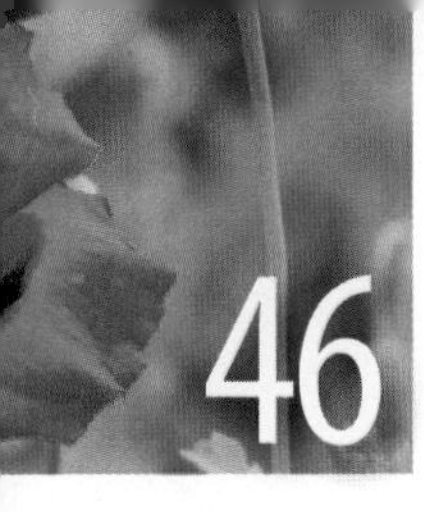

# 46 AMPHETAMINES

## HISTORY AND EPIDEMIOLOGY

Amphetamine was first synthesized in 1887 but was essentially lost until the 1920s, when concerns arose regarding the supply of ephedrine for asthma therapy. Both amphetamine and methamphetamine were supplied as stimulants for soldiers and prisoners of war during World War II. Amphetamine tablets were available in 1935 for the treatment of narcolepsy and were advocated as anorexiants in 1938. Abuse was reported as early as 1940 and benzedrine inhalers were banned by the United States (US) Food and Drug Administration (FDA) in 1959. Over the subsequent decades, there were sporadic periods of widespread amphetamine use and abuse in the US. As products became restricted, derivatives of amphetamine and methamphetamine surfaced and circumvented existing regulations. Still today, the ease and low cost of methamphetamine synthesis encourage establishment of illegal clandestine laboratories.

## PHARMACOLOGY

The term "amphetamine" is representative of a broad group of compounds with a shared phenylethylamine structure. Numerous substitutions on the phenylethylamine backbone are possible, resulting in a variety of xenobiotics, some with unique properties. For the purposes of this chapter, all phenylethylamines, even those that are not actually amphetamines, will be called *amphetamines* for simplicity, and the name *amphetamine* specifically refers to β-phenylisopropylamine, the original compound.

The primary mechanism of action of amphetamines is the release of the biogenic amines dopamine, norepinephrine, and serotonin as described in Figure 46–1. Binding selectivity to the neurotransmitter transporters largely determines the range of pharmacologic effects for a particular amphetamine. The affinity of 3,4-methylenedioxymethamphetamine (MDMA) for serotonin transporters, for example, is 10 times greater than that for dopamine and norepinephrine transporters. With this high affinity for serotonin transporters, MDMA produces primarily serotonergic effects. Other predominantly serotonergic amphetamines include *para*-methoxyamphetamine and bromo-dragonFLY (Table 46–1).

### Structure Modification

Specific substitutions made to the phenylethylamine backbone have led to the wide variety of novel drugs. Substitutions at different positions of the phenylethylamine molecule alter the general pharmacology and clinical effects of amphetamines. Table 46–2 describes the pharmacology of specific substitutions. Addition of a halogen group (eg, iodine or bromine) increases the potency and neurotoxicity of the compound.

## PHARMACOKINETICS AND TOXICOKINETICS

### Absorption

Amphetamines can be absorbed by intravenous, oral, intranasal, and inhalational routes. Amphetamines are rapidly absorbed, with bioavailability that ranges between 60% and 90% depending on the route of administration. Peak serum concentrations are variable and are substance and route dependent.

### Distribution

After absorption, amphetamines are distributed to most compartments of the body. Most amphetamines are also relatively lipophilic and readily cross the blood–brain barrier. Amphetamines have large volumes of distribution, varying from 3 to 5 L/kg for amphetamine, 3 to 4 L/kg for methamphetamine and phentermine, and 11 to 33 L/kg for methylphenidate. Some amphetamines such as pemoline have a small volume of distribution (0.2–0.6 L/kg).

### Metabolism

Amphetamines are metabolized via multiple pathways, including diverse routes of hepatic transformation and renal elimination. In general, because multiple enzymes and elimination pathways (including renal) are involved in amphetamine metabolism, it is less likely that polymorphisms or drug interactions alone will significantly increase toxicity.

### Elimination

Renal elimination of the parent compound is substantial for many amphetamines. Amphetamines are bases with a typical $pK_a$ range of 9 to 10, and renal elimination increases as pH decreases. The half-life of amphetamines varies significantly, from 2.5 to over 34 hours. Repetitive administration, which occurs typically during binge use, leads to drug accumulation and prolongation of the apparent half-life and duration of effect.

## PATHOPHYSIOLOGY

Most complications associated with amphetamines are a result of an uncontrolled hyperadrenergic condition similar to that which occurs with other sympathomimetics such as cocaine, except the duration of effect is typically longer. Most patients with acute amphetamine toxicity manifest effects in the central nervous system (CNS) and cardiovascular system. The majority of the specific effects are from excessive catecholamine release as opposed to direct effects from the amphetamines themselves.

## CLINICAL MANIFESTATIONS

The general acute and chronic toxicities of amphetamines are shown in Table 46–3. Effects specific to individual amphetamines follow. Complications can result from intravenous (IV) drug use and from the associated contaminants. Contamination with blood and bodily fluids leads to human

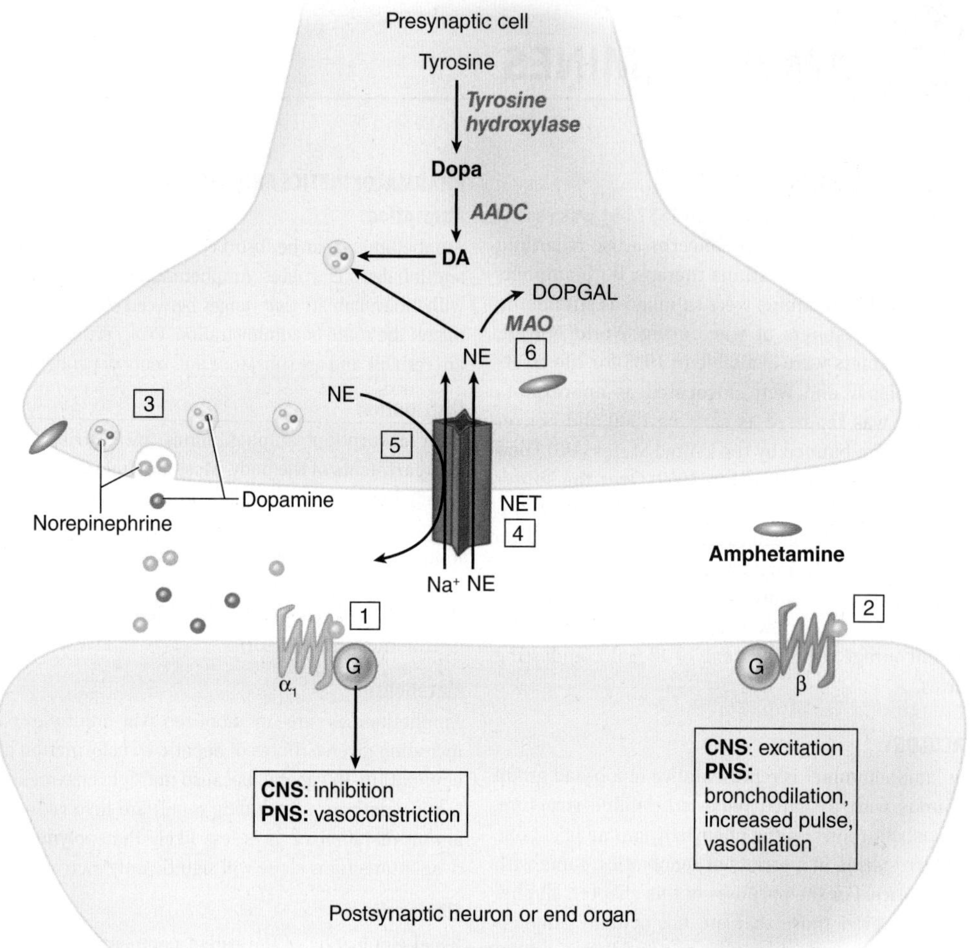


**FIGURE 46–1.** Noradrenergic nerve ending. The postsynaptic membrane represents an end organ or another neuron in the central nervous system (CNS). The primary mechanism of action of amphetamine is the release of catecholamines, particularly dopamine (DA) and norepinephrine (NE), from the presynaptic terminals. Two storage pools exist for DA in the presynaptic terminals: the vesicular pool and the cytoplasmic pool. The vesicular storage of DA and other biogenic amines is maintained by the acidic environment within the vesicles and the persistence of a stabilizing electrical gradient with respect to the cytoplasm. *(1, 2)* Activating or antagonizing postsynaptic α- and β-adrenoceptors. *(3)* Amphetamines release DA or NE from the cytoplasmic pool by exchange diffusion at the DA uptake transporter site in the membrane. *(4)* Amphetamines diffuse through the presynaptic terminal membrane and interact with the neurotransmitter transporter on the vesicular membrane to cause exchange release of DA or NE into the cytoplasm. DA is subsequently released into the synapse by reverse transport at the DA uptake site. *(5)* Amphetamine diffuses through the cellular and vesicular membranes, alkalinizing the vesicles, and permitting dopamine release from the vesicles and delivery into the synapse by reverse transport. *(6)* Inhibiting monoamine oxidase (MAO) to prevent NE degradation; or inhibiting catechol-*O*-methyltransferase (COMT) to prevent NE degradation. AADC = aromatic L-amino acid decarboxylase; DOPGAL = 3,4-dihydroxyphenylglycoaldehyde; G = G protein; NET = membrane norepinephrine uptake transporter; NME = normetanephrine; PNS = peripheral nervous system.

immunodeficiency virus infection, hepatitis, and malaria. Bacterial and foreign body contamination results in endocarditis, tetanus, wound botulism, osteomyelitis, and pulmonary and soft tissue abscesses.

## DIAGNOSTIC TESTING

The choice and extent of diagnostic tests should be guided by the history and physical examination. In all patients with altered mental status, blood specimens should be sent for glucose, blood urea nitrogen, and electrolyte assays. An electrocardiogram should be obtained in all patients to screen for tachydysrhythmias and coingestants, and continuous cardiac monitoring should be initiated. A complete blood count, urinalysis, coagulation profile, creatine phosphokinase, chest radiograph, computed tomography scan of the head, echocardiogram of the heart, and lumbar puncture will be necessary, depending on the clinical presentation.

Qualitative urine immunoassays are available for amphetamines, but these tests rarely contribute to management in the acute setting. A major limitation is the high rate of false-positive and false-negative results common to the amphetamine immunoassay.

**TABLE 46–1 Examples of Amphetamines**

| *Xenobiotic* | *Clinical Manifestations* | *Structure* |
|---|---|---|
| 4-Bromo-2,5-dimethoxyamphetamine (DOB) | Marked psychoactive effect, potency > mescaline<br>Fantasy, mood altering<br>Agitation, sympathetic excess<br>Sold as impregnated paper, like LSD | 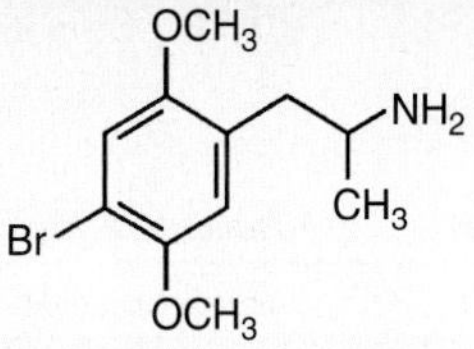 $OCH_3$, $NH_2$, $CH_3$, Br, $OCH_3$ |
| 4-Bromo-2,5-methoxyphenylethylamine (2CB, MFT) | Relaxation<br>Sensory distortion<br>Agitation<br>Hallucinations<br>Potency > mescaline | 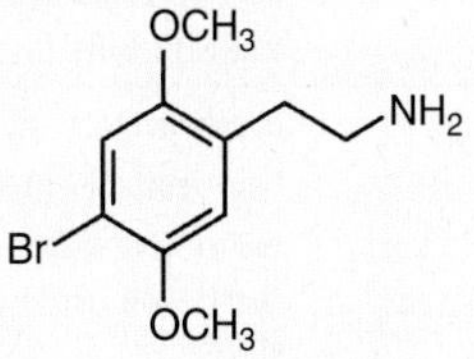 $OCH_3$, $NH_2$, Br, $OCH_3$ |
| Methcathinone (cat, Jeff, khat, ephedrone) | Hallucinations<br>Sympathetic excess | 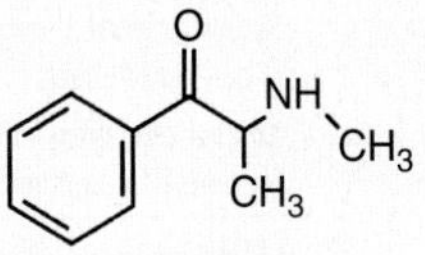 O, NH, $CH_3$, $CH_3$ |
| 4-Methyl-2,5-dimethoxyamphetamine (DOM/STP) (serenity, tranquility, peace) | Narrow therapeutic index<br>Euphoria, perceptual distortion<br>Hallucinations, sympathetic excess | 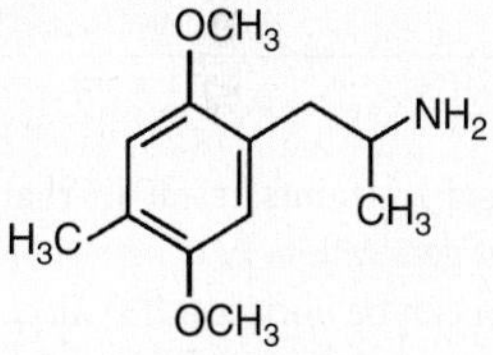 $OCH_3$, $NH_2$, $CH_3$, $H_3C$, $OCH_3$ |
| 3,4-Methylenedioxyamphetamine (MDA, love drug) | Empathy, euphoria<br>Agitation, delirium, hallucinations, sympathetic excess | 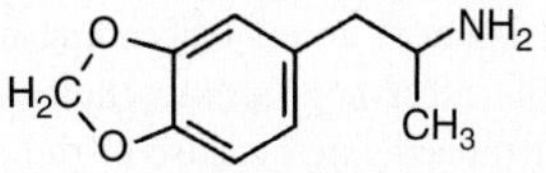 O, $H_2C$, O, $NH_2$, $CH_3$ |
| 3,4-Methylenedioxyethamphetamine (MDEA, Eve) | Comparable to MDMA<br>Sympathetic excess | 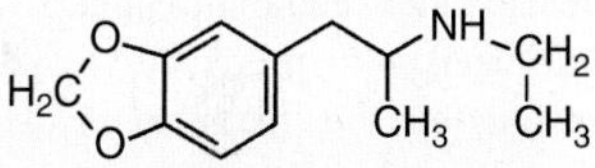 O, $H_2C$, O, NH, $CH_2$, $CH_3$, $CH_3$ |
| 3,4-Methylenedioxymethamphetamine (MDMA, Adam, molly, ecstasy, XTC) | Psychotherapy "facilitator"<br>Euphoria, empathy, nausea, anorexia, anxiety, insomnia<br>Sympathetic excess | 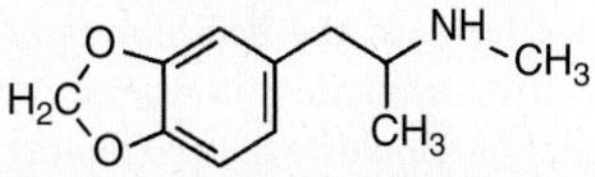 O, $H_2C$, O, NH, $CH_3$, $CH_3$ |
| *para*-Methoxyamphetamine (PMA) | Potent hallucinogen<br>Sympathetic excess | 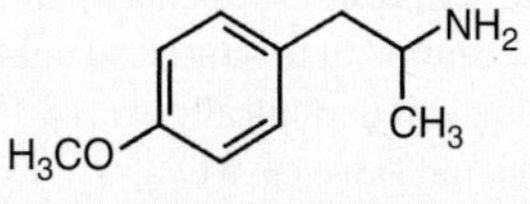 $NH_2$, $CH_3$, $H_3CO$ |
| 2,4,5-Trimethoxyamphetamine | Similar to mescaline | 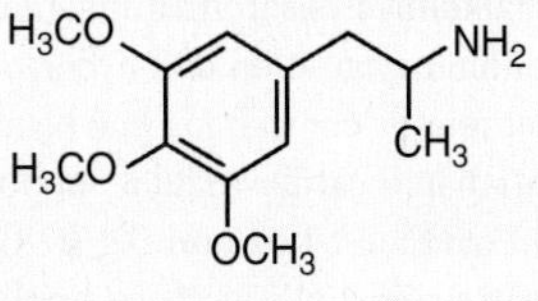 $H_3CO$, $NH_2$, $CH_3$, $H_3CO$, $OCH_3$ |

LSD = lysergic acid diethylamide.

## MANAGEMENT

The initial medical assessment of the agitated patient must include vital signs, a rapid glucose determination, and a complete physical examination. Determination of core body temperature is essential to diagnose the presence and degree of hyperthermia, which is a frequent and rapidly fatal manifestation in patients with drug-induced delirium. Significant hyperthermia necessitates immediate interventions to achieve rapid cooling. Some patients require temporary physical restraints to gain pharmacologic control and prevent personal harm to themselves or others. Physical restraints should be discontinued as soon as possible;

**TABLE 46–2 Specific Substitutions on Phenylethylamine**

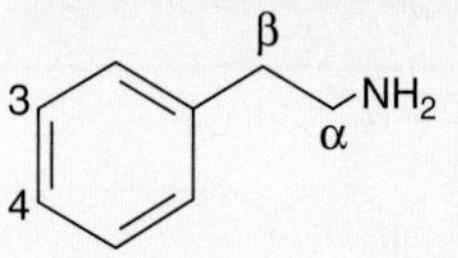

| Substitution | Pharmacologic Effect |
|---|---|
| α-Carbon | Indirect acting; resists oxidation by monoamine oxidase |
| β-Carbon | Decreases central nervous system penetration<br>Whereas hydroxyl (–OH): increases adrenergic activity |
| Amino group | No substitution: α-adrenergic > β-adrenergic effects<br>Larger group: β-adrenergic > α-adrenergic effects<br>t-Butyl group: $\beta_2$-adrenergic selective<br>Methyl ($-CH_3$) group: maximum α- and β-adrenergic effects |
| 3-, 4- of aromatic ring | Hydroxylation at 3- and 4-: increased α- and β-adrenergic effects<br>Absence of hydroxylation (at one or both positions) prevents degradation by catechol-*O*-methyltransferase. |
| Halogenation | Enhances potency of neurotoxic properties of amphetamines by selective action on the serotonin system |

prolonged restraints result in rhabdomyolysis and continued heat generation. IV access should be obtained so that IV sedation can be initiated. If IV access cannot be obtained, it is necessary to attempt to administer intramuscular sedation until definitive access is accomplished.

The most appropriate choice of chemical sedation is a benzodiazepine because of the characteristic high therapeutic index, good antiepileptic activity, and predictable pharmacokinetic properties. Benzodiazepines are effective not only for the treatment of delirium induced by acute overdose of cocaine, amphetamines, and other xenobiotics but also the delirium associated with ethanol and sedative–hypnotic withdrawal (Antidotes in Brief: A26). Sedation should be titrated rapidly until the patient is calm. In our clinical experience, cumulative benzodiazepine doses required in the initial 30 minutes to achieve adequate sedation will periodically exceed 100 mg of diazepam or its equivalent (Table 46–4).

Rhabdomyolysis from amphetamines usually results from psychomotor agitation and hyperthermia. Sedation prevents further muscle contraction and heat production. Adequate IV hydration and cardiovascular support should maintain urine output of at least 1 to 2 mL/kg/h. Although urinary acidification can significantly increase amphetamine elimination, urinary pH manipulation does not decrease toxicity and instead increases the risk of acute kidney injury from rhabdomyolysis.

Amphetamine body packers, although uncommon, should be treated similarly to those who transport cocaine (Special Considerations: SC4).

## INDIVIDUAL AMPHETAMINES

### Methamphetamine

Methamphetamine is known by many names, including, but not limited to, "yaba," "speed," "go," "crack," "uppers," and "dexies." The terms "crystal," "shard," and "ice" refer to the crystalline form of methamphetamine. The production of methamphetamine is relatively simple, requiring minimal equipment and chemicals. Because methamphetamine laboratories use many potentially toxic xenobiotics, including phosphine gas, methylamine gas, chloroform, and hydrochloric acid, they pose a significant health risk to law enforcement officers and the general public. Methamphetamine is notable for its long half-life (19–34 hours), and the duration of its acute effects is often greater than 24 hours.

**TABLE 46–3 Clinical Manifestations of Amphetamine Toxicity**

***Acute***

***Cardiovascular System***
- Aortic dissection
- Dysrhythmias
- Hypertension
- Myocardial ischemia
- Tachycardia
- Vasospasm

***Central Nervous System***
- Agitation
- Anorexia
- Bruxism
- Choreoathetoid movements
- Euphoria
- Headache
- Hyperreflexia
- Hyperthermia
- Intracerebral hemorrhage or infarction
- Paranoid psychosis
- Seizures

***Other Sympathomimetic Symptoms***
- Diaphoresis
- Mydriasis
- Nausea
- Tachypnea
- Tremor

***Other Organ System Manifestations***
- Acute respiratory distress syndrome
- Ischemic colitis
- Muscle rigidity
- Rhabdomyolysis

***Laboratory Abnormalities***
- Creatine phosphokinase elevated
- Hyperglycemia
- Hyponatremia
- Leukocytosis
- Liver enzymes elevated
- Myoglobinuria

***Chronic***
- Aortic and mitral regurgitation
- Cardiomyopathy
- Dopaminergic and serotonergic neuron damage
- Pulmonary hypertension
- Vasculitis

**TABLE 46–4 Management of Patients With Amphetamine Toxicity**

| |
|---|
| ***Agitation*** |
| Benzodiazepines (usually adequate for the cardiovascular manifestations) |
| Diazepam 10 mg (or equivalent) intravenously; repeat rapidly until the patient is calm (cumulative dose periodically can be as high as 100 mg of diazepam). An equivalent titrated dose of IM midazolam is recommended if IV access is not available. |
| ***Seizures*** |
| Benzodiazepines |
| Barbiturates |
| Propofol for status epilepticus (typically will require endotracheal intubation) |
| ***Hyperthermia*** |
| External cooling |
| Control agitation rapidly |
| ***Gastric Decontamination and Elimination*** |
| Activated charcoal for recent ingestions |
| ***Hypertension*** |
| Control agitation first |
| α-Adrenergic antagonist (phentolamine)[a] |
| Vasodilators (IV nitroglycerin or nicardipine) |
| ***Delirium or Hallucinations With Abnormal Vital Signs*** |
| If agitated: benzodiazepines |

[a]Avoid β-adrenergic antagonists, especially with suspected cocaine toxicity.
IM = intramuscular; IV = intravenous.

## 3,4-Methylenedioxymethamphetamine

3,4-Methylenedioxymethamphetamine, also known as MDMA, "ecstasy," "E," "Adam," "XTC," "Molly," and "MDM," is commonly abused. 3,4-Methylenedioxymethamphetamine and similar analogs are so-called *entactogens* (meaning "touching within"), capable of producing euphoria, inner peace, and a desire to socialize. People who use MDMA report that it enhances pleasure, heightens sexuality, and expands consciousness without the loss of control. Negative effects reported with acute use included ataxia, restlessness, confusion, poor concentration, and impaired memory. Unlike amphetamine and methamphetamine, MDMA is a potent stimulus for the release of serotonin. The sympathetic effects of MDMA are mild in low doses. However, when a large amount of MDMA is taken, the clinical presentation is similar to that of other amphetamines. Dysrhythmias, hyperthermia, rhabdomyolysis, disseminated intravascular coagulation (DIC), and deaths are reported. Hyponatremia is also reported with MDMA use. 3,4-Methylenedioxymethamphetamine and its metabolites increase the release of vasopressin (antidiuretic hormone), and this is thought to be related to the serotonergic effects. Furthermore, substantial free water intake combined with sodium loss from physical exertion increases the risk of the development of hyponatremia.

A major concern with MDMA is its long-term effects on the brain. In numerous animal models, acute administration of MDMA leads to the decrease in SERT function and number. Recovery of SERT function takes several weeks. Repetitive administration of MDMA ultimately may result in permanent damage to serotonergic neurons, typically causing injury to the axons and the terminals while sparing the cell bodies.

## *Para*-Methoxyamphetamine and *Para*-Methoxymethamphetamine-Monomethoxy Derivatives

*Para*-methoxyamphetamine (PMA) is the 4-methoxylated analog of amphetamine, and *para*-methoxy-*N*-methylamphetamine (PMMA; methyl-MA) is the 4-methoxy analog of methamphetamine. Although the effects of PMA and PMMA mimic some aspects of MDMA and methamphetamine, unique properties of PMA and PMMA make them considerably more lethal, earning the street name "death." Methoxy ring substitution of amphetamine or methamphetamine at the 3 or 4 positions (*para* substitution is the most common) yields PMA and PMMA derivatives that have significantly less sympathomimetic activity than amphetamine but very potent serotonergic activity.

## Cathinones (Methcathinone, Methylenedioxypyrovalerone, and Mephedrone); "Bath Salts"

Cathinone (2-amino-1-phenyl-1-propanone) is a naturally occurring substance found in the leaves of the *Catha edulis* (khat) plant. Also known as guat and gat, the fresh leaves and stems are commonly used as a stimulant in Africa and the Middle East. The plant form contains numerous amphetamines in minute quantities, but the primary active ingredient is cathinone. As the leaves age, cathinone is degraded to cathine, which has about one-tenth the stimulant effect of D-amphetamine. The primary effects of khat are increased alertness, insomnia, euphoria, anxiety, and hyperactivity. Khat chewing is linked to cardiac and gastrointestinal (GI) disease.

Methcathinone, the methyl derivative of cathinone, was used in Russia as an antidepressant in the 1930s and 1940s. Also known as "Cat" and "Jeff," cathinone was used recreationally, historically most often in countries formerly part of the Soviet Union. Various synthetic cathinones, including mephedrone and methylenedioxypyrovalerone (MDPV), gained popularity in both the US and Europe. Many other synthetic cathinones produced include methylone, mephedrone, butylone, MDPV, dimethylcathinone, ethcathinone, ethylone, 3-,4-fluoromethcathinone, and α-pyrrolidinovalerophenone. α-Pyrrolidinovalerophenone (1-phenyl-2-(pyrrolidin-1)-ylpentan-1-one), are popular drugs of abuse.

Cathinones possess amphetamine-like properties and have sympathomimetic effects, although as a group, they are considered less potent. Common adverse effects include agitation, tachycardia, hallucinations, and a general sympathomimetic toxidrome. Some synthetic cathinones cause hyponatremia, although the mechanism is not clear.

## Bromo-dragonFLY

Bromo-dragonFLY (BDF) is a member of a newer class of benzodifurans, which were used as potent tools for investigation of the serotonin receptor family. Structurally, BDF is closely related to other phenylethylamines such as DOB and 2C-B but contains two furan rings on either side of the benzene ring, creating a fully aromatic tricyclic structure. There are several similar compounds to BDF, differing by substitution of the bromine atom with other entities. These drugs have a potent hallucinogenic effect mediated primarily through the

5-HT$_{2A}$ receptor (also with affinity for the 5-HT$_{2B}$ and 5-HT$_{2C}$ receptors). Bromo-dragonFLY use is associated with deaths in Europe and the US. Reports demonstrate delayed complications owing to severe peripheral vasoconstriction and limb ischemia. Such complications likely result from the potent serotonergic properties of BDF.

### 2,5-Dimethoxy-4-Methylamphetamine and 2,5-Dimethoxy-4-Iodoamphetamine

2,5-Dimethoxy-4-methylamphetamine (DOM) is also known as STP, which stands for "serenity, tranquility, and peace." Because of its delayed onset of action and duration of effect, it was not very popular. 2,5-Dimethoxy-4-iodoamphetamine (DOI) is another potent hallucinogen, previously sold as a substitute for lysergic acid diethylamide (LSD). Dimethoxy amphetamine derivatives are serotonin receptor agonists with selectivity at the 5-HT$_{2A}$, 5-HT$_{2B}$, and 5-HT$_{2C}$ receptor subtypes. Potent hallucinogenic effects and dysphoria characterize the use of DOB and DOI, with minimal sympathomimetic effects. These symptoms can often be delayed with a prolonged duration of effect, sometimes refractory to the use of benzodiazepines. Reversible vasospasm with the use of dimethoxy amphetamine derivatives is reported.

### The 2C-Series and *N*-2-Methoxybenzylphenylethylamines

The 2C-series and its derivatives are similar in structure and function to DOM and DOI as all are dimethoxy phenylethylamine derivatives with potent hallucinogenic properties. The first of this series, 2C-B, was initially intended for psychotherapy; however, it fell out of favor because of GI side effects and limited entactogenic effects. Multiple other 2C compounds have been developed by altering substitutions at positions 2, 4, and 5 on the phenyl ring. Reported clinical effects of this series include sympathomimetic effects, delirium, hallucinations, and psychosis. 2-(4-Iodo-2,5-dimethoxyphenyl)-*N*-[(2-methoxyphenyl)methyl]ethanamine (2C-I-NBOMe, *N*-Bomb) was discovered in 2003, along with other similar NBOMe compounds. They possess strong 5-HT$_{2A}$ agonism and are highly potent, which allows for microgram doses. NBOMes are used by all routes, but poor oral bioavailability limits oral use. Reported clinical effects include euphoria, hallucinations, and sympathomimetic effects. Deaths are reported.

# 47 CANNABINOIDS

## HISTORY AND EPIDEMIOLOGY

Cannabis has been used for more than 4,000 years. The earliest documentation of the therapeutic use of marijuana is the fourth century B.C. in China. Cannabis use spread from China to India to North Africa, reaching Europe around A.D. 500. In colonial North America, cannabis was cultivated as a source of fiber. Pure δ-9-tetrahydrocannabinol (hereafter called THC) was subsequently isolated from hashish extract in 1964, and the structure was elucidated in 1967. In 1970, the United States (US) Controlled Substances Act classified marijuana as a Schedule I drug. Currently, marijuana is the most commonly used illicit xenobiotic in the US; however, it is rapidly becoming legalized.

Synthetic cannabinoids (SCs) have been targeted as potential therapeutics for decades. Development of these compounds promoted the discovery of central and peripheral cannabinoid receptors ($CB_1$ and $CB_2$) in the 1980s. In the 1990s, the endogenous cannabinoids were discovered and were subsequently synthesized. These free fatty acids are quickly hydrolyzed in vivo, a fact that previously limited potential for pharmaceutical development.

In 2004, SC-laced herbal incense blends became available over the Internet and through smoke shops in Western Europe. The incidence of SC exposure in the US increased, and in November 2010, the US Drug Enforcement Administration (DEA) began the process of listing selected SCs as Schedule I drugs on a temporary basis. Toxicologists face a new era in the field of cannabinoids: Research continues to advance understanding of the cannabinoid system, and a myriad of new and discrete SCs emerge every year. Even marijuana is found with higher potency and changing phytocannabinoid ratios that may affect patients in unanticipated ways.

## MEDICAL USES

Cannabis has been used medicinally for thousands of years to treat a seemingly endless array of conditions. However, modern medicine is supported by an evidence-based system rather than the belief-based medicine of the past. Although smoked marijuana and THC preparations have not typically proven acutely dangerous, efficacy is questionable. Several issues must be considered when examining the body of evidence both for and against the medical use of cannabinoids. Marijuana is not the same entity as, nor is it interchangeable with, THC. Multiple additional cannabinoids present in marijuana are biologically active and must be considered. Second, significant study design flaws limit the conclusions that can be drawn from existing studies. Finally, poor overall understanding of cannabinoid physiology may hamper future study design.

### Pain

Studies examining the efficacy of cannabis in the setting of induced acute pain showed no improvement. These studies were limited by the lack of a positive control and examined only extremes of induced pain. Smoked marijuana failed to attenuate thermal pain in volunteers, and an oral THC analog had no effect on postsurgical pain. When used for the treatment of chronic and neuropathic pain, cannabinoids have had some favorable outcomes, although design flaws severely limit the quality of medical evidence.

### Nausea and Vomiting

Trials of cannabinoids for treatment of chemotherapy-induced nausea and vomiting demonstrate superiority over placebo, but compared with serotonin and dopamine antagonists, this difference is not statistically significant.

### Glaucoma

Trials investigating the efficacy of cannabinoids for the treatment of glaucoma demonstrate the inferiority to longer acting traditional therapeutics, which have more significant effects on intraocular pressure (IOP) and longer durations of effect.

### Summary of Medical Use

In 2003, the Institute of Medicine undertook an extensive review of the evidence supporting the medical use of marijuana. It concluded that in some circumstances, cannabinoids show promise for use as therapeutics, but the quality of current studies necessitated further research specifically for the treatment of chronic pain. In addition, smoking marijuana provides a crude and unpredictable delivery mechanism, and safer, more precise methods of administration are needed. Similarly, a meta-analysis in 2015 composed of randomized clinical trials (RCTs) showed only moderate evidence to support the efficacy of cannabinoids in treating chronic pain and spasticity related to multiple sclerosis. Currently, US Food and Drug Administration approval is for the control of chemotherapy-related nausea and vomiting that are resistant to conventional antiemetics, for breakthrough postoperative nausea and vomiting, and for appetite stimulation in patients with human immunodeficiency virus (HIV) with anorexia-cachexia syndrome. The claims of benefit in the other medical conditions are not clearly supported by evidence.

## PHARMACOLOGY AND PATHOPHYSIOLOGY

The term *cannabinoid* refers to compounds that bind to the cannabinoid receptors regardless of whether they are derived from plants (phytocannabinoids), synthetic processes (SCs), or endogenous sources (endocannabinoids). The *terms cannabinoid, cannabinometic,* and *cannabinoid receptor agonist* are interchangeable. *Cannabis* is a collective term referring to the bioactive substances from the cannabis plant. The *Cannabis* genus (species *sativa* and *indica*) produces more than 60 chemicals called cannabinoids. The major cannabinoids are cannabinol, cannabidiol (CBD), and tetrahydrocannabinol. The principal psychoactive cannabinoid is THC. *Marijuana* is the common name for a mixture of dried leaves and flowers of the *C. sativa* plant. Hashish and hashish oil are the pressed resin and the oil expressed from the pressed resin, respectively. The concentration of THC varies from 1% in low-potency marijuana up to 50% in hash oil. THC extracted from marijuana using butane (butane hash oil or BHO) approaches THC concentrations of 100%. Pure THC and several pharmaceutical SCs are available by prescription with the generic names of dronabinol and nabilone, respectively. Nabiximol is the generic name for an oral mucosal spray containing THC and cannabidiol, which is approved for medical use in Canada, the United Kingdom, and parts of Europe. Some newer products contain $\Delta^8$ THC, although the clinic effects seem largely indistinguishable from $\Delta^9$ THC at this time.

Cannabinoid receptors are G protein–linked neuromodulators that inhibit adenyl cyclase in a dose-dependent and stereospecific manner. Although historically the cannabinoid receptor system is described as having a central $CB_1$ and a peripheral $CB_2$ receptor, $CB_2$ receptors are also found in the central nervous system (CNS). These two currently identified cannabinoid receptors are distinguished largely by their anatomic distribution and mechanisms of cellular messaging (Fig. 47–1).

### $CB_1$ Receptors and the Psychogenic Effects of Cannabis

The $CB_1$ receptors are the most numerous G protein–coupled receptors in the mammalian brain, accounting for the multiple and varied effects of cannabinoids on behavior, learning, and mood as well as suggesting the enormous complexity of the endocannabinoid system. The highest concentration of $CB_1$ receptors is located in areas of the brain associated with movement and higher functions of cognition and emotions. A relative lack of $CB_1$ receptors in the brainstem also explains lack of coma and respiratory depression that occurs with *Cannabis* use. Interactions with the $CB_2$ receptors are less well defined with regard to acute toxicity.

### Mechanism of Cellular Signaling

Figure 47–1 summarizes the mechanism of cellular signaling of endogenous cannabinoids. Exogenous cannabinoids act similarly to endogenous cannabinoids upon receptor binding, except that binding affinity and metabolism will vary among exogenous ligands and endogenous cannabinoids. $CB_1$ receptors are located either presynaptically or postsynaptically, and their activation can inhibit or enhance the release of acetylcholine, L-glutamate, γ-aminobutyric acid, noradrenaline, dopamine, and 5-hydroxytryptamine.

## PHARMACOKINETICS AND TOXICOKINETICS

### Absorption

Inhalation of smoke containing THC results in the onset of psychoactive effects within minutes typically reaching peak serum concentration before finishing the cigarette. From 10% to 35% of available THC is absorbed during smoking. Peak serum concentrations depend on the dose. A marijuana cigarette containing 1.75% THC produces a peak serum THC concentration of approximately 85 ng/mL.

Ingestion of cannabis results in an unpredictable onset of psychoactive effects in 1 to 3 hours. Only 5% to 20% of available THC reaches the systemic circulation after ingestion. Peak serum THC concentrations usually occur 2 to 4 hours after ingestion, but delays up to 6 hours are described. Dronabinol has an oral bioavailability of approximately 10% with high interindividual variability. Nabilone has an oral bioavailability estimated to be greater than 90% and reaches peak serum concentrations 2 hours after ingestion.

### Distribution

THC has a steady-state volume of distribution of approximately 2.5 to 3.5 L/kg. Cannabinoids are lipid soluble and accumulate in fatty tissue. After administration is stopped, the cannabinoids are slowly released from fat stores during adipose tissue turnover. THC crosses the placenta and enters the breast milk.

### Metabolism

THC is nearly completely metabolized by hepatic microsomal hydroxylation and oxidation (primarily CYP2C9 and CYP3A4). The primary metabolite (11-OH-THC) is active and is subsequently oxidized to the inactive 11-nor-THC carboxylic acid metabolite (THC-COOH) and many other inactive metabolites. Time course for parent compound and metabolites is shown in Figure 47–2.

### Excretion

Reported elimination half-lives of THC and its major metabolites vary considerably. After IV doses of THC, the mean elimination half-life ranges from 1.6 to 57 hours. Elimination half-lives are expected to be similar after inhalation. The elimination half-life of 11-OH-THC is 12 to 36 hours, and that of THC-COOH ranges from 1 to 6 days. In the 72 hours after ingestion, approximately 15% of a THC dose is excreted in the urine, and roughly 50% is excreted in the feces. After IV administration, approximately 15% of a THC dose is excreted in the urine, and only 25% to 35% is excreted in the feces.

## CLINICAL MANIFESTATIONS

The clinical effects of THC use, including time of onset and duration of effect, vary with the dose, the route of administration (ingestion is slower in onset than inhalation), the experience of the user, the vulnerability of the user to psychoactive effects, and the setting in which the THC is used.

### Psychological Effects

The most commonly self-reported effect is relaxation. Other commonly reported effects are perceptual alterations (heightened sensory awareness, slowing of time), a feeling of well-being (including giddiness or laughter), and increased appetite.

### Physiological Effects

Use of cannabis is associated with physiologic effects on cerebral blood flow, the heart, the lungs, and the eyes. Marijuana and THC increase cerebral blood flow, blood pressure, and heart rate and decrease vascular resistance. Inhalation or ingestion of THC produces a dose-related short-term decrease in airway resistance and an increase in airway conductance in both normal individuals and individuals with asthma. The principal ocular effects of cannabis are conjunctival injection and a transient decrease in IOP.

## ACUTE TOXICITY

In addition to the physiological and psychological effects described, acute toxicity includes decreases in coordination, muscle strength, and hand steadiness. Lethargy, sedation,

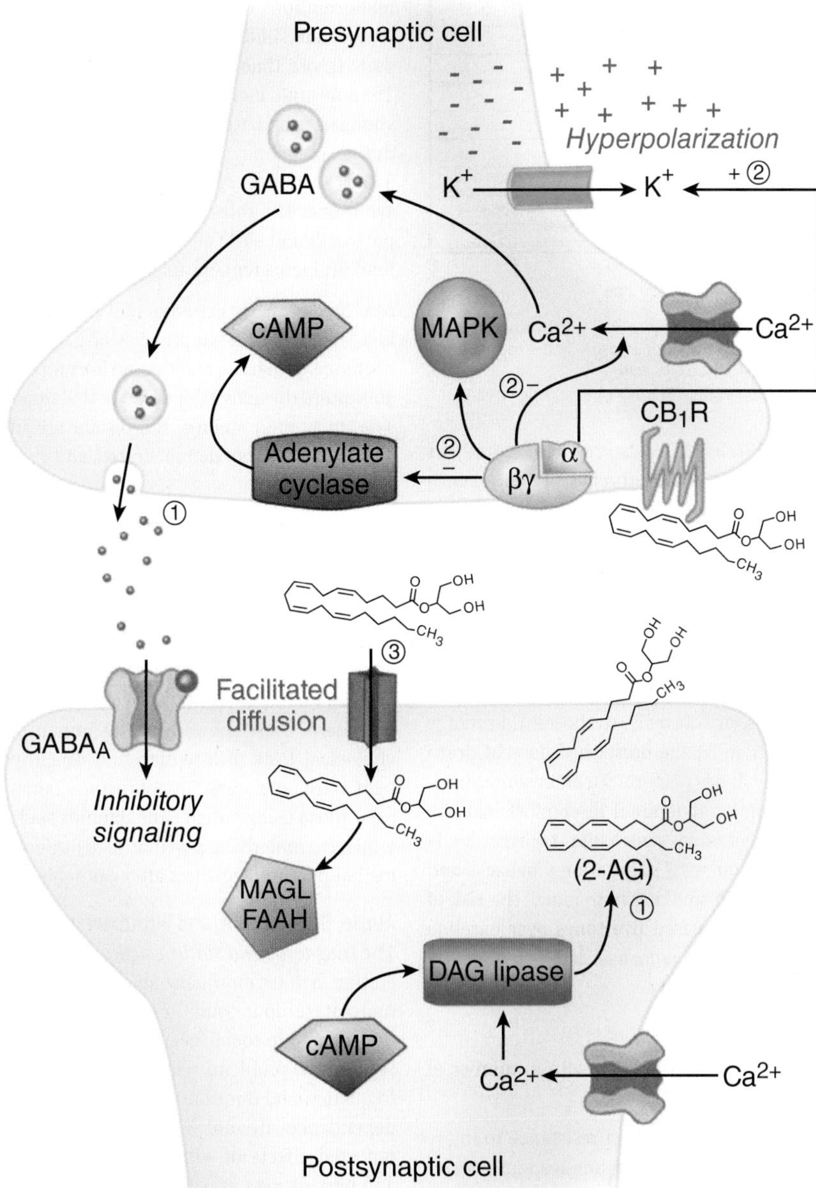


**FIGURE 47–1.** Endocannabinoids act as allosteric cellular messengers. ① In response to presynaptic γ-aminobutyric acid (GABA) release and postsynaptic binding resulting in increased cyclic adenosine monophosphate (cAMP), endocannabinoids are synthesized on demand and bind to presynaptic cannabinoid receptors. ② Activation of these G protein receptors results in decreased presynaptic adenylate cyclase, decreased cAMP, decreased calcium ion influx, and increased potassium efflux. The net results are hyperpolarization of the presynaptic cell and decreased neurotransmitter release. ③ After binding, endocannabinoids diffuse back to the postsynaptic area, where they undergo degradation by monoacylglycerol lipase (MAGL) and fatty acid amide hydrolase (FAAH). 2-AG = 2-arachidonoylglycerol; $CB_1R$ = cannabinoid type$_1$ receptor; DAG lipase = diacylglycerol lipase; MAPK = mitogen-activated protein kinase. *(Adapted from Seely KA, Prather PL, James LP, et al. Marijuana-based drugs: innovative therapeutics or designer drugs of abuse? Mol Interv. 2011 Feb;11(1):36-51.)*

postural hypotension, inability to concentrate, decreased psychomotor activity, slurred speech, and slow reaction time also occur. In young children, the acute ingestion produces obtundation that is sometimes accompanied by apnea, cyanosis, bradycardia, hypotonia, and opisthotonus.

The acute toxicity profile of nonclassical SCs stands in stark contrast to the relatively mild effects of smoked or ingested phytocannabinoid products. Agitation and seizures are reported. Psychosis (new onset, acute exacerbation of existing psychiatric disorders, and increased risk of psychosis relapse) and anxiety have resulted after a single dose. Tachycardia is common and some tachydysrhythmias require cardioversion. Chest pain and increased troponin concentrations also occur. Diffuse pulmonary infiltrates and dyspnea requiring intubation and mechanical ventilation were reported in a habitual SC user. Case reports of acute kidney injury

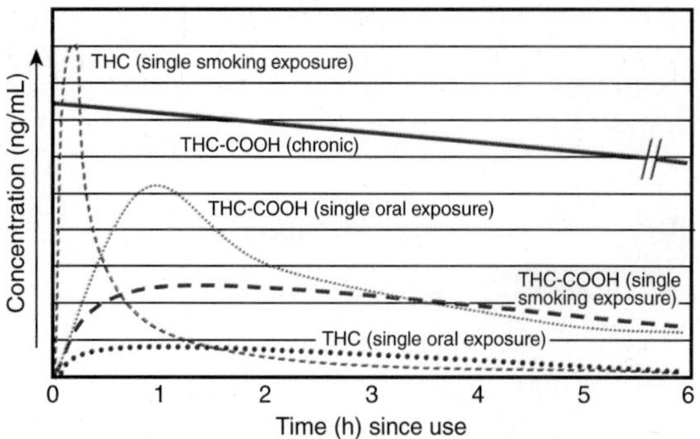


**FIGURE 47–2.** Estimated relative time course of Δ⁹-tetrahydrocannabinol (THC) and its major metabolite in the urine based on the route of exposure. THC-COOH = Δ⁹ THC carboxylic acid.

are described. Cerebral ischemia is also reported. Some SCs are likely responsible for several outbreaks of somnolence and bradycardia. This stands in contrast to earlier generations of SCs users who presented with sympathomimetic-like symptoms.

## ADVERSE REACTIONS

### Acute Use

Cannabis users occasionally experience distrust, dysphoria, fear, panic reactions, or transient psychoses. Commonly reported adverse reactions at the prescribed dose of dronabinol or nabilone include postural hypotension, dizziness, sedation, xerostomia, abdominal discomfort, nausea, and vomiting. Life-threatening ventricular tachycardia is reported. Atrial fibrillation with palpitations, nausea, and dizziness is associated with smoking marijuana. The risk of myocardial infarction is increased five times over baseline in the 60 minutes after marijuana use, but subsequently declines rapidly to baseline risk levels.

### Chronic Use

Long-term use of cannabis is associated with a number of adverse effects.

***Immune System.*** Cannabinoids affect host resistance to infection by modulating the secondary immune response (macrophages, T and B lymphocytes, acute phase and immune cytokines). However, an immune-mediated health risk from using cannabis is not currently recognized.

***Respiratory System.*** Chronic use of smoked marijuana is associated with clinical findings compatible with obstructive lung disease. Smoking marijuana delivers more particulates to the lower respiratory tract than does smoking tobacco, and marijuana smoke contains carcinogens similar to tobacco smoke. It is unclear whether marijuana use is associated with respiratory cancer.

***Cardiovascular System.*** Marijuana use is a risk for individuals with coronary artery disease. Patients who use marijuana are at significantly increased risk for cardiovascular and noncardiovascular mortality.

***Reproductive System.*** Reduced fertility in chronic users is a result of oligospermia, abnormal menstruation, and decreased ovulation. No definitive patterns of congenital malformations are recognized. No detrimental effects were reported in children born to women who smoked marijuana daily (more than 21 cigarettes per week) in rural Jamaica. Tremors and increased startling were reported in infants younger than 1 week of age whose mothers used cannabis during pregnancy. These findings, which persisted beyond 3 days, were not associated with other signs of a withdrawal syndrome. The role of secondhand exposure to cannabis on postnatal and early childhood development of neurobehavioral problems remains unstudied.

***Endocrine System.*** In experimental animals, cannabis exposure is associated with suppression of gonadal steroids, growth hormone, prolactin, and thyroid hormone. In addition, cannabis alters the activity of the hypothalamic-pituitary-adrenal axis. In human studies, the results are inconsistent, long-term effects are not demonstrated, and clinical consequences are undefined.

***Neurobehavioral Effects.*** There is a concern that chronic cannabis use results in deficits in cognition and learning that last well after cannabis use has stopped. Adults who used cannabis more than seven times per week had impairments in math skills, verbal expression, and memory retrieval processes; people who used cannabis one to six times per week showed no impairments. After 1 day of abstinence, 65 heavy marijuana users showed greater impairment on neuropsychological tests of attention and executive functions than light marijuana users. Patients using cannabinoids at younger ages, those using potent cannabinoids such as SCs, and those who have underlying psychiatric disorders are more likely to exhibit psychotic features after cannabinoid exposure.

### Abuse, Dependence, and Withdrawal

The *Diagnostic and Statistical Manual of Mental Disorders*, 5th edition, defines marijuana abuse as repeated instances of use under hazardous conditions; repeated, clinically meaningful impairment in social, occupational, or educational functioning; or legal problems related to marijuana use. The amount, frequency, and duration of cannabis use required to develop dependence are not well established. The most reliably reported effects of withdrawal are irritability, restlessness, and nervousness as well as appetite and sleep disturbances. The duration of withdrawal manifestations, without treatment, is not clearly established.

***Cannabinoid Hyperemesis Syndrome.*** Chronic, heavy marijuana use is associated with a clinical syndrome cannabinoid hyperemesis syndrome (CHS) composed of abdominal discomfort, nausea, and hyperemesis. Symptoms are often refractory to opioids and antiemetics. Patients typically have multiple visits to the emergency department and are subjected to a host of diagnostic and therapeutic modalities ranging from computed tomography scans and endoscopy to cholecystectomy. Many patients report an almost immediate relief of symptoms with bathing or showering in hot water. The pathophysiology of this syndrome is unclear. Endogenous cannabinoids demonstrate increased binding affinity for other G protein receptors such as transient receptor potential cation channel subfamily V member 1 ($TPRV_1$). Relief with hot water may indicate dysfunction of pain perception, excess substance P release, and involvement of $TRPV_1$, and these factors may assist in elucidating the mechanism for this syndrome as well as providing new treatment modalities. This hypothesis is supported by reports of successful treatment of CHS with topical capsaicin. Ultimately, resolution of this syndrome depends on cessation of marijuana use.

Reports also exist of successful CHS treatment with benzodiazepines, dopamine antagonists, and substance P inhibitors. Current evidence suggests that haloperidol is superior to these other therapies. Upon discharge, patients should be educated that the syndrome will likely return if the individual continues to use cannabinoids, and full resolution of symptoms should take place in 10 to 14 days.

## CANNABIS AND DRIVING

In experimental driving studies, cannabis impairs driving ability, but cannabis-using drivers recognize their impairment and compensate for it by driving at slower speeds and increasing following distance. However, the slower reaction time caused by cannabis results in impaired emergency response behavior. One study comparing past driving records of subjects entering a drug treatment center with control participants found that a self-reported history of cannabis use was associated with a statistically significant increase in adjusted relative risk for all crashes (relative risk, 1.49; 95% confidence interval {CI}, 1.17–1.89) and for "at fault" crashes (relative risk, 1.68; 95% CI, 1.21–2.34).

## DIAGNOSTIC TESTING

Cannabinoids can be detected in plasma or urine. Immunoassays are routinely available; gas chromatography–mass spectrometry (GC-MS) is the most specific assay and is considered the reference method. Enzyme-multiplied immunoassay technique (EMIT) is a qualitative urine test that is often used for screening purposes. Enzyme-multiplied immunoassay technique identifies the metabolites of THC. The US National Institute on Drug Abuse guidelines for urine testing specify test cutoff concentrations of 50 ng/mL for screening and 15 ng/mL for confirmation. Qualitative urine test results do not indicate or measure toxicity or degree of exposure.

Using GC-MS, metabolites are typically detected in the urine up to 7 days after the use of a single marijuana cigarette. The length of time between stopping cannabis use and a negative EMIT urine test result (< 20 ng/mL) depends on the extent of use. Release of THC from adipose tissue is important in drug test interpretation because many chronic users release cannabinoids in quantities sufficient to result in positive urine test results for several weeks. In light users being tested daily under observed abstinence, the mean time to the first negative urine test result is 8.5 days (range, 3–18 days), and the mean time to the last positive urine is 18.2 days (range, 7–34 days). In heavy users being tested under the same conditions, the mean time to the first negative urine test result (EMIT assay < 20 ng/mL) was 19.1 days (range, 3–46 days), and the mean time to the last positive urine sample was 31.5 days (range, 4–77 days).

Immunoassays give false-negative and false-positive test results (Table 47–1). To help identify evidence tampering, negative urine immunoassays should be accompanied by examining the urine for clarity and measuring urinary specific gravity, pH, temperature, and creatinine. Immunoassays for THC will not detect nonclassical SCs or their metabolites.

**TABLE 47–1 Xenobiotics or Conditions Reported to Produce Inaccurate Screening Test Results for Tetrahydrocannabinol**

| *False Negative*[a] | *False Positive* |
|---|---|
| Bleach (NaOCl) | Dronabinol |
| Citric acid | Efavirenz |
| Detergent additives | Ethacrynic acid |
| Dettol | Hemp seed oil |
| Dilution | Nonsteroidal antiinflammatory drugs |
| Glutaraldehyde | Promethazine |
| Lemon juice | Riboflavin |
| Niacin | |
| Potassium nitrite ($KNO_2$) | |
| Table salt (NaCl) | |
| Tetrahydrozoline | |
| Vinegar (acetic acid) | |
| Water | |

[a]Xenobiotics "possibly" producing false-negative urine test results are usually added to a urine sample, not ingested.

### Passive Inhalation

Multiple studies demonstrate that under tightly controlled conditions in fixed spaces with large amounts of smoke, passive inhalation can result in a positive urine test. However, in real-world scenarios, passive inhalation of marijuana smoke is unlikely to result in positive urine test results unless the exposure is substantial.

### Saliva

Saliva samples are used to establish the presence of cannabinoids and time of cannabis consumption. Cannabinoids (THC, THC-COOH, 11-OH-THC) in saliva are derived from either the smoke of the marijuana or hashish or from a preliminary metabolism in the mouth. Saliva THC concentrations above 10 ng/mL are consistent with recent use and correlate with subjective toxicity and heart rate changes.

### Hair

Hair sample analysis is not useful in identifying THC or its metabolites. Only small quantities of non–nitrogen-containing substances, such as cannabinoids, are found in hair pigments.

### Sweat

Perspiration deposits drug metabolites on the skin, and these are renewed even after the skin is washed. Detection threshold is reported to be 10 ng/mL, but forensic confirmation by alternative means is required.

### Estimating Time of Exposure

A measurable serum concentration of THC is consistent with recent exposure and toxicity, but there is poor correlation between serum THC concentrations and actual clinical effects. The ratio of THC to THC-COOH is used to estimate time of smoking marijuana. Similar concentrations of each indicate cannabis use within 20 to 40 minutes and imply toxicity. In naïve users, a concentration of THC-COOH that is greater than THC indicates that use probably occurred more than 30 minutes ago. The high background concentrations of THC-COOH in habitual users make estimations of time of exposure unreliable in this population.

## MANAGEMENT

Gastrointestinal (GI) decontamination is not recommended for patients who ingest cannabis products, nabilone, dronabinol, or nonclassical SCs because clinical toxicity is rarely serious and responds to supportive care. In addition, a patient with a significantly altered mental status, such as somnolence, agitation, or anxiety, has risks associated with GI decontamination that outweigh the potential benefits of the intervention.

There are no specific antidotes for cannabis or SC toxicity. We recommend that agitation, anxiety, seizures, or transient psychotic episodes be treated with a low-sensory environment, reassurance, and benzodiazepines (midazolam 1–2 mg either intramuscularly or intravenously, or diazepam 5–10 mg intravenously) as needed. The management of patients exposed to SCs should not be expected to mirror that of THC or prescription THC-based cannabinoids. Symptomatic and supportive care is often necessary.

Laboratory evaluation should be initiated for signs of electrolyte disturbances and direct toxicity of the CNS, cardiovascular, renal, and musculoskeletal systems. Appropriate crystalloid fluid resuscitation should be given for rhabdomyolysis and acute kidney injury.

Antipsychotics are not recommended at this time during any phase of undifferentiated agitated delirium. If psychotic features persist after the resolution of sympathomimetic features, a quiet space with close observation is indicated, and antipsychotic medications are reasonable if resolution is prolonged. Patients should be observed until asymptomatic.

# 48 COCAINE

## HISTORY AND EPIDEMIOLOGY

Cocaine is contained in the leaves of *Erythroxylum coca* (coca plant), a shrub that grows abundantly in Colombia, Peru, Bolivia, the West Indies, and Indonesia. As early as the sixth century, the inhabitants of Peru chewed or sucked on the leaves for social and religious reasons. In the 1100s, the Incas used cocaine-filled saliva as local anesthesia for ritual trephinations of the skull. In 1859, Albert Niemann isolated cocaine as the active ingredient of the plant. Europeans were introduced to cocaine in 1884, when the Austrian ophthalmologist Karl Koller described cocaine as an effective local anesthetic for eye surgery. Koller's colleague, Sigmund Freud, wrote extensively on the psychoactive properties of cocaine. Within a few years, reports of cocaine toxicity appeared in medical journals. Recreational cocaine use was legal in the United States (US) until the passage of the Harrison Narcotics Act of 1914. Currently, cocaine is an approved pharmaceutical with limited use in otolaryngology.

## PHARMACOLOGY

The alkaloid form of cocaine, benzoylmethylecgonine, is a weak base that is relatively insoluble in water. It is extracted from the leaf by mechanical degradation in the presence of a hydrocarbon, such as gasoline. The resulting product is converted into a hydrochloride salt to yield a white powder, cocaine hydrochloride, which is very water soluble. Cocaine hydrochloride is used by insufflation, application topically to mucous membranes, injection after dissolution in water, or ingestion; however, it degrades rapidly when pyrolyzed. Smokable cocaine (crack) is formed by dissolving cocaine hydrochloride in water and adding a strong base, such as sodium bicarbonate. A hydrocarbon solvent is added, the cocaine base is extracted into the organic phase, and then evaporated. The term "free-base" refers to the use of cocaine base in solution.

Cocaine is rapidly absorbed after all routes of exposure. Bioavailability when smoking cocaine exceeds 90% and is approximately 80% after nasal application. Table 48–1 lists the typical onsets and durations of action for various routes of cocaine use. After absorption, cocaine is approximately 90% bound to plasma proteins, primarily $\alpha_1$-acid glycoprotein, and reaches a final volume of distribution of 1.6 to 2.7 L/kg. The metabolism of cocaine is complex and dependent on both genetic and acquired factors. Three major pathways of cocaine metabolism are well described (Fig. 48–1). Cocaine undergoes *N*-demethylation in the liver to form norcocaine, a minor metabolite in humans that rarely accounts for more than 5% of drug. Norcocaine readily crosses the blood–brain barrier and produces clinical effects in animals that are quite similar to cocaine. Nearly half of a dose of cocaine is both nonenzymatically and enzymatically hydrolyzed to form benzoylecgonine (BE). BE is most likely a potent vasoconstrictor with limited ability to traverse the blood–brain barrier. Finally, plasma cholinesterase (PChE) and other esterases metabolize cocaine to ecgonine methyl ester (EME). In normal individuals, between 32% and 49% of cocaine is metabolized to EME. Similar to BE, EME crosses the blood–brain barrier poorly and in animals is a vasodilator, sedative, anticonvulsant, and protective metabolite against lethal doses of cocaine. Genetic or acquired alterations in PChE activity modulate the effects of cocaine. Patients with low PChE activity demonstrate increased sensitivity to cocaine, findings that are corroborated in multiple animal models.

Ethanol has a unique pharmacologic interaction with cocaine. A transesterification reaction between the two drugs produces ethylbenzoylecgonine, which is also called "ethyl cocaine" or "cocaethylene" (CE). In human volunteers given cocaine and ethanol, CE accounted for approximately 17% of

**TABLE 48–1 Pharmacology of Cocaine by Various Routes of Administration**

| *Route of Exposure* | *Onset of Action (min)* | *Peak Action (min)* | *Duration of Action (min)* |
|---|---|---|---|
| Intravenous | < 1 | 3–5 | 30–60 |
| Nasal insufflation | 1–5 | 20–30 | 60–120 |
| Smoking | < 1 | 3–5 | 30–60 |
| Gastrointestinal | 30–60 | 60–90 | 30–140 |

Data from Jeffcoat AR, Perez-Reyes M, Hill JM, et al. Cocaine disposition in humans after intravenous injection, nasal insufflation (snorting), or smoking. *Drug Metab Dispos*. 1989;17(2):153-159 and Van Dyke C, Jatlow P, Ungerer J, et al. Oral cocaine: plasma concentrations and central effects. *Science*. 1978;200(4338):211-213.

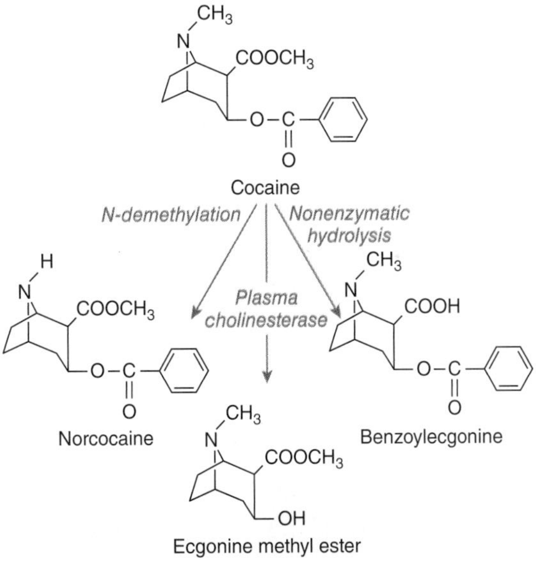

**FIGURE 48–1.** Metabolism of cocaine. The three principal metabolic pathways of cocaine are depicted.

the metabolites. Cocaethylene has a longer duration of action than cocaine and similar neurotoxic and cardiotoxic effects.

## PATHOPHYSIOLOGY

### Neurotransmitter Effects

Cocaine blocks the reuptake of biogenic amines such as serotonin and the catecholamines dopamine, norepinephrine, and epinephrine. Based on animal models, dopamine is responsible for psychomotor agitation, tachycardia emanates from adrenally derived epinephrine, and hypertension results from neuronally derived norepinephrine. Serotonin is an important modulator of dopamine and has a role in cocaine addiction, reward, and seizures.

Although much emphasis is placed on the reuptake blockade of these biogenic amines, it is clear that this effect is insufficient to account for the clinical manifestations of cocaine toxicity. Rather, the primary effect is central nervous system (CNS) excitation mediated through excitatory amino acids. Because experimental evidence in animals and clinical experience in humans demonstrate that sedation treats both the central effects of cocaine and the peripheral effects of biogenic amines, the model in Figure 48–2 best explains acute toxicity.

### Cardiovascular Effects

Cocaine use is associated with myocardial ischemia and myocardial infarction (MI). The increased risk of MI results from several different mechanisms, including hypertension and tachycardia with resultant increase in myocardial oxygen demand, vasospasm resulting in decreased coronary artery blood flow, oxidative stress, accelerated atherogenesis, and hypercoagulability.

***Vasospasm.*** Although increased myocardial oxygen demand is sufficient to cause ischemia in some individuals, it is clear that cocaine also produces profound vasoconstriction. Nicotine, which is simultaneously used by many cocaine users, has additive, if not synergistic, effects with cocaine.

***Oxidative Stress.*** Chronic exposure to elevated concentrations of catecholamines in the context of repetitive cocaine use results in the formation of reactive oxygen species and oxidation products known as "aminochromes" that directly damage myocardial cells. Evidence suggests that this pathophysiologic pathway is important in the development of cocaine-induced cardiomyopathy.

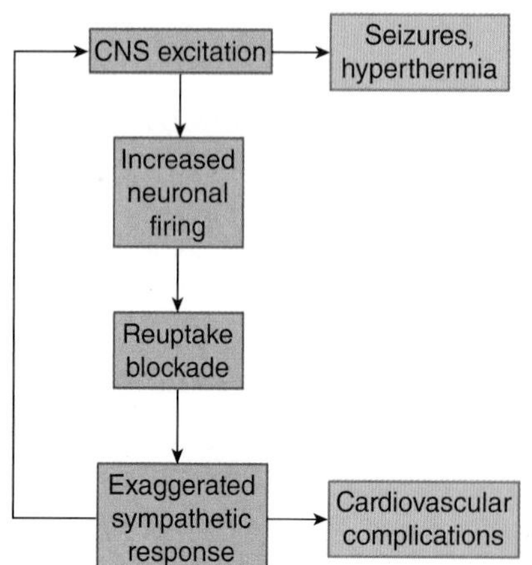


**FIGURE 48–2.** Cocaine-induced central nervous system (CNS) effects modulate peripheral events.

***Atherogenesis.*** Cocaine use accelerates atherosclerosis in experimental animals. In human endothelial cells, cocaine directly increases the permeability to lipids by altering tight junctions, which is hypothesized to promote the formation of subendothelial atherosclerotic plaques.

***Dysrhythmias.*** Like other local anesthetics (Chap. 37), cocaine blocks neuronal sodium channels, thereby preventing saltatory conduction. Because of homology between neuronal and cardiac sodium channels, cocaine also inhibits the rapid inward $Na^+$ current responsible for phase 0 depolarization of the cardiac action potential (Chap. 41). Like many sodium channel blockers, binding is both pH and use dependent such that binding increases as pH falls or heart rate increases (Chap. 41). Consequently, cocaine can be characterized as a Vaughan-Williams class 1C antidysrhythmic (Chap. 30). Cocaine and CE also block cardiac potassium channels. This results in QT interval prolongation and increases the risk of torsade de pointes.

### Hematologic Effects

Enhanced coagulation and impaired thrombolysis compound the effects of accelerated atherogenesis and vasospasm. Cocaine activates human platelets to initiate clotting and enhances the activity of plasminogen activator inhibitor type 1 (PAI-1), thereby impairing clot lysis.

### Pulmonary Effects

***Bronchospasm.*** The association between cocaine use and asthma was not recognized until smoking cocaine became prevalent. Although it is possible that bronchospasm results from direct administration of cocaine to the airways, inhaled contaminants of cocaine, or thermal insult are also possible causes. Additionally, the unique pyrolytic metabolite of cocaine, anhydroecgonine methyl ester, is a muscarinic agonist that produces bronchospasm in experimental animals.

## CLINICAL MANIFESTATIONS

Immediate clinical effects are associated with the sympathetic overactivity, and their duration of effect is predictable based on the pharmacokinetics of cocaine use. Other manifestations, such as those associated with tissue ischemia, often present in a delayed fashion, with a clinical latency of hours to even days after last cocaine use. The reasons for this delay are not clear but may relate to the presence of an altered sensorium associated with acute cocaine use.

Varying degrees of hypertension, tachycardia, tachypnea, and hyperthermia occur. Although any of these vital sign abnormalities can be life threatening, experimental and clinical evidence suggests that hyperthermia is the most critical. Initially with any dose and after a massive dose, apnea, hypotension, and bradycardia can result, all from direct suppression (anesthesia) of brainstem centers. These effects are fleeting and rarely noted when patients present to a healthcare facility as either the sympathetic overdrive rapidly ensues or sudden death results. Additional sympathomimetic findings include mydriasis, diaphoresis, and neuropsychiatric manifestations.

### Central Nervous System

Seizures, coma, headache, focal neurologic signs or symptoms, or behavioral abnormalities that persist longer than the predicted duration of effect of cocaine should alert the clinician to a potential catastrophic CNS event. Hemorrhage occurs at any anatomic site in the CNS. Both vasospastic infarction and transient ischemic attack are reported in association with cocaine use.

### Eyes, Nose, and Throat

Sympathetic excess produces mydriasis through stimulation of the dilator fibers of the iris with characteristic retention of the ability to respond to light. Like other mydriatics, cocaine produces acute narrow angle-closure glaucoma. Vasospasm of the retinal vessels causes both unilateral and bilateral loss of vision. Cocaine also produces corneal anesthesia but is highly toxic to the corneal epithelium. The loss of eyebrow and eyelash hair from thermal injury associated with smoking crack cocaine is called madarosis.

Chronic intranasal insufflation of cocaine produces perforation of the nasal septum. Angioedema and oropharyngeal burns, located as far distally as the esophagus, are associated with smoking crack cocaine.

### Pulmonary

Pneumothorax, pneumomediastinum, and pneumopericardium are reported after both smoked and intranasal cocaine use. After insufflation or inhalation, the user commonly performs a Valsalva maneuver in an attempt to retain the drug. Bearing down against a closed epiglottis increases intrathoracic pressure, and an alveolar bleb ruptures against the pleural, mediastinal, or pericardial surfaces.

Cocaine use exacerbates reversible airways disease, and it is common for patients to present with shortness of breath and wheezing. "Crack lung" is the term given to an acute pulmonary syndrome that occurs after inhalational use of crack cocaine. The syndrome is a poorly defined constellation of symptoms, including fever, hemoptysis, hypoxia, acute respiratory distress syndrome, and respiratory failure. It is associated with diffuse alveolar and interstitial infiltrates on chest radiography.

Vasospasm and subsequent thrombosis of the pulmonary artery or its branches can produce pulmonary infarction. Patients present with shortness of breath and pleuritic chest pain characteristic of a pulmonary embolus.

### Cardiovascular

Chest pain or discomfort is a common emergency department complaint in cocaine users. Cocaine use is associated with cardiac ischemia and infarction in young people and reportedly accounts for as much as 25% of MIs in patients younger than 45 years of age. Although MI is of concern, only approximately 6% of patients with complaints referable to the heart manifest biochemical evidence of myocardial injury. The cardiovascular differential diagnosis also includes aortic dissection, coronary artery dissection, and dysrhythmias.

Catecholamine-induced direct myocardial toxicity contributes to both acute and chronic cardiac disease. Takotsubo cardiomyopathy is thought to result from catecholamine toxicity on the myocardium during high levels of stress and is also reported after cocaine use. Chronic cocaine use is associated with a dilated cardiomyopathy, which is presumed to be the result of repeated subclinical ischemic events. Patients typically present with signs and symptoms of congestive heart failure or pulmonary edema.

### Abdominal

Cocaine users have a disproportionate incidence of perforated ulcers. Vasospasm produces ischemic colitis that presents with abdominal pain or bloody stools. More severe vasospasm, with or without thrombosis, leads to intestinal infarction with associated hypotension and metabolic acidosis. Signs and symptoms of bowel obstruction, such as vomiting or distension, might suggest body packing (gastrointestinal drug smuggling). Although less common, splenic and renal infarctions also occur.

### Musculoskeletal

Rhabdomyolysis is common in all conditions that produce an agitated delirium and/or hyperthermia; cocaine is no exception. Unlike most other toxicologic disorders, however, psychomotor agitation is not a prerequisite for cocaine-associated rhabdomyolysis. Muscle injury also results from either vasospasm or direct muscle toxicity; however, the exact mechanism remains unclear.

### Neuropsychiatric

The neuropsychiatric effects of cocaine are most likely dose dependent. Low-dose administration produces alertness, exhilaration, and hypersexual. As the cocaine dose increases, agitation, aggressive behavior, confusion, disorientation, and hallucinations develop. Other possible manifestations include a variety of movement disorders that most likely result from dysregulation of dopamine. Some patients develop acute dystonias or choreoathetoid movements that are referred to as "crack dancing."

### Obstetric

Acute cocaine use during pregnancy is associated with abruptio placentae, causing patients to present with abdominal pain and vaginal bleeding. The remaining maternal and fetal complications comprise every possible complication described in nonpregnant patients.

## DIAGNOSTIC TESTING

Cocaine and BE, its principal metabolite, can be detected in blood, urine, saliva, hair, and meconium. Routine drug of abuse testing relies on urine testing using a variety of immunologic techniques. Although cocaine is rapidly eliminated within just a few hours of use, BE is easily detected in the urine for 2 to 3 days after last use. When more sophisticated testing methodology is applied to chronic users, cocaine metabolites are identified for 2 to 3 weeks after the last use.

Urine testing, even using rapid point-of-care assays, offers little to clinicians managing patients with presumed cocaine toxicity because it cannot distinguish recent from remote cocaine use. The greatest benefit for cocaine testing is in cases of unintentional poisoning or suspected child abuse and neglect. Here confirmation of a clinical suspicion is essential to support a legal argument. In addition, there is a role for urine testing of body packers, especially when the concealed xenobiotic is unknown. Although many body packers have negative urine throughout their hospitalizations, a positive urine test result is suggestive of the concealed drug but obviously not confirmatory. More important, a conversion from a negative study on admission to a positive study not only confirms the substance ingested but also suggests packet leakage, which could be a harbinger of life-threatening toxicity (Special Considerations: SC4). Another indication for urine testing for cocaine occurs in young patients with chest pain syndromes in whom the history of drug use, specifically cocaine, is not forthcoming.

Routine diagnostic tests such as a bedside rapid reagent glucose, electrolytes, renal function tests, and markers of skeletal muscle and cardiac muscle injury are more likely to be useful than urine drug screening. Occasionally, the electrocardiogram (ECG) will show signs of ischemia or infarction or dysrhythmias that require specific therapy. Because the ECG has poor sensitivity and specificity, cardiac markers are always required adjuncts when considering myocardial ischemia or MI.

## CESSATION OF USE

A cocaine withdrawal syndrome is not reported. After binge use of cocaine, a "washed-out" syndrome occurs that is best explained by dopamine depletion. Patients complain of anhedonia and lethargy, and they have trouble initiating and sustaining movement. However, they are arousable with minimal stimulation and usually remain cognitively intact.

Symptoms typically associated with cocaine toxicity sometimes present in a delayed fashion after cessation of cocaine use. The reasons for this delay are multifactorial and not entirely apparent but are presumed to be related to prolonged elimination of metabolites such as CE; changes in receptor regulation; or effects on platelets, coagulation, and thrombolysis that stimulate a slow cascade, leading to thrombosis.

## MANAGEMENT

### General Supportive Care

As in the case of all poisoned patients, the initial emphasis should be on stabilization and control of the patient's airway, breathing, and circulation. If tracheal intubation is required, it is important to recognize that cocaine toxicity is a relative contraindication to the use of succinylcholine. Specifically, in the setting of rhabdomyolysis, hyperkalemia will be exacerbated by succinylcholine administration, and life-threatening dysrhythmias may result (Chap. 39). Additionally, PChE metabolizes both cocaine and succinylcholine. Thus, their simultaneous use will either prolong cocaine toxicity, paralysis, or both. If hypotension is present, the initial approach should be intravenous (IV) infusion of 0.9% sodium chloride solution because many patients are volume depleted as a result of poor oral intake and excessive fluid losses from uncontrolled agitation, diaphoresis, and hyperthermia. Administration of IV fluids and caloric supplementation are also important in patients with rhabdomyolysis secondary to cocaine-associated agitation and hyperthermia.

Determination of the core temperature is an essential element of the initial evaluation, even when patients are severely agitated. When hyperthermia is present, rapid cooling with ice water immersion is required to normalize core body temperature. Sedation or paralysis and intubation are often necessary to facilitate the rapid cooling process. We recommend not to use antipyretics, drugs that prevent shivering (chlorpromazine or meperidine), and dantrolene because they are ineffective and have the potential for adverse drug interactions such as serotonin toxicity (meperidine) (Chap. 9) or seizures (chlorpromazine).

Sedation remains the mainstay of therapy in patients with cocaine-associated agitation. Both animal models and extensive clinical experience in humans support the central role of benzodiazepines. Although the choice among individual benzodiazepines is not well studied, the goal is to use parenteral therapy with a drug that has a rapid onset and a rapid peak of action, making titration easy. Using this rationale, we recommend midazolam (IV or IM) and diazepam (only IV) over lorazepam. Drugs should be administered in initial doses that are consistent with routine practices and increased incrementally based on an appropriate understanding of their pharmacology. This may result from cocaine-induced alterations in benzodiazepine receptor function (Antidotes in Brief: A26). On the rare occasion when benzodiazepines fail to achieve an adequate level of sedation, it is reasonable to administer either a rapidly acting barbiturate or propofol.

After sedation is accomplished, often no additional therapy is required. Specifically, patients with hypertension and tachycardia usually respond to sedation and volume resuscitation. In the uncommon event that hypertension or tachycardia persists, a direct-acting vasodilator such as nitroglycerin, nicardipine, or an $\alpha$-adrenergic antagonist (eg, phentolamine) is recommended. The use of a $\beta$-adrenergic antagonist or a mixed $\alpha$- and $\beta$-adrenergic antagonists (eg. labetalol) in patients with acute cocaine toxicity is contraindicated because of unopposed $\alpha$-adrenergic agonism.

### Decontamination

The majority of patients who present to the hospital after cocaine use do not require GI decontamination because the most popular methods of cocaine use are smoking, IV, and intranasal administration. Less commonly, patients ingest cocaine unintentionally or in an attempt to conceal evidence during an arrest (body stuffing) or transport large quantities of drug across international borders (body packing). These patients often require intensive decontamination and possibly surgical removal (Special Considerations: SC4).

### Specific Management

In patients with end-organ manifestations of vasospasm that does not resolve with sedation, cooling, and volume resuscitation we recommend treatment with vasodilators (eg, phentolamine). Phentolamine is dosed IV in increments of 1 to 2.5 mg and repeated as necessary until symptoms resolve or systemic hypotension develops.

*Acute Coronary Syndrome.* In the setting of hypoxia, high-flow oxygen therapy is clearly indicated because it will help overcome some of the supply–demand mismatch that occurs with coronary insufficiency. Aspirin is likely safe in patients with cocaine-associated chest pain and is recommended for routine use. In addition, administration of morphine is likely to be effective because it relieves cocaine-induced vasoconstriction. Nitroglycerin is recommended because it reduces cocaine-associated coronary constriction of both normal and diseased vessels and relieves chest pain and associated symptoms. Interestingly, benzodiazepines are at least as effective or superior to nitroglycerin. Although the reasons for this are unclear, possible etiologies include blunting of central catecholamines or direct effects on cardiac benzodiazepine receptors. Either or both drugs are recommended in standard dosing.

Several studies in both animals and humans underscore the potential risks of β-adrenergic antagonism in the setting of acute cocaine toxicity. Mixed α- and β-adrenergic antagonists do not appear to offer any advantage in the treatment of patients with cocaine-associated coronary artery vasospasm. Despite these studies, β-adrenergic antagonists are frequently administered in the context of cocaine-associated chest pain for a variety of reasons, and several authors have argued in favor of their safety. They often fail to distinguish acute toxicity from chronic or remote use by including patients based on urine drug testing, suggest that adverse events are extremely rare, and point to the absence of any documented cases of severe adverse events with the administration of combined α- and β-adrenergic antagonists. Even if the frequency of severe adverse events is rare, no quality data currently support the efficacy of β-adrenergic antagonism in the context of acute cocaine use. Thus, we feel that in the setting of acute cocaine toxicity, β-adrenergic antagonism is contraindicated. The 2008 American Heart Association (AHA) guidelines for the treatment of cocaine-associated chest pain and MI state that use of β-adrenergic antagonists should be avoided in the acute setting. The 2014 AHA guidelines on the management of non–ST-segment elevation MI list β-adrenergic antagonists as class III (harm) because of the risk of potentiating coronary artery vasospasm.

There are no data on the use of unfractionated heparin (UFH) or low-molecular-weight heparins (LMWHs), glycoprotein IIb/IIIa inhibitors, or clopidogrel. The recent AHA guidelines recommend the administration of UFH or LMWH in patients with cocaine-associated MI. When acute thrombosis is likely, angiography and mechanical approaches to patency are recommended but thrombolytic therapy is reasonable if interventional cardiology is unavailable. Standard contraindications such as persistent hypertension, aortic dissection, trauma, and altered mental status must be considered before thrombolysis.

*Dysrhythmias.* Most patients present with sinus tachycardia that resolves after sedation, cooling, rehydration, and time to metabolize the drug. Other stable dysrhythmias should be treated similarly and often spontaneously revert because of the short duration of effect of cocaine. However, cocaine use is associated with atrial, supraventricular, and ventricular dysrhythmias, including torsade de pointes. Most notably, wide-complex tachycardias result from sodium channel blockade.

When approaching patients with cocaine-associated dysrhythmias, there are several important points to consider. The first is that β-adrenergic antagonism is contraindicated. Furthermore, class IA and IC antidysrhythmics are also contraindicated because of their ability to exacerbate cocaine-induced sodium and potassium channel blockade. Additionally, although popular in many advanced cardiac life support dysrhythmia algorithms, the effects of amiodarone are largely unknown in the setting of cocaine toxicity. Because of the lack of data demonstrating a benefit for amiodarone and because of concerns about its β-adrenergic antagonist effects, the use of this medication is not recommended at this time. Thus, for rapid atrial fibrillation and narrow-complex reentrant tachycardias, a calcium channel blocker such as diltiazem is reasonable. For wide-complex dysrhythmias, a trial of hypertonic sodium bicarbonate is recommended (Antidotes in Brief: A5). When the use of hypertonic sodium bicarbonate fails to treat the dysrhythmia, lidocaine is recommended.

*Ischemic Stroke.* The safety of thrombolysis in cocaine-associated ischemic stroke is uncertain. One study found no increase in intracerebral hemorrhage after administration of tissue plasminogen activator in patients who had recently used cocaine, although acute cocaine toxicity was not specifically investigated. When thrombosis is confirmed highly likely the use of thrombectomy or thrombolytic therapy is reasonable in cocaine-related stroke.

*Limb and Bowel Ischemia.* Only limited case reports address the management of patients with limb and bowel ischemia. Imaging is essential because it is important to try to distinguish thrombosis or embolus from vasospasm. If a discrete lesion is found, either angioplasty or thrombolysis is reasonable depending on institutional resources. Vasodilators such as phentolamine, nitroglycerin, and nicardipine and anticoagulation are also reasonable in an attempt to improve the low-flow state and prevent clot.

## ADULTERANTS

A variety of adulterants, contaminants, and diluents, collectively called "cutting agents," are present in cocaine. Adulterants are pharmacologically active substances intentionally added to enhance or mimic the effects of a drug. Diluents describe inert substances added to increase bulk, and contaminants describe unintentional by-products present as a result of impure manufacturing processes or drug storage. Historically, common cocaine adulterants included sympathomimetics and other local anesthetics. The adulterant levamisole is worth special mention. It is postulated that the addition of levamisole acts to both enhance and potentially lengthen the duration of effects of cocaine. Levamisole toxicity is associated with neutropenia, agranulocytosis, vasculitis, purpura, and more uncommonly, a multifocal inflammatory leukoencephalopathy characterized by cerebral demyelination and white matter lesions.

## DISPOSITION

Patients who present to healthcare facilities with classic sympathomimetic signs and symptoms that resolve spontaneously in the absence of signs of end-organ damage can be safely discharged after 4-6 hours of observation. When hyperthermia, rhabdomyolysis, or other signs of end-organ damage are evident, hospital admission is usually required. Patients with chest pain and clearly diagnostic or evolving ECGs suggestive of ischemia or infarction, positive cardiac biomarkers, dysrhythmias other than sinus tachycardia, congestive heart failure, or persistent pain require admission. Patients who become pain free and whose ECGs remain unchanged are candidates for discharge if a single cardiac marker obtained at least 8 hours after the onset of chest pain is normal. It is essential to provide a referral for substance use counseling. Repeated cocaine use is the greatest risk factor for future cardiovascular complications.

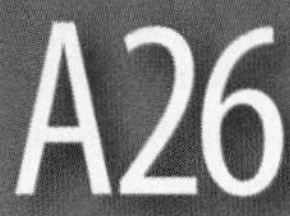

Antidotes in Brief

# A26 BENZODIAZEPINES

Benzodiazepines are sedative–hypnotics that are used broadly for a range of clinical indications, including xenobiotic-induced seizures, xenobiotic-induced psychomotor agitation, withdrawal from ethanol and other sedative–hypnotics, cocaine-associated myocardial ischemia, chloroquine overdose, and to induce muscle relaxation in serotonin toxicity, neuroleptic malignant syndrome, strychnine poisoning, and black widow spider envenomation. This Antidotes in Brief provides a summary of the clinical pharmacology of benzodiazepines and a review of their use in specific clinical scenarios, with an emphasis on specific drug selection and safe administration.

## HISTORY

The first benzodiazepine, chlordiazepoxide, was discovered serendipitously in 1957 as part of a search to develop safer and more marketable sedatives. The introduction of chlordiazepoxide in 1960 represented a major breakthrough in the field of psychopharmacology and ushered in an era of rapid development and widespread use of numerous other benzodiazepines.

## CHEMISTRY

All benzodiazepines share a common chemical structure. Modification of side chains of the structure leads to differences in lipophilicity, central nervous system (CNS) penetration, duration of action, potency, and rate of elimination. The nonbenzodiazepine hypnotics (zolpidem, zopiclone, and zaleplon) lack the typical benzodiazepine structure but have similar pharmacologic effects.

## γ-AMINOBUTYRIC ACID TYPE A RECEPTORS

Benzodiazepines bind to a specific site on the postsynaptic γ-aminobutyric acid type A ($GABA_A$) receptor. The $GABA_A$ receptor is a ligand-gated chloride channel that, when bound by the inhibitory neurotransmitter GABA, opens to allow an inward flux of negatively charged chloride ions. This results in membrane hyperpolarization and subsequent inhibition of neuronal excitability. When benzodiazepines bind to the $GABA_A$ receptor, the frequency of channel opening is increased in the presence of GABA, resulting in increased chloride ion influx and enhanced neuronal inhibition. In the absence of GABA, the benzodiazepines have no effect on chloride conductance.

The $GABA_A$ receptor is formed by five polypeptide subunits coded as either α, β, γ, δ, ε, θ, λ, or ρ, and at least 19 isoforms of these subunits (eg, $\alpha_{1-5}$) are identified. The most common pentamer is composed of two α subunits; two β subunits; and an additional subunit, most commonly $\gamma_2$. Different $GABA_A$ receptor subunit isoforms predominate in different areas of the CNS and confer distinct functional effects and pharmacologic properties.

## BENZODIAZEPINE RECEPTORS

### Central

The term "central benzodiazepine receptors" is used to refer to benzodiazepine binding sites on GABAergic neurons of the nervous system. The benzodiazepine binding site is located at the interface of an α and a γ subunit, most commonly an $\alpha_1$ and a $\gamma_2$ subunit (Fig. A26–1). The $\alpha_1$ isoform, located in the sensory and motor areas of the brain, mediates sedative and hypnotic effects. The $\alpha_2$, $\alpha_3$, and $\alpha_5$ isoforms are dispersed throughout the subcortical and limbic areas of the brain and mediate anxiolytic and antiepileptic effects. γ-Aminobutyric acid type A receptors that contain $\alpha_4$ and $\alpha_6$ subunits are insensitive to benzodiazepines and are of low prevalence in the brain.

Most benzodiazepines have substantial affinity for the $\alpha_1$, $\alpha_2$, $\alpha_3$, and $\alpha_5$ isoforms, which explains their combined sedative–hypnotic, anxiolytic, and anticonvulsant effects. In contrast, the nonbenzodiazepine hypnotics (eg, zolpidem) have high affinity for $\alpha_1$, intermediate affinity for $\alpha_2$ and $\alpha_3$, and low affinity for $\alpha_5$ isoforms, which explains their lack of antiepileptic effects.

### Peripheral (Tryptophan-Rich Sensory Protein)

The term "peripheral benzodiazepine receptor" (PBR) was originally used to define benzodiazepine binding sites

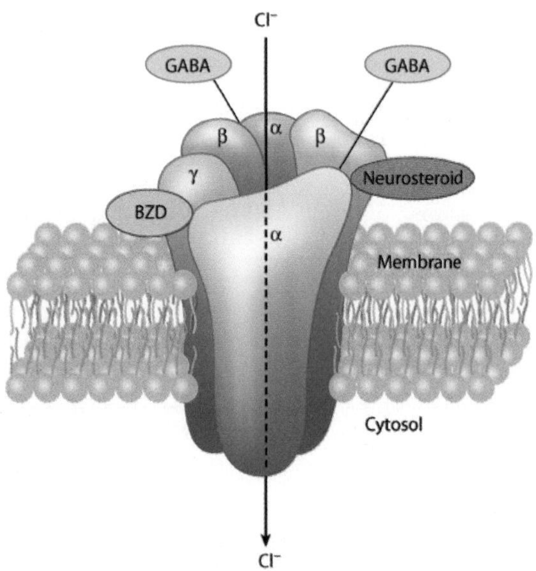


**FIGURE A26–1.** The γ-aminobutyric acid type A ($GABA_A$) chloride ($Cl^-$) channel. The figure demonstrates a typical configuration of the $GABA_A$ $Cl^-$ channel, which consists of two α, two β, and one γ isoforms. The benzodiazepine (BZD) receptor is located between an α and a γ subunit. Neurosteroid binding at the opposite side of the α isoform is a positive allosteric modulator.

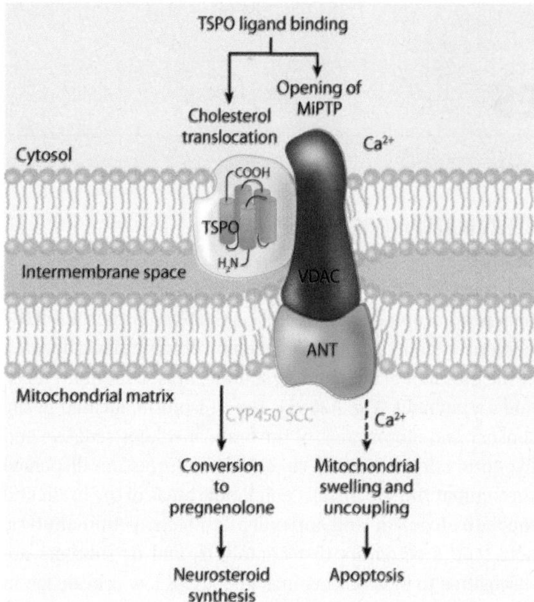


**FIGURE A26–2.** The "peripheral benzodiazepine receptor" has three main components: the tryptophan-rich sensory protein (TSPO; 18-kDa translocator protein), a voltage-dependent anion channel (VDAC), and an adenine nucleotide transporter (ANT), which are shown on the mitochondrial membrane. Stimulation of the TSPO can trigger influx of $Ca^{2+}$ or cholesterol across the mitochondrial membrane. MiPTP = mitochondrial permeability transition pore; SCC = side chain cleavage.

outside of the nervous system. However, it was subsequently discovered that this receptor was also expressed in CNS tissues and that it was the binding site for numerous other nonbenzodiazepine ligands. The PBR is currently called the "tryptophan-rich sensory protein" or TSPO. The TSPO, shown in Fig. A26–2, is hypothesized to have two major roles: opening of the mitochondrial permeability transition pore, leading to calcium influx and apoptosis, and, synthesis of neurosteroids that modulate $GABA_A$ function.

## PHARMACOKINETICS AND PHARMACODYNAMICS

This Antidotes in Brief focuses on the most commonly used parenteral benzodiazepines: diazepam, lorazepam, and midazolam. Clinically important pharmacologic parameters of these three benzodiazepines are listed in Table A26–1.

The intravenous (IV) route is preferred in critically ill patients because it guarantees immediate and complete absorption with a relatively rapid onset of action. Intraosseous (IO) delivery and the intramuscular (IM) route are usually acceptable when no IV access is present; however, the absorption of IM diazepam is slow, incomplete, and erratic, and therefore, it is recommended not to use IM injection of diazepam unless no other alternatives exist. These and other pharmacodynamic properties are outline in Table A26–2.

After being absorbed, benzodiazepines distribute into the CNS to produce their sedative and antiepileptic effects. Electroencephalographic (EEG) analysis was used as a surrogate for the pharmacodynamic effects of sedation. Peak EEG effects were present immediately at the end of the

**TABLE A26–1 Pharmacologic Properties of Select Benzodiazepines**

| *Parameter* | *Diazepam* | *Midazolam* | *Lorazepam* |
|---|---|---|---|
| Molecular weight (g/mol) | 284.7 | 325.78 | 321.2 |
| Oral bioavailability | > 90% | 40% | > 90% |
| Volume of distribution (healthy adults) (L/kg) | 0.89 ± 0.18 | 0.80 ± 0.19 | 1.28 ± 0.34 |
| Protein binding (%) | 97–99 | 96 | 85 |
| Lipid solubility (LogD; octanol/water at pH 7) | 3.86 | 3.68 | 2.48 |
| Hepatic metabolism | Phase 1 | Phase 1 | Phase 2 |
| Active metabolites | Yes (desmethyldiazepam and others) | Yes: α-hydroxymidazolam (10% of parent, but accumulates with chronic dosing) | No |
| Average dose (mg) in a 70-kg adult[a] | | | |
| Sedation | 10 mg IV over 2 min<br>Wait 2 min before redosing | 2 mg IV over > 2 min (maximum, 1.5 mg over > 2 min in older adult or debilitated patients), or 5–10 mg IM<br>Wait 2 min before IV redosing | 2 mg IV over 1 minute (dilute with equal volume of NS or $D_5W$ before injection)<br>Wait 15 min before redosing |
| Status epilepticus (initial dose) | 10 mg IV | 10 mg IM | 4 mg IV |
| Diluent(s) | Alcohol 10%<br>Benzyl alcohol 1.5%<br>Propylene glycol 40% | Benzyl alcohol 1%<br>Sodium edetate 1% | Benzyl alcohol 2%<br>Propylene glycol 80% |
| Formulations | 5 mg/mL<br>5 mg/mL (rectal gel) | 1 mg/mL<br>5 mg/mL | 2 mg/mL<br>4 mg/mL |

[a]Avoid intraarterial administration because severe spasm may occur with resulting ischemia or gangrene. Also avoid extravasation.

$D_5W$ = 5% dextrose in water; IV = intravenous; NS = 0.9% NaCl.

**TABLE A26–2 Relative Pharmacodynamic Properties of Benzodiazepines in Humans**

| | *Diazepam* | *Midazolam* | *Lorazepam* |
|---|---|---|---|
| ***Anticonvulsant*** | | | |
| Onset of action | | | |
| IV | Rapid (minutes) | Rapid (minutes) | Rapid (minutes) |
| IM | Not advisable | ~3 min | 9 min |
| IN | 3–5 min | 5 min | ~10 min |
| PR | 5–10 min | 10–20 min | 20 min |
| Duration of action | | | |
| IV | 1–2 h | 30–80 min | Many hours |
| IM | Unpredictable | 1–2 h | Many hours |
| ***Sedative*** | | | |
| Onset of action | | | |
| IV | 1–2 min | 1–2 min | 5–20 min |
| IM | Unpredictable | 5–10 min | 20–30 min |
| IN | 3–5 min | 5–10 min | ~10 min |
| Relative duration of action | | | |
| Single dose | Short | Short | Long |
| Repeated doses | Long (secondary to active metabolites) | Intermediate (secondary to active metabolites) | Long |

IM = intramuscular; IN = intranasal; IV = intravenous; PR = per rectum.

diazepam infusion but were delayed for 5 to 10 minutes after midazolam administration and 30 minutes after lorazepam administration (Table A26–3).

The presence of pharmacologically active metabolites prolongs the duration of action of select benzodiazepines, especially when repeated doses are administered. Diazepam, midazolam, and chlordiazepoxide produce active metabolites that prolong the clinical duration of effect. For older adult patients and those with hepatic failure, lorazepam is recommended to avoid prolonged effects of these active metabolites.

## ROLE OF BENZODIAZEPINES IN SELECT CLINICAL SCENARIOS

Many chapters in this text discuss the use of benzodiazepines as $GABA_A$ agonists in the management of poisoned patients (Chaps. 42, 46, 48, 50, 52, and 56). In contrast, the use of benzodiazepines as modulators of TSPOs for the treatment of poisoned patients is a more speculative but evolving field. As such, focused discussions of two additional xenobiotics, chloroquine (Chap. 28) and cocaine (Chap. 48), are warranted.

**TABLE A26–3 Selected Pharmacokinetic and Pharmacodynamic Properties of Intravenous Benzodiazepines**

| *Parameter* | *Diazepam (0.15 mg/kg)* | *Midazolam (0.1 mg/kg)* | *Lorazepam (0.045 mg/kg)* |
|---|---|---|---|
| Onset of EEG effect | Immediate | Immediate | Slow |
| Time to peak EEG effect (min) | 1 | 5–10 | 30 |
| Duration of EEG effect (h) | 5–6 | 2 | 8 |
| Elimination half-life (h) | 33 ± 5 | 2.8 ± 0.5 | 12 ± 2 |

EEG = electroencephalographic.

### Xenobiotic-Induced Seizures

Benzodiazepines are well-established as the initial treatment of choice for xenobiotic-induced seizures. Non—sedative–hypnotic antiepileptics such as phenytoin are ineffective in treating most xenobiotic-induced seizures and sometimes exacerbate toxicity, and therefore, they should be avoided.

Current data and clinical guidelines indicate that IV lorazepam or IM midazolam is preferred for rapid seizure cessation. A large multicenter, randomized, double-blind trial demonstrated that a dose of IM midazolam (10 mg) was at least as, if not more, effective than IV lorazepam (4 mg) for seizure cessation in the prehospital setting. If seizure control is not achieved promptly with rapidly escalating doses of benzodiazepines, second-line sedative–hypnotics such as phenobarbital or propofol are recommended along with appropriate management of airway, ventilation, and circulation. In refractory status epilepticus or if overdose of isoniazid or other hydrazine-containing compounds are suspected, high-dose pyridoxine should be administered (Chap. 29 and Antidotes in Brief: A15).

### Sedative–Hypnotic Withdrawal

Benzodiazepines were established almost 50 years ago as the first-line treatment of alcohol withdrawal. Since then, the benzodiazepines have also been used as the primary management of withdrawal from benzodiazepines, γ-hydroxybutyric acid (GHB) and GHB precursors 1,4-butanediol and γ-butyrolactone, as well as important adjuncts in the treatment of withdrawal from baclofen, gabapentin, and the nonbenzodiazepine hypnotics (eg, zolpidem, zopiclone).

Diazepam has favorable properties that make it a desirable first-line treatment for moderate to severe sedative–hypnotic withdrawal in which prolonged agitation is expected. The presence of active diazepam metabolites also confers a longer duration of therapeutic effect and an auto-tapering effect at the end of therapy. Oral chlordiazepoxide is commonly used in early uncomplicated alcohol withdrawal because of its long duration of action and active metabolites (Chap. 50).

### Psychomotor Agitation

In patients with extreme psychomotor agitation caused by sympathomimetic or other xenobiotic toxicity, IV diazepam or midazolam is recommended because of their rapid onset and rapid peak effects. When a short duration of sedation is anticipated, such as when treating a patient with toxicity after IV or inhaled use of cocaine, midazolam is recommended over diazepam because the duration of the effects of midazolam better matches the duration of effects of cocaine, thereby limiting oversedation when cocaine is rapidly metabolized. When difficult axis precludes rapid safe IV access, we recommend IM midazolam for the treatment of undifferentiated agitation.

### Chloroquine

Although chloroquine overdose is uncommon, case fatality rates are extremely high, and ingestion of 5 g or more was once considered universally fatal. However, in 1988, a case series was reported of patients with chloroquine overdose who survived with the use of a regimen consisting of early endotracheal intubation, high-dose epinephrine infusion, and IV diazepam (2 mg/kg over 30 minutes).

The mechanism of the beneficial cardiovascular effect of diazepam in chloroquine toxicity is unclear, but peripheral TSPO agonism possibly plays a role. Benzodiazepines, chloroquine, and experimental TSPO agonists share some structural elements, suggesting a receptor-based mechanism. Although the ideal regimen has not been defined, for patients with severe chloroquine or hydroxychloroquine toxicity, it is reasonable to administer high-dose diazepam at a dose of 2 mg/kg IV over 30 minutes followed by 1 to 2 mg/kg/day for 2 to 4 days.

### Cocaine-Associated Chest Pain

Patients who use cocaine frequently present to emergency departments with chest pain or signs or symptoms that could represent myocardial ischemia or infarction. Unlike most patients with acute cocaine toxicity, however, these patients often present hours after their last drug use and without the classic sympathomimetic findings of acute cocaine toxicity. Although the pathophysiology of cocaine-induced myocardial ischemia is complex and multifactorial (Chap. 48), one component of delayed myocardial ischemia likely results from the vasoconstrictive actions of benzoylecgonine, the principal long-acting metabolite of cocaine.

Chronic cocaine use is associated with an increased number of TSPOs on human platelets. Also, in experimental models of cardiac ischemia and reperfusion injury, TSPO agonists limit myocardial infarction size and improve cardiac function. This effect most likely occurs through inhibition of the opening of the mitochondrial permeability transition pore. Additionally, TSPO agonists directly antagonize the vasoconstrictive effects of norepinephrine in rat aortic tissue.

Benzodiazepines are commonly used to treat the agitation associated with sympathomimetic overdose (Chaps. 46 and 48). Although it is assumed that the normalization of vital signs results from a decrease in CNS stimulation and psychomotor agitation, it is reasonable to believe that the effects on TSPOs are contributory. In two randomized controlled studies, benzodiazepines were equivalent to nitroglycerin in improving chest pain. Thus, it is reasonable to administer IV lorazepam or diazepam as an adjunct to nitroglycerin therapy in patients with chest pain in the setting of recent cocaine use.

## ADVERSE EFFECTS AND SAFETY ISSUES

The most common adverse effects of benzodiazepines are CNS and respiratory depression. Although this is unavoidable in some cases, it is limited by selecting the optimal drug and the proper dose and dosing interval. Extra caution is advised in older adult patients because they are more sensitive, particularly to the sedative and respiratory depressant effects of midazolam. Additionally, patients with hepatic failure are at increased risk of adverse effects with diazepam or midazolam because of decreased drug clearance. For this reason, we recommend lorazepam in patients with cirrhosis. In contrast, paradoxical reactions rarely occur in which some patients become more agitated after benzodiazepine administration, particularly children. These infrequent reactions probably result from disinhibition and typically respond to larger doses of benzodiazepines. Although paradoxical agitation also responds to flumazenil (Antidotes in Brief: A25), we recommend against reversal when benzodiazepines are used for most toxicologic indications.

### Pregnancy and Lactation

Diazepam, lorazepam, and midazolam are labeled as United States Food and Drug Administration Pregnancy Category D. Since the risk to a fetus is likely negligible from short-term benzodiazepine administration in emergent situations, we recommend that benzodiazepines not be withheld in critically ill poisoned patients because of pregnancy status. Benzodiazepines are excreted into breast milk in very small quantities. It is thus reasonable to forgo breastfeeding (by discarding pumped breast milk, ie, "pumping and dumping") for several hours after a single IV dose or for 24 hours after repeated benzodiazepine dosing.

## DOSING AND ADMINISTRATION

When selecting a benzodiazepine, the pharmacokinetics and pharmacodynamics should be considered, along with existing clinical data. Onset of effect, peak effect, and duration of effect should be weighed in the context of the anticipated clinical course. Intravenous dosing is recommended for critically ill patients, although other routes such as IM, intranasal, or intraosseous are effective when IV access is unavailable or impractical. Benzodiazepines with rapid onset of action, such as diazepam or midazolam, are recommended when rapid symptom control is necessary. A long-acting benzodiazepine with active metabolites, such as diazepam, is recommended in cases of sedative–hypnotic withdrawal and ethanol withdrawal when prolonged symptoms are anticipated. Lorazepam is reasonable in patients with hepatic failure because of its relatively preserved clearance and lack of active metabolites.

Common equivalent initial IV doses in adults are: lorazepam 1 mg, diazepam 5 mg, and midazolam 2 mg. When repeated administration is necessary, appropriate spacing between doses is crucial to avoid oversedation and respiratory depression. Intravenous diazepam and midazolam can be safely administered every 2 to 5 minutes, but we recommend delaying lorazepam redosing by 15 minutes because of its slower time to peak effect.

## FORMULATION AND ACQUISITION

Multiple forms of parenteral benzodiazepines are available. Some formulations contain significant diluents (Table A26–1) large doses of which may result in toxicity (Chap. 19).

# 49 ETHANOL

## HISTORY AND EPIDEMIOLOGY

Ethanol, or ethyl alcohol, is commonly referred to as "alcohol." This term is somewhat misleading because there are numerous other alcohols. However, ethanol is one of the most commonly used and abused xenobiotics in the world. Its use is pervasive among adolescents and adults of all ages and socioeconomic groups and represents a tremendous financial and social cost. The ethanol content of alcoholic beverages is expressed by volume percent or by proof. In the United States (US), a proof spirit (100 proof) is one containing 50% ethanol by volume. The derivation of proof comes from the days when sailors in the British Navy suspected that the officers were diluting their rum (grog) ration and demanded "proof" that this was not the case. They achieved this by pouring a sample of grog on black granular gunpowder. If the gunpowder ignited by match or spark, the rum was up to standard, 100% proof that the liquor was at least 50% ethanol. This became shortened to 100 proof.

In addition to beverages, ethanol is present in hundreds of medicinal preparations used as a diluent or solvent. Consumption of illicitly produced ethanol ("moonshine") can result in methanol, lead, or arsenic poisoning, or botulism. Of historic interest is that the addition of cobalt salts to beer to stabilize the "head" (foam) led to outbreaks of congestive cardiomyopathy among heavy beer drinkers (Chap. 64).

Alcoholism is a leading cause of morbidity and mortality in the US. The prevalence of ethanol dependence in the US is around 6% for men and 2% for women. The overall estimated annual cost of excessive drinking in the US for 2010 was $249 billion. The Global Burden of Disease Study identified three effects of ethanol: harmful impact of traumatic injuries, a risk factor for muliple diseases, and the dose dependent protective effect in relation to ischemic heart disease. Overall, ethanol accounted for 3.5% of mortality and disability, 1.5% of all deaths, 2.1% of all life years lost, and 6% of all the years lived with disability.

## PHARMACOKINETICS AND TOXICOKINETICS

Ethanol is rapidly absorbed from the gastrointestinal (GI) tract, with approximately 20% absorbed from the stomach and the remainder from the small intestine. Factors that enhance absorption include rapid gastric emptying, ethanol intake without food, the absence of congeners, dilution of ethanol (maximum absorption occurs at a concentration of 20%), and carbonation. Under optimal conditions for absorption, 80% to 90% of an ingested dose is fully absorbed within 60 minutes. Factors that delay or decrease ethanol absorption include high concentrations of ethanol (by causing pylorospasm), the presence of food, the coexistence of GI disease, and coingestion of xenobiotics such as aspirin and anticholinergics. When any of these factors is present, absorption may be delayed for 2 to 6 hours. The relative amount of ethanol that is absorbed from the stomach is determined by the presence of an alcohol dehydrogenase (ADH) enzyme in the gastric mucosa, which oxidizes a proportion of the ingested ethanol, thus reducing the amount available for absorption. This effect is more pronounced in men than in women and in nonalcoholics than in alcoholics. However, this gender difference is undetectable after age 50 years. After complete distribution, ethanol is present in body tissues in a concentration proportional to that of the tissue water content. Table 49–1 shows some simple pharmacokinetic calculations based on these principles.

**TABLE 49–1 Basic Information and Calculations**

Ethanol MW: 46 Da

$$\text{mmol} = \frac{\text{mg}}{\text{MW}} = \frac{\text{mg}}{46}$$

$$\text{mmol/L} = \frac{\text{mg/dL}}{4.6}$$

Specific gravity:[a] 0.7939 (~0.8) g/mL

Volume of distribution ($V_d$): 0.6 L/kg

$$\text{Serum ethanol concentration (mg/dL)}^{b} = \frac{\text{Dose (mg)}}{V_d\ \text{(L/kg)} \times \text{Body weight (kg)} \times 10}$$

Average reduction in serum ethanol concentration (elimination phase):

Nontolerant adults: 3.26–4.35 mmol/L/h (15–20 mg/dL/h, 100–125 mg/kg/h)

Tolerant adults: 6.52–8.70 mmol/L/h (30–40 mg/dL/h, 175 mg/kg/h)

For a 70-kg individual:

| *Dose of Ethanol* | *Serum Ethanol Concentration*[b] |
|---|---|
| 10 mL/kg of 10% (20 proof) | 153 mg/dL (36.30 mmol/L) |
| 3 mL/kg of 10% (20 proof) | 46 mg/dL (10.87 mmol/L) |
| 1.5 mL/kg of 10% (20 proof) | 23 mg/dL (5.43 mmol/L) |
| 150 mL (5 "shots") of 40% (80 proof) | 125 mg/dL (31.09 mmol/L) |
| 30 mL (1 "shot") of 40% (80 proof) | 25 mg/dL (5.87 mmol/L) |
| One "standard drink" (~0.6 fluid (fl) oz or 14 grams of "pure" ethanol): 1.5 fl oz of 80-proof distilled spirits or "hard liquor" (eg, whiskey, gin, rum, vodka, and tequila), 2–3 fl oz of cordial, liqueur, or aperitif (24% ethanol), 3–4 fl oz of fortified wine (eg, sherry or port, 14% ethanol), 5 fl oz of table wine (12% ethanol), 8–9 fl oz of malt liquor (7% ethanol), or 12 fl oz of regular beer (5% ethanol) | 25 mg/dL (9.11 mmol/L) |

[a]Specific gravity of ethanol is dependent on its water content and temperature. The specific gravity of 100% ethanol at temperature between 20° and 35°C ranges from 0.78934 to 0.77641 (~0.8) g/mL. [b]This is the theoretical maximum concentration, based on instantaneous and complete ethanol absorption and no distribution or metabolism. Concentration consistent with legal intoxication = 10.87–17.39 mmol/L (50–80 mg/dL or 0.05–0.08 g/dL %). The legal breath ethanol concentration to serum ethanol concentration ratio has been set at 1:2,100; the amount of ethanol in 1 mL of blood is the same amount in 2,100 mL of exhaled air: Measured breath ethanol concentration (mmol/L) × 2,100 = (Calculated) serum ethanol concentration (mmol/L).

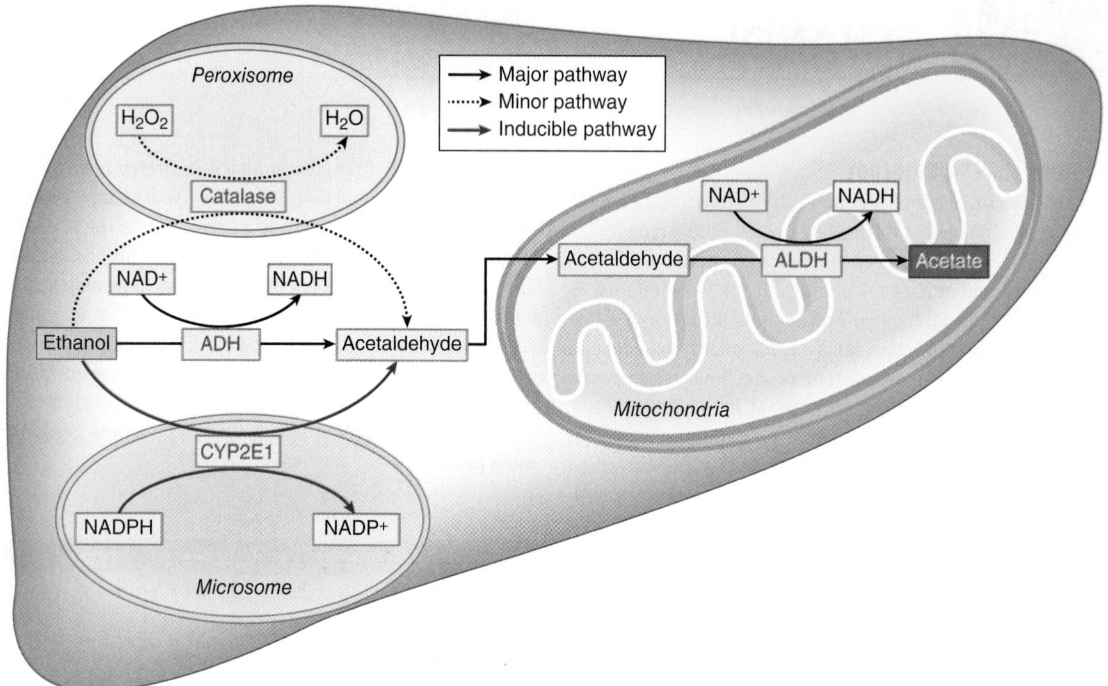


**FIGURE 49–1.** Ethanol is metabolized in the cytoplasm of hepatocytes to acetaldehyde through major, minor, and inducible pathways. Acetaldehyde is metabolized in the mitochondria to acetic acid.

Ethanol is primarily eliminated by the liver, with 2% to 5% excreted unchanged by the kidneys, lungs, and sweat (Fig. 49–1). The alcohol dehydrogenase (ADH) system is the rate-limiting step. Under normal conditions, acetate is converted to acetylcoenzyme A (acetyl-CoA), which enters the citric acid cycle and is metabolized to carbon dioxide and water. The entry of acetyl-CoA into the citric acid cycle is thiamine dependent (Antidotes in Brief: A27). Cytochrome P450 2E1 is responsible for very little ethanol metabolism in the nontolerant drinker but becomes more important as the ethanol concentration rises or as ethanol use becomes chronic. The ability of ethanol to induce CYP2E1 forms the basis for the well-established interactions between ethanol and a host of other xenobiotics metabolized by this system.

Alcohol dehydrogenase is saturated at relatively low serum ethanol concentrations and elimination changes from first-order to zero-order kinetics. In adults, the average rate of ethanol metabolism is 100 to 125 mg/kg/h (21.7–27.1 mmol/h) in occasional drinkers and up to 175 mg/kg/h in habitual drinkers. As a result, the average-sized adult metabolizes 7 to 10 g/h, and the serum ethanol concentration falls 15 to 20 mg/dL/h (3.26–4.35 mmol/L/h). Tolerant drinkers, by recruiting CYP2E1, increase their clearance of ethanol to 30 mg/dL/h (6.52 mmol/L/h) or even higher.

## XENOBIOTIC INTERACTIONS

Ethanol interacts with a variety of xenobiotics (Table 49–2). The most frequent ethanol–drug interactions occur as a result of ethanol-induced increase in hepatic enzyme activity. By contrast, acute ethanol use inhibits metabolism of other

**TABLE 49–2 Ethanol–Xenobiotic Interactions**

| *Xenobiotics* | *Adverse Effects* |
|---|---|
| Carbamates, cephalosporins,[a] chloramphenicol, chlorpropamide, *Coprinus* mushrooms, griseofulvin, metronidazole, nitrofurantoin, thiram derivatives | Disulfiramlike effect |
| Antihistamines ($H_1$), chloral hydrate, cyclic antidepressants, opioids, phenothiazines | Additive sedative effect |
| Aspirin | Enhances antiplatelet effect |
| Disulfiram (Antabuse) | Nausea, vomiting, abdominal pain, flushing, diaphoresis, chest pain, headache, vertigo, palpitations |
| Isoniazid | Increased incidence of hepatitis; increased metabolism[b] |
| Methadone | Increased methadone metabolism[b] |
| Oral hypoglycemics | Potentiates hypoglycemic effect |
| Phenytoin | Increased phenytoin metabolism[b] |
| Ranitidine, cimetidine | Increased ethanol concentration |
| Sedative–hypnotics | Additive sedative effect or respiratory depression |
| Vasodilators | Potentiates vasodilator effect |
| Warfarin | Increased warfarin metabolism[b] |

[a]Those containing a *N*-methylthiotetrazole side chain.

[b]Effect possibly associated with chronic ethanol consumption.

xenobiotics due to competitive inhibition of hepatic enzyme activity or a reduction in hepatic blood flow. The interaction between ethanol and disulfiram is well described and it can be life threatening (Chap. 51).

## PATHOPHYSIOLOGY

No specific receptor for ethanol is identified, and the mechanism of action leading to inebriation remains the subject of debate. The major actions of ethanol involve enhancing the inhibitory effects of γ-aminobutyric acid (GABA) at $GABA_A$ receptors and blockade of the *N*-methyl-D-aspartate (NMDA) subtype of glutamate, an excitatory amino acid (EAA) receptor. Chronic ethanol administration also results in tolerance, dependence, and an ethanol withdrawal syndrome mediated in part by desensitization and/or downregulation of $GABA_A$ receptors and upregulation of NMDA receptors (Chap. 50).

Chronic alcoholism has multiorgan system effects (Table 49–3). In addition to the harmful effects of ethanol itself such as impairment of protein synthesis, its metabolite, acetaldehyde, is inherently toxic to biologic systems. Acetaldehyde directly impairs cardiac contractile function, disrupts cardiac excitation–contractile coupling, inhibits myocardial protein synthesis, interferes with phosphorylation, causes structural and functional alterations in mitochondria and hepatocytes, and inactivates acetyl-coenzyme A. Acetaldehyde also reacts with intracellular proteins to generate adducts. Acetaldehyde-protein and DNA adducts promote oxidative stress, lipid peroxidation, hepatic stellate cell activation–associated inflammation and fibrosis, and mutagenesis. Acetaldehyde adducts are believed to be important in the early phase of alcoholic liver disease, and in advanced liver disease, they contribute to the development of hepatic fibrosis as well as hepatocellular carcinoma.

Oxidation of ethanol generates an excess of acetyl-CoA and reducing potential in the cytosol in the form of NADH with the ratio of NADH to $NAD^+$ being dramatically increased. This ratio, also known as the redox potential, determines the ability of the cell to carry on various oxidative processes. The excess acetyl-CoA and the unfavorable change in redox potential caused by ethanol metabolism contribute to the development of metabolic disorders such as impaired gluconeogenesis, alterations in fatty acid metabolism, fatty liver, hyperlipidemia, hypoglycemia, elevated lactate concentration, hyperuricemia (gouty attacks), increased collagen and scar tissue formation, and alcoholic ketoacidosis (AKA) (Fig. 49–2).

**TABLE 49–3 Systemic Effects Associated With Alcoholism**

| | |
|---|---|
| ***Cardiovascular*** | ***Genitourinary*** |
| Cardiomyopathy | Hypogonadism |
| "Holiday heart" (dysrhythmias) | Impotence |
| "Wet" beriberi or high-output heart failure (thiamine deficiency) | Infertility |
| ***Endocrine and Metabolic*** | ***Hematologic*** |
| Hypoglycemia | Coagulopathy |
| Hypokalemia | Folate, $B_{12}$, iron-deficiency anemias |
| Hypomagnesemia | Hemolysis (Zieve syndrome, stomatocytosis, spur-cell anemia) |
| Hypophosphatemia | Leukopenia |
| Hypothermia | Thrombocytopenia |
| Hypertriglyceridemia | ***Neurologic*** |
| Hyperuricemia | Alcohol amnestic syndrome |
| Metabolic acidosis | Alcoholic hallucinosis |
| Malnutrition | Alcohol withdrawal |
| ***Gastrointestinal*** | Cerebellar degeneration |
| Mouth | Cerebral atrophy (dementia) |
| Cancer of the mouth, pharynx, larynx | Cerebrovascular accident (hemorrhage, infarction) |
| Cheilosis | Inebriation |
| Stomatitis (nutritional) | Korsakoff psychosis |
| Esophagus | Marchiafava-Bignami disease |
| Boerhaave syndrome | Myopathy |
| Cancer of the esophagus | Osmotic demyelination syndrome |
| Esophageal spasm (diffuse) | Pellagra |
| Esophagitis | Polyneuropathy |
| Mallory-Weiss tear | Subdural hematoma |
| Stomach and duodenum | Wernicke encephalopathy |
| Diarrhea | ***Ophthalmic*** |
| Gastritis (acute) | Tobacco–ethanol amblyopia |
| Gastritis (chronic hypertrophic) | ***Psychiatric*** |
| Hematemesis | Animated behavior |
| Malabsorption | Loss of self-restraint |
| Peptic ulcer | Manic-depressive illness |
| Liver | Suicide and depression |
| Cirrhosis | ***Respiratory*** |
| Hepatitis | Atelectasis |
| Steatosis | Pneumonia |
| Pancreas | Respiratory acidosis |
| Pancreatitis (acute or chronic) | Respiratory depression |

## ACUTE CLINICAL FEATURES

Ethanol is a selective central nervous system (CNS) depressant at low doses and a general depressant at high doses. Initially, it depresses the areas of the brain involved with highly integrated functions. Cortical release leads to animated behavior and the loss of restraint. This paradoxical CNS stimulation is due to disinhibition. Patients are energized and loquacious, expansive, emotionally labile, increasingly gregarious or appear to have lost self-control, exhibit antisocial behavior, and are ill tempered. As the degree of inebriation increases, inhibition and impairment of neuronal activity occur. Patients become irritable, abusive, aggressive, violent, dysarthric, confused, disoriented, or lethargic. With severe inebriation, there is loss of airway protective reflexes, coma, and increasing risk of death from respiratory depression. An ethanol-naïve adult with a serum ethanol concentration of greater than 250 mg/dL (54 mmol/L) is usually comatose.

Tolerance shifts the dose–response curve to the right but does not change the clinical effects. Tolerance is metabolic (pharmacokinetic) and functional (pharmacodynamic). Metabolic tolerance to ethanol is based on enhanced elimination by CYP2E1. Functional tolerance occurs through alterations in $GABA_A$ and NMDA receptors. Acute ethanol tolerance is demonstrated by the Mellanby effect, in which impairment is greater at a given serum ethanol concentration when it is

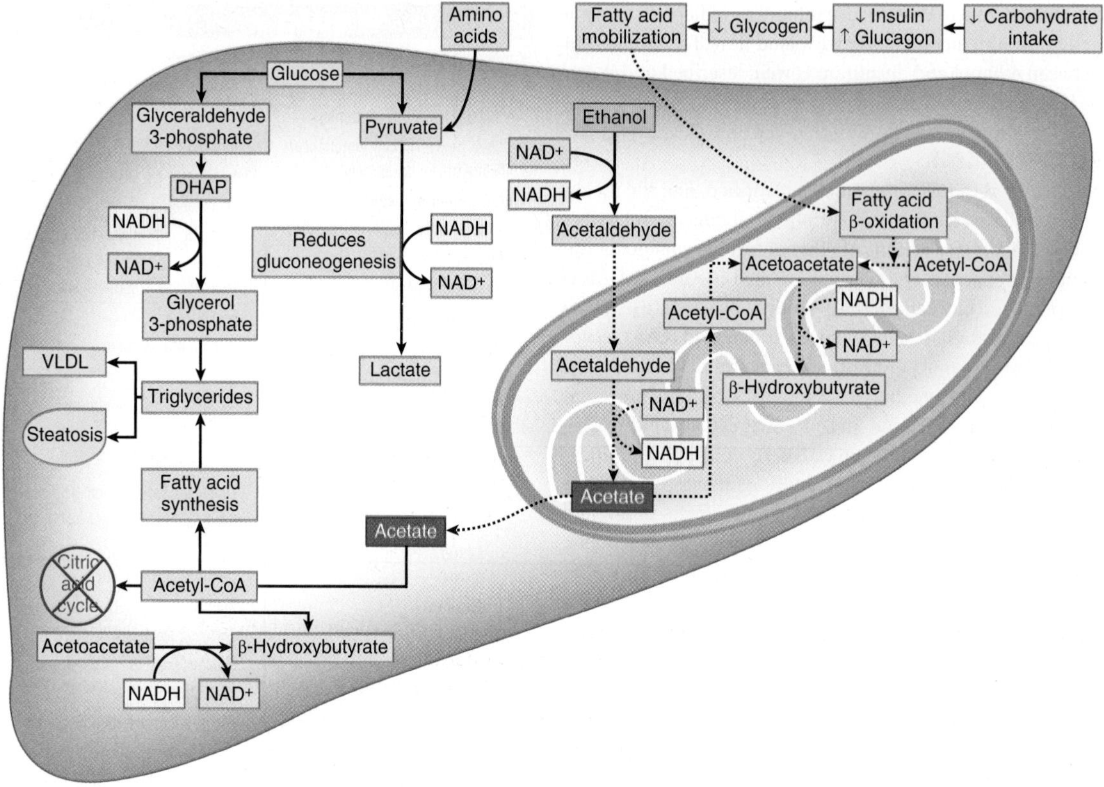


**FIGURE 49–2.** Ethanol metabolism drives reactions toward NADH and acetate. The high cytoplasmic redox state favors the reduction of pyruvate to lactate and diverts pyruvate from being a substrate for gluconeogenesis, favors the reduction of dihydroxyacetone phosphate (DHAP) to glycerol 3-phosphate, and serves as substrate for triglycerides formation. The high cytoplasmic redox state and acetate load limit the citric acid cycle, thus decreasing the supply of NADH for oxidative phosphorylation, resulting in a decrease in adenosine triphosphate (ATP) production and favoring conversion of acetyl-CoA to ketone bodies and fatty acid synthesis. Abrupt discontinuation of ethanol and starvation result in mobilization and oxidation of fatty acids. Fatty acid metabolism results in the formation of acetyl-CoA, which combines with the excess acetate, in the form of acetyl-CoA, that is generated from ethanol metabolism to form acetoacetate. Most of the acetoacetate is reduced to β-hydroxybutyrate because of the high cellular redox state.

increasing than for the same serum ethanol concentration when it is falling.

Many patients present with obvious signs and symptoms consistent with inebriation that include flushed facies, diaphoresis, tachycardia, hypotension, hypothermia, hypoventilation, mydriasis, nystagmus, vomiting, dysarthria, muscular incoordination, ataxia, altered consciousness, and coma. However, a presumed inebriated patient presenting to an emergency department (ED) has a broad range of diagnostic possibilities and should prompt a careful evaluation for a variety of occult clinical and metabolic disorders. The presence or absence of an odor of ethanol on the breath is an unreliable means of ascertaining whether a person is inebriated or whether ethanol was recently consumed. Diplopia, visual disturbances, and nystagmus are caused by either the toxic effects of ethanol or may represent Wernicke encephalopathy. Inebriation impairs cardiac output in patients with preexisting cardiac disease and induces dysrhythmias such as atrial fibrillation, atrioventricular block, and nonsustained ventricular tachycardia. The association between ethanol use and cardiac dysrhythmias, particularly supraventricular tachydysrhythmias, in apparently healthy people is called "holiday heart syndrome." The most common dysrhythmia is atrial fibrillation, which usually reverts to normal sinus rhythm within 24 hours. Ethanol-related seizures occur as a consequence of ethanol dependence. Most commonly these seizures are caused by alcohol withdrawal and are classically characterized by generalized tonic-clonic activity followed by a brief postictal period. However, a significant percentage of patients with ethanol-related seizures have other identifiable causes, and they include head trauma (eg, intracranial hemorrhage or contusion), idiopathic generalized epilepsy, cerebrovascular accident, intracranial lesions (eg, tumors, infection, and gliosis), and toxic-metabolic causes (eg, hypoglycemia).

## DIAGNOSTIC TESTS

Hospital laboratory analysis of blood samples for ethanol concentration is usually based on serum (liquid portion of whole blood after the cellular components and clotting factors are removed) or rarely plasma (acellular liquid portion of unclotted whole blood). By contrast, forensic casework expresses ethanol concentration in terms of ethanol concentration in whole blood (Special Considerations: SC10). All patients with altered mental status should have a rapid reagent glucose test. Additionally, when there is concern for disorders other than acute ingestion, laboratory investigations recommended potentially include a complete blood count, electrolytes, blood urea nitrogen, creatinine, urine ketones, acetone, lipase, liver enzymes, ammonia, calcium, and magnesium. Patients with an anion gap metabolic acidosis should have urine ketones and a serum lactate concentration determined (Chap. 79). When alcoholic ketoacidosis (AKA) is suspected, acetone and acetoacetate concentrations in either serum or urine are often low or absent and β-hydroxybutyrate will be elevated. This occurs because of the altered redox state mentioned above (Fig. 49–2).

When the serum ethanol concentration is inconsistent with the patient's clinical condition, prompt reevaluation of the patient is indicated to elucidate the etiology of the altered mental status. The threshold for head computed tomography (CT) imaging should be low in comatose patients with concentrations below 300 mg/dL (65 mmol/L) and those with values in excess of 300 mg/dL (65 mmol/L) who fail to improve clinically during a limited period of close observation.

## MANAGEMENT OF POSSIBLY INEBRIATED PATIENTS

Occasionally, an extremely inebriated or comatose patient will have severe respiratory depression, necessitating endotracheal intubation and ventilatory support. Any patient with an acute altered mental status mandates immediate investigation and treatment of reversible causes such as hypoxia, hypoglycemia, and opioid toxicity. In addition, treatment for presumed thiamine depletion is recommended. Abnormal vital signs should be addressed and stabilized. Patients who are combative and violent should be both physically restrained and then chemically sedated (Special Considerations: SC3). The choice of sedatives is controversial. In general, when ethanol inebriation is highly suspected, we recommend an antipsychotic because of the low risk of further respiratory compromise. However, when the diagnosis is unclear or vital signs suggest either withdrawal or a sympathomimetic, we recommend a benzodiazepine (Antidotes in Brief: A26). Caution should be taken because of additive effects of ethanol and benzodiazepine on respiratory depression.

A variety of therapies are advocated either to reverse the intoxicating effects of ethanol or to enhance its elimination. Those proven to be either ineffective or unreliable include caffeine, naloxone, flumazenil, and rapid IV saline loading. Hemodialysis is an effective means of enhancing the systemic elimination of ethanol because of the small volume of distribution and low molecular weight of ethanol. In severe ethanol poisoning resulting in respiratory failure or coma, hemodialysis is a reasonable adjunct treatment to supportive care. However, the risks of hemodialysis such as precipitation of acute and severe withdrawal usually exceed its benefit.

## INDICATIONS FOR HOSPITALIZATION

A patient with uncomplicated inebriation can be safely discharged after a careful observation with social service or psychiatric counseling. An individual should not be discharged while impairment of cognitive and motor function persists. However, it is reasonable to discharge a mildly intoxicated patient to a protected environment under the supervision of a responsible, not intoxicated adult. In all cases **except** allowing a person to drive, the clinical assessment of the patient is more important than the serum ethanol concentration. Indications for hospital admission include persistently abnormal vital signs, persistently abnormal mental status with or without an obvious cause, an overdose with intended self-harm, concomitant serious trauma, consequential ethanol withdrawal, and those with an associated serious disease process such as pancreatitis or GI hemorrhage. All patients should be offered referrals to substance use counseling programs.

### Ethanol-Associated Hypoglycemia

Hypoglycemia associated with ethanol consumption occurs when ethanol metabolism increases the cellular redox ratio. The higher redox state favors the conversion of pyruvate to lactate, diverting pyruvate from being a substrate for gluconeogenesis (Fig. 49–2). Hypoglycemia typically occurs when there is a reduced caloric intake and only after the hepatic glycogen stores are depleted, as in an overnight fast. The mechanism by which hypoglycemia is associated with ethanol consumption in the well-nourished individual is less well defined. Although the conditions associated with hypoglycemia in adults are also present in infants and children, children with their smaller livers have less glycogen stores than adults and are more likely to develop hypoglycemia.

***Clinical Features.*** Patients with ethanol-associated hypoglycemia usually present with an altered consciousness 2 to 10 hours after ethanol ingestion. Other physical findings include hypothermia and tachypnea. Laboratory findings, in addition to hypoglycemia, usually include a positive serum ethanol concentration, ketonuria without glucosuria, and mild metabolic acidosis.

***Management.*** Acute treatment of ethanol-associated hypoglycemia is similar to other causes of hypoglycemia (Chap. 20 and Antidotes in Brief: A8) and should prompt a systematic evaluation for coexisting clinical and metabolic disorders. Hospital admission is reasonable in severe or resistant cases, because this represents serious metabolic impairment that cannot be rapidly rectified.

### Alcoholic Ketoacidosis

The development of AKA requires a combination of physical (eg, starvation and abrupt discontinuation of ethanol) and physiologic events to occur. The normal response to starvation and depletion of hepatic glycogen stores is for amino acids to be converted to pyruvate. Pyruvate serves as a substrate for gluconeogenesis and is converted to acetyl-CoA, which can enter the citric acid cycle or is used in various biosynthetic pathways (eg, fatty acids, ketone bodies, cholesterol, and acetylcholine). As described earlier, ethanol metabolism generates an excess of acetate and a high cellular redox potential. This excess acetate is converted to acetyl-CoA by cytoplasmic and mitochondrial adenosine triphosphate (ATP)–dependent acetyl-CoA synthetases (Fig. 49–2). The consequences of increased cellular acetyl-CoA and a shift in the cellular redox potential include inhibition of pyruvate dehydrogenase complex thus inhibition of entry of pyruvate into the citric acid cycle, inhibition of the citric acid cycle itself, and enhanced formation of the ketone bodies (ie, acetoacetate, β-hydroxybutyrate, and acetone). The high redox state also favors the conversion of pyruvate to lactate, diverting pyruvate from being a substrate for gluconeogenesis. To compensate for the lack of normal metabolic substrates, the body mobilizes fat from adipose tissue and increases fatty acid metabolism as an alternative source of energy. This response is mediated by a decrease in insulin and an increase in glucagon, catecholamines, growth hormone, and cortisol. Fatty acid metabolism results in the formation of acetyl-CoA. Two molecules of acetyl-CoA condense to form acetoacetyl-CoA, which is metabolized to acetoacetate via the 3-hydroxy-3-methylglutaryl CoA (HMG-CoA) pathway. Most of the acetoacetate is reduced to β-hydroxybutyrate because of the excess reducing potential or high redox state of the cell. Volume depletion interferes with the renal elimination of acetoacetate and β-hydroxybutyrate and contributes to the metabolic acidosis. An elevated lactate concentration results from shunting from pyruvate or from hypoperfusion or infection that may coexist with the underlying ketoacidosis.

***Clinical Features.*** Patients with AKA are typically chronic ethanol users, presenting after a few days of "binge" drinking, who become acutely starved because of cessation in oral intake due to binging itself or because of nausea, vomiting, abdominal pain from gastritis, hepatitis, pancreatitis, or a concurrent acute illness. The patient usually appears acutely ill with salt and water depletion, tachypnea, tachycardia, and hypotension. Medical conditions such as sepsis, meningitis, pyelonephritis, or pneumonia that may occur simultaneously should be excluded, and ethanol withdrawal should be anticipated.

The serum ethanol concentration is usually low or undetectable because ethanol intake substantially decreased earlier in the clinical course. The hallmarks of AKA include an elevated anion gap metabolic acidosis with an elevated serum lactate concentration. The nitroprusside test used to detect the presence of ketones in serum and urine is negative or mildly positive in patients with AKA because the nitroprusside reaction only detects molecules containing ketone moieties. This includes acetoacetate and acetone but not β-hydroxybutyrate. Reliance on the nitroprusside test alone underestimates the severity of ketoacidosis. Specific assays for β-hydroxybutyrate are performed in some hospital laboratories and are available as point-of-care testing at bedside.

***Management.*** Treatment should begin with adequate crystalloid fluid replacement, dextrose, thiamine and folic acid. Supplemental multivitamins, potassium, and magnesium are recommended on an individual basis. The administration of dextrose will stimulate the release of insulin, decrease the release of glucagon, and reduce the oxidation of fatty acids. Exogenous glucose also facilitates the synthesis of ATP, which reverses the pyruvate-to-lactate and $NAD^+$/NADH ratios. The provision of thiamine facilitates pyruvate entry into the citric acid cycle, thus increasing ATP production. Volume replacement restores glomerular filtration and improves excretion of ketones and organic acids. Administration of either insulin or sodium bicarbonate in the management of AKA is usually unnecessary.

Patients presenting with AKA are manifesting serious metabolic impairment and frequently require hospital admission. They often succumb to other precipitating or coexisting medical or surgical disorders such as occult trauma, pancreatitis, GI hemorrhage or hepatorenal dysfunction, and infections. However, death is rare from isolated ethanol-induced ketoacidosis.

| TABLE 49–4 *DSM-5* Alcohol Use Disorder |
|---|
| Drinking more or longer than intended? |
| Desire or unsuccessful efforts to control alcohol use? |
| A lot of time drinking or to recover from alcohol effects? |
| Craving to use alcohol? |
| Drinking or sick from drinking interfering with obligations at work, home, or school? |
| Continued drinking even though it is causing social or interpersonal problems? |
| Alcohol use reducing social, occupational, or recreational activities? |
| Recurrent alcohol use in situations where it is physically hazardous? |
| Continued drinking in spite of physical or psychological problems? |
| Need for increased drinking to achieve desired effect? |
| Drinking to relieve or avoid withdrawal symptoms? |

Data from American Psychiatric Association: *Diagnostic and Statistical Manual of Mental Disorders*, 5th ed. Arlington, VA: American Psychiatric Association; 2013.

## ALCOHOLISM

Alcoholism is traditionally defined as a chronic, progressive disease characterized by tolerance and physical dependence to ethanol and pathologic organ changes and is recognized to be a multifactorial, genetically influenced disorder. The most recent edition of the American Psychiatric Association's *Diagnostic and Statistical Manual of Mental Disorders* (*DSM-5*) integrated alcohol abuse and alcohol dependence into a single disorder called *alcohol use disorder* (AUD) with mild, moderate, and severe subclassifications. The presence of at least two of the symptoms (Table 49–4) within 12 months indicates an AUD. The severity of AUD is defined by the number of symptoms present (ie, mild, two or three symptoms; moderate, four or five symptoms; and severe, six or more symptoms).

Screening is a preliminary procedure to assess the likelihood that an individual has a substance use disorder or is at risk of negative consequences from alcohol or other xenobiotics use. Whereas screening tools, such as the Brief Michigan Alcoholism Screening Test (MAST) and the CAGE questions (Table 49–5), were initially developed to identify people with active alcohol dependence for referral to treatment, the screening, brief intervention, and referral to treatment (SBIRT) was developed to provide universal screening; secondary prevention in detecting risky or hazardous substance use before the onset of abuse or dependence; early intervention; and treatment for people who have problematic or hazardous alcohol problems within healthcare settings.

| TABLE 49–5 The CAGE Questions |
|---|
| 1. Have you ever felt you should **c**ut down on your drinking? |
| 2. Have people **a**nnoyed you by criticizing your drinking? |
| 3. Have you ever felt bad or **g**uilty about your drinking? |
| 4. Have you ever had a drink first thing in the morning to steady your nerves or to get rid of a hangover (**e**ye opener)? |

Two or more affirmatives = probable diagnosis of alcoholism.

Mayfield D, et al. The CAGE questionnaire: validation of a new alcoholism screening instrument. *Am J Psychiatry*. 1974;131:1121-1126.

The Alcohol Use Disorders Identification Test (AUDIT) was developed from a six-country World Health Organization collaborative project as a screening instrument to identify heavy drinkers and explicitly addresses alcohol-related problems and symptoms of dependence over the past year (Table 49–6). A modified version of the AUDIT instrument, the AUDIT-C, is used to help identify patients who are hazardous drinkers or have active alcohol use disorders and might benefit from brief primary care interventions. The AUDIT-C uses the first three questions from AUDIT and is scored on a scale of 0 to 12 points. In men, a score of 4 points or more is considered positive for alcohol misuse; in women, a score of 3 points or more is considered positive.

Various strategies are used to treat alcoholism, including psychosocial interventions, pharmacologic interventions, or both. Pharmacologic treatment of ethanol dependence that is of potential collateral toxicologic consequence includes opioid antagonists such as naltrexone and nalmefene, disulfiram, serotonergic agents, gabapentin, and topiramate.

**TABLE 49–6 Screening for alcohol abuse using the Alcohol Use Disorder Identification Test (AUDIT)**

(Scores for response categories are given in parentheses. Added together, Total Scores range from 0 to 40, with scores of 1 to 7 suggesting low-risk drinking; 8 to 14, hazardous or harmful drinking; and > 15, alcohol dependence.)

| | | | | |
|---|---|---|---|---|
| 1. How often do you have a drink containing alcohol? | | | | |
| (0) Never | (1) Monthly or less | (2) Two to four times a month | (3) Two or three times a week | (4) Four or more times a week |
| 2. How many drinks containing alcohol do you have on a typical day when you are drinking? | | | | |
| (0) 1 or 2 | (1) 3 or 4 | (2) 5 or 6 | (3) 7 to 9 | (4) 10 or more |
| 3. How often do you have six or more drinks on one occasion? | | | | |
| (0) Never | (1) Less than monthly | (2) Monthly | (3) Weekly | (4) Daily or almost daily |
| 4. How often during the past year have you found that you were not able to stop drinking once you had started? | | | | |
| (0) Never | (1) Less than monthly | (2) Monthly | (3) Weekly | (4) Daily or almost daily |
| 5. How often during the past year have you failed to do what was normally expected of you because of drinking? | | | | |
| (0) Never | (1) Less than monthly | (2) Monthly | (3) Weekly | (4) Daily or almost daily |
| 6. How often during the past year have you needed a first drink in the morning to get yourself going after a heavy drinking session? | | | | |
| (0) Never | (1) Less than monthly | (2) Monthly | (3) Weekly | (4) Daily or almost daily |
| 7. How often during the past year have you had a feeling of guilt or remorse after drinking? | | | | |
| (0) Never | (1) Less than monthly | (2) Monthly | (3) Weekly | (4) Daily or almost daily |
| 8. How often during the past year have you been unable to remember what happened the night before because you had been drinking? | | | | |
| (0) Never | (1) Less than monthly | (2) Monthly | (3) Weekly | (4) Daily or almost daily |
| 9. Have you or has someone else been injured as a result of your drinking? | | | | |
| (0) No | | (2) Yes, but not in the past year | | (4) Yes, during the past year |
| 10. Has a relative or friend or a doctor or other health worker been concerned about your drinking or suggested you cut down? | | | | |
| (0) No | | (2) Yes, but not in the past year | | (4) Yes, during the past year |

Reproduced with permission from *AUDIT: The Alcohol Use Disorders Identification Test. Guidelines for use of primary health care.* Geneva: World Health Organization, 2001. WHO does not endorse any specific companies, products or services.

Antidotes in Brief

# A27 THIAMINE HYDROCHLORIDE

## INTRODUCTION

Thiamine (vitamin $B_1$) is a water-soluble vitamin found in organ meats, yeast, eggs, and green leafy vegetables that is essential in the creation and utilization of cellular energy. Although there is no toxicity associated with thiamine excess, thiamine deficiency is responsible for "wet" beriberi (high output congestive heart failure) and "dry" beriberi (Wernicke encephalopathy and the Wernicke-Korsakoff syndrome).

## HISTORY

Kanehiro Takaki first established the relationship between a nutritional deficiency and beriberi in 1884. It was not until 1901 that Gerrit Grijns determined that the nutrient was contained in the outer coat of rice and was lost during the polishing process. Ten years later, Casimir Funk isolated thiamine. In 1881, Carl Wernicke reported three patients with alcoholism who died after developing confusion, ataxia, and ophthalmoplegia. A few years later, Sergei Korsakoff reported amnesia and confabulation that were preceded in many patients with alcoholism by the clinical findings reported by Wernicke.

## PHARMACOLOGY

### Biochemistry

As a coenzyme in the pyruvate dehydrogenase complex, thiamine diphosphate (thiamine pyrophosphate), the active form of thiamine, facilitates the conversion of pyruvate to acetyl-coenzyme A (acetyl-CoA). This overall process links pyruvate production from anaerobic glycolysis to the citric acid cycle, in which the sum of anaerobic and aerobic metabolism produces the equivalent of 36 moles of adenosine triphosphate (ATP) from each mole of glucose (Fig. A27–1). Within the citric acid cycle, thiamine is also required as a cofactor for the α-ketoglutarate dehydrogenase complex to catalyze the reaction of α-ketoglutarate to succinyl-CoA (Fig. A27–2), and in the pentose phosphate pathway for transketolase, an enzyme in which nicotinamide adenine dinucleotide phosphate (NADPH) is formed for subsequent use in reductive biosynthesis.

Thiamine requirements are determined by total caloric intake and energy demand, with 0.33 mg of thiamine required for every 4,400 kJ (1,000 kcal) of energy. The recommended daily consumption is 0.5 mg/1,000 kcal to provide a margin of safety, or about 1.2 mg/day for adults.

### Pharmacokinetics

Thiamine is well absorbed from the human gastrointestinal (GI) tract by a complex process. At low concentrations, absorption occurs through a saturable mechanism. As thiamine concentrations increase, however, the majority of absorption occurs through simple passive diffusion. In volunteers, intravenous administration peaks rapidly and has an apparent elimination half-life of 96 minutes. By contrast, oral administration peaks in a mean of 53 minutes, is only 5.3% bioavailable, and has an apparent elimination half-life of 154 minutes. Whereas rapid IV infusions produce higher peak concentrations, urinary elimination significantly increases. In contrast, a slower IV infusion increases the area under the curve (AUC) and decreases the urinary elimination. Synthesized analogs such as thiamine propyl disulfide, benfotiamine, and fursultiamine have enhanced bioavailability, but their use remains largely experimental.

Chronic liver disease, folate deficiency, steatorrhea, hyperemesis gravidarum, and other forms of malabsorption all significantly decrease the absorption of thiamine. Bariatric surgery also predisposes patients to thiamine deficiency. Malabsorption has even greater clinical relevance in patients

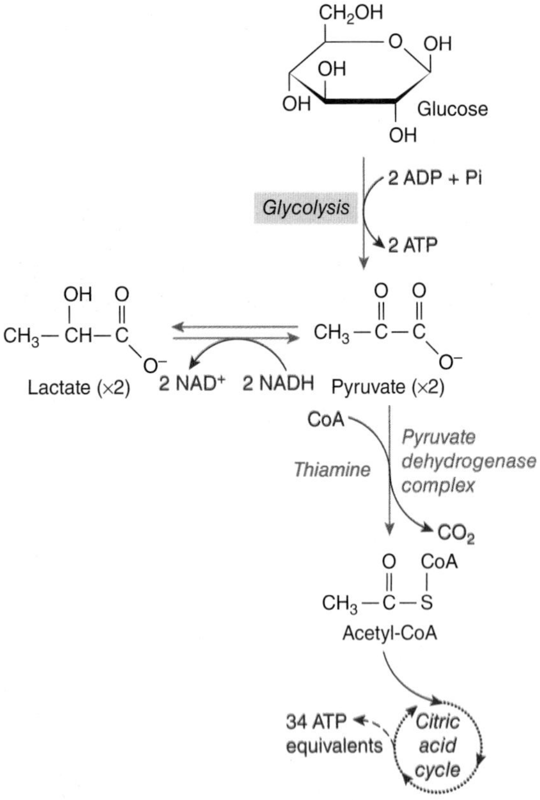

**FIGURE A27–1.** Thiamine links anaerobic glycolysis to the citric acid cycle. Anaerobic glycolysis only yields 2 moles of adenosine triphosphate (ATP) as each mole of glucose is metabolized to 2 moles of pyruvate. To obtain the 34 additional ATP equivalents that can be derived as the citric acid converts pyruvate to $CO_2$ and $H_2O$, pyruvate must first be combined with coenzyme A (CoA) to form acetylcoenzyme A (acetyl-CoA) and $CO_2$. This process is dependent on the thiamine-requiring enzyme system known as pyruvate dehydrogenase complex.

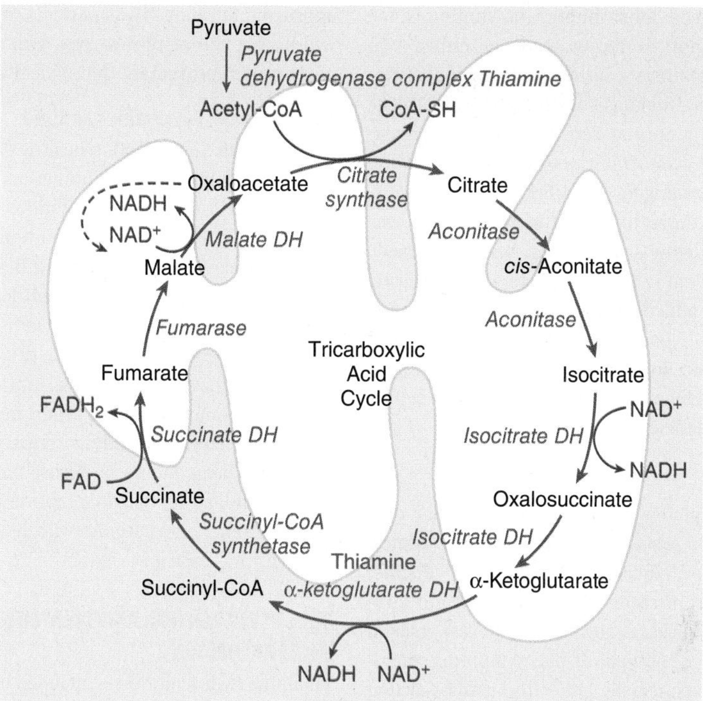


**FIGURE A27–2.** Thiamine is essential for α-ketoglutarate dehydrogenase activity, which is a rate-limiting step within the citric acid cycle. Thiamine deficiency leads to an accumulation of α-ketoglutarate, which is shunted to glutamate and causes excitatory neurotoxicity.

with alcoholism. In experimental studies, when healthy volunteers were given small amounts of ethanol, a 50% reduction in GI thiamine absorption resulted.

Thiamine is eliminated from the body largely by renal clearance. In an animal model, furosemide, acetazolamide, chlorothiazide, amiloride, mannitol, and salt loading all significantly increased urinary elimination of thiamine. Spironolactone use is associated with higher thiamine concentrations.

## THIAMINE DEFICIENCY

### Pathophysiology

Rodents develop signs of encephalopathy 10 days after being rendered thiamine deficient and demonstrate deterioration of the blood–brain barrier with hemorrhage into the mammillary bodies and other areas of the brain. This pattern is similar to findings described in humans with Wernicke encephalopathy (Fig. A27–3). Although there are no controlled trials of thiamine deprivation in humans, several unfortunate events support this time course. One report describes three patients who were given total parenteral nutrition (TPN) without multivitamins; signs and symptoms developed in 7, 10, and 14 days, respectively.

The proximate cause of Wernicke encephalopathy is unclear. In several models, excitatory amino acid–induced alterations in calcium transport led to thiamine-deficient encephalopathy. Additional investigations demonstrate roles for triggered mast cell degranulation, histamine, and nitric oxide in the generation of neuronal injury. The final common pathway is localized cerebral edema, which appears to result from altered expression of aquaporin.

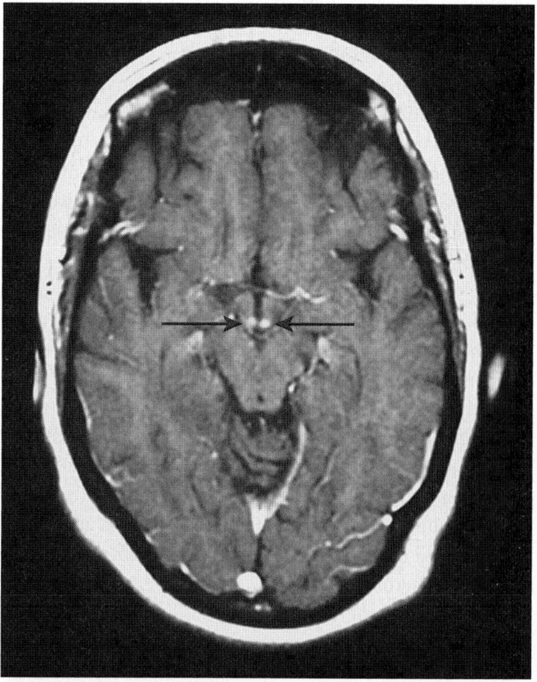

**FIGURE A27–3.** Postgadolinium axial and coronal T1-weighted magnetic resonance image of a patient with Wernicke encephalopathy showing pronounced enhancement of the mammillary bodies (arrows). *(Used with permission from Dr. Alexander Baxter, Department of Radiology, New York University Grossman School of Medicine.)*

In what may be the most important finding since Wernicke's original report, a recent study described two healthy nonalcoholic brothers who developed signs, symptoms, and neuroimaging findings consistent with Wernicke encephalopathy despite normal serum thiamine concentrations. Both brothers were confirmed to have compound mutations of a gene encoding for low-affinity thiamine transporter (THTR2). High-dose thiamine (up to 600 mg) was clinically effective. As demonstrated by magnetic resonance imaging, vasogenic edema is a characteristic finding during the acute crises. When added to the cases in which thiamine was excluded from TPN or infant formula, these findings definitively relate intracellular thiamine concentrations to clinical and anatomical manifestations of Wernicke encephalopathy and thiamine deficiency.

### Clinical Manifestations

When thiamine is completely removed from the human diet, tachycardia is often the first sign of deficiency. The clinical symptoms of thiamine deficiency present as two distinct patterns: "wet" beriberi or cardiovascular disease and "dry" beriberi, the neurologic disease known as Wernicke-Korsakoff syndrome. Although some patients display symptoms consistent with both disorders, usually either the cardiovascular or the neurologic manifestations predominate. A genetic variant of transketolase activity, combined with low physical activity and low-carbohydrate diet, predisposes to neurologic symptoms, but high-carbohydrate diets and increased physical activity lead to cardiovascular symptoms. Thus, cardiovascular disease is more common in the Asian population, and neurologic disease predominates in the northern European population.

Wet beriberi results from high-output cardiac failure induced by peripheral vasodilation and the formation of arteriovenous fistulae secondary to thiamine deficiency. These patients complain of fatigue, decreased exercise tolerance, shortness of breath, and peripheral edema. Patients with congestive heart failure seem to have an analogous worsening cardiac function caused by diuretic-associated thiamine use, which improves with thiamine supplementation.

The classic triad of oculomotor abnormalities, ataxia, and global confusion defines dry beriberi or Wernicke encephalopathy. Other manifestations include hypothermia and the absence of deep-tendon reflexes. Vomiting and anorexia are common and are presumed to be related to increases in intracranial pressure. Additionally, patients develop a peripheral neuropathy with paresthesias, hypesthesias, and an associated myopathy, all related to axonal degeneration. Laboratory studies may reflect a metabolic acidosis with elevated lactate concentration brought on by excessive anaerobic glycolysis resulting from blocked entry of substrate into the citric acid cycle. Korsakoff psychosis, a frequently irreversible disorder of learning and processing of new information characterized by a deficit in short-term memory and confabulation, often occurs with Wernicke encephalopathy. A 10% to 20% mortality rate is associated with Wernicke encephalopathy, with survivors having an 80% risk of developing Korsakoff psychosis. Even with treatment, approximately only 21% of patients with Korsakoff psychosis will have a complete recovery, with others having variable degrees of improvement that typically take months.

### Epidemiology: Populations at Risk

In the United States (US), a healthy diet and mandatory thiamine supplementation of numerous food products protect most people from the manifestations of thiamine deficiency. Alcoholic patients, whose consumption of ethanol is their major source of calories, are the best described and most easily recognized patients at risk for thiamine deficiency. Consequential thiamine deficiency is also described in the following settings: incarceration, drug rehabilitation, hemodialysis, hyperemesis gravidarum, parenteral nutrition, acquired immunodeficiency syndrome (AIDS), malignancies, institutionalized older adults, critically ill children, sepsis, congestive heart failure on furosemide therapy, malabsorption secondary to diarrhea, eating disorders, the refeeding syndrome, and patients who have undergone bariatric surgery.

## ROLE IN PREVENTION AND TREATMENT OF WERNICKE ENCEPHALOPATHY

Thiamine hydrochloride is included in the initial therapy for any patient with an altered mental status, potentially acting as both treatment and prevention of Wernicke encephalopathy. Glucose loading increases thiamine requirements, which can exacerbate marginal thiamine deficiencies, elevate lactate concentrations, or precipitate coma over hours in the absence of parenteral thiamine supplementation. Although it was commonly believed that acute glucose loading, in the form of a bolus of hypertonic dextrose, can precipitate Wernicke encephalopathy over several hours in normal individuals, there is evidence to support this effect only in rare patients who already had grave manifestations of thiamine deficiency or exaggerated delay in the provision of thiamine. Previously healthy patients require prolonged dextrose administration over several hours in the absence of thiamine to develop Wernicke encephalopathy. Because the morbidity and mortality associated with Wernicke encephalopathy are so severe and underdiagnosed and treatment is both benign and inexpensive, parenteral thiamine hydrochloride is recommended in the initial therapy for all patients who receive dextrose, all patients with altered consciousness, and every potential alcoholic or nutritionally deprived individual who presents to the emergency department or other clinical setting.

## ROLE IN THE TREATMENT OF OTHER DISORDERS

A supplementary indication for the administration of thiamine hydrochloride occurs in patients with ethylene glycol poisoning. As shown in Fig. 79–2, a minor pathway for the elimination of glyoxylic acid involves its conversion to α-hydroxy-β-ketoadipate by α-ketoglutarate: glyoxylate carboligase, a thiamine and magnesium-requiring enzyme. Because therapy is benign and inexpensive, it is reasonable to administer standard doses of thiamine to patients with suspected or confirmed metabolic acidosis from ethylene glycol poisoning. Standard doses of thiamine are also recommended for patients with alcoholic ketoacidosis (AKA) and starvation ketoacidosis. It is also reasonable to include routine thiamine administration in patients with congestive heart failure treated with long-term use of loop diuretics.

## ADVERSE EFFECTS

Very few complications are associated with the parenteral administration of thiamine. A single case of repeated angioedema was reported with oral thiamine. The safety of thiamine use was evaluated in a large case series in which nearly 1,000 patients received parenteral doses of up to 500 mg of thiamine without significant complications. This study suggests that if anaphylaxis to thiamine exists, its occurrence is exceedingly rare, permitting the safe IV administration of thiamine to most patients.

## PREGNANCY AND LACTATION

Thiamine hydrochloride is listed as Pregnancy Category A and is also considered safe for use in lactating mothers.

## DOSING AND ADMINISTRATION

For prevention of Wernicke encephalopathy, initial therapy usually consists of the immediate parenteral administration of 100 mg of thiamine hydrochloride. This can be given either intramuscularly or intravenously, but the oral route should be avoided because of its unpredictable and poor absorption. Although there are no dose-finding studies, some authorities recommend daily doses as high as 250 mg/day in high-risk patients without signs and symptoms of Wernicke encephalopathy. Current recommendations also exist for patients on TPN (3–3.5 mg/day), enteral feeding (2.2–2.9 mg/1,500 kcal), and renal replacement therapy (100 mg/day).

The practice of requiring the administration of parenteral thiamine before hypertonic dextrose in patients with altered consciousness is illogical. Besides the fact that the first dose of dextrose is unlikely to cause thiamine deficiency, thiamine uptake into cells and activation of enzyme systems is slower than that of glucose uptake, which suggests that even pretreatment with thiamine offers little benefit over posttreatment. Despite these limitations, it is prudent to administer at least 100 mg of parenteral thiamine whenever dextrose administration is required in patients at risk for Wernicke encephalopathy.

For treatment of Wernicke encephalopathy, we agree with current guidelines recommended by the British National Formulary and the Royal College of Physicians, British Association for Psychopharmacology, the European Federation of Neurological Societies (EFNS), and the National Institute for Health and Clinical Excellence (NICE), all of which suggest that the initial thiamine regimen for patients with clinical Wernicke encephalopathy is 500 mg intravenously 3 times daily for 2 to 3 days and 250 mg intravenously daily for the next 3 to 5 days. As stated earlier, because there is pharmacokinetic evidence favoring slow infusions over bolus therapy, this practice is reasonable after the first dose. Additionally, because data suggest that transketolase activity is improved when magnesium supplementation is routinely added to thiamine administration, we recommend administering 2 g of magnesium sulfate IV to patients with known or suspected hypomagnesemia and normal kidney function. Because of the safety of thiamine hydrochloride and the urgency to correct the manifestations of thiamine deficiency, up to 1,000 mg of thiamine hydrochloride is reasonable for use in the first 12 hours if a patient demonstrates persistent neurologic abnormalities.

Dosing in other disorders is less well defined. In patients with congestive heart failure, regimens have varied from 100 mg twice per week to 300 mg/day, but for sepsis, single doses of 200 mg were given. For ethylene glycol poisoning and AKA, we recommend a dose of 100 mg intravenously daily. For all these disorders, strong evidence to favor one regimen over alternatives is lacking.

## FORMULATION AND ACQUISITION

Multiple manufacturers formulate thiamine hydrochloride for IV or IM administration. Typical concentrations are either 50 or 100 mg/mL. Thiamine available in the US is formulated in 0.5% (5 mg/mL) chlorobutanol as a preservative. In the United Kingdom, the formulation Pabrinex is chlorobutanol free. Chlorobutanol is a sedative with a long elimination half-life, but doses of 600 mg were given to human volunteers without complication. Thus, following United Kingdom and EFNS recommendations of 1,500 mg/day of thiamine would only deliver 75 to 150 mg of chlorobutanol depending on which preparation was used.

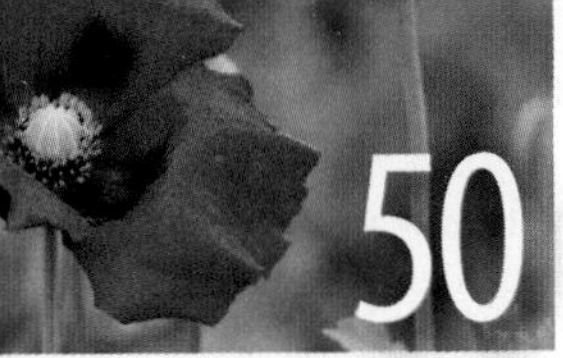

# 50 ALCOHOL WITHDRAWAL

## HISTORY AND EPIDEMIOLOGY

The medical problems associated with alcoholism and alcohol withdrawal were initially described by Pliny the Elder in the first century B.C. Initial treatments as described by Osler at the turn of the 20th century were focused on supportive care, including confinement to bed, cold baths to reduce fever, and judicious use of potassium bromide, chloral hydrate, hyoscine, and possibly opium. Some of the initial large series of alcohol-related complications in the early 20th century describe alcohol use as a major public health concern. The mortality rate among patients with delirium tremens (DTs) was 52%. It wasn't until 1955 when Isbell and colleagues (in an unethical study) proved abstinence from alcohol was responsible for DTs.

Currently, ethanol is responsible for approximately 3.8% of all deaths worldwide (6.3% of men and 1.1% of women) and accounts for 4.6% of the global burden of disease (7.6% of men and 1.4% of women). The lifetime risk of alcohol use disorders in men is more than 20%, with a risk of about 15% for alcohol abuse and 10% for alcohol dependence. Alcohol-related complications accounted for 21% of all medical intensive care unit (ICU) admissions. The presence of any alcohol use disorder (alcohol abuse, dependence, or harmful alcohol use) was associated with a twofold increase in mortality among intensive care unit (ICU) patients with organ failure and a nearly threefold increase in mortality in postsurgical patients.

## PATHOPHYSIOLOGY

Alcohol withdrawal syndrome is a neurologic disorder with a continuum of progressively worsening effects caused by the reduction or discontinuation of ethanol in a person who has developed ethanol dependence following chronic and heavy ethanol use. The effects of chronic alcohol consumption on neurotransmitter function best explain the clinical findings. Persistent stimulation of the inhibitory γ-aminobutyric acid (GABA) receptor chloride channel complex by ethanol leads to downregulation. This allows the alcohol user to function relatively normally despite the presence of sedative concentrations of ethanol in the brain. A converse series of events occurs at the *N*-methyl-D-aspartate (NMDA) subtype of glutamate receptor. Binding of ethanol to the glycine binding site of this receptor inhibits the NMDA receptor function, resulting in compensatory quantitative upregulation of these excitatory receptors. Thus, withdrawal of alcohol is associated with both a decrease in GABAergic activity and an increase in glutamatergic activity. Stated another way, it is a concomitant loss of inhibition and an increase in excitation.

## CLINICAL MANIFESTATIONS

Alcohol withdrawal is defined in the *Diagnostic and Statistical Manual of Mental Disorders*, 5th edition (*DSM-5*) as the cessation of heavy or prolonged alcohol use resulting, within a period of a few hours to several days, in the development of two or more of the clinical findings listed in Table 50–1. The clinical course of alcohol withdrawal varies widely among patients, and progression of individual patients through these different stages is also highly variable.

One of the more commonly used means for accurately assessing the severity of alcohol withdrawal is the Clinical Institute Withdrawal Assessment of Alcohol Scale, Revised (CIWA-Ar) score. However, its use is limited by the requirement of subjective assessments by the patient. For these reasons, we prefer the use of a general alertness scale such as the Richmond Agitation Sedation Scale (RASS), which is observer based.

### Early Uncomplicated Withdrawal

Alcohol withdrawal begins as early as 6 hours after the cessation of drinking. Early withdrawal is characterized by autonomic hyperactivity, including tachycardia, hypertension, fine tremor, and diaphoresis, as well as psychological changes such as emotional lability, anxiety, insomnia, and psychomotor agitation. This constellation of findings is sometimes called *alcoholic tremulousness*. Most patients who ultimately develop severe manifestations of alcohol withdrawal syndrome initially develop these findings.

### Alcoholic Hallucinosis

Alcoholic hallucinosis is characterized by vivid hallucinations that are generally transient. Although classically these hallucinations are tactile or visual ("pink elephants"), other types of hallucinations, particularly auditory and persecutory, are described. Tactile hallucinations include formications, or the sensation of ants crawling on the skin, which can result in repeated itching and excoriations. However, as opposed to DTs, patients with alcoholic hallucinosis have a clear sensorium.

**TABLE 50–1 Diagnostic Criteria for Alcohol Withdrawal Syndrome**

A. Cessation of or reduction in alcohol intake, which has previously been prolonged or heavy.
B. Criterion A, plus any 2 of the following symptoms developing within several hours to a few days:
   - Anxiety
   - Autonomic hyperactivity
   - Hallucinations
   - Insomnia
   - Nausea and vomiting
   - Psychomotor agitation
   - Seizures (generalized tonic–clonic)
   - Tremor (worsening)
C. The above symptoms cause clinically significant distress or impairment in social, occupational, or other important areas of functioning.
D. The above symptoms are not attributable to other causes; for example, another mental disorder, intoxication, or withdrawal from another substance.
E. Specify if hallucinations (usually visual or tactile) occur with intact reality testing, or if auditory, visual, or tactile illusions occur in the absence of a delirium.

### Alcohol Withdrawal Seizures

Approximately 10% of patients with alcohol withdrawal develop seizures, or "rum fits." For many patients, a generalized seizure is the first manifestation of the alcohol withdrawal often occurring in the first 24 hours. These seizures often occur in the absence of other signs of alcohol withdrawal and are characteristically brief, generalized, tonic–clonic events with a short postictal period. Rapid recovery and normal mental status initially minimize the seriousness of alcohol withdrawal seizures. However, for approximately one-third of patients with DTs, the sentinel event is an isolated alcohol withdrawal seizure.

### Delirium Tremens

Delirium tremens is the most serious manifestation of alcohol withdrawal and generally occurs between 48 and 96 hours after the cessation of drinking. Many of the clinical characteristics of DTs are similar to those of uncomplicated early alcohol withdrawal, differing only in severity, and include tremors, autonomic instability (hypertension and tachycardia), and psychomotor agitation. However, unlike the other forms of alcohol withdrawal, DTs is defined by a disturbance of consciousness. Unlike the early manifestations of alcohol withdrawal, which typically last for 3 to 5 days, DTs often lasts for up to 2 weeks.

## RISK FACTORS FOR THE DEVELOPMENT OF ALCOHOL WITHDRAWAL

The strongest predictor for the development of alcohol withdrawal is a history of prior episodes of withdrawal or DTs or a family history of alcoholic withdrawal. These factors, in addition to a select number of clinical and biochemical variables, were combined to create the Prediction of Alcohol Withdrawal Severity Scale (PAWSS), which demonstrated a 93% sensitivity for predicting complicated alcohol withdrawal among hospitalized patients.

## DIAGNOSTIC TESTING

### Clinical and Biochemical Predictors

Although consistent abnormalities in readily obtained laboratory values are observed in patients with alcohol withdrawal, their role in predicting the severity is poorly understood. The single best predictor is the onset of clinical symptoms with an elevated blood ethanol concentration (variably defined as greater than 150–200 mg/dL {32.6–43.4 mmol/L}).

## MANAGEMENT

### Alcohol Withdrawal Seizures

Alcohol withdrawal seizures are perhaps the most rigorously studied complication of alcohol withdrawal. They are generally self-limited, and if treatment is needed, benzodiazepines are preferred. There is no role for phenytoin in either treatment or prevention of alcohol withdrawal seizures. Many patients with alcohol use disorders develop underlying seizure foci from repeated head trauma. Those patients should be maintained on antiepileptics in consultation with neurology, and have neuroimaging as clinically indicated.

### Alcohol Withdrawal

Among those who seek medical attention, many patients with alcohol withdrawal can be safely managed as outpatients. In one study, patients who were not clinically intoxicated, had no history of either DTs or alcohol withdrawal seizures, had no comorbid psychiatric or medical disorders, and had a CIWA-Ar score of less than 8 (out of a potential maximal total of 67) were safely managed as outpatients.

For all patients with alcohol withdrawal, the initial stages of therapy remain the same and should include a thorough assessment to identify a coexisting medical, psychiatric, or toxicologic disorder. In particular, an assessment for central nervous system (CNS) trauma and infection should include the use of computed tomography and lumbar puncture as indicated. Patients with altered cognition and an elevated body temperature should receive antibiotics, pending the results of a lumbar puncture.

Chronic ethanol consumption leads to severe vitamin and nutritional deficiencies and electrolyte disturbances that should be corrected. Specifically, thiamine is recommended for all patients to prevent the development of Wernicke encephalopathy. We recommend an initial dose of parenteral thiamine of 100 mg in the management of the patient with alcohol withdrawal (Antidotes in Brief: A27). In addition, there is a high incidence of intravascular volume depletion among people with alcoholism, and volume resuscitation is recommended in patients with clinically significant alcohol withdrawal. Finally, for patients with alcohol withdrawal syndrome, prevention of nosocomial complications is paramount for reducing hospital stays. Currently, in addition to adequate volume replacement, we recommend (1) that all patients be kept with the head of the bed elevated to prevent aspiration and (2) that deep vein thrombosis prophylaxis be given if the patient is bed bound for more than 24 hours.

Oral benzodiazepine administration is generally effective in patients with early or mild alcohol withdrawal, although initial rapid titration with an intravenous (IV) regimen may be more efficient in patients with more severe symptoms. Intravenous diazepam offers a rapid time to peak clinical effects, which limits the oversedation that may occur after rapid readministration of lorazepam (Antidotes in Brief: A26). Midazolam is recommended intramuscularly if IV access is not available. Other pharmacokinetic factors and experience confirm that diazepam is the preferred benzodiazepine for initial IV use in patients with moderate to severe alcohol withdrawal. Diazepam has a long half-life and two active metabolites (desmethyldiazepam and oxazepam). The prolonged half-life (48–72 hours) of desmethyldiazepam further extends the effective duration of action of the initial dose of diazepam. For patients with advanced liver disease, the use of diazepam may result in a very prolonged period of sedation because of impaired clearance of the parent compound and its metabolites. In these patients, a benzodiazepine without active metabolites, such as oxazepam or lorazepam, is recommended.

The goal of therapy is to have the patient sedated but breathing spontaneously, with normal vital signs. Although normalization of vital signs is not a mandatory therapeutic endpoint, abnormal vital signs despite adequate sedation should prompt a search for comorbidities. In many patients, attaining complete sedation using a loading protocol allows for autotitration; that is, as alcohol withdrawal resolves, the blood concentrations of the benzodiazepine decrease, allowing gradual clinical recovery. In practicality, most patients need periodic symptom-triggered redosing with benzodiazepines to maintain adequate sedation. This is particularly important in patients who develop alcohol withdrawal with a concomitantly elevated blood alcohol concentration.

Multiple studies suggest that if additional doses are required, they should be administered based on symptoms ("symptom triggered") as opposed to on a fixed dosing schedule. Typical symptom-triggered dosing is initiated in patients with a CIWA-Ar score that remains greater than 8 or a RASS score of +1 or greater. For patients with moderate or severe alcohol withdrawal, symptom-triggered doses of IV diazepam 10 to 20 mg usually suffice. For less symptomatic patients, oral chlordiazepoxide 50 to 100 mg is recommended.

### Resistant Alcohol Withdrawal and Delirium Tremens

There is a subgroup of patients with alcohol withdrawal who require very large doses of diazepam or another comparable drug to achieve initial sedation. Patients with resistant alcohol withdrawal and DTs often have benzodiazepine requirements that exceed 2,600 mg of diazepam within the first 24 hours and generally require admission to an ICU or step-down unit. We recommend beginning with administration of benzodiazepines in a symptom-triggered fashion. In instances of extreme benzodiazepine resistance, patients often receive a second GABAergic drug because of "failure" of benzodiazepine therapy. Phenobarbital, given in combination with a benzodiazepine, in individual IV doses of 65 to 260 mg to a maximum of 10 to 15 mg/kg, is recommended. Caution is required to avoid stacking doses of phenobarbital because the onset of clinical effect takes approximately 20 to 40 minutes. Alternatively, propofol, either as individual bolus or as an infusion (in standard ICU dosing regimens, 10–50 μg/kg/min), can serve as an adjunct to benzodiazepines for patients with resistant alcohol withdrawal. Although propofol has a rapid onset, it is difficult to titrate and usually requires endotracheal intubation.

### Ethanol

Ethanol consumption is a common and effective means by which people with alcohol use disorder can self-medicate to treat or prevent mild alcohol withdrawal. Consequently, some hospitals still administer ethanol. Despite its widespread use, little randomized controlled data supports its use. The necessity for frequent blood alcohol monitoring, unpredictable elimination kinetics, potential for significant hepatic complications, postulated adverse effects of ethanol on wound healing, and difficulty in safely administering this therapy make it inappropriate to recommend the use of ethanol for the medical treatment of alcohol withdrawal.

### Adrenergic Antagonists

Numerous studies have investigated the use of sympatholytics to control the autonomic symptoms of alcohol withdrawal. Both β-adrenergic antagonists and clonidine reduced blood pressure and heart rate in randomized, placebo-controlled trials. However, the inability of these xenobiotics to address the underlying pathophysiologic mechanism of alcohol withdrawal and subsequently control the neurologic manifestations makes them suboptimal as the sole therapeutic. Additionally, by altering the physiologic parameters that serve as classic markers for the severity of withdrawal, there is a risk of underadministering necessary amounts of benzodiazepines. There are a growing number of reports documenting the use of the central α-adrenergic agonist dexmedetomidine as an adjuvant to benzodiazepines for treatment of alcohol withdrawal. The impact on global outcomes remains mixed, with studies reporting increased or decreased duration of hospitalization with dexmedetomidine use. Consequently, with the unclear efficacy and the potential for bradycardia, we recommend not to use it for the routine primary treatment of alcohol withdrawal. In the setting in which standard therapies, such as escalating doses of benzodiazepines and barbiturates, fail to provide adequate sedation (eg, RASS) or control of the alcohol withdrawal (eg, CIWA), a trial of dexmedetomidine seems reasonable while continuing the therapies.

### Magnesium

The theoretical benefits of magnesium supplementation are based on the high prevalence of magnesium deficiency in people with alcohol use disorder, its ability to block NMDA receptors, and its usefulness in preventing seizures in other disorders, including eclampsia. However, in a randomized, placebo-controlled trial, magnesium had no effect on either the incidence of withdrawal seizures or severity of alcohol withdrawal. Aside from repletion of electrolyte abnormalities as part of routine patient care, we recommend against the routine administration of magnesium for the treatment of alcohol withdrawal in patients with a normal serum magnesium concentration.

### Antiepileptics

Carbamazepine has been used in multiple trials for treatment of mild alcohol withdrawal, more commonly in Europe, where an IV preparation is available. However, there are insufficient data to recommend its use. Valproic acid appears to have a benzodiazepine-sparing effect in patients with mild withdrawal, but the true clinical benefit is unclear. Thus we recommend against using antiepileptics as monotherapy or primary therapy for treatment of patients with moderate or severe alcohol withdrawal.

### Gabapentin

Gabapentin, originally introduced as an antiepileptic, has been used extensively for treatment of neuropathic pain and delirium. An extensive literature demonstrates that gabapentin, administered in doses up to 2,400 mg/day, is extremely effective in treatment of alcohol dependence. However, literature related to its use for the treatment of established alcohol withdrawal remains mixed. Therefore, although it may be appropriate for mild outpatient alcohol withdrawal, its use, especially as monotherapy or in routine inpatient care, cannot be recommended.

### Other Therapeutics

Recently there has been growing attention toward the use of baclofen, a $GABA_B$ receptor agonist, because of its purported ability to reduce alcohol cravings and treat alcohol withdrawal. However, because data from three randomized controlled clinical studies have failed to demonstrate clinical benefit and because baclofen therapy was associated with increased deaths, we recommend against using baclofen for monotherapy at this time, although its use as an adjunctive therapy deserves further study.

Ketamine is also proposed as an adjunct for treatment of severe alcohol withdrawal or DTs. Like so many other studies, a retrospective study of the use of ketamine in a small number of ICU patients with alcohol withdrawal found that it was associated with a reduction in the need for diazepam without demonstrating any patient-centered outcomes. Pending more controlled clinical data, ketamine is only reasonable in patients with severe benzodiazepine-resistant alcohol withdrawal for whom other more established adjuncts, including phenobarbital and possibly propofol, have either failed or are unable to be tolerated.

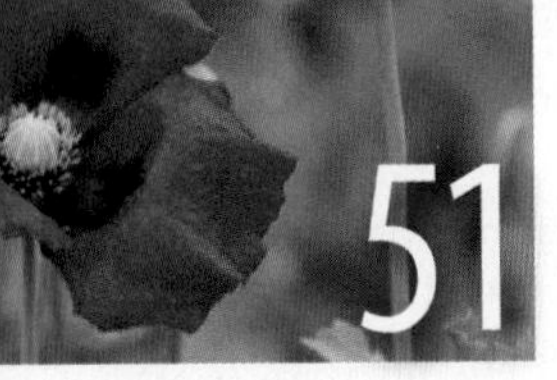

# 51 DISULFIRAM AND DISULFIRAM-LIKE REACTIONS

## HISTORY AND EPIDEMIOLOGY

Disulfiram was synthesized from thiocarbamide in the 1880s to accelerate the vulcanization (stabilization) of rubber. Sixty years later, it was the first Western medication used to treat alcohol dependence. Disulfiram was never widely used clinically, and its use further declined after several studies revealed no significant difference in drinking outcomes between unsupervised disulfiram administration and placebo. A distinction must be made between the clinical manifestations of a disulfiram–ethanol reaction and the toxic effects of disulfiram itself. Although life-threatening effects associated with disulfiram are rare, clinicians should be aware of proper diagnosis and management of patients with disulfiram-associated toxicity.

## PHARMACOLOGY AND PHARMACOKINETICS OF DISULFIRAM

Approximately 70% to 90% of an ingested therapeutic dose of disulfiram is absorbed as a bis(diethyldithiocarbamate)–copper complex, with peak serum concentrations achieved 8 to 10 hours following a 250-mg dose. Subsequent conversion to diethylamine and carbon disulfide occurs rapidly (Fig. 51–1). Disulfiram is highly lipid soluble and approximately 80% protein bound. The hepatic metabolites of disulfiram are mostly excreted renally, and an estimated 5% to 20% is not metabolized and is excreted unchanged in the feces. The volume of distribution is not described. Disulfiram has a half-life estimated at 60 to 120 hours. Diethyldithiocarbamate (DDC) is estimated to have a half-life of 13.9 hours and carbon disulfide 8.9 hours. Both disulfiram and DDC are selective inhibitors of CYP2E1.

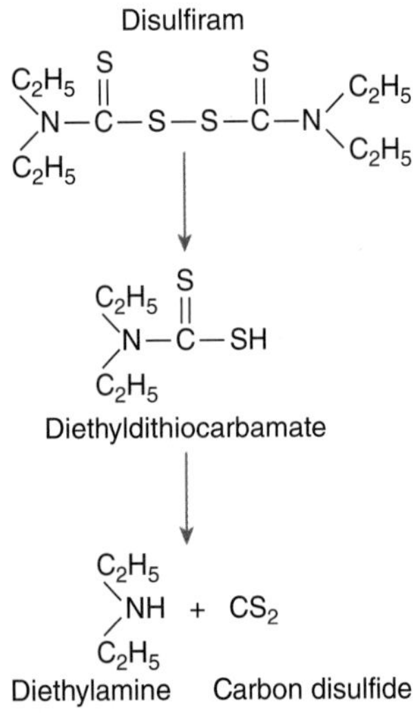

Disulfiram

$(C_2H_5)_2N{-}C({=}S){-}S{-}S{-}C({=}S){-}N(C_2H_5)_2$

↓

$(C_2H_5)_2N{-}C({=}S){-}SH$

Diethyldithiocarbamate

↓

$(C_2H_5)_2NH + CS_2$

Diethylamine    Carbon disulfide

**FIGURE 51–1.** Disulfiram metabolism occurs in the liver and in the erythrocyte. The most consequential metabolites are diethyldithiocarbamate and carbon disulfide.

## OTHER ENZYMES INHIBITED BY DISULFIRAM

In addition to aldehyde dehydrogenase (ALDH), disulfiram and its active metabolites have many other effects. DDC is a potent metal chelator, which explains interest in the treatment of nickel poisoning (Chap. 69). DDC also inhibits dopamine β-hydroxylose (DBH), which converts dopamine to norepinephrine. Inhibition of DBH leads to increased concentrations of dopamine in the brain and periphery and decreased concentrations of norepinephrine and epinephrine, which may relate to its hypotensive effects.

## DISULFIRAM–ETHANOL REACTION

### Pharmacology and Pharmacokinetics

The primary indication for disulfiram is as an avoidant and aversive treatment for alcohol dependence. Disulfiram inhibits ALDH, the enzyme that catalyzes the oxidation of acetaldehyde to acetate (Fig. 51–2). The increased concentration of acetaldehyde is responsible for the symptoms produced by the disulfiram–ethanol reaction. Aldehyde dehydrogenase inhibition develops over 12 hours and is mainly irreversible. Recovery of enzymatic activity depends on de novo ALDH synthesis that takes place in 6 or more days. The metabolites of disulfiram, including DDC and its sulfoxide and sulfone metabolites, also inhibit ALDH. The disulfiram–ethanol reaction occurs up to 3 weeks after the cessation of disulfiram therapy. Disulfiram–ethanol reactions occur after exposure to the ethanol contained in many household products (Table 51–1).

### Clinical Manifestations

Symptoms of the disulfiram–ethanol reaction often begin within 15 minutes of ethanol ingestion, peak at 30 to 60 minutes, and gradually resolve over the next several hours. Symptoms are diverse and include flushing, pruritus,

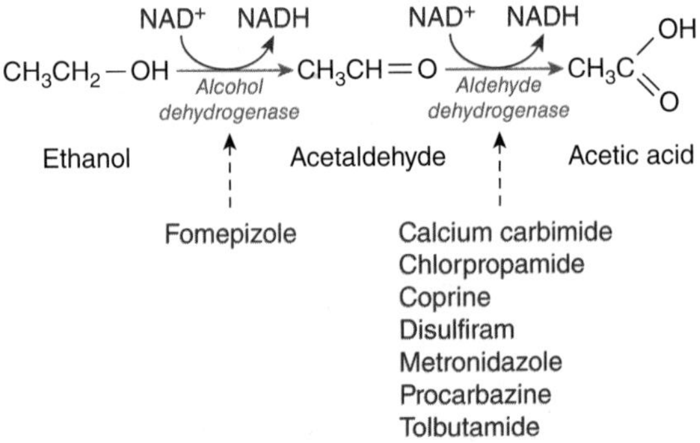

$CH_3CH_2{-}OH$ (Ethanol) → [Alcohol dehydrogenase; $NAD^+$ → NADH] → $CH_3CH{=}O$ (Acetaldehyde) → [Aldehyde dehydrogenase; $NAD^+$ → NADH] → $CH_3COOH$ (Acetic acid)

Inhibitor of alcohol dehydrogenase: Fomepizole

Inhibitors of aldehyde dehydrogenase: Calcium carbimide, Chlorpropamide, Coprine, Disulfiram, Metronidazole, Procarbazine, Tolbutamide

**FIGURE 51–2.** The site of action of disulfiram and other xenobiotics. The irreversible inactivation of aldehyde dehydrogenase results in an increased acetaldehyde concentration after ethanol is administered. $NAD^+$ = nicotinamide adenine dinucleotide (oxidized); NADH = nicotinamide adenine dinucleotide (reduced).

**TABLE 51–1 Common Household Products That Contain Ethanol and May Cause a Reaction with Disulfiram**

| |
|---|
| Adhesives |
| Alcohols: denatured alcohol, rubbing alcohol |
| Detergents |
| Foods: liquor-containing desserts, fermented vinegar, some sauces |
| Nonprescription xenobiotics: analgesics, antacids, antidiarrheals, cough and cold preparations, topical anesthetics, vitamins |
| Personal hygiene products: aftershave lotions, colognes, contact lens solutions, deodorants, liquid soaps, mouthwashes, perfumes, shampoos, skin liniments, and lotions |
| Solvents |

diaphoresis, lightheadedness, headache, nausea, vomiting, and abdominal pain. Disulfiram-like reactions occur when ethanol is ingested with xenobiotics other than disulfiram (Table 51–2). Healthcare providers should warn patients of such reactions when prescribing certain medications that cause this adverse effect.

**TABLE 51–2 Xenobiotics Reported to Cause a Disulfiram-like Reaction With Ethanol**

| |
|---|
| Antimicrobials |
|   Cephalosporins, especially those that contain an nMTT side chain, such as cefotetan, cefoperazone, cefamandole, and cefmenoxime |
|   Metronidazole |
|   Moxalactam |
|   Trimethoprim–sulfamethoxazole |
|   Possible reactions with chloramphenicol, furazolidone, griseofulvin, nitrofurantoin, procarbazine quinacrine, sulfonamides |
| Calcium carbimide (citrated) |
| Carbon disulfide |
| Carbon tetrachloride |
| Chloral hydrate |
| Dimethylformamide |
| Mushrooms |
|   *Coprinus* mushrooms, including *C. atramentaria*, *C. insignis*, *C. variegatus*, and *C. quadrifidus*; *Boletus luridus*, *Clitocybe clavipes*, *Polyporus sulphureus*, *Pholiota squarosa*, *Tricholoma aurantum*, *Verpa bohemica* |
| Nitrefazole |
| Phentolamine |
| Procarbazine |
| Sulfonylurea oral hypoglycemics |
|   Chlorpropamide |
|   Tolbutamide |
| Tacrolimus |
| Thiram analogs (fungicides) |
|   Copper, mercuric, and sodium diethyldithiocarbamate |
|   Zinc and ferric dimethyldithiocarbamate |
|   Zinc and disodium ethylenebis (dithiocarbamate) |
| Thiuram analogs |
|   Tetraethylthiuram monosulfide and disulfide (disulfiram) |
|   Tetramethylthiuram disulfide (thiram) |
| Tolazoline |
| Trichloroethylene |

nMTT = *N*-methylthiotetrazole.

## MANAGEMENT OF DISULFIRAM–ETHANOL REACTIONS

The duration of the disulfiram–alcohol reaction varies from 30 to 60 minutes in mild cases to several hours and is largely dependent on the amount of alcohol absorbed and its metabolism. Because of vomiting and volume depletion, serum glucose, electrolytes, and kidney function should be evaluated. Because only small amounts of ethanol precipitate the reaction, it is useful to quantify the presence of ethanol with a blood concentration. Patients with cardiovascular instability should have an electrocardiogram (ECG) performed and be attached to continuous cardiac monitoring. Symptomatic and supportive care is the mainstay of treatment. Most patients with hypotension respond to intravenous (IV) 0.9% sodium chloride. Refractory hypotension is rare, but if necessary, a vasopressor should be administered. A direct-acting adrenergic agonist such as norepinephrine is recommended because disulfiram inhibits DBH, an enzyme necessary for norepinephrine synthesis. For further symptomatic care, antiemetics are reasonable, and for cutaneous flushing, a histamine ($H_1$) receptor antagonist, such as diphenhydramine, is useful. Fomepizole reduces the accumulation of acetaldehyde by blocking alcohol dehydrogenase (Fig. 51–2) and is only recommended for patients experiencing a severe disulfiram–ethanol reaction leading to cardiogenic or distributive shock (Antidotes in Brief: A33).

## CLINICAL MANIFESTATIONS OF DISULFIRAM TOXICITY

### Acute Disulfiram Overdose

Reported cases of acute disulfiram overdose are infrequent and typically do not cause life-threatening toxicity. Most patients develop gastrointestinal (GI) symptoms within 1 to 2 hours that include nausea, vomiting, and abdominal pain. Neurologic symptoms develop after large acute disulfiram overdoses and include lethargy and coma. Dysarthria and movement disorders, including myoclonus, ataxia, dystonia, and akinesia, usually take three or more days to develop, occur rarely, and are related to direct effects of carbon disulfide on the basal ganglia. Persistent neurologic abnormalities, such as paresis, myoclonus, and neuropathy, are rare but can last weeks to months.

### Chronic Disulfiram Therapy

The toxic effects of disulfiram alone, including depression, lethargy, loss of libido, psychosis, delirium, meningeal signs, unilateral weakness, optic neuritis, and peripheral neuropathy, are often overlooked or misattributed to alcoholism. In aggregate adverse drug reaction data, hepatic reactions were the most frequent (34%) followed by neurologic (21%), cutaneous (15%), psychiatric (4%), and other (26%). Asymptomatic elevations in aminotransferase concentrations, up to three times the upper limits of normal, associated with disulfiram therapy are reported to range from 6% to 30%. The incidence of disulfiram-induced fatal hepatitis is reportedly 1 in 30,000 patients treated per year.

### Disulfiram and Pregnancy

There is a paucity of information regarding the teratogenic effects, if any, of disulfiram in humans or animals. There are no human data on the safety in breastfeeding.

## DIAGNOSTIC TESTING

### Acute Disulfiram Toxicity

Serum concentrations of disulfiram and its metabolites can be measured but are not useful when managing most patients with suspected acute or chronic disulfiram overdose, disulfiram toxicity, or a disulfiram–ethanol reaction. Elevated acetaldehyde concentrations in the blood will occur but are not readily available and thus also are not clinically useful in managing patients.

### Chronic Disulfiram Toxicity

The development of hepatotoxicity is a concern with chronic disulfiram administration. Two common strategies used for detecting and preventing severe hepatotoxicity include routine clinical monitoring for signs or symptoms of hepatic injury as well as periodic monitoring of alanine aminotransferase, aspartate aminotransferase, alkaline phosphatase, and total bilirubin.

The development of an aminotransferase concentration greater than three times the upper limit of the normal in combination with evidence of impaired hepatic synthetic function, elevated total bilirubin greater than two times the upper limit of the reference range, or international normalized ratio greater than 1.5 is suggestive of more severe drug-induced liver injury. In such situations, the mortality rate may be 16% or higher and necessitates discontinuing disulfiram.

## MANAGEMENT OF DISULFIRAM TOXICITY

### Acute Disulfiram Toxicity

There is no antidote for acute disulfiram overdose. No specific studies have evaluated GI decontamination for acute overdose. Unless otherwise contraindicated, activated charcoal at a dose of 1 g/kg is recommended for patients with recent ingestions.

### Chronic Disulfiram Toxicity

Periodic monitoring of function tests should be performed, and therapy should be discontinued with symptoms of hepatic injury such as jaundice, abdominal pain, nausea, vomiting, or fever. Treatment of hepatotoxicity is supportive and usually resolves after discontinuation of disulfiram therapy.

# 52 HALLUCINOGENS

## HISTORY

A "hallucination" is defined as a false perception that has no basis in the external environment. Hallucinations differ from illusions, which are distorted perceptions of objects based in reality. Although the term *psychedelic* has been used for years to refer to the recreational and nonmedical effects of hallucinogens, other terms, such as *entheogen* and *entactogen*, frequently appear in discussions. Entheogens are "substances that generate the god or spirit within," and entactogens create an awareness of "the touch within." These terms all refer to the same xenobiotics, used with differing intent or in varying settings.

Hallucinogens are a diverse group of xenobiotics that alter and distort perception, thought, and mood without clouding the sensorium. Hallucinogens are categorized by their chemical structures (Table 52–1). This chapter focuses on lysergamides, tryptamines, phenylethylamines, and the aforementioned "unclassified" hallucinogens. The other classes are found in Chaps. 44, 46, 47, and 56. Hallucinogens have been used for thousands of years by many different cultures, largely during religious ceremonies. From medieval times through recent years, several large-scale epidemics of vasospastic ischemia, gangrene, and hallucinations (collectively called ergotism) resulted from *Claviceps purpurea* contamination of cereal crops. Synthetic hallucinogen use is often said to have begun in 1938 when Albert Hofmann, a Swiss chemist, synthesized lysergic acid diethylamide (LSD). Designer hallucinogens exploit a loophole in United States (US) drug enforcement laws by modifying existing illegal drugs into novel substances.

The Internet is now a vehicle for the rapid and facile sharing of information on the synthesis of emerging drugs, user experiences, and adverse effects. All-night dance clubs host "rave parties" at which emerging hallucinogens are popular. Although the impact of these parties on the growth of hallucinogens in the US is unclear, many of the newer hallucinogens are christened "club drugs" because of this association. A survey of dance club patrons in South London suggests that novel psychoactive substances supplement established recreational drugs like 3,4-methylenedioxymethamphetamine (MDMA).

**TABLE 52–1 Structural Classifications of Hallucinogens**

| |
|---|
| **Lysergamides** |
| D-Lysergic acid diethylamide (LSD) |
| Lysergic acid hydroxyethylamide |
|   Morning glory (*Ipomoea violacea*) |
|   South American morning glory (*Ololiuqui*) |
| Ergine |
|   Woodrose (*Argyreia nervosa*) |
| **Indolealkylamines and Tryptamines** |
| 5-Methoxy-*N,N*-dimethyltryptamine (5-MeO-DiPT, Foxy Methoxy) |
| *N,N*-Dimethyltryptamine (DMT) |
| α-methyltryptamine (AMT) |
| Psilocin |
| Psilocybin |
| **Phenylethylamines** |
| Mescaline |
| 3,4-Methylenedioxymethamphetamine (MDMA) |
| 2C-B |
| 2C-T-7 |
| **Tetrahydrocannabinoids** |
| Marijuana |
| Hashish |
| **Belladonna Alkaloids** |
| Jimsonweed (*Datura stramonium*) |
| Henbane (*Hyoscyamus niger*) |
| Deadly nightshade (*Atropa belladonna*) |
| *Brugmansia* spp |
| **Miscellaneous** |
| Kava Kava (*Piper methysticum*) |
| Kratom (*Mitragyna speciose korth*) |
| Nutmeg (*Myristica fragrans*)-myristicin, elemicin, safrole |
| Phencyclidine (PCP), ketamine |
| *Salvia divinorum* |

## EPIDEMIOLOGY

Resurgence in LSD use was reported among US high school teens in the late 1990s, with more prevalent use in the suburbs than the cities. From 2006 to 2015, the National Survey on Drug Use and Health (NSDUH) reported increases in lifetime use trends for LSD, MDMA, ketamine, α-methyltryptamine (AMT), dimethyltryptamine (DMT), and 5-methoxydimethyl tryptamine (5-MeO-DMT).

## LYSERGAMIDES

Lysergamides are derivatives of lysergic acid, a substituted tetracyclic amine based on an indole nucleus (Fig. 52–1). Naturally occurring lysergamides are found in several species of morning glory (*Rivea corymbosa, Ipomoea violacea*) and Hawaiian baby woodrose (*Argyreia nervosa*). The synthetic lysergamide, LSD, is derived from an ergot alkaloid of the fungus, *Claviceps purpurea*. Lysergic acid diethylamide users experience heightened awareness of auditory and visual stimuli with size, shape, and color distortions. Auditory and visual hallucinations occur, as well as synesthesia, a confusion of the senses, in which users report "hearing colors" or "seeing sounds." A "bad trip" or dysphoric reaction is said to occur when LSD use produces anxiety, bizarre behavior, and combativeness.

## INDOLEALKYLAMINES (TRYPTAMINES)

Indolealkylamines, or tryptamines, represent a class of natural and synthetic compounds that structurally share a substituted monoamine group (Fig. 52–2). Naturally occurring exogenous tryptamines include psilocybin, bufotenine and *N,N*-dimethyltryptamine (DMT). Psilocybin is found

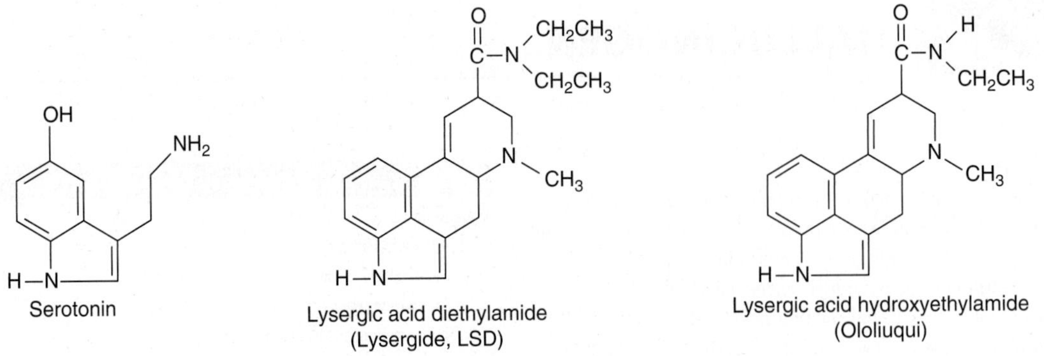

**FIGURE 52–1.** Hallucinogens of the lysergamide chemical class and their chemical similarity to serotonin.

in three major genera of mushrooms: *Psilocyba, Panaelous,* and *Conocybe.* Hallucinogenic mushrooms are discussed at length in Chap. 90. *N,N*-dimethyltryptamine a 5-$HT_{2A}$, 5-$HT_{2C}$, and 5-$HT_{1A}$ receptor agonist, is a potent short-acting hallucinogen found naturally in the bark of the Yakee plant (*Virola calophylla*), which grows in the Amazon basin. In ayahuasca, DMT-containing plants (eg, *Psychotria viridis*) are combined with plants containing harmine alkaloids (eg, *Banisteriopsis caapi*), which inhibit hepatic monoamine oxidases to increase the oral bioavailability of DMT (Chap. 44). All species of the toad genus *Bufo* have parotid glands on their backs that produce a variety of xenobiotics, including dopamine, epinephrine, and serotonin. One species of toad, *Bufo alvarius* (Sonoran Desert toad or Colorado River toad) also secretes 5-methoxydimethyl tryptamine (5-MeO-DMT), a psychoactive substance. Two of the more important synthetic tryptamines include *N,N*-diisopropyl-5-methoxytryptamine (5-MeO-DiPT, Foxy Methoxy) and α-methyltryptamine (AMT, IT-290), which are often sold surreptitiously as MDMA.

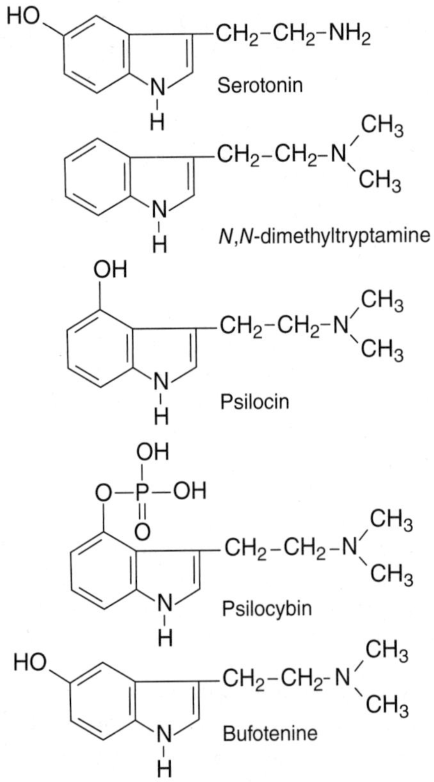

**FIGURE 52–2.** Hallucinogens of the indolealkylamine chemical class and their chemical similarity to serotonin.

## PHENYLETHYLAMINES (AMPHETAMINES)

Dopamine, norepinephrine, and tyrosine are endogenous phenylethylamines. Exogenous phenylethylamines stimulate catecholamine release and cause a variety of physiologic and psychiatric effects, including hallucinations. The best recognized of the naturally occurring psychoactive phenylethylamines is mescaline, which is found in the peyote (*Lophophora williamsii*) cactus. Substitution on the phenylalkylamine structure has important effects on both the hallucinogenic and stimulant potential of the drug. The presence of a methyl group in the side chain of the phenylethylamines is associated with a higher degree of hallucinogenic effect (Fig. 52–3). 3,4-Methylenedioxymethamphetamine,

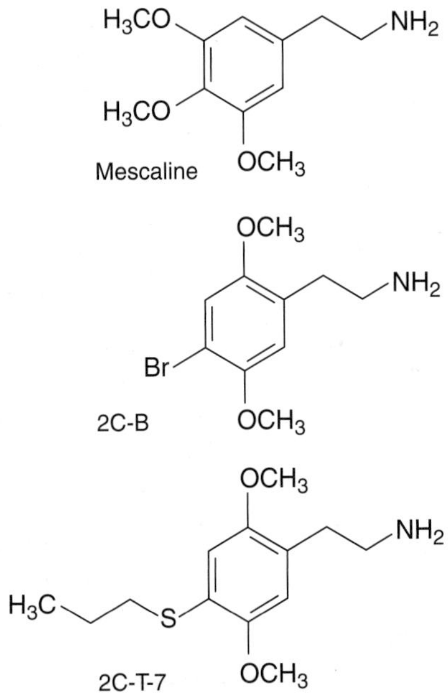

**FIGURE 52–3.** Hallucinogens of the phenylethylamine chemical class.

amphetamine, and methamphetamine are well-known members of this family and are discussed in detail in Chap. 46.

The synthesis and effects of hundreds of other hallucinogenic amphetamines are well described, including 4-bromo-2,5-dimethoxyphenethylamine (2C-B, Nexus, Bromo, Spectrum) and 2,5-dimethoxy-4-*N*-propylthiopheneethylamine (2C-T-7, Blue Mystic).

## *SALVIA DIVINORUM*

*Salvia divinorum* is a perennial herbaceous member of the mint family recognized for its hallucinogenic properties. Since the 16th century, the Mazatec Indians have used *S. divinorum* as a hallucinogen in religious rites as a means of producing "visions." There is wide variability among state laws against *S. divinorum*, and there continues to be widespread marketing of this hallucinogen on the Internet as a "legal hallucinogen."

## KRATOM

Kratom, or *Mitragyna speciosa Korth*, is derived from the leaves of a tree native to Asia and Africa. Kratom has dual properties, producing stimulant effects and opioidlike analgesic effects. The kratom alkaloids mitragynine and 7-hydroxymitragynine are reported to activate μ-, δ-, and κ-opioid receptors. It is used as a substitute for opium; although hallucinogenic effects are uncommon, they are reported after heavy use.

## NUTMEG

Nutmeg is derived from *Myristica fragrans*, an evergreen tree native to the Spice Islands. The fruits of the tree contain a central kernel called the nutmeg; the surrounding red aril is used to produce a spice called mace. It is a recreational herbal that is used to produce euphoria and hallucinations; it is more likely to be abused by adolescents because of its low cost and accessibility.

## BELLADONNA ALKALOIDS

The belladonna alkaloids, including atropine, hyoscyamine, and scopolamine, are isolated from a number of plants including deadly nightshade (*Atropa belladonna*) and jimson weed (*Datura stramonium*). Given their wide availability, in the wild and over the Internet, these plants are frequently used as hallucinogens by adolescents.

## TOXICOKINETICS

The toxicokinetics of many common hallucinogens are shown in Table 52–2.

## PHARMACOLOGY

Although the lysergamide, indolealkylamine, and phenylethylamine hallucinogens are structurally distinct, the similarities in their effects on cognition support a common site of action on central serotonin receptors. Serotonin modulates many psychological and physiological processes, including mood, personality, affect, appetite, motor function, sexual activity, temperature regulation, pain perception, sleep induction and antidiuretic hormone (ADH) release. The lysergamide, indolealkylamine, and phenylethylamine hallucinogens all bind to the 5-$HT_2$ class of receptors. There is a good correlation between the affinity of both indolealkylamine and phenylethylamine hallucinogens for 5-$HT_2$ receptors in vitro and hallucinogenic potency in humans. Other potential mechanisms include enhanced release of glutamate, modulation of NMDA receptor-mediated effects, and modulation of thalamic filtering.

The effect of salvinorin A occurs via binding at the κ-opioid receptor, making it structurally and mechanistically unique

**TABLE 52–2 Pharmacology of Selected Hallucinogens**

| *Drug Name or Source* | *Psychoactive Component (if Different)* | *Typical Oral Dose* | *Onset* | *Duration* |
|---|---|---|---|---|
| *Bufo* species toads | 5-MeO-DMT | 5–15 mg (smoked) | Immediate (smoked) | 5–20 min (smoked) |
| DMT | — | 15–60 mg | 5–20 min | 30–60 min |
| "Foxy Methoxy" | 5-MeO-DiPT | 6–10 mg | 20–30 min | 3–6 h |
| Woodrose (*Argyreia nervosa*) | Ergine | 5–10 seeds | Minutes | 6–8 h |
| Jimson weed (*Datura stramonium*) | Atropine, hyoscyamine, scopolamine | 10 seeds | 20–30 min | 2–3 h |
| Kratom (*Mitragyna speciosa Korth*) | Mitragynine, 7-hydroxy-mitragynine | 2–6 g (stimulant); > 7 g (sedative) | 10–15 min | 4–6 h |
| LSD | Lysergic acid diethylamide | 50–100 μg | 30–60 min | 10–12 h |
| "Magic mushrooms" (*Psilocybe* spp) | Psilocybin, psilocin | 5 g mushrooms | 30 min–2 h | 4 h |
| Nutmeg (*Myristica fragrans*) | Myristicin, elemicin | 20 g | 1 h | 24 h |
| Peyote (*Lophophora williamsii*) | Mescaline | 6–12 buttons, 270–540 mg mescaline | 1–3 h | 10–12 h |
| *Salvia divinorum* | Salvinorin A | — | 30 min (inhaled); 1 h (PO) | 15–20 min (inhaled); 2 h (PO) |
| 2C-B | — | 16–30 mg | 1 h | 6–10 h |

PO = oral.

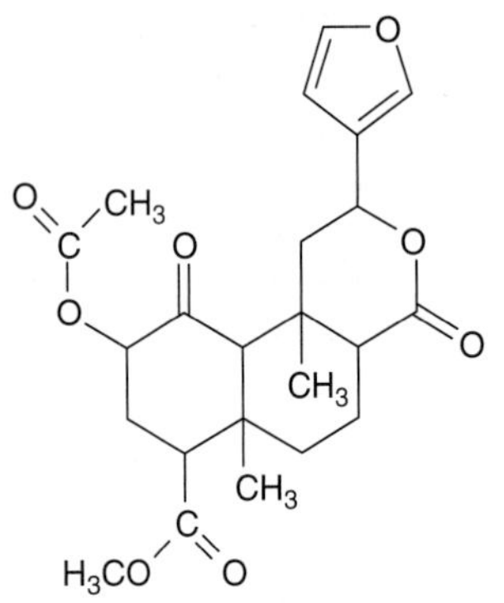

**FIGURE 52–4.** Structure of salvinorin A.

(Fig. 52–4). The κ-opioid receptor is distinct from the μ-opioid receptor, the stimulation of which generally causes euphoria and analgesia (Chap. 9). Salvinorin A does not have any serotonergic activity. The opioid effects of kratom are attributed to mitragynine, which is active at both supraspinal opioid δ and μ receptors. Additionally, mitragynine activates noradrenergic and serotonergic pathways. Nutmeg contains a number of purportedly psychoactive compounds, including myristicin, elemicin, and safrole (Fig. 52–5). The psychoactive components of nutmeg include terpenes and alkyl benzyl derivatives (myristicin, elemicin, and safrole), which are weak monoamine oxidase inhibitors that also demonstrate serotonergic activity.

## CLINICAL EFFECTS

Physiologic changes accompany and often precede the perceptual changes induced by lysergamides, tryptamines, and phenylethylamines. The physical effects are caused by direct drug effect or by a response to the disturbing or enjoyable hallucinogenic experience. Sympathetic effects include mydriasis, tachycardia, hypertension, tachypnea, hyperthermia, and diaphoresis. Other clinical findings that are reported include piloerection, dizziness, hyperactivity, muscle weakness, ataxia, altered mental status, coma, and hippus (rhythmic pupillary dilation and constriction). Nausea and vomiting often precede the psychedelic effects produced by psilocybin and mescaline. Potentially life-threatening complications, such as hyperthermia, hypertension, tachycardia, coma, respiratory arrest, and coagulopathy, are reported with massive LSD overdose. Similar sympathetic symptoms are described after the use of 2C-B and 2C-T-7. An analog of 2C-B, called 2C-B-FLY, or Bromo-dragonFLY, is implicated in finger necrosis requiring amputation secondary to potent peripheral vasospastic activity and sudden cardiac death.

The vast majority of morbidity from hallucinogen use stems from trauma. Hallucinogen users frequently report lacerations and bruises sustained during their "high." Additionally, dysphoria drives patients to react to stimuli with unpredictable and occasionally aggressive behavior. Many websites regarding hallucinogen use advise readers to take hallucinogens only while under the supervision of an observer.

The psychological effects of hallucinogens are dose related and cause changes in arousal, emotion, perception, thought process, and self-image. The person experiencing the effects of a hallucinogen is usually fully alert, oriented, and aware that he or she is under the influence of a drug. Euphoria, dysphoria, and emotional lability occur. Illusions are common, typically involving distortion of body image and alteration in visual perceptions. Many people report an intensification of their sensory perceptions. Synesthesias, or sensory misperceptions, such as "hearing colors" or "seeing sounds," are commonly described. Hallucinations are visual, auditory, tactile, or olfactory.

## LABORATORY

Routine urine drug-of-abuse immunoassay screens do not detect LSD or other hallucinogens. Although LSD can be detected by radioimmunoassay of the urine, confirmation by high-performance liquid chromatography (HPLC) or gas chromatography is necessary for reliability. False-positive urine immunoassay test results for LSD are reported after exposure to several medications, including fentanyl, sertraline, haloperidol, and verapamil. Depending on their structure, phenylethylamines cause positive qualitative urine test results by immunoassay for amphetamines. Urine immunoassays do not detect 5-Meo-DiPT, DMT, AMT, 2C-T-7, and 2CB, but gas chromatography–mass spectrometry testing methods for detection of these compounds is available. Routine urine drug immunoassay screens do not detect salvinorin A, mitragynine, or myristicin. Myristicin testing is not widely available.

## TREATMENT

Hallucinogen users rarely seek medical attention because either they experience only the desired effect of the drug or they minimize or cannot perceive the adverse effects. For any hallucinogen user presenting to the emergency department, initial treatment must begin with attention to airway, breathing, circulation, level of consciousness, and abnormal vital signs. Even in those in whom exposure to a hallucinogen is suspected, the basic approach for altered mental status

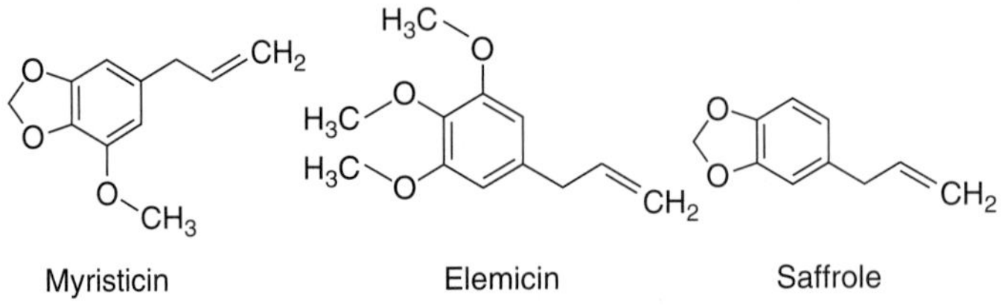

Myristicin Elemicin Saffrole

**FIGURE 52–5.** Structure of myristicin.

should include the administration of dextrose, naloxone, and oxygen as clinically indicated, and a vigorous search for other etiologies. Because of their rapid absorption, gastrointestinal decontamination with activated charcoal is of little value after clinical symptoms appear, and attempts may lead to further agitation. Sedation with benzodiazepines is usually sufficient to treat the hypertension, tachycardia, and hyperthermia that occur. We recommend avoiding use of physical restraints when possible to prevent hyperthermia and rhabdomyolysis. Hyperthermia resulting from agitation or muscle rigidity requires urgent sedation with benzodiazepines and rapid ice bath cooling. Seizures that occur with tryptamine or phenylethylamine use should be initially treated with benzodiazepines. Seizures also result from hyponatremia in MDMA users, and treatment with 3% (hypertonic) saline is recommended (Chap. 46).

The treatment of anticholinergic toxicity from the belladonna alkaloids involves several critical components: correction of abnormal vital signs, management of delirium, and rapid intervention for seizures or dysrhythmias. Physostigmine is recommended for patients with evidence of anticholinergic delirium or agitation if there are no contraindications (Antidotes in Brief: A11). Treatment of serotonin toxicity from phenylethylamine use is largely supportive and includes the avoidance of further administration of serotonergic medications. Specific therapy with cyproheptadine is recommended (Chap. 42).

## LONG-TERM EFFECTS

Long-term consequences of LSD use include prolonged psychotic reactions, severe depression, and exacerbation of preexisting psychiatric illness. When LSD was initially popularized, some patients behaved in a manner similar to schizophrenia and required admission to psychiatric facilities. Flashbacks are reported in up to 15% to 80% of LSD users. These perceptions are triggered during times of stress, illness, and exercise and are often a virtual recurrence of the initial hallucinations. Hallucinogen persisting perception disorder (HPPD) is a chronic disorder in which flashbacks lead to impairment in social or occupational function. According to the *Diagnostic and Statistical Manual of Mental Disorders*, fifth edition, the diagnosis of HPPD requires the recurrence of perceptual symptoms that were experienced while intoxicated with the hallucinogen that causes functional impairment and is not due to a medical condition. Lysergic acid diethylamide causes psychological but not physical dependence; therefore, it does not cause any physical withdrawal symptoms.

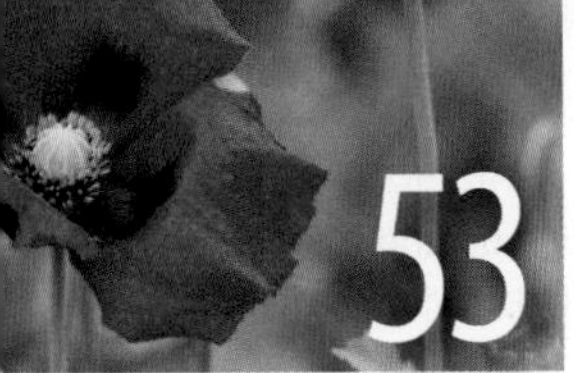

# 53 γ-HYDROXYBUTYRIC ACID

Since its scientific discovery as a γ-aminobutyric acid (GABA) mimetic neurochemical, γ-hydroxybutyric acid (GHB) has been transformed from a drug of investigational importance and licit medical uses to the toxic ingredient in banned nutritional supplements and illicit recreational drugs. GHB and its numerous chemical precursors and structural analogs, most notably γ-butyrolactone (GBL) and 1,4-butanediol (1,4-BD), represent a group of drugs among the broad class of recreational drugs known as "club drugs." Like most other "club drugs," GHB, GBL, and 1,4-BD are physically and psychologically addictive with acute and chronic toxicity that may be severe or lethal.

## HISTORY AND EPIDEMIOLOGY

γ-Hydroxybutyric acid was discovered in 1960 while searching for analogs of the inhibitory neurotransmitter GABA. Three years later, GHB was determined to be a naturally occurring neurochemical in the mammalian brain. GHB found its first clinical application as an anesthetic in the early 1960s. In 1966, the first associations of the effects of 1,4-BD with GHB were made, and later extended to other analogs such as GBL. GHB later became popular as a sports supplement and "natural" soporific. In the late 1980s, GHB was introduced to the health and dietary supplement market with dubious claims that it could metabolize fat, enhance muscle building, and improve sleep. However, it was quickly associated with severe adverse effects and deaths. The United States Food and Drug Administration (FDA) intervened in 1990 to prohibit further nonprescription sale of GHB in nutritional supplements but was circumvented by substitution of GBL for GHB as the active ingredient in dietary supplements. Subsequently, the FDA issued a voluntary recall of GBL-containing health supplements in 1999. As was the case with the initial recall of GHB, GBL was substituted by yet another GHB precursor, 1,4-BD. Predictably, the consequences of 1,4-BD misuse and abuse were clinically similar to those of GHB and GBL, including death. In 2002 GHB was approved by the FDA for the treatment of narcolepsy. In 2007, 1,4-BD was identified in the sticky surface material of toy beads marketed under the names Bindeez or Aquadots and caused inadvertent toxicity in children ingesting these beads.

Illicit use of GHB and its analogs occurs primarily at the: recreational setting of raves or night clubs; athletic setting of bodybuilding gyms and fitness centers; home consumer setting of individuals seeking its "natural health benefits"; and criminal setting of drug-facilitated sexual assault.

## PHARMACOLOGY

γ-Hydroxybutyrate is both a precursor and degradation product of GABA. It has a dual pharmacologic profile, with the intrinsic neuropharmacology of endogenous GHB being distinct and divergent from that of exogenously administered GHB. The principal difference is that the intrinsic neuropharmacologic activity of endogenous GHB is mediated by the GHB receptor, whereas the neuropharmacologic activity of exogenously administered GHB is likely mediated by the $GABA_B$ receptor.

### Endogenous GHB

GHB is formed from GABA as shown in Figure 53–1. Endogenous GHB acts as a neurotransmitter by binding to GHB-specific receptors that modulate other neurotransmitter systems. The GHB receptor has no affinity for typical $GABA_A$ or $GABA_B$ agonists. Rather, GHB receptors are highly associated with dopaminergic neurons and increase the concentration of dopamine by stimulating synthesis. GHB is also a neuromodulator of dopamine, acetylcholine, serotonin, endogenous opioids, and glutamate. Through an unclear mechanism, GHB increases the release of growth hormone by promoting slow-wave sleep without affecting total sleep time. GHB acid activity is terminated by active uptake from the synaptic cleft for metabolism.

### Exogenous GHB

Exogenous GHB is directly ingested or internally transformed from GBL or 1,4-BD. The resultant stimulation of the $GABA_B$ receptor signals adenylate cyclase to activate calcium channels and G protein–coupled inwardly rectifying $K^+$ channels, thereby decreasing dopamine and acetylcholine concentrations.

## γ-HYDROXYBUTYRIC ACID ANALOGS

Although GBL and 1,4-BD exist in the mammalian brain, their pharmacologic properties are only evident after conversion to GHB occurs. Table 53–1 lists the common synonyms for GHB an its analogs.

## PHARMACOKINETICS AND TOXICOKINETICS

The endogenous production and metabolism of GHB is shown in Figure 53–1. Oral bioavailability of exogeneous GHB is approximately 60% in animals. It is rapidly absorbed from the gastrointestinal (GI) tract in 15 to 45 minutes and has a final volume of distribution 0.6 L/kg.

It is lipid soluble and crosses the blood–brain barrier rapidly. It does not bind significantly to any plasma proteins. In adult volunteers, the elimination half-life is 20 to 53 minutes. Less than 5% of GHB is excreted unchanged in the urine. Compared with GHB, GBL is more rapidly absorbed from the GI tract and has a longer duration of action, both of which result from higher lipid solubility. Because 1,4-BD exerts its effects after conversion to GHB by alcohol dehydrogenase, coingestion of ethanol delays the onset of clinical effects.

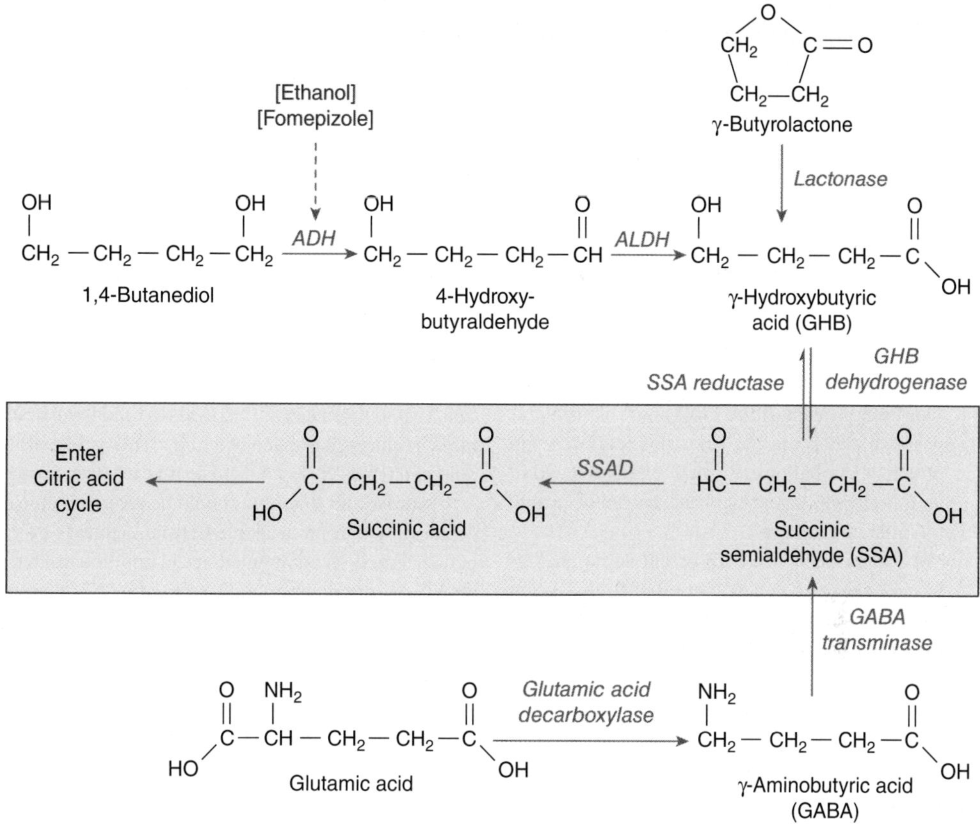


**FIGURE 53–1.** The synthesis and metabolism of γ-hydroxybutyric acid (GHB). ADH = alcohol dehydrogenase; ALDH = aldehyde dehydrogenase; SSAD = succinic semialdehyde dehydrogenase.

## CLINICAL MANIFESTATIONS

In volunteers undergoing sleep studies, a clear oral dose–response effect for GHB was noted: doses of 20 to 30 mg/kg create euphoria, memory loss, and drowsiness, and doses of 40 to 60 mg/kg result in coma. Vital signs typically reveal hypotension, bradycardia, bradypnea, and hypothermia. Bradypnea is the most consequential of these effects, and apnea is the most likely cause of death. Pupils are typically miotic and poorly responsive to light. Salivation and vomiting are common, especially when central nervous system

**TABLE 53–1** Common Synonyms for γ-Hydroxybutyric Acid and Analogs

| GHB (γ-Hydroxybutyrate) | GBL (γ-Butyrolactone) | 1,4-BD (1,4-Butanediol) | GHV (γ-Hydroxyvaleric Acid) | GVL (γ-Valerolactone) | THF (Tetrahydrofuran) |
|---|---|---|---|---|---|
| 4-Hydroxybutanoic acid | 1,4-Butanolide | 1,4-Butylene glycol | γ-Methyl-GHB | 4,5-Dihydro-5-methyl-2(3H)-furanone | No other synonyms |
| 4-Hydroxybutyric acid sodium salt | 4-Butanolide | 1,4-Dihydroxybutane | | 4-Hydroxypentanoicacid lactone | |
| γ-Hydroxybutyric acid | Butyric acid lactone | 1,4-Tetramethylene glycol | | γ-Methyl-GHB | |
| γ-Hydroxybutyric acid sodium salt | Butyrolactone | | | | |
| Sodium 4-hydroxybutyrate | Butyrolactone-γ | | | | |
| Sodium oxybate | 4-Butyrolactone | | | | |
| | Butyryl lactone | | | | |
| | 4-Deoxytetronic acid | | | | |
| | Dihydro-2(3H)-furanone | | | | |
| | 2(3H)-Furanone | | | | |
| | 2(3H)-Furanone dihydro | | | | |
| | Tetrahydro-2-furanone | | | | |
| | 4-Hydroxbutyric acid lactone | | | | |
| | γ-Hydroxybutyric acid lactone | | | | |
| | 1,4-Lactone | | | | |

(CNS) depression is prominent. These effects compound bradypnea and hypoventilation in that they increase the risk for aspiration.

Central nervous system effects can range from hallucinations, disorientation, and agitation to lethargy followed by stupor and coma. These findings most likely represent disinhibition of higher cortical areas and are consistent with other sedative–hypnotics. Motor abnormalities are also common, and there is debate about whether they represent seizures, myoclonus, or both. In animal models, GHB can produce seizures, yet electroencephalogram monitoring in humans suggests that repetitive movements most likely represent myoclonus.

The duration of effect is characteristically short. Many patients will abruptly awaken within 1 to 3 hours of presentation and appear completely normal. Even those patients who require endotracheal intubation are usually extubated within 8 hours. As long as aspiration and hypoxia have not occurred, most patients suffer no sequelae.

Patients who continually use GHB or one of its analogs every 2 to 4 hours over a prolonged period of time develop both tolerance and dependence. In these patients, withdrawal symptoms occur after discontinuation or a reduction in dose (see later).

## DIAGNOSTIC TESTING

The presence of GHB or its analogs can be determined quantitatively and qualitatively, in both serum and urine, using a variety of analytical techniques. The most important caveat is that appropriate cutoff values must be selected to distinguish use and overdose from endogenous concentrations. Because of rapid metabolism and elimination, concentrations return to baseline shortly after drug-naïve patients become clinically normal. Normal urinary concentrations of endogenous GHB are less than 5 to 10 μg/mL, and serum concentrations of endogenous GHB are less than 5 μg/mL. Attempts to relate concentrations to clinical effects in any individual might not be valid because of the potential for tolerance. In general, unconsciousness occurs when serum concentrations reach 50 μg/mL, and concentrations above 260 μg/mL typically produce deep coma in naïve patients. Because most clinical hospital laboratories do not routinely test for the presence of GHB analogs and recovery is typically rapid, results of analytical testing are not useful for clinical care. Other recommended routine tests in patients with depressed levels of consciousness include a rapid evaluation of blood glucose and an ethanol concentration. Electrocardiogram findings include sinus bradycardia and prominent U waves, which may be related to the bradycardia. When intentional self-harm is suspected, a determination of serum acetaminophen concentration is also recommended.

## MANAGEMENT

The provision of good supportive care remains the mainstay of therapy. The decision to perform endotracheal intubation should be made at the bedside and be based on a clinical assessment of oxygenation and ventilation. Despite deep coma, many patients will have adequate respirations and airway protective reflexes. As the duration of unconsciousness is relatively brief, coma in and of itself should not be considered an absolute indication for endotracheal intubation. Hypotension usually responds to fluids, and bradycardia rarely requires pharmacologic intervention. Hypothermia is mild and typically responds to passive external rewarming.

Dextrose and thiamine should be given as clinically indicated. Although no available GHB antagonists exist, a trial of naloxone is recommended in the undifferentiated patient based on the findings of small pupils and CNS and respiratory depression. However, naloxone administration to GHB-toxic humans is usually unsuccessful.

There is no role for GI decontamination in patients with isolated GHB toxicity because GHB is rapidly absorbed from the GI tract. The increased risk of vomiting and aspiration also limits any beneficial role. If a coingestant is present, decontamination with activated charcoal is reasonable if there are no contraindications (Chap. 3).

## GHB WITHDRAWAL

GHB withdrawal is similar to ethanol and benzodiazepine withdrawal and can be severe and potentially life threatening. The onset of withdrawal typically occurs 1 to 6 hours after last use. Manifestations of withdrawal include tachycardia, hypertension, tremors, agitation, dysphoria, nausea, vomiting, auditory and visual hallucinations, and seizures. Benzodiazepines and supportive care are the recommended mainstays of therapy (Antidotes in Brief: A26). Rapid cooling, IV fluids, and evaluation for other medical or traumatic illnesses should be performed. Some patients require large doses of benzodiazepines to control symptoms. In patients with withdrawal symptoms refractory to benzodiazepines, barbiturates and propofol are reasonable. Baclofen, a $GABA_B$ receptor agonist, is also a reasonable treatment in patients with severe GHB withdrawal, although research is needed determine appropriate dosing.

# 54 INHALANTS

## HISTORY AND EPIDEMIOLOGY

Inhalant use is defined as the deliberate inhalation of vapors for the purpose of changing one's consciousness or becoming "high." It is also referred to as volatile substance use, which was first described in medical literature in 1951. Initially, inhalant use was viewed as physically harmless, but reports of "sudden sniffing death" began to appear in the 1960s. Shortly thereafter, evidence surfaced of other significant morbidities, including organic brain syndromes, peripheral neuropathy, and withdrawal.

In the United States, the problem is greatest among children of lower socioeconomic groups. Inhalants are appealing to adolescents because they are inexpensive, readily available, and sold legally. Inhalant use includes sniffing, huffing, and bagging. *Sniffing* entails the inhalation of a volatile substance directly from a container. *Huffing* involves pouring a volatile liquid onto fabric. *Bagging* refers to instilling a solvent into a plastic or paper bag and rebreathing from the bag several times.

## COMMON INHALANTS

There are myriad xenobiotics used as inhalants (Table 54–1). The most commonly inhaled hydrocarbons are fuels, such as gasoline, and solvents, such as toluene. The choice of xenobiotic used likely reflects its availability: cases from the 1970s frequently reported use of antiperspirants and typewriter correction fluid; computer and electronics cleaners have largely replaced these products. *Dusting* refers to the inhalation of compressed air cleaners containing halogenated hydrocarbons like 1,1-difluoroethane, marketed for cleaning dust from computer and electronics equipment.

## PHARMACOLOGY AND PHARMACOKINETICS

Although chemically heterogeneous, inhalants are generally highly lipophilic and gain rapid entrance into the central nervous system (CNS). Little is known about the cellular basis of the effects of inhalants. Evidence to date shows the most commonly used hydrocarbons have molecular mechanisms similar to those of other classic CNS depressants, frequently with common cellular sites of action. Their effects are probably best represented by the model for ethanol in which multiple different cellular mechanisms explain diverse pharmacologic and toxicologic effects.

### Volatile Hydrocarbons

The clinical effects of the volatile hydrocarbons are likely mediated through stimulation of inhibitory neurotransmission and antagonism of excitatory neurotransmission within the CNS. Like ethanol, toluene, trichloroethane (TCE), and trichloroethylene enhance γ-aminobutyric acid type A ($GABA_A$) receptor activity to hyperpolarize neuronal cell membranes and inhibit excitability. Like inhaled anesthetics, these inhalants act presynaptically on the GABA nerve terminals. Toluene-induced increases in inhibitory synaptic currents are blocked by dantrolene and ryanodine, suggesting toluene effects release of calcium from intracellular nerve terminal stores. Despite very different molecular structures, ethanol, enflurane, chloroform, toluene, and TCE compete for binding sites at glycine receptors thereby interfering with glutamate-mediated excitatory neurotransmission. Chronic exposure leads to upregulation of excitatory neurotransmission as occurs with ethanol.

Most research on inhalants has focused on the neural basis of their effects, yet it is the cardiotoxicity that is responsible for the majority of their lethal effects. Toluene reversibly inhibits myocardial voltage-activated sodium channels and, to a lesser extent, muscle sodium channels. Toluene also inhibits cardiac potassium channels. The combined inhibition of the sodium channels and the inwardly rectifying potassium channels is postulated to play a role in cardiac dysrhythmias and sudden sniffing death associated with the aromatic and halogenated hydrocarbons.

There are scant data on the pharmacokinetics of the inhalants but analogies to inhalational anesthetics provide some insight. Factors determining pharmacokinetic and

**TABLE 54–1 Common Inhalants and the Constituent Xenobiotics**

| *Inhalant* | *Chemical* |
|---|---|
| Carburetor cleaner | Methanol, methylene chloride, toluene, propane |
| Cigarette lighter fluid | Butane |
| Computer keyboard dust remover | Difluoroethane, tetrafluoroethane |
| Deodorizers (room) | Butyl nitrite, isobutyl nitrite, cyclohexyl nitrite |
| Dry cleaning agents, spot removers, degreasers | Tetrachloroethylene, trichloroethane, trichloroethylene |
| DVD and video cassette recorder head cleaner | Ethyl chloride |
| Freon (refrigerants) | Hydrofluorocarbons |
| Gasoline | Aliphatic and aromatic hydrocarbons |
| Glues and adhesives | Toluene, *n*-hexane, benzene, xylene, trichloroethane, trichloroethylene, tetrachloroethylene, ethyl acetate, methylethyl ketone, methyl chloride |
| Hair spray, deodorants, air fresheners | Butane, propane, fluorocarbons |
| Nail polish remover | Acetone |
| Paint thinner | Toluene, methylene chloride, methanol |
| "Poppers" | Amyl nitrite, isobutyl nitrite |
| Paints, lacquers, varnishes | Trichloroethylene, toluene, *n*-hexane |
| Spray paint | Toluene, butane, propane |
| Typewriter correction fluid | Trichloroethane, trichloroethylene |
| Whipped cream dispensers, "whippits" | Nitrous oxide |

pharmacodynamic effects of a given inhalational anesthetic include its concentration in inspired air; partition coefficient; interaction with other inhaled substances, ethanol, and drugs; the patient's respiratory rate and blood flow; percent body fat; and individual variation in drug metabolism (Chap. 38). Partition coefficients measure the relative affinity of a gas for two different xenobiotics at equilibrium and are used to predict the rate and extent of uptake of an inhaled xenobiotic. The blood:gas partition coefficient is most commonly referenced. The higher the number, the more soluble the xenobiotic is in blood. Inhalants with a low blood:gas partition coefficient, like $N_2O$, are rapidly taken up by the brain and, conversely, are rapidly eliminated from the brain once exposure is ended (Table 54–2). Most inhalants are eliminated unchanged by the lungs, undergo hepatic metabolism, or both.

Reward and reinforcement effects of inhalants are readily demonstrated. Although the mechanisms underlying their reinforcement behavior remain poorly studied, activation of the dopaminergic neurons of the ventral tegmental area is thought to play an important role in solvent use, similar to more commonly studied xenobiotics.

### Volatile Alkyl Nitrites

Little still is known about the molecular basis of use of the volatile alkyl nitrites. Their effects are thought to be mediated through smooth muscle relaxation in the central and peripheral vasculature, and they share a common cellular pathway with other nitric oxide (NO) donors similar to nitroglycerin and sodium nitroprusside.

### Nitrous Oxide

The pharmacokinetics and pharmacodynamics of $N_2O$ use are derived from its use as an inhalational anesthetic (Chap. 38). In contrast to other used volatile solvents, $N_2O$ mediates its stimulant effects through inhibition of excitatory NMDA-activated currents and has no effect on GABA-activated currents.

## CLINICAL MANIFESTATIONS

Signs and symptoms of inhalant use are often subtle, tend to vary widely among individuals, and generally resolve within several hours of exposure. After acute exposure, there is often a distinct odor of the used inhalant on the patient's breath or clothing. Depending on the inhalant used and the method, there may be discoloration of skin around the nose and mouth. Mucous membrane irritation causes sneezing, coughing, and tearing. Patients may complain of dyspnea and palpitations. Gastrointestinal complaints include nausea, vomiting, and abdominal pain. After an initial period of euphoria, patients have residual headache and dizziness.

**TABLE 54–2 Blood:Gas Partition Coefficients, Routes of Elimination, and Important Metabolites of Selected Inhalants**

| *Xenobiotic* | *Blood:Gas Partition Coefficient (98.6°F {37°C})* | *Routes of Elimination* | *Important Metabolites* |
|---|---|---|---|
| Acetone | 243–300 | Largely unchanged via exhalation 95% and urine 5% | None |
| *n*-Butane | 0.019 | Largely unchanged via exhalation | Metabolized to 2-butanol and 2-butanone |
| Carbon tetrachloride | 1.6 | 50% unchanged via exhalation; 50% hepatic metabolism and urinary excretion | CYP2E1 to trichloromethyl radical, trichloromethyl peroxy radical, phosgene |
| *n*-Hexane | 2 | 10%–20% exhaled unchanged; hepatic metabolism and urinary excretion | CYP2E1 to 2-hexanol, 2,5-hexanedione, γ-valerolactone |
| Methylene chloride | 5–10 | 92% exhaled unchanged; hepatic metabolism and urinary excretion | 1. CYP2E1 to CO and $CO_2$<br>2. Glutathione transferase to $CO_2$, formaldehyde, and formic acid |
| Nitrous oxide | 0.47 | > 99% exhaled unchanged | None |
| Toluene | 8–16 | < 20% exhaled unchanged;<br>> 80% hepatic metabolism and urinary excretion | CYP2E1 to benzoic acid, then<br>1. Glycine conjugation to form hippuric acid (68%)<br>2. Glucuronic acid conjugation to benzoyl glucuronide (insignificant pathway except after large exposure) |
| 1,1,1-Trichloroethane | 1–3 | 91% exhaled unchanged; hepatic metabolism and urinary excretion | CYP2E1 to trichloroethanol, then<br>1. Conjugated with glucuronic acid to formurochloralic acid or<br>2. Further oxidized to trichloroacetic acid |
| Trichloroethylene | 9 | 16% exhaled unchanged; 84% hepatic metabolism and urinary excretion | CYP2E1 to epoxide intermediate (transient); chloral hydrate (transient); trichloroethanol (45%), trichloroacetic acid (32%). Urinary trichloroacetic acid peaks 2–3 days postexposure |
| 1,2-Dichloro-1,1-difluoroethane | NA | NA | CYP2E1 to 2-chloro-2,2-difluoroethyl glucuronide, 2-2chloro-2,2-difluoroethyl sulfate, chlorodifluoroacetic acid, chlorodifluoroacetaldehyde hydrate, chlorodifluoroacetaldehyde-urea adduct, and inorganic fluoride; no covalently bound metabolites to liver proteins |

NA = not applicable.

### Volatile Hydrocarbons

Initial CNS effects include euphoria and hallucinations, which are both visual and auditory, as well as headache and dizziness. As toxicity progresses, CNS depression worsens, and patients develop slurred speech, confusion, tremor, and weakness. Transient cranial nerve palsies are reported. Further CNS depression is marked by ataxia, lethargy, seizures, coma, and respiratory depression. These effects generally resolve spontaneously. Chronic users demonstrate impaired executive function compared with control participants. Toluene leukoencephalopathy, characterized by dementia, ataxia, nystagmus and other eye movement disorders, and anosmia, is the prototypical manifestation of chronic inhalant neurotoxicity. Neuroimaging in patients with toluene leukoencephalopathy demonstrates white matter abnormalities confirmed on autopsy.

Acute cardiotoxicity associated with hydrocarbon inhalation is manifested most dramatically in "sudden sniffing death." In witnessed cases, sudden death occurred when sniffing was followed by some physical activity. It is thought that the inhalant "sensitizes the myocardium" by blocking the potassium current (Ikr), thereby prolonging repolarization. This produces a substrate for dysrhythmia propagation; the activity or stress then causes a catecholamine surge that initiates the dysrhythmia.

The most significant respiratory complication of inhalational use is hypoxia, which is either caused by displacement of inspired oxygen with the inhalant, reducing the fraction of inspired oxygen ($FiO_2$), or by rebreathing of exhaled air, as occurs with bagging. Direct pulmonary toxicity associated with inhalants is most often a result of inadvertent aspiration of a liquid hydrocarbon. Aspiration injury is associated with acute respiratory distress syndrome (ARDS). Irritant effects on the respiratory system are frequently transient, but some patients progress to chemical pneumonitis. This syndrome is characterized by tachypnea, fever, tachycardia, crackles, rhonchi, leukocytosis, and radiographic abnormalities, including perihilar densities, bronchovascular markings, increased interstitial markings, infiltrates, and consolidation. Barotrauma, from deep inhalation or breath-holding, presents as pneumothorax, pneumomediastinum, or subcutaneous emphysema.

Hepatoxicity is associated with exposure to halogenated hydrocarbons, particularly carbon tetrachloride ($CCl_4$), but also chloroform, trichloroethane, trichloroethylene, and toluene. Intentional inhalation of ($CCl_4$) is rarely reported, but its toxic metabolite, the trichloromethyl radical, created by the cytochrome CYP2E1, can covalently bind to hepatocyte macromolecules and cause lipid peroxidation.

Most reported kidney toxicity is associated with toluene inhalation. Prolonged toluene inhalation was said to cause a distal renal tubular acidosis (RTA), resulting in hypokalemia. However, whereas distal RTA is typically associated with a hyperchloremic metabolic acidosis and a normal anion gap, toluene use is associated with both normal and increased anion gap acidosis. Production of hippuric acid, a toluene metabolite, plays an important role in the genesis of the metabolic acidosis. The excretion of abundant hippurate in the urine unmatched by ammonium mandates an enhanced rate of excretion of sodium and potassium cations. Continued loss of potassium in the urine leads to hypokalemia. Toluene using patients often present with profound hypokalemic muscle weakness.

Acute dermatologic and upper airway toxicity is associated with the inhalation of fluorinated hydrocarbons. This is caused by the cooling of the gas as it rapidly expands on release from its pressurized container. First- and second-degree burns of the face, oropharynx, neck, shoulder, and chest are reported.

Bone mineral density was significantly lower in 25 adolescent chronic glue sniffers compared with that of healthy control participants. In a mouse model, chronic exposure to toluene significantly reduced bone mineral density. Skeletal fluorosis, manifested clinically by pain in affected bones and joints, hypertrophic nodules (Fig. 54–1), and decreased joint mobility, is reported following use of fluoride-containing inhalants.

Methylene chloride (dichloromethane), most commonly found in paint removers and degreasers, is unique among the halogenated hydrocarbons in that it undergoes metabolism in the liver by CYP2E1 to carbon monoxide (CO). In addition to acute CNS and cardiac manifestations, inhalation of methylene chloride is associated with delayed onset and prolonged duration of signs and symptoms of CO poisoning. The CO metabolite is generated 4 to 8 hours after exposure and its

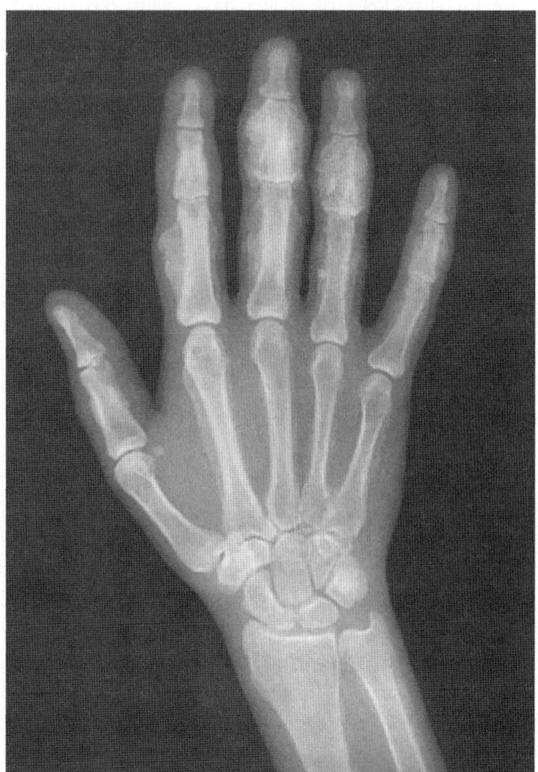

**FIGURE 54–1.** Radiograph of the hand from a patient with skeletal fluorosis. *(Used with permission from William Eggleston, PharmD, Department of Emergency Medicine, State University of New York, Upstate Medical University, Syracuse, NY.)*

apparent half-life is 13 hours, significantly longer than that of CO following inhalation (Chap. 95).

Chronic inhalation of the solvent *n*-hexane, a petroleum distillate found, for example, in rubber cement, causes a sensorimotor peripheral neuropathy. Toxicity is mediated via a metabolite, 2,5-hexanedione, which interferes with glyceraldehyde-3-phosphate dehydrogenase–dependent axonal transport, resulting in axonal death. Numbness and tingling of the fingers and toes is the most common initial complaint; progressive, ascending loss of motor function with frank quadriparesis may ensue (Chap. 78).

### Teratogenicity

Fetal solvent syndrome (FSS) was first reported in 1979. The authors described a 20-year-old primigravida with a 14-year history of solvent use defined as "daily" and "heavy" who gave birth to an infant exhibiting facial dysmorphia, growth retardation, and microcephaly, a constellation of findings that resembles fetal alcohol syndrome (FAS). Subsequent case reports and series support this observation. Craniofacial abnormalities common to both FAS and FSS include small palpebral fissures, a thin upper lip, and midfacial hypoplasia. Features of FSS that distinguish it from FAS include micrognathia, low-set ears, abnormal scalp hair pattern, large anterior fontanelle, and downturned corners of the mouth. Hypoplasia of the philtrum and nose is more characteristic of FAS. Compared with matched control participants, infants born to mothers who report inhalant use are more likely to be premature, have low birth weight, have smaller birth length, and have a small head circumference. Follow-up studies show developmental delay compared with children matched for age, race, sex, and socioeconomic status.

***Withdrawal.*** Observed similarities in the acute effects of inhalants compared with other CNS depressants suggest similar patterns of tolerance and withdrawal. Withdrawal symptoms, including irritability, both hypersomnia and insomnia, fatigue, craving, nausea, tremor, and dry mouth lasting 2 to 5 days after last use, are described.

### Volatile Alkyl Nitrites

Methemoglobinemia caused by inhalation of amyl, butyl, and isobutyl nitrites is well reported. Patients with methemoglobinemia present with signs and symptoms that include shortness of breath, cyanosis, tachycardia, and tachypnea (Chap. 97). "Poppers retinopathy" characterized by eye pain; transient increased intraocular pressure; and central, bilateral visual loss is reported after use of alkyl nitrites.

### Nitrous Oxide

Reported deaths associated with use of $N_2O$ include asphyxiation and motor vehicle collisions while under the influence, and not a direct toxic effect. Investigations after deaths associated with $N_2O$ have found many of the dead were discovered with plastic bags over their heads in an apparent attempt to both prolong the duration of effect and increase the concentration of the inhalant.

Chronic use of $N_2O$ is associated with neurologic toxicity mediated via irreversible oxidation of the cobalt ion of cyanocobalamin (vitamin $B_{12}$). Oxidation blocks formation of methylcobalamin, a coenzyme in the production of methionine and *S*-adenosylmethionine, required for methylation of the phospholipids of the myelin sheaths. Additionally, cobalamin oxidation inhibits the conversion of methylmalonyl to succinyl coenzyme A. The resultant accumulation of methylmalonate and propionate results in synthesis of abnormal fatty acids and their subsequent incorporation into the myelin sheath (Chap. 38). Patients develop a myeloneuropathy resembling the subacute combined degeneration of the dorsal columns of the spinal cord of classic vitamin $B_{12}$ deficiency. Presenting signs and symptoms reflect varying involvement of the posterior columns, the corticospinal tracts, and the peripheral nerves. Numbness and tingling of the distal extremities is the most common presenting complaint. Physical examination reveals diminished sensation to pinprick and light touch, vibratory sensation and proprioception, gait disturbances, the Lhermitte sign (electric shock sensation from the back into the limbs with neck flexion), hyperreflexia, spasticity, urinary and fecal incontinence, and extensor plantar response. Magnetic resonance imaging may reveal symmetric enhancement and edema of the dorsal columns, referred to as the inverted V-sign.

## LABORATORY AND DIAGNOSTIC TESTING

Routine urine toxicology screens do not detect inhalants or their metabolites. Specialized testing is not readily available at most institutions, and the need to send the specimen to a reference laboratory limits the clinical utility in most situations. A thorough history and physical examination and careful questioning of the patient's friends and family are more helpful in cases of suspected inhalant use. Depending on the patient's signs and symptoms, additional diagnostic testing is recommended, including an electrocardiogram, radiograph, electrolytes, liver enzymes, methemoglobin, carboxyhemoglobin, and blood pH. Inhalation of some xenobiotics presents unique diagnostic considerations (Table 54–3). Routine laboratory testing, including cerebrospinal fluid analysis, is unremarkable in patients with inhalant-induced leukoencephalopathy.

**TABLE 54–3 Inhalants With Unique Clinical Manifestations**

| *Inhalant* | *Clinical Manifestations* |
|---|---|
| Toluene | Hypokalemia<br>Hepatotoxicity<br>Leukoencephalopathy (chronic) |
| Difluoroethane, tetrafluoroethane | Frostbite<br>Skeletal fluorosis (chronic) |
| 1,1,1-Trichloroethane, trichloroethylene | Hepatotoxicity |
| Methylene chloride | Carbon monoxide poisoning |
| Carburetor cleaner | Methanol poisoning |
| *n*-Hexane | Peripheral neuropathy (chronic) |
| Alkyl nitrites (amyl, butyl, isobutyl) | Methemoglobinemia<br>Vision loss |
| Nitrous oxide | Myeloneuropathy (chronic)<br>Megaloblastic anemia (chronic)<br>Skin hyperpigmentation (chronic) |

A computed tomography (CT) scan of the head is generally normal until late in the disease, when diffuse hypodensity of white matter becomes evident. T2-weighted magnetic resonance imaging with its superior resolution of white matter is the diagnostic study of choice.

## MANAGEMENT

Management begins with assessment and stabilization of the patient's airway, breathing, and circulation (the "ABCs"). The patient should be attached to a pulse oximeter and cardiac monitor. Oxygen should be administered if indicated. Early consultation with a regional poison center or medical toxicologist is recommended to assist with identification of the xenobiotic and patient management.

Cardiac dysrhythmias associated with inhalant use carry a poor prognosis. An evaluation for life-threatening electrolyte abnormalities is indicated and rapid correction is recommended in patients presenting with dysrhythmias. Patients with nonperfusing rhythms should be managed with standard management with defibrillation. There are no evidence-based treatment guidelines for the management of inhalant-induced cardiac dysrhythmias, but β-adrenergic antagonists are thought to offer some cardioprotective effects to the sensitized myocardium. Treatment with either propranolol or esmolol is a reasonable choice in managing ventricular dysrhythmias that result from inhalant use.

Other complications, including methemoglobinemia, elevated carboxyhemoglobin, and methanol toxicity, should be managed with the appropriate antidotal therapy when present. Patients with respiratory symptoms that persist beyond the initial complaints of gagging and choking should be evaluated for hydrocarbon pneumonitis and treated supportively (Chap. 78).

Cessation of use is the most important therapeutic intervention in patients with *n*-hexane–induced neuropathy. For patients with $N_2O$-induced myeloneuropathy, in addition to cessation, vitamin $B_{12}$ is recommended by either (1) intramuscular injection of 1,000 μg vitamin $B_{12}$ daily for 1 week followed by weekly injection of 1,000 μg for 4 to 9 weeks and then monthly injection of 1,000 μg until clinical resolution or (2) daily oral administration of 1,000 to 2,000 μg of vitamin $B_{12}$ until clinical resolution. Methionine was also successfully used when vitamin $B_{12}$ treatment alone failed to improve neurologic effects. There is no guideline for dosing methionine for patients with nitrous oxide toxicity, although case reports have used a 3-g daily oral regimen. In addition to the therapy above, patients with bone marrow abnormalities associated with nitrous oxide toxicity should be treated with a single 30-mg intravenous (IV) dose of folinic acid (Antidotes in Brief: A12).

Agitation, either from acute effects of the inhalant or from withdrawal, is safely managed with a benzodiazepine. In the vast majority of patients, symptoms resolve quickly, and hospitalization is not required. The potential toxicity of inhalants should be reinforced, and patients should be referred for counseling. Subsets of users, meeting the criteria for inhalant dependence and inhalant-induced psychosis, require inpatient psychiatric care. Pharmacotherapy with carbamazepine or the antipsychotics haloperidol, risperidone, and aripiprazole is reasonable for some patients with an inhalant-induced psychotic disorder. Drug use treatment programs for inhalant use are scarce, and few providers have special training in this area.

# 55 NICOTINE

## HISTORY AND EPIDEMIOLOGY

Nicotine is the principal alkaloid derived from plants of the genus *Nicotiana*, collectively known as the tobacco plant, in the family *Solanaceae*. Other fruits and vegetables from the Solanaceae family, such as tomatoes, potatoes, eggplant, and cauliflower, also contain comparatively small amounts of nicotine ranging from 3.8 to 100 ng/g. The tobacco plant is native to the Americas, and its use most likely predates the Mayan empire. In 1492, Christopher Columbus and his crew were given tobacco by the Arawaks but reportedly threw it away, not knowing any use for it. Ramon Pane, a monk who accompanied Columbus on his second voyage to America, is credited with introducing tobacco to Europe. Because of the highly addictive properties of nicotine, the global disease burden related to cigarette use today is staggering. Cigarette smoking increases rates of illnesses, such as chronic obstructive pulmonary disease (COPD), cardiovascular disease, pulmonary infections, macular degeneration, and cancers, and tobacco use causes more than 5 million deaths worldwide per year.

Although the long-term effects of tobacco dependency are significant, this chapter is concerned with the sources, effects, and management of acute toxicity. The epidemiology of nicotine poisoning is changing with the rise of e-cigarette use as concentrated liquid products are now common in many homes with children. Other smoking cessation products containing nicotine or nicotinelike compounds are also increasingly available. Some of the more novel smokeless tobacco products have the appearance and flavor of candy, raising concern about the potential for unintentional poisoning of young children, in particular.

## PHARMACOLOGY AND PHARMACOKINETICS

The pharmacologic characteristics of nicotine are listed in Table 55–1. Peak plasma concentrations of nicotine and its principal metabolite cotinine are influenced most strongly by individual variations in clearance. Hepatic nicotine metabolism is inducible and nicotine-dependent individuals metabolize the drug more rapidly than naïve ones. Nicotine metabolism is also linked to race and sex. The half-life of nicotine is 1 to 4 hours. In contrast, the elimination half-life of cotinine is approximately 20 hours, and therefore, urinary cotinine is a more useful marker of nicotine exposure.

The $LD_{50}$ of nicotine is usually estimated at 0.5 to 1 mg/kg in adults but is much higher at about 6.5 to 13 mg/kg according to some reports. Severe toxicity is reported with ingestion of less than 2 mg in a child, and this dose is sufficient to produce mild symptoms in an unhabituated adult.

**TABLE 55–1 Pharmacology of Nicotine**

| | |
|---|---|
| Absorption | Lungs, oral mucosa, skin, intestinal tract; increased in more alkaline environments |
| Volume of distribution | 2.6 L/kg |
| Protein binding | 5% |
| Metabolism | 80%–90% hepatic via CYP2A6 and CYP2D6, aldehyde oxidase, flavin monooxygenase, and by glycosylation; remainder in lung, kidney; principal (inactive) metabolite is cotinine |
| Half-life | Nicotine: 1–4 h, decreases with repeated exposure<br>Cotinine: 20 h |
| Elimination | 2%–35% excreted unchanged in urine |

## SOURCES AND USES OF NICOTINE

### Cigarettes and Cigars

The amount of nicotine contained in a single cigarette is highly variable, ranging from less than 10 mg in a "low-nicotine" cigarette to 30 mg in some European cigarettes (Table 55–2). The potential for nicotine toxicity from smoking is limited because peak effects by this route occur within seconds and tend to limit further intake of drug. Most reports of acute nicotine toxicity referable to cigarette exposure are associated with cigarette and cigarette butt ingestion, usually by young children.

### Waterpipes, Hookah, and Shisha

Although the use of cigarettes has decreased in the United States (US), waterpipe use has become popular especially among college students, with hookah bars opening all around the country. A container holding 10 to 20 g of tobacco, often fruit flavored, is connected to the pipe and covered with aluminum foil. Coal is used as a heat source and placed on top of the foil. Toxins associated with waterpipe use include carbon monoxide and nicotine. In a study including 16 participants who smoked only a waterpipe with up to 32 mg of nicotine for a mean of 39 minutes and mixed tobacco users,

**TABLE 55–2 Commercial Sources of Nicotine**

| Source | Content (mg) | Delivered (mg) |
|---|---|---|
| 1 cigarette | 10–30 | 0.05–3 |
| 1 cigarette butt | 5–7 | — |
| 1 cigar | 15–40 | 0.2–1 |
| 1 g snuff (wet) | 12–16 | 2–3.5 |
| 1 g chewing tobacco | 6–8 | 2–4 |
| 1 piece nicotine gum | 2 or 4 | 1–2 |
| 1 nicotine patch | 8.3–114 | 5–22 over 16–24 h |
| 1 nicotine lozenge | 2 or 4 | 2–4 |
| 1 nicotine nasal spray | 0.5 | 0.2–0.4 |
| 30-mL bottle of 3.6% nicotine liquid refill for e-cigarette cartridges (30-, 50-, and 100-mL bottles also sold) | 36 mg/mL | < 43.2 μg/100 mL "puff" of nicotine mist |

plasma nicotine concentrations peaked to 11.7 ng/mL and 28.4 ng/mL, respectively, 45 minutes after use. Several reports demonstrate overt carbon monoxide poisoning associated with waterpipes.

### Oral Tobacco

Snuff and chewing tobacco are still widely used as smokeless tobacco products despite clear associations with periodontal disease, dental cavities, and up to a 48 times greater risk of oropharyngeal cancers compared with people who do not use tobacco products.

### Gum

Nicotine gum has been available without a prescription as an aid to smoking cessation in the US since 1996. It is sold in 2-mg and 4-mg strengths per piece. Approximately 53% to 72% of the nicotine in the gum is absorbed. If the gum is swallowed whole, then serum concentrations rise even more slowly because the acidic environment of the stomach delays absorption.

### Lozenges

Nicotine lozenges containing 2 mg and 4 mg of nicotine are available for purchase without a prescription in the US. The potential for rapid absorption of nicotine as a bolus dose from chewing the lozenge is a concern.

### Transdermal Patches

Nicotine patches have been Food and Drug Administration (FDA) approved for purchase without prescription in the US since 1996. Most nicotine transdermal delivery systems are designed to deliver 7, 14, or 21 mg of nicotine over 24 hours. Several reports document consequential nicotine toxicity related to nicotine patch misuse. Children developed symptoms after exploratory self-application of one or more patches to the skin, and concurrent use of multiple patches is a means of suicide. Severe toxicity also occurs if patches are punctured—for example, by biting or tearing—thus allowing delivery of excessive quantities of nicotine. The patch reservoirs contain an estimated 36 to 114 mg per patch.

### Spray or Inhaler

A nicotine spray has been available in the US since 1996 to aid efforts at smoking cessation. The most commonly reported adverse effects during initiation of therapy are due to local irritation and include rhinorrhea, lacrimation, sneezing, and nasal and throat irritation. No report of acute nicotine toxicity from nicotine inhalers has been published to date.

### Electronic Cigarettes

Electronic cigarettes, or e-cigarettes, are a relatively new nicotine delivery product now widely available in various strengths and flavors. Liquid nicotine is sold in different formulations with the highest strength preparations (3.6% nicotine) containing more than 1 g of nicotine per 30 mL bottle. This raises serious concerns about the risk of both unintentional and intentional toxic exposures. Additionally, large-volume liquid nicotine replacement fluid bottles (used to refill e-cigarette cartridges) are available, augmenting the potential for harm. Deaths from unintentional and intentional ingestion of e-cigarette liquid are reported.

### Partial Nicotine Receptor Agonists (Varenicline, Cytisine)

Partial nicotine receptor agonists are used to aid smoking cessation. Theoretically, they work by reducing smoking satisfaction (agonist/antagonist effect) while helping to maintain moderate concentrations of central dopamine release (partial agonist effect). Cytisine is a plant-derived xenobiotic with a chemical structure similar to nicotine that is used in Eastern and Central Europe as a smoking cessation drug since the 1960s. Despite its widespread use, the safety, efficacy, pharmacokinetics, and pharmacodynamics of cytisine in humans are not well studied. Varenicline was approved by the US FDA as a prescription-only aid to smoking cessation in 2006. Several randomized controlled trials demonstrated efficacy in diminishing nicotine cravings, and evidence suggests that varenicline increases the probability of successful abstinence from smoking. In 2009, the US FDA mandated a black box warning due to an association with increased risk of depression or suicidal behavior. There is now increasing experience with acute varenicline overdose, including effects such as nausea, vomiting, tachycardia, and hypertension, and one reported fatality after intentional overdose.

### Plants and Leaves

Green tobacco sickness (GTS) refers to nicotine-induced symptoms, including nausea, vomiting, headache, and dizziness, that occur when nicotine is topically absorbed during the handling of tobacco plants. Residual moisture or dew drops on tobacco leaves contain as much as 9 mg of nicotine per 100 mL. Tobacco workers are most at risk when their clothing comes in contact with moisture on the tobacco plants.

### Miscellaneous

In the pre-Columbian Americas, many tribes used tobacco extract and tobacco smoke enemas for both medicinal and spiritual purposes. They are still recommended by some naturopaths and folk healers as remedies for constipation, urinary retention, pinworm, and "hysterical convulsions." Toxicity is reported from this practice.

## PATHOPHYSIOLOGY

Nicotine mimics the effects of acetylcholine by binding to nicotinic receptors (nAChRs) in the brain, spinal cord, autonomic ganglia, adrenal medulla, neuromuscular junctions, and chemoreceptors of the carotid and aortic bodies. Activation of nAChRs in the central nervous system (CNS) directly stimulates neurotransmitter release.

At doses generally produced by cigarette smoking, there is stimulation of the reticular activating system and an alerting pattern on the electroencephalogram. Nicotine-stimulated release of dopamine is an important mediator of nicotine addiction. Nicotine also stimulates glutaminergic activation and the GABA ($\gamma$-aminobutyric acid)-ergic inhibition of dopaminergic neurons in the hippocampus, basal forebrain, and ventral tegmental area of the midbrain. These pathways, along with endogenous cannabinoid and opioid systems, are important neuromodulatory pathways for drug-induced reward, dependence, and withdrawal. Norepinephrine, acetylcholine, GABA, serotonin, glutamate, and endorphins are all released by nicotine and are associated with cognitive and mood enhancement as well as appetite suppression, increased basal energy expenditures, and anxiety reduction.

The clinical effects of nicotine are dose dependent. Low doses of nicotine and related compounds stimulate nicotinic receptors centrally and in autonomic and somatic motor nerve fibers, resulting in sympathetic agonism. At toxic concentrations, prolonged or excessive nicotinergic stimulation ultimately leads to receptor blockade (Chap. 39), with parasympathetic and neuromuscular-blocking effects. At very high doses, nicotine induces seizures.

**TABLE 55–3 Signs and Symptoms of Acute Nicotine Poisoning**

| | *Gastrointestinal* | *Respiratory* | *Cardiovascular* | *Neurologic* |
|---|---|---|---|---|
| Early (0.25–1 h) | Nausea<br>Vomiting<br>Salivation<br>Abdominal pain | Bronchorrhea<br>Hyperpnea | Hypertension<br>Tachycardia<br>Pallor | Agitation<br>Anxiety<br>Dizziness<br>Blurred vision<br>Headache<br>Hyperactivity<br>Confusion<br>Tremors<br>Fasciculations<br>Seizures |
| Late (0.5–4 h) | Diarrhea | Hypoventilation<br>Apnea | Bradycardia<br>Hypotension<br>Dysrhythmias<br>Shock | Lethargy<br>Weakness<br>Paralysis |

## CLINICAL MANIFESTATIONS

Patients with nicotine exposure rarely display more than mild symptoms and typically have a benign course. Exposure to nicotine in low doses comparable to cigarette smoking in nicotine-naïve patients produces fine tremor; cutaneous vasoconstriction; increased gastrointestinal motility; nausea; and increases in heart rate, respiratory rate, and blood pressure. Low-dose nicotine also increases mental alertness and produces euphoria. Because nicotine is poorly absorbed in the acid environment of the stomach, symptom onset occurs 30 to 90 minutes after ingestion of nicotine-containing products.

Early signs and symptoms of nicotine toxicity are referable to nicotinic cholinergic excess; increased salivation, nausea, vomiting, diaphoresis, and diarrhea all occur within minutes of systemic absorption. Vasoconstriction manifests with pallor and hypertension. Tachycardia also occurs, and nicotine gum chewing is implicated in the development of atrial fibrillation in several cases. Neurologic signs and symptoms include headache, dizziness, ataxia, confusion, and perceptual distortions. Nicotine is an irritant, and ingestion of nicotine, including use of nicotine gum, causes a burning sensation and pain in the mouth, and constriction of the pharyngeal muscles. Similarly, application of nicotine patches generally results in dermal irritation.

Vomiting is the most common adverse effect reported, although agitation also commonly occurs. The relative rarity of life-threatening symptoms is caused in part by autodecontamination from vomiting. In addition, because most reported cases involve unintentional tobacco ingestion by young children, there is significant selection bias.

Data from poison centers in the US suggest that the increased availability of e-cigarettes and liquid nicotine is associated with an increased incidence of consequential poisoning. Most liquid nicotine exposures occur in children younger than 5 years of age, and children exposed to liquid nicotine have 2.6 times higher odds of having severe outcomes than children exposed to traditional cigarettes, including one reported death. This is likely caused by larger nicotine concentrations available in liquid nicotine. Although less common, ingestion of novel smokeless tobacco preparations, such as gums and lozenges, is more likely to produce symptoms compared to cigarette ingestion because these are buffered to promote more rapid nicotine release.

Because nicotine is rapidly metabolized, patients who develop only mild symptoms are expected to recover quickly. Most patients recover fully within 12 hours. An important exception to this rule is noted in patients with symptoms of nicotine toxicity after transdermal nicotine patch application because a reservoir of drug persists in the subcutaneous tissue after patch removal and can serve as a source of ongoing absorption. Removal of the patch and decontamination of these patients should remain paramount to limiting further absorption.

Clinical manifestations of severe poisoning are classically biphasic, reflecting early central stimulation followed by depression. Initial signs include cardiac dysrhythmias, seizures, and muscle fasciculations in addition to the cholinergic features described earlier. Bradycardia, hypotension, coma, and neuromuscular blockade with respiratory failure from muscular paralysis are a more delayed development (Table 55–3).

Exposure to fresh tobacco leaves produces GTS, which is likened to the experience of seasickness typically occurring within 3 to 17 hours after exposure. This syndrome, characterized by dizziness, headache, weakness, nausea, vomiting, diarrhea, abdominal cramps, chills, and in severe cases, signs of autonomic instability, often has a duration of several days.

## DIAGNOSTIC TESTING

Determination of serum or urinary concentrations of nicotine or its metabolites is unlikely to be helpful in the management of the acutely poisoned patient. Measurement can be made for confirmation purposes using various chromatographic techniques. Cigarette smokers typically maintain serum nicotine concentrations between 30 and 50 ng/mL during the day but can achieve concentrations as high as 100 ng/mL. Postmortem analyses of nicotine concentrations in blood after fatal acute toxicity range from 5.5 to 800 mg/L.

The presence of measurable concentrations of nicotine or cotinine in biologic samples often reflects coincidental or chronic exposure and does not necessarily imply acute toxicity. Urinary cotinine has a longer detection window than nicotine and is often used to document exposure to nicotine-containing products, including exposure to secondhand smoke, or to guide dosage adjustments in nicotine replacement therapy. Conversely, the absence of cotinine in the urine is used to document abstinence from tobacco products.

## MANAGEMENT

Most patients with unintentional or low-dose nicotine exposures do not require medical treatment. Patients should be immediately referred for evaluation if they are symptomatic or have ingested any amount of nicotine-containing liquid. Children who ingest one or more cigarettes or three or more cigarette butts should also be referred for evaluation without delay. Patients with mild or no symptoms can be observed for several hours and safely discharged home if there are no complicating circumstances such as significant comorbid cardiovascular illness or intent to self-harm.

Patients with dermal exposure to wet tobacco leaves or pesticides should be undressed completely and the skin washed thoroughly with soap and copious amounts of water. Medical staff charged with handling both clothing and patients before decontamination should wear personal protective gear and dispose of materials safely. Symptomatic patients should have any nicotine dermal patches removed immediately and the skin washed with soap and water.

Vomiting is the most commonly reported adverse effect in patients with acute nicotine toxicity and limits absorption in some cases. Induction of emesis is not recommended because it is unlikely to be of added benefit and has the potential for harm. Orogastric lavage is reasonable in patients who present immediately after large intentional and potentially life-threatening ingestions of nicotine-containing products with the exception of liquid nicotine. Liquid nicotine formulations are more rapidly absorbed, making orogastric lavage less useful. Activated charcoal adsorbs nicotine and can reduce absorption, and therefore, we recommend it for patients with consequential ingestions.

There is no specific antidote for nicotine toxicity. Treatment of acute nicotine toxicity is symptomatic and supportive. The first priority is to ensure airway protection and respiratory support. Atropine is used to treat symptoms associated with parasympathetic stimulation such as excess salivation, wheezing, or bradycardia. Endotracheal intubation is required for airway protection or to assist ventilation in severely poisoned patients. Seizures are treated with a benzodiazepine. Hypotension is treated with fluid boluses and infusion of 0.9% NaCl initially. Patients who fail to respond to volume infusion require treatment with a vasopressor such as norepinephrine. Dysrhythmias should be treated according to standard advanced cardiac life support protocols. Nicotine elimination is enhanced in acidic urine, but the potential risks outweigh the benefits of this elimination strategy, so we recommend against this approach.

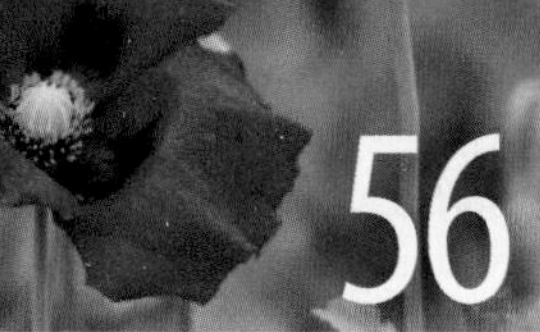

# 56 PHENCYCLIDINE AND KETAMINE

## HISTORY AND EPIDEMIOLOGY

Phencyclidine (PCP) was discovered in 1926 but was not developed as a general anesthetic until the 1950s. Phencyclidine was marketed under the name Sernyl because it rendered an apparent state of serenity when administered to laboratory monkeys. Its human surgical use began in 1963, but it was rapidly discontinued when a 10% to 30% incidence of postoperative psychoses and dysphoria was documented over the subsequent 2-year period. Simultaneously, in the 1960s, PCP emerged as a street drug called "the PeaCe Pill." Numerous street names have since been given to PCP including "angel dust," PCP, "crystal," "crystal joints" (CJs), "the sheets," "Hog," or "elephant tranquilizer."

Phencyclidine abuse became widespread during the 1970s, and by the late 1970s, PCP abuse reached epidemic proportions. The manufacture of PCP was ultimately prohibited in 1978 when it was added to the list of federally controlled substances. Classifying PCP as a Schedule II drug led to its decrease in availability and, consequently, a decrease in its use. The United States (US) Controlled Substances Act of 1986 made these derivatives illegal and established that the use of the precursor of PCP, piperidine, necessitated mandatory reporting.

Laboratory investigation of PCP derivatives led to the discovery of ketamine, which was introduced for general clinical practice in 1970. Decades of clinical experience have established that ketamine provides adequate surgical anesthesia, a rapid recovery, and less prominent emergence reactions than PCP. In the US, abuse of ketamine was first noted in urban areas on the West Coast in 1971. During the 1980s, there were reports of its abuse internationally, including among physicians. The nonmedical use of dissociative anesthetics has continued to increase throughout the 1990s and into the 2000s despite the common complications associated with their use. Because of its abuse potential, ketamine was placed in Schedule III of the US Controlled Substances Act in 1999.

In more recent years, several other PCP and ketamine analogs (eg, arylcyclohexylamines) were manufactured for their psychoactive effects (Table 56–1). These designer drugs have been synthesized as a means of evading law enforcement. There are several reports of toxicity and fatalities from the ketamine analog methoxetamine (2-{3-methoxyphenyl}-2-{ethylamino} cyclohexanone or 3-MeO-2-oxo-PCE) since its production in 2010 by an underground pharmaceutical chemist. It is advertised as having less renal and hepatic adverse effects than ketamine. Toxicity and fatalities from methoxetamine have been reported throughout Europe and Asia (Hong Kong, Taiwan, Korea, and Japan). The ban of arylcyclohexylamines in the United Kingdom in 2013 led to the use diarylethylamines as the next class of dissociatives to be abused.

## PHARMACOLOGY

### Chemistry

The chemical name of PCP, 1-(1-phenylcyclohexyl)piperidine, provided the basis for its street acronym PCP. During the unlawful chemical synthesis of PCP, more than 60 analogs are made that have similar effects on the central nervous system (CNS) and are used as PCP substitutes. Ketamine and tiletamine, two legal analogs of PCP, are used clinically for sedation and anesthesia.

The molecular structure of ketamine contains a chiral center, producing a racemic mixture of two resolvable optical isomers or enantiomers, the S(+) isomer and R(−) isomer. Commercially available injectable preparations of ketamine contain equal concentrations of the two enantiomers. These two molecules differ in their pharmacodynamic effects, with the S(+) isomer being a more effective anesthetic but also producing a higher incidence of psychotic emergence reactions than the R(−) isomer. In other studies, the S(+) isomer caused a greater increase in both blood pressure and pulse than the R(−) isomer and had more bronchodilatory effects. The R(−) ketamine enantiomers produce longer lasting antidepressant effects than the S(+) enantiomers.

Ketamine analogs are "designer" dissociatives made by clandestine chemists. Methoxetamine is a derivative of ketamine that is suggested to have a decreased anesthetic effect because of its 3-methoxy group. The addition of an ethyl group to its cyclic ring is thought to diminish urologic toxicity. However, because it is not a legally manufactured pharmaceutical, the only human experience is derived from its nonmedical reports.

### Pharmacokinetics and Toxicokinetics

Phencyclidine is weak base with a pKa between 8.6 and 9.4 and a high lipid-to-water-partition coefficient (log D = 3.63). It is rapidly absorbed from the respiratory system

**TABLE 56–1 Common Phencyclidine (PCP) and Ketamine Analogs**

| *Name* | *Chemical Name* | *Other Name* |
|---|---|---|
| ***PCP Analogs*** | | |
| PCE | *N*-Ethyl-1-phenylcyclohexylamine | Cyclohexamine |
| TCP | (1-{1-(Thiophen-2-yl)cyclohexyl} piperidine) | Tenocyclidine |
| PCPy | 1-(1-Phenylcyclohexy)pyrrolidine | Rolicyclidine, PHP |
| ***Ketamine Analogs*** | | |
| 3-MeO-2-oxo-PCE | 2-(3-Methoxyphenyl)-2-(ethylamino) cyclohexanone | Methoxetamine |
| 3-MeO-PCE | 2-(3-Methoxyphenyl)-2-(ethylamino) cyclohexane | Methoxieticyclidine |
| 2-MK | 2-(2-Methylphenyl)-2-(methylamino) cyclohexanone | 2-MeO-ketamine |
| N-EK | 2-(2-Chlorophenyl)-2-(ethylamino) cyclohexanone | *N*-Ethylnorketamine |

and the gastrointestinal (GI) tracts; as such, it is typically self-administered by the oral, nasal, inhalational, IV, or subcutaneous routes. The effects of PCP are dependent on routes of delivery and dose. Its onset of action is most rapid from the IV and inhalational routes (2–5 minutes) and slowest (30–60 minutes) after GI absorption. Sedation is commonly produced by doses of 0.25 mg/kg intravenously; ingestion typically requires 1 to 5 mg to produce similar sedation. Signs and symptoms of toxicity usually last 4 to 6 hours, and large overdoses generally resolve within 24 to 48 hours. However, in PCP-toxic patients, the relationships between dose, clinical effects, and serum concentrations are neither reliable nor predictable.

There are several explanations for the protracted CNS effects of PCP. The large volume of distribution of 6.2 L/kg and high lipid solubility account for its entry and storage in adipose and brain tissue. Also, on reaching the acidic cerebrospinal fluid (CSF), PCP becomes ionized, producing CSF concentrations approximately 6 to 9 times greater than those of serum. Phencyclidine undergoes first-order elimination over a wide range of doses. It has an apparent terminal elimination half-life of 21 ± 3 hours under both control and overdose settings. Ninety percent of PCP is metabolized in the liver and 10% is excreted in the urine unchanged. In acidic urine, PCP becomes ionized and then cannot be reabsorbed. Acidification of the urine increased renal clearance of PCP from 1.98 ± 0.48 L/h to 2.4 ± 0.78 L/h. Although this accounts for a 23% increase in the renal clearance, it only represents a 1.1% increase of the total clearance.

Ketamine is water soluble and has a high lipid solubility (log D = 2.01) that enables it to distribute to the CNS readily. It has a pKa of 7.5 and a volume of distribution of 1.8 ± 0.7 L/kg. Ketamine has approximately 10% of the potency of PCP. Human trials demonstrate that similar to PCP, the clinical effects of ketamine are both route and dose dependent. Peak blood concentrations occur within 1 minute of IV administration and within 5 minutes of a 5-mg/kg intramuscular (IM) injection. Ketamine distributes rapidly into the CNS with the duration of its hypnotic and anesthetic effects extended by its slow redistribution from the brain to other tissues. Recovery time averages 15 minutes for IV administration but is 30 and 120 minutes after IM administration. Oral and rectal doses are not well absorbed and undergo substantial first-pass metabolism. In contrast to oral administration of ketamine in which clinical effects persist for 4 to 8 hours, after nasal administration, they last for 45 to 90 minutes.

Ketamine is extensively metabolized in the liver by CYP2B6 and to a lesser extent by CYP3A4 and CYP2C9. The elimination half-life is 2.3 ± 0.5 hours and is prolonged when xenobiotics requiring hepatic metabolism are coadministered. Because of the enzymatic metabolism, both tolerance and enzyme induction are reported after chronic administration.

Pharmacokinetic data for methoxetamine are obtained from in vivo animal studies and from in vitro studies with human hepatocytes and microsomes. The major metabolic pathway of methoxetamine is *N*-deethylation by cytochromes CYP2B6 and CYP3A4 into normethoxetamine.

### Available Forms

Phencyclidine is available illicitly in a variety of forms, including powder, liquid, tablets, leaf mixtures, and rock crystal. Because of its uncontrolled illegal manufacture, the contents of products sold as PCP vary considerably, with powder often the purest form. A typical dose consumed contains approximately 5 mg.

On the street and on the Internet, ketamine is known as "vitamin K," "Special K," "Super K," "Ket," or simply "K." It is available in a liquid form that is dried into a pure white crystalline powder and is typically self-administered by ingestion or insufflation in a fashion similar to PCP. It is rarely injected IV or IM in aqueous form. Common sedating doses are 75 to 300 mg orally (30–75 mg for insufflation). Higher doses, ranging between 300 and 450 mg orally (100–250 mg for insufflation), result in substantial CNS toxicity.

New designer dissociatives (methoxetamine, 2-MK, and N-EK) are currently sold through the Internet internationally as powders that are ingested, insufflated, or injected. Methoxetamine is used extensively in the United Kingdom and is referred to by various names, including MXE, M-ket, Kmax, Mexxy, Special-M, MEX, legal ketamine, and Minx.

## PATHOPHYSIOLOGY

The arylcyclohexylamines are a group of anesthetics that functionally and electrophysiologically "dissociate" the somatosensory cortex from higher centers. The precise mechanisms by which they achieve these effects are complex and not fully understood; however, investigation of the nature of PCP-induced psychosis has led to a substantial identification of the various sites of PCP activity.

Most studies demonstrate that arylcyclohexylamines block the NMDA receptors at serum concentrations encountered clinically. Binding to the NMDA receptor occurs at a site independent of glutamate. This site is located within the ionotropic channel, partially overlapping the $Mg^{2+}$ binding site, and it is often termed the PCP binding site. As such, they antagonize the action of glutamate on this channel and noncompetitively block $Ca^{2+}$ influx.

Arylcyclohexylamines also bind to the biogenic amine reuptake complex but with 10% to 20% of the affinity to which they bind to the NMDA receptor. This weak inhibition of the catecholamine reuptake accounts for the observed increase in blood pressure and heart rate.

In large overdoses, arylcyclohexylamines also stimulate σ receptors at concentrations generally associated with coma, although with lower affinity than NMDA receptors. Both $D_2$ and σ receptors have an inhibitory effect on the cholinergic receptor pathways. At the higher concentrations, typically associated with death, arylcyclohexylamines bind to the nicotinic, opioid, and muscarinic cholinergic receptors.

In humans, although the dissociatives induce excitatory activity in the thalamus and limbic areas, they do not affect cortical regions. Excitation, muscle twitching, posturing, and tonic–clonic motor activity with or without electroencephalogram (EEG) changes are reported with these subcortical EEG alterations. In the clinical setting, many report ketamine to possess antiepileptic properties at clinically relevant doses that may be explained by an NMDA inhibitory effect. This effect is used to treat patients with refractory status epilepticus in the critical care setting.

Treatment of depression with low-dose ketamine is based on the premise that by blocking presynaptic disinhibition of glutamatergic neurons, a glutamine surge occurs through a cascade of cellular events (involving postsynaptic α-amino-3-hydroxy-5-methyl-4-isoxazoleproprionic acid {AMPA} receptors, extrasynaptic NMDA receptors and brain-derived neurotrophic factors {BDNF}, and mammalian target of rapamycin {mTORC1}) that restore prefrontal connectivity.

## CLINICAL MANIFESTATIONS

The reported signs and symptoms of arylcyclohexylamine toxicity are variable. The variations are a result of differences in dosage, the multiple routes of administration, concomitant xenobiotic use, and other associated medical conditions. Also, individual differences in xenobiotic susceptibility, the development of tolerance in chronic users, and contaminants in the drug manufacture account for erratic clinical findings.

### Vital Signs

Body temperature is rarely affected directly by arylcyclohexylamines. When hyperthermia does occur from agitation, all the known complications, including encephalopathy, rhabdomyolysis, myoglobinuria, acute kidney injury, electrolyte abnormalities, and liver failure, occur.

Most arylcyclohexylamine toxic patients demonstrate mild sympathomimetic effects secondary to their monoamine reuptake inhibition. Phencyclidine consistently increases both the systolic blood pressure (SBP) and diastolic blood pressure (DBP) in a dose-dependent fashion. Ketamine also produces mild increases in blood pressure, heart rate, and cardiac output via this same mechanism.

### Cardiopulmonary

Cardiovascular catastrophes are rarely encountered in patients with PCP toxicity. These complications result from direct vasospasm, causing severe systemic hypertension, pulmonary edema, hypertensive encephalopathy, and cerebral hemorrhage. Hypertension, along with abnormal behavior, miosis, and nystagmus in children, strongly suggest toxicity caused by a dissociative anesthetic.

Because these dissociative anesthetics were designed to retain normal ventilation, hypoventilation is uncommon. In clinical studies, PCP increased the minute ventilation, tidal volume, and respiratory rate of volunteers. Clinically, in PCP-toxic patients, irregular respiratory patterns occur, with tachypnea occurring much more often than bradypnea. Hypoventilation, when present, is usually secondary to the use of particularly high doses of PCP. Although respiratory depression in humans is an uncommon event, it is reported with fast or high-dose infusions of ketamine. Ketamine relaxes bronchial smooth muscles, decreases mean airway pressure and $PaCO_2$, and increases $PaO_2$.

## NEUROPSYCHIATRIC

Most patients with arylcyclohexylamine toxicity who are brought to medical attention manifest diverse psychomotor abnormalities. These xenobiotics impair responses to external stimuli by separating various elements of the mind. Consciousness, memory, perception, and motor activity appear dissociated from each other. This dissociation prevents the user from attaining cognition and properly assembling all information to construct "reality." Clinically, the person appears inebriated, either calm or agitated, and sometimes violent. In patients with large overdose, the anesthetic effect causes patients to develop stupor or coma. In recreational use, "dissociatives" are not taken for these effects but rather for out-of-body experiences.

Volunteers who took oral doses of up to 7.5 mg/day of PCP or 0.1 mg/kg of ketamine exhibited clinical toxicity, but higher doses (PCP > 10 mg/day; ketamine 0.5 mg/kg) generally caused a more severe impairment of mental function. Intravenous doses of 0.1 mg/kg of PCP or 0.5 mg/kg of ketamine diminish all sensory modalities (pain, touch, proprioception, hearing, taste, and visual acuity) in a dose-dependent fashion. Both xenobiotics also cause feelings of apathy, depersonalization, hostility, isolation, and alterations in body image. The deficits in sensory modalities are evident before the development of the psychological effects of PCP, with pain perception disappearing first. This alteration in analgesic perception is caused by a blocking action on the thalamus and midbrain (Fig. 56–1). The reaction to the misperceived or disconnected reality results in unintentional actions and violent behavior. The hallmark of PCP toxicity is the recurring delusion of superhuman strength and invulnerability resulting from both its anesthetic and dissociative properties.

Typical neurologic signs include horizontal, vertical, or rotatory nystagmus; ataxia; and altered gait. Initially, except for ataxia, movement is not impaired until the patient becomes unconscious. On physical examination, use of

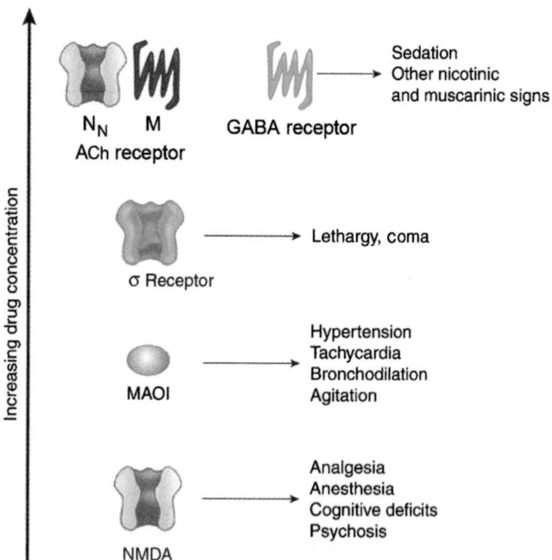


**FIGURE 56–1.** Clinical effects of the arylcyclohexylamines. The arylcyclohexylamines bind to different receptors in the central nervous system with varying degrees of affinity; that is, an increasing concentration is necessary to achieve the various clinical effects. ACh = acetylcholine; GABA = γ-aminobutyric acid; MAOI = monoamine oxidase inhibitor; $N_N$ = nicotinic receptor; M = muscarinic receptor; NMDA = *N*-methyl-D-aspartate.

dissociative anesthetics typically produces relatively small pupils, nystagmus, and diplopia. Other cerebellar symptoms are also encountered, most notably dizziness, ataxia, dysarthria, and nausea.

Larger doses of PCP produce loss of balance and confusion, the latter characterized by inability to repeat a set of objects, frequent loss of ideas, blocking, lack of concreteness, and disordered linguistic expression. Similarly, ketamine users report a high incidence of incoordination, confusion, unusual thought content, and an inability to speak. In general, dissociative anesthetics stimulate the CNS, but seizures rarely occur, except at high doses. The largest case series of PCP-toxic patients reported a 3.1% incidence of seizures.

Although arylcyclohexylamine-toxic patients also present with motor disturbances, it is unclear to what extent these dissociative drugs are actually responsible for these manifestations. The most common of the reported disturbances are dystonic reactions: opisthotonos, torticollis, tortipelvis, and risus sardonicus (facial grimacing). Myoclonic movements, tremor, hyperactivity, athetosis, stereotypies, and catalepsy also occur.

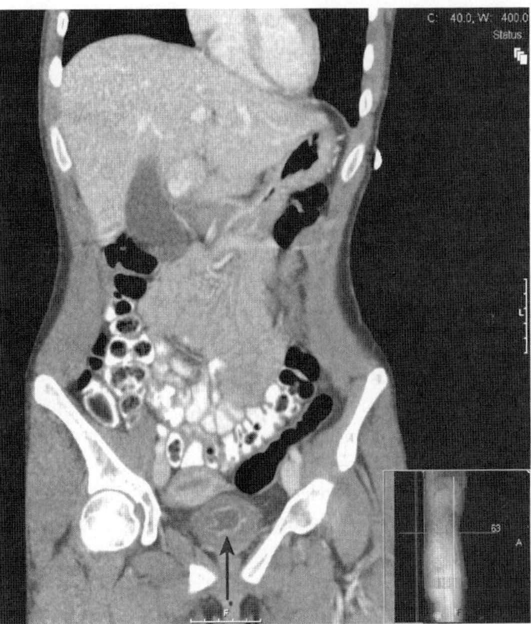

**FIGURE 56–2.** Ketamine-associated lower urinary tract syndrome. This abdominal-pelvic computed tomography (CT) scan was obtained in an 18-year-old girl who presented to the hospital with complaints of severe abdominal pain and hematuria. The image demonstrates a small bladder (red arrow) volume with an irregular thickened mucosal surface that enhances with contrast. *(Used with permission from the Fellowship in Medical Toxicology, New York University School of Medicine, New York City Poison Center.)*

### Cholinergic and Anticholinergic Effects

Both cholinergic and anticholinergic clinical manifestations occur in patients manifesting arylcyclohexylamine toxicity. Miosis or mydriasis, blurred vision, profuse diaphoresis, hypersalivation, bronchospasm, bronchorrhea, and urinary retention are reported. Ketamine stimulates salivary and tracheobronchial secretions, both of which are equally and effectively inhibited by atropine and glycopyrolate.

### Urologic and Hepatobiliary

Intense abdominal and pelvic pain is regularly reported in habitual ketamine users. In the majority of cases, the cause is urologic. The first case series describing ketamine-associated urologic dysfunction was reported in 2007. Symptoms consisted of a severe lower urinary tract syndrome (LUTS), including dysuria, frequency, urgency, urge incontinence, and painful hematuria (Fig. 56–2). When investigated by cystoscopy, patients with hematuria were frequently found to have ulcerative cystitis. The symptoms of ketamine-induced urologic dysfunction are secondary to an inflammatory process that reduces bladder size. Patients develop diminished voiding capacity of 20 to 200 mL, decreased bladder compliance, and detrusor overactivity as measured by urodynamic testing. A thickened bladder wall, a small bladder volume, and perivesicular stranding are usually detected by ultrasonography and computed tomography (CT) of the lower urologic tract. Cystoscopy demonstrates an erythematous bladder mucosa with various degrees of ulcerations. Bladder biopsies confer epithelium denudation and ulcerative cystitis. Intravenous urography and urography by CT reveal unilateral or bilateral ureteric narrowing. Bilateral hydronephrosis was reported in 44% to 50% of patients, and renal impairment is also described.

Intense abdominal pain in frequent ketamine users is also suggestive of hepatobiliary dysfunction. Case series of patients who used ketamine illicitly or therapeutically report abnormal liver function test results and biliary tract abnormalities. Computed tomography revealed common bile duct dilation with a smooth, tapered end, a condition that mimics benign cystic dilation of the bile ducts.

### Emergence Reaction

The acute psychosis observed during the recovery phase of PCP anesthesia limited its clinical use. This bizarre behavior, characterized by confusion, vivid dreaming, and hallucinations, is termed an "emergence reaction." These same postanesthetic reactions also limit the clinical use of ketamine. The incidence of emergence reactions after ketamine administration is approximately 50% in adults and 10% in children. The origin of these altered visual experiences is thought to be the depressive action of ketamine on auditory (inferior colliculus) and visual (medial geniculate) relay centers. Feelings of floating in space or body detachment and ataxia and dizziness occur because of a decreased perception to gravity.

### Tolerance and Withdrawal

Phencyclidine induces modest tolerance in animals. Dependence was observed in monkeys who self-administered PCP over 1 month and manifested by the appearance of dramatic withdrawal signs when access was denied. Signs included vocalizations, bruxism, oculomotor hyperactivity, diarrhea, piloerection, difficulty remaining awake, tremors, and in one case convulsions. When either PCP or ketamine (2.5 mg/kg/h) was readministered to the animals, PCP withdrawal symptoms were ameliorated, indicating cross-dependence between PCP and ketamine.

Physiologic dependence in humans is not formally studied. It is implied to occur by the observation that chronic PCP users developed depression, anxiety, irritability, lack of energy, sleep disturbance, and disturbed thoughts after 1 day of abstinence from use. Additionally, neonates whose mothers used PCP developed jitteriness, vomiting, and hypertonicity that lasted for at least 2 weeks. There are a few cases of ketamine tolerance in which patients report a need to use an increased quantity of drug to achieve the same effects. Ketamine-using patients characterized their withdrawal symptoms as anxiety, shaking, sweating, and palpitations.

## DIAGNOSTIC TESTING

If it is necessary to confirm the suspicion of PCP usage, urine is most commonly used for analysis. Qualitative testing is more important than a quantitative determination as serum concentrations do not correlate closely with the clinical effects. Although nonspecific, laboratory findings associated with PCP use include leukocytosis, hypoglycemia, and elevated concentrations of muscle enzymes (creatine phosphokinase), myoglobin, blood urea nitrogen (BUN), and creatinine. There is no commercially available quantitative immunoassay for ketamine or methoxetamine.

## MANAGEMENT

### Agitation

Conservative management is indicated for patients with arylcyclohexylamine toxicity and includes maintaining adequate respiration, circulation, and thermoregulation. The psychobehavioral symptoms observed during acute dissociative reactions and during the emergence reaction are similar. To prevent self-injury, a common form of PCP-induced morbidity and mortality, the patient must be safely restrained, initially physically, and then medically sedated. An IV catheter should be inserted and blood drawn for electrolytes, glucose, BUN, and creatinine concentrations. The use of 0.5 to 1.0 g/kg of body weight of dextrose and 100 mg of IV thiamine should be administered as clinically indicated.

Hyperthermia occurs secondary to psychomotor agitation and should be rapidly identified. Treatment should be accomplished immediately with adequate sedation to control motor activity. Rapid immersion in an ice water bath is recommended when body temperatures are greater than 106°F (41.1°C).

Benzodiazepines are recommended as the first-line sedatives. A benzodiazepine such as diazepam or midazolam administered in titrated doses every 5 to 10 minutes until agitation is controlled is usually safe and effective. By contrast, phenothiazines lower the seizure threshold, and both phenothiazines and butyrophenones cause acute dystonic reactions. Phenothiazines also cause significant hypotension because of their $\alpha$-adrenergic blocking effects on the vasculature, worsen hyperthermia, and exacerbate any anticholinergic effects, and they should therefore be avoided.

### Decontamination

Patients with a history of recent oral use of arylcyclohexylamines are candidates for gastrointestinal decontamination. Although there is rarely, if ever, an indication for orogastric lavage, decontamination is indicated if potentially lethal coingestants are suspected. Activated charcoal (1 g/kg) is recommended as soon as possible and repeated in 4 hours for two doses as long as no contraindications exist. Activated charcoal effectively adsorbs PCP and increases its nonrenal clearance even without prior gastric evacuation.

Theoretically, xenobiotics that are weak bases, such as PCP, can be eliminated more rapidly if the urine is acidified. Although urinary acidification with ammonium chloride was previously recommended, we do not recommend this approach. The risks associated with acidifying the urine, which simultaneously induces an acidemia increasing urinary myoglobin precipitation, outweigh any perceived benefits (Chap. 4).

Most patients rapidly regain normal CNS function within 45 minutes to several hours after its use. However, those who have taken exceedingly high doses or who have an underlying psychiatric disorder may remain comatose or exhibit bizarre behavior for days or even weeks before returning to normal. Those who rapidly regain normal function should be monitored for several hours and then, after a psychiatric consultation, should receive drug counseling and additional social support as indicated. Patients whose recovery is delayed should be treated supportively and monitored carefully in an intensive care unit.

The major toxicity of PCP appears to be behaviorally related: self-inflicted injuries, injuries resulting from exceptional physical exertion, and injuries sustained as a result of resisting the application of physical restraints are frequent. Patients appear to be unaware of their surroundings and sometimes even oblivious to pain because of the dissociative anesthetic effects. In addition to major trauma, rhabdomyolysis and resultant myoglobinuric acute kidney injury account in large measure for the high morbidity and mortality associated with PCP. Early fluid therapy should be used to avoid deposition of myoglobin to the kidneys. Urinary alkalinization as part of the treatment regimen for rhabdomyolysis would theoretically increase PCP reabsorption and deposition in fat stores and is not recommended given its unproven role (Antidotes in Brief: A5).

### Cystitis

The objectives of the management of ketamine-induced cystitis are establishing the diagnosis, decreasing symptoms, and maintaining kidney function. Urinalysis should be obtained on all symptomatic patients to exclude urinary tract infection, and a serum creatinine should be obtained to evaluate kidney function. However, initial urinalyses are typically sterile. For patients whose symptoms are mild, abstinence from ketamine use will be enough to reverse symptoms and pathology. Several therapeutic regimens have been tried with little success. They include antibiotics, nonsteroidal antiinflammatory drugs (NSAIDs), corticosteroids, and anticholinergics. Urologic evaluation and follow-up are necessary. For patients with moderate and severe symptoms, urologic consultation and repeated kidney function monitoring are essential.

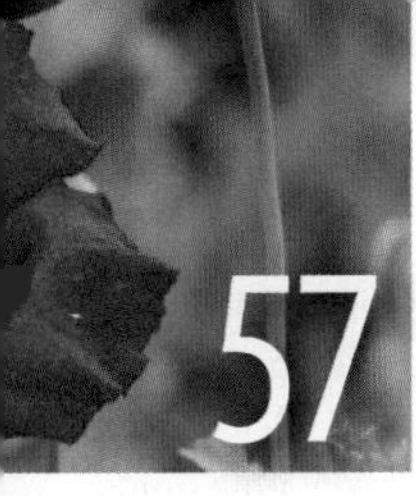



# 57 ALUMINUM

Normal concentrations

| | |
|---|---|
| Serum | 2 μg/L (0.074 μmol/L) |
| Whole blood | 12 μg/L (0.445 μmol/L) |
| Urine (24-hour collection) | 4–12 μg/g creatinine (0.148–0.445 μmol/g creatinine) |

## CHEMISTRY

Aluminum (Al), the most abundant metal in the crust of the earth, is a nonessential element and a trace metal with a single oxidation state, $Al^{3+}$. Aluminum ores are converted to alumina and then reduced to aluminum metal. The first step usually involves refining bauxite at high temperature and pressure in a caustic soda to form alumina (aluminum oxide, $Al_2O_3$). The second step occurs by the Hall–Heroult process in potrooms and uses electrolytic reduction to form aluminum. In this chapter, aluminum metal is discussed as an occupational toxin with mainly lung manifestations. Aluminum salts, the more common form discussed in human toxicity, primarily act as neurotoxins, with both acute and chronic toxicity.

## HISTORY AND EPIDEMIOLOGY

The first case of aluminum toxicity with neurologic findings was reported in 1921. Subsequently, a case series described occupational asthma in Norwegian aluminum (potroom) workers ("potroom asthma"). In 1947, 26% of German potroom workers exposed to high concentrations of aluminum dust mixed with mineral oil–based lubricants developed pulmonary fibrosis or "aluminosis." Some potroom workers also developed neurologic findings later termed "potroom palsy". In the 1970s, encephalopathy in patients with chronic kidney disease (CKD), called "dialysis dementia," was attributed to using aluminum salt–containing phosphate binders or, more rarely, to aluminum-contaminated dialysis fluid. Later, the relationship between aluminum and microcytic anemia and osteomalacia in dialysis patients was recognized. In 1982, alum (potassium aluminum sulfate or ammonium aluminum sulfate) was first used in the treatment of hemorrhagic cystitis.

Although aluminum was linked to the spongiform leukoencephalopathy that was rarely reported in heroin users who inhaled the pyrolysate of heroin heated on aluminum or tin foil (called "chasing the dragon"), a causal relationship was never established. Similarly, while there are concerns over the relation between aluminum and Alzheimer disease, to date no studies have proven that aluminum is the cause of the disease. Regardless, regulatory agencies in the United States (US) and Canada decreased the amount of aluminum allowable in food and water products.

## ALUMINUM-CONTAINING XENOBIOTICS

Patients take antacids containing aluminum hydroxide for symptomatic control of dyspepsia and gastroesophageal reflux disease. Aluminum hydroxide is usually packaged with magnesium hydroxide to counteract the induced delay of gastric emptying and constipation caused by aluminum hydroxide. These antacids are poorly absorbed and exit the stomach in about 30 minutes. Sucralfate, an aluminum-containing salt with sucrose sulfate, is also used for symptomatic control of ulcer disease, to accelerate healing of peptic ulcer disease, and as a protectant against stress ulcer formation. This sucrose aluminum complex is poorly absorbed from the gastrointestinal (GI) tract, and the little that is absorbed is excreted by the kidney unchanged. Alum is usually a 1% solution of potassium aluminum sulfate salt $\{KAl(SO_4)_2 * 12H_2O\}$ or an ammonium aluminum sulfate salt $\{NH_4Al(SO_4)_2 * 12H_2O\}$, and is uncommonly used as an astringent for hemorrhagic cystitis administered by bladder irrigation. It is poorly absorbed, although toxicity occurs.

## TOXICOKINETICS

### Absorption

The daily intake of aluminum in the US is estimated to be 2 to 25 mg from food and beverages, depending on the diet studied. Gastrointestinal absorption, which mainly occurs in the proximal small bowel, occurs by both diffusion and active transport via transferrin and calcium transporters. Absorption increases in the presence of citrate, other small organic acids, uremia, and iron deficiency anemia, and decreases in the presence of phosphorus and silicon. Dermal absorption from deodorants is negligible. Pulmonary absorption of inhaled aluminum particulates in workers is 1.5% to 2%.

### Distribution

The initial volume of distribution of aluminum is 0.06 L/kg, equally distributed between plasma and red blood cells. Aluminum then becomes 90% bound to transferrin, with approximately 10% bound to citrate. From the blood, approximately 50% distributes to the bone, and approximately 1% to the brain. The remainder of the aluminum distributes variably to the heart, liver, kidney, and other organ systems. Intracellularly, aluminum localizes in the lysosomes of brain neurons, liver, spleen, kidney epithelial tubules and glomerular mesangium cells, cardiac myocytes, and the mitochondria of osteoblasts.

### Metabolism/Excretion

Aluminum is not metabolized in the body and is considered to be greater than 95% excreted unchanged in the urine. Less than 2% of aluminum is excreted by the bile. Because aluminum is primarily excreted in the urine, patients with CKD have decreased aluminum excretion. There is no normal reference point for elimination half-life. The elimination half-life is approximately 85 days in patients receiving dialysis. Based on urinary excretion in workers (with preserved kidney function), the apparent half-life is extended to years, possibly as a result of deposits in the lungs.

## PATHOPHYSIOLOGY

Little is known about the pathophysiology of aluminum toxicity. The information that follows is based on a summary of limited research.

### Pulmonary System

Rats exposed to alumina and aluminum through intratracheal injection develop epithelialization of alveoli, focal fibrosis occurring in the respiratory bronchioles and alveolar ducts, and alveolar proteinosis.

### Central Nervous System

The primary site of aluminum entry into the brain appears to be the cerebral microvasculature. Following IV administration in animals, aluminum concentrations are higher in the frontal cortex than in the lateral ventricles. The mechanisms of entry are postulated to be transferrin mediated, endocytosis, and other active processes. Aluminum decreases acetylcholine activity, possibly through a decrease in choline acetyltransferase.

### Hematologic System

Aluminum toxicity results in a microcytic hypochromic anemia, likely through inhibition of δ-aminolevulinic acid dehydrogenase in the heme synthesis pathway.

### Musculoskeletal System

Aluminum concentrates in the mitochondria of the osteoblasts at the mineralization front where it competes and replaces other cations in the bone, leading to osteomalacia that is resistant to vitamin D.

## MANIFESTATIONS

### Acute Toxicity

Patients with acute aluminum toxicity typically develop encephalopathy, myoclonus, and seizures. The encephalopathy manifests as disorientation, confusion, and coma. All symptoms appear to develop within days to a few weeks of receiving massive systemic aluminum exposure (usually to an aluminum salt), usually in the presence of CKD. Aluminum concentrations range from barely elevated to extremely elevated. Although recovery occurs in patients promptly treated with deferoxamine and/or hemodialysis (HD), patients with a delay to treatment often remain debilitated or die.

### Chronic Toxicity

Two distinct types of chronic aluminum toxicity are reported: occupationally related lung disease, and a multisystem syndrome most often noted in HD patients.

***Pulmonary.*** Potroom asthma is characterized by dyspnea, cough, wheezing, bronchitis, and chest tightness. These symptoms develop after only a few months of exposure to the metal fumes of aluminum and aluminum dust. The asthma often improves on cessation of exposure, although some workers never fully recover. Pulmonary fibrosis, termed aluminosis, is very similar to the other pneumoconiosis and develops in workers exposed to aluminum dust. Patients experience cough, shortness of breath, and dyspnea on exertion, and they eventually develop restrictive lung disease. Abnormal chest radiographic findings include increased pulmonary markings, distortion of pleura and diaphragms, and irregular opacities. Recovery of lung function does not occur, and patients die from complications of pulmonary disease such as pneumonia.

***Multisystem Toxicity.*** The other form of chronic aluminum toxicity primarily affects the hematopoietic, nervous, and musculoskeletal systems. In patients with CKD, the toxicity occurs after months to years of exposure to aluminum salt–contaminated dialysate and/or aluminum salt–containing phosphate binders. Although toxicity occurs uncommonly following other exposures, modern preparation of dialysate using reverse osmosis of water has virtually eliminated this disease. The microcytic hypochromic anemia of aluminum poisoning is unresponsive to iron replacement therapy and usually precedes encephalopathy and osteomalacia. The encephalopathy is characterized by speech disturbances, electroencephalogram abnormalities, myoclonic jerks, and dementia. Osteomalacia can lead to bone pain and fractures. Death is common in these patients when aluminum toxicity is not recognized and treated.

## DIAGNOSTIC TESTS

Aluminum concentrations can be measured in the serum, whole blood, and urine. Toxicity has occurred in patients with a wide range of serum and urine concentrations, with some dying of severe clinical manifestations with concentrations only slightly above normal. Pulmonary function testing can be performed to evaluate for restrictive lung function in exposed workers.

## MANAGEMENT

Patients with symptoms or with elevated aluminum concentrations should be removed from any aluminum exposure if identified. Patients with occupational asthma should be treated with bronchodilators and steroids. The only chelator with proven benefit is deferoxamine (DFO) (Antidotes in Brief: A7). Deferoxamine chelates the aluminum to form aluminoxamine, which is excreted in the urine or removed by HD.

### Acute Toxicity

A DFO dose of 15 mg/kg/day intravenously is recommended. Chelation mobilizes aluminum from its storage sites in blood and increases its renal elimination. In dialysis-dependent patients, DFO alone is reported to precipitate aluminum encephalopathy and death, either from DFO redistribution of aluminum to brain tissue or aluminum oxide redistribution across the blood–brain barrier. It is recommended that in patients with stage 5 CKD 3 to 4 hours of HD be performed 6 to 8 hours after chelation in order to clear the aluminoxamine and prevent redistribution to vital tissues. Patients with normal kidney function and urine output do not require HD.

### Chronic Toxicity

Prompt chelation therapy with DFO reverses encephalopathy, osteomalacia, and anemia. The National Kidney Foundation provides guidelines for the treatment of dialysis encephalopathy. These guidelines for nephrologists recommend 4 months of once-weekly DFO at 5 mg/kg over 1 hour given 5 hours before a regularly scheduled HD session in patients with serum aluminum concentrations greater than 300 μg/L. In patients with serum aluminum concentrations between 50 and 300 μg/L, DFO 5 mg/kg is recommended during the last hour of HD, once a week for 2 months. Therapy is repeated as needed based on kidney function and neurologic symptoms.

### Other Treatments

Treatments with reported benefit in experimental models include zinc, copper, pomegranate peel, vitamin E, selenium, taurine, melatonin, coenzyme Q10, and fish oil, although there is not enough evidence to recommend the routine use of any of these xenobiotics at this time.

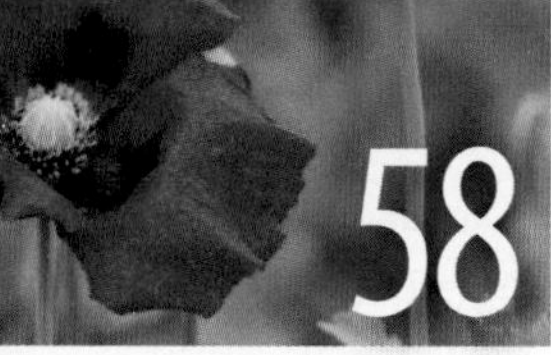

# 58 ANTIMONY

| Normal concentrations | |
|---|---|
| Serum | < 3 μg/L (24.6 nmol/L) |
| Urine (24 hour) | < 6.2 μg/L (50.1 nmol/L) |
| | < 3.5 μg/g creatinine (28.7 nmol/g creatinine) |

## HISTORY AND EPIDEMIOLOGY

Antimony (Sb) and its compounds are among the oldest known remedies in the practice of medicine. The medicinal use of antimony for the treatment of syphilis, whooping cough, and gout dates to the medieval period. Various antimony compounds were also used as topical preparations for the treatment of herpes, leprosy, mania, and epilepsy. Orally administered tartar emetic (antimony potassium tartrate) was used for treatment of fever, pneumonia, inflammatory conditions, and as a decongestant, emetic, and sedative, but it was abandoned because of its significant toxicity. The use of antimony as a homicidal agent continued well into the 20th century. The current medical use of antimony is limited to the treatments of leishmaniasis and schistosomiasis and to sporadic use as aversive therapy for alcohol use disorder.

In developed countries, antimony poisoning rarely occurs following intentional ingestion, or occupational exposures in the glass workers, miners, or during metal working. Most recent descriptions of antimony toxicity result from parenteral exposures to sodium stibogluconate during the treatment of schistosomiasis and leishmaniasis. Oral exposures usually occur following the use of antimonials containing potassium tartrate compounds. Several cases were described after the use of old porcelain houseware or after the use of antimonials as home remedies.

## CHEMISTRY

Antimony is found in the same group on the periodic table as arsenic (As), and as such, it has many similar chemical, physical, and toxicologic properties. Pure antimony is a lustrous, silver-white, brittle, hard metal that is extremely rare to find in nature because of its ability to rapidly convert to either antimony oxide or antimony trioxide. Thus, for the purposes of this chapter, the term *antimony* refers to antimony ions.

Like arsenic, antimony forms both organic and inorganic compounds with trivalent ($3^+$) and pentavalent ($5^+$) oxidation states. Common inorganic trivalent antimony compounds include antimony potassium tartrate ($C_8H_4K_2O_{12}Sb_2$), antimony trichloride ($SbCl_3$), antimony trioxide ($Sb_2O_3$), antimony trisulfide ($Sb_2S_3$), and stibine ($SbH_3$). Antimony pentasulfide ($Sb_2S_5$) and pentoxide ($Sb_2O_5$) are inorganic compounds that can act as oxidizing agents. Antimony pentachloride ($SbCl_5$) is used as a chemical reagent with acidic properties. It reacts with water, forming hydrochloric acid causing a direct corrosive effect on skin and mucous membranes. From an industrial perspective, the most important application of antimony is the use of antimony oxychloride ($Sb_6O_6Cl_4$) as a flame retardant.

Tartar emetic (antimony potassium tartrate) is an odorless trivalent antimony compound with a sweet metallic taste and a potent emetic effect. Antimony potassium tartrate is considered to be one of the most toxic antimony compounds, with minimal lethal doses reported between 200 mg and 1,200 mg.

## PHARMACOLOGY

One proposed mechanism for the antiparasitic mechanism of action of antimony is the inhibition of phosphofructokinase leading to energy failure from impaired adenosine triphosphate (ATP) synthesis. Another possible mechanism is selective targeting of guanosine diphosphate–mannose pyrophosphorylase, which interferes with nucleoside and mannose metabolism and results in the inability to synthesize purines. A more recently proposed mechanism involves the inhibition of trypanothione reductase.

## TOXICOKINETICS

### Absorption

Absorption from the gastrointestinal tract begins immediately following ingestion, and the oral bioavailability of antimony ranges from 15% to 50%. This poor gastrointestinal absorption in humans, in addition to the concomitant emesis, necessitates parenteral administration of many antimony-based pharmaceuticals. Pulmonary absorption of many inorganic antimony compounds is very slow and limited by low water solubility. In contrast, animal data suggest that inhaled trivalent antimony is well absorbed from the lungs, distributed to various organs, and subsequently excreted in the feces and urine. Transdermal absorption of antimony trioxide in humans is negligible.

### Distribution

Distribution depends on the oxidation state of antimony. In animals, more than 95% of trivalent antimony is incorporated into the red blood cells within 2 hours of exposure, whereas in a similar time frame, 90% of pentavalent antimony remains in the serum. When administered intravenously or orally, antimony is predominantly distributed among highly vascular organs, including the liver, kidneys, thyroid, and adrenals. The antimony that is detected in the liver and spleen is predominantly in the pentavalent form, whereas the thyroid accumulates trivalent forms. After inhalation, antimony accumulates predominantly in red blood cells and to a significantly lesser extent in the liver and spleen.

After intramuscular (IM) administration of sodium stibogluconate, the antimony concentration-versus-time profile suggests a two-compartment open model, with the rapid distribution phase and slower elimination half-life in the range of 10 hours.

### Metabolism

In humans, metabolic transformation of antimony is limited. Antimony is converted by binding to macromolecules, incorporation into lipids, and covalent interactions with sulfhydryl groups and phosphates. Pentavalent antimony is converted to trivalent compounds either in the liver or in the acidic intracellular environment of *Leishmania*-infected cells.

### Excretion

Trivalent antimony is excreted in the bile after conjugation with glutathione. A significant proportion of excreted antimony undergoes enterohepatic recirculation. The remainder is excreted in urine. The overall elimination is very slow, with only 10% of a given dose cleared in the first 24 hours and 30% in the first week. Pentavalent antimony is much more rapidly excreted by the kidneys than trivalent antimony (50%–60% versus 10% over the first 24 hours). Renal excretion of sodium stibogluconate is as high as 90% within 6 hours of an IM administration. However, urine and serum antimony concentrations remain elevated for several years following therapeutic use. The clearance of tartar emetic has a biphasic pattern, with 90% being excreted within 24 hours after acute exposure, followed by a second slower phase with an estimated half-life of approximately 16 days.

The renal elimination half-life of inhaled stibine is estimated at approximately 4 days following occupational exposure.

## PATHOPHYSIOLOGY

Antimony has no known biological functions and is considered to be toxic even at very low concentrations. Like other toxic metals, antimony binds to sulfhydryl groups to inhibit a variety of metabolic functions. Trivalent antimony compounds are more toxic than the pentavalent compounds because of their higher affinity for erythrocytes and sulfhydryl groups. Tartar emetic and other antimony salts are gastrointestinal irritants. One proposed mechanism for this local effect is the activation of enterochromaffin cells, which produce and secrete serotonin (5-$HT_3$). Released serotonin acts on the 5-$HT_3$ receptors, stimulating vagal sensory fibers and activating the vomiting center. In addition, there is an apparent direct central medullary action, particularly after the administration of higher doses of antimony.

## CLINICAL MANIFESTATIONS

Serious adverse events and deaths resulting from treatment with sodium stibogluconate are very rare and include cardiac dysrhythmias and pancreatitis. Patients older than 50 years are at an increased risk for more serious reactions to meglumine antimonate used for the treatment of visceral leishmaniasis (Table 58–1).

Workers with occupational exposures usually present with subtle delayed clinical symptoms as chronic toxicity develops. Patients with acute ingestions usually present with symptoms mimicking the toxicity of arsenic and other metal and metalloid salts.

### Local Irritation

The most common manifestations of antimony toxicity involve local irritation. In sufficient concentration, antimony acts as an irritant to the eyes, skin, and mucosa. Antimony pentachloride is very irritating and causes local dermal and mucosal burns, as it reacts with water, releasing hydrochloric acid, heat, and antimony pentoxide ($Sb_2O_5$). Following ingestion, contact with the water in saliva produces sufficient hydrochloric acid to result in gastrointestinal burns. Ophthalmic exposure to $Sb_2O_5$ can causes a typical caustic injury, resulting in blepharospasm, lacrimation, photophobia, and corneal burns. Thrombophlebitis is common after the intravenous (IV) use of antimony.

***Gastrointestinal.*** Following acute ingestion, antimony rapidly produces anorexia, nausea, vomiting, abdominal pain, and diarrhea. Some patients report a metallic taste. A garlic odor on the breath is often recognized, but this may be due to concomitant arsenic exposure. In severe overdose, gastrointestinal irritation progresses to hemorrhagic gastritis. Many patients develop pancreatitis following treatment with pentavalent antimonial salts.

***Cardiovascular.*** In animals, antimony decreases myocardial contraction; lowers coronary vascular resistance, producing decreased systolic pressure; and causes bradycardia. The majority of reported human cardiac effects are related to the electrocardiographic (ECG) changes. Prolongation of the QT interval, inversion or flattening of T waves, and ST segment changes are frequently described during treatment of visceral leishmaniasis with pentavalent antimonial compounds (sodium stibogluconate and meglumine antimonate). Torsade de pointes is reported in patients treated with pentavalent antimonial preparations. Chronic antimony exposure resulting in elevated concentrations of antimony in urine is associated with an increase in composite cardiovascular and cerebrovascular disease.

***Respiratory.*** Local irritation from antimony trioxide produces laryngitis, tracheitis, and pneumonitis. Pneumonitis is usually reversible after exposure ceases and can be followed radiologically. Acute respiratory distress syndrome was reported after acute exposure to antimony pentachloride. Workers chronically exposed to antimony compounds are at risk for developing "antimony pneumoconiosis."

***Renal.*** Patients treated with sodium stibogluconate develop varied manifestations of nephrotoxicity ranging from renal cell casts, proteinuria, and increased blood urea nitrogen concentration to acute kidney injury (AKI). Some patients also develop renal tubular acidosis and acute tubular necrosis. Older age and underlying chronic kidney disease are risk factors for the development of AKI that can progress to death. Antimonials also cause drug-induced acute interstitial nephritis that is responsive to treatment with steroids.

***Hepatic.*** Acute exposure to antimony results in severe acute liver injury. Chronic therapeutic use of antimony compounds for the treatment of leishmaniasis causes liver toxicity that ranges from reversible elevations of aminotransferase concentrations to hepatic necrosis. Elderly patients are at an increased risk for the development of significant hepatic failure.

***Hematologic.*** Severe anemia was reported in HIV-positive patients during treatment with sodium stibogluconate. Bone marrow biopsy documented transient severe marrow

**TABLE 58–1 Clinical Manifestations of Antimony Compound Poisoning**[a]

| *Antimony Compound* | *Stibine* | *Antimony Potassium Tartrate* | *Antimony Trioxide* | *Antimony Pentachloride/Pentoxide* | *Meglumine Antimoniate* | *Sodium Stibogluconate* |
|---|---|---|---|---|---|---|
| **Formula** | $SbH_3$ | $C_8H_{10}K_2O_{15}Sb_2$ | $Sb_2O_3$ | $SbCl_5Sb_2O_5$ | $C_7H_{18}NO_8Sb$ | $C_{12}H_{38}Na_3O_{26}Sb_2$ |
| **Brand/common name** | | Tartar emetic | | | Glucantime | Pentostan |
| **Common use** | | | Flame retardant | | Antileishmanial | Antileishmanial |
| **Oxidation state** | $3^+$ | $3^+$ | $3^+$ | $5^+$ | $3^+/5^+$ | $3^+/5^+$ |
| CLINICAL EFFECTS | | | | | | |
| **Local Irritation** | | | | | | |
| Conjunctival/mucosal irritant | ++ | | | ++ | | |
| Corneal burns | + | + | + | + | | + |
| Thrombophlebitis | | | | | + | + |
| **Gastrointestinal** | | | | | | |
| Anorexia | + | + | + | + | + | + |
| N/V/D | + | + | + | + | + | + |
| Abdominal pain | + | + | + | + | + | + |
| Pancreatitis | | | | | + | + |
| **Cardiovascular** | | | | | | |
| Prolonged QT interval | | | | | + | + |
| ST segment and T wave changes | | | | | + | + |
| Torsade de pointes | | | | | + | + |
| Ventricular dysrhythmias | | | | | + | + |
| Pericarditis | | | | | + | |
| **Respiratory** | | | | | | |
| Laryngitis | | | + | | | |
| Tracheitis | | | + | | | |
| Pneumonitis | | | | | | |
| ARDS | | | | + | | |
| Pneumoconiosis | | | + | + | | |
| Metal fume fever | | | + | + ($Sb_2O_5$) | | |
| **Renal** | | | | | | |
| Renal cell casts | | | | | + | + |
| Proteinuria | | | | | + | + |
| Increased BUN | | | | | + | + |
| Acute interstitial nephritis | | | | | + | + |
| Hematuria | + | | | | | |
| **Hepatic** | | | | | | |
| Abnormal LFTs | + | | | | + | + |
| Hepatic necrosis | + | | | | + | + |
| **Hematologic** | | | | | | |
| Anemia | + | | | | + | + |
| Hemolysis | + | | | | | |
| Thrombocytopenia | | | | | + | + |
| Leukopenia/lymphopenia | | | | | + | + |
| **Dermatologic** | | | | | | |
| Antimony spots | + | | + | | | |
| Contact dermatitis | + | | + | | + | |
| Severe cutaneous reactions | | | | | | |
| **Neurologic** | | | | | | |
| Vestibular-cochlear toxicity | | | | | + | |
| Tinnitus | | | | | + | |
| Rotatory dizziness | | | | | + | |
| Peripheral sensory neuropathy | | | | | | + |
| Cerebellar ataxia | | | | | | + |
| **Musculoskeletal** | | | | | | |
| Muscle and joint pain | | | | | + | + |
| Rhabdomyolysis | | | | | | |
| **Genotoxicity** | + | | | | | |
| **Carcinogenicity** | | | + | | | |

[a]The absence of a + indicates the absence of reported or recognized clinical manifestation.

ARDS = acute respiratory distress syndrome; BUN = blood urea nitrogen; LFTs = liver function tests; N/V/D = nausea, vomiting, and diarrhea.

dyserythropoiesis, followed by complete recovery on discontinuation of the therapy. Patients treated with sodium stibogluconate for visceral leishmaniasis occasionally develop thrombocytopenia. Leukopenia is frequently observed in patients treated with antimonial compounds.

***Dermatologic.*** Antimony spots are papules and pustules that develop around sweat and sebaceous glands and may resemble varicella. Chronically exposed patients develop eczema and lichenification of the arms, legs, and joint creases with sparing of the face, hands, and feet that more commonly occur in the summer.

***Neurologic.*** Patients treated with sodium stibogluconate developed a reversible, peripheral sensory neuropathy and cerebellar ataxia in temporal association with exposure. Reversible cochlear vestibular toxicity associated with tinnitus and severe rotatory dizziness was also reported.

***Musculoskeletal.*** The therapeutic use of parenteral antimonials is associated with diffuse musculoskeletal pain. The symptoms are sometimes so severe that they require treatment interruption in about one-third of patients.

***Immunologic.*** A case-control study of 100 patients and 300 controls showed a marked association between systemic sclerosis and antimony exposure in both male and female patients. The use of meglumine antimoniate was reported to cause two different subsets of cutaneous hypersensitivity reactions: IgE-mediated allergic reactions (type I) that present immediately and can range from localized and generalized urticaria to anaphylaxis and delayed (type IV) allergic reactions including eczematous lesions and persistent subcutaneous nodules.

***Reproductive.*** In animal studies, antimony causes ovarian atrophy, uterine metaplasia, and impaired conception. An association was found with spontaneous abortion and premature births reported in women who were occupationally exposed to antimony salts.

***Carcinogenicity.*** The International Agency for Research on Cancer classified antimony trioxide as possibly carcinogenic to humans (group 2B).

## STIBINE

Antimony compounds react with nascent hydrogen, forming an extremely toxic gas, stibine ($SbH_3$), which resembles arsine ($AsH_3$) (Chap. 59). Historically, stibine release was reported during the charging of lead storage batteries. Stibine, probably the most toxic antimony compound, is a colorless gas with a very unpleasant smell that rapidly decomposes at temperatures above 302°F (150°C). In addition to gastrointestinal symptoms that include nausea, vomiting, and abdominal pain, stibine has strong oxidative properties that may result in massive hemolysis. Severe stibine exposure results in hematuria, rhabdomyolysis, and death.

## DIAGNOSTIC TESTING

Standard laboratory testing to assess volume depletion and AKI is indicated for patients with acute antimony toxicity. A complete blood count, electrolytes, kidney function studies, and a urinalysis should be obtained. When there is a known or suspected exposure to stibine, additional studies should include tests for hemolysis, such as determinations of bilirubin and haptoglobin. Blood should also be obtained for a blood type and crossmatch, as transfusions are likely to be required.

An ECG should be obtained to evaluate for QT interval prolongation and dysrhythmias. Patients with known myocardial disease should have frequent evaluations of cardiac function, and continuous ECG monitoring is recommended for all patients with significant symptoms or abnormal cardiovascular status. A chest radiograph should be performed in patients with respiratory symptoms and evidence of hypoxia after significant inhalation exposure. In addition, an abdominal radiograph is reasonable in patients with ingestion to evaluate gastrointestinal antimony load and help guide decontamination.

An antimony concentration in a 24-hour urine collection is used for the assessment of the intensity of exposure to either trivalent or pentavalent antimony. A serum antimony concentration should be sent, but cannot be used for treatment decisions as it is unlikely to be determined in a timely fashion.

## TREATMENT

### Decontamination

Following a significant acute ingestion, the majority of patients develop vomiting. Gastric lavage is reasonable only if performed before the onset of spontaneous emesis. Although it is unknown whether antimony is adsorbed to activated charcoal, based on experience with salts of arsenic, thallium, and mercury, administration of activated charcoal is recommended. Additionally, because antimony has a documented enterohepatic circulation, multiple-dose activated charcoal is reasonable if the patient can tolerate it. Based on experience with arsenic poisoning, whole-bowel irrigation (WBI) is also recommended in patients with severe ingestions who are able to tolerate it, especially if radiographs confirm radiopaque material.

Patients with dermal exposures, particularly to antimony tri- or pentachloride, should be decontaminated with soap and water. Prompt removal from the contaminated area is important for patients exposed to stibine. Rescuers need to take appropriate precautions to ensure their own safety (Chap. 101).

### Supportive Care

The mainstay of treatment for patients with antimony poisoning is good supportive care. Clinicians should anticipate massive volume depletion and begin rehydration with isotonic crystalloid solutions. Electrolytes, urine output, and kidney and liver function should be followed closely. Antiemetics are recommended both for patient comfort and to facilitate the administration of activated charcoal, but caution is advised as many antiemetics will contribute to QT interval prolongation. Following stibine exposure, the hemoglobin concentration should be followed closely and blood should be transfused based on standard criteria.

### Chelation

Human experience with regard to chelation of antimony is limited. Most of the available data are based on animal experimentation. Dimercaprol, succimer, and dimercaptopropane–sulfonic acid (DMPS) all improve the survival of experimental animals. A single case series documented survival in three of four patients exposed to tartar emetic who were treated with intramuscular dimercaprol at a dose of 200 to 600 mg/day. All four patients had increased urinary excretion of antimony. In another case report, a patient survived after chelation with dimercaprol but without evidence of enhanced urinary excretion of antimony. Although specific recommendations are difficult to make, it is reasonable to begin therapy with IM dimercaprol until it is certain that antimony is removed from the gastrointestinal tract, at which time the patient can be switched to oral succimer. If the patient experiences cardiac or respiratory symptoms with associated ECG changes during administration of dimercaprol, treatment should be stopped. Because chelation doses for antimony poisoning are not established, chelators should be administered in doses and regimens that are determined to be safe and effective for other metals (Antidotes in Brief: A28 and A29).

# 59 ARSENIC

| Normal concentration | |
|---|---|
| Whole blood | < 5 μg/L (0.067 μmol/L) |
| Urine (24-hour) | < 50 μg/L (0.67 μmol/L) |
| | < 100 μg/g creatinine (1.33 μmol/g creatinine) |

## HISTORY/EPIDEMIOLOGY

Arsenic poisoning can be unintentional, suicidal, homicidal, occupational, environmental, or iatrogenic. Contaminated soil, water, and food are the primary sources of arsenic for the general population. Pentavalent arsenic is the most common inorganic form in the environment. Enviromental contamination results from emissions from foundries and other industries. The consumption of contaminated water has emerged as the primary cause of large-scale outbreaks of chronic arsenic toxicity. In 2001, the United States (US) Environmental Protection Agency (EPA) decreased the maximum permissible concentration of arsenic in drinking water to 10 parts per billion (ppb, or 10 μg/L), after statistical modeling indicated an increased risk of lung and bladder cancer from water contaminated with arsenic at the formerly acceptable concentration of 50 ppb. The World Health Organization uses the same 10 ppb standard.

## CHEMISTRY

Arsenic exists in multiple forms: elemental, gaseous (arsine), organic, and inorganic ($As^{3+}$, trivalent, or arsenite and $As^{5+}$, pentavalent, or arsenate). Arsenic metal is nonpoisonous because of its insolubility in water and, therefore, bodily fluids. Arsine, which is highly toxic, is discussed in Chap. 94. Trivalent arsenicals are more toxic than pentavalent arsenicals. Also, organic arsenicals vary in toxicity. Arsenobetaine and arsenosugars, which are synthesized by fish and crustaceans, have very low toxicity. By contrast, the organoarsenical medication melarsoprol, used for African trypanosomiasis, is highly toxic and similar to inorganic arsenite.

## PHARMACOLOGY/PHYSIOLOGY

Arsenic trioxide ($As_2O_3$) is administered therapeutically in oncology at conventional doses of 0.15 to 0.16 mg/kg per day either intravenously or orally. The beneficial effects in acute promyelocytic leukemia occur from initiating cellular apoptosis when arsenic concentrations reach 0.5 to 2.0 μmol/L. The trivalent arsenic ion binds to mitochondrial membrane sulfhydryl (SH) groups, damaging mitochondrial membranes and collapsing membrane potentials. Melarsoprol, the arsenoxide derivative of an organic arsenical, is used to treat the meningoencephalitic stage of West African (Gambian) and East African (Rhodesian) trypanosomiasis. The drug concentrates in trypanosomes via a purine transporter. Its target is trypanothione, the primary reducing agent in trypanosomes. The resulting decrease in trypanothione leads to a loss of reducing capacity with subsequent lysis of the parasite.

## TOXICOLOGY/PATHOPHYSIOLOGY

The primary biochemical lesion of $As^{3+}$ is inhibition of the pyruvate dehydrogenase (PDH) complex (Fig. 59–1). This decreases acetyl-coenzyme A (CoA) formation, which decreases citric acid cycle activity and subsequently impairs adenosine triphosphate (ATP) production. Specifically, arsenic blocks the dihydrolipoamide–lipoamide recycling. In addition, arsenic inhibits thiolase, the catalyst for the final step in fatty acid oxidation, which further decreases ATP. Trivalent arsenic also inhibits glutathione synthetase, glucose-6-phosphate dehydrogenase (required to produce nicotinamide adenine dinucleotide phosphate {NADPH}), and glutathione reductase.

Arsenic blocks cardiac delayed rectifier channels $I_{Ks}$ and $I_{Kr}$, which are responsible for cardiac repolarization. Toxicity results in ventricular dysrhythmias, including torsade de pointes. Inhibition of glucose transport plus the

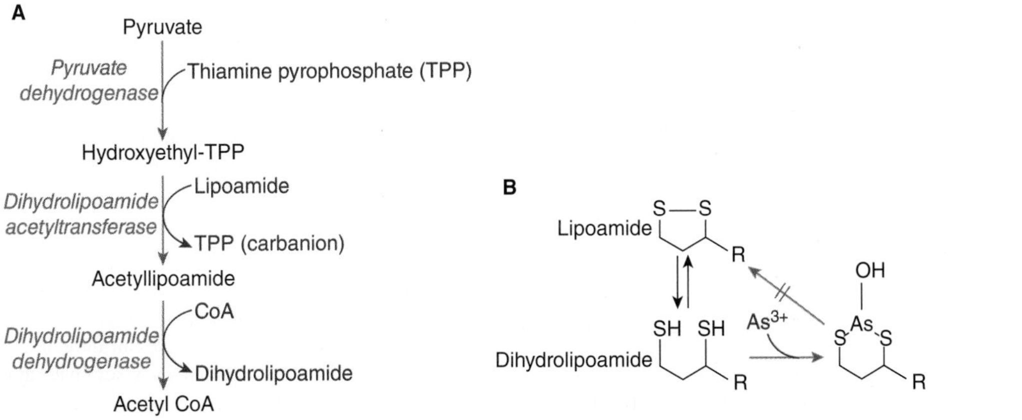

**FIGURE 59–1.** Effect of trivalent arsenicals ($As^{3+}$) on pyruvate dehydrogenase (PDH) complex. (**A**) The PDH complex is composed of three enzymes, which use thiamine pyrophosphate (TPP) and lipoamide as cofactors to decarboxylate pyruvate and form acetyl CoA. (**B**) Arsenic interferes with the regeneration of lipoamide from dihydrolipoamide, thereby altering the function of the PDH complex.

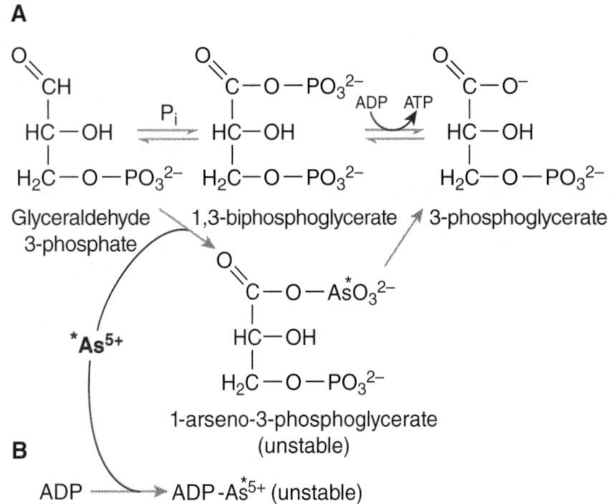


**FIGURE 59–2.** Pathophysiologic effects of $As^{5+}$ (arsenate). (**A**) Arsenate (chemical formula $AsO_4^{3-}$) substitutes for inorganic phosphate ($P_i$; the asterisk indicates substitutions), bypassing the formation of 1,3-bisphosphoglycerate (1,3-BPG), and thus losing the ATP formation that occurs when 1,3-PBG is metabolized to 3-phosphoglycerate. (**B**) Energy loss also occurs if arsenate substitutes for $P_i$ and blocks the formation of ATP from ADP. ADP = adenosine diphosphate; ATP = adenosine triphosphate.

inhibited gluconeogenesis can lead to glycogen depletion and hypoglycemia.

Some toxicity from $As^{5+}$ results from its transformation to $As^{3+}$. It also inhibits oxidative phosphorylation by substituting for inorganic phosphate ($P_i$) in the glycolysis reaction catalyzed by glyceraldehyde 3-phosphate dehydrogenase (Fig. 59–2). Chronic arsenic exposure is associated with cardiovascular disease, hepatic portal fibrosis, and cancer.

## PHARMACOKINETICS/TOXICOKINETICS

### Absorption

Inorganic arsenic is tasteless and odorless and is well absorbed by the gastrointestinal (GI), respiratory, intravenous, and mucosal routes. Poorly soluble trivalent compounds such as $As_2O_3$ are less well absorbed than more soluble trivalent and pentavalent compounds. Systemic absorption via the respiratory tract depends on the particulate size, as well as the arsenic compound and its solubility. Large, nonrespirable particles are cleared from the airways by ciliary action and swallowed, allowing GI absorption to occur. Respirable particles lodging in the lungs can be absorbed over days to weeks or remain unabsorbed for years. Dermal penetration of arsenic through intact skin does not pose a risk for toxicity.

### Pharmacokinetics

Intravenous administration of a single 10-mg dose of $As_2O_3$ resulted in a maximum plasma concentration ($Cp_{max}$) of 6.85 μmol/L and a β elimination half-life ($t_{1/2}\beta$) of 12.13 ± 3.31 hours. A study in humans receiving intravenous radioarsenic isotope ($^{74}As$) showed arsenic clearing from the blood in three phases:

*Phase 1 (2–3 hours)*—Arsenic is rapidly cleared with a half-life of 1 to 2 hours; more than 90% may be cleared during this phase.

*Phase 2 (3 hours–7 days)*—A more gradual decline occurs, with an estimated half-life of 30 hours; by 10 hours postinfusion, the arsenic is concentrated in red blood cells (RBCs) by a 3:1 ratio compared to plasma.

*Phase 3 (10 or more days)*—Clearance continues slowly with an estimated half-life of 300 hours.

Metabolism occurs primarily in the liver but also in the kidneys, testes, and lungs. If the arsenic is pentavalent, approximately 50% to 70% will first be reduced to trivalent arsenic. Addition of one methyl group produces $MMA^{5+}$; adding a second methyl group produces $DMA^{5+}$. The estimated human $LD_{50}$ (median lethal dose for 50% of test subjects) doses are reported to be as follows: arsenic trioxide, 1.43 mg/kg; monomethylarsonic acid ($MMA^{5+}$), 50 mg/kg; and dimethylarsinic acid ($DMA^{5+}$), 500 mg/kg. Thus these monomethylation and dimethylation steps were previously thought to detoxify arsenic. However, this concept is now questioned because the generation of these trivalent intermediates ($MMA^{3+}$ and $DMA^{3+}$) creates metabolites that are more toxic than the parent compounds.

Urinary elimination of ionic arsenic and its methylated metabolites occurs via glomerular filtration and tubular secretion; active reabsorption does occur. In the first 4 to 5 days after ingestion, 46% to 68.9% is eliminated. Approximately 30% is eliminated with a half-life of greater than 1 week, while the remainder is slowly excreted with a half-life of greater than 1 month.

Arsenobetaine (AsB) is also well absorbed orally and is excreted unchanged in the urine. Elimination occurs more rapidly than with inorganic arsenic. In human volunteers 25% was excreted within 2 to 4 hours, 50% by 20 hours, and 70% to 83.7% after 166 hours.

## CLINICAL MANIFESTATIONS

### Inorganic Arsenicals

Toxic manifestations vary depending on the amount and form of arsenic ingested and the chronicity of ingestion. Larger doses of a potent compound such as arsenic trioxide rapidly produce manifestations of acute toxicity, whereas chronic ingestion of substantially lower amounts of pentavalent arsenic in groundwater slowly result in a different clinical picture. Manifestations of subacute toxicity can develop in patients who survive acute poisoning, as well as in patients who are slowly poisoned environmentally.

### Acute Toxicity

Gastrointestinal signs and symptoms of nausea, vomiting, abdominal pain, and diarrhea are the earliest manifestations of acute poisoning by the oral route. They occur minutes to several hours following ingestion. The diarrhea resembles cholera in that it looks like "rice water." Severe multisystem illness can result both from volume depletion and direct toxic effects. Cardiovascular signs ranging from sinus tachycardia and orthostatic hypotension to shock can develop. A prolonged QT interval can be followed by ventricular dysrhythmias. Acute encephalopathy can develop and progress over several days, with delirium, coma, and seizures attributed to cerebral edema and microhemorrhages. Acute respiratory distress syndrome (ARDS), hepatitis, hemolytic anemia, acute kidney injury, rhabdomyolysis, and death can occur. Acute kidney injury occurs secondary to ischemia caused by hypotension, hypovolemia, tubular deposition of myoglobin or hemoglobin, renal cortical necrosis, and direct renal tubular toxicity.

In the days and weeks following an acute exposure, prolonged or additional signs and symptoms in the nervous, GI, hematologic, dermatologic, pulmonary, and cardiovascular systems occur. Encephalopathic symptoms of headache, confusion, decreased memory, personality change, irritability, hallucinations, delirium, and seizures develop and persist. Sixth cranial nerve palsy and bilateral sensorineural hearing loss are reported. Peripheral neuropathy typically develops 1 to 3 weeks after acute poisoning, although it can occur earlier. Superficial touch of the extremities sometimes elicits severe or deep aching pains, a finding that also occurs with thallium poisoning (Chap. 72). Motor weakness often develops. The most severely affected patients manifest an ascending flaccid paralysis that mimics Guillain-Barré syndrome. Respiratory findings include dry cough, crackles, hemoptysis, chest pain, and patchy interstitial infiltrates. Leukopenia and, less commonly, anemia and thrombocytopenia occur from days to 3 weeks after an acute exposure but resolve as bone marrow function returns. Dermatologic lesions can include patchy alopecia, oral herpetiform lesions, a diffuse pruritic macular rash, and a brawny nonpruritic desquamation. Mees lines, transverse striate leuconychia of the nails, are 1 to 2 mm wide and rarely occur in arsenic poisoning (Fig. 59–3). Other possible toxic manifestations of inorganic arsenic toxicity include nephropathy, fatigue, anorexia with weight loss, and torsade de pointes, and persistence of GI symptoms.

### Chronic Toxicity

Chronic low-level exposure to inorganic arsenicals typically occurs from occupational or environmental sources. Gastrointestinal symptoms of nausea, vomiting, and diarrhea are less likely than with acute toxicity, but can occur. Malignant and nonmalignant skin lesions, hypertension, diabetes mellitus, peripheral vascular disease, and several internal malignancies are associated with consumption of arsenic in drinking water. The skin is very susceptible to the toxic effects of arsenic. Multiple lesions are reported, including hyperpigmentation, hyperkeratosis, squamous and basal cell carcinomas, and Bowen disease. Population studies show an increased prevalence of diabetes mellitus, restrictive lung disease, and vascular disease. Blackfoot disease, an obliterative arterial disease of the lower extremities occurring in Taiwan, is linked with chronic arsenic exposure. Encephalopathy and peripheral neuropathy are the neurologic manifestations most commonly reported.

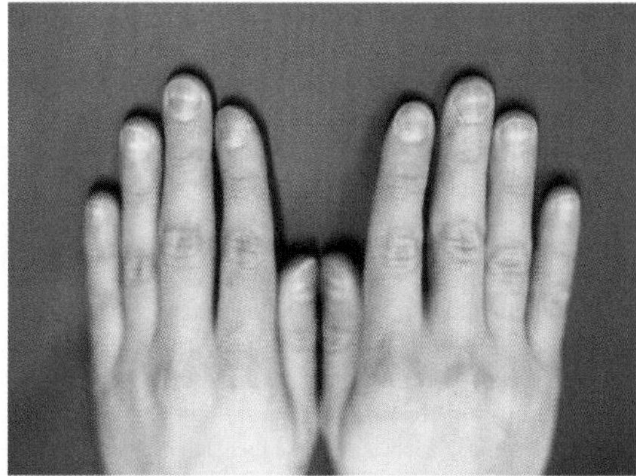

**FIGURE 59–3.** Mees lines, parallel white bands across the nails, result from exposures to metals, radiation, and chemotherapeutics, among others. *(Used with permission from the Fellowship in Medical Toxicology, New York University Grossman School of Medicine, New York City Poison Center.)*

Arsenic is classified as a definite carcinogen by the International Agency for Research on Cancer (IARC, Group 1) and the National Toxicology Program (NTP). Cancers known to develop include lung, skin, and bladder.

### Adverse Drug Effects: Arsenic Trioxide

The most common adverse effects are dermatologic (skin dryness, pigmentary changes, and maculopapular eruptions with or without pruritus); GI (nausea, vomiting, anorexia, diarrhea, and dyspepsia); hematologic (leukemoid reactions); hepatic (elevation of aminotransferase concentrations typically less than or equal to 10 times the upper limit of normal values, with a reported incidence of 20% with low-dose and 31.9% with conventional-dose therapy); cardiac (prolonged QT interval in 40%–63% of patients, first-degree atrioventricular block, ventricular ectopy, monomorphic nonsustained ventricular tachycardia, torsade de pointes, asystole, and death); facial edema; and neurologic (paresthesias, peripheral neuropathy, and headache). Leukemoid reactions (white blood cell counts greater than $50 \times 10^9$/L) develop in nearly 50% of patients between 14 and 42 days of beginning treatment. Such patients are at risk for intracerebral hemorrhage or infarction.

## DIAGNOSTIC TESTING

Timing of testing for arsenic must be correlated with the clinical course of the patient, whether the poisoning is acute, subacute, chronic, or remote with residual clinical effects. Confounding factors, such as food-derived organic arsenicals or accumulated arsenic (DMA and arsenobetaine) in patients with chronic kidney disease, must be evaluated to prevent erroneous diagnoses.

### Urine and Blood

Diagnosis ultimately depends on finding an elevated urinary arsenic concentration in a 24 hour collection. In an emergency, a spot urine sample for arsenic should be sent prior to beginning chelation therapy.

A markedly elevated arsenic concentration verifies the diagnosis in a patient with characteristic history and clinical findings, whereas a low concentration does not exclude arsenic toxicity. In acutely symptomatic patients, initial spot urine arsenic concentrations ranged from 192 to 198,450 μg/L. Because urinary excretion of arsenic is intermittent, definitive diagnosis hinges upon finding a 24-hour urinary concentration ≥50 μg/L, 100 μg/g creatinine, or 100 μg total arsenic.

When interpreting slightly elevated urinary arsenic concentrations, laboratory findings must also be correlated with the history and clinical findings, as seafood ingestion has been reported to transiently elevate urinary arsenic excretion up to 1,700 μg/L. When seafood arsenic is a consideration, speciation of arsenic can be accomplished to distinguish harmless arsenobetaine from other more toxic forms of arsenic. If arsenic speciation cannot be done, the patient can be retested after a 1-week abstinence from fish, shellfish, and algae food products.

Diagnostic evaluation of chronic toxicity should include laboratory parameters that typically become abnormal within days to weeks following an acute exposure. Tests should include a complete blood count (CBC), kidney and liver function tests, urinalysis, and 24-hour urinary arsenic determinations. Complete blood count findings can include a normocytic, normochromic, or megaloblastic anemia, an initial leukocytosis followed by development of leukopenia with neutrophils depressed more than lymphocytes, a relative eosinophilia, thrombocytopenia, and a rapidly declining hemoglobin indicative of hemolysis or a GI hemorrhage. Basophilic stippling of RBCs also occurs. Elevated serum creatinine, aminotransferases, and bilirubin as well as depressed haptoglobin concentrations develop. Urinalysis reveals proteinuria, hematuria, and pyuria. Urinary arsenic excretion in subacute and chronic cases varies inversely with the postexposure time period, but low concentration excretion is reported to continue for months after exposure.

### Hair and Nail Testing

In cases of suspected arsenic toxicity, in which the urinary arsenic measurements fall to less than toxic concentrations, analysis of hair and nails may yield the diagnosis. Arsenic is detected in the proximal portions of hair within 30 hours of ingestion. The Society of Hair Testing has made the following recommendations for collection of hair specimens: (1) collect approximately 200 mg of hair from the posterior vertex region of the scalp using scissors to cut as close to the scalp as possible, and (2) tie the hairs together, wrap in aluminum foil to protect from environmental contamination, and store at room temperature. Although these recommendations are only validated for testing drugs of abuse, it is reasonable to follow them for hair testing of arsenic. Like hair, nails grow slowly, at approximately 0.1 mm per day. Total replacement of a fingernail requires 3 to 4 months, whereas toenails require 6 to 9 months of growth. Blood and urine tests are the standard analysis for arsenic poisoning. However, when remote toxicity is highly suspected, hair and nail arsenic concentrations are occasionally of value.

### Other Tests

Abdominal radiographs demonstrate radiopaque material in the GI tract soon after ingestion. Because the sensitivity and specificity of abdominal radiographs are unknown, a negative radiograph does not exclude arsenic ingestion. Electrocardiographic changes reported include QRS complex widening, QT interval prolongation, ST-segment depression, T-wave flattening, ventricular premature contractions, nonsustained monomorphic ventricular tachycardia, and torsade de pointes. Nerve conduction studies can confirm or diagnose clinical or subclinical axonopathy.

## MANAGEMENT

### General

Acute arsenical toxicity is life-threatening and mandates immediate treatment. Advanced life support monitoring and therapies should be initiated when necessary, with a few caveats. Careful attention to fluid balance is important, because cerebral and pulmonary edema occur. Xenobiotics that prolong the QT interval, such as the class IA, IC, and III antidysrhythmics, should be avoided whenever possible. Potassium, magnesium, and calcium concentrations should be maintained within normal range to avoid exacerbating a prolonged QT interval. Glucose concentrations and glycogen stores should be maintained with oral or parenteral nutrition as needed.

Arsenic is poorly adsorbed to activated charcoal in vitro and significant poisoning is associated with nausea and vomiting and altered mental status, which make activated charcoal administration difficult. Despite these concerns, activated charcoal, in conjunction with airway protection if necessary, is recommended. If radiopaque material is present in the GI tract, whole-bowel irrigation is reasonable. Arsenic can be readily removed from skin with soap, water, and vigorous scrubbing.

### Chelation Therapy

***Chelators.*** The initiation of chelation therapy depends on the clinical condition of the patient as well as the arsenic concentration. A severely ill patient with known or suspected acute poisoning should be chelated immediately, even before laboratory confirmation is received. Cases of subacute and chronic toxicity can await rapid laboratory confirmation prior to beginning chelation, unless the clinical condition deteriorates. Dimercaprol is the initial chelator of choice in the US. Dosing regimens and adverse effects are discussed in Antidotes in Brief: A28. However, because of its narrow therapeutic index, most patients should be switched to succimer (Antidotes in Brief: A29) once their GI tract has been decontaminated and they are hemodynamically stable. D-Penicillamine has not demonstrated efficacy in chelating or reversing the biochemical toxicity of arsenic and is not recommended.

### Hemodialysis

Hemodialysis removes negligible amounts of arsenic, with or without concomitant dimercaprol therapy, and is not indicated in patients with normal kidney function. In patients with acute kidney injury, although hemodialysis clearance rates have ranged from 76 to 87.5 mL/min, a 4-hour dialysis session is only reported to remove on the order of 3 to 5 mg of arsenic, which is inconsequential when compared to normal renal elimination. Hemodialysis is therefore not recommended.

# A28 DIMERCAPROL (BRITISH ANTI-LEWISITE OR BAL)

## INTRODUCTION

British anti-Lewisite (BAL) (2,3-dimercaptopropanol; dimercaprol) is a metal chelator used with edetate calcium disodium ($CaNa_2EDTA$) for lead encephalopathy and severe lead poisoning as well as other metals and metalloids. In severe lead poisoning, dimercaprol should precede the first dose of $CaNa_2EDTA$ by 4 hours to prevent redistribution of lead to the central nervous system (CNS). Because $CaNa_2EDTA$ mobilizes lead from soft tissues other than the CNS, the acute rise in blood lead concentration can exacerbate CNS toxicity. Dimercaprol protects against this rise. The role of dimercaprol in aluminum toxicity (Chap. 57) remains, while the role in arsenic and mercury poisoning has diminished since the development of oral succimer. Dimercaprol remains indicated when the gastrointestinal tract is compromised and administration of oral succimer is impossible.

## HISTORY

Investigation into the use of sulfur donors as antidotes was precipitated by the World War II threat of chemical warfare with Lewisite and mustard gas. The investigations of Stocken and Thompson at Oxford led to the discovery of the dithiol 2,3-dimercaptopropanol (or BAL) that combines with Lewisite to form a stable five-membered ring.

## PHARMACOLOGY

### Chemistry

Dimercaprol is an oily liquid with a disagreeable odor that is only available dissolved in peanut oil.

### Mechanism of Action

The sulfhydryl groups of dimercaprol form chelates with certain metals, which are then excreted in the urine. Lead, arsenic, and inorganic mercury salts are the metals most amenable to chelation with dimercaprol.

### Pharmacokinetics

Following intramuscular (IM) administration, blood concentrations of dimercaprol peak in about 30 minutes, distribution occurs quickly, and blood concentrations begin to fall within 2 hours. Urinary excretion of dimercaprol metabolites accounts for nearly 45% of the dose within 6 hours and 81% of the dose within 24 hours. Dimercaprol is also found in the feces, suggesting that an enterohepatic circulation exists. Hemodialysis is useful in removing the dimercaprol–metal chelate in cases of kidney failure.

## ROLE OF DIMERCAPROL IN ARSENIC POISONING

### Animal Studies

In a rodent model, low concentrations of topical dimercaprol were very effective both in preventing Lewisite-induced toxicity and in reversing toxicity when administered within 1 hour of skin exposure. In rabbits, ophthalmic application of dimercaprol proved effective in preventing corneal destruction if applied within 20 minutes of exposure. When begun within 2 hours of Lewisite exposure, dimercaprol injections of 4 mg/kg every 4 hours led to a 50% survival of exposed rabbits. Although dimercaprol increases the $LD_{50}$ (median lethal dose for 50% of test subjects) of sodium arsenite, the therapeutic index of dimercaprol is low and arsenic redistribution to the brain occurs. In these same models succimer increases the LD50 with no redistribution to the brain.

### Human Studies

In human volunteers given minute amounts of arsenic dimercaprol, urinary arsenic concentration increased by approximately 40%, with maximum excretion occurring 2 to 4 hours after administration. In patients with arsenical dermatitis, dimercaprol (IM) produced both subjective and objective improvement, limited the duration of dermatitis, and increased urinary arsenic elimination. In patients with inorganic arsenic poisoning, maximal efficacy and minimal toxicity were achieved when 3 mg/kg of dimercaprol was administered IM every 4 hours for 48 hours and then twice daily for 7 to 10 days. This regimen resulted in complete recovery in six of seven patients with severe arsenical encephalopathy. Other cases support the effectiveness of dimercaprol in treating arsenic-induced agranulocytosis, encephalopathy, dermatitis, and probably arsenical fever. When dimercaprol first became widely available, 42 children were treated following arsenic ingestions, and their results were compared with a historical group of 111 untreated children who had also ingested arsenic. Treated children had fewer deaths (zero vs three), a shorter average hospital length of stay (1.6 vs 4.2 days), and fewer cases of persistent symptoms at 12 hours (0% vs 29.3%).

## ROLE OF DIMERCAPROL IN MERCURY POISONING

Thirty-eight patients ingesting more than 1 g of mercuric chloride who were treated with dimercaprol within 4 hours of exposure were compared with historical controls. There were no deaths in the 38 treated patients as compared to 27 deaths in the 86 untreated patients. Dimercaprol is particularly useful for patients who ingest a mercuric salt, as the associated gastrointestinal toxicity of the mercuric salt limits the potential of an orally administered antidote such as succimer.

Animal models demonstrate that when dimercaprol is administered following poisoning from elemental mercury vapor or short-chain organic mercury compounds, brain concentrations of mercury increase. As a result, dimercaprol therapy is not recommended in these circumstances (Chap. 68).

## ROLE OF DIMERCAPROL IN LEAD POISONING

Dimercaprol is used in combination with $CaNa_2EDTA$ to treat patients with severe lead poisoning, as the combined use increases lead binding sites without increasing toxicity from either treatment. Additionally, the combined use protects against any exacerbation of CNS toxicity, as noted above. In all other cases, succimer is the chelator of choice. When treating patients with lead encephalopathy, it is essential to administer the dimercaprol first, followed 4 hours later by $CaNa_2EDTA$ with a second dose of dimercaprol. This regimen prevents the $CaNa_2EDTA$ from redistributing lead into the brain.

## ADVERSE EFFECTS AND SAFETY ISSUES

The toxicity of dimercaprol is dose-dependent. Less than 1% of 700 IM injections resulted in minor reactions, such as pain, among patients who received 2.5 mg/kg of dimercaprol every 4 to 6 hours for four doses. When doses of 4 mg/kg and 5 mg/kg are given, the incidence of adverse effects rises to 14% and 65%, respectively. At these higher doses, reported symptoms include, in decreasing order of frequency, nausea and vomiting; headache; burning sensation of lips, mouth, throat, and eyes; lacrimation; rhinorrhea; salivation; muscle aches; burning and tingling of extremities; tooth pain; diaphoresis; chest pain; anxiety; and agitation. Elevations in systolic and diastolic blood pressure and tachycardia commonly occurred and correlated with increasing doses. Thirty percent of children given dimercaprol may develop a fever that can persist throughout the treatment period.

An acidic urine allows dissociation of the dimercaprol–metal chelate. Because dissociation of the dimercaprol–metal chelate will occur in acidic urine, we recommend that the urine of patients receiving dimercaprol be alkalinized with sodium bicarbonate to a pH of 7.5 to 8.0 to prevent liberation of the metal (Antidotes in Brief: A5). Dimercaprol should be used with caution in patients with glucose-6-phosphate dehydrogenase (G6PD) deficiency, as it may cause hemolysis. Because dimercaprol is formulated in peanut oil, patient with known peanut allergies should receive alternative therapies (such as succimer and $CaNa_2EDTA$) if available. Unintentional IV infusion of dimercaprol could theoretically produce fat embolism, lipoid pneumonia, chylothorax, and associated hypoxia.

### Pregnancy and Lactation

Dimercaprol is Pregnancy Category C. There are no data in human poisoning in pregnancy, and dimercaprol should only be administered to a pregnant woman after addressing a risk–benefit analysis with the patient. No data address whether dimercaprol or its chelates are excreted in human breast milk. However, in the 2010 United States (US) Centers for Disease Control and Prevention (CDC) guidelines for the identification and management of lead exposure in pregnant and breastfeeding women, the CDC suggests allowing breastfeeding for mothers with blood lead concentrations of less than or equal to 40 μg/dL (1.93 μmol/L). Mothers with blood lead concentrations of greater than 40 μg/dL are encouraged to pump and discard their breast milk until their blood lead concentrations drop to less than 40 μg/dL. Because dimercaprol is only indicated for BLLs greater than 40, we encourage the latter.

## DOSING AND ADMINISTRATION

Dimercaprol should only be administered by deep IM injection. The dose of dimercaprol for lead encephalopathy is 75 $mg/m^2$ IM every 4 hours for 5 days. As noted earlier, we recommend that the first dose of dimercaprol precede the first dose of $CaNa_2EDTA$ by 4 hours. The dose of dimercaprol for severe inorganic arsenic poisoning has not been established. We recommend the use of 3 mg/kg IM every 4 hours for 48 hours and then twice daily for 7 to 10 days. The dose of dimercaprol for patients exposed to inorganic mercury salts is 5 mg/kg IM initially, followed by 2.5 mg/kg every 8 to 12 hours for 1 day, followed by 2.5 mg/kg every 12 to 24 hours until the patient appears clinically improved, up to a total of 10 days. We recommend that the urine be alkalinized to avoid dissociation of the dimercaprol–metal chelate.

## FORMULATION AND ACQUISITION

Dimercaprol is available in 3-mL ampules containing 100 mg/mL of dimercaprol, 200 mg/mL of benzyl benzoate, and 700 mg/mL of peanut oil.

# 60 BISMUTH

| Normal concentrations | |
|---|---|
| Blood | < 5 µg/dL (239.5 nmol/L) |
| Serum | < 1 µg/dL (<47.9 nmol/L) |
| Urine | < 20 µg/L (<95.7 nmol/L) |

## HISTORY AND EPIDEMIOLOGY

Elemental bismuth is nontoxic; thus, the term bismuth in this chapter refers to bismuth salts. Nearly 300 years ago, bismuth was recognized as medicinally valuable. It was included in topical salves and oral preparations for various gastrointestinal disorders. Nephrotoxicity was described as early as 1802. In the early 20th century, cases of kidney failure were reported in children administered intramuscular bismuth salts for the treatment of gingivostomatitis. Syphilis was also once treated with intramuscular bismuth. A diffuse macular rash of the trunk and extremities known as "erythema of the 9th day" occasionally occurred. More recently, bismuth-induced encephalopathy occurred sporadically among patients with ileostomies or colostomies who were taking excessive doses or developed impaired kidney function.

## CHEMISTRY AND TOXICOLOGY

Bismuth is present in nature in both trivalent and pentavalent forms. The trivalent bismuthyl (BiO) form is employed for all medicinal uses. Most of orally administered bismuth remains in the gastrointestinal (GI) tract, being excreted in the feces, and only 0.2% is systemically absorbed. Absorption of some bismuth preparations, such as colloidal bismuth subcitrate, increases as gastric pH increases. The time to peak absorption usually ranges between 15 and 60 minutes. The distribution and elimination of orally administered bismuth follow a complex, multicompartmental model. The volume of distribution in humans is unknown.

Once in the circulation, bismuth binds to $\alpha_2$-macroglobulin, IgM, β-lipoprotein, and haptoglobin. Bismuth rapidly enters the liver, kidney, lungs, and bone. Bismuth can cross the placenta and enter the amniotic fluid and fetal circulation. It also readily crosses the blood–brain barrier. Ninety percent of absorbed bismuth is eliminated through the kidneys, where it induces the production of its own metal-binding protein.

Three different half-lives describe the pharmacokinetics of orally administered bismuth: the distribution half-life is approximately 1 to 4 hours; the plasma half-life lasts 5 to 11 days; and the half-life of urinary excretion lasts between 21 and 72 days, with urinary bismuth detected as long as 5 months after the last oral dose.

## PATHOPHYSIOLOGY

Bismuth salts and their toxicities can be categorized into four groups based upon solubility and GI absorption (Table 60–1). Bismuth-induced encephalopathy likely results from sulfhydryl binding. The factors predisposing some individuals to encephalopathy from group II bismuth salts, however, are not well defined. Age, gender, and duration of therapeutic use do not predict the likelihood of developing encephalopathy.

**TABLE 60–1 The Characteristics of Bismuth Salts**

| *Group* | *Chemistry* | *Primary Toxicity* | *Examples* |
|---|---|---|---|
| I | Inorganic, insoluble in water | Minimal | Bismuth subnitrate, bismuth subcarbonate |
| II | Organic, lipid soluble | Neurologic | Bismuth subsalicylate, bismuth subgallate |
| III | Organic, water soluble | Renal | Bismuth triglycollamate, bismuth dicitratobismuthate |
| IV | Organic, water soluble, hydrolyzable | Minimal | Bicitropeptide |

## CLINICAL MANIFESTATIONS

### Acute

Acutely, massive overdoses result in abdominal pain and oliguria or anuria. Acute kidney injury usually occurs following exposure to the water-soluble bismuth salts (group III). Bismuth causes degeneration of the proximal renal tubule, similar to other metals. Neurotoxicity following acute overdose is uncommon but hearing loss, tinnitus, and altered mental status are reported.

### Chronic

Repeated doses of oral bismuth produce a diffuse, progressive encephalopathy. Patients exhibit apathy and irritability followed by difficulty concentrating, diminished short-term memory, and, occasionally, visual hallucinations. Muscle twitching, myoclonus, ataxia, and tremors are characteristic. Weakness and, rarely, seizures advance to immobility. With continued bismuth administration, these patients develop coma and die.

Fractures are caused by severe neuromuscular manifestations such as myoclonus. Like several other metals, bismuth can cause a generalized pigmentation of skin. Deposition of bismuth sulfide into the mucosa causes a blue-black discoloration of gums. Formation of bismuth sulfide in the GI tract causes blackening of the stool.

## DIAGNOSIS

The diagnosis of bismuth-induced encephalopathy is based on a history of exposure coupled with diffuse neuropsychiatric and motor findings. Other causes of encephalopathy should be entertained and excluded (Table 60–2). An abdominal radiograph will likely demonstrate radiopacities of bismuth in the intestines. Stool will be black but will test negative for occult blood. Blood bismuth concentrations confirm exposure but correlate poorly with morbidity.

| TABLE 60–2 Differential Diagnosis of Bismuth Encephalopathy |
|---|
| Akinetic status epilepticus |
| Creutzfeldt–Jacob disease |
| Delirium tremens |
| Hyperglycemic hyperosmolar syndrome |
| Lithium toxicity (chronic) |
| Malignant catatonia |
| Myxedema coma |
| Neurodegenerative leukoencephalopathies |
| NMDA receptor antibody encephalitis |
| Paradichlorobenzene encephalopathy |
| Postanoxic and posthypoglycemic encephalopathies |
| Progressive multifocal ataxia |
| Tetanus/strychnine |
| Viral encephalopathies |

NMDA = *N*-methyl-D-aspartate.

Although patients with encephalopathy typically have a blood concentration > 10 μg/dL (with the majority between 10 and 100 μg/dL), encephalopathy with blood concentrations below 10 μg/dL is also rarely reported. The electroencephalographic (EEG) findings of patients with bismuth encephalopathy generally demonstrate nonspecific slow wave changes. In encephalopathic patients with blood concentrations > 200 μg/dL cortical hyperdensities of the gray matter are reported on computed tomography. These findings tend to resolve with recovery. Magnetic resonance imaging was normal in one encephalopathic patient.

## TREATMENT

Usually, supportive care results in a complete recovery. Administration of polyethylene glycol electrolyte lavage solution is recommended until the rectal effluent is clear. Although evidence for activated charcoal is lacking, one dose, especially in patients with severe encephalopathy from oral exposure, is reasonable once the airway it protected.

## CHELATION

It is uncertain whether different chelators affect the clinical course of patients with bismuth encephalopathy. Chelation therapy with dimercaprol is beneficial in experimental models, reportedly beneficial in humans, and often recommended by others, although clear evidence of efficacy is lacking. Dimercaprol undergoes biliary elimination, offering a major advantage over other chelators in patients with acute kidney injury. Based on the limited data available, it is reasonable to administer dimercaprol in encephalopathic patients with kidney failure in whom no neurologic improvement is noted within 48 hours of whole-bowel irrigation and cessation of bismuth administration (Antidotes in Brief: A28). In human volunteers following colloidal bismuth subcitrate exposure, succimer and dimercaptopropane sulfonate (DMPS) increased urinary elimination of bismuth by 50-fold. The availability of DMPS and indications for use are limited. Although succimer can be used for severely poisoned patients, there are no current data that outcomes are changed once the offending source of bismuth is withheld or removed (Antidotes in Brief: A29).

## BISMUTH DRUG INTERACTIONS AND REACTIONS

The coadministration of proton pump inhibitors (PPIs) increases the absorption of some bismuth preparations, and long courses of combined therapy should be avoided if possible. In the United States, where bismuth subsalicylate is the most common oral bismuth-containing compound, up to 90% of the salicylate is absorbed. Salicylate toxicity is reported, and salicylate concentrations should be performed in both acute and chronic exposures. Methemoglobinemia from subnitrate salt of bismuth is rarely described.

# 61 CADMIUM

Normal Concentrations

| | |
|---|---|
| Whole blood | < 5 μg/L (44.5 nmol/L) |
| Urine | < 3 μg/g creatinine |
| | < 26.7 nmol/g creatinine |

## HISTORY AND EPIDEMIOLOGY

Cadmium, a bluish solid at room temperature, is readily oxidized to a divalent ion, $Cd^{2+}$. Naturally occurring cadmium commonly exists as cadmium sulfide (CdS), a trace contaminant of zinc-containing ores. When combined with other metals, cadmium forms alloys of relatively low melting points, which accounts for its extensive use in solders and brazing rods. Today, cadmium is primarily used as a reagent in electroplating and in the production of nickel-cadmium batteries.

Environmental exposure to cadmium generally occurs through the consumption of foods grown in cadmium-contaminated areas. Environmental cadmium poisoning in Japan resulted in an epidemic of painful osteomalacia. The afflicted developed pathologic fractures and called out "itai-itai" ("ouch-ouch") as they walked because of the severity of their pain. Smokers have higher blood cadmium concentrations than nonsmokers, probably as a result of contamination of soil where the tobacco is grown. Cadmium and tobacco are synergistic causes of chronic pulmonary disease. Welders, solderers, and jewelry workers who use cadmium-containing alloys are at risk for developing acute cadmium toxicity due to inhalation of cadmium oxide fumes.

## TOXICOKINETICS

There is no known biologic role for cadmium. Ingested cadmium salts are poorly bioavailable (5%–20%), whereas inhaled cadmium fumes (cadmium oxide) are readily bioavailable (up to 90%). After exposure, cadmium is absorbed into the bloodstream, where it is bound to $\alpha_2$-macroglobulin and albumin. It is then quickly and preferentially redistributed to the liver and kidney and, to a lesser extent, the pancreas, spleen, heart, lung, and testes.

After incorporation into the liver and kidney, cadmium forms a complex with metallothionein (MT), which binds and sequesters cadmium. Circulating Cd-MT is filtered by the glomerulus but reabsorbed and concentrated in proximal tubular cells, explaining why the kidney is a principal target organ in cadmium toxicity. The volume of distribution (Vd) of cadmium is unknown. The slow release of cadmium from metallothionein-complexed hepatic stores accounts for its very long biologic half-life of 10 or more years.

## PATHOPHYSIOLOGY

### Cellular Pathophysiology

Cadmium toxicity results from interactions of the free cations with target cells. Complexation with metallothionein is cytoprotective, and metallothionein functions as a natural chelator for cadmium. Cadmium binds to sulfhydryl groups, denaturing proteins and/or inactivating enzymes. The mitochondria are severely affected, resulting in an increased susceptibility to oxidative stress. Cadmium also affects processes involved in DNA repair, generation of reactive oxygen species, and induction of apoptosis. Cadmium also interferes with calcium transport mechanisms, leading to intracellular hypercalcemia and, ultimately, apoptosis.

### Specific Organ System Injury

Table 61–1 lists the specific organ system toxicities of cadmium.

## CLINICAL MANIFESTATIONS

### Acute Poisoning

***Pulmonary/Cadmium Fumes.*** Cadmium pneumonitis results from inhalation of cadmium oxide fumes. The acute phase mimics metal fume fever (Chap. 94), but the two entities are distinctly different. Whereas metal fume fever is benign and self-limited, acute cadmium pneumonitis progresses to hypoxia, respiratory insufficiency, and death. Within 6 to 12 hours of exposure, patients typically develop constitutional symptoms, such as fever and chills, as well as a cough and respiratory distress.

At this stage, the physical examination, oxygenation, and chest radiograph are normal, leading to an underestimation of the severity of illness. As the pneumonitis progresses to acute respiratory distress syndrome (ARDS), crackles and rhonchi develop, oxygenation becomes impaired, and the chest radiograph develops a pattern consistent with alveolar filling. In fulminant cases, death usually occurs within 3 to 5 days.

### Oral/Cadmium Salts

Acute ingestions are rare, with gastrointestinal (GI) injury the most significant initial clinical finding. When severe, hemorrhagic necrosis of the upper GI tract leads to multisystem organ failure and death.

### Nephrotoxicity

The most common finding in chronic cadmium poisoning is proteinuria, which precedes glomerular dysfunction. In most cases, proteinuria is considered to be irreversible even

**TABLE 61–1 Major Acute and Chronic Organ System Effects of Cadmium**

| *Organ* | *Acute* | *Chronic* |
|---|---|---|
| Kidney | | Proteinuria<br>Nephrolithiasis |
| Bone | | Osteomalacia |
| Lung | Pneumonitis | Cancer |
| Gastrointestinal system | Caustic injury | |

after removal from exposure, but improvement is sometimes reported. It is unclear whether kidney dysfunction progresses after removal from exposure.

### Pulmonary Toxicity

Workers chronically exposed to relatively low concentrations of cadmium fail to demonstrate consistent effects on the lung, with some evidence of both restrictive lung disease and changes on pulmonary function tests. In one study, patients with restrictive lung disease improved after cadmium exposure was reduced. Cadmium exposure is associated with lung cancer and designated as a human carcinogen by the International Agency for Research on Cancer.

### Musculoskeletal Toxicity

Osteomalacia is generally only a prominent feature of environmental toxicity. Victims of the original itai-itai epidemic were mostly older women, whereas occupational cadmium exposures typically occur in younger men. In addition, differences in cumulative dosing and in route of exposure (oral vs pulmonary) partly account for the unique prominence of osteomalacia in patients with environmental exposures.

### Other Organ Systems

Although the liver stores as much cadmium as any other organ, hepatotoxicity is not a prominent feature in humans, probably because hepatic cadmium is usually complexed to metallothionein. Cadmium exposure is linked to olfactory disturbances, impaired higher cortical function, and parkinsonism. Cadmium induces hypertension in rats, but human studies have only yielded unconvincing and conflicting results. Cadmium is associated with atherosclerotic plaques and heart failure.

## DIAGNOSTIC TESTING

Cadmium concentrations have limited usefulness in the management of the acutely exposed patient. Diagnosis and treatment are based on the history, physical examination, and symptoms, and in acute exposures, ancillary tests (such as pulse oximetry and chest radiography) are more useful than actual cadmium concentrations.

In the patient chronically exposed to cadmium, both cadmium concentrations and ancillary testing are recommended. Urinary cadmium concentrations are a better reflection of the total-body cadmium burden than are whole blood concentrations.

## MANAGEMENT

### Acute Exposure

***Oral Exposure/Cadmium Salts.*** After the patient's airway, breathing, and circulation are secured, attention should be given to GI decontamination. Although large ingestions of soluble cadmium salts are rare, they are potentially fatal, with the lowest reported human lethal dose being 5 g. If a significant ingestion occurs but emesis has not occurred, gastric lavage is recommended. In this situation, a small nasogastric tube should suffice, as inorganic cadmium salts are powders, not pills. All patients with known exposures and/or abnormal findings consistent with cadmium should be admitted to the hospital for supportive care, monitoring of renal and hepatic function, and possibly evaluation of the GI tract for injury.

The benefits of chelation in acute cadmium exposure are unproven. Multiple chelators have been studied, all in animal models, with inconsistent results. In a patient thought to have acutely ingested potentially lethal amounts of cadmium, treatment with succimer is reasonable but unproven. Doses that are well tolerated (10 mg/kg/dose 3 times a day) are reasonable. Most other chelators are either ineffective or detrimental.

***Pulmonary/Cadmium Fumes.*** The patient's airway should be assessed, and appropriate oxygenation ensured, although hypoxia is commonly delayed. Corticosteroids are used in most reported cases (although there are no studies to support their efficacy), and a standard dose of methylprednisolone (1 mg/kg up to 60 mg) is reasonable. All patients with acute inhalational exposures to cadmium should be admitted to the hospital for observation and supportive care until respiratory symptoms have resolved.

Chelation is not recommended as an option for patients with single acute exposures to cadmium fumes, as these patients do not appear to develop extrapulmonary injury.

### Chronic Exposure

Patients chronically exposed to cadmium frequently come to attention during routine screening, as those who work with cadmium are under close medical surveillance. These patients may have developed proteinuria or, less commonly, chronic pulmonary complaints.

Management is challenging. Cessation of cadmium exposure is the first intervention.

We recommend against chelation for chronic cadmium toxicity.

# 62 CESIUM

**Cesium**

Normal concentrations

| | |
|---|---|
| Whole blood or serum | = < 10 μg/L (75.42 nmol/L) |
| Urine | = < 20 μg/L (150.48 nmol/L) |

## HISTORY AND EPIDEMIOLOGY

The name "cesium" derives from Latin word for "sky" (*caelum*). Cesium (Cs) is among the most rare and reactive alkali metals. Elemental cesium ($Cs^0$) is silvery white, soft, and malleable. Elemental cesium ($Cs^0$) ignites violently when exposed to moist air or water but forms stable salt complexes. Since $Cs^0$ is so highly reactive and short lived, the term "cesium" will refer to cesium salts in the following discussion, unless specifically noted otherwise.

Radioactive cesium isotopes are products of nuclear fission of uranium and plutonium. Both $^{134}Cs$ and $^{137}Cs$ decay via β particle emission; however, only $^{137}Cs$ emits γ rays. Since $^{137}Cs$ has a long half-life of 30 years, it is a radiological hazard as it deposits and complexes in earth and water. Several releases of radioactive cesium have occurred in the past century, resulting in large-scale contamination and human exposure, the most recent of which were the critical nuclear power plant malfunctions in Chernobyl and Fukushima Daiichi.

Occupational exposure to radiocesium occurs routinely in nuclear power plant employees and people who live and work in close proximity to a nuclear facility. Both $^{137}Cs$ and $^{131}Cs$ are used as sources of external and internal radiation. Internal radiotherapy with $^{131}Cs$ seed implantation, called brachytherapy, is approved for treatment of numerous malignancies.

Nonradioactive cesium chloride is promoted as a supplement and alternative treatment for cancer, despite no scientific support for this claim.

## PHARMACOLOGY

Cesium resembles potassium and it either mimics or antagonizes potassium in cellular processes. Since cesium blocks the delayed rectifier ($I_{kR}$) channel in the cardiac myocyte and prolongs repolarization (QT interval) it is used as a model to induce torsade de pointes. Radiocesium is indistinguishable from nonradioactive cesium in biological and chemical reactions.

### Pharmacokinetics and Toxicokinetics

Pharmacokinetic data are derived from radiotracer studies in animals and a few human volunteers. Exposure to cesium occurs through ingestion, inhalation, injection, and dermal contact. Animal studies demonstrate rapid absorption via inhalation, intraperitoneal injection, and ingestion. Human volunteer studies demonstrate 98% to 99% absorption of ingested cesium. Absorption through intact skin is minimal but may be as much as 20% through burned skin.

Data from human volunteers suggest that once ingested, cesium is absorbed from the small intestine and distributes to the blood compartment and various organs. Volunteer radiotracer studies demonstrate rapid initial accumulation in the liver and the salivary glands following ingestion with subsequent distribution to the myocardium, spleen, adrenals, gastrointestinal (GI) tract, bone, lungs, and skeletal muscle over days after exposure.

Cesium undergoes enterohepatic circulation, limiting fecal elimination. As such, urinary excretion accounts for 80% to 90% and fecal excretion for 2% to 10% of elimination of an ingested dose. Only a small amount of cesium is eliminated through sweat or respiratory secretions.

$^{137}Cs$ elimination follows first-order kinetics using a two-compartment model. The biological elimination half-life ranges from 45 to 200 days. The biological half-life increases with age and male sex and decreases with pregnancy. Radiocesium transfers to placenta and maternal breast milk.

## PATHOPHYSIOLOGY

β Particles have very limited dermal penetration, and effects from external exposure are limited to dermal irritation and burns. Release of β particles within the body, as typically occurs after inhalation, ingestion, or dermal absorption, may harm internal organs. γ Rays can penetrate the skin with external exposure and cause organ toxicity.

Cardiotoxicity is the principal and most dangerous clinical effect of nonradioactive cesium. QT interval prolongation occurs rapidly and predisposes individuals to torsade de pointes (TdP) and ventricular dysrhythmias. Cesium-induced ventricular dysrhythmias are potentiated by bradycardia. This is explained by either potentiation of early afterdepolarization (EAD) formation or increase in temporal variability of the refractory period throughout the cardiac muscle. In addition to bradycardia, EADs are induced by hypokalemia and metabolic acidosis and suppressed by calcium channel blockers, such as verapamil. Sodium channel modulation also may be contributory in cesium-induced ventricular dysrhythmias. Experimentally, low concentrations of tetrodotoxin, a sodium channel antagonist, terminates EADs induced by cesium chloride, but is not recommended for human use.

## CLINICAL MANIFESTATIONS

Radiation injuries are discussed in detail in Chap. 100. The following discussion focuses on nonradioactive cesium toxicity.

### Cardiovascular Toxicity

Based on case reports of cardiovascular toxicity, the most common ingested dose was 3 g/day, although doses of 9 g/day and 10 g/day are reported. Time from daily oral cesium exposure to development of dysrhythmias ranged from 1 week to 3 months. Rapid onset of dysrhythmias is reported following injection of cesium chloride into breast mass tissue. Most patients with ventricular ectopy, TdP, or ventricular dysrhythmias reported a chief complaint of syncope or "seizure-like" activity. Prolonged QT interval was universally present and either did not correct or was challenging to correct with potassium repletion. Serum cesium concentrations ranged from 2400 μg/dL to 28,000 μg/dL, and urine cesium concentration ranged from 130,000 μg/L to 360,000 μg/L. Whole blood cesium concentrations were reported in two cases; 100,000 μg/L and 160,000 μg/L.

### Gastrointestinal Effects

Nausea, vomiting, diarrhea, and abdominal cramping are described in patients who ingest 3 to 10 g of cesium chloride per day.

### Electrolyte Abnormalities

Some patients taking cesium chloride in an attempt to treat cancer develop hypokalemia and hypomagnesemia. Electrolyte imbalance likely reflects GI loss through vomiting and/or diarrhea. Serum potassium concentration ranged from 2.7 mEq/L to 3.4 mEq /L, and serum magnesium concentrations were reported as low as 1.4 mg/dL.

### Neurologic Effects

A heightened sense of perception as well as facial and acral tingling are described following self-administration of 6 g of cesium chloride daily for 36 consecutive days. Reports of syncope and "seizures" should be interpreted with caution since a nonperfusing cardiac rhythm is the most likely etiology.

## DIAGNOSTIC TESTING

Radioactive cesium is detected by whole-body counters using γ ray spectrometry and β counting. Urine and feces are analyzed for $^{137}Cs$ and/or $^{134}Cs$ in a similar manner. Analysis of nonradioactive cesium in blood, urine, feces, or tissue samples is performed by spectrometric methods such as flame atomic emission spectrometry, inductively coupled plasma mass spectrometry (ICP-MS), or instrumental neutron activation analysis.

## MANAGEMENT

### Radiocesium

Patient management following radiation exposure is outlined in detail in Chap. 100 and Antidotes in Brief: A31. Gastrointestinal decontamination is likely of limited value and is not recommended following cesium ingestion. Cesium is not well adsorbed to activated charcoal, and patients who present with significant cesium toxicity often have vomiting or altered mental status. Administration of antiemetics and repletion of volume loss are advised but caution to avoid antiemetics that prolong the QT interval is required. Correction of electrolyte imbalances is essential in patients who present with nausea and vomiting.

All patients with suspected cesium salt ingestion should have an electrocardiogram (ECG) and be attached to a continuous cardiac monitor. We recommend serial determinations of the QT intervals. If TdP occurs, it is an unstable rhythm requiring cardioversion, but intravenous magnesium infusion and/or overdrive pacing are recommended for recurrent episodes. Lidocaine is efficacious in animal models and is a reasonable second-line drug. We recommend against the routine use of amiodarone given its propensity to prolong the QT interval.

### Prussian Blue

In 2003, the insoluble form of Prussian blue was approved by the United States Food and Drug Administration for oral treatment of thallium and cesium toxicity (Antidotes in Brief: A31). The insoluble crystal lattice adsorbs cesium in the intestinal lumen, enhances both elimination and gut dialysis, and thereby reduces the half-life of radiocesium by as much as 43%. Since laboratory confirmation will be substantially delayed, Prussian blue is recommended upon suspicion of cesium toxicity. Although the optimal dose and interval are unknown, the manufacturer's recommended dose of 3 g orally three times per day, for a total daily dose of 9 g in adults and adolescents, is reasonable. A dose of 1 g orally three times per day is recommended in children for a total daily dose of 3 g. The recommended duration of therapy is 30 days for radiocesium poisoning. Patients with nonradioactive cesium poisoning should ideally be treated until their blood concentrations fall within the normal range, or at least until their cardiovascular system stabilizes and their QT interval normalizes.

# 63 CHROMIUM

Normal concentrations

| | |
|---|---|
| Whole blood | = 20–30 μg/L (385–577 nmol/L) |
| Serum | = 0.05–2.86 μg/L (1–54 nmol/L) |
| Urine | = < 1 μg/g creatinine (< 0.22 nmol/mmol creatinine) |

## INTRODUCTION

Chromium toxicity results from occupational exposure, environmental exposure, or a combination of both routes. Like many metals, the clinical manifestations of chromium toxicity depend upon whether the exposure is acute or chronic and on the chemical form of chromium. Acute toxicity is more likely to involve multiple-organ failure, whereas chronic exposure is more likely to lead to cancer.

## HISTORY AND EPIDEMIOLOGY

Chromium (Cr) is a naturally occurring element found in compounds with oxidation states of −2 to +6, but primarily in the trivalent ($Cr^{3+}$) and hexavalent ($Cr^{6+}$) forms (Table 63–1). Elemental chromium ($Cr^0$) does not exist naturally.

Elemental chromium is added to steel to form stainless steel. Chromium is also plated onto machine parts such as crankshafts, printing rollers, ball bearings, and cutting tools to create hard, smooth surfaces. Hexavalent chromium was first recognized as a carcinogen in the late 1800s, producing nasal tumors in Scottish chrome pigment workers. In the 1930s, the pulmonary carcinogenicity of chromium was described in German chromate workers.

## PHARMACOLOGY

Chromium is an essential element involved in glucose metabolism, by either facilitation of insulin binding to insulin receptors or by amplification of the effects of insulin. The chemical properties and health risks of chromium depend mostly on its oxidative state, and on the solubility of the chromium compound. Reduction of $Cr^{6+}$ to $Cr^{3+}$ occurs by abstraction of electrons from cellular constituents such as proteins, lipids, DNA, RNA, and plasma transferrin. During reduction, several other oxidative states transiently occur (namely $Cr^{4+}$ and $Cr^{5+}$) and contribute to the cytotoxicity, genotoxicity, and carcinogenicity of $Cr^{6+}$ chromium compounds.

**TABLE 63–1 Common Forms of Chromium**

| *Name* | *Chemical Formula* | *Oxidation State* | *Uses* |
|---|---|---|---|
| Barium chromate | $BaCrO_4$ | $6^+$ | Safety matches, anticorrosive, paint pigment |
| Calcium chromate | $CaCrO_4$ | $6^+$ | Batteries, metallurgy |
| Chromic acid | $H_2CrO_4$ | $6^+$ | Electroplating, oxidizer |
| Chromic chloride | $CrCl_3$ | $3^+$ | Supplement in total parenteral nutrition |
| Chromic fluoride | $CrF_3$ | $3^+$ | Mordant in dye industry, mothproofing for wool |
| Chromic oxide | $Cr_2O_3$ | $3^+$ | Metal plating, wood treatment |
| Chromite ore | $FeCr_2O_4$ | $3^+$ | Water tower treatment |
| Chromium picolinate | $C_{18}H_{12}CrN_3O_6$ | $3^+$ | Nutritional supplement |
| Lead chromate | $PbCrO_4$ | $6^+$ | Yellow pigment for paints and dye |
| Potassium dichromate | $K_2Cr_2O_7$ | $6^+$ | Oxidizer of organic compounds, leather tanning, porcelain painting |

### Environmental Exposure

Processing of chromium ores releases $Cr^{3+}$ into the environment. The most significant environmental sources of $Cr^{6+}$ are chromate production, ferrochrome pigment manufacturing, chrome plating, and some types of welding. People are exposed to chromium via drinking water, food and food supplements (eg, chromium picolinate), joint arthroplasty, and cigarettes. CCA (copper, chromate, and arsenate)-treated lumber was voluntarily removed from the United States consumer market in December 2003 because of health concerns with regard to the arsenic and chromium constituents.

### Occupational Exposure

Workers in industries that use chromium are exposed to 100 times greater concentrations of chromium than the general population. Chromium pigmentation production and leather tanning use significantly more $Cr^{6+}$ compounds, whereas metal finishing, wood preservation, and cooling towers use $Cr^{3+}$ compounds. A meta-analysis of occupational exposures demonstrated a statistically significant increase in both lung and stomach cancer in workers with exposure to hexavalent chromium.

### Medical Device Exposure

The use of metal-on-metal (MoM) implants for total hip arthroplasty and surface refinishing releases metal ions into the blood of patients. Although some patients with MoM hip implants report memory difficulties, chronic pain, and pain in the implanted hip, the true incidence and nature of adverse health outcomes due to release of chromium ions and particles from these implants are not yet established. Currently, there is insufficient evidence to conclusively demonstrate that with regard to chromium, MoM hip implants produce side effects beyond those that occur at the site of implantation. There is no consensus on the significance of elevated blood chromium concentrations, nor are there data to specify the concentration of chromium necessary to produce adverse systemic effects. Further discussion of orthoprosthetic cobaltism is found in the chapter on cobalt effects in MoM hip implants (Chap. 64).

## PHARMACOKINETICS AND TOXICOKINETICS

Because they possess significantly different properties, $Cr^{3+}$ and $Cr^{6+}$ must be evaluated separately.

### Absorption

***Trivalent Chromium Compounds.*** Oral absorption is limited, with approximately 98% of ingested $Cr^{3+}$ recovered in the feces, just 0.1% excreted in the bile, and 0.5% to 2.0% excreted in the urine. Absorption by other routes except through burns and other disrupted mucosal or epithelial surfaces is also poor.

***Hexavalent Chromium Compounds.*** Epidemiologically, inhalation of $Cr^{6+}$ is the most consequential route of exposure. The exact rate of absorption is unknown, but in animal studies, roughly 50% to 85% of small (< 5 μm) inhaled $Cr^{6+}$ potassium dichromate particles are absorbed. Hexavalent chromium is modestly absorbed after ingestion. In human volunteers, approximately 10% of an ingested dose of sodium chromate was absorbed; duodenal administration increased this to roughly 50%. This difference likely relates to the reduction of the hexavalent chromium to trivalent chromium in the acidic environment of the stomach. Hexavalent chromium compounds are generally not well absorbed after dermal exposure.

### Distribution

Because most of the $Cr^{6+}$ is rapidly reduced on absorption, $Cr^{3+}$ accounts for virtually the entire body burden of chromium. Trivalent chromium accumulates to the greatest extent in the kidneys, bone marrow, lungs, lymph nodes, liver, spleen, and testes. The kidneys and liver alone account for approximately 50% of the total body burden.

### Elimination

Urinary excretion of trivalent chromium occurs rapidly. Roughly 80% of parenterally administered $Cr^{6+}$ is excreted as $Cr^{3+}$ in the urine and 2% to 20% in the feces. The urinary excretion half-life of $Cr^{6+}$ ranges from 15 to 41 hours. Because $Cr^{3+}$ is concentrated in red blood cells (RBCs), an apparent slow compartment is created, with the elimination half-life dependent on the life span of the RBCs.

## PATHOPHYSIOLOGY

### Trivalent Chromium

Chromium picolinate is a popular $Cr^{3+}$ dietary supplement. There is no strong evidence of any significant end-organ toxicity as a consequence of exposure to $Cr^{3+}$, perhaps because $Cr^{3+}$ is so poorly absorbed. Animal data and epidemiologic studies of workers exposed to $Cr^{3+}$ compounds have failed to demonstrate a statistically significant increased incidence of cancer.

### Hexavalent Chromium

Hexavalent chromium is a powerful oxidizing agent that has corrosive and irritant effects. However, the greatest toxicity from $Cr^{6+}$ lies in its ability to produce oxidative DNA damage. Although the exact mechanisms whereby $Cr^{6+}$ is genotoxic are unknown, transient toxic chromium intermediates such as $Cr^{4+}$ and $Cr^{5+}$ formed during the intracellular reduction of $Cr^{6+}$ to $Cr^{3+}$ are probably responsible.

## CLINICAL MANIFESTATIONS

The clinical manifestations of chromium poisoning depend on the valence of the element, the source and route of exposure, and the duration of exposure. The clinical manifestations of chromium exposure are best divided into acute and chronic (low-level exposure) effects.

### Acute

Manifestations of acute, massive $Cr^{6+}$ ingestions are similar to other corrosive metal ingestions. Gastrointestinal hemorrhage with or without bowel perforation occurs. Dermal chromic acid ($H_2CrO_4$) burns lead to severe systemic toxicity with as little as 10% body surface area involvement. Because of the strong oxidative properties of $Cr^{6+}$, intravascular hemolysis with disseminated intravascular coagulation also develops. Renal effects include acute tubular necrosis leading to acute kidney injury. Metabolic abnormalities after acute, massive exposure include metabolic acidosis with elevated lactate concentration, hyperkalemia, and uremia. Although $Cr^{6+}$ is generally not well absorbed after dermal exposure, it is a corrosive that causes inflammation and ulceration.

### Chronic

The respiratory tract is the organ most affected after chromium exposure. When inhaled, $Cr^{6+}$ is a respiratory tract irritant that causes inflammation and, with continued exposure, ulceration (including nasal septal perforation). Furthermore, the sensitizing effects of $Cr^{6+}$ lead to chronic cough, shortness of breath, occupational asthma, bronchospasm, and anaphylactoid reactions. Chronic deposition of $Cr^{6+}$ particles is associated with pulmonary fibrosis and pneumoconiosis. Chromate workers have a significantly increased risk of lung cancer with a latency between 13 and 30 years after exposure.

Because $Cr^{3+}$ is a sensitizing agent, occupational exposure to $Cr^{3+}$ is associated with contact dermatitis (dermatitis toxicosis) in 10% to 20% of chromium workers. Similarly, chromium-containing gaming table felt has led to hand dermatitis referred to as "blackjack disease," and to painless, scarring skin ulcerations ("chrome holes").

## DIAGNOSTIC TESTING

Chromium is detectable in blood, urine, and hair of exposed individuals. Because of the great difficulty in speciation, differentiation between $Cr^{3+}$ and $Cr^{6+}$ is generally not performed; instead, the total chromium concentration is generally reported. Hair and nail samples are not reliable indicators of exposure to chromium because of the difficulty distinguishing between chromium contamination of the hair sample and chromium incorporated into the hair during protein synthesis.

### Ancillary Tests

After confirmed or suspected acute chromium exposure, complete blood count, serum electrolytes, blood urea nitrogen, creatinine, urinalysis, and liver enzymes testing should be performed. If signs of systemic toxicity are evident, serial determination of coagulation function and disseminated intravascular coagulation may be useful to guide therapy.

## MANAGEMENT

Acute chromium ingestions are infrequent, but often severe, with significant morbidity and mortality. Consequently, after adequate airway, breathing, and circulatory support are addressed, attention should be given to decontamination.

### Decontamination

Ingestion of $Cr^{3+}$ compounds is unlikely to require decontamination. Decontamination with soap and water is recommended after skin contact. No specific pulmonary decontamination is required. Lavage using a standard nasogastric tube is reasonable after $Cr^{6+}$ ingestions if the patient presents to the emergency department within several hours of exposure and no vomiting has occurred. Because endoscopic evaluation is likely to be needed and there are no data to suggest adsorption to activated charcoal is useful, we recommend against using activated charcoal. The administration of oral *N*-acetylcysteine as an anti-oxidant is reasonable based on animal studies. The routine use of ascorbic acid cannot be recommended at this time.

### Chelation Therapy

At this time, there is no evidence to support the use of any chelation therapy after acute $Cr^{6+}$ or $Cr^{3+}$ poisoning.

### Extracorporeal Elimination

Hemodialysis, hemofiltration, and peritoneal dialysis do not efficiently remove chromium. Therefore, in patients with normal kidney function, extracorporeal elimination is not recommended. In the setting of acute kidney injury or chronic kidney disease, hemodialysis is a reasonable therapeutic choice to attempt to reduce serum chromium concentrations, although there are no data that clinical outcomes are affected.

# 64 COBALT

Normal concentrations

| | |
|---|---|
| Serum | = 0.1–1.2 µg/L (1.7–20.4 nmol/L) |
| Urine | = 0.1–2.2 µg/L (1.7–37.3 nmol/L) |

## HISTORY AND EPIDEMIOLOGY

The main industrial use of cobalt (Co) is the formation of hard, high-speed, high-temperature cutting tools. When aluminum and nickel are blended with cobalt, an alloy (alnico) with magnetic properties is formed. Other uses for cobalt include electroplating because of its resistance to oxidation and as an artist's pigment because of its bright blue color.

Cobalt chloride was combined with iron salts and marketed in the 1950s for the treatment of anemia, a practice that continued until the 1970s. The radioactive isotope, cobalt-60 ($^{60}Co$), is used in radiotherapy. Epidemics of cardiomyopathy and goiter termed "beer drinkers' cardiomyopathy" and "cobalt-induced goiter" occurred in the 1960s and the 1970s when cobalt sulfate was added to beer as a foam stabilizer.

## CHEMISTRY

Cobalt occurs in elemental, inorganic, and organic forms. Elemental cobalt ($Co^0$) toxicity occurs through both inhalational and oral exposures. Inorganic cobalt salts most commonly occur in one of two oxidation states: cobaltous ($Co^{2+}$) or cobaltic ($Co^{3+}$). Cobaltous salts were used for the treatment of anemia and were associated with the "beer drinkers' cardiomyopathy." Organic cobalt exposure results from cyanocobalamin (vitamin $B_{12}$) ingestion, but because of its limited oral absorption and its rapid renal elimination, it is considered of low toxicity. By contrast, little is known cobaltic salts.

## TOXICOKINETICS

Oral absorption of cobalt oxides, salts, and metals is highly variable, with a reported bioavailability of 5% to 45%. Both iron deficiency and iron overload enhance radiolabeled $^{57}CoCl_2$ absorption from the small bowel. Inhaled cobalt oxide is approximately 30% bioavailable. The volume of distribution and elimination half-life are not defined. Most (50%–88%) absorbed cobalt (organic and inorganic) is eliminated renally, and the remainder is eliminated in the feces.

## PATHOPHYSIOLOGY

Like most other metals, cobalt is a multiorgan toxin. Divalent cobalt inhibits several key enzyme systems and interferes with initiation of protein synthesis. Polynucleotide phosphorylase, an essential enzyme in RNA synthesis, functions at 50% of normal in the presence of cobalt sulfate. Cobalt salts also interfere with the citric acid cycle mitochondrial enzyme, α-ketoglutarate dehydrogenase. Because divalent cobalt increases the rate of glycolysis while it decreases oxygen consumption, it inhibits aerobic metabolism. Although divalent cobalt is a weak inhibitor of this process, it is capable of almost entirely inhibiting the reaction when nicotinamide adenine dinucleotide (NADH) is added. Moreover, cobalt salts are capable of inhibiting dihydrolipoic acid by complexing with its sulfhydryl groups. These reactions result in the inability to convert both pyruvate into acetyl-coenzyme A (CoA) and α-ketoglutarate into succinyl-CoA, both of which are thiamine requiring processes. These combined interactions offer explanations as to why chronic ethanol use and cobalt exposure result in cardiomyopathy. Additionally, as cobalt is capable of accepting an electron, it can participate in oxidation-reduction (redox) cycling and produce free radicals in the lung. Divalent cobalt also inhibits tyrosine iodinase, the enzyme responsible for combining iodine ($I_2$) with tyrosine to form monoiodotyrosine in the first step in the synthesis of thyroid hormone. Thus inhibition of tyrosine iodinase results in a decrease in triiodothyronine ($T_3$) and thyroxine ($T_4$).

Multiple animal models demonstrate that cobalt chloride administration results in reticulocytosis, polycythemia, and erythropoiesis. Although the pathogenesis of these events remains largely unknown, one theory is that cobalt binds to iron-binding sites such as transferrin, resulting in impaired oxygen transport to renal cells, which, in turn, induces erythropoietin production.

## TOXICITY

The minimal acute toxic dose of cobalt compounds is not well defined. Patients with "beer drinkers' cardiomyopathy" received an average daily dose of 6 to 8 mg of cobalt sulfate (over weeks to months), whereas infants being treated for anemia who received much higher daily cobalt doses of an iron-cobalt preparation (40 mg of cobalt chloride and 75 mg of ferrous sulfate) for 3 months did not develop toxic effects. The inconsistency suggests that multiple factors are responsible including a specific role for the NADH excess associated with ethanol metabolism.

## CLINICAL MANIFESTATIONS

### Acute Exposure

Organ systems affected by acute cobalt poisoning include endocrine, gastrointestinal, central and peripheral nervous system, hematologic, cardiovascular, ophthalmic, and metabolic. Chronic inhalational exposures affect the pulmonary system and dermatologic system.

### Cardiovascular

Patients with "beer drinkers' cardiomyopathy" presented with tachycardia, dyspnea, and metabolic acidosis with elevated lactate concentrations and congestive heart failure. Other clinical findings included polycythemia and low-voltage electrocardiograms (ECGs). The mortality rate for these cases was 38% and 46% (Nebraska and Quebec, respectively) and death occurred rapidly, often within 72 hours of presentation.

Most of the survivors responded immediately to supportive care and thiamine supplementation. Common postmortem findings were dilated cardiomyopathy and cellular degeneration with vacuolization and edema with a lack of inflammation or fibrosis. After extensive investigation, it was determined that the etiology was cobalt sulfate, which was added to specific brands of beer as a foam stabilizer.

### Endocrine

Both acute and chronic cobalt exposures are associated with thyroid hyperplasia and goiter. Occupational data also suggest that inhalational exposure to cobalt metals, salts, and oxides is associated with abnormalities in thyroid function. Among decedents from beer drinker's cardiomyopathy, 11 of 14 had abnormal thyroid histology consisting of follicular cell abnormalities and colloid depletion.

### Hematologic

Patients receiving cobalt chloride have increased hemoglobin, hematocrit, and red blood cells.

### Renal

A single report associates reversible acute kidney injury with the chronic administration of cobalt chloride as treatment for anemia. Some animal models of cobalt cardiomyopathy demonstrate cellular changes in renal tissue. However, based on studies of occupational exposures and patients with orthopedic implants, it appears that acute and chronic exposure to cobalt has little effect on the kidneys.

### Reproduction

In pregnant rats, cobalt chloride exposure results in neither teratogenicity nor fetal toxicity. In mice, chronic exposure to cobalt results in impaired spermatogenesis and decreased fertility without affecting follicular-stimulating hormone or luteinizing hormone, whereas acute exposures did not demonstrate similar reproductive effects. Despite these findings, there are no reported human cases that associate cobalt exposure with teratogenicity or impaired fertility.

### Carcinogenesis

The International Agency for Research on Cancer (IARC) considers cobalt metal without tungsten carbide, cobalt sulfate, and other soluble cobalt (II) salts probably carcinogenic to humans (group 2A). Cobalt metal associated with tungsten carbide is possibly carcinogenic to humans (group 2B).

### Other

Gastrointestinal distress is reported following the ingestion of "therapeutic" doses of cobalt salts, as well as elemental cobalt. Decreased proprioception, impaired cranial nerve VIII function, and nonspecific peripheral nerve findings are reported with acute oral cobalt chloride exposures.

### Arthroprosthetic Cobaltism

Metal-on-metal alloy orthopedic implants result in elevations of the associated metal concentration in blood, urine, and hair. Serum cobalt concentrations become elevated 3 weeks after surgery and remain elevated. Despite the elevation of both chromium and cobalt in measured samples, the constellation of clinical findings is more consistent with cobalt.

The association of having a cobalt-containing prosthetic, an elevated cobalt burden, and findings of end-organ toxicity has been coined "arthroprosthetic cobaltism." Before these clinical manifestations occur, cobalt ions are deposited in the soft tissue, which is termed metallosis and is accompanied by discoloration of synovial fluid and pseudotumor formation.

### Chronic Occupational Exposure

***Pulmonary.*** Two pulmonary diseases are associated with cobalt exposure: asthma and "hard-metal disease." Occupational asthma is reported in hard metal workers with a prevalence of 2% to 5%. Cobalt-associated pulmonary toxicity was first noted in tungsten-carbide workers and was subsequently referred to as "hard-metal disease." Signs and symptoms of hard-metal disease include upper respiratory tract irritation, exertional dyspnea, severe dry cough, wheezing, and interstitial lung disease ranging from alveolitis to progressive fibrosis. Despite the progressive and debilitating nature of hard-metal disease, most signs and symptoms improve with cessation of exposure.

***Dermatologic.*** In a study of 1,782 construction workers, 23.6% developed dermatitis and 11.2% developed oil acne while using cobalt-containing cement, fly ash, or asbestos. As in hard-metal disease, it is difficult to isolate cobalt as the sole contributor to the development of dermatitis.

## DIAGNOSTIC TESTING

Body fluid cobalt concentrations are not readily available and therefore cannot be used to direct emergent clinical care. Adjunctive testing that might support a clinical diagnosis of cobalt toxicity should include complete blood count (CBC), reticulocyte count, erythropoietin (EPO) concentration, and thyroid-stimulating hormone (TSH) concentration. The results of these tests might reflect the level of exposure or potential toxicity discussed above.

### Cardiac Studies

Electrocardiogram, echocardiogram, and radionuclide angiocardiography with $^{99}$Tc are useful screening tests for detecting abnormalities associated with cobalt cardiomyopathy and/or pulmonary hypertension caused by hard-metal disease. Magnetic resonance imaging (MRI) is used to exclude other causes of cardiomyopathy.

### Pulmonary Testing

Patients with hard-metal lung disease may demonstrate bilateral upper lobe interstitial lung disease on chest radiograph. Pulmonary function testing may show decreased vital capacity and a decrease in transfer factor for carbon monoxide, both of which are useful for identifying patients at risk for pulmonary fibrosis. A definitive diagnosis of hard-metal disease requires a tissue sample with findings of multinucleated giant cells in the setting of interstitial pulmonary fibrosis.

### Soft Tissue Imaging

Although screening with plain radiography is reasonable, ultrasonography combined with metal artifact reduction sequence MRI has come to the forefront as the more sensitive and specific radiologic study for cobalt-containing implants, revealing soft tissue reactions, metallosis, and pseudotumor, and assisting in revision planning. These tests, however, do not assist in the diagnosis of cobalt toxicity, but merely reveal the presence of local reactions that would place the patient at risk of systemic toxicity. It is advised that the reader refer to their regional medical device oversight body (eg, US Food and Drug Administration, Medicines and Healthcare Products Regulatory Agency) for current recommendations on the frequency of screening and implications of testing results.

### Cobalt Testing

Published literature on "normal concentrations" in blood and urine is fraught with variability, which likely reflects differences in the population under study and the techniques for measurement. Concentrations in clinically poisoned patients are usually at least 1 to 2 or more orders of magnitude greater than published normal concentrations.

## TREATMENT

### Acute Management

Patients with acute cobalt poisoning require coordinated therapy. There are no studies examining the benefit of gastric emptying, activated charcoal, or whole-bowel irrigation (WBI) following acute ingestion. It is reasonable to attempt WBI for radiopaque solid forms of cobalt prior to attempted endoscopic or surgical removal. We recommend against chelation therapy until the gastrointestinal cobalt source is removed. After decontamination, reduction of tissue burden and prevention of end organ toxicity are the next crucial steps.

The data on chelation therapy are unfortunately limited to animal models and human case reports. In a series of animal models of acute cobalt toxicity, succimer and calcium disodium edetate (CaNa2EDTA) enhanced fecal elimination, and glutathione and DTPA were able to enhance urinary elimination; *N*-acetylcysteine (NAC) was able to enhance elimination by both routes. Succimer, NAC, DTPA, and $CaNa_2EDTA$ were effective in reducing mortality in different models. In human case reports, $CaNa_2EDTA$ seems the best choice to enhance the renal elimination of cobalt.

Based on human case reports, several animal studies, and safety profiles, $CaNa_2EDTA$ and NAC are reasonable chelating choices. Despite a paucity of data, reasonable indications for chelation include patients who demonstrate end-organ manifestations of toxicity. This includes acidemia and cardiac failure. Other manifestations of severe cobalt toxicity such as pericardial effusion, clinically significant goiter, and hyperviscosity syndrome should be treated as are patients with other etiologies—pericardiocentesis, airway protection, and phlebotomy, respectively. Based on years of experience with lead, we recommend the regimen for $CaNa_2EDTA$ at doses of 1,000 mg/m$^2$/day by continuous infusion for 5 days. If the diagnosis is confirmed and signs of cardiac failure and acidemia persist after 5 days, an alternate chelator (succimer or DTPA) can be started. Similarly, we recommend NAC dosing based on the acetaminophen (APAP) experience. The 21-hour intravenous NAC protocol should be initiated and continued as in the case of fulminant hepatic failure (Antidotes in Brief: A3) for as long as the patient can tolerate therapy, or continued if cardiac failure or acidemia persists. Thiamine hydrochloride should be administered to all patients independent of whether the patient has alcohol use disorder or heart failure or is malnourished. We recommend the administration of 500 mg intravenously of thiamine 3 times daily for 2 to 3 days and 250 mg intravenously daily for the next 3 to 5 days for life-threatening manifestations (cardiac failure and acidemia) (Antidotes in Brief: A27).

### Arthroprosthetic Cobaltism

The key to treatment is early clinical suspicion with the constellation of findings of cardiomyopathy, hypothyroidism, polycythemia, and peripheral and central nervous system impairment. Early arthroprosthetic revision supports the decontamination tenets within this text and published in case reports. However, emergent revisions may not be practical in a patient who is acutely ill or too high a risk for anesthesia. Therefore, the only modality of treatment other than a supportive one is chelation. However, based on the limited literature, it is unclear if chelation eliminates significant quantities of cobalt in the presence of a large reservoir of metal.

### Occupational/Chronic Exposure

As is always the case of occupational poisonings, prevention is of paramount importance. The use of skin and respiratory protection and improvement of personal hygiene reduces exposure and subsequently the amount of urinary cobalt in occupationally exposed workers.

# 65 COPPER

Normal concentrations

| | |
|---|---|
| Whole blood | = 70–140 μg/dL (11–22 mmol/L) |
| Total serum | = 120–145 μg/dL (18.8–22.8 mmol/L) |
| Free serum | = 0.1–7 μg/dL (0.02–1.1 mmol/L) |
| Ceruloplasmin | = 20–50 mg/dL (1–4 mmol/L) |
| Urine | = 25–50 μg/day (0.4–0.8 mmol/day) |

## HISTORY AND EPIDEMIOLOGY

Copper is available in nature as elemental copper or as one of its sulfide or oxide ores. The smelting, or separation, of copper ores began about 7,000 years ago; copper gradually assumed its current level of importance at the start of the Bronze Age, around 3000 B.C. Important copper compounds are shown in Table 65–1. Although acute copper poisoning is uncommon in the United States, it still occurs in other countries. In addition to intentional ingestion, acute or chronic copper poisoning occurs when the metal is leached from copper pipes or copper containers.

## CHEMICAL PRINCIPLES

Elemental (metalic) copper ($Cu^0$) is not poisonous. Ingestion of large amounts of metallic copper, for example as coins, rarely produces acute copper poisoning. Poisoning under these circumstances is a result of the release of copper ions by acidic gastric contents. The majority of patients suffering from acute copper poisoning are directly exposed to ionic copper. In copper sulfate, the copper atom is in the +2 oxidation state. Cuprous salts, containing copper in the +1 oxidation state, are unstable in water and readily oxidize to the +2 (cupric) form. These water-soluble salts are more likely to be toxic.

## PHARMACOLOGY AND PHYSIOLOGY

Copper is an essential metal with total-body stores in milligram amounts (100–150 mg). Copper is absorbed by an active process involving a Cu-adenosine triphosphatase (ATPase) in the small intestinal mucosal cell membrane. The gastrointestinal absorption varies with the copper intake and source and is as low as 12% in patients with high copper intake. In the presence of damaged mucosa, the fractional absorption is likely to be significantly higher. Once absorbed, copper is rapidly bound to carriers such as albumin, ceruloplasmin, and amino acids for transport to the liver and other tissues. In acute overdose, a high fraction of the plasma copper remains bound to albumin, and thus is biologically active. The volume of distribution of copper is 2 L/kg.

After being released locally in the reduced (2+) form from its carrier, copper uptake by the hepatic cells occurs via a specific uptake pump. Some copper is released from the liver, bound primarily to ceruloplasmin. Ceruloplasmin-bound

**TABLE 65–1 Important Copper Compounds**

| *Chemical Name* | *Chemical Structure* | *Common Name* | *Notes* |
|---|---|---|---|
| Chalcopyrite | $CuFeS_2$ | Copper iron sulfide | Copper ore; source of 80% of world's copper |
| Chromated cupric arsenate | 35% CuO<br>20% $CrO_3$<br>45% $As_2O_5$ | CCA | Wood preservative[a] |
| Copper octanoate | $Cu\{CH_3(CH_2)_6COO\}_2$ | Copper soap | Fungicide in home garden products, paint, rot-proof rope, and roofing |
| Copper triethanolamine complex | $Cu\{(HOCH_2CH_2)_3N\}_2$ | Chelated copper | Algicide |
| Cupric acetoarsenite | $Cu(C_2H_3O_2)_2 \cdot 3Cu(AsO_2)_2$ | Paris or Vienna green | Insecticide, wood preservative, pigment[a] |
| Cupric arsenite | $CuHAsO_3$ | Swedish or Scheele green | Wood preservative, insecticide[a] |
| Cupric chloride | $CuCl_2$ | | Catalyst in petrochemical industry |
| Cupric chloride, basic | $CuCl_2 \cdot 3Cu(OH)_2$ | Basic copper chloride; copper oxychloride | Fungicide |
| Cupric hydroxide | $Cu(OH)_2$ | Copper hydroxide | Fungicide |
| Cupric oxide | CuO | Black copper oxide; tenorite | Glass pigment, flux, polishing agent |
| Cupric sulfate | $CuSO_4$ | Roman vitriol, blue vitriol, bluestone, hydrocyanite | Fungicide, plant growth regulator, white wash, homegrown crystals |
| Cupric sulfate, basic | $CuSO_4 \cdot 3Ca(OH)_2 \cdot 3CaSO_4$ | Bordeaux solution | Fungicide |
| Cuprous cyanide | CuCN | Cupricin | Electroplating solutions |
| Cuprous oxide | $Cu_2O$ | Red copper oxide, cuprite | Antifouling paint |

[a]No longer used in the United States.

copper accounts for approximately 90% to 95% of serum copper. Copper bound to this carrier has a plasma half-life of approximately 24 hours. The amount of unbound copper in the blood under normal circumstances is well below 1%.

Copper is predominantly biliary eliminated. Biliary excretion approximates gastrointestinal absorption and averages 2,000 μg/24 h. Under normal conditions, renal elimination is trivial, accounting for approximately 5 to 25 μg/24 h. The elimination half-life of erythrocyte copper is 26 days.

## TOXICOLOGY AND PATHOPHYSIOLOGY

### Redox Chemistry

Copper is capable of assuming one of several different oxidation states and is an active participant in redox reactions. In particular, participation in the Fenton reaction and the Haber–Weiss reaction explains the toxicologic effects of copper as a generator of oxidative stress and inhibitor of several key metabolic enzymes. In the presence of sulfhydryl-rich cell membranes, cupric ions are reduced to cuprous ions, which are capable of generating superoxide radicals in the presence of oxygen. The mitochondrial electron transport chain and lipid membranes serve as ready sources of electrons for copper reduction, which ultimately leads to mitochondrial or membrane dysfunction, respectively.

### Erythrocytes

Cupric ion inhibits sulfhydryl groups on enzymes in important antioxidant systems, including glucose-6-phosphate dehydrogenase and glutathione reductase, leading to depletion of glutathione in poisoning. The importance of hemoglobin-derived reactive oxygen species is demonstrated by the lack of hemolysis in the presence of copper under anaerobic conditions.

### Liver

Although most of the accumulated copper ions in hepatocytes are rapidly complexed with metallothionein, unsequestered copper ions participate in redox reactions. Copper ions also generate hydroxyl radicals, which are potent inducers of both lipid peroxidation and other reactive oxygen species. These effects are most pronounced in mitochondria, perhaps as a consequence of the reduction of cupric to cuprous ion in these organelles. Histologically, liver damage follows a centrilobular pattern of necrosis.

### Kidney

Reactive oxygen species are probably also responsible for the nephrotoxic effects of unbound copper. Pathologic analyses of the kidneys of copper-poisoned patients typically reveal acute tubular necrosis and demonstrate hemoglobin casts. These findings suggest that kidney failure results indirectly from the hemoglobinuria induced by the massive release of free extracellular hemoglobin.

### Central Nervous System

Since copper ions do not readily cross the blood–brain barrier, accumulation is accomplished through carrier-mediated transport of albumin-bound, not ceruloplasmin-bound, ionized copper into the central nervous system. Once in the central nervous system, oxidative damage, as occurs in other tissues, results in cellular dysfunction and destruction.

## CLINICAL MANIFESTATIONS

### Acute Copper Salt Poisoning

The acute lethal ingested dose of copper sulfate is estimated to be 0.15 to 0.3 g/kg. Gastrointestinal effects are the most common initial manifestations of poisoning and include the rapid onset of emesis and abdominal pain, followed by hemorrhage, ulceration, or perforation. Other common symptoms include retrosternal chest pain and a metallic taste. Copper-induced hemolysis occurs rapidly following exposure. In most reported cases, significant methemoglobinemia occurs early in the clinical course and is rapidly followed by hemolysis. Because free methemoglobin is filterable, methemoglobinuria occurs. In patients with more severe poisoning, hepatotoxicity is a frequent manifestation and jaundice results from either hepatocellular necrosis or hemolysis or both. Kidney and lung toxicities occur occasionally and represent extra-erythrocytic manifestations of the oxidative effects of the copper ions. In spite of massive intravascular hemolysis, hemoglobinuric acute kidney injury is uncommon in patients who receive adequate volume-replacement therapy. Hypotension and cardiovascular collapse occur in those most severely poisoned and are likely multifactorial in origin. Depressed mental status, which ranges from lethargy to coma, or seizures following acute poisoning are likely epiphenomena related to damage to other organ systems.

Intravenous injection of copper sulfate produces a clinical syndrome identical to that which occurs following ingestion, although the gastrointestinal findings are less pronounced. Inhalation of copper oxide fumes, generated during welding or other industrial processes, can produce metal fume fever. Patients present with cough, chills, chest pain, and fever that are most likely immunologic, and not toxicologic, in origin (Chap. 94).

### Chronic Copper Poisoning

Chronic exogenous copper poisoning is uncommon in adults but occurs in children in some parts of the world. This condition, commonly called childhood cirrhosis in India and idiopathic copper toxicosis elsewhere, generally occurs in the setting of excessive dietary intake of copper as a result of copper-contaminated water from brass vessels used to store milk.

"Vineyard sprayer's lung," first described in 1969, refers to the occupational pulmonary disease that occurred among Portuguese vineyard workers applying Bordeaux solution, a 1% to 2% copper sulfate solution neutralized with hydrated lime. The patients developed interstitial pulmonary fibrosis and histiocytic granulomas containing copper. Many of these workers also developed lung adenocarcinoma, hepatic angiosarcoma, and micronodular cirrhosis, raising the possibility of a carcinogenic effect of chronic copper exposure.

Ophthalmic effects of copper salts, primarily following occupational exposure, include irritation of the corneal, conjunctival, or adnexal structures.

## DIAGNOSTIC TESTING

Real-time analytical testing for copper is impractical, and management decisions must be based on clinical criteria. Copper concentrations are often obtained for confirmatory or investigative purposes. Although never adequately studied, whole-blood copper concentrations appear to correlate better with clinical findings than serum copper concentrations. Unfortunately, there is little correlation between clinical findings at any given copper concentration. Reported serum copper concentrations in patients with hemolysis range from 96 to 747 μg/dL. Copper concentrations in patients with copper-induced acute kidney injury ranged from 115 to 390 μg/dL. Concentrations in severe poisoning are often above 5,000 μg/dL. Occasionally, serum copper concentrations reveal a secondary rise, likely because of release during hepatocellular necrosis.

Routine laboratory testing following acute copper poisoning should include an assessment of fluid and electrolyte status, hemolysis, and hepatotoxicity. Differentiation between hepatotoxicity and hemolysis as a cause for jaundice is made by comparison of the bilirubin fractions and an assessment of the hepatic enzymes and hemoglobin; that is, indirect bilirubin is proportionally elevated in patients with hemolysis, whereas the direct fraction rises in patients with hepatocellular necrosis. A prolonged prothrombin time in the absence of liver injury or disseminated intravascular coagulopathy is likely the result of a direct effect of copper ions on the coagulation cascade.

## MANAGEMENT

Optimal supportive care is the cornerstone to the effective management of patients with acute copper poisoning. Attention to antiemetic therapy, fluid and electrolyte correction, and normalization of vital signs are the critical steps before consideration of chelation therapy. Gastrointestinal decontamination is not a concern as the onset of emesis generally occurs within minutes of ingestion and is often protracted and adsorption to activated charcoal has not been well studied. Hemodialysis is indicated for patients with acute kidney injury using standard criteria. For patients with life-threatening hepatic failure, liver transplantation is a reasonable option.

### Chelation Therapy

Chelation therapy is recommended when hepatic or hematologic compromise or other concerning or severe manifestations of poisoning are present. Three chelators are clinically available, and most data regarding dosing and efficacy are derived either from their use in the treatment of patients with Wilson disease or from their effects on copper elimination during chelation of patients manifesting toxicity from other metals. d-Penicillamine is an orally bioavailable chelator that is effective in preventing copper-induced hemolysis in patients with Wilson disease. The d-penicillamine–copper complex undergoes rapid renal clearance in patients with competent kidneys. The recommended dose is 1 to 1.5 g/day given orally in four divided doses. d-Penicillamine is also indicated for the treatment of chronic copper poisoning. The major risk of d-penicillamine is hypersensitivity reactions, which occur in 25% of patients who are penicillin allergic. Trientine, another orally bioavailable chelator, is the second-line treatment for patients with Wilson disease, but its use in acute copper salt poisoning is unstudied. Although intramuscular dimercaprol is likely to be less effective than d-penicillamine, its use is appropriate when vomiting or gastrointestinal injury prevents oral d-penicillamine administration. Furthermore, because the dimercaprol–copper complex primarily undergoes biliary elimination, whereas d-penicillamine undergoes renal elimination, dimercaprol should be used in patients with acute kidney injury (Antidotes in Brief: A28). Succimer triples the baseline copper elimination in a murine model. Given its ease of use, ready availability, relative safety, and benefit in experimental models, succimer can be used in lieu of d-penicillamine in patients with less consequential poisoning, particularly when there is difficulty in obtaining d-penicillamine, using a standard lead poisoning regimen (Antidotes in Brief: A29).

### Extracorporeal Elimination

Exchange transfusion is of undefined but probably limited benefit in patients with acute copper sulfate poisoning. Hemodialysis and peritoneal dialysis appear to be of little clinical use and are not routinely recommended.

# 66 LEAD

Normal concentration
Whole blood < 5 µg/dL (< 0.24 µmol/L)

## HISTORY AND EPIDEMIOLOGY

The low melting point and high malleability of lead made it one of the first metals smelted and used by humans. Ancient Egyptians and Hebrews used lead, and the Phoenicians established lead mines in Spain circa 2000 B.C. The Greeks and Romans released lead during the process of extracting silver from ore. Postindustrial lead use increased dramatically, and today, lead is used widely for its waterproofing and electrical- and radiation-shielding properties. Use of both lead-based paint for house paint and leaded gasoline has been essentially eliminated by regulation in the United States (US) since the 1980s, but is still a concern in many nations, and persistence of lead paint in older US homes and water-supply systems still constitutes an enormous environmental challenge.

Recognition of the clinical effects of excess lead exposure can be traced back to antiquity. Dioscorides, a Greek physician in the second century B.C., observed adverse cognitive effects, and Pliny cautioned the Romans of the danger of inhaled fumes from lead smelting. With the 19th-century Industrial Revolution, lead poisoning became a common occupational disease. The reproductive effects of lead poisoning were recognized by the turn of the 20th century.

The majority of health effects that occur today in the US concern childhood lead poisoning due to residential house paint. From the 1970s to the present, the research thrust in childhood lead poisoning has centered on the recognition and quantification of more subtle neurocognitive impairment caused by subclinical lead poisoning. Over this time period, the US Centers for Disease Control and Prevention (CDC) has steadily revised downward the definitions of an elevated blood lead concentration or thresholds of concern in children, from 60 µg/dL in the early 1960s to 3.5 µg/dL today. Environmental exposures affect the entire population, particularly young children. Most environmental lead poisoning of consequence in the US still results from exposure to residential lead paint (Table 66–1). The CDC reported in 2000 that children enrolled in Medicaid had a prevalence of elevated blood lead concentrations 3 times greater than those not enrolled. Refugee, immigrant, and foreign-born adopted children remain at particularly high risk, and remarkable cases of extremely elevated blood lead concentrations (> 100 µg/dL) are still being detected on routine screening.

Adults with occupational exposures to lead constitute another large group of persons at risk. It is estimated that more than 3 million workers in the US, employed in more than 100 occupations, are exposed to lead. Some types of lead-related work are more hazardous than others (Table 66–2).

Finally, numerous additional sources of lead exposure are also reported, including contaminated folk medications or cosmetics, imported food, ingested lead foreign bodies, and retained bullets. Ayurveda and other folk medicine, specifically "rasa shastra," in which heavy metals are incorporated into products for their medicinal value, is a frequent source of lead exposure in children and adults. In 2010, an outbreak of lead encephalopathy from artisanal gold mining was first reported in Nigeria and has claimed hundreds of lives.

## CHEMICAL PRINCIPLES

Lead is a silvery-gray, soft metal with a low melting point. Metallic lead is relatively insoluble in water and dilute acids but dissolves in nitric, acetic, and hot, concentrated sulfuric acids. Inorganic lead compounds are often brightly colored and vary widely in water solubility; several are used extensively as pigments in paints such as lead chromate (yellow) and lead oxide (red). Lead also forms organic compounds, of which two, tetramethyl and tetraethyl lead (TEL), were used commercially as gasoline additives. Lead complexes with ligands containing sulfur, oxygen, or nitrogen as electron donors. There is no known physiologic role for lead, and thus any lead presence in human tissue represents contamination.

## PHARMACOLOGY

### Inorganic and Metallic Lead

***Absorption.*** Adults absorb an estimated 10% to 15% of ingested lead in food, and children have a higher gastrointestinal (GI) absorption rate, averaging 40% to 50%. Fasting and diets deficient in iron, calcium, and zinc enhance GI absorption of lead. Swallowed metallic lead (fishing weights, bullets, etc) is also absorbed, albeit less readily than most lead compounds.

**TABLE 66–1 Environmental Lead Sources**

| *Source* | *Comment* |
|---|---|
| Air | Leaded gasoline (pre-1976 US; still prevalent worldwide), industrial emissions |
| Dust | House dust from deteriorated lead paint |
| Food | Lead solder in cans (pre-1991 US; still prevalent in imported canned foods); "natural" dietary supplements; "moonshine" whiskey and lead foil–covered wines; contaminated flour, paprika, other imported foods and candy; lead leached from leaded crystal, ceramics, vinyl lunch boxes |
| Other | Complementary and alternative medicines, children's toys and jewelry (especially imported products), cosmetics, leaded ink, vinyl mini-blinds |
| Paint | Especially pre-1978 homes |
| Soil | From yards contaminated by deteriorated lead paint, lead industry emissions, artisanal mining, roadways with high leaded gasoline usage |
| Water | Leached from leaded plumbing (pipes, solder), cooking utensils, water coolers |

**TABLE 66–2 Occupational and Recreational Lead Sources**

| |
|---|
| **High-Risk Occupations** |
| Automobile radiator repairers |
| Crystal glass makers |
| Firing range instructors, bullet salvagers |
| Lead smelters, refiners |
| Metal welders, cutters (includes bridge and highway reconstruction workers) |
| Painters, construction workers (sanding, scraping, or spraying of lead paint; demolition of lead-painted sites) |
| Polyvinyl chloride plastic manufacturers |
| Shipbreakers |
| Storage battery manufacturers, repairers, recyclers |
| **Moderate-Risk Occupations** |
| Automobile factory workers and mechanics |
| Enamelers |
| Glass blowers |
| Lead miners |
| Plumbers |
| Pottery glazers |
| Ship repairers |
| Shot makers |
| Solderers |
| Type founders |
| Varnish makers |
| Wire and cable workers |
| **Possible Increased-Risk Occupations** |
| Electronics manufacturers |
| Jewelers |
| Pipefitters |
| Printers |
| Rubber product manufacturers |
| Traffic police officers, taxi drivers, garage workers, turnpike tollbooth operators, gas station attendants (exposed to leaded gasoline exhaust fumes; unlikely now in the US but still a hazard in resource poor countries) |
| **Recreational and Hobby Sources** |
| Ceramic crafts |
| Furniture refinishing, restoring |
| Home remodeling, refinishing |
| Painting (fine artist's pigments) |
| Repair of automobiles, boats |
| Stained-glass making |
| Target shooting, recasting lead for bullets |
| **Additional Sources** |
| Ingested lead foreign bodies and retained lead bullets |
| Illicit substance abuse (heroin, methamphetamine, leaded gasoline "huffing") |
| Burning batteries, leaded paper, or wood for fuel |
| Hand–mouth contact with pool cue chalk, glazes, leaded ink |

The overall absorption of inhaled lead averages 30% to 40%. Cutaneous absorption of inorganic lead is traditionally considered low. Soft tissue absorption of metallic lead from retained bullets depends on particle size, total surface area, and location; multiple small shot and location in which particles are bathed by synovial, serosal, or spinal fluid favor a more rapid increase in blood lead concentration. Transplacental lead transfer is critical in fetal and neonatal lead exposure. Lead readily crosses the placental barrier throughout gestation, and lead uptake is cumulative until birth. Breast milk also contains lead in relatively low concentration but is a significant source of neonatal exposure at maternal blood lead concentrations of approximately 40 μg/dL or greater.

***Distribution.*** Absorbed lead is at least 99% bound to erythrocytes. From blood, lead is distributed into both a relatively labile soft tissue pool and into a more stable bone compartment. In adults, approximately 95% of the body lead burden is stored in bone versus only 70% for children. The remainder is distributed to the major soft tissue lead-storage sites, including the liver, kidney, bone marrow, and brain. Most of the toxicity associated with lead is a result of soft tissue uptake, especially the brain.

***Excretion.*** Absorbed lead that is not retained is primarily excreted in urine (approximately 65%) and bile (approximately 35%). Children excrete less of their daily uptake than adults. Biologic half-lives for lead are estimated as follows: blood, 25 days (adults, short-term experiments) and 10 months (children, natural exposure); soft tissues (adults, short-term exposure), 40 days; bone (labile, trabecular pool), 90 days; and cortical bone, 10 to 20 years.

### Organic Lead

Alkyl lead compounds are lipid soluble and have unique pharmacokinetics that are less well characterized than those of inorganic lead. Tetraethyl lead is absorbed through ingestion, inhalation, and intact skin, with subsequent distribution to lipophilic tissues, including the brain. Tetraethyl lead (TEL) is metabolized to triethyl lead, which is likely the major toxic compound. Alkyl lead also slowly releases lead as the inorganic form, with subsequent kinetics as noted above.

## PATHOPHYSIOLOGY

### General Mechanisms

The affinity of lead for biologic electron-donor ligands, especially sulfhydryl groups, allows it to bind and impact numerous enzymatic, receptor, and structural proteins. Lead is also chemically similar to the divalent cations calcium, magnesium, and zinc, and it interferes with numerous calcium and perhaps magnesium- and zinc-mediated metabolic pathways, particularly in mitochondria and in second-messenger systems regulating cellular energy metabolism.

### Neurotoxicity

Lead-induced neurotransmitter dysfunction is linked to its calcium-mimetic properties. Through blockade of calcium influx at voltage-sensitive calcium channels, lead inhibits depolarization-triggered release of acetylcholine, dopamine, and γ-aminobutyric acid (GABA) but augments the background rate of spontaneous release. The dampening of the evoked neurotransmitter response in conjunction with enhanced background release results in a decreased "signal-to-noise" ratio. In addition, lead decreases calcium currents at the *N*-methyl-D-aspartate (NMDA) glutamate receptor and directly activates the intracellular second-messenger protein kinase C. These effects on neurotransmitter release, receptor activity, and intracellular signaling adversely affect "synaptic pruning" in the developing brain, a process by which the volume of excessive synaptic connections is selectively reduced. This disruption results in suboptimal cortical microarchitecture and function, and it particularly affects the hippocampus, an important locus of learning and memory.

### Hematologic Toxicity

Lead is a potent inhibitor of several enzymes in the heme biosynthetic pathway most notably ferochelatase. It also induces a defect in erythropoietin function secondary to associated kidney damage. A shortened erythrocyte life span is caused by increased membrane fragility with resultant hemolysis. The inhibition of pyrimidine-5′-nucleotidase underlies the appearance of basophilic stippling in erythrocytes, representing clumping of degraded RNA, which is normally eliminated by this enzyme (Fig. 66–1). The clumped RNA serves as lead points for hemolysis as red cells move through the reticuloendothelial system.

### Nephrotoxicity

Functional changes associated with acute lead nephropathy include decreased energy-dependent transport, resulting in a Fanconi-like syndrome of aminoaciduria, glycosuria, and phosphaturia. The association of plumbism with gout ("saturnine gout") was noted more than 100 years ago. Lead competitively decreases uric acid excretion in the distal tubule, resulting in elevated blood urate concentrations and urate crystal deposition in joints. Kidney function is virtually always impaired in patients with saturnine gout.

### Cardiotoxicity

The most important manifestation of lead toxicity on the cardiovascular system is hypertension. This is likely caused by altered calcium-activated changes in contractility of vascular smooth muscle cells secondary to decreased $Na^+$,$K^+$-ATPase activity and stimulation of the $Na^+$-$Ca^{2+}$ exchange pump.

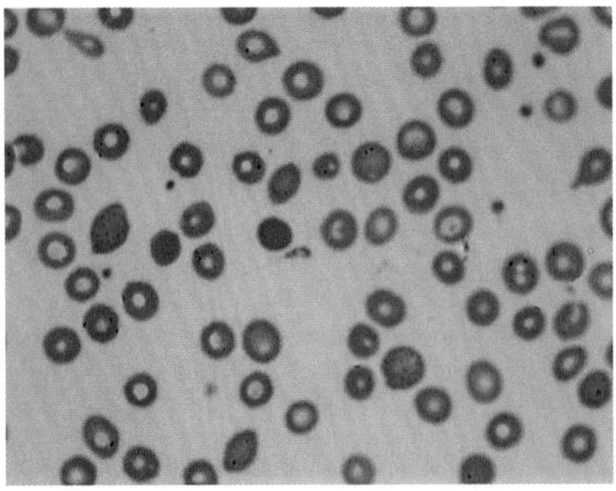

**FIGURE 66–1.** This peripheral smear of blood examined under high-power microscopy demonstrates the classic basophilic stippling associated with lead poisoning. The patient's blood lead concentration was > 100 μg/dL. *(Used with permission from the Fellowship in Medical Toxicology, New York University Grossman School of Medicine, New York City Poison Center.)*

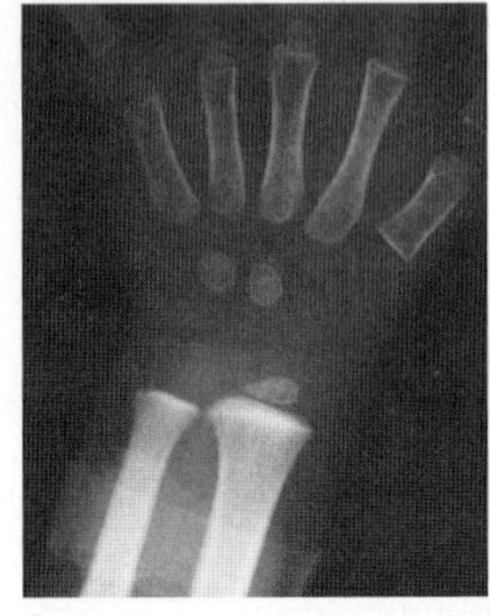

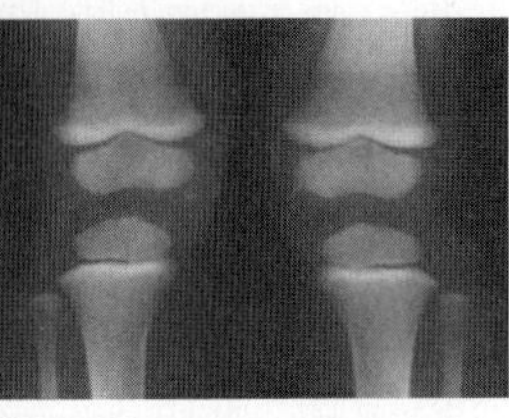

**A** **B**

**FIGURE 66–2.** (**A**) Radiograph of the wrist reveals increased bands of calcification ("lead lines"). (**B**) Similar radiographic findings in another patient at the knee. *(Reproduced with permission from Wells RG. Diagnostic imaging of infants and children. McGraw Hill LLC, 2013.)*

### Reproductive Toxicity

Impairment of both male and female reproductive function is associated with overt plumbism.

### Endocrine Toxicity

Reduced thyroid and adrenopituitary function are found in adult lead workers. Children with elevated blood lead concentrations have a depressed secretion of human growth hormone and insulin-like growth factor.

### Skeletal Toxicity

In addition to the importance of the skeletal system as the largest repository of lead body burden, bone metabolism is also adversely affected by lead. Both new bone formation and coupling of normal osteoblast and osteoclast function are impaired. Bands of increased metaphyseal density on radiographs of long bones ("lead lines") in young children with heavy lead exposure represent increased calcium deposition (not primarily lead) in the zones of provisional calcification (Fig. 66–2). Impaired bone growth and shortened stature are associated with childhood lead poisoning.

### Gastrointestinal Toxicity

Lead toxicity causes constipation, anorexia, and colicky abdominal pain. Although the mechanisms are not fully elucidated, theories include impaired intestinal motility, alterations in luminal ion transport, and spasmodic contraction of intestinal wall smooth muscle.

## CLINICAL MANIFESTATIONS

### Inorganic Lead

The manifestations of lead toxicity are characterized into distinct acute and chronic syndromes (Tables 66–3 and 66–4). In general, children are considered to be more susceptible

**TABLE 66–3 Clinical Manifestations of Lead Poisoning in Children**

| *Clinical Severity* | *Typical Blood Lead Concentrations (μg/dL)* |
|---|---|
| **Severe** | > 70–100 |
| CNS: Encephalopathy (coma, altered sensorium, seizures, bizarre behavior, ataxia, apathy, incoordination, loss of developmental skills, papilledema, cranial nerve palsies, signs of increased ICP) | |
| GI: Persistent vomiting | |
| Hematologic: Pallor (anemia) | |
| **Moderate** | 50–70 |
| CNS: Hyperirritable behavior, intermittent lethargy, decreased interest in play, "difficult" child | |
| GI: Intermittent vomiting, abdominal pain, anorexia | |
| **Mild** | ≤ 49 |
| CNS: Impaired cognition, behavior, balance, fine-motor coordination | |
| Miscellaneous: Impaired hearing, impaired growth | |

CNS = central nervous system; GI = gastrointestinal; ICP = intracranial pressure.

**TABLE 66–4 Clinical Manifestations of Lead Poisoning in Adults**

| *Clinical Severity* | *Typical Blood Lead Concentrations (μg/dL)* |
|---|---|
| **Severe** | > 100 |
| CNS: Encephalopathy (coma, seizures, obtundation, delirium, focal motor disturbances, headaches, papilledema, optic neuritis, signs of increased ICP) | |
| PNS: Foot drop, wrist drop | |
| GI: Abdominal colic | |
| Hematologic: Pallor (anemia) | |
| Renal: Nephropathy | |
| **Moderate** | 70–100 |
| CNS: Headache, memory loss, decreased libido, insomnia | |
| PNS: Peripheral neuropathy | |
| GI: Metallic taste, abdominal pain, anorexia, constipation | |
| Kidney: Arthritis due to saturnine gout (impaired urate excretion) | |
| Miscellaneous: Mild anemia, myalgias, muscle weakness, arthralgias | |
| **Mild** | 20–69[a] |
| CNS: Fatigue, somnolence, moodiness, lessened interest in leisure activities | |
| Miscellaneous: Adverse effects on cognition, reproduction, kidney function, or bone density; hypertension and cardiovascular disease; possible increased risk of bladder, lung, and stomach cancer | |

[a]Chronic lead exposure at lower blood lead concentrations leads to cumulative body burdens of lead associated with these clinical findings.

CNS = central nervous system; GI = gastrointestinal; ICP = intracranial pressure; PNS = peripheral nervous system.

than adults to toxicity for a given measured blood lead concentration, a distinction that applies primarily to central nervous system (CNS) effects.

***Asymptomatic Children.*** Children with *elevated body lead burdens but without overt symptoms* represent the largest group of persons at risk for chronic lead toxicity. The subclinical toxicity of lead in this population centers around subtle effects on growth, hearing, and neurocognitive development. Numerous population-based studies report significant inverse associations with blood lead concentration and IQ.

***Symptomatic Children.*** Subencephalopathic symptomatic plumbism usually occurs in children 1 to 5 years of age and is associated with blood lead concentrations greater than 70 μg/dL but may occur with concentrations as low as 50 μg/dL. Unfortunately, common behavioral and abdominal manifestations in well children of this age, including the "terrible twos" temperamental outbursts, functional constipation, abdominal pain, and not eating as much as parents expect, often overlap with the milder range of reported symptoms of lead poisoning. Other uncommon clinical presentations are described, including isolated seizures without encephalopathy (indistinguishable from idiopathic epilepsy), chronic hyperactive behavior disorder, isolated developmental delay, progressive loss of cortical function simulating degenerative cerebral disease, peripheral neuropathy (reported particularly in children with sickle cell hemoglobinopathy), and the occurrence of GI effects (colicky abdominal pain, vomiting, constipation) with myalgias of the trunk and proximal girdle muscles.

Acute lead encephalopathy is the most severe presentation of pediatric plumbism (Table 66–3). Encephalopathy usually occurs in children ages 15 to 30 months; is associated with blood lead concentrations greater than 100 μg/dL; and is characterized by severe vomiting and apathy, bizarre behavior, loss of recently acquired developmental skills, ataxia, incoordination, seizures, altered sensorium, or coma. Physical examination often reveals papilledema, oculomotor or facial nerve palsy, diminished deep tendon reflexes, or other evidence of increased intracranial pressure (ICP) (Fig. 66–3). Milder findings that portend incipient encephalopathy include anorexia, constipation, intermittent abdominal pain, sporadic vomiting, hyperirritable or aggressive behavior, periods of lethargy interspersed with lucid intervals, and decreased interest in play activities. Patients frequently brought to medical attention for vomiting and lethargy during the 2 to 7 days before onset of frank encephalopathy. The incidence of permanent neurologic sequelae, including intellectual disability, seizure disorder, blindness, and hemiparesis, is 25% to 30% in patients who develop encephalopathic symptoms before the onset of chelation (Fig. 66–4).

***Adults.*** Most adult plumbism is related to chronic occupational respiratory exposure and typically manifests as signs and symptoms representing disorders of several organ systems (Table 66–4). True acute poisoning occurs rarely, after very high inhalational, large oral, or intravenous (IV) exposures. Clinical manifestations in such patients include colicky abdominal pain, hepatitis, pancreatitis, hemolytic anemia, and encephalopathy over days or weeks. Mild plumbism

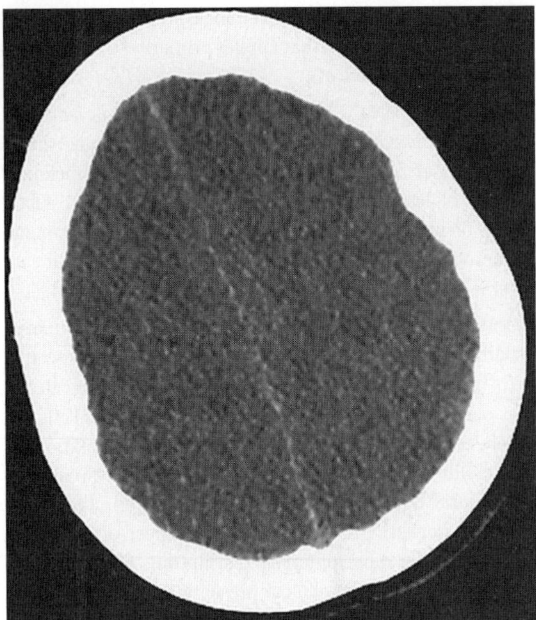

**FIGURE 66–3.** Computed tomography scan of the brain at the vertex shows loss of the gray-white differentiation, sulci, and diffuse cerebral edema. *(Reproduced with permission from Block J, Jordanov MI, Stack LB, Thurman RJ: The Atlas of Emergency Radiology. McGraw Hill LLC, 2013.)*

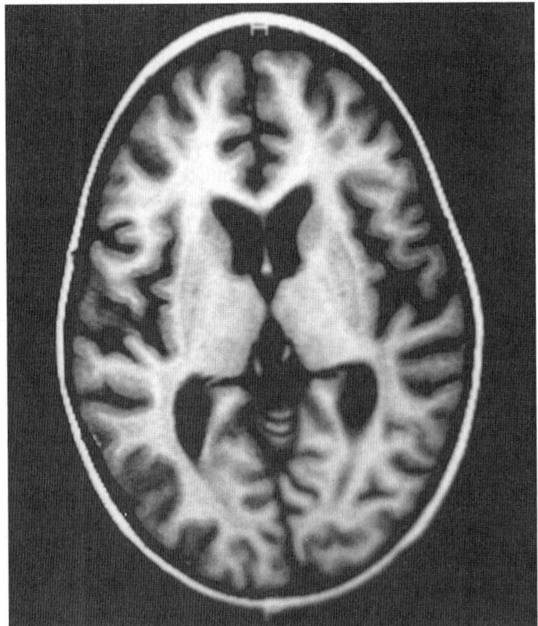

**FIGURE 66–4.** Magnetic resonance image of the brain reveals cortical atrophy and multiple areas of cerebral infarction, done on hospital day 22. At this time, the child's clinical status was notable for choreoathetoid movements and generalized hypotonia, inability to localize visual or auditory stimuli, and nonpurposeful movements of the extremities. *(Used with permission from Eric Faerber, MD, Department of Radiology, St. Christopher's Hospital for Children, Philadelphia, PA.)*

manifests as minor CNS findings, such as changes in mood and cognition. In patients with severe plumbism, the hallmark of toxicity is acute encephalopathy, which has been rarely reported in adults since the 1920s. Encephalopathy in adults is usually associated with very high blood lead concentrations (typically > 150 μg/dL) and is manifested by seizures (75% of cases), obtundation, confusion, focal motor disturbances, papilledema, headaches, and optic neuritis.

Increased blood pressure is probably the most prevalent adverse health effect observed from lead toxicity in adults. Epidemiologic studies document significant associations between hypertension and body lead burdens. Additional studies correlate body lead burden with several other disorders of aging, including a decline in cognitive ability, essential tremor, cardiac and cerebrovascular events, electrocardiographic abnormalities, chronic kidney disease, osteoporosis, cataract prevalence, and all-cause and cardiovascular mortality.

### Organic Lead

Clinical symptoms of TEL toxicity are usually nonspecific initially and include nausea, vomiting, anorexia, insomnia, and emotional instability. Patients exhibit tremor and increased deep tendon reflexes, as well as liver or kidney injury. In more severe cases, these symptoms progress to encephalopathy with delusions, hallucinations, and hyperactivity, which resolve or deteriorate to coma and, occasionally, death. In contrast to inorganic lead poisoning, patients with significant TEL toxicity do not consistently manifest hematologic abnormalities or elevations of heme synthesis pathway biomarkers. In addition, significant neurotoxicity occurs at blood lead concentrations considerably lower than those typically associated with inorganic lead poisoning.

## DIAGNOSTIC TESTING

### Clinical Diagnosis in Symptomatic Patients

The medical evaluation should first include a comprehensive medical history. Further inquiry should elicit environmental, occupational, or recreational sources of exposure as detailed earlier (Tables 66–1 and 66–2). Plumbism is more likely in a child between the ages of 1 and 5 years with prior plumbism or noted elevated blood lead concentrations; history of pica or acute unintentional ingestions; aural, nasal, or esophageal foreign bodies; history of iron-deficiency anemia; residence in a pre-1960s–built home in the US only, especially with deteriorated paint, or one that has undergone recent remodeling; family history of lead poisoning; or foreign-born status. In adults, the history should focus on occupational and recreational activities involving lead exposure (Table 66–2), a history of plumbism, and gunshot wounds with retained bullets.

An emergency department patient with potential lead encephalopathy presents the physician with a dilemma: severe lead toxicity requires urgent diagnosis, but confirmatory blood lead assays are not usually rapidly available. For adults, a history of occupational exposure is often available from medical records or family members, and lead encephalopathy can be strongly considered with positive supportive laboratory findings such as anemia, basophilic stippling, elevated erythrocyte protoporphyrin (especially > 250 μg/dL), sometimes available on an urgent basis, and abnormal urinalysis. In this context, it is reasonable to institute presumptive chelation therapy while awaiting a blood lead concentration. In children, a similar indication for presumptive treatment would be suggested by a constellation of clinical features and ancillary studies, such as age 1 to 5 years, a prodromal illness of several days' to weeks' duration (suggestive of milder lead-related symptoms), history of pica and source of lead exposure, the laboratory features noted above (which are equally helpful in young children), and suggestive radiologic findings (detailed below) such as dense metaphyseal "lead lines" or ingested foreign bodies. In both adults and children, the decision to institute empiric chelation treatment should not deter additional emergent diagnostic efforts to exclude or to confirm other important entities while blood lead concentrations are pending. Lumbar puncture should be generally avoided in patients with suspected lead encephalopathy because of the risk of cerebral herniation. If there is a significant suspicion of a CNS infection, we recommend empiric treatment be instituted while awaiting blood lead concentration results and that lumbar puncture be delayed until the blood lead concentration is determined to be normal.

## Laboratory Evaluation

In any patient suspected of symptomatic plumbism, whole blood should be collected by venipuncture into special lead-free evacuated tubes. For asymptomatic children, blood lead concentration screening is often performed by capillary blood testing for convenience; however, venous confirmation of elevated capillary lead concentrations, unless extremely high (eg, ≥ 70 μg/dL) or unless the patient is clearly symptomatic, is still warranted before chelation or other significant interventions. The erythrocyte protoporphyrin concentration reflects inhibition of the heme synthesis pathway and is useful for tracking response to therapy and in distinguishing acute from chronic lead poisoning. Routine serum chemistries, kidney function tests, liver function tests, urinalysis, and complete blood count are recommended in patients who are symptomatic or about to undergo chelation therapy. Radiographic studies should be obtained according to relevant history to determine the presence of ingested foreign bodies, retained bullets, or shrapnel (Figs. 66–5, 66–6, 66–7). In addition, the presence of "lead lines" can strengthen the clinical diagnosis of childhood plumbism before blood lead concentrations are available (Fig. 66–2).

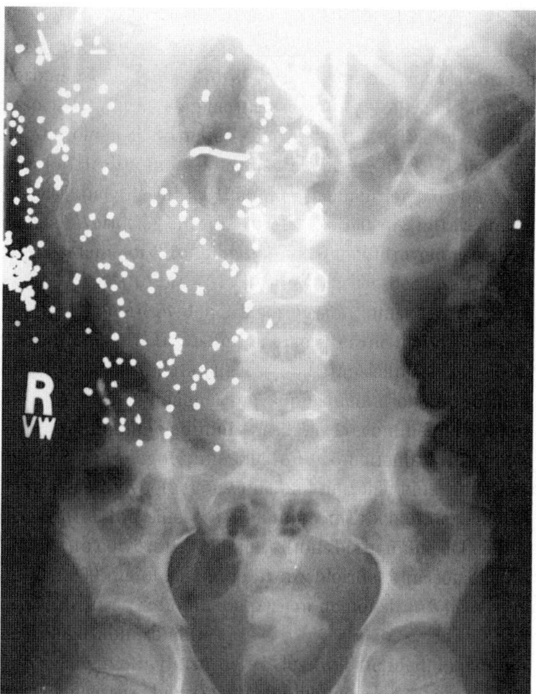


**FIGURE 66–5.** Abdominal radiograph of an 8-year-old child who sustained a shotgun wound to the right paraspinal area, with resultant paraplegia and multiple visceral injuries. The blood lead concentration was found to be 60 μg/dL at 11 weeks after injury, and chelation therapy was commenced. *(Used with permission from Children's Hospital of Philadelphia, Department of Radiology, Philadelphia, PA.)*

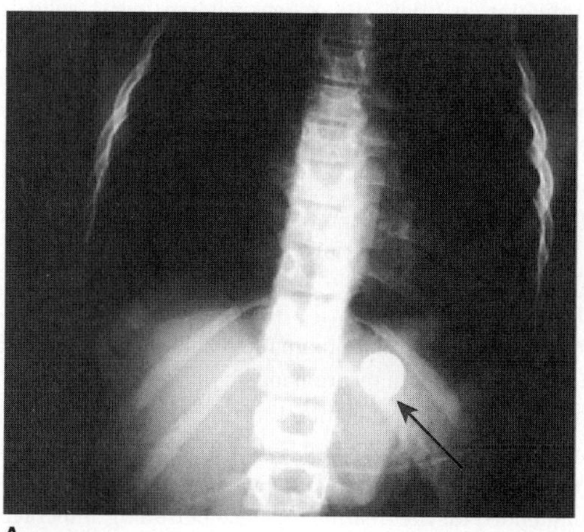
A

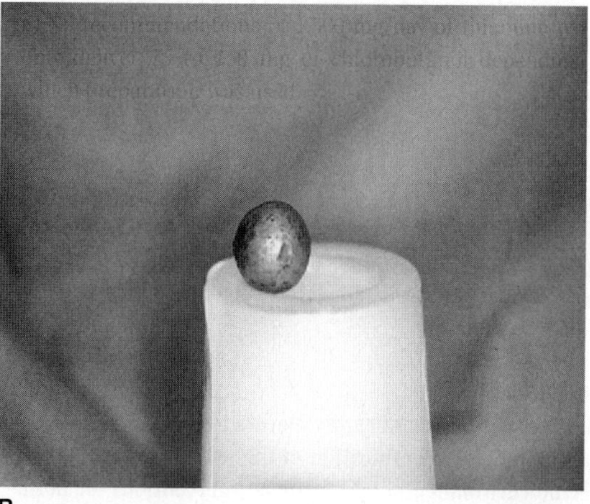
B

**FIGURE 66–6.** An unusual source of lead poisoning. (**A**) Radiograph of the abdomen reveals (↑) ingested metallic foreign body. (**B**) The ingested foreign body was a Civil War–era musketball from the collection of the patient's father. *(Used with permission from Evaline Alessandrini, MD, Division of Emergency Medicine, Children's Hospital of Philadelphia, Philadelphia, PA.)*

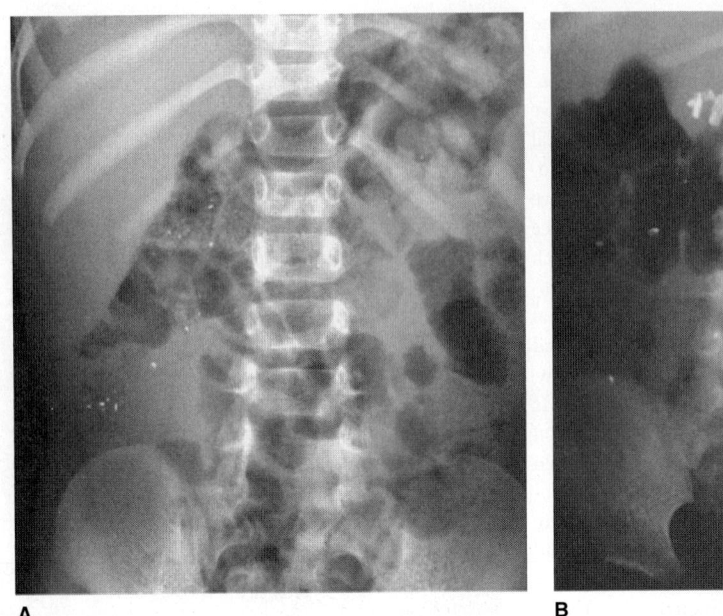
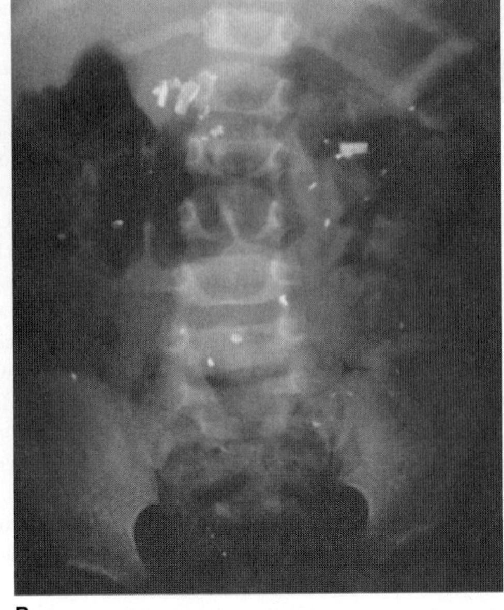

A B

**FIGURE 66–7.** Different appearances of lead-containing paint chips as seen on abdominal radiography. *(Reproduced with permission from Wells RG. Diagnostic imaging of infants and children. McGraw Hill LLC, 2013.)*

## SCREENING

Screening is an essential public health practice for the prevention of severe plumbism in children, pregnant women, and other adults from high-risk settings. Table 66–5 outlines the US CDC pediatric guidelines, which also are endorsed by the American Academy of Pediatrics and by us as well. Table 66–6A summarizes the Occupational Safety and Health Administration (OSHA) mandated action blood lead concentration values for worker notification, removal, and reinstatement. An expert panel convened by the Association of Occupational and Environmental Clinics (AOEC) published an alternative set of health-based management recommendations for lead-exposed workers, which we support (Table 66–6B).

## MANAGEMENT

The most important aspect of treatment is removal from further exposure to lead. In children for whom some residual lead exposure potentially continues, optimization of nutritional status is vital in order to minimize absorption. Unfortunately, although pharmacologic therapy with chelators is the mainstay of therapy for symptomatic patients, it is an inexact science.

### Decreasing Exposure

All patients with significantly elevated blood lead concentrations warrant identification of the lead exposure source, specific environmental and medical interventions, or both. In adults, this usually involves worksite changes. Remedial actions include improvements in ventilation, modification of personal hygiene habits, and optimal use of respiratory apparatus. It is vital to prohibit smoking, eating, and drinking in a lead-exposed work area. Work clothes should be changed after each shift and should not be placed in a locker together with street clothes. In patients with plumbism or consequential elevated blood lead concentrations believed due to retained bullets, surgical removal of this lead source is recommended when anatomically feasible. Table 66–7 also summarizes several specific educational guidelines that should be offered to parents of lead-exposed children.

Occasionally, children require urgent GI decontamination to reduce ongoing acute lead exposure. We recommend the prompt institution of whole-bowel irrigation (WBI) for those patients with large burdens of lead paint chips (Fig. 66–7) (Antidotes in Brief: A2). When children ingest solid lead foreign bodies, such as fishing sinkers, bullets, or curtain weights, we recommend prompt endoscopic removal when anatomically feasible. For foreign bodies in the small bowel, a trial of WBI is reasonable but has not been uniformly successful. Surgical removal is recommended for such foreign bodies if there is delayed passage, failure of WBI, or rapid elevations in blood lead concentrations.

### Chelation Therapy

Decisions about chelation are often complex, and consultation with experts is recommended. In brief, the indications for and specifics of chelation therapy are determined by the age of the patient, the blood lead concentration, and clinical symptoms (Table 66–8). Three chelators are currently recommended for the treatment of lead poisoning: dimercaprol (Antidotes in Brief: A28) and edetate calcium disodium ($CaNa_2EDTA$) (Antidotes in Brief: A30), which are used parenterally for more severe cases, and oral succimer (Antidotes in Brief: A29).

**TABLE 66–5 Pediatric Screening and Follow-Up Guidelines**

*Screening*

1. Screening is recommended for all children who are Medicaid eligible at age 1 and 2 years (and those ages 3–6 years who have not been screened previously). Children who may not be Medicaid eligible but whose families participate in any poverty assistance program should also be screened.
2. Certain local health departments (eg, New York, Chicago, and Philadelphia) recommend screening at younger ages or more frequently. Such recommendations include starting at age 6–9 months, testing every 6 months for children younger than 2 years, and provision of additional education and more rapid follow-up testing for children younger than 12 months whose blood lead concentrations are 6–9 μg/dL.
3. In addition, children who are not Medicaid eligible but are designated high-risk by their state or local health departments should be screened as per these local policies.[a]
4. For children who are neither Medicaid eligible nor live in areas with locale-specific health department guidelines, recommendations are less clear. The AAP supports universal screening of such children as well.[b]
5. Recent immigrants, refugees, or international adoptee children should be screened on arrival to the US.

*Follow-Up*

| *Blood Lead Concentration (μg/dL)* | *Recommended Action and Confirmatory Testing Schedule* |
|---|---|
| < 3.5 | Retest in 1 year, or more frequently if at high risk for lead exposurec; anticipatory guidance |
| 3.5–9 | Confirmatory testing within 3 months; education, environmental history, nutritional counseling and assess for iron deficiency, developmental assessment; report to local health department, environmental investigation of the home[6] |
| 10–19 | Confirmatory testing within 1 month; perform steps as described above for blood lead concentrations 3.5–9 μg/dL |
| 20–44 | Confirmatory testing within 2 weeks; perform steps as described above for blood lead concentrations 3.5–9 μg/dL; clinical evaluation, refer to lead hazard reduction program; consider abdominal radiograph, obtain iron studies and hemoglobin/hematocrit[30]; contact the Poison Control Center or a Pediatric Environmental Health Specialty Unit (PEHSU) for guidance |
| 45–69 | Confirmatory testing within 48 hours; perform steps as described above for blood lead concentrations 20–44 μg/dL; clinical evaluation and case management within 48 hours; consider admitting patient to the hospital if symptomatic, the home is not lead-safe, and/or there is potential for further lead exposure; chelation therapy[6,19] |
| ≥ 70 | Hospitalize child; perform steps as described above; immediate chelation therapy |

[a]Many relevant state and city health department contacts may be located at: http://www.cdc.gov/nceh/lead/about/program.htm. [b]The 1997 CDC guidance allowed for targeted screening of some children of low-risk geographic and demographic background based on a personal risk questionnaire. A listing of potential risk factors is instructive and is summarized here. [c]Screening was recommended if a child had any of the following high-risk factors:

*Housing:* Lives in or regularly visits a home built before 1960; lives in or regularly visits a home built before 1978 undergoing remodeling or renovation (or renovated within 6 months).

*Medical history:* Pica for paint chips or dirt; iron deficiency.

*Personal, family, and social history:* Personal, family, or playmate history of lead poisoning; parental occupational, industrial, hobby exposures; live in proximity to major roadway; use of hot tap water for consumption; use of complementary remedies, cosmetics, ceramic food containers; trips or residence outside US; parents are migrant farm workers, receive poverty assistance.

Educational interventions as per **Table 66–7**.

Chelation therapy as per **Table 66–8**.

AAP = American Academy of Pediatrics; CDC = Centers for Disease Control and Prevention.

**TABLE 66–6A Occupational Safety and Health Administration General Industry[a] Standards for Various Blood Lead Concentrations**

| *Number of Tests* | *Blood Lead Concentration (μg/dL)* | *Action Required* |
|---|---|---|
| 1 | ≥ 40 | Notification of worker in writing; medical examination of worker and consultation |
| 3 (average) | ≥ 50 | Removal of worker from job with potential lead exposure |
| 1 | ≥ 60 | Removal of worker from job with potential lead exposure |
| 2 | < 40 | Reinstatement of worker in job with potential lead exposure |

[a]The construction industry standard is similar for worker notification (at 40 μg/dL) and reinstatement (< 40 μg/dL twice) but requires worker removal for a single value ≥ 50 μg/dL.

Data from US Department of Labor, Occupational Safety and Health Administration: Medical Surveillance Guidelines—1910.1025 App C.

http://www.osha.gov/pls/oshaweb/owadisp.show_document?p_table=STANDARDS&p_id=10033 and US Department of Labor, Occupational Safety and Health Administration: Medical Surveillance Guidelines. Lead—1926.

## Children

Lead encephalopathy is an acute life-threatening emergency and should be treated under the guidance of a multidisciplinary team in the intensive care unit of a hospital experienced in the management of critically ill children. The recommended treatment for encephalopathy is combination parenteral chelation therapy with maximum-dose dimercaprol and $CaNa_2EDTA$ along with meticulous supportive care. Dimercaprol is always given first to reduce the

**TABLE 66–6B Health-Based Occupational Surveillance Recommendations[a]**

| *Blood Lead Concentration (μg/dL)* | *Recommendation* |
|---|---|
| < 10 | Check every month for 3 months and then every 6 months (unless exposure increases); if blood lead concentration increases > 4 μg/dL, exposure evaluation or reduction effort; exposure evaluation or reduction if blood lead concentration 5–9 μg/dL for women who are or may become pregnant |
| 10–19 | As for blood lead concentration < 10 μg/dL and check every 3 months; exposure evaluation and reduction effort; consider removal if no improvement with exposure reduction or complicating medical condition;[b] resume check every 6 months if 3 blood level concentrations < 10 μg/dL |
| ≥ 19 | Remove from exposure if blood lead concentration > 30 μg/dL or repeat blood lead concentration in 4 weeks; check every month; consider return to work after blood lead concentration < 15 μg/dL twice |

[a]All potentially lead-exposed workers warrant preemployment clinical evaluation, baseline blood lead concentration, and serum creatinine concentration. [b]Such conditions include chronic kidney disease, hypertension, neurologic disorders, and cognitive dysfunction.

Data from Kosnett MJ, Wedeen RP, Rothenberg SJ, et al. Recommendations for medical management of adult lead exposure. *Environ Health Perspect*. 2007;115(3):463-471.

**TABLE 66–7 Evaluation and Management of Patients With Lead Exposure**

| |
|---|
| **Adults** |
| Implement careful lead exposure monitoring (Table 66–6A and 6B) |
| Improve ventilation |
| Use a respiratory protective apparatus |
| Wear protective clothing; change from work clothes before leaving worksite |
| Modify personal hygiene habits |
| Prohibit eating, drinking, and smoking at the worksite |
| Evaluate possible sources beyond occupational setting (Tables 66–1 and 66–2) |
| **Children** |
| Notify the local health department to initiate home inspection and abatement as needed |
| Home lead paint abatement (professional contractors if possible; use plastic sheeting, low dust-generating paint removal; replacement of lead-painted windows, floor treatment; final cleanup with high-efficiency particle air vacuum, wet mopping) |
| Avoid most hazardous areas of the home and yard |
| Dust control: Wet mopping, sponging with high-phosphate detergent; frequent hand, toy, and pacifier washing |
| Soil lead exposure reduction by planting grass and shrubs around the house |
| Use only cold, flushed tap water for consumption |
| Optimize nutrition to reduce lead absorption: avoid fasting; give an iron-, calcium-, vitamin C–sufficient diet; supplement iron and calcium as necessary |
| Avoid food storage in open cans |
| Avoid imported ceramic containers for food and beverage use |
| Evaluate parental occupations and hobbies and eliminate high-risk activity |
| Evaluate possible sources beyond lead paint exposure (Tables 66–1 and 66–2) |

CNS burden of lead. Cerebral edema should be managed in a standard fashion.

The presence of radiopaque material in the GI tract on radiography has raised concern that parenteral chelation might enhance absorption of residual gut lead. This issue is not settled fully, but we recommend the initiation of parenteral chelation without delay in seriously symptomatic patients. Careful provision of adequate IV fluids optimizes kidney function while avoiding overhydration and the risk of exacerbating cerebral edema. The occurrence of the syndrome of inappropriate secretion of antidiuretic hormone (SIADH) is associated with lead encephalopathy, so urine volume, urine osmolarity, specific gravity, and serum electrolytes should be closely monitored, especially as fluids are gradually liberalized with clinical improvement.

Chelation regimens for less severe manifestations of lead poisoning and asymptomatic children with elevated lead concentrations are summarized in Table 66–8. When dimercaprol is unavailable, succimer plus $CaNa_2EDTA$, or even succimer alone in resource-limited locales, is reasonable. After initial chelation therapy, decisions to repeat treatment are based on clinical symptoms and follow-up blood lead concentrations. For patients with encephalopathy or any severe symptoms or with an initial blood lead concentration greater than 100 μg/dL, we recommend repeated courses of treatment. It is reasonable that at least 2 days elapse before restarting chelation. A third course of chelation is rarely necessary sooner than 5 to 7 days after the second course ends.

## Adults

***General Considerations.*** The first principle in the treatment of adults with lead poisoning is that chelation therapy is not a substitute for adherence to OSHA lead standards at the worksite and should never be given prophylactically. Table 66–8 outlines recommended chelation therapy regimens for adults. For encephalopathic adult patients, we recommend combined dimercaprol and $CaNa_2EDTA$ therapy, just as for children. Recent reports support the use of succimer in adult patients with mild to moderate plumbism after environmental and occupational remedies are instituted. Chelation therapy using similar clinical and blood lead concentration–based guidelines is recommended in the perioperative period for patients undergoing surgical removal of retained bullets or débridement of adjacent lead-contaminated tissue. Treatment of patients with acute TEL toxicity is largely supportive, with sedation as necessary. For patients evaluated soon after a large-volume ingestion, nasogastric suction is recommended with airway protection performed as needed. In general, chelation therapy for TEL toxicity is associated with enhanced lead excretion but has not been found to be clinically efficacious. However, for symptomatic, especially encephalopathic, patients (in whom there may be a significant component of metabolically derived inorganic lead toxicity) or those with very elevated blood lead concentrations, we do recommend chelation therapy.

## Pregnancy, Neonatal, and Lactation Issues

Lead freely passes the placental barrier and accumulates in the fetus throughout gestation. Maternal bone stores are also a potential endogenous source of elevated blood lead concentrations in pregnancy and contribute to modest increases in blood lead concentration during the third trimester, particularly in women with low calcium intake. Screening should be conducted at prenatal visits and blood lead concentration obtained if any concern arises. In general, any pregnant woman with a blood lead concentration of greater than 5 μg/dL requires close follow-up testing, along with careful environmental and occupational exposure investigation and nutritional counseling. Appropriate calcium intake (2,000 mg/day) through adequate diet or supplementation should be ensured because its use is associated with decreased bone resorption during pregnancy, which likely lessens fetal lead exposure. Adequate maternal iron intake is also associated with lower neonatal blood lead concentration. Women with blood lead concentrations greater than 10 μg/dL should be reported to the lead poisoning program of the local health department, and if an occupational source is suspected, a consult to an occupational medicine specialist should be obtained. Pregnant patients with blood lead concentrations greater than 45 μg/dL should undergo medical toxicology and high-risk pregnancy consultation.

Chelation therapy during early pregnancy poses theoretical problems of teratogenicity, particularly that caused by enhanced excretion of potentially vital trace elements, or translocation of lead from mother to fetus (Antidotes in Brief: A28, A29, and A30). In general, there currently seems

**TABLE 66–8 Chelation Therapy Guidelines for Initial Course of Treatment[a]**

| *Condition, Blood Lead Concentration (μg/dL)* | *Dose* | *Regimen/Comments* |
|---|---|---|
| **Adults** | | |
| Encephalopathy | Dimercaprol 450 mg/m²/day[a,b] and | 75 mg/m² IM every 4 hours for 5 days |
| | $CaNa_2EDTA$ 1,000–1,500 mg/m²/day[a] | Continuous infusion or 2–4 divided IV doses for 5 days (start 4 hours after dimercaprol) |
| Symptoms suggestive of encephalopathy or > 100 | Dimercaprol 300–450 mg/m²/day[a,b] and | 50–75 mg/m² IM every 4 hours for 3–5 days (base dose, duration on blood lead concentration, severity of symptoms; see text) |
| | $CaNa_2EDTA$ 1,500 mg/m²/day[a] | Continuous infusion or 2–4 divided IV doses for 5 days (start 4 hours after dimercaprol) |
| | | Lab: Baseline CT scan; CBC, $Ca^{2+}$, blood lead concentration, BUN, Cr, LFTs, U/A; repeat CBC, $Ca^{2+}$, BUN, Cr, LFTs, U/A daily; blood lead concentration on days 3 and 5 |
| Mild symptoms or 70–100 | Succimer 700–1,050 mg/m²/day | 350 mg/m² 3 times per day orally for 5 days, then twice per day for 14 days. Remove from exposure (Table 66–7) |
| | | Lab: CBC, blood lead concentration, BUN, Cr, LFTs, U/A; repeat CBC, LFTs, blood lead concentration on days 7 and 21 |
| Asymptomatic and < 70 | Usually not indicated | – |
| **Children** | | |
| Encephalopathy | Dimercaprol 450 mg/m²/day[a] and | 75 mg/m² IM every 4 hours for 5 days |
| | $CaNa_2EDTA$ 1,500 mg/m²/day[a] | Continuous infusion or 2–4 divided IV doses for 5 days (start 4 hours after dimercaprol) |
| | | Lab: Baseline AXR, CT scan, CBC, $Ca^{2+}$, $Na^{+}$, blood lead concentration, BUN, Cr, LFTs, U/A; repeat CBC, $Ca^{2+}$, $Na^{+}$, BUN, Cr, LFTs, U/A daily; blood lead concentration on days 3 and 5 |
| Symptomatic (without encephalopathy) or > 69 | Dimercaprol 300–450 mg/m²/day[a] and | 50–75 mg/m² IM every 4 hours for 3–5 days (base dose, duration on blood lead concentration, severity of symptoms; see text) |
| | $CaNa_2EDTA$ 1,000–1,500 mg/m²/day[a] | Continuous infusion or 2–4 divided IV doses for 5 days (start 4 hours after dimercaprol) |
| | | Lab: Baseline AXR, CBC, $Ca^{2+}$, blood lead concentration, BUN, Cr, LFTs, U/A; repeat CBC, $Ca^{2+}$, BUN, Cr, LFTs, U/A on days 3 and 5 and blood lead concentration day 5 |
| Asymptomatic: 45–69 | Succimer 700–1,050 mg/m²/day[a] or | 350 mg/m² 3 times per day orally for 5 days and then twice per day for 14 days |
| | | Lab: Baseline AXR, CBC, blood lead concentration, LFTs; repeat CBC, LFTs, blood lead concentration days 7 and 21 |
| | $CaNa_2EDTA$, 1,000 mg/m²/day[a] | Continuous infusion or 2–4 divided IV doses for 5 days (see text) |
| | | Lab: Baseline AXR, CBC, $Ca^{2+}$, blood lead concentration, BUN, Cr, LFTs, U/A; repeat $Ca^{2+}$, BUN, Cr, LFTs, U/A on days 3 and 5 and blood lead concentration on day 5 |
| 20–44 | Routine chelation not indicated (see text) | If succimer used, same regimen as per above group (Table 66–7) |
| < 20 | Chelation not indicated | (Table 66–7) |

[a]Subsequent treatment regimens should be based on post-chelation blood lead concentration and clinical symptoms (see text). Approximate equivalent doses are expressed in milligrams per kilogram of body weight: dimercaprol 450 mg/m²/day (~24 mg/kg/day); 300 mg/m²/day (~18 mg/kg/day). $CaNa_2EDTA$ 1,000 mg/m²/day (~25–50 mg/kg/day); 1,500 mg/m²/day (~50–75 mg/kg/day); adult maximum dose 2–3 g/day; succimer 350 mg/m² (~10 mg/kg). [b]Some clinicians recommend $CaNa_2EDTA$ alone in these contexts (see text).

AXR = abdominal radiography; BUN = blood urea nitrogen; Ca = calcium; $CaNa_2EDTA$ = edetate calcium disodium; CBC = complete blood count; Cr = creatinine, CT scan = computed tomography scan of the brain; IM = intramuscular; IV = intravenous; Lab = suggested laboratory and radiologic evaluation; LFTs = hepatic aminotransferases; U/A = urinalysis with microscopy (frequent monitoring of urine dipstick analysis for hematuria and proteinuria also advised during $CaNa_2EDTA$ therapy).

to be little support for routine chelation therapy in asymptomatic pregnant women with only moderate increases in blood lead concentration (eg, < 45 μg/dL), particularly during the first-trimester period of fetal organogenesis. Symptomatic women and those with blood lead concentrations greater than or equal to 70 μg/dL should undergo chelation, regardless of trimester. For pregnant patients whose blood lead concentrations are 45 to 69 μg/dL, medical toxicology and high-risk obstetric consultations are recommended, as well as for women with lower blood lead concentrations for whom substantial questions exist about the source of lead exposure or for whom blood lead concentrations are rising significantly during their pregnancy on follow-up testing.

Postnatally, infant blood lead concentrations usually decline over time without chelation, but this occurs very slowly, and the course is variable. Thus, postpartum chelation therapy should be conducted for neonates, according to blood lead concentrations, as per the guidelines described above for older children. For overtly symptomatic neonates or those with extremely elevated blood lead concentrations, both chelation therapy and exchange transfusion are reasonable treatment modalities. Lastly, breast milk from heavily exposed mothers is a potential source of lead exposure. For mothers with blood lead concentrations of less than or equal to 40 μg/dL, breastfeeding should be encouraged with close follow-up of maternal and infant blood lead concentrations (Table 66–9). We also recommend maternal calcium supplementation (1,200 mg/day of elemental calcium as calcium carbonate), a simple intervention that reduces breast milk lead content by 5% to 10%.

**TABLE 66–9 Summary of Guidelines for Breastfeeding With Perinatal Lead Exposure[a]**

**Recommendations for Initiation of Breastfeeding[b]**

- Measurement of concentrations of lead in breast milk is not recommended.
- Mothers with blood lead concentrations < 40 μg/dL should breastfeed if there are no other contraindications. Mothers should supplement their diets with calcium.
- Mothers with confirmed blood lead concentrations ≥ 40 μg/dL should begin breastfeeding when their blood lead concentrations drop below 40 μg/dL. Until then, they should pump and discard their breast milk *(chelation therapy of mother with blood lead concentration ≥ 45 μg/dL is reasonable[b])*
- These recommendations are likely not appropriate in countries where infant mortality from infectious diseases is high.

**Recommendations for Continuation of Breastfeeding[b]**

- Breastfeeding should continue for infants with blood level concentrations below 5 μg/dL.
- Infants born to mothers with blood lead concentration ≥ 5 μg/dL but < 40 μg/dL can continue to breastfeed unless there are indications that the breast milk is contributing to elevating blood lead concentrations. These infants should have blood lead concentration tests at birth and be followed according to the following schedule:

  Infant blood lead concentration 5–24 μg/dL: Follow-up test, within 1 month *(we recommend at 1 and 3 weeks until trend established)[b]*

  Infant blood lead concentration 25–44 μg/dL: Follow-up blood lead concentration within 2 weeks *(we recommend at 1 week, then weekly during first month)[b]*

  Infant blood lead concentration ≥ 45 μg/dL: Follow-up test within 24 hours and then frequently *(also see above if maternal blood lead concentrations > 40 μg/dL)[b]*

For infants whose blood lead concentrations are rising or failing to decline by 5 μg/dL or more, environmental and other sources of lead exposure should be evaluated. If no external source is identified, and maternal blood lead concentrations are > 20 μg/dL and infant blood lead concentration is ≥ 5 μg/dL, then breast milk should be suspected as the source, and breastfeeding should be temporarily interrupted until maternal blood lead concentrations decline.[b]

[a]Data from Centers for Disease Control and Prevention. Guidelines for the identification and management of lead exposure in pregnant and lactating women. http://www.cdc.gov/nceh/lead/publications/LeadandPregnancy2010.pdf. Published 2010. Comments in italics are the opinions of the authors. It should be noted that these guidelines were developed at a time when the CDC threshold of concern for infant blood lead concentration was 10 μg/dL. In light of the new lowered threshold to 5 μg/dL, more conservative guidelines may be developed in the foreseeable future. [b]Owing to the complexity of these cases and varied data regarding the contribution of maternal blood lead concentration and breast milk to infant exposure and clinical effects, pediatric toxicology consultation is advised to assist with risk assessment, interpretation, and management.

Antidotes in Brief

# A29 SUCCIMER (2,3-DIMERCAPTOSUCCINIC ACID) AND DMPS (2,3-DIMERCAPTO-1-PROPANESULFONIC ACID)

## INTRODUCTION

Succimer is an orally active metal chelator that is approved by the United States (US) Food and Drug Administration (FDA) for the treatment of lead poisoning in children with blood lead concentrations greater than 45 μg/dL (2.17 μmol/L). Succimer is also used to treat patients poisoned with arsenic, cadmium, and mercury. Succimer has a wider therapeutic index and exhibits many advantages over dimercaprol and calcium disodium ethylenediaminetetraacetic acid ($CaNa_2EDTA$).

## HISTORY

Succimer was initially synthesized in 1949 in England. Chinese investigators subsequently demonstrated the ability of succimer to increase the 50% lethal dose ($LD_{50}$) of tartar emetic in mice (Chap. 58). An early review of the Chinese experience with intravenous (IV) succimer for occupational lead and mercury poisoning suggested efficacy similar to IV $CaNa_2EDTA$ and to intramuscular (IM) DMPS (racemic-2,3-dimercapto-1-propanesulfonic acid) for mercury. The US FDA approved succimer for the treatment of lead-poisoned children in 1991.

2,3-Dimercapto-1-propanesulfonic acid (DMPS) has been used in the Soviet Union since the late 1950s and continues to be used in Russia and Eastern Europe. In the US, DMPS is an investigational drug.

## PHARMACOLOGY

### Chemistry

Succimer is the highly polar and water-soluble analog of 2,3-dimercapto propanol (dimercaprol).

### Related Chelators

Racemic-2,3-dimercapto-1-propanesulfonic acid (DMPS) is a chelator that, like succimer, is another water-soluble analog of dimercaprol. A dose of 15 mg/kg of DMPS is equimolar to 12 mg/kg of succimer but is infrequently used in the US because of a risk of developing Stevens-Johnson syndrome.

### Mechanisms of Action

Lead and cadmium bind to the adjoining sulfur and oxygen atoms, whereas arsenic and mercury bind to the two sulfur moieties, forming pH-dependent water-soluble complexes (Fig. A29–1).

## PHARMACOKINETICS AND PHARMACODYNAMICS

Succimer is highly protein bound to albumin and is eliminated almost exclusively via the kidney. Only approximately 20% of the administered oral dose is recovered in the urine, presumably reflecting the low bioavailability of the drug. Following oral administration, succimer is rapidly and extensively metabolized primarily to a mixed disulfide with two molecules of l-cysteine to one molecule of succimer.

The use of succimer in both children and adults with chronic lead poisoning demonstrates consistent findings. During the first 5 days of succimer chelation (1,050 mg/m$^2$/day in children and 30 mg/kg/day in adults, both in three divided doses), the blood lead concentration rapidly dropped by approximately 60% to 70%. This blood lead concentration remained unchanged during the next 14 to 23 days of continued therapy. Increases in urinary lead excretion are concurrent with the reduction in blood lead concentration, with maximal excretion occurring on day 1. Typically, 2 weeks after the completion of succimer, the blood lead concentration rebounds to values 20% to 40% lower than pretreatment values.

## ROLE IN LEAD POISONING

In animals, succimer prevents the deleterious effect of lead on heme synthesis, blood pressure, and behavior. The 2001 Treatment of Lead-Exposed Children (TLC) trial compared succimer to placebo in children with lead concentrations between 20 and 44 μg/dL (0.97–1.93 μmol/L). The largest reduction in blood lead occurred within the first week of therapy with succimer and then rebounded somewhat. However, at the end of 1 year, there was no difference in the blood lead concentrations and no difference in test scores on cognition, behavior, or neuropsychological function between the two groups.

## ROLE IN LEAD ENCEPHALOPATHY

The experience with succimer in severely lead-poisoned patients, including those with encephalopathy, is limited to case studies and a large retrospective analysis. Three children with mean blood lead concentrations higher than 70 μg/dL (3.38 μmol/L) who were treated with 5 days of succimer achieved comparable declines in blood lead concentration to two similar children who had been treated previously with a combination of dimercaprol for 3 days and $CaNa_2EDTA$ for 5 days. Three adult patients with encephalopathy achieved significant improvement following succimer chelation. A retrospective analysis was performed of more than 3,000

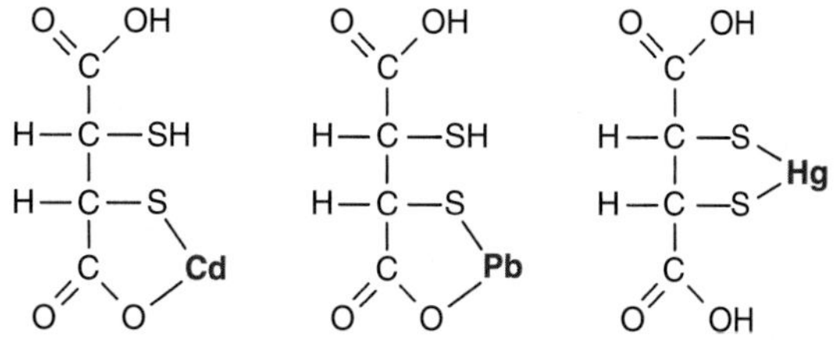

O OH C H—C—SH H—C—S Cd C O O | O OH C H—C—SH H—C—S Pb C O O | O OH C H—C—S H—C—S Hg C O OH

**FIGURE A29–1.** The chelation of cadmium, lead, and mercury with succimer.

children with moderate to severe lead poisoning in Nigeria who were treated with succimer alone. About one-third of the children had lead concentrations greater than 80 μg/dL (3.86 μmol/L), 6% had concentrations greater than 120 μg/dL (5.79 μmol/L), and 24 had lead encephalopathy. Treatment in children with a blood lead concentration greater than 120 μg/dL (5.79 μmol/L) resulted in a 68% reduction. In the 3 months before the institution of succimer, there were 400 fatalities attributed to lead compared with 6 deaths during the 13 months during which succimer was used.

## ROLE IN ARSENIC POISONING

Succimer has been used for arsenic toxicity in China and the Soviet Union since 1965. Animal studies with sodium arsenite and lewisite demonstrate the ability of succimer to improve the $LD_{50}$ with a good therapeutic index, lack of redistribution of arsenic to the brain as compared to dimercaprol, and reduced kidney and liver arsenic concentrations. A comparison of dimercaprol, succimer, and DMPS as arsenic antidotes demonstrated higher therapeutic indices for succimer and DMPS over dimercaprol in patients with chronic arsenic poisoning.

## ROLE IN MERCURY POISONING

Succimer enhances the elimination of mercury and has been used to treat patients poisoned with inorganic, elemental, and methylmercury. It improves survival, decreases kidney damage, and enhances the elimination of mercury in animals following exposure to inorganic mercury and methylmercury. However, one study in mice subjected to intraperitoneal mercuric chloride demonstrated an enhanced deposition of mercury in motor neurons following chelation with succimer or DMPS. Of 53 construction workers who were exposed to mercury vapor, 11 received succimer and *N*-acetyl-D,L-penicillamine in a crossover study. Mercury elimination was increased during the period of succimer administration compared with the period of *N*-acetyl-D,L-penicillamine administration. When succimer was given to victims of an extensive Iraqi methylmercury exposure, blood methylmercury half-life decreased from 63 days to 10 days.

## ADVERSE EFFECTS AND SAFETY ISSUES

Succimer is generally well tolerated, with few serious adverse events reported. Commonly reported adverse effects include nausea, vomiting, flatus, diarrhea, and a metallic taste in 10% to 20% of patients. Mild elevations in aspartate aminotransferase (AST) and alanine aminotransferase (ALT) are reported.

In the Nigeria experience, ALT did not exceed 500 U/L and no hepatic failure was noted. Rarely, chills, fever, urticaria, reversible neutropenia, and eosinophilia are reported. Because neutropenia was observed in some patients taking succimer and because bone marrow effects are reported with other drugs in the same chemical class, we recommend a complete blood count with a differential and a platelet count before initiating treatment and weekly during treatment. Therapy should be discontinued if the absolute neutrophil count drops to less than 1,200/μL. A number of studies with succimer demonstrate no rise in urinary zinc, copper, iron, or calcium elimination. An obvious limitation concerning the safety of succimer is that there is still relatively limited clinical experience with the drug, particularly with regard to administration longer than the standard 19-day protocol.

One concern with administering succimer orally is that outpatient management might permit continued unintentional lead exposure and the possibility for succimer-facilitated lead absorption. A radiolabeled lead tracer administered to adult volunteers suggested that succimer increased the net absorption of lead from the gastrointestinal tract and may distribute it to other tissues. Two children with environmental exposure to lead had dramatic rises in blood lead concentrations while receiving succimer at home. In the event of unintentional exposure to a new lead source, decontamination of the gastrointestinal tract should complement (or even precede) oral succimer. A case report describes a 3-year-old patient who reportedly ingested 185 mg/kg of succimer and remained asymptomatic.

## PREGNANCY AND LACTATION

Succimer is US FDA Pregnancy Category C. There was a dose-dependent effect of succimer on early and late fetal resorption and on fetal body weight and length when succimer was administered to pregnant mice during organogenesis. Large doses of succimer administered to pregnant mice during organogenesis are teratogenic and fetotoxic. The use of succimer during pregnancy should only be undertaken if the potential benefit to the mother justifies the potential risk to the fetus. It is not known whether succimer is excreted in human milk, but breastfeeding is a contraindication in some sources and is discouraged in the package insert. However, the US Centers for Disease Control and Prevention (CDC) guidelines for the identification and management of lead exposure in pregnant and breastfeeding women, the CDC suggests allowing breastfeeding for mothers with blood lead concentrations of less than or equal to 40 μg/dL (1.93 μmol/L). Mothers with blood lead concentrations of greater than 40 μg/dL are encouraged to pump and discard their breast milk until their blood lead concentrations are reduced to less than 40 μg/dL.

## COMBINED CHELATION THERAPY

Succimer can be combined with $CaNa_2EDTA$ to take advantage of the ability of succimer to remove lead from soft tissues, including the brain, while capitalizing on the ability of $CaNa_2EDTA$ to mobilize lead from bone. This combination is recommended in patients in whom dimercaprol would be indicated but is not available. A retrospective review comparing dimercaprol plus $CaNa_2EDTA$ to succimer plus $CaNa_2EDTA$ in children with blood lead concentrations greater than 45 μg/mL (> 2.17 μmol/L) demonstrated a similar reduction in blood lead concentrations. The succimer plus $CaNa_2EDTA$ combination was better tolerated.

## DOSING AND ADMINISTRATION

The recommended dosage is 350 mg/$m^2$ in children, 3 times a day for 5 days, followed by 350 mg/$m^2$ twice a day for 14 days. In adults, the recommended dosage is 10 mg/kg 3 times a day for

5 days followed by 10 mg/kg twice a day for 14 days. Repeated courses may be needed depending on the blood lead concentration. However, a minimum of 2 weeks between courses is recommended unless blood lead concentrations are initially greater than 100 μg/dL (4.83 μmol/L) or the patient has lead encephalopathy. For patients who cannot swallow the capsule, it can be separated immediately prior to use and the contents sprinkled into a small amount of juice or on apple sauce, ice cream, or any soft food, or placed on a spoon and followed by a fruit drink.

## FORMULATION AND ACQUISITION

Succimer is available as 100-mg bead-filled capsules.

Antidotes in Brief

# A30 EDETATE CALCIUM DISODIUM ($CaNa_2EDTA$)

## INTRODUCTION

Edetate calcium disodium ($CaNa_2EDTA$) is a chelator that is primarily used for patients with severe lead poisoning in conjunction with dimercaprol. In a clinical trial, disodium EDTA ($Na_2EDTA$) reduced adverse cardiovascular outcomes in patients with a history of myocardial infarction. We recommend against using $Na_2EDTA$ for chelation because of the potential for life-threatening hypocalcemia.

## HISTORY

Ethylenediaminetetraacetic acid (EDTA) was discovered and synthesized in the 1930s and approved by the United States (US) Food and Drug Administration (FDA) as a food additive in the 1940s. Investigations on $CaNa_2EDTA$ for lead toxicity began in the 1950s.

## PHARMACOLOGY

### Chemistry

Edetate calcium disodium is an ionic, water-soluble compound that is also referred to as calcium disodium versenate, calcium disodium EDTA, or calcium disodium ethylenediaminetetraacetic acid.

### Mechanism of Action

Edetate calcium disodium ($CaNa_2EDTA$) is capable of chelating many metals, although it is currently used almost exclusively in the management of patients with lead poisoning. When $CaNa_2EDTA$ chelates lead, the calcium in the chelator is displaced by lead, forming a stable-ring compound that is eliminated in the urine.

## PHARMACOKINETICS AND PHARMACODYNAMICS

Edetate calcium disodium has a small volume of distribution (0.05–0.23 L/kg) that approximates the extracellular fluid compartment. It penetrates erythrocytes poorly, and less than 5% gains access to the spinal fluid. The half-life is about 20 to 60 minutes, and renal elimination approximates the glomerular filtration rate. As a result, 50% of a given dose of $CaNa_2EDTA$ is excreted in the urine in 1 hour and more than 95% is excreted in 24 hours. Following $CaNa_2EDTA$ administration, urinary lead excretion is increased 20- to 50-fold in the form of a stable, soluble, nonionized compound.

## ROLE IN LEAD EXPOSURE

### Animals

In animals, although $CaNa_2EDTA$ decreases tissue lead stores, it transiently increases brain lead concentrations. Additional doses are then able to enhance lead elimination, reduce blood lead concentrations, and subsequently reduce brain lead concentrations. This offers an explanation as to why some human case reports demonstrate worsening lead encephalopathy when $CaNa_2EDTA$ is used without antecedent initiation of dimercaprol therapy.

### Humans

The $CaNa_2EDTA$ mobilization test was once widely recommend as a diagnostic aid for assessing the potential benefits of chelation therapy. Currently, it is considered obsolete and is no longer recommended. In humans, $CaNa_2EDTA$ reduces blood lead concentrations, enhances renal excretion of lead, and reverses the effects of lead on hemoglobin synthesis. With chronic lead exposure, blood lead concentrations rebound considerably days to weeks following the cessation of $CaNa_2EDTA$. Although $CaNa_2EDTA$ has been used clinically since the 1970s, no rigorous clinical studies have ever been performed to evaluate whether $CaNa_2EDTA$ is capable of reversing the neurobehavioral effects of lead. Based on the treatment of over 3,000 patients in an outbreak in Nigeria, succimer has become the chelator of choice in lead-poisoned children without encephalopathy and lead concentration less than 70 μg/dL (3.38 μmol/L) in the US.

## ADVERSE EFFECTS AND SAFETY ISSUES

The principal toxicity of $CaNa_2EDTA$ is related to the metal chelated. When $CaNa_2EDTA$ is given to patients with lead poisoning, renal toxicity results from the release of lead in the kidneys during excretion. Because lead toxicity causes kidney damage independent of chelation, it is important to monitor kidney function closely during $CaNa_2EDTA$ administration and to adjust the dose and schedule appropriately. Nephrotoxicity is minimized by limiting the total daily dose of $CaNa_2EDTA$ to 1 g in children or 2 g in adults, which limits the daily renal lead release, although higher doses are recommended to treat patients with lead encephalopathy. Continuous infusion seems to increase efficacy and decrease toxicity when compared to intermittent dosing. Other uncommon adverse effects include malaise, fatigue, thirst, chills, fever, myalgia, dermatitis, headache, anorexia, urinary frequency and urgency, sneezing, nasal congestion, lacrimation, glycosuria, anemia, transient hypotension, increased prothrombin time, and inverted T waves on the electrocardiogram. Mild reversible increases in alanine aminotransferase (ALT) and aspartate aminotransferase (AST) (usually less than three times the upper limit of normal) and decreases in alkaline phosphatase are frequently reported. Depletion of endogenous metals, particularly zinc, iron, and manganese, can result from chronic therapy but requires no monitoring with acute dosing used in poisoning.

## PREGNANCY AND LACTATION

Although $CaNa_2EDTA$ is US FDA Pregnancy Category B, there are no adequate and well-controlled studies in pregnant women and a risk-to-benefit analysis must be made prior to use. Lead encephalopathy is life threatening, and chelation should be commenced regardless of the trimester. It is not known whether $CaNa_2EDTA$ is excreted in human milk. The 2010 US Centers for Disease Control and Prevention (CDC) guidelines suggest allowing breastfeeding for mothers with blood lead concentrations of less than or equal to 40 μg/dL. Mothers with higher blood lead concentrations are encouraged to pump and discard their breast milk until their blood lead concentrations drop to less than 40 μg/dL.

## DOSING AND ADMINISTRATION

The dose of $CaNa_2EDTA$ is determined by the patient's body surface area or weight (up to a maximum dose) and the severity of the poisoning and kidney function. For patients with lead encephalopathy, the dose of $CaNa_2EDTA$ is 1,500 $mg/m^2/day$ (approximately 50–75 mg/kg/day) by continuous IV infusion starting 4 hours *after* the first dose of dimercaprol and after an adequate urine flow is established. Concurrent dimercaprol and $CaNa_2EDTA$ therapies are administered for 5 days, followed by a rest period of at least 2 to 4 days, which permits lead redistribution. Careful attention to total fluid requirements in children and patients who have or who are at risk for lead encephalopathy is paramount, as rapid intravenous infusions may increase intracranial pressure and cerebral edema. Dosage adjustments limiting the daily dose to 50 mg/kg (about 1000 $mg/m^2$) are necessary for adults with lead nephropathy, and the following dosage regimen is recommended: 500 $mg/m^2$ every 24 hours for 5 days for patients with a serum creatinine of 2 to 3 mg/dL; every 48 hours for three doses for a serum creatinine of 3 to 4 mg/dL; and one dose for a serum creatinine concentration greater than 4 mg/dL. A blood lead concentration should be measured 1 hour after the $CaNa_2EDTA$ infusion is discontinued to avoid falsely elevated blood lead concentration determinations.

In symptomatic children without manifestations of lead encephalopathy, the dose of $CaNa_2EDTA$ is 1000 $mg/m^2/day$ (approximately 25–50 mg/kg/day) in addition to dimercaprol at 50 $mg/m^2$ every 4 hours. If $CaNa_2EDTA$ is to be administered IM to avoid the use of an IV and fluid overload, then procaine is added to the $CaNa_2EDTA$ in a dose sufficient to produce a final concentration of 0.5%. This can be accomplished by mixing 1 mL of a 1% procaine solution for each milliliter of chelator. The procaine minimizes pain at the injection site.

## COMBINATION THERAPY WITH SUCCIMER

The combination of $CaNa_2EDTA$ with succimer appears more potent than either individual drug in promoting urine and fecal lead excretion and in decreasing blood and liver lead concentrations. However, this approach increases nephrotoxicity and zinc depletion and is not routinely recommended at this time unless dimercaprol is unavailable.

## FORMULATION

Edetate calcium disodium EDTA is available as calcium disodium versenate in 5-mL ampules containing 200 mg of $CaNa_2EDTA$ per milliliter (1 g per ampule).

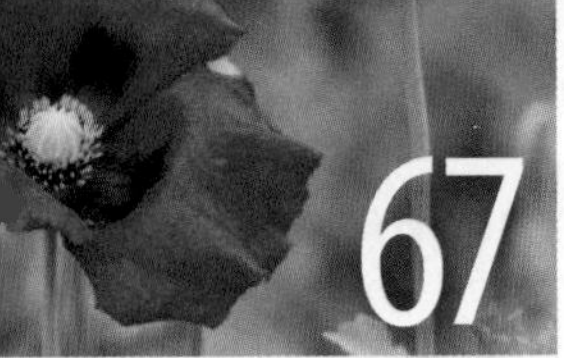

# 67 MANGANESE

Normal concentrations

| | |
|---|---|
| Whole blood | = 4–15 μg/L (72.8–273 nmol/L) |
| Serum | = 0.9–2.9 μg/L (7.3–15.5 nmol/L) |
| Urine | < 10 μg/L (< 182 nmol/L) |

## HISTORY AND EPIDEMIOLOGY

Manganese (Mn) is the 12th most abundant element in the Earth's crust (0.106%). The name manganese derives from *Magnesia*, a prefecture of Thessaly in ancient Greece. Manganese salts are brightly pigmented, and the earliest known uses were artisanal. Adding manganese to iron produces a stronger metal alloy, and by the early 19th century, manganese became an important component in the manufacture of steel. Manganese is used in batteries and glass production, ceramics, fungicides, pesticides, and catalysts.

Most reported cases of manganese toxicity, or manganism, are associated with chronic occupational exposure. Manganism was first described in 1837, when the development of a characteristic neuropsychiatric syndrome in French pyrolusite mill workers was linked with exposure to high concentrations of manganese oxide dusts. Inhalation of inorganic manganese compounds also occurs during smelting, welding, or burning of coal, oil, or fuel containing manganese compounds. A neuropsychiatric syndrome in welders is attributed to the inhalation of manganese oxide fumes. Manganism is also described in several nonoccupational settings. Manganese chloride and manganese sulfate are used as nutritional supplements, and manganese toxicity is well documented in patients receiving excessive dosing in total parenteral nutrition. Also, epidemic manganese toxicity was reported from the use of intravenous psychostimulant drugs such as methcathinone when potassium permanganate was used during synthesis.

Environmental exposure to excessive manganese in drinking water is linked to neurodevelopmental deficiencies in children, including effects on cognition, behavior, memory, and motor function. The potential environmental health risks of methylcyclopentadienyl manganese tricarbonyl (MMT), an antiknock agent added to gasoline as an alternative to lead, are concerning with regard to its contribution to the environmental burden of manganese and to human health.

Permanganates were first discovered to be strong oxidizers in the 18th century. Weak solutions of potassium permanganate 0.01% are still used in medicine as topical drying and antiseptic skin preparations.

## CHEMISTRY

Manganese is a dark-gray, brittle, paramagnetic, transition metal that occurs in several mineral forms. Most manganese in the environment is found complexed to oxygen, carbon, or chloride. Manganese can exist in oxidation states from −3 to +7. Divalent manganese ($Mn^{2+}$) is the most common, the most bioavailable, and the most physiologically important form. $Mn^{3+}$ is also biologically important and is, for example, the form of manganese in superoxide dismutase.

## PHARMACOLOGY AND PHYSIOLOGY

Manganese is considered an essential dietary element because it is a cofactor in many human enzyme systems, including superoxide dismutase, hexokinase, xanthine oxidase, arginase, hydroxy-methyl-glutaryl (HMG) coenzyme a (CoA) reductase, and glutamine synthase. It is found in nuts, grains, legumes, black tea, fruits, and vegetables, and most people consume 2 to 9 mg of manganese compounds per day. Manganese salts—usually manganese sulfate or manganese chloride—are added to infant formulas, processed foods, and dietary supplements, but these are less well absorbed. Although deficiency in humans is not reported, experimental manganese restriction produced a scaling, erythematous, pruritic rash, alterations in calcium homeostasis (eg, hypercalcemia, hyperphosphatemia), and increased alkaline phosphatase in healthy volunteers.

Normally, less than 5% of dietary manganese is absorbed throughout the length of the small intestine. Because manganese competes with iron for binding sites on transferrin, the absorption of manganese is dependent on iron status, increasing in the presence of iron deficiency and decreasing when iron stores are adequate. Manganese absorption from the gastrointestinal tract is also inversely proportional to the amount of calcium in the diet, most likely because of competition between divalent cations for transport.

About 85% of manganese in the whole blood is bound to hemoglobin in erythrocytes, and normal measured whole blood concentrations are as much as five times greater than those measured in serum. The remaining manganese in plasma is mostly bound to transferrin, $\beta_1$-globulin, and albumin. Manganese is widely distributed to all tissues and crosses both the placental and the blood–brain barriers.

Manganese is primarily eliminated via the bile in feces, which requires normal hepatic function for healthy manganese homeostasis. It accumulates in bile against a concentration gradient, which suggests an active transport mechanism. Renal excretion is negligible. The elimination half-life of manganese from the body is approximately 40 days, but this value is highly variable among individuals.

## PATHOPHYSIOLOGY

Manganese toxicity results either from overexposure or impaired elimination. Because of its low enteral absorption, excessive dietary ingestion of manganese is unlikely to cause toxicity in adults with normal elimination. However, parenteral administration of either nutritional supplements or xenobiotics containing manganese presents a greater toxicologic risk.

The major occupational route of exposure is inhalation of manganese dusts or fumes. Whereas normal liver function protects against accumulation of manganese in soft tissue, patients with hepatic disease are at risk for manganese bioaccumulation and toxicity from normal dietary intake.

Manganese is deposited throughout cerebral tissue but concentrates in the basal ganglia structures, most notably the globus pallidus and, to a lesser extent, in the caudate and putamen. The specific mechanisms of manganese neurotoxicity are also not well established, although oxidative stress, mitochondrial dysfunction, neuroinflammation, and alterations in neurotransmitter metabolism are all likely implicated. Manganese concentrates in mitochondria and inhibits both mitochondrial F1-ATPase and complex I in the electron transport chain, thereby disrupting oxidative phosphorylation and contributing to energy failure and cytotoxicity. Like other transition metals, manganese causes local damage by generating reactive oxygen species during redox cycling between the divalent ($Mn^{2+}$) and trivalent ($Mn^{3+}$) forms. The participation of manganese in Fenton reactions results in oxidative tissue damage. Manganese also promotes sustained inflammatory neuronal injury by activating microglia and astrocytes potentiating the release of nitric oxide, prostaglandin E1, TNF-α, NF-κB, and other inflammatory mediators from activated glial cells.

## CLINICAL MANIFESTATIONS

Early reports of manganism in manganese workers and miners described an acute phase characterized by psychiatric symptoms known as "manganese madness" that included visual hallucinations, behavioral changes, anxiety, impotence, and decreased libido. However, classic manganism is best typified by a late-presenting syndrome of extrapyramidal movement abnormalities, including marked bradykinesia, rigidity, postural instability, loss of facial expression, impaired speech, and pronounced gait disturbance. Signs and symptoms vary with duration and extent of exposure, may be insidious in onset, and may not become apparent for several years (Table 67–1). More work is needed to describe the disease evolution, as well as to understand the relevance of subtle preclinical neuropsychological signs for predicting sequelae.

Although the movement disorder that typically occurs in patients with manganism is similar to that seen in cases of idiopathic Parkinson disease, including a typical "cock walk" on the balls of the feet, there are several distinguishing clinical features, including a lack of or atypical tremor, a particular tendency to fall backward, and an absence of severe progressive dementia. Cognitive impairment or vestibular–auditory dysfunction is usually mild, if present at all, and Lewy bodies are absent in patients with manganism. Although symptomatic improvement with levodopa therapy is reported in some patients, most evidence indicates that dopamine supplementation does not improve signs and symptoms in patients with manganese-induced parkinsonism.

Acute inhalational exposure to high concentrations of manganese oxides can cause metal fume fever (Chap. 94), with characteristic fever, chills, nausea, headache, myalgias, and arthralgias. Chronic occupational exposure to manganese oxide fumes is also associated with chemical pneumonitis and increased rates of bronchitis and pneumonia, but it does not cause pulmonary fibrosis.

**TABLE 67–1 Typical Features of Chronic Manganism**

| *System* | *Early Manifestations* | *Late Manifestations* |
|---|---|---|
| Constitutional | Asthenia, lethargy | — |
| Gastrointestinal | Anorexia | — |
| Neurologic | Fine intention tremor<br>Headaches | Coarse intention tremor<br>Visual hallucinations<br>Cognitive impairment<br>Loss of facial expression<br>Dysphagia<br>Micrographia<br>Gait instability[a]<br>Low-volume speech |
| Psychiatric | Apathy<br>Irritability<br>Emotional lability | Decreased libido or impotence<br>Anxiety<br>Additional behavioral changes |
| Musculoskeletal | Arthralgias | Muscle rigidity |

[a]Decreased arm swing, toe walking, and inability to turn or walk backward without falling.

## DIAGNOSTIC TESTING

Manganism is often difficult to differentiate from other neurodegenerative disorders. Several tests help establish the diagnosis, but each has important limitations. Careful evaluation of plausible sources of exposure, findings on neurologic and neuropsychologic examinations, and determining hepatic function and iron reserve status are important. If movement abnormalities are present, then failure of sustained response to levodopa therapy is highly suggestive of manganism.

Although normal reference values for manganese in blood and urine are published, concentrations are poorly correlated with total body manganese burden. Whole blood manganese concentrations are the most reliable values for biomonitoring purposes, although they only correlate with group and not with individual exposures. Additionally, manganese concentrations vary with age, gender, and during pregnancy. Neonates have concentrations up to three times the traditional upper limit of normal, likely to due to concomitant iron status and erythropoiesis. Manganese concentrations in whole blood are most commonly determined by flame or furnace atomic absorption spectrophotometry. Whole blood manganese concentrations should be elevated after acute overexposure, but abnormal concentrations are neither sensitive nor specific for chronic manganese toxicity because manganese is rapidly cleared from the blood. Signs and symptoms of manganism are insidious and typically occur long after concentrations in urine or blood have normalized.

Urine manganese concentrations are not well correlated with either symptoms or extent of exposure. Increased urinary elimination of manganese after chelation challenge with calcium disodium edetate ($CaNa_2EDTA$) occurs but cannot be interpreted. The utility of hair, nail clippings, and saliva as biomarkers of chronic manganese exposure is not clearly established.

Patients with manganese-associated movement disorders often have a characteristic pattern of abnormalities on magnetic resonance imaging (MRI) that includes a bilateral, symmetric, hyperintense signal in the basal ganglia, particularly in the globus pallidus, on T1-weighted images. This pattern is also reported in patients with iatrogenic manganism from long-term parenteral nutrition and is sometimes seen in cirrhotic patients with impaired dietary manganese elimination. While highly suggestive of manganism in the correct clinical context, an increased T1-weighted signal in the basal ganglia is a nonspecific finding that may also reflect iron, copper, or lipid deposition; hemorrhage; or neurofibromatosis.

By contrast to these radiographic abnormalities, MRI findings in patients with Parkinson disease typically demonstrate a hypointense signal in the substantia nigra on T2-weighted images. Some evidence suggests that single-photon emission computed tomography and positron emission tomography are helpful to differentiate these two clinical entities. For example, molecular imaging studies of patients with chronic manganese exposure and extrapyramidal symptoms have largely failed to demonstrate abnormal nigrostriatal dopaminergic activity and projections, although these are clearly abnormal in patients with Parsinson disease.

## TREATMENT

Treatment for patients with manganese toxicity is primarily supportive. Removal from the source of exposure is paramount, although clinical manifestations often still progress as manganese body stores fall. Antiparkinsonian therapy is generally ineffective or has limited benefit in relieving motor symptoms. Antioxidant therapy is proposed by some authors, based on the hypothesis that oxidant stress and mitochondrial dysfunction contribute to manganese-induced cellular damage, but because human data are lacking, these therapies are reasonable but not recommended at this time. Iron supplementation in addition to chelation therapy improved neurologic symptoms in one patient and is reasonable in patients with iron deficiency or acute exposures.

The clinical utility of chelation therapy in patients with manganese toxicity has not been well studied and remains controversial. Treatment with $CaNa_2EDTA$ was reportedly useful in some cases (Antidotes in Brief: A30). More often, however, chelation improves urinary excretion of manganese without affecting neurologic manifestations of toxicity. Chelation with succimer had no effect on either manganese concentrations in blood and urine or on clinical signs of manganism in two patients. Thus, these chelators are not routinely recommended at this time. Iron supplementation is another therapy proposed to reduce manganese concentrations in blood and lower total body burden. Because hemodialysis was not beneficial in a case of massive intravenous manganese overdose, we recommend against attempts at extracorporeal removal.

# 68 MERCURY

Normal concentrations

| | |
|---|---|
| Whole blood | < 10 μg/L (50 nmol/L) |
| Urine | < 20 μg/L (100 nmol/L) |

## HISTORY AND EPIDEMIOLOGY

The toxicologic manifestations of mercury are well known as a result of thousands of years of medicinal applications, industrial use, and environmental disasters. Mercury occurs naturally in small amounts as the elemental silver-colored liquid (quicksilver); as inorganic salts such as mercuric sulfide (cinnabar), mercurous chloride (calomel), mercuric chloride (corrosive sublimate), and mercuric oxide; and as organic compounds (methylmercury and dimethylmercury).

In the 1800s, the United States witnessed an epidemic of "hatters' shakes" in hat industry workers from mercury used in felt production. In the early 1900s, acrodynia, or "pink disease," was described in children who received calomel for ascariasis or teething discomfort. In the 1940s, the Minamata Bay event occurred when methylmercury was dumped in the sea and poisoned the inhabitants of the local fishing community. The largest outbreak of methylmercury poisoning to date occurred in Iraq in late 1971 when grain treated with a fungicide was baked into bread. Approximately 6,530 hospital admissions and more than 400 deaths resulted. Mercury derived from seafood is rarely a health concern in non-pregnant patients with normal diets.

## FORMS OF MERCURY AND KINETICS

The three important classes of mercury compounds (elemental, inorganic, and organic) differ with respect to toxicodynamics and toxicokinetics (Table 68–1).

**TABLE 68–1 Differential Characteristics of Mercury Exposure**

| | *Elemental* | *Inorganic* | *Organic* |
|---|---|---|---|
| Primary route of exposure | Inhalation | Oral | Oral |
| Primary tissue distribution | CNS, kidney | Blood (transient, acute)<br>Kidney<br>CNS (delayed) | CNS, kidney, liver, blood, hair |
| Clearance | Kidney, GI | Kidney, GI | Methyl: GI<br>Aryl: kidney, GI |
| *Clinical effects* | | | |
| CNS | Tremor | Tremor, erethism | Paresthesias, ataxia, tremor, tunnel vision, dysarthria |
| Pulmonary | +++ | – | – |
| Gastrointestinal | + | +++ (caustic) | + |
| Renal | + | +++ (ATN) | + |
| Acrodynia | + | ++ | – |
| Therapy | Dimercaprol, succimer | Dimercaprol, succimer | Succimer (early) |

ATN = acute tubular necrosis; CNS = central nervous system; GI = gastrointestinal; + to +++ = present with increasing importance; – = absent.

### Absorption

***Elemental Mercury.*** Elemental mercury ($Hg^0$) found in old thermometers and sphygmomanometers, is absorbed primarily via inhalation of vapor, although slow absorption following aspiration, subcutaneous deposition, and direct intravenous embolization are reported. Elemental mercury is negligibly absorbed from a normally functioning gut and therefore usually considered nontoxic when ingested. Abnormal gastrointestinal (GI) motility prolongs mucosal exposure to elemental mercury and increases subsequent ionization to more readily absorbed forms.

***Inorganic Mercury Salts.*** The principal route of absorption for inorganic mercury salts is the GI tract. Inorganic mercury salts are also absorbed across skin and mucous membranes, as evidenced by urinary excretion of mercury following the dermal application of mercurial ointments and powders containing HgCl.

***Organic Mercury Compounds.*** Organic mercury compounds are primarily absorbed from the GI tract. Although both dermal and inhalational absorption of organic mercury compounds are reported, precise quantitation and exclusion of concomitant absorption by ingestion are difficult to determine.

### Distribution and Biotransformation

Following absorption, mercury distributes widely to all tissues, but predominantly to the kidneys, liver, spleen, and central nervous system (CNS). The initial distributive pattern into nervous tissue of elemental and organic mercury differs from that of the inorganic salts because of their greater lipid solubility.

***Elemental Mercury.*** Although peak concentrations are delayed in the CNS, significant accumulation occurs following an acute, intense exposure to elemental mercury vapor. Conversion of elemental mercury to the charged mercuric cation within the CNS favors retention and local accumulation of the metal.

***Inorganic Mercury Salts.*** The greatest concentration of mercuric ions is found in the kidneys, particularly within the renal tubules. Very little mercury is found as free mercuric ions. In blood, mercuric ions are found both within the red blood cells (RBCs) and bound to plasma proteins in approximately equal proportions. Penetration of the blood–brain barrier is poor because of low lipid solubility, but slow elimination and prolonged exposure contribute to consequential CNS accumulation.

***Organic Mercury Compounds.*** Once absorbed, aryl and long-chain alkyl mercury compounds differ from the short-chain organic mercury compounds (ie, methylmercury). The former possess a labile carbon-mercury bond, which is subsequently cleaved, releasing the inorganic mercuric ion. Thus, the distribution pattern and toxicologic manifestations produced by the aryl and long-chain alkyl compounds are comparable to those of the inorganic mercury salts, but organification facilitates absorption and reduces the local caustic effects. In contrast, short-chain alkyl mercury compounds possess relatively stable carbon–mercury bonds that survive the absorptive phase. Because it is lipophilic, methylmercury readily distributes across all tissues, including the blood–brain barrier and placenta. Methylmercury also concentrates in RBCs to a much greater degree than do mercuric ions.

### Elimination

***Elemental Mercury and Inorganic Mercury Salts.*** Mercuric ions are excreted through the kidney by both glomerular filtration and tubular secretion, and in the GI tract by transfer across mesenteric vessels into feces. The total-body half-life of elemental mercury and inorganic mercury salts is estimated at approximately 30 to 60 days.

***Organic Mercury Compounds.*** The elimination of short-chain alkyl mercury compounds is predominantly fecal. Enterohepatic recirculation contributes to its somewhat longer half-life of about 70 days. Less than 10% of methylmercury is excreted in urine and feces as the mercuric cation.

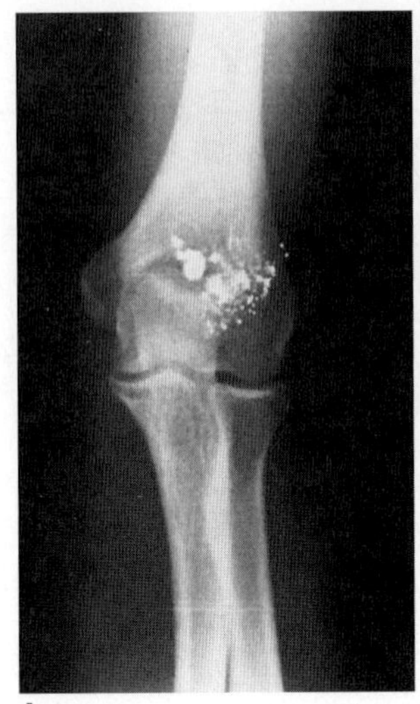


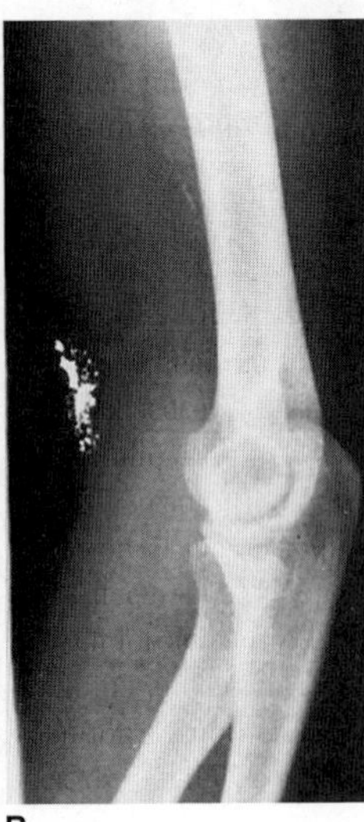


**FIGURE 68–1.** Anteroposterior (**A**) and lateral (**B**) views of the elbow after an unsuccessful suicidal gesture involving an attempted intravenous injection of elemental mercury in the antecubital fossa. Note the extensive subcutaneous mercury deposition, which was partially removed by surgical intervention. (*Used with permission from Diane Sauter, MD.*)

## PATHOPHYSIOLOGY

Toxicity arises largely from covalent binding to sulfur, replacing the hydrogen ion in the body's ubiquitous sulfhydryl groups. This results in widespread dysfunction of enzymes, transport mechanisms, membranes, and structural proteins. Necrosis of the GI mucosa and proximal renal tubules, which occurs shortly after mercury salt poisoning, is thought to result from direct oxidative effect of mercuric ions. An immune mechanism is attributed to the membranous glomerulonephritis and acrodynia associated with the use of mercurial ointments. Neuronal cytotoxicity of methylmercury may result in part from muscarinic receptor-mediated calcium release from smooth endoplasmic reticulum of cerebellar granule cells. Animal evidence suggests that methylmercury triggers reactive oxygen species and inhibits astrocyte uptake of cysteine, the rate-limiting step in the production of glutathione, a major antioxidant.

## CLINICAL SYNDROMES

### Elemental Mercury

Symptoms of *acute elemental mercury inhalation* occur within hours of exposure and consist of cough, chills, fever, and shortness of breath. Gastrointestinal complaints include nausea, vomiting, and diarrhea, accompanied by a metallic taste, dysphagia, salivation, weakness, headaches, and visual disturbances. Chest radiography during the acute phase reveals interstitial pneumonitis and both patchy atelectasis and emphysema. Symptoms may resolve or progress to acute respiratory distress syndrome and death.

Subacute inorganic mercury poisoning manifested by tremor, acute kidney injury, and gingivostomatitis can also occur during the acute phase. Massive endobronchial hemorrhage followed by death has occurred secondary to direct *aspiration of metallic mercury* into the tracheobronchial tree. There is no evidence to support the development of clinically significant disease from dental amalgams. Unusual cases of chronic toxicity have resulted from intentional *subcutaneous or intravenous injection of elemental mercury* (Fig. 68–1).

### Inorganic Mercury Salts

Acute *ingestion of mercuric salts* produces a characteristic severe irritant to outwardly caustic gastroenteritis. Immediately following oropharyngeal pain, nausea, vomiting, and diarrhea develop, which are followed by abdominal pain, hematemesis, and hematochezia. The lethal dose of mercuric chloride is estimated at 30 to 50 mg/kg. The life-threatening manifestations of severe acute mercuric salt ingestion are hemorrhagic gastroenteritis, massive fluid loss resulting in shock, and acute kidney failure.

*Subacute or chronic mercury poisoning* occurs after (a) inhalation, aspiration, or injection of elemental mercury; (b) ingestion or dermal application (from skin lightening creams) of inorganic mercury salts; or (c) ingestion of aryl or long-chain alkyl mercury compounds. Slow in vivo oxidation of elemental mercury and dissociation of the carbon-mercury bond of aryl or long-chain alkyl mercury compounds result in the production of the inorganic mercurous and mercuric ions. Gastrointestinal symptoms consist of a metallic taste and burning sensation in the mouth, loose teeth and gingivostomatitis, hypersalivation (ptyalism), and nausea. The neurologic manifestations of chronic inorganic mercurialism include tremor, as well as the syndromes of neurasthenia and erethism. Neurasthenia is a symptom complex that includes fatigue, depression, headaches, hypersensitivity to stimuli, psychosomatic complaints, weakness, and loss of concentrating ability. Erethism, derived from the Greek word *red*, describes the easy blushing and extreme shyness of the afflicted. Other symptoms of erethism include anxiety, emotional lability, irritability, insomnia, anorexia, weight loss, and delirium. The mercurial tremor is a central intention tremor that is abolished during sleep. In the most severe forms of mercury-associated tremor, choreoathetosis and spasmodic ballismus are noted. Other neurologic manifestations of inorganic mercurialism include a mixed sensorimotor neuropathy, ataxia, concentric constriction of visual fields ("tunnel vision"), and anosmia.

Chronic poisoning with mercuric ions is associated with renal dysfunction, which ranges from asymptomatic, reversible proteinuria to nephrotic syndrome with edema and hypoproteinemia. An idiosyncratic hypersensitivity to mercury ions is thought to be responsible for acrodynia or "pink disease," which is an erythematous, edematous, and hyperkeratotic induration of the palms, soles, and face, and a pink papular rash, described as morbilliform, urticarial, vesicular, and hemorrhagic. This symptom complex also includes excessive sweating, tachycardia, irritability, anorexia, photophobia, insomnia, tremors, paresthesias, decreased deep-tendon reflexes, and weakness. The acral rash may progress to desquamation and ulceration. Thimerosal (ethylmercury thiosalicylate) was widely used as a preservative in the pharmaceutical industry (Chap. 19). The claim that thimerosal-containing vaccines cause autism has been refuted by numerous studies and meta-analyses. No causal association with early thimerosal exposure and adverse neuropsychological outcomes was shown in children tested at 7 to 10 years of age.

### Organic Mercury Compounds

In contrast to the inorganic mercurials, methylmercury produces an almost purely neurologic disease that is permanent except in the mildest of cases. Although the predominant syndrome associated with methylmercury is that of a delayed neurotoxicity, acutely, GI symptoms, tremor, respiratory distress, and dermatitis occur.

Characteristically, manifestations follow a latent period of weeks to months. Infants exposed prenatally to methylmercury were the most severely affected individuals in Minamata. Often born to mothers with little or no manifestation of methylmercury toxicity themselves, exposed infants exhibited decreased birth weight and muscle tone, profound developmental delay, seizure disorders, deafness, blindness, and severe spasticity. In Iraq, several weeks after methylmercury-contaminated grain was ingested, paresthesias involving the lips, nose, and distal extremities developed, as did headaches, fatigue, and tremor. More serious cases progressed to ataxia, dysarthria, visual field constriction, and blindness.

The extreme toxicity of dimethylmercury was demonstrated by the delayed fatal neurotoxicity that developed in a chemist who spilled dimethylmercury on her gloved hands. Progressive difficulty with speech, vision, and gait preceded her death.

## DIAGNOSTIC TESTING

Demonstration of mercury in blood, urine, or tissues is necessary for confirmation of exposure. Table 68–2 highlights the differences in various diagnostic tests for mercury. Blood should be collected into a special trace-element collection tube. Urine should be collected for 24 hours into an acid-washed container with a plastic cap. Spot collections must be adjusted for creatinine concentration. Patients undergoing testing for chronic conditions should be advised to have a seafood free diet for 1 to 2 weeks before specimen collection. Because organic mercury is eliminated via the fecal route, urine mercury concentrations are not useful in methylmercury poisoning. Because mercury accumulates in the hair, hair analysis has been used as a tool for measuring mercury burden. However, because metal incorporation reflects past exposure and hair avidly binds to noningested environmental mercury, the reliability of this method is questionable and is not recommended.

**TABLE 68–2 Diagnostic Testing for Mercury**

| | *Whole Blood* | *24-Hour Urine* | *Hair* | *Clinical* |
|---|---|---|---|---|
| **Elemental/ Inorganic** | (+) | (++) | (+) | (+) |
| | Acute, transient | Confirm exposure | Reflects past exposure and external adsorption | Poor correlation to TBB |
| | | Monitor chelation | | Early detection |
| | | Poor correlation to TBB | | |
| **Organic** | (++) | (–) | (+) | (+) |
| | Best reflects TBB | Fecal elimination | Reflects past exposure and external adsorption | Poor correlation to TBB |
| | | | | Reflects irreversible CNS toxicity |
| | | | | Early detection |

CNS = central nervous system; TBB = total-body burden; + to ++ = useful testing specimen; – = lack of utility.

## GENERAL MANAGEMENT

After initial assessment and stabilization, the early toxicologic management of patients with mercury poisoning includes termination of exposure by removal from vapors; washing exposed skin; GI decontamination; supportive measures such as hydration and humidified oxygen; baseline diagnostic studies such as complete blood count, serum chemistries, blood gases, radiographs, and electrocardiogram; specific analysis of blood and urine for mercury; consideration of possible coingestants; and meticulous monitoring.

### Elemental Mercury

Inhalation of mercury vapors or aspiration of metallic mercury may result in life-threatening respiratory failure, and in this situation, stabilization of cardiorespiratory function is the initial priority. Postural drainage and endotracheal suction are a reasonable technique to remove aspirated metallic mercury. Parenteral deposition of subcutaneous or intramuscular mercury is amenable to surgical excision if well localized.

Spilled mercury compounds should not be vacuumed because vacuuming could volatilize the mercury. Guidance for decontamination of major spills and disposal of materials can be provided by local and federal hazardous materials agencies.

### Inorganic Mercury Salts

Ingestion of inorganic mercuric salts may lead to cardiovascular collapse caused by severe gastroenteritis and third-space fluid loss. Fluid resuscitation is a priority. Although GI decontamination is particularly problematic because of their causticity and risk for perforating injury, unless there is high suspicion for a perforating GI mucosal injury, removal of mercury from absorptive surfaces should take priority over endoscopic evaluation. The prominence of vomiting makes gastric lavage unnecessary for most patients with inorganic mercury poisoning. Because inorganic mercuric salts have substantial adsorption to activated charcoal (800 mg mercuric chloride can be absorbed to 1 g activated charcoal in vitro), administration is reasonable. Whole-bowel irrigation with polyethylene glycol solution is also a reasonable adjunct to remove residual mercury and should be considered, following its progress with serial radiographs.

### Organic Mercury Compounds

Because organic mercury exposures do not typically present as single, acute ingestions, but rather as chronic or subacute ingestion of contaminated food, GI decontamination is unnecessary.

## CHELATION

Early chelation minimizes or prevents the widespread effects of poisoning. A history of significant mercury exposure combined with the presence of typical symptoms of mercury poisoning is an appropriate indication for the institution of chelation therapy, even if laboratory confirmation is pending (Antidotes in Brief: A28 and A29). Provocative chelation, in which urinary mercury excretion before and after a chelating dose is compared to determine the degree of mercury poisoning, is of no value and therefore not recommended.

### Elemental Mercury and Inorganic Mercury Salts

For clinically significant acute inorganic mercury poisoning, dimercaprol should be administered for 10 days in decreasing dosages of 5 mg/kg/dose every 4 hours IM for 48 hours, then 2.5 mg/kg every 6 hours for 48 hours, then 2.5 mg/kg every 12 hours for 7 days. When a patient is able to take oral medications and the GI tract is clear, succimer at 10 mg/kg orally 3 times a day for 5 days, then twice a day for 14 days, is recommended as a substitute for dimercaprol.

### Organic Mercury Compounds

The neurotoxicity of methylmercury and other organic mercury compounds is resistant to treatment, and therapeutic options are less than satisfactory. We recommend against using dimercaprol because animal evidence suggests that it increases mercury mobilization into the brain. Although clinical improvement was not evident, 2,3-dimercapto-1-propanesulphonate, d-penicillamine, *N*-acetyl-d, l-penicillamine, and a thiolated resin all led to a marked reduction of blood half-life of mercury during the outbreak of methylmercury poisoning in Iraq in 1971. At this time, succimer is the most reasonable treatment for patients with methylmercury poisoning because of its apparently low toxicity and reported efficacy in animal models.

# 69 NICKEL

Normal concentrations

| | |
|---|---|
| Serum | < 1.1 µg/L (17 nmol/L) |
| Urine | < 6 µg/L (102 nmol/L) |

## HISTORY AND EPIDEMIOLOGY

Nickel is a white, lustrous metal first identified in 1751 that has been used as a component in a variety of metal alloys for more than 1,700 years. The ability of nickel to form naturally occurring alloys with iron has made it useful for many centuries in the production of coins, tools, and weapons. Today, most nickel is used in the production of stainless steel, a highly corrosion-resistant alloy containing 8% to 15% nickel by weight.

Occupational exposure to nickel and nickel-containing compounds occurs in a variety of industries, including nickel mining, refining, reclaiming, and smelting. Chemists, magnet makers, jewelry makers, oil hydrogenator workers, battery manufacturers, petroleum refinery workers, electroplaters, stainless steel and alloy workers, and welders may be at increased risk for exposure to nickel and nickel-containing compounds. Nickel carbonyl is responsible for the majority of acute occupational nickel toxicity. There have been two notable occupational disasters associated with exposure to nickel carbonyl. The Gulf Oil Company refinery incident in Port Austin, Texas, in 1953 resulted in more than 100 workers being exposed, with 31 hospitalizations and 2 deaths. The Toa Gosei Chemical company incident in Nagoya, Japan, in 1969, resulted in 156 male workers being exposed to nickel carbonyl, with 137 developing signs and symptoms but no fatalities reported. In contrast, the most common health issue related to nickel is the development of allergic dermatitis from jewelry and clothing. Nickel ranks behind poison ivy and poison oak as the second most common cause of allergic contact dermatitis.

## TOXICOKINETICS

Diet is a source of nickel exposure for humans. Foods high in nickel include nuts, legumes, cereals, and chocolate. Nickel is also present in the air, soil, and drinking water. Nickel is not considered an essential element for human health, and dietary recommendations for nickel have not been established. Although estimates vary widely, the total-body burden for a 70-kg reference human is about 10 mg of nickel. Nickel carbonyl is a highly volatile, deadly, liquid nickel compound used in nickel refining and petroleum processing and as a chemical reagent.

### Absorption

Depending on the form, nickel can enter the body through the skin, lungs, and gastrointestinal tract. Following inhalational exposure, nickel tends to accumulate in the lungs, and only 20% to 35% of nickel deposited in the human lung is absorbed. The remainder of the inhaled material is swallowed, expectorated, or deposited in the upper respiratory tract. Subsequent systemic absorption from the respiratory tract is dependent on the solubility of the specific nickel compound in question. Soluble nickel salts (nickel sulfate or nickel chloride) are more easily absorbed, whereas the less soluble oxides and sulfides of nickel have much lower levels of absorption.

Following ingestion, approximately 27% of the total nickel in divalent nickel sulfate given to humans in drinking water is absorbed, whereas only approximately 1% is absorbed when given in food. Serum nickel concentrations peak from 1.5 to 3 hours following ingestion of nickel. Several nickel compounds are capable of penetrating the skin. However, it has not been determined if nickel is simply absorbed into the deep layers of the skin or if it actually reaches the bloodstream. Once absorbed, nickel exists in the body primarily as the divalent cation.

### Distribution

In human serum, the exchangeable pool of primarily divalent nickel is bound to albumin, L-histidine, and $\alpha_2$-macroglobulin. A nonexchangeable pool of nickel also exists and is tightly bound to a transport protein known as nickeloplasmin. Nickel is also concentrated in various solid organs with the highest concentrations in the lungs, followed by the thyroid, adrenals, kidneys, heart, liver, brain, spleen, and pancreas.

### Elimination

Most ingested nickel is excreted in the feces; however, as more than 90% of ingested nickel does not leave the gut, most nickel found in feces represents this unabsorbed fraction rather than the elimination of previously absorbed nickel. Regardless of the route of exposure, absorbed nickel is excreted in the urine. The half-life of elimination of nickel depends on the source of exposure. Following unintentional ingestion of contaminated water, the mean serum half-life of nickel is reported to be 60 hours. This half-life decreased substantially (to 27 hours or less) following treatment with intravenous fluids.

## CLINICAL MANIFESTATIONS

### Acute

The most important source of acute, nondermatologic nickel toxicity is nickel carbonyl. Exposure to this compound is associated with pulmonary, neurologic, and hepatic dysfunction. Inhalation of nickel-containing aerosolized particles tends to affect the lungs and upper airways directly, whereas ingestion and intravenous administration may result in systemic toxicity, usually involving the neurologic system. By far the most common disorder associated with acute exposure to nickel is an allergic dermatitis.

***Nickel Allergy and Dermatitis.*** According to the North American Contact Dermatitis Group, nickel has been the most frequently positive of the 65 tested allergens in patch-testing since 1992. The five-fold greater prevalence of nickel allergy

| TABLE 69–1 Findings Suggestive of Nickel Dermatitis |
|---|
| Previous history of allergic response to jewelry |
| Multiple body piercings |
| Eruptions at the site of metal contact, or flexor areas if generalized |
| Eruptions following placement of orthodontic appliances containing high concentrations of nickel (unusual) |
| Seasonal dermatitis in warm months (increased metal–skin contact and increased sweating) |
| Facial dermatitis in mobile phone users |

in women is presumably a consequence of their higher rates of body piercing and more frequent wearing of jewelry. Nickel dermatitis may be classified into primary and secondary types. The more common primary dermatitis presents as a typical eczematous reaction in the area of skin that is in contact with nickel. It is characterized initially by erythematous papules that may proceed to lichenification with repeated scratching. Areas typically involved include sites of contact with nickel-containing jewelry, buttons on jeans, and nickel-containing belt buckles. The secondary form involves a more widespread dermatitis as a result of other exposures such as ingestion, transfusion, inhalation, or implantation of metal medical devices, and may be regarded as a systemic contact dermatitis elicited by nickel. Secondary eruptions are typically symmetrically distributed and may localize in the elbow flexure and on the eyelids, sides of the neck, and face, and may sometimes become widespread. The diagnosis of nickel allergy is suggested by specific historical findings (Table 69–1).

### Inhalational Exposure

***Nickel Carbonyl.*** Nickel carbonyl is the most harmful form of nickel and is responsible for the majority of acute occupational nickel exposures. Nickel carbonyl is described as having a "musty" or "sooty" odor, although thresholds for detection vary considerably and potentially harmful exposures cannot be excluded simply by a reported lack of odor. Nickel carbonyl exposure causes both immediate and delayed symptoms (Table 69–2). In patients who developed symptoms shortly following exposure, the initial manifestations involved nonspecific complaints, including respiratory tract irritation, chest pain, cough, dyspnea, frontal headache, dizziness, weakness, and nausea. Patients manifesting only these initial signs are categorized as mildly toxic. Manifestations of severe acute nickel carbonyl poisoning generally develop over the course of several hours to days and are associated with acute respiratory distress syndrome and interstitial pneumonitis and/or myocarditis. Altered mental status, seizures, and extreme weakness that sometimes necessitates mechanical ventilation can occur. Deaths from nickel carbonyl are typically caused by interstitial pneumonitis and cerebral edema occurring within 2 weeks of initial exposure. Survivors usually recover completely, although in some cases, the development of a prolonged neurasthenic syndrome occurs that lasts for months.

***Noncarbonyl Nickel.*** There are few human cases of inhalational nickel poisoning. However, from the available data, the

**TABLE 69–2 Symptoms and Signs of Nickel Carbonyl Poisoning**

| *Symptoms and Signs in 179 Cases* | *Frequency, %* |
|---|---|
| Chest pain/tightness | 67 |
| Dizziness | 66 |
| Nausea | 64 |
| Weakness | 54.8 |
| Headache | 54 |
| Cough | 43.6 |
| Dyspnea | 8.9 |
| Vomiting | 7.3 |
| Fever | 6.7 |
| Somnolence | 5.1 |
| Abdominal pain | 1.7 |

primary concerns appear to be pulmonary, neurologic, and, perhaps, renal.

### Parenteral Administration

Acute parenteral toxicity from nickel-containing compounds occurred when water used in hemodialysis was heated in a nickel-plated tank. Patients developed nonspecific symptoms, including headache, nausea, and vomiting, similar to nickel carbonyl poisoning, although no respiratory complaints are reported. The effects resolved after several hours, and recovery was without sequelae.

### Ingestion

Acute ingestion of water contaminated with nickel salts causes nausea, vomiting, diarrhea, weakness, and headache, as well as pulmonary symptoms, including cough and dyspnea, which may persist for 48 hours.

### Dermal Absorption

Although transdermal absorption is typically of minor clinical significance, disruption of the normal integument likely allows for more efficient systemic absorption. A metal refinery worker suffered a 40% body surface area partial-thickness chemical injury resulting from exposure to a chemical mixture that included nickel carbonate and nickel sulfate. Serial blood tests confirmed nickel absorption and he was treated with chelation.

### Chronic Nickel Exposure

Chronic inhalational exposure to nickel is associated with injury as well as specific histologic changes in the nasopharynx and upper respiratory tract, including atrophy of the olfactory epithelium rhinitis, sinusitis, nasal polyps, and septal damage. Pulmonary effects include asthma and pulmonary fibrosis. The International Agency for Research on Cancer classifies nickel compounds as a group 1 carcinogen (carcinogenic to humans).

## DIAGNOSTIC TESTING

Even though nickel is widely distributed to many body fluids and tissues, urine and blood are the most commonly analyzed samples. Urine and blood nickel concentrations primarily reflect exposure in the past 2 days. Concentrations among workers occupationally exposed to nickel are substantially higher than unexposed populations but do not correlate directly with adverse health effects. Testing for allergic contact dermatitis due to nickel is performed using "strip" patch testing, as for other types of contact dermatitis.

## TREATMENT

The first step in treatment of nickel-related medical problems is eliminating the exposure. This includes detection and removal of the source. In the case of acute exposures to nickel carbonyl, removal of clothing to prevent continued exposure and thorough skin decontamination are recommended.

Symptomatic treatment for pulmonary symptoms can include the administration of supplemental oxygen for hypoxia. The use of bronchodilators and corticosteroids is reasonable for the treatment of concomitant bronchospasm. Mechanical ventilation is required in the most severe cases.

The administration of intravenous fluids to promote diuresis reduces the half-life of ingested nickel chloride by approximately 50%. Hemodialysis does not effectively remove nickel from the serum.

### Chelation

Because there are no controlled human trials, specific recommendations for the use of chelation to treat nickel toxicity are not currently supported by the literature. As a result, extrapolation from animal studies and case reports form the basis for most treatment regimens. Most studies and reports involving treatment focused on workers exposed to nickel carbonyl.

Although dimercaprol was used in the past, the most recent literature has focused on the use of diethyldithiocarbamate (DDC) (Chaps. 51 and 72). Patients with suspected severe poisonings are typically given the first gram of DDC in divided oral doses. When less-severe exposures are suspected, treatment decisions are based on the urinary nickel concentration. At urinary concentrations less than 100 μg/L, no initial therapy is recommended as delayed symptoms are unlikely to develop. At urinary concentrations between 100 and 500 μg/L, an oral regimen consisting of 1 g DDC initially, 0.8 g at 4 hours, 0.6 g at 8 hours, and 0.4 g at 16 hours is used. Diethyldithiocarbamate is continued at a dose of 0.4 g every 8 hours until there is symptomatic improvement and urine nickel concentration is normal regardless of severity. Critically ill patients should be given parenteral DDC starting at a dose of 12.5 mg/kg if available. Although typically well-tolerated, DDC induces a disulfiram reaction (Chap. 51) if taken with ethanol. Disulfiram is metabolized into two molecules of DDC. Given that DDC is not pharmaceutically available in the United States, there is some interest in the use of disulfiram as an antidote for nickel carbonyl. Although disulfiram cannot be considered standard care because of the lack of convincing evidence, it would be reasonable because of its theoretical efficacy. One suggested treatment regimen is 750 mg given orally every 8 hours for 24 hours, followed by 250 mg every 8 hours.

Contact dermatitis from nickel is treated with standard measures, including avoidance, topical steroids, and antihistamines for pruritis.

# 70 SELENIUM

Normal concentrations

| | |
|---|---|
| Whole blood | 0.1–0.34 mg/L (1.27–4.32 μmol/L) |
| Serum | 0.04–0.6 mg/L (0.51–7.6 μmol/L) |
| Urine | < 0.03 mg/L (0.38 μmol/L) |
| Hair | 5.1–17.7 nmol/g |

## HISTORY AND EPIDEMIOLOGY

Selenium was discovered in 1817. It has unusual light-sensitive electrical conductive properties, leading to its use throughout industry. It is both an essential component of the human diet and a potentially deadly poison. In the 1970s, selenium was found to be an essential cofactor of the enzyme glutathione peroxidase. Deficiency occurs when daily intake falls below 20 μg/day. Keshan disease, an endemic cardiomyopathy associated with multifocal myonecrosis, periacinar pancreatic fibrosis, and mitochondrial disruption, occurs in patients who consume a selenium-poor diet over years. The recommended daily allowance (RDA) for selenium was established in 1980 in the United States (US) as 55 μg/day. Dietary selenium is easily obtained through meats, grains, and cereals; Brazil nuts, grown in the foothills of the highly seleniferous Andes Mountains, contain the highest concentration measured in food.

Chronic selenium toxicity, or selenosis, occurs endemically from dietary exposure in seleniferous areas of China and Venezuela and manifests as dermatitis, hair loss, and nail changes at an intake more than 100 times the US RDA. Sporadic outbreaks of chronic selenium toxicity resulted from improperly formulated dietary supplements.

Selenium sulfide is the active ingredient in many antidandruff shampoos. Gun-bluing solution, used to care for the exterior surface of firearms, is composed of selenious acid, as well as other compounds, such as cupric sulfate in hydrochloric acid, nitric acid, copper nitrate, and methanol. Table 70–1 lists commonly encountered of selenium compounds.

## CHEMICAL PRINCIPLES

Selenium is a nonmetal element that is found in abundance throughout the earth's crust, usually as a metal selenide in sulfide ores such as marcasite, arsenopyrite, and chalcopyrite. Selenium exists in elemental, organic and inorganic forms, with important oxidation states of 0 (elemental), $2^+$ (selenide [$Se^{2+}$]), $4^+$ (selenite [$SeO_3^{2+}$]), and $6^+$ (selenate [$SeO_4^{2+}$]). Water solubility generally increases with oxidation state, so elemental selenium and metal selenides are insoluble, whereas alkali selenites and selenates are highly water soluble. In general, toxicity from elemental selenium is rare and only occurs from long-term exposure. The organic alkyl compounds (dimethylselenide, trimethylselenide) are the next least toxic; in fact, they are by-products of endogenous selenium detoxification (methylation). Selenious acid ($H_2SeO_3$) is the most toxic form of selenium.

## PHARMACOLOGY

Selenium exists in one of three forms in the body. First, selenium-specific proteins, or selenoproteins, contain selenocysteine residues and play specific roles, primarily in oxidation-reduction (redox) physiology. Second, a number of nonspecific proteins contain selenium, such as albumin and selenomethionine, in which selenium appears to have no specific role but which may represent a storage form of selenium. Third, selenium has several inorganic forms throughout the body, such as selenate, alkyl selenides, and elemental selenium ($Se^o$).

## PHARMACOKINETICS AND TOXICOKINETICS

Gastrointestinal absorption varies with the species of selenium, and human data are limited. Elemental selenium is the least bioavailable (up to 50%); inorganic selenite and selenate salts are 75% bioavailable; and selenious acid is quite well absorbed in the lungs and gastrointestinal tract, at approximately 85% in animal studies. Organic selenium compounds are the best absorbed at approximately 90%, as determined by isotope tracers in human volunteer studies. Dermal absorption appears to be limited, and selenium disulfide shampoos are not systemically absorbed when used as recommended.

The toxic dose of selenium varies widely between selenium compounds and parallels gastrointestinal bioavailability. Elemental selenium has no reported adverse effects in acute overdose, although long-term exposure can be harmful. The selenium salts, particularly selenite, are more acutely toxic,

**TABLE 70–1 Selenium Compounds**

| *Name* | *Chemical Formula* | *Oxidation State* | *Uses* |
|---|---|---|---|
| Selenium (elemental) | Se | 0 | Photography, catalyst, dietary supplement, xerography |
| Selenium sulfide | $SeS_2$ | $2^-$ | Antidandruff shampoo, fungicide |
| Hydrogen selenide | $H_2Se$ | $2^-$ | A by-product of metal selenides reaction with water; no commercial use |
| Dimethylselenide | $CH_3SeCH_3$ | $2^-$ | Metabolite, garlic odor |
| Selenium dioxide | $SeO_2$ | $4^+$ | Catalyst, photography, glass decolorizer, vulcanization of rubber, xerography |
| Selenium oxychloride | $SeOCl_2$ | $4^+$ | Solvent, plasticizer |
| Selenious acid | $H_2SeO_3$ | $4^+$ | Gun-bluing solution |
| Sodium selenite | $Na_2SeO_3$ | $4^+$ | Glass and porcelain manufacture |
| Selenium hexafluoride | $SeF_6$ | $6^+$ | Gaseous electrical insulator |
| Sodium selenate | $Na_2SeO_4$ | $6^+$ | Glass manufacture, insecticide |

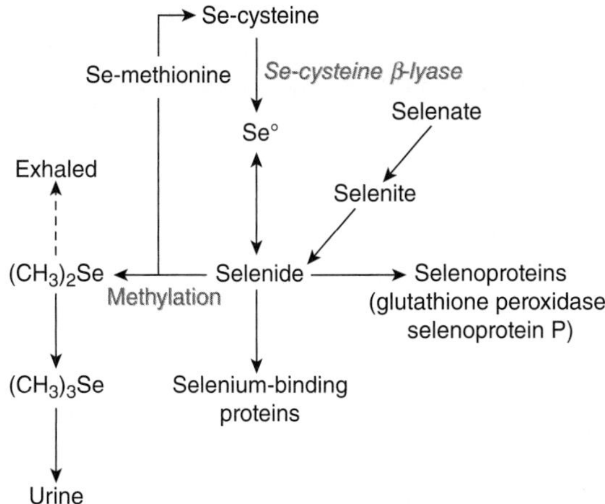


**FIGURE 70–1.** Metabolism of selenium. The selenide anion is central in selenium metabolism. Organic selenocysteine is converted via the β-lyase enzyme to elemental selenium and then to selenide. Selenomethionine either undergoes transsulfuration to selenocysteine or methylation to excretable metabolites. The selenate and selenite salts are reduced to selenide. Selenide then undergoes one of three processes: methylation, incorporation into selenoproteins, or binding by nonspecific plasma proteins.

as is selenium oxide ($SeO_2$), through its conversion to selenious acid in the presence of water. Selenious acid may be lethal from as little as a tablespoon of 4% solution in children.

The metabolic fate of selenium centers on the selenide anion, which has one of three final fates: (a) incorporation into selenoproteins such as glutathione peroxidase and triiodothyronine; (b) binding by nonspecific plasma proteins such as albumin or globulins; or (c) hepatic methylation into nontoxic excretable metabolites. Trimethylselenide is the primary metabolite and is excreted by the kidneys, the major elimination pathway for selenium. Some fecal elimination also occurs (Fig. 70–1).

## PATHOPHYSIOLOGY

In selenium deficiency, glutathione peroxidase activity is decreased, and glutathione (GSH) and glutathione *S*-transferases are increased. As a result, selenium-deficient rats are more resistant to substances detoxified by glutathione *S*-transferase, such as acetaminophen and aflatoxin B, and less resistant to other prooxidants, such as nitrofurantoin, diquat, and paraquat. Excess selenium causes oxidative stress, presumably as a result of prooxidant selenide ($R\text{-}Se^-$) anions. In addition, the replacement of sulfur by selenium in enzymes of cellular respiration causes mitochondrial disruption, and the substitution of selenomethionine in place of methionine interferes with protein synthesis. Integumentary effects most likely result from selenium interpolation into disulfide bridges of structural proteins such as keratin.

## CLINICAL MANIFESTATIONS

### Acute Overdose

Dermal exposure to selenium dioxide, which is converted to selenious acid, and to selenium oxychloride causes painful caustic burns through generation of hydrochloric acid. Excruciating pain results from accumulation under fingernails. Corneal injury with severe pain, lacrimation, and conjunctival edema are reported after exposure to selenium dioxide sprayed unintentionally into the face.

***Inhalational Exposure.*** When inhaled, all selenium compounds are respiratory irritants. In general, inhaled elemental selenium dusts are less systemically toxic than those compounds that are converted to selenious acid. Acute exposure to high concentrations of hydrogen selenide gas produces throat and eye pain, rhinorrhea, wheezing, and pneumomediastinum, with residual restrictive and obstructive disease. In contrast, selenium dioxide and selenium oxide fumes form selenious acid in the presence of water in the respiratory tract. Initial symptoms include bronchospasm with upper respiratory irritation and burning. Chemical pneumonitis with fever, chills, headache, vomiting, and diarrhea can develop later. Selenium hexafluoride is a caustic gas used in industrial settings as an electrical insulator. In the presence of water, it is converted to elemental selenium and hydrofluoric acid. Signs and symptoms are consistent with hydrofluoric acid (HF) exposure (Chap. 77).

***Oral Exposure.*** Following ingestion of elemental selenium and organic selenium compounds, acute toxicity is not expected. However, ingestion of even small quantities of inorganic selenium compounds, such as selenium oxide, selenium dioxide, or selenious acid, is almost invariably fatal. The onset of symptoms is within minutes and, in some cases, death occurs within 1 hour of ingestion. Gastrointestinal symptoms include abdominal pain, diarrhea, nausea, and vomiting. Patients frequently have a garlic odor. Skeletal muscle involvement is characterized by weakness, hyporeflexia, myoclonus, fasciculations, and elevated creatine phosphokinase concentrations. Acute kidney injury presumably results from myoglobinuria and hemolysis. More severely poisoned patients exhibit lethargy, delirium, and coma. Circulatory failure is the hallmark of serious inorganic selenium toxicity. Patients present with dyspnea, chest pain, tachycardia, and refractory hypotension. Pulmonary edema, ventricular dysrhythmias, myocardial and mesenteric infarction, and metabolic acidosis all contribute to poor outcome in these patients.

### Chronic

Outside of seleniferous areas, chronic elemental selenium toxicity, is most commonly reported as a result of improperly formulated selenium-containing dietary supplements. Selenosis is similar to arsenic toxicity, with its most consistent manifestations being nail and hair abnormalities. The hair becomes very brittle, breaking off easily at the scalp, with regrowth of discolored hair, and the development of an intensely pruritic scalp rash. The nails are also brittle with white or red ridges that can be either transverse or longitudinal; the thumb is usually involved first, and paronychia can develop. The skin becomes erythematous, swollen, and blistered, slow to heal, and with a persistent red discoloration. An increase in dental caries can occur. Neurologic manifestations include memory loss, hyperreflexia, peripheral paresthesias, anesthesia, and hemiplegia.

## DIAGNOSTIC TESTING

Over time, selenium is incorporated into blood and erythrocyte proteins, making serum the best measure of acute toxicity and whole blood preferable for the assessment of chronic exposure. Whereas normal blood values are known, there is no predictable relationship between selenium concentrations and exposure, toxicity, or time course. Urine concentrations reflect very recent exposure because urinary excretion of selenium is maximal within the first 4 hours. Although hair concentrations have been used, the usefulness of hair selenium is limited in countries such as the US where the use of selenium sulfide shampoos is widespread. In general paired blood and urine specimens are recommended.

Other ancillary tests to assess selenium toxicity include an electrocardiogram, thyroid function, platelet counts, aminotransferases, creatinine, and creatine phosphokinase concentrations.

## MANAGEMENT

Standard pain management strategies are required for patients with burns. Anecdotal reports suggest benefit of a 10% sodium thiosulfate solution or ointment but are not recommended. For workers exposed to selenium hexafluoride, it is reasonable to treat affected areas with calcium gluconate gel. This is the same treatment as for hydrofluoric acid exposures (Chap. 77).

As with any toxic exposure, prompt removal from the source is required, if possible. Patients with dermal exposure should have immediate copious irrigation. There are limited data to support the use of gastrointestinal decontamination following the ingestion of most selenium substances as there is little expected acute toxicity. However, in compounds associated with systemic toxicity, such as the selenite salts, decontamination with orogastric lavage or activated charcoal is reasonable. Special mention should be made of the ingestion of selenious acid. Given its toxicity, the judicious use of small nasogastric lavage would be reasonable based on the time since ingestion, the amount and concentration ingested, the presence or absence of spontaneous emesis, the likelihood of caustic esophageal injury, and the clinical condition of the patient.

There are no proven antidotes for selenium toxicity. Animal studies and scant human data suggest that chelation with dimercaprol, edetate calcium disodium ($CaNa_2EDTA$), or succimer forms nephrotoxic complexes with selenium, does not speed clinical recovery, and may, in fact, worsen toxicity and is therefore unadvisable. Extracorporeal removal techniques such as hemodialysis or hemofiltration decrease selenium concentrations in patients undergoing the procedure regularly, so theoretically, this could be effective in lowering toxic serum selenium concentrations. However, because of extensive protein binding, this benefit is likely minor and only relevant to patients undergoing frequent dialysis. Nonetheless, although there are only scant reports of hemodialysis in acute selenium poisoning, it would be reasonable in patients with severe toxicity.

Supportive care is the mainstay of therapy in selenium poisoning. In particular, patients with selenious acid toxicity will require intensive monitoring and multisystem support to survive.

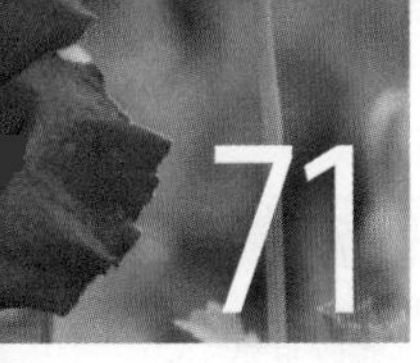

# 71 SILVER

| Normal concentrations | |
|---|---|
| Serum | < 0.5 μg/L (< 10 nmol/L) |
| Urine (24-hour) | < 1 μg/L (< 20 nmol/L) |

## HISTORY AND EPIDEMIOLOGY

Silver is a precious metal that has been used for thousands of years as coinage, a financial standard, a chemical catalyst, an electrical conductor, and a medicine. Silver poisoning is rare and results from occupational exposure or self-administration of silver-containing products for unproven medicinal purposes.

Colloidal silver protein (CSP), a suspension of finely divided metallic silver made from mixing silver nitrate, sodium hydroxide, and gelatin, was used in oral medications in the late 19th and early 20th centuries to treat a variety of ailments, including syphilis, epilepsy, and nasal allergies. While banned from routine administration by intravenous, intramuscular, and oral routes in the United States, silver salts are approved for use in topical medications, primarily as a caustic to stop bleeding and as a component of burn care. Silver sulfadiazine added to burn dressings kills bacteria and increases the rate of reepithelialization across partial-thickness wounds. Central venous catheters impregnated with silver sulfadiazine and silver-impregnated Foley catheters are used to lower infection rates (Table 71–1). Silver is also used in water filtration cartridges and as a low-cost non-filtration point-of-use-water-treatment technology.

## EPIDEMIOLOGY

A number of occupations expose humans to varying amounts of silver on a daily basis. Workplace exposure is often via transdermal, transmucosal, or inhalational routes as silver particles are liberated during various mining, refining, and manufacturing processes. The estimated oral intake of silver for humans not working in silver-related industries ranges from 10 to 88 μg/day.

**TABLE 71–1 Medicinal Silver-Containing Products**

| *Product Name/Device* | *Route of Administration/ Exposure* | *Applications* |
|---|---|---|
| Silver nitrate (1% $AgNO_3$) | Ophthalmic | Prevention of gonorrheal ophthalmia neonatorum |
| Silver nitrate (10% $AgNO_3$) | Cutaneous | Chemical cautery of nasal mucosa and exuberant granulations |
| Silver sulfadiazine (0.2% or 1% micronized silver sulfadiazine) | Cutaneous | Antimicrobial adjunct for prevention and treatment of wound infection in burn patients |
| Silver-impregnated catheters and tubes | Nanoparticle coating | Antimicrobial adjunct for use in catheters and tubes |
| Silver acetate | Mucocutaneous (oral) | Used as a smoking cessation adjunct. Silver combined with smoke creates an unpleasant metallic taste. |

## PHARMACOLOGY

Silver is excreted in the bile and eliminated in the feces (30–80 μg/day) and urine (10 μg/day). Fecal elimination occurs in two phases. In the rapid phase, the elimination half-life varies with route of administration from 24 hours with oral exposure to 2.4 days following intravenous administration. A slower phase has a half-life of 48 to 52 days and is thought to represent mobilization of hepatic stores. A study of one human documented that 18% of a single dose of orally administered silver was still retained after 30 weeks. Metallic silver binds to reactive groups of proteins (sulfhydryl, amine, carboxyl, phosphate, and imidazole) to provoke protein denaturation and precipitation. Its antimicrobial effects are also thought to result from inhibition of fungal DNAse and complexation with bacterial DNA.

## PATHOPHYSIOLOGY

Acutely, intravenous administration of 50 mg or more of silver is fatal in humans, leading to acute respiratory distress syndrome, hemorrhage, and necrosis of bone marrow, liver, and kidneys. Although the exact mechanism is unknown, in animal models, silver blocks $Na^+$,$K^+$-ATPase activity. At nonlethal doses given by any route, essentially the only toxic manifestation of silver exposure is the development of argyria, a permanent bluish-gray discoloration of skin resulting from silver deposition throughout the integument (Fig. 71–1). This skin discoloration of argyria comes from the silver itself and from the induction of increased melanin production. Ingested silver dissolves in the acidic environment of the stomach, forming silver ions that are transported by glutathione and other biomolecules to the dermis. These ions are reduced by sunlight and sulfur. Subsequently, selenium ions align or collocate alongside silver atoms, creating blue discoloration.

## CLINICAL MANIFESTATIONS

When medicinal silver products are used as intended, silver is generally not considered to be toxic. In large enough quantities, however, silver toxicity occurs (Table 71–2). For the vast majority of cases, the only clinical manifestation is argyria, which can result from either direct mechanical impregnation of skin by silver particles as occurs in industry or from systemic absorption of silver through the conjunctiva or oral mucous membranes after prolonged topical treatment with silver salts, acupuncture, intravenous administration, or ingestion of colloidal silver protein. Argyria occurs at exposure doses much lower than those associated with acutely toxic effects of silver; the degree of discoloration is directly proportional to the amount of silver absorbed or ingested. Although 8 g of silver accumulation is typically necessary

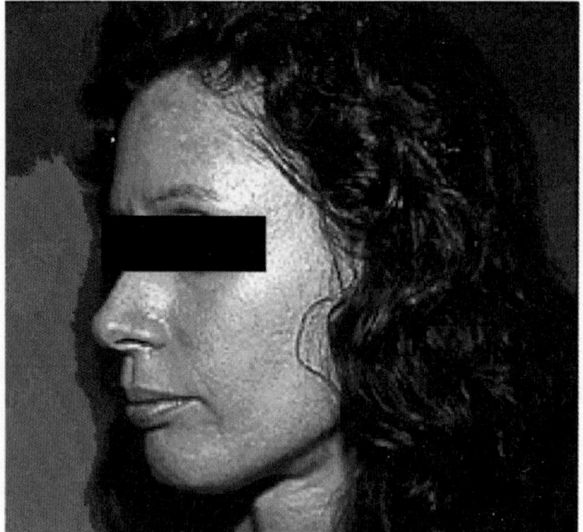

**FIGURE 71–1.** Argyria, the slate or silver discoloration of the skin that results from silver overexposure is demonstrated in this image of Rosemary Jacobs, who developed the condition after use of colloidal silver nasal drops for 3 years as a teenager. *(Used with permission from Rosemary Jacobs. We thank Ms. Rosemary Jacobs for her support and her permission to use the featured photographs.)*

| TABLE 71–2 | Clinical Manifestations of Silver Toxicity |
|---|---|
| Cardiovascular | Animals given silver in their drinking water developed ventricular hypertrophy that was not attributable to silver deposition in the heart. |
| Dermatologic | Generalized argyria, localized argyria, and argyrosis (silver deposition in the eyes) develops in humans chronically exposed to silver. |
| Hematologic | Topical application of silver in humans is rarely associated with bone marrow depression with subsequent leukopenia or aplastic anemia. |
| Hepatic | Vitamin E and selenium-deficient rats given silver salts developed hepatic necrosis. |
| Neurologic | Silver deposits in peripheral nerves, basal membranes, macrophages, and elastic fibers were found in a 55-year-old woman with progressive vertigo, cutaneous hypoesthesia, and weakness after self-administration of silver salts for 9 years. Seizures were reported in another patient who ingested > 20 mg silver daily for 40 years and resolved when ingestion ceased. |
| Renal | Tubular lesions are demonstrated in animals, and acute tubular necrosis is rarely reported in humans. |

before argyria is noted, the lowest known dose of silver resulting in argyria was 1 g of metallic silver administered as 4 g of silver arsphenamine intravenously. Argyria progresses in stages beginning with characteristic gray-brown staining of gingiva, then moving to hyperpigmentation and discoloration in sun-exposed areas. Later, sclerae, nail beds, and mucous membranes become hyperpigmented, and on autopsy, viscera are noted to be blue.

## DIAGNOSTIC TESTING

Silver concentrations in the urine or serum can confirm exposure. Patients with argyria alone have had serum concentrations of silver as high as 500 μg/L. Confirmation of the diagnosis of argyria is through skin biopsy.

## TREATMENT

Ingestion of silver salts is potential caustic and should be treated as such (Chap. 76). Chelators such as dimercaprol and D-penicillamine are ineffective in treating both toxicity and argyria. Hydroquinone 5% reduces the number of silver granules in the upper dermis and around sweat glands, as well as diminishes the number of melanocytes. Sunscreens and opaque cosmetics are used to prevent further pigmentation darkening from sun exposure. Successful treatment of argyria using laser technology is also reported and appears promising. Although supplementation with vitamin E and selenium is beneficial in experimental animals and sulfur supplementation has been suggested, there are no recommendations for any of these therapies at this time.

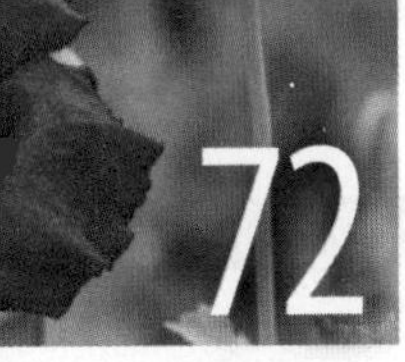

# 72 THALLIUM

| | |
|---|---|
| Normal concentrations | |
| Whole blood | < 2 μg/L (9.78 nmol/L) |
| Urine (24-hour) | < 5 μg/L (24.5 nmol/L) |

## HISTORY AND EPIDEMIOLOGY

Elemental thallium is a soft, pliable metal that is essentially nontoxic. Thallium forms univalent thallous ($Tl^{1+}$) and trivalent thallic ($Tl^{3+}$) salts, which are highly toxic. In the early 1900s, thallium salts were used medicinally to treat syphilis, gonorrhea, and tuberculosis, and as a depilatory for ringworm of the scalp. Many cases of severe thallium poisoning (thallotoxicosis) resulted from this treatment. Because thallium sulfate is odorless, tasteless, and highly toxic, it became commercially available as a rodenticide. After numerous reports of unintentional poisonings, the use of thallium salts as a household rodenticide was restricted in the United States (US) in 1965 and totally abandoned in 1972. Life-threatening unintentional poisoning continues to occur in other countries, especially where thallium salts are still commonly used as rodenticides. Additional cases occur in the US and other countries as a result of suicide, homicide, and contamination of herbal products and illicit drugs. The small amounts of thallium salts used as radioactive contrast are insignificant and pose no risk for thallium toxicity.

## TOXICOKINETICS

Exposures usually occur via one of three routes: inhalation, ingestion, and absorption through intact skin. Thallium salts are rapidly absorbed following all routes of exposure. Bioavailability is greatest after ingestion and exceeds 90%. The volume of distribution is estimated as 3.6 L/kg, with the highest concentrations found in the large and small intestine, liver, kidney, heart, brain, and muscle. The toxicokinetics of thallium are described in the following three-phase model. The first phase occurs within 4 hours after ingestion, during which time thallium is distributed to the central compartment and to well-perfused peripheral organs such as the kidney, liver, and muscle. In the second phase, which lasts between 4 and 48 hours, thallium is distributed into the central nervous system (CNS). The third or elimination phase usually begins within 24 hours after ingestion. The primary mechanism of thallium elimination is secretion into the intestine, but enteral reabsorption of thallium that is present in the bile subsequently reduces the fecal elimination. Thallium is excreted primarily via the feces (51.4%) and the urine (26.4%). Unlike many other metals, thallium does not have a major anatomic reservoir. For this reason, reported elimination half-lives are as short as 1.7 days in humans with thallium poisoning.

## PATHOPHYSIOLOGY

Thallium behaves biologically in a manner similar to potassium because both have similar ionic radii. Thallium replaces potassium in the activation of potassium-dependent enzymes. In low concentrations, thallium is stimulatory, but in high concentrations, inhibition occurs. Examples include pyruvate kinase and sodium-potassium adenosine triphosphatase ($Na^+,K^+$-ATPase). The dermatologic, neurologic, and cardiovascular effects of thallium toxicity mirror the manifestations of thiamine deficiency (beriberi), highlighting the inhibitory effect of thallium on glycolytic enzymes. Complexation with riboflavin reduces the flavin containing coenzyme, flavin adenine dinucleotide (FAD), disrupting the electron transport chain and leading to failure of energy production. In the CNS, damage is also caused by activation of glutaminergic transmission. Thallium also has a high affinity for the sulfhydryl groups present in many other enzymes and proteins. Disruption of crosslinking of keratin leads to abnormal hair and nail growth. Additionally, the complexation of sulfhydryl groups decreases both the production of glutathione and the reduction of oxidized glutathione, increasing susceptibility to oxidative damage. Thallium also adversely affects protein synthesis by damaging ribosomes.

Pathologic studies of the CNS in patients with thallium poisoning reveal localized areas of edema in the cerebrum and brainstem. The peripheral nervous system, which is usually clinically affected before the CNS, develops a diffuse axonopathy in a classic dying back or Wallerian degeneration pattern.

## CLINICAL MANIFESTATIONS

Many of the effects of thallium poisoning are nonspecific and occur throughout the acute and chronic phases of an exposure. When combined, however, a clear toxic syndrome is defined (Table 72–1). Alopecia and a painful ascending peripheral neuropathy are the most characteristic findings. Because of the delayed development of alopecia, the diagnosis of thallotoxicosis is often delayed. Neurologic effects usually appear 2 to 5 days after exposure. Patients develop severely painful, rapidly progressive, ascending peripheral neuropathies. When death occurs, it is usually the result of coma with loss of airway protective reflexes, respiratory paralysis, and cardiac arrest.

### Teratogenicity

In animal models, thallium is teratogenic. A case–control study evaluating more than 1,000 infants born in a region of China with high environmental concentrations of thallium demonstrated an association between thallium exposure and low birth weight. Thallium slowly traverses the placenta, and findings consistent with thallium poisoning are described both in the fetus after abortion and in the neonate after viable delivery. However, normal infants are also reported despite being born to mothers with significant maternal toxicity. It is reasonable to conclude that a fetus exposed to thallium during organogenesis has the potential for permanent injury. Those exposed later in pregnancy often recover

**TABLE 72–1 Clinical Manifestations of Thallium Poisoning**

| | *Onset of Effects* | | | |
|---|---|---|---|---|
| ***Organ System*** | ***Immediate (< 6 hours)*** | ***Intermediate (rarely in the first few days; within 2 weeks)*** | ***Late (> 2 weeks)*** | ***Residual Effects‡*** |
| Gastrointestinal | | | | |
| Nausea | † | | | |
| Vomiting | † | | | |
| Diarrhea | † | | | |
| Constipation | † | † | | |
| Cardiovascular | | | | |
| Nonspecific electrocardiogram changes | † | † | | |
| Hypertension | | † | | |
| Sinus tachycardia | | † | | |
| Pleural and pericardial effusions | | † | | |
| Respiratory | | | | |
| Pleuritic chest pain | † | † | | |
| Respiratory depression | | † | † | |
| Renal | | | | |
| Albuminuria | | † | | |
| Acute kidney injury | | † | | † |
| Dermatologic | | | | |
| Dry skin | | † | | |
| Alopecia | | † | | † |
| Mees lines | | | † | † |
| Neurologic | | | | |
| Sensory neuropathy (painful ascending with paresthesias and numbness) | | † | † | † |
| Motor neuropathy (distal and ascending) | | † | † | † |
| Cranial nerve abnormalities (ptosis, bulbar dysfunction) | | † | | |
| Delirium, psychosis, coma | | † | | † |
| Memory and cognitive deficits | | | † | † |
| Optic neuritis | † | † | | † |

† = Typical onset of clinical effects. The predicted time course if often accelerated with extremely large doses. When † appears in two adjacent columns, the time course is highly variable and likely dose dependent. With small ingestions, many of the effects listed above are evident. ‡ = Effects that persist long after exposure, possibly permanently.

without deficit if their exposures are limited and the mother recovers. When a viable child is delivered, it is important to note that thallium is eliminated in breast milk and that ongoing evaluation of maternal toxicity is essential because nursing will result in continued exposure for the child.

## ASSESSMENT

Most patients with acute thallium toxicity seek health care soon after exposure because of alterations in their gastrointestinal (GI), cardiovascular, or neurologic function. Many patients with small acute or chronic exposures usually seek care because of alopecia or neuropathy. The differential diagnosis of the neuropathy includes poisoning by arsenic, colchicine, or vinca alkaloids, and disorders such as botulism, thiamine deficiency, and Guillain-Barré syndrome. Both the sensory neuropathy and the preservation of reflexes help differentiate thallium-induced neuropathy from Guillain-Barré syndrome and most other causes of acute neuropathy. When GI manifestations are present in addition to a neuropathy and other end-organ manifestations, possible poisoning with metal salts such as arsenic and mercury should be evaluated (Chaps. 59 and 68). The differential diagnosis of rapid-onset alopecia is more restricted and includes arsenic, selenium, colchicine, and vinca alkaloid poisoning as well as radiation injury. When present, Mees lines indicate past exposure to metals, mitotic inhibitors, or antimetabolites and, as such, are nonspecific for thallium poisoning (Chaps. 59 and 68).

### Diagnostic Testing

Radiographs of tampered food products or of the abdomen can document the presence of a metal such as thallium, which is radiopaque. Routine studies, such as the complete blood count, electrolytes, urinalysis, and electrocardiogram, are often normal or, at most, merely demonstrate nonspecific abnormalities. Although microscopic inspection of the hair is intriguing, this test is unlikely to be conclusive for inexperienced observers. The definitive clinical diagnosis of thallium poisoning can only be established by demonstrating elevated thallium concentrations in various body fluids or organs. Thallium can be recovered in the hair, nails, feces, saliva, cerebrospinal fluid, blood, and urine. Blood and urine are the most common matrices.

## MANAGEMENT

The treatment goals for a patient with thallium poisoning are initial stabilization, prevention of absorption, and enhanced elimination. After the initial assessment and stabilization of the patient's airway, breathing, and circulatory status, GI decontamination is recommended in all patients with suspected thallium ingestions because of the morbidity and mortality associated with a significant exposure.

### Decontamination

Orogastric or nasogastric lavage is recommended for patients who have not had spontaneous emesis and present within 1 to 2 hours after ingestion (Chap. 3). Thallium salts are substantially adsorbed to activated charcoal (AC) in vitro. Additionally, because thallium undergoes enterohepatic recirculation, AC will be useful both to prevent absorption after a recent ingestion and also to enhance elimination of thallium in patients who present in the postabsorptive phase. In some patients with severe thallium toxicity, constipation will be prominent, so the addition of oral mannitol or another cathartic to the first dose of AC is reasonable. Although no studies address the efficacy of whole-bowel irrigation with polyethylene glycol electrolyte lavage solution, we recommend this technique when radiopaque material is demonstrated in the GI tract (Antidotes in Brief: A2).

### Potassium

Parenteral potassium administration is associated with an increase in urinary thallium elimination. Potassium administration is believed to both block tubular reabsorption of thallium and mobilize thallium from tissue stores, thereby increasing thallium concentrations available for glomerular filtration. However, the mobilization of the thallium is of concern. Many authors report either the development of acute neurologic symptoms or the significant exacerbation of neurologic manifestations during potassium administration. Additionally, animal models demonstrate that potassium loading enhances lethality and permits thallium redistribution into the CNS. For these reasons, we recommend against the use of potassium loading. Likewise, the similarities between thallium and potassium might suggest a role for administration of sodium polystyrene sulfonate (SPS) as a sodium–thallium exchange resin. Despite excellent in vitro binding of thallium by SPS, it is unlikely to be clinically useful because of preferential binding between potassium and SPS and a comparatively large reservoir of potassium in the body, and SPS is therefore not recommended.

### Prussian Blue

Prussian blue is approved by the US Food and Drug Administration for thallium toxicity (Antidotes in Brief: A31). Prussian blue interferes with the enterohepatic recirculation of thallium by exchanging potassium ions from its lattice for thallium ions in the GI tract. This results in the formation of a concentration gradient, causing an increased movement of thallium into the GI tract. Humans with thallium exposure are routinely given Prussian blue, with apparent clinical benefits, enhanced fecal elimination, and decreasing thallium concentrations. The dose of Prussian blue is 250 mg/kg/day orally via a nasogastric tube in two to four divided doses. For patients who are constipated, the Prussian blue can be dissolved in 50 mL of 15% mannitol.

### Chelation

Patients with thallium toxicity do not respond to traditional chelation therapy. Studies demonstrate that the use of EDTA and diethylenetriamine pentaacetic acid is without benefit. Dimercaprol (British anti-Lewisite) and D-penicillamine also fail to enhance thallium excretion in experimental models. Although succimer improved survival in one animal model, the benefit was less than that achieved for Prussian blue and was at the cost of an increase in brain thallium concentrations.

### Extracorporeal Drug Removal

Extracorporeal drug removal has at most a limited beneficial role in patients with thallium exposure, especially if initiated shortly after the initial exposure while serum concentrations remain high before effective tissue distribution. Although extracorporeal therapy alone is probably insufficient for patients with significant poisoning and unnecessary in those with small exposures, some benefit seems likely when used in combination with other therapies, especially in patients with either underlying chronic kidney disease or acute kidney injury from thallium poisoning, and those with early massive, and presumed lethal, exposures. Intermittent hemodialysis is the preferred modality.

# A31 PRUSSIAN BLUE

## INTRODUCTION

Poisoning with salts of thallium or cesium is an uncommon cause of life-threatening toxicity. Radioactive cesium is either released as part of a nuclear incident or dispersed as a "dirty bomb." Prussian blue enhances the elimination of thallium and cesium.

## HISTORY

Prussian blue was discovered unintentionally by Diesbach in 1704 while attempting to make another pigment, cochineal red lake. It took approximately 250 years to recognize that Prussian blue attracted monovalent alkali metals into its crystal lattice. In 2003, the United States (US) Food and Drug Administration (FDA) approved Prussian blue for the treatment of thallium and radioactive cesium poisoning. The Prussian blue literature is complicated by many confusing chemical and physical terms. The product synthesized by Diesbach, $Fe_4\{Fe(CN_6)\}_3$, iron(III) hexacyanoferrate(II), commonly known as insoluble Prussian blue, is the US FDA-approved product. Many synonyms exist for Prussian blue that are unfortunately used interchangeably to refer to both insoluble Prussian blue and a soluble (colloidal) Prussian blue that either has the molecular formula $KFe\{Fe(CN)_6\}_3$ or $K_3Fe\{Fe(CN)_6\}_3$. For the purpose of clarity, general statements that follow use the term "Prussian blue." In many instances, the terms "insoluble" and "soluble" are chosen to highlight differences between the compounds. The currently available pharmaceutical preparation was likely selected preferentially for its efficacy in cesium poisoning.

## PHARMACOLOGY

The crystal lattice of Prussian blue binds cationic potassium ions from the surrounding environment. However, because its affinity increases as the ionic radius of the monovalent cation increases, Prussian blue preferentially binds cesium (ionic radius: 1.69 Å) and thallium (ionic radius: 1.47 Å) over potassium (ionic radius: 1.33 Å). Oral Prussian blue binds thallium or cesium in the gastrointestinal (GI) tract enhances elimination through both enteroenteric circulation (GI dialysis) and enterohepatic circulation. Insoluble Prussian blue remains almost exclusively (99%) in the GI tract and is eliminated nearly entirely in feces at a rate determined by GI transit time. In contrast, soluble Prussian blue is slightly absorbed based on the clinical finding of a blue discoloration that develops in the sweat and tears of patients undergoing prolonged therapy.

## THALLIUM

### In Vitro Adsorption

The in vitro adsorptions of both soluble and insoluble Prussian blue are similar when thallium concentrations remain low, but as thallium concentrations increase, the soluble form has greater adsorptive capacity. In vitro analysis of the US FDA-approved antidote demonstrated that pH and hydration state greatly influenced adsorption, with the maximal adsorptive capacity (MAC) predicted to be as high as 1,400 mg of thallium/g at pH 7.5.

### In Vitro Comparison of Prussian Blue and Activated Charcoal

Thallium is well adsorbed to activated charcoal. One investigation determined that the maximal adsorptive capacity (MAC) of activated charcoal was 124 mg of thallium/g, whereas the MAC for Prussian blue was only 72 mg of thallium/g. In another study, a MAC of only 59.7 mg of thallium/g was calculated for activated charcoal, compared with a higher MAC for insoluble Prussian blue of 72.7 mg of thallium/g.

### Animal Data: Kinetics, Tissue Concentrations, and Survival

Control animals eliminated 53% of the administered dose of thallium, versus 93% of the dose in animals given activated charcoal, and 82% in animals given insoluble Prussian blue. Multiple studies demonstrate that Prussian blue not only decreases the half-life of thallium in animals but also lowers thallium content in critical organs such as the brain and the heart. Half-lives are typically reduced by approximately 50% when Prussian blue is given. Also, a statistically significant survival advantage is shown in thallium-poisoned animals treated with Prussian blue.

### Radioactive Thallium

There is no published experience describing human poisoning with radioactive thallium. In one small study, insoluble Prussian blue decreased the biologic half-life of radioactive thallium in rats by approximately 40%. In vitro evidence suggests that Prussian blue has a MAC of 5,000 MBq/g. In a controlled trial, in which Prussian blue was given to a patient after myocardial scintigraphy, radioactivity was reduced 18% and 30% after 24 and 48 hours, respectively.

### Thallium Poisoning in Humans

In 1971, three patients were the first to receive Prussian blue as a treatment for thallium poisoning. A seven-fold increase in fecal thallium elimination was noted in the one patient who could be studied. Subsequently, many humans with thallium poisoning have received Prussian blue, with or without a cathartic and other treatments, as part of their therapy. One of the largest series was composed of 11 thallium-poisoned patients who were treated with soluble Prussian blue. In all individuals studied, fecal elimination remained high, even when urinary elimination decreased, suggesting selective redistribution of thallium into the gut. Although the authors commented on clinical improvement in these patients, the lack of controlled data makes these subjective observations difficult to interpret. Similarly, a substantial reduction in thallium half-life was demonstrated when Prussian blue was compared with no therapy at all in patients with thallium poisoning.

### Dosage and Administration

The dosage of Prussian blue has never been investigated systematically in humans. In most of the reports, a total dose of 150 to 250 mg/kg/day was administered orally or via a nasogastric tube in two to four divided doses. Because constipation or obstipation is often present or expected, Prussian blue is generally administered dissolved in 50 mL of 15% mannitol. The manufacturer recommends a total dose of 9 g divided daily (3 g every 8 hours) for adults and adolescents and 3 g divided daily (1 g every 8 hours) in children along with a high-fiber diet. Because Prussian blue is well tolerated, the editors of this text continue to recommend the 150- to 250-mg/kg/day dosing. If patients cannot tolerate swallowing large numbers of capsules, it is recommended to open the capsules and mix them with food or liquids when needed. The use of a cathartic is reasonable when constipation is significant or symptomatic. By convention, Prussian blue is continued until total urinary thallium concentrations decrease below 0.5 mg/day. In patients who remain significantly symptomatic, it is reasonable to continue Prussian blue therapy for a short period past the 0.5 mg/day endpoint.

## CESIUM

The radioactive isotope of cesium ($^{137}Cs$), a common by-product of nuclear fission reactions, is a strong β and γ emitter with a physical half-life of more than 30 years and a biologic half-life of about 110 days. Another isotope ($^{134}Cs$) is only produced by neutron activation of the stable isotope ($^{133}Cs$) and has a physical half-life of about 2 years and a biologic half-life comparable to $^{137}Cs$. Cesium is absorbed in the small bowel, distributes like potassium, and undergoes enteric recirculation in a manner comparable to thallium. Approximately 80% of a given dose of cesium is eliminated in the urine, with 20% cleared in the feces. The isotope $^{137}Cs$ is used as a radiotherapy source in nuclear medicine and to irradiate banked blood and is a by-product of radiologic disasters and a potential threat in the form of a dirty bomb. Toxicity from nonradioactive cesium is also reported (Chap. 62).

### In Vitro Adsorption

Unlike thallium, the adsorption of cesium to activated charcoal is negligible. When the US FDA-approved antidote was analyzed, like thallium, pH and hydration introduced significant variations in binding, with a MAC of 715 mg of cesium/g noted at pH 7.5.

### Animal Data: Kinetics, Tissue Concentrations, and Survival

Small animal investigations with either $^{134}Cs$ or $^{137}Cs$ consistently demonstrate that Prussian blue therapy reverses the urine-to-stool elimination ratio from 8:1 to 0.3:1 and reduces the biologic half-life and the total-body area under the curve by as much as 60%. When dogs were contaminated with $^{137}Cs$, Prussian blue reduced the total-body burden by as much as 51%.

### Human Volunteer Studies

Two human volunteers ingested meals contaminated with $^{134}Cs$ to compare the efficacy of both the soluble and insoluble forms of Prussian blue with controls. At 14 days after exposure and without therapy, the volunteers retained 94.7% of the ingested dose, compared with retention of only 5.1% following therapy with insoluble Prussian blue and 4.9% following soluble Prussian blue. In another study, when Prussian blue was given daily at a dose of 0.5 g every 8 hours in the postabsorptive phase, the biologic half-life of $^{134}Cs$ was reduced from 106 to 44 days.

### Radioactive Cesium Poisoning in Humans

There are no controlled trials of Prussian blue in radioactive cesium poisoning. Experience is derived exclusively from treating disaster victims. In 1987, in Brazil, 37 patient who were incorporated with radioactive cesium from a discarded radiotherapy unit were given insoluble Prussian blue in doses ranging from 3 g/day in children up to 10 g/day in adults. Therapy with insoluble Prussian blue reduced half-lives by a mean of 32% and reduced the retained cesium dose from between 51% and 84% of the total dose. In another trial, insoluble Prussian blue was given to three victims of radioactive cesium incorporation many weeks after Chernobyl. The reported reduction in biologic half-life ranged from 12% to 52%. Kinetic modeling based on all available data suggests that Prussian blue is most effective if given nearly immediately after exposure. However, administration as late as 30 days after exposure, and perhaps even 1 year after exposure, will substantially reduce the biological half-life of $^{137}Cs$.

### Nonradioactive Cesium Poisoning in Humans

In a patient with syncope and QT interval prolongation from ingested cesium as naturopathic treatment, the apparent half-life of cesium was reported as 7.9 days during Prussian blue therapy in comparison to 86.6 days after therapy. In another patient who ingested cesium chloride and had multiple episodes of torsade de pointes, therapy with insoluble Prussian blue (3 g/day) was associated with a reduction in the apparent half-life for cesium from 61.7 to 29.4 days.

### Dosage and Administration

We agree with the manufacturer's recommendation that for radioactive cesium poisoning, adults and adolescents 13 years or older receive a total daily dose of 9 g divided into 3 g, 3 times per day. Children aged 2 through 12 years should receive a total daily dose of 3 g divided into 1 g, 3 times per day. Although the manufacturer offers no recommendation in children under the age of 2 years, administering 150 to 250 mg/kg/day in divided doses is appropriate. For patients with non-radioactive cesium poisoning the duration of treatment is usually based on clinical symptoms and the ECG. Therapy for radioactive cesium poisoning should be continued for at least 30 days. Since constipation does not commonly occur with either radioactive or nonradioactive cesium poisoning, neither routine cathartic administration nor the use of a high-fiber diet is recommended.

## ADVERSE EFFECTS AND SAFETY ISSUES

Animal studies show no adverse effects of therapeutic doses. The only significant adverse effects reported in humans receiving therapeutic doses are constipation and hypokalemia, and the constipation is likely to be related more to the thallium toxicity than to Prussian blue. Cyanide release from soluble Prussian blue is trivial.

## PREGNANCY AND LACTATION

Insoluble Prussian blue is listed as US FDA Pregnancy Category C. Because of the severe consequences of poisoning from radioactive cesium and thallium, both of which cross the placenta, and the lack of systemic absorption of insoluble Prussian blue, a risk-to-benefit analysis would favor the use of the antidote in all poisoned pregnant patients. Both cesium and thallium are excreted in breast milk. The confinement of Prussian blue in the GI tract would make excretion in breast milk unlikely. In any event, women contaminated with cesium or thallium should not breastfeed.

## FORMULATION AND ACQUISITION

Insoluble Prussian blue is available as a 0.5-g blue powder in gelatin capsules for oral administration manufactured from Haupt Pharma Berlin GmbH for distribution by HEYL Chemisch-pharmazeutische Fabrik GmbH & Co. KG, Berlin (281-395-7040; fax 281-395-2320; see information at www.heyltex.com). Prussian blue is part of the US Strategic National Stockpile, which can be accessed at CDC emergency response hotline: 770-488-7100; and is also stored at REAC/TS, Oak Ridge: emergency number 865-576-1005.

# 73 ZINC

Normal concentrations

| | |
|---|---|
| Blood | 600–1,000 μg/dL (91.8–153 mmol/L) |
| Serum | 109–130 μg/dL (16.7–19.9 mmol/L) |
| Urine (24-hour) | < 500 μg/day (< 7.65 mmol/day) |

## HISTORY AND EPIDEMIOLOGY

The Babylonians used zinc alloys more than 5,000 years ago. Zinc oxide and zinc sulfate were used in Western Europe during the late 1700s and early 1800s for gleet (urethral discharge), vaginal exudates, and convulsions. In the late 1800s, brass workers who inhaled zinc oxide fumes developed "zinc fever," "brass founders' ague," or "smelter shakes," all of which are now recognized as metal fume fever (Chap. 94).

Zinc salts enhance the solubility of pharmaceuticals such as insulin and are used in baby powders, sun blocks, and topical burn preparations (zinc oxide). Zinc gluconate–containing lozenges are marketed to shorten the duration of the common cold. The United States (US) Food and Drug Administration (FDA) approved zinc acetate in 1997 for maintenance therapy of Wilson disease, a disorder of copper metabolism (Chap. 65).

Zinc is used in industry to enhance the durability of iron and steel alloys (galvanization) and is commonly used in construction. Inhalational zinc oxide exposures occur commonly in those who weld galvanized steel. Hematologic and neurologic impairment is associated with large unintentional exposures to zinc denture creams.

## CHEMISTRY

Zinc is among the most abundant elements comprising the earth's crust. It has two common oxidation states: $Zn^0$ (elemental or metallic) and $Zn^{2+}$. The pure element exists as a blue to white shiny metal, but it also combines with other elements to form many familiar compounds: zinc chloride ($ZnCl_2$), zinc oxide (ZnO), zinc sulfate ($ZnSO_4$), and zinc sulfide (ZnS). Once the metal is exposed to moisture, it gets coated with zinc oxide or carbonate ($ZnCO_3$). Like other transition metals, zinc is involved in reactions that generate reactive oxygen species with resultant tissue toxicity.

## PHARMACOLOGY AND PHYSIOLOGY

Zinc is an essential nutrient and acts as a cofactor for more than 200 metalloenzymes (including acid phosphatase, alkaline phosphatase, alcohol dehydrogenase, carbonic anhydrase, superoxide dismutase, and both DNA and RNA polymerase), contributes to gene expression, and has a role in membrane stabilization, vitamin A metabolism, and the development and maintenance of the nervous system. Zinc and copper concentrations generally have an inverse relationship in the plasma (Chap. 65). Zinc is also important in maintaining olfactory and gustatory function and normal fetal growth. The average daily intake of zinc in the US is 5.2 to 16.2 mg; foods that contain zinc include leafy vegetables (2 ppm) as well as meats, fish, and poultry (29 ppm). The recommended daily allowance is 11 mg/day for men and 8 mg/day for women. Pregnant and nursing women require 12 mg/day.

## TOXICOKINETICS AND PATHOPHYSIOLOGY

The main site of oral zinc absorption is the jejunum, although it occurs throughout the intestine by either metallothionein binding or zinc-protein complex in the luminal cells. Metallothioneins are specific metal-binding proteins that have diverse functions but are involved in essential metal homeostasis. Albumin binds about two-thirds of zinc in the plasma, and the remainder is bound to $\alpha_2$-globulins. The primary route of zinc excretion is fecal.

## CLINICAL MANIFESTATIONS

The metallic form of zinc ($Zn^0$) is not toxic per se, and only the salt forms are considered here unless otherwise specifically mentioned. The hallmark of acute zinc toxicity is gastrointestinal (GI) distress, including nausea, vomiting, abdominal pain, and GI bleeding. Zinc chloride, which is used in soldering flux in concentrations greater than 20%, is particularly caustic when ingested. Partial and full-thickness burns to the oral mucosa, pharynx, esophagus, and stomach, as well as the laryngotracheal tree, occur even following small ingestions. In contrast, certain zinc salts (such as zinc oxide), as found in baby powders, lotions, and calamine lotion, are nonirritating when applied to the skin and nontoxic when ingested.

Acute inhalation of zinc chloride from smoke bombs produces lacrimation, rhinitis, dyspnea, stridor, and retrosternal chest pain. Upper respiratory tract inflammation progresses to acute respiratory distress syndrome (ARDS), generally with no manifestations of systemic absorption. Inhalation of zinc oxide is associated with metal fume fever and not pneumonitis despite similar ambient zinc concentrations. This is likely related to relative water solubility of the two zinc salts.

There are rare reports of renal complications, hyperamylasemia, pancreatitis, and jaundice and death that follow intentional intravenous administration.

Chronic zinc toxicity can produce a reversible sideroblastic anemia and a reversible myelodysplastic syndrome. Both anemia and granulocytopenia occur, with the bone marrow showing vacuolated precursors and ringed sideroblasts. The mechanism appears to be a zinc-induced copper deficiency. A neurologic syndrome of progressive myeloneuropathy called "swayback" is defined by a spastic gait, usually a prominent sensory ataxia, and hematologic manifestations that is associated with elevated zinc concentrations and copper deficiency. Similar findings of hyperzincemia, hypocupremia, and the development of this progressive myeloneuropathy are associated with excessive use of zinc-containing denture creams. To date, neither the International Agency for Research on Cancer (IARC) nor the US Environmental Protection Agency (EPA) has classified zinc as carcinogenic.

### Metal Fume Fever

Metal fume fever typically occurs within 12 hours after an exposure to zinc fumes. Patients develop fever, chills, cough, chest pain, dyspnea, dry throat, and a metallic taste in the mouth. Although exposure to zinc oxide fumes is the most common exposure associated with this syndrome, exposure to zinc compounds and other metal oxides are also implicated. The chest radiograph is commonly normal, although infiltrates are sometimes noted. Hypoxia and tachycardia are rare. Overall, however, the syndrome is relatively benign with tolerance developing within days. An immune mechanism is suggested, and chronic exposure is needed for sensitization (Chap. 94).

## DIAGNOSTIC TESTING

Because zinc is ubiquitous in the environment and laboratory, great care must be taken to avoid contamination of the samples. Since elevated zinc concentrations occur in the setting of copper deficiency, a serum copper concentration should always be obtained simultaneously. Whole blood zinc concentrations exceed plasma concentrations by a ratio of approximately 6–7:1 because the metal accumulates in erythrocytes. Urine zinc concentrations are not well defined. In the US, normal urine concentrations are generally accepted as less than 0.5 mg/day. Clinicians should consult their laboratory for specific collection protocols.

Abdominal radiographs have limited utility in determining the GI burden of zinc, except following ingestions of pennies. Findings should be used to guide the decision to continue GI decontamination only in certain circumstances. Magnetic resonance imaging in patients with chronic zinc exposure and secondary copper deficiency reveals increased T2 signal in the dorsal columns of the cervical spinal cord similar to that found in $B_{12}$ deficiency.

## MANAGEMENT

Treatment for acute oral zinc toxicity is primarily supportive. Efforts should be focused on hydration as well as antiemetic therapy. Esophageal foreign bodies containing zinc need to be removed if they do not pass spontaneously. We recommend whole-bowel irrigation (WBI) for GI decontamination after acute zinc salt ingestion. The data regarding the efficacy of chelation therapy for zinc are limited in humans. Edetate calcium disodium ($CaNa_2EDTA$) was used successfully in several cases, as was the combination of $CaNa_2EDTA$ and dimercaprol. Limited experience exists with regard to treatment of patients; however, it is reasonable to give 1,000 mg/m$^2$/day IV $CaNa_2EDTA$ divided every 6 hours to patients with severe neurologic toxicity or hemodynamic compromise.

For less severely toxic patients, many of the clinical manifestations and metabolic effects of zinc toxicity are due to its ability to cause copper deficiency. In patients with zinc overload–related copper deficiency, the supplementation of oral copper alone improved the hematopoietic effects and prevented further neurologic deterioration without chelation therapy. Initial recommended starting doses are 2 mg intravenously or 6 mg orally of elemental copper once per day. A decrease in oral dose by 2 mg each week is recommended with the goal of eventually giving 2 mg orally once per day until complete resolution of toxicity and normalization of blood concentrations occur.

Supportive care for patients with inhalational zinc exposures includes oxygen therapy and bronchodilators as clinically indicated. Ventilatory support may be required in severe cases. As metal fume fever is typically self-limited, nonsteroidal anti-inflammatory drugs should be sufficient to relieve the transient discomfort.

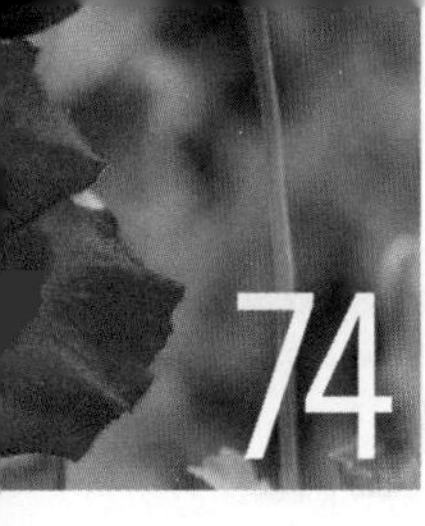



# 74 ANTISEPTICS, DISINFECTANTS, AND STERILANTS

## HISTORY AND EPIDEMIOLOGY

Joseph Lister, often considered the father of modern surgery, revolutionized surgical treatment and dramatically reduced surgical mortality by introducing the concept of antisepsis to the surgical theatre. Lister demonstrated that phenol, a chemical that was used to treat foul-smelling sewage, could be used to clean dirty wounds of patients with compound fractures and dramatically increase survival rates.

Antiseptics, disinfectants, and sterilants are a diverse group of germicides used to prevent the transmission of microorganisms to patients (Table 74–1). Although these terms are sometimes used interchangeably, the distinguishing characteristics between the groups are important to emphasize. An *antiseptic* is a chemical that is applied to living tissue to kill or inhibit microorganisms. A *disinfectant* is a chemical that is applied to inanimate objects to kill microorganisms. A *sterilant* is a chemical that is applied to inanimate objects to kill all microorganisms as well as spores. The choice of disinfectant or sterilant depends on the degree of risk for infection involved in use of medical and surgical instruments and patient care items.

## ANTISEPTICS

### Chlorhexidine

This cationic biguanide has had extensive use as an antiseptic since the early 1950s. It is found in a variety of skin cleansers, usually as a 4% emulsion, and is also found in some mouthwashes.

*Clinical Effects.* Few cases of deliberate ingestion of chlorhexidine are reported. Symptoms are usually mild, and gastrointestinal (GI) irritation is the most likely effect after ingestion. Intravenous administration of chlorhexidine is associated with acute respiratory distress syndrome (ARDS) and hemolysis. Inhalation of vaporized chlorhexidine causes methemoglobinemia, likely as a consequence of the conversion of chlorhexidine to *p*-chloraniline. In one patient, the rectal administration of 4% chlorhexidine resulted in acute colitis with ulcerations.

Topical absorption of chlorhexidine is negligible. Contact dermatitis is reported in up to 8% of patients who received repetitive topical applications of chlorhexidine. More ominously, anaphylactic reactions, including shock, are associated with dermal application. Eye exposure results in corneal damage.

*Management.* Treatment guidelines for chlorhexidine exposure are similar to those for other potential caustics (Chap. 76). Patients with significant symptoms after ingestion should undergo endoscopy, but the need for such extensive evaluation is uncommon.

### Hydrogen Peroxide

Hydrogen peroxide, an oxidizer with weak antiseptic properties, has a long history of use as an antiseptic and a disinfectant. This oxidizer is generally available in several concentrations: dilute, for home use with a concentration of 3% to 9% by weight (usually 3%); and concentrated for industrial purposes, with a concentration greater usually than 10%.

Toxicity from hydrogen peroxide occurs after ingestion, inhalation, injection, wound irrigation, rectal administration, dermal exposure, and ophthalmic exposure. Hydrogen peroxide has two main mechanisms of toxicity: local tissue injury and gas formation. The extent of local tissue injury and amount of gas formation are determined by the concentration of the hydrogen peroxide. Dilute hydrogen peroxide is an irritant, and concentrated hydrogen peroxide is a caustic. Gas formation results when hydrogen peroxide interacts with tissue catalase or gastric contents, liberating molecular oxygen, and water. At standard temperature and pressure, 1 mL of 3% hydrogen peroxide liberates 10 mL of oxygen, whereas 1 mL of 35% hydrogen peroxide liberates more than 100 mL of oxygen. Gas formation results in life-threatening embolization. Gas embolization is a result of dissection of gas under pressure into the tissues or of liberation of gas in the tissue or blood following absorption. The use of hydrogen peroxide in partially closed spaces, such as operative wounds, or its use under pressure during wound irrigation increases the likelihood of embolization.

*Clinical Effects.* Following ingestion of concentrated hydrogen peroxide, airway compromise manifested by stridor, drooling, apnea, and radiographic evidence of subepiglottic narrowing occurs. The combination of local tissue injury and gas formation from the ingestion of concentrated hydrogen peroxide causes abdominal bloating, abdominal pain, vomiting, and hematemesis. Endoscopy shows esophageal edema and erythema and significant gastric mucosal erosions. Symptoms consistent with sudden oxygen embolization include rapid deterioration in mental status, cyanosis, respiratory failure, seizures, ischemic electrocardiogram (ECG) changes, and acute paraplegia. Portal vein gas, seen on computed tomography (CT) scans, is also a prominent feature in some cases. Arterialization of oxygen gas embolization results in cerebral infarction. Death from intravenous injection of 35% hydrogen peroxide is reported.

Clinical sequelae from the ingestion of dilute hydrogen peroxide are usually much more benign. Nausea and vomiting are the most common symptoms. A whitish discoloration is noted in the oral cavity. Gastrointestinal injury is usually limited to superficial mucosal irritation, but multiple gastric and duodenal ulcers, accompanied by hematemesis, and diffuse hemorrhagic gastritis are reported. Portal venous gas embolization occurs as a result of the ingestion of 3% hydrogen peroxide and is usually only associated with abdominal pain.

However, the use of 3% hydrogen peroxide for wound irrigation results in significant complications. Extensive subcutaneous emphysema occurred after a dog bite to a human's face was irrigated under pressure with 60 mL of 3% hydrogen peroxide.

**TABLE 74–1 Antiseptics, Disinfectants, Sterilants, and Related Xenobiotics**

| *Xenobiotic* | *Commercial Product* | *Use* | *Toxic Effects* | *Therapeutics and Evaluation* |
|---|---|---|---|---|
| **Acids** | | | | |
| Boric acid | Borax<br>Sodium perborate<br>Dobell solution | Antiseptic<br>Mouthwash<br>Eyewash<br>Roach powder | Blue-green emesis and diarrhea<br>Boiled lobster appearance of skin<br>Central nervous system (CNS) depression; kidney failure | Orogastric lavage<br>Hemodialysis (rare) |
| **Alcohols**<br>(Chaps. 49 and 79) | | | | |
| Ethanol | Rubbing alcohol (70% ethanol) | Antiseptic<br>Disinfectant | CNS depression<br>Respiratory depression<br>Dermal irritant | Supportive |
| Isopropanol | Rubbing alcohol (70% isopropanol) | Antiseptic<br>Disinfectant | CNS depression<br>Respiratory depression<br>Ketonemia, ketonuria<br>Gastritis/hemorrhage<br>Hemorrhagic tracheobronchitis | Supportive<br>Hemodialysis (rare) |
| **Aldehydes** | | | | |
| Formaldehyde | Formalin<br>(37% formaldehyde, 12%–15% methanol) | Disinfectant<br>Fixative<br>Urea-formaldehyde insulation | Caustic<br>CNS depression<br>Carcinogen | Orogastric lavage<br>Hemodialysis<br>Sodium bicarbonate<br>Endoscopy<br>Folinic acid |
| Glutaraldehyde | Cidex (2% glutaraldehyde) | Sterilant | Mucosal and dermal irritant | Supportive |
| *ortho*-Phthalaldehyde (OPA) | Cidex OPA (< 1% OPA) | Sterilant | Mucosal and dermal irritant | Supportive |
| **Chlorinated Compounds** | | | | |
| Chlorhexidine | Hibiclens | Antiseptic | GI irritation | Supportive |
| Chlorates | Sodium chlorate<br>Potassium chlorate | Antiseptic (obsolete)<br>Matches<br>Herbicide | Hemolysis<br>Methemoglobinemia<br>Kidney failure | Exchange transfusion<br>Hemodialysis |
| Chlorine | | Disinfectant | Irritant | Supportive |
| Chlorophors (sodium hypochlorite) | Household bleach (5% NaOCl)<br>Dakin solution (1 part 5% NaOCl, 10 parts $H_2O$) | Disinfectant<br>Decontaminating solution | Mild GI irritation | Endoscopy (rare) |
| **Ethylene Oxide** | | Sterilant<br>Plasticizer | Irritant<br>CNS depression<br>Peripheral neuropathy<br>Carcinogen, mutagen | Supportive |
| **Mercurials**<br>(Chaps. 19 and 68) | Merbromin 2% (Mercurochrome)<br>Thimerosal (Merthiolate) | Antiseptic (obsolete) | CNS<br>Kidney | Orogastric lavage, activated charcoal, dimercaprol, succimer |
| **Iodinated Compounds** | | | | |
| Iodine | Tincture of iodine (2% iodine, 2% sodium iodide, and 50% ethanol)<br>Lugol solution (5% iodine) | Antiseptic | Caustic | Orogastric lavage, milk, starch, sodium thiosulfate<br>Endoscopy |
| Iodophors | Povidone-iodine (Betadine) (0.01% iodine) | Antiseptic | Limited | Same as iodine |
| **Oxidants** | | | | |
| Hydrogen peroxide | $H_2O_2$ 3%—household<br>$H_2O_2$ 35%—industrial | Disinfectant | Oxygen emboli<br>Caustic | Orogastric lavage<br>Radiographic evaluation<br>Endoscopy |
| Potassium permanganate | Crystals, solution | Antiseptic | Oxidizer, caustic, increased serum manganese | Decontamination<br>Endoscopy |

(*Continued*)

**TABLE 74–1 Antiseptics, Disinfectants, Sterilants, and Related Xenobiotics (*Continued*)**

| *Xenobiotic* | *Commercial Product* | *Use* | *Toxic Effects* | *Therapeutics and Evaluation* |
|---|---|---|---|---|
| **Phenols** | | | | |
| Nonsubstituted | Phenol | Disinfectant | Caustic<br>Dermal burns<br>Cutaneous absorption<br>CNS effects | Decontamination: polyethylene glycol 400 or water<br>Endoscopy |
| Substituted | Hexachlorophene | Disinfectant | CNS effects | Supportive |
| **Quaternary Ammonium Compounds** | | | | |
| Benzalkonium chloride | Zephiran | Disinfectant | Caustic | Endoscopy |

CNS = central nervous system; GI = gastrointestinal.

Systemic oxygen embolism, causing hypotension, cardiac ischemia, and coma, resulted from the intraoperative irrigation of an infected herniorrhaphy wound. Multiple cases of acute colitis are reported as a complication of administering 3% hydrogen peroxide enemas.

***Diagnosis.*** In patients with significant symptoms, a careful examination should be performed to detect any evidence of gas formation such as crepitus. A chest radiograph is recommended to assess for gas in the cardiac chambers, mediastinum, or pleural space. Likewise, an abdominal radiograph of computed tomography (CT) scan is also recommended to assess for gas in the GI tract or portal system and define the extent of bowel distension. Magnetic resonance imaging and CT imaging are reasonable to detect brain and spinal cord lesions secondary to gas embolism and should be obtained if the patient experiences neurologic effects. For those with clinical presentations consistent with esophageal, gastric, or intestinal injury, endoscopic evaluation is recommended.

***Management.*** The treatment of patients with hydrogen peroxide ingestions depends, to a large degree, on whether the patient has ingested a diluted or concentrated solution. We recommend home observation for asymptomatic patients who unintentionally ingest small amounts of 3% hydrogen peroxide. There is not enough evidence to support the dilution with milk or water. Nasogastric or orogastric aspiration of hydrogen peroxide is reasonable if the patient presents within 30 minutes after ingestion. Continuous gastric suctioning for patients with abdominal distension from gas formation is recommended. Place patients with clinical or radiographic evidence of gas in the heart in the Trendelenburg position to prevent gas from blocking the right ventricular outflow tract. Careful aspiration of intracardiac air through a central venous line is recommended in patients in extremis if hyperbaric therapy is not immediately available. Hyperbaric therapy is recommended in cases of life-threatening gas embolization after hydrogen peroxide ingestion.

## Iodine and Iodophors

Iodine usually refers to molecular iodine, also known as $I_2$, free iodine, and elemental iodine, which is the active ingredient of iodine-based antiseptics. The use of ethanol as the solvent, such as in tincture of iodine, allows substantially more concentrated forms of $I_2$ to be available. Iodine ($I_2$) and tincture of iodine ingestions are much less common than in the past as a result of the change in antiseptic use from iodine to iodophor antiseptics.

Iodophors have molecular iodine compounded to a high-molecular-weight carrier or to a solubilizing xenobiotic. Povidone-iodine, a commonly used iodophor, consists of iodine linked to polyvinylpyrrolidone (povidone). Iodophors limit the release of molecular iodine and are generally less toxic. The most common preparation is a 10% povidone-iodine solution that contains 1% "available" iodine (referring to all oxidizing iodine species), but only 0.001% free iodine (referring only to molecular iodine).

Significant systemic absorption of iodine from topical iodine or iodophor preparations is rare. Markedly elevated iodine concentrations occur in patients who receive topical iodophor treatments to areas of dermal breakdown, such as burn injuries. Significant absorption occurs when iodophors are applied to the vagina, perianal fistulas, umbilical cords, and the skin of low-birth-weight neonates. Several cases of kidney failure or death following intraoperative irrigation of a hip wound with povidone-iodine are reported.

***Clinical Effects.*** Problems associated with the use of iodine include unpleasant odor, skin irritation, allergic reactions, and clothes staining. Ingestion of iodine causes abdominal pain, vomiting, diarrhea, GI bleeding, delirium, hypovolemia, anuria, and circulatory collapse. Severe caustic injury of the GI tract occurs. The ingestion of approximately 45 mL of a 10% iodine solution resulted in death from multisystem failure 67 hours after ingestion. In another case, the ingestion of 200 mL of tincture of iodine containing 60 mg/mL iodine and 40 mg/mL potassium iodide in 70% v/v ethanol resulted in acute kidney injury (AKI) and severe hemolysis.

Reports of adverse consequences from iodophor ingestions are rare. In one case report, a 9-week-old infant died within 3 hours after receiving 15 mL of povidone-iodine mixed with 135 mL of polyethylene glycol by nasogastric tube over a 3-hour period for the treatment of infantile colic. Postmortem examination showed an ulcerated and necrotic intestinal tract.

Metabolic acidosis occurred in several burn patients after receiving multiple applications of povidone-iodine ointment. These patients had elevated serum iodine concentrations and normal lactate concentrations. Metabolic acidosis associated with an elevated lactate concentration after iodine ingestion likely reflects tissue destruction. Electrolyte abnormalities also occur following the absorption of iodine. A patient with decubitus ulcers who received prolonged wound care with povidone-iodine–soaked gauze developed hypernatremia, hyperchloremia, metabolic acidosis, and AKI. The hyperchloremia was thought to be caused by a spurious elevation of measured chloride ions from interference of iodine with the chloride assay. Other problems associated with topical absorption of iodine-containing preparations are hypothyroidism (particularly in neonates), hyperthyroidism, elevated liver enzyme concentrations, neutropenia, anaphylaxis, and hypoxemia.

***Management.*** The patient who ingests iodine requires expeditious evaluation, stabilization, and decontamination. If signs of perforation are absent, it is reasonable to proceed with careful nasogastric or orogastric aspiration and lavage to limit the caustic effect of the iodine. In symptomatic patients, irrigation with a starch solution, such as corn starch, is recommended to convert iodine to the much less toxic iodide and, in the process, turn the gastric effluent dark blue-purple. If starch is not available, milk or 100 mL of a solution of 1% to 3% sodium thiosulfate is a reasonable alternative to convert iodine to iodide. We recommend early endoscopy in patients with significant symptoms to help assess the extent of the GI injury. Hemodialysis and continuous venovenous hemodiafiltration were used successfully to enhance elimination of iodine in a patient with chronic kidney disease with iodine toxicity who developed worsening renal function after undergoing continuous mediastinal irrigation with povidone-iodine. The benefit of hemodialysis or continuous venovenous hemodiafiltration is unknown in patients with normal kidney function and therefore not routinely recommended at this time.

### Potassium Permanganate

Potassium permanganate ($KMnO_4$) is a violet water-soluble xenobiotic that is usually sold as crystals or tablets or as a 0.01% dilute solution. Currently, potassium permanganate is most often used in baths and wet bandages as a dermal antiseptic, particularly for patients with eczema.

Potassium permanganate is a strong oxidizer, and poisoning results in local and systemic toxicity. Upon contact with mucous membranes, potassium permanganate reacts with water to form manganese dioxide, potassium hydroxide, and molecular oxygen. Local tissue injury is the result of contact with the nascent oxygen, as well as the caustic effect of potassium hydroxide. A brown-black staining of the tissues occurs from the manganese dioxide. Systemic toxicity occurs from free radicals generated by absorbed permanganate ions.

***Clinical Effects.*** Following ingestion, initial symptoms include nausea and vomiting. Laryngeal edema and ulceration of the mouth, esophagus, and, to a lesser extent, the stomach result from the caustic effects. Airway obstruction and fatal GI perforation and hemorrhage are reported. Esophageal strictures and pyloric stenosis are potential late complications. Systemic effects include hepatotoxicity, AKI, methemoglobinemia, hemolysis, hemorrhagic pancreatitis, airway obstruction, ARDS, disseminated intravascular coagulation, and cardiovascular collapse.

Chronic ingestion of potassium permanganate results in classic manganese poisoning (manganism) characterized by behavioral changes, hallucinations, and delayed onset of parkinsonian-like symptoms (Chap. 67).

***Management.*** Immediate assessment for evidence of airway compromise should be performed. Corticosteroids are recommended if laryngeal edema is present. In the absence of airway compromise, dilution with milk or water is reasonable. Patients with symptoms consistent with caustic injury should undergo early upper–GI tract endoscopy. We recommend methylene blue for clinically significant methemoglobinemia (Antidotes in Brief: A43).

## OTHER ANTISEPTICS

### Alcohols

Ethanol and isopropanol (Chaps. 49 and 79) are commonly used as skin antiseptics.

### Chlorine and Chlorophors

Chlorine, one of the first antiseptics, is still used in the treatment of the community water supply and in swimming pools. Chlorine is a potent pulmonary irritant that can cause severe bronchospasm and ARDS. Chapter 94 contains a further discussion of chlorine.

Sodium hypochlorite (NaOCl), found in household bleaches and in Dakin solution, remains a commonly used disinfectant. The ingestion of large amounts of household liquid bleach (5% NaOCl) on rare occasions can result in esophageal burns with subsequent stricture formation. However, the vast majority of household bleach ingestions do not cause significant GI injuries. Endoscopy is reasonable in symptomatic patients only. Endoscopy is recommended in symptomatic patients who ingest a more concentrated "industrial strength" (35% NaOCl) preparations, because of the increased likelihood of local tissue injury (Chap. 76).

### Mercurials

Both inorganic mercurials, such as mercuric bichloride ($HgCl_2$), and organic mercurials, such as merbromin (mercurochrome) and thimerosal (merthiolate), which both contain 49% mercury, were previously used as topical antiseptics. The usefulness of mercurials is significantly limited because of their relatively weak bacteriostatic properties and the many concerns associated with mercury toxicity despite there being no causal link between vaccinations containing thimerosal and autism (Chap. 68).

## DISINFECTANTS

### Formaldehyde

Formaldehyde is a water-soluble, highly reactive gas at room temperature. Formalin consists of an aqueous solution of formaldehyde, usually containing approximately 37% formaldehyde and 12% to 15% methanol. Formaldehyde is irritating to the upper airways, and its odor is readily detectable at low concentrations. Lethality in adults follows ingestion of as little as 30 to 60 mL of formalin.

Exposure to formaldehyde, a potent tissue fixative, results in both local and systemic symptoms, causing coagulation necrosis, protein precipitation, and tissue fixation. Ingestion of formalin results in significant gastric injury, including hemorrhage, diffuse necrosis, perforation, and stricture.

The most extensive damage appears in the stomach, with only occasional involvement of the small intestine and colon. Chemical fixation of the stomach occurs. Esophageal involvement is not very prominent and, if present, is usually limited to its distal segment.

The most striking and rapid systemic manifestation of formaldehyde poisoning is anion gap metabolic acidosis, resulting both from tissue injury and from the conversion of formaldehyde to formic acid. Although the methanol component of the formalin solution is readily absorbed and produces methanol concentrations reportedly as high as 40 mg/dL, the rapid metabolism of formaldehyde to formic acid is responsible for much of the metabolic acidosis (Chap. 79).

***Clinical Effects.*** Patients presenting after formalin ingestions complain of the rapid onset of severe abdominal pain, vomiting, and diarrhea. Altered mental status and coma usually follow rapidly. Physical examination demonstrates epigastric tenderness, hematemesis, cyanosis, hypotension, and tachypnea. Profound hypotension is due to decreased myocardial contractility, as well as hypovolemic shock. Early endoscopic findings include ulceration, necrosis, perforation, and hemorrhage of the stomach, with infrequent esophageal involvement. Chemical pneumonitis occurs after significant inhalational exposure. Intravascular hemolysis is described in hemodialysis patients whose dialysis equipment contained residual formaldehyde after undergoing routine cleaning.

Occupational and environmental exposure to formaldehyde receives considerable attention. In particular, there is concern over the potential off-gassing of formaldehyde from the widely used urea formaldehyde in building insulation and particle board. Headache, nausea, skin rash, sore throat, nasal congestion, and eye irritation are associated with the use of these polymers.

Formaldehyde exposure is associated with an increased incidence of nasopharyngeal carcinoma and is classified as a Group 1, known, carcinogen by the International Agency for Research on Cancer (IARC).

***Management.*** Dilution with water is reasonable for the immediate management of a patient who has ingested formalin. Gastric aspiration with a small-bore nasogastric or orogastric tube is also reasonable to limit systemic absorption. Significant acidemia is treated with sodium bicarbonate and folinic acid (Chap. 79). Immediate hemodialysis removes the accumulating formic acid as well as the parent molecules formaldehyde and methanol and is reasonable in refractory acidemia. The empiric use of ethanol or fomepizole is also reasonable to block metabolism of methanol (Antidotes in Brief: A33 and A34). Early endoscopy is recommended for all patients with significant GI manifestations to assess the degree of burn injury. Surgical intervention is required for those with suspected severe burns, tissue necrosis, and/or perforation.

### Phenol

The concentration of phenol in consumer products can vary significantly, from 0.1% to 4.7% in various lotions, ointments, gels, gargles, lozenges, and throat sprays to up to 89% in nail cauterizer solution. Although many cases of phenol poisoning were reported in the past, acute oral overdoses of phenol-containing solutions are uncommon today.

Phenol acts as a caustic, causing cell wall disruption, protein denaturation, and coagulation necrosis. It also acts as a central nervous system (CNS) stimulant. The lethal oral dose is as little as 1 g. Phenol also demonstrates excellent skin penetrance and causes severe dermal burns, resulting in potentially fatal systemic toxicity within minutes to hours. Deaths from parenteral administration of phenol are reported.

***Clinical Effects.*** Central nervous system effects include CNS stimulation, seizures, lethargy, and coma. Cardiac signs and symptoms from phenol include tachycardia, bradycardia, and hypotension. Parenteral administration of 10 mL of 89% phenol resulted in hypoxemia, ARDS, pulmonary nodular opacities, and AKI requiring intubation and hemodialysis. Other systemic effects include hypothermia, metabolic acidosis, methemoglobinemia, and extrapyramidal movement disorders.

Local toxicity to the GI tract from the ingestion of phenol results in nausea, painful oral lesions, vomiting, severe abdominal pain, bloody diarrhea, and dark urine. Serious GI burns are uncommon, and strictures are rare. Dermal exposures to phenol usually result in a light-brown staining of the skin. Excessive dermal absorption of phenol during chemical peeling procedures is associated with dysrhythmias and many of the other toxic manifestations.

***Management.*** When phenol is mixed with water, a bilayer with unique properties is created that makes it difficult to remove from tissues. Either low-molecular-weight PEG, for example, PEG 300 or 400 (not to be confused with high-molecular-weight PEG 3350 that is used for whole-bowel irrigation), or high-flow water is reasonable for dermal irrigation and careful gastric decontamination. Endoscopic evaluation is recommended for symptomatic patients to determine the extent of GI injury.

### Substituted Phenols and Other Related Compounds

Hexachlorophene is considered generally less tissue-toxic than phenol. During the 1970s, an association was observed between repetitive whole-body washing of premature infants with 3% hexachlorophene and the development of vacuolar encephalopathy and cerebral edema. There are also multiple reports of significant neurologic toxicity and death in children who ingested hexachlorophene. In addition, fatalities occurred after patients absorbed substantial amounts of hexachlorophene during the treatment of burns. The use of hexachlorophene has declined significantly. Currently used substituted phenols include a sodium solution of octylphenoxyethoxyethyl ether sulfonate, chloroxylenol, and cresol.

***Clinical Effects.*** A sodium solution of octylphenoxyethoxyethyl ether sulfonate and lanolin is a safe antiseptic. Irritative effects such as nausea, vomiting, and diarrhea are the main adverse effects following ingestion.

***Management.*** Treatment is supportive care.

### Quaternary Ammonium Compounds

Quaternary ammonium compounds, positively charged compounds in which four organic groups are linked to a nitrogen atom ($NH_4^+$), are cationic surfactants (surface-active agent) that are used as disinfectants, detergents, and sanitizers.

Other cationic surfactants include the pyridinium compounds and the quinolinium compounds.

*Clinical.* Quaternary ammonium compounds are usually less toxic than phenol or formaldehyde. Most of the infrequent complications that are described result from ingestions of benzalkonium chloride. Complications of these ingestions include burns to the mouth and esophagus, CNS depression, elevated liver enzyme concentrations, metabolic acidosis, and hypotension. Paralysis is also occasionally described as a complication of these ingestions and is presumably a result of cholinesterase inhibition at the neuromuscular junction. Topical use of the quaternary ammonium compounds causes contact dermatitis.

Ingestions of other cationic surfactants, such as the pyridinium-derived cetrimonium bromide, are associated with corrosive burns to the mouth, lips, and tongue. Peritoneal irrigation with cetrimonium bromide produces metabolic abnormalities, hypotension, and methemoglobinemia. Intravenous administration of cetrimonium bromide leads to hemolysis, muscle paralysis, and cardiac arrest.

*Management.* Treatment recommendations following the ingestion of the quaternary ammonium compounds and other cationic surfactants are similar to those for other potentially caustic ingestions. Emergency department evaluation is recommended for all patients who ingest more than a taste of a dilute (< 1%) solution. Therapy is mainly supportive care. Endoscopy is indicated if signs and symptoms suggest the possibility of a burn.

## STERILANTS

### Ethylene Oxide

Ethylene oxide ($C_2H_4O$) is a gas that is commonly used to sterilize heat-sensitive material in healthcare facilities. Unlike antiseptics and disinfectants, which generally do not exhibit full sporicidal activity, sterilants, such as ethylene oxide, inactivate all organisms. Medical attention regarding ethylene oxide toxicity has centered on its mutagenic and possible carcinogenic effects. Ethylene oxide is classified as IARC group 1—carcinogenic to humans. Retrospective studies suggest an excess incidence of leukemia and gastric cancer in ethylene oxide–exposed workers.

Also, an increased incidence of spontaneous abortions is associated with occupational exposure to ethylene oxide.

*Clinical Effects.* The acute toxicity of ethylene oxide is mainly the result of its irritant effects, including conjunctival, upper respiratory tract, GI, and dermal irritation. Dermal burns from acute exposure to ethylene oxide are reported. Rare cases of syncope, seizures, coma, and parkinsonism are reported following inhalation. Chronic exposure to high concentrations of ethylene oxide causes mild cognitive impairment and motor and sensory neuropathies and an increase rate of spontaneous abortions.

*Management.* Treatment for patients with ethylene oxide exposure is supportive.

### Glutaraldehyde

Glutaraldehyde is a liquid solution used in the cold sterilization of nonautoclavable endoscopic, surgical, and dental equipment. The sterilant ability of glutaraldehyde results from the alkylation of sulfhydryl, hydroxyl, carboxyl, and amino groups, within microbes interfering with RNA, DNA, and protein synthesis. It is prepared as a 2% alkaline solution in 70% isopropanol. Healthcare workers are exposed to glutaraldehyde vapors when equipment is processed in poorly ventilated areas or in open immersion baths or after spills.

*Clinical.* Clinical signs and symptoms are comparable to those of formaldehyde exposure, although human toxicity data are limited. Glutaraldehyde is a mucosal irritant. Coryza, epistaxis, headache, asthma, chest tightness, palpitations, tachycardia, and nausea are all associated with glutaraldehyde vapor exposure. Occupational asthma, contact dermatitis, and ocular inflammation also occur. Colitis is reported following the use of endoscopes contaminated with residual glutaraldehyde solution.

*Management.* Treatment recommendations are similar to those for patients with formaldehyde exposure. Prompt removal from the exposure is essential. Copious irrigation with water is recommended for dermal decontamination. Severe inhalational exposures require hospital admission for observation, supportive care, and treatment of bronchospasm.

## OTHER PRODUCTS

### Boric Acid

Boric acid is an odorless, transparent crystal, although it is most commonly available as a finely ground white powder. It is also available as a 2.5% to 5% aqueous solution. Although once used extensively for antisepsis and irrigation, boric acid is only weakly bacteriostatic. As a result of its germicidal limitations and its inherent toxicity, boric acid is nearly obsolete in modern antiseptic therapy. Boric acid is also employed in the treatment of cockroach infestation and as a soap, contact lens solution, toothpaste, and food preservative.

Boric acid is readily absorbed through the GI tract, wounds, abraded skin, and serous cavities. Absorption does not occur through intact skin. Boric acid is predominantly eliminated unchanged by the kidney. The exact mechanism of action of toxicity remains unclear. Local effects are limited to tissue irritation.

Over the years, boric acid developed a reputation as an exceptionally potent toxin. These cases date predominantly from the first half of the 20th century when boric acid was widely used as an irrigant. Routes of exposure to boric acid, resulting in fatalities, include wound irrigation, pleural irrigation, rectal washing, bladder irrigation, and vaginal packing.

*Clinical Effects.* Boric acid poisoning usually involves multiple exposures over a period of days. The initial effects—nausea, vomiting, diarrhea, and occasionally crampy abdominal pain—are frequently confused with an acute gastroenteritis. At times, the emesis and diarrhea are greenish blue. Following the onset of GI signs and symptoms, the majority of patients develop a characteristic intense generalized erythroderma. This rash, described as producing a "boiled lobster" appearance, appears indistinguishable from toxic epidermal necrolysis or staphylococcal scalded skin syndrome in the neonate. The rash is especially noticeable on the palms, soles, and buttocks. Extensive desquamation takes place within

1 to 2 days. At the time of development of the erythroderma, patients, particularly young infants, develop prominent signs of CNS irritability, resembling meningeal irritation. Seizures, delirium, and coma occur. Acute kidney injury is common, both as a result of the renal elimination of this compound and prerenal azotemia from GI losses. Other complications of boric acid poisoning include hepatic injury, hyperthermia, and cardiovascular collapse. A marked decrease in the incidence of significant boric acid poisoning is attributed to the abandonment of boric acid as an irrigant and particularly its removal from the nursery setting.

Two retrospective studies on boric acid ingestions suggest that a single acute ingestion of boric acid is generally quite benign. Symptoms, when present, primarily consist of nausea and vomiting. None of the 1,184 patients in these two studies manifested the generalized erythroderma so commonly described in previous reports. Central nervous system manifestations of acute overdose were infrequent and limited to occasional lethargy and headache. Kidney injury did not occur following single acute ingestions. However, fatalities from massive acute ingestion of boric acid are still reported in both unintentional ingestions in children and intentional ingestions in adults. Long-term chronic exposure to boric acid results in alopecia in adults and seizures in children.

***Management.*** Treatment of boric acid toxicity is supportive care. Because boric acid has a low molecular weight and relatively small volume of distribution, in cases of massive oral overdose or AKI, hemodialysis, or perhaps exchange transfusion in infants, is reasonable in shortening the half-life of boric acid.

### Chlorates

Sodium chlorate is a strong oxidizer. Although their use as local antiseptics is obsolete, chlorates are used as herbicides and in the manufacture of matches, explosives, and dyestuffs. More recent cases of chlorate poisoning continue to result from the ingestion of sodium chlorate–containing weed killers and industrial chemicals. Sodium chlorate is rapidly absorbed from the GI tract and eliminated predominantly unchanged from the kidneys. The major mechanism of toxicity of chlorate is its ability to oxidize hemoglobin and increase red blood cell membrane rigidity. Consequently, methemoglobinemia and hemolysis result. Methemoglobinemia occurs prior to or after the development of hemolysis. The hemolysis and the resultant hemoglobinuria secondarily cause disseminated intravascular coagulation and potential renal toxicity, respectively. Chlorates are also directly toxic to the proximal renal tubule. The worsening kidney function is especially problematic because of its adverse effect on chlorate elimination.

***Clinical.*** Clinical signs and symptoms of chlorate poisoning usually begin 1 to 4 hours after ingestion. The earliest manifestations are nausea, vomiting, diarrhea, and crampy abdominal pain. Subsequently, patients exhibit cyanosis from the methemoglobinemia and black-brown urine from the hemoglobinuria. Obtundation and anuria ensue. Laboratory studies demonstrate methemoglobinemia, anemia, Heinz bodies, ghost cells, fragmented spherocytes, metabolic acidosis, thrombocytopenia, and abnormal coagulation. Hyperkalemia is particularly problematic if the patient ingests potassium chlorate preparations.

***Management.*** In symptomatic patients with chlorate ingestions, it is reasonable to pursue GI decontamination with activated charcoal. The utility of methylene blue in the treatment of symptomatic chlorate-induced methemoglobinemia has been questioned as a consequence of the inactivation by chlorates of glucose-6-phosphate dehydrogenase, an enzyme that is required for methylene blue to effectively reduce methemoglobin. Nevertheless, more recent experience suggests that early use of methylene blue prior to the onset of hemolysis is beneficial due to the necessity of the intact erythrocyte for methylene blue to be efficacious and thus a reasonable treatment. Exchange transfusion and hemodialysis are reasonable in the treatment of patients with severe chlorate poisoning. Because the chlorate ion is easily dialyzable, hemodialysis will be effective in removal of chlorate as well as in treating concomitant AKI.

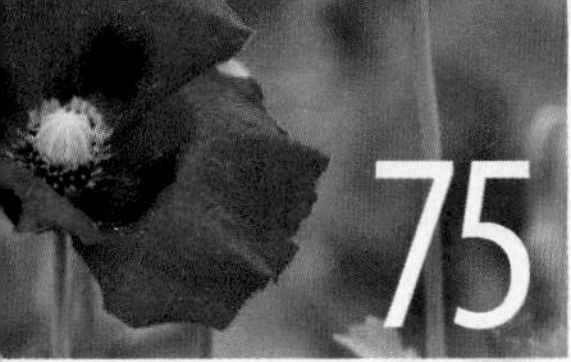

# 75 CAMPHOR AND MOTH REPELLENTS

Many different products have been used as moth repellents. In the United States (US), paradichlorobenzene has largely replaced both camphor and naphthalene as the most common component of mothballs and moth flakes because it is less toxic. However, both naphthalene and camphor are still available.

## CAMPHOR

### History and Epidemiology

Camphor has been used as an aphrodisiac, contraceptive, abortifacient, suppressor of lactation, analeptic, cardiac stimulant, antiseptic, cold remedy, muscle liniment, and drug of abuse. Camphorated oil and camphorated spirits contain varying concentrations. Historically, most camphorated oil was 20% weight (of solute) per weight (of solvent) (w/w) camphor with cottonseed oil and most camphorated spirits contained 10% w/w camphor with isopropyl alcohol. Today, based on a 1983 US Food and Drug Administration (FDA) ruling, nonprescription camphor products may not contain greater than an 11% concentration of camphor. Camphorated oil is still used as an herbal remedy and muscle liniment, and products containing more than 11% camphor can be purchased legally outside of the US.

### Pharmacology

The pharmacologic activity of camphor is not well studied, and its mechanism of action remains unclear.

### Pharmacokinetics and Toxicokinetics

There are limited data on the pharmacokinetics and toxicokinetics of camphor. Camphor toxicity is reported following ingestion, dermal application, inhalation, intranasal instillation, intraperitoneal administration, and transplacental transfer. Ingestion of solid camphor also causes toxicity. Liquid camphor preparations are rapidly absorbed from the gastrointestinal tract. The volume of distribution is estimated at 2 to 4 L/kg with protein binding of approximately 61%. Camphor is predominantly metabolized in the liver where it undergoes hydroxylation followed by conjugation with glucuronic acid. Inactive metabolites are excreted by the kidneys.

Although the toxic dose is not well delineated, as little as 1 teaspoon (1 g) of 20% camphorated oil has been reported to cause death in an infant. A potential lethal dose of 50 to 500 mg/kg of camphor is often cited for humans.

### Pathophysiology

The mechanism of toxicity of camphor is unknown. Camphor is an irritant. Pathologic changes following ingestion include cerebral edema, neuronal degeneration, fatty changes in the liver, centrilobular congestion of the liver, and hemorrhagic lesions in the skin, gastrointestinal tract, and kidneys.

### Clinical Manifestations

Exposure can often be detected by its characteristic aromatic odor. Ingestion typically produces oropharyngeal irritation, nausea, vomiting, and abdominal pain. Generalized tonic-clonic seizures usually occur within 1 to 2 hours postingestion. Most seizures are brief and self-limited, although some patients have a more protracted course. Other neurologic manifestations include headache, lightheadedness, transient visual changes, confusion, myoclonus, and hyperreflexia. Psychiatric manifestations include agitation, anxiety, and hallucinations. Transient elevations of hepatic aminotransferases are reported. Chronic administration can cause altered mental status and elevated hepatic aminotransferase concentrations suggestive of Reye syndrome. Camphor crosses the placenta. Both fetal demise and delivery of healthy neonates are reported in mothers experiencing camphor toxicity within 24 hours of term delivery. Inhalation and dermal exposure usually produce mucous membrane irritation and dermal irritation, respectively.

### Diagnostic Testing

No specific diagnostic test is available or indicated when managing patients with camphor toxicity. Camphor and its metabolites can be identified in blood and urine, but these tests are not clinically useful.

### Management

Following an acute ingestion, patients who have ingested more than 30 mg/kg of camphor or have signs and symptoms consistent with camphor toxicity should be evaluated in a health care facility. Gastric lavage is not recommended because of the rapidity of absorption and the risk of seizures. It remains reasonable to administer activated charcoal following a large recent ingestion if no contraindications exist. Case reports suggest that most patients who develop life-threatening camphor toxicity develop symptoms within a few hours postexposure. Based on this, we recommend an observation period of at least 4 hours following a potentially toxic ingestion. Patients with camphor-induced seizures should be treated with benzodiazepines and/or barbiturates. If repeat doses of benzodiazepines fail to control seizures, phenobarbital or propofol should be administered.

## NAPHTHALENE

### History and Epidemiology

Naphthalene is a bicyclic aromatic hydrocarbon that is pure white and has a noxious odor that is found in moth repellants, toilet-bowl and diaper-pan deodorizers, and soil fumigants. Most unintentional exposures to naphthalene-containing mothballs occur in children and do not cause life-threatening toxicity.

### Pharmacology, Pharmacokinetics, and Toxicokinetics

Naphthalene toxicity is reported following ingestion, dermal application, and inhalation. Naphthalene absorption is not well studied. Once absorbed, it is slowly metabolized in the liver to multiple metabolites including 1-naphthol ($\alpha$-naphthol), 1,2-naphthoquinone, and 1,4-naphthoquinone.

These cytotoxins deplete intracellular glutathione stores and are responsible for the oxidative stress that lead to naphthalene-induced hemolysis and methemoglobinemia. While the reported toxic dose is highly variable, it is generally accepted that as little as one naphthalene mothball can produce toxicity in a glucose-6-phosphate dehydrogenase (G6PD) deficient child.

### Pathophysiology

Oxidant stress can cause methemoglobinemia and/or hemolysis. When oxidant stress causes iron on hemoglobin to be converted from the ferrous state ($Fe^{2+}$) to the ferric state ($Fe^{3+}$) state, methemoglobin is formed (Chap. 97). When oxidant stress causes hemoglobin denaturation, the heme groups and the globin chains dissociate and precipitate in the erythrocyte, forming Heinz bodies. An erythrocyte with denatured hemoglobin is more susceptible to hemolysis and to removal by the reticuloendothelial system.

Hemolysis and methemoglobinemia can occur independently or simultaneously in patients with either normal or deficient G6PD activity. Patients with G6PD deficiency are at much greater risk of hemolysis rather than methemoglobinemia because of their decreased glutathione stores.

### Clinical Manifestations

Acute and chronic exposures to naphthalene result in similar toxicity. Ingestion and inhalational exposures to naphthalene commonly cause headache, nausea, vomiting, diarrhea, abdominal pain, fever, and altered mental status. Hemolysis and/or methemoglobinemia usually do not become clinically evident before 1 to 2 days postexposure because of the slow generation of $\alpha$-naphthol. Anemia secondary to hemolysis often does not reach its nadir until 3 to 5 days postexposure.

Signs and symptoms of hemolysis and methemoglobinemia are nonspecific and include tachycardia, tachypnea, shortness of breath, generalized weakness, decreased exercise tolerance, and altered mental status. Methemoglobinemia produces cyanosis, whereas hemolysis produces pallor, jaundice, and dark urine.

### Diagnostic Testing

Both naphthalene and its metabolites can be identified in blood and urine but provide no valuable information for managing acute exposures because of long turn-around times and a lack of correlation between concentrations and symptoms. Blood should be sent for cooximetry if methemoglobinemia is suspected. Hemoglobin, bilirubin, lactate dehydrogenase, haptoglobin, and urinalysis will help diagnosis hemolysis. Examination of a peripheral blood smear can reveal evidence of hemolysis before a patient develops clinical or laboratory evidence of anemia. Testing for G6PD activity is not recommended during an acute episode of hemolysis because young erythrocytes have higher G6PD activity than do older red blood cells possibly resulting in a false-negative test.

### Management

Most patients with an unintentional exposure to one or part of one naphthalene-containing mothball do not require evaluation. Patients who should be evaluated include those who recently ingested more than one naphthalene-containing mothball, anyone with signs or symptoms of hemolysis and/or methemoglobinemia, patients with known or suspected G6PD deficiency, all intentional ingestions, and patients with large inhalational exposures, especially those occurring in an occupational setting.

Most patients with unintentional exposures do not require gastrointestinal decontamination. Administration of activated charcoal, 1 g/kg, although not of proven efficacy, is reasonable for patients with large ingestions.

Patients with laboratory evidence of hemolysis should be closely observed and only transfused for life-threatening anemia. Most patients typically recover quickly as young erythrocytes are resistant to hemolysis. Patients with significant methemoglobinemia should receive intravenous methylene blue, 1 to 2 mg/kg (Antidotes in Brief: A43).

## PARADICHLOROBENZENE

### History and Epidemiology

Paradichlorobenzene is the most common component of moth repellents and is also found in deodorizers and disinfectants. Low-level exposure to paradichlorobenzene in the US is extremely common as a result of environmental contamination from release of paradichlorobenzene into air by industrial facilities.

### Pharmacology, Pharmacokinetics, Toxicokinetics, and Pathophysiology

Paradichlorobenzene is pure white and has a noxious odor. The mechanism for the effects of paradichlorobenzene, its pharmacology, and its toxicokinetics are not well studied. Paradichlorobenzene is well absorbed via ingestion, inhalation, and dermal exposure. Following absorption, it rapidly distributes to tissues, particularly adipose. Paradichlorobenzene undergoes hepatic metabolism by several CYP450 enzymes.

### Clinical Manifestations

Inhalation of paradichlorobenzene may cause nausea and vomiting, headache, and mucous membrane irritation. Most patients who ingest paradichlorobenzene develop only self-limited gastrointestinal distress.

Case reports associate chronic exposure to paradichlorobenzene with weight loss, ataxia, pulmonary granulomatosis, dyspnea, hepatotoxicity, anemia, and fixed drug eruptions. More importantly, significant neuropsychiatric dysfunction, specifically cerebellar dysfunction, motor weakness, behavioral changes, and cognitive decline, is reported following chronic intentional and occupational exposure.

### Diagnostic Testing

Both paradichlorobenzene and its metabolite, 2,5-dichlorophenol, can be identified in blood and urine following exposure, but have no role in acute poisoning. Quantifying the amount of paradichlorobenzene in the urine of workers may be useful for monitoring occupational exposures. Structural central nervous system abnormalities, including toxic leukoencephalopathy, are occasionally noted on imaging studies such as magnetic resonance imaging that demonstrate

**TABLE 75–1 Moth Repellents: Laboratory Differentiation**

| *Characteristic* | *Camphor* | *Naphthalene* | *Paradichlorobenzene* |
|---|---|---|---|
| Water solubility (g/L) | 1.2 | 0.03 | 0.08 |
| Buoyancy in water | Floats | Sinks | Sinks |
| Buoyancy in water saturated with table salt | Floats | Floats | Sinks |
| Radiopacity | Radiolucent | Faintly radiopaque | Densely radiopaque |
| Melting point | 350.6°F (177°C) | 176°F (80°C) | 127.4°F (53°C) |
| Boiling point | 399.2°F (204°C) | 424.4°F (218°C) | 345.2°F (174°C) |
| In chloroform | Untested | Blue color | No reaction |
| Place on copper wire in a flame | Untested | Flame is yellow-orange | Initially flame is yellow-orange then bright green |
| Solubility in turpentine | Untested | Fast | Slow |

hyperintense signals in the periventricular white matter, corpus callosum, deep cerebellar nuclei, the parieto-occipital region, and internal capsule.

## Management

Because most unintentional exposures to paradichlorobenzene do not cause significant toxicity, evaluation by health professionals is unnecessary. Likewise, routine gastrointestinal decontamination should be considered to be potentially more harmful than beneficial. However, administration of activated charcoal, 1 g/kg, is reasonable for patients with large, intentional ingestions. Laboratory testing is generally not helpful in the acute setting unless there is clinical evidence for hemolysis or methemoglobinemia. Transfusion of packed red blood cells is recommended for symptomatic anemia resulting from acute hemolysis. Methylene blue is recommended for symptomatic methemoglobinemia.

# MOTHBALL RECOGNITION

Healthcare providers occasionally must determine whether a mothball is made of naphthalene, paradichlorobenzene, or camphor because management and prognosis for each are different. When the container is unavailable, as is often the case, mothballs are difficult to distinguish based on appearance, odor, texture, or size. Identifying a moth repellent as paradichlorobenzene often permits outpatient management, saving both hospital resources and unnecessary concern. Of tests described in Table 75–1 and shown in Fig. 75–1, the easiest to accomplish is to compare buoyancy in water and a saturated salt solution.

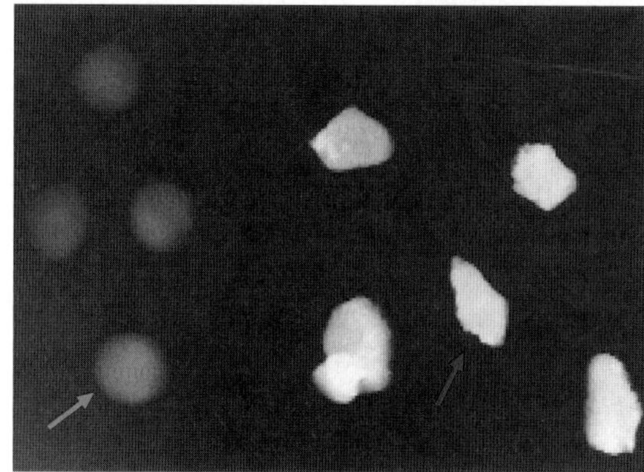

**FIGURE 75–1.** Radiograph of mothballs. Paradichlorobenzene (→) is densely radiopaque, whereas naphthalene (→) is faintly radiopaque.

# 76 CAUSTICS

## HISTORY AND EPIDEMIOLOGY

A caustic is a xenobiotic that causes both functional and histologic damage on contact with tissue surfaces. As early as 1927, legislation in the United States (US) governing the packaging of alkali- and acid-containing products mandated that warning labels be placed on these products. In response to the recognition that caustic exposures were more frequent in children, the US Federal Hazardous Substances Act and US Poison Prevention Packaging Act were passed in 1970. These acts mandated that all caustics with a concentration greater than 10% be sold in child-resistant containers. By 1973, the household concentration triggering mandatory child-resistant packaging was lowered to 2%. In addition, the subsequent development of poison prevention education dramatically decreased the incidence of unintentional caustic injuries in children in the US. The positive impact of both regulatory legislation and public health intervention is evident when observing the decreasing number of significant exposures in the US compared to the number of exposures in resource-poor nations that lack these policies.

Caustic exposures follow a bimodal age distribution pattern with peak occurrences in the pediatric population age 1 to 5 years and again in adulthood. In children, exposures usually consist of household products and occur most often in an unsupervised setting. In adults, exposures to household or industrial products result from occupational exposure, suicide attempts, and assaults. Although less frequent, intentional exposures by adults are invariably more significant. One study noted that although children comprised 39% of admissions for caustic ingestions, adults comprised 81% of patients requiring treatment.

Table 76–1 lists common caustics and the products that contain them. This chapter reviews the pathophysiology and approach to patients with potentially serious exposures.

**TABLE 76–1 Sources of Common Caustics**

| *Caustic* | *Common Applications* |
|---|---|
| Acetic acid | Permanent hair curl neutralizers, photographic stop bath, concentrated solution for food purposes |
| Ammonia (ammonium hydroxide) | Toilet bowl cleaners, metal cleaners and polishes, hair dyes and tints, antirust products, jewelry cleaners, floor strippers, glass cleaners, wax removers |
| Benzalkonium chloride | Detergents |
| Boric acid | Roach powders, water softeners, germicides |
| Formaldehyde, formic acid | Deodorizing tablets, plastic menders, fumigants, embalmers |
| Hydrochloric acid (muriatic acid) | Metal and toilet bowl cleaners |
| Hydrofluoric acid | Antirust products, glass etching, microchip etching |
| Iodine | Antiseptics |
| Mercuric chloride ($HgCl_2$) | Preservatives |
| Methylethyl ketone peroxide | Industrial synthetic intermediate |
| Oxalic acid | Disinfectants, household bleaches, metal polishes, antirust products, furniture refinishers |
| Phenol (creosol, creosote) | Antiseptics, preservatives |
| Phosphoric acid | Toilet bowl cleaners |
| Phosphorus | Matches, fireworks, rodenticides, methamphetamine synthesis |
| Potassium permanganate | Illicit abortifacients, antiseptic solutions |
| Potassium hydroxide | Oven cleaners, hair products, manufacture of biodiesel, soaps |
| Selenious acid | Gun-bluing agents |
| Sodium hydroxide (lye) | Detergents, paint removers, drain cleaners and openers, oven cleaners |
| Sodium borates, carbonates, phosphates, and silicates | Detergents, electric dishwasher preparations, water softeners |
| Sodium hypochlorite | Bleaches, cleansers |
| Sulfuric acid | Automobile batteries, drain cleaners |
| Zinc chloride | Soldering flux |

## PATHOPHYSIOLOGY

An acid is a proton donator and causes significant injury, generally at a pH below 3. An alkali is a proton acceptor and causes significant injury, generally when the pH is above 11. The extent of injury is modulated by duration of contact; ability of the caustic to penetrate tissues; volume, pH, and concentration; the presence or absence of food in the stomach; and a property known as titratable acid/alkaline reserve (TAR). Titratable acid/alkaline reserve quantifies the amount of neutralization needed to bring the pH of a caustic to that of physiologic tissues. Beyond tissue damage, some caustics have the potential to cause systemic toxicity.

### Alkalis

Following exposure, dissociated hydroxide ions ($OH^-$) penetrate tissue surfaces, producing a histologic pattern of liquefactive necrosis. This process includes protein dissolution, collagen destruction, fat saponification, cell membrane emulsification, transmural thrombosis, and cell death. Erythema and edema of the mucosa occur within seconds followed by an inflammatory reaction extending to the submucosa and muscular layers (Figs. 76–1 and 76–2).

Although federal regulations have lowered the maximal available household concentration of many caustics, two industrial-strength products seem to be readily available and therefore warrant special mention: ammonium hydroxide and sodium hypochlorite. Ammonia (ammonium hydroxide) products are weak bases—partially dissociated in water—that cause significant esophageal burns, depending on the

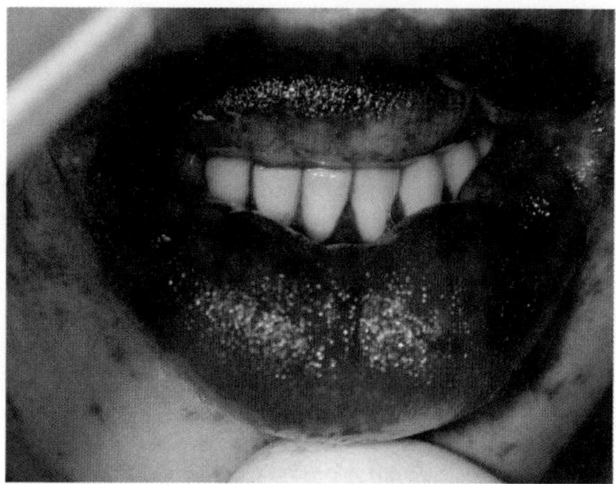

**FIGURE 76–1.** Photograph demonstrating burns to the lips and tongue of a 20-year-old man following ingestion of sodium hydroxide. *(Used with permission from the Fellowship in Medical Toxicology, New York University Grossman School of Medicine, New York City Poison Center.)*

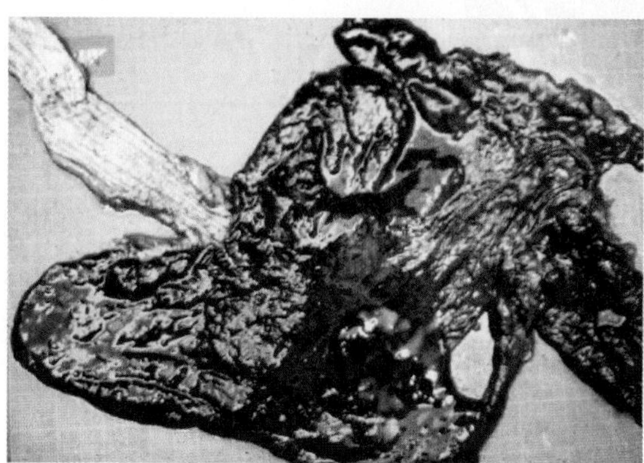

**FIGURE 76–3.** Postmortem specimen from a man with an intentional ingestion of a mixture of phosphoric and hydrochloric acid that was used as a brick cleaner. Note the relative sparing of the esophagus in contrast to full-thickness injury with perforation of the stomach. *(Used with permission from the Fellowship in Medical Toxicology, New York University Grossman School of Medicine, New York City Poison Center.)*

concentration and volume ingested. Household ammonium hydroxide ranges in concentration from 3% to 10%. Strictures are reported in patients who ingested 28% solutions. Sodium hypochlorite is the major component in most industrial and household bleaches. Severe injuries typically only occur in patients with large-volume ingestions of concentrated products and most other patients do well with supportive care.

As wound healing of gastrointestinal tract tissue occurs, neovascularization and fibroblast proliferation take place, laying down new collagen and replacing the damaged tissue with granulation tissue. This process typically persists for up to 8 weeks as remodeling takes place and is often followed by esophageal shortening. If the initial injury penetrates deeply, there is progressive narrowing of the esophageal lumen. The dense scar formation presents clinically as a stricture. Strictures can evolve over a period of weeks to months, leading to dysphagia and significant nutritional deficits.

### Acids

Following exposure, hydrogen ions ($H^+$) desiccate epithelial cells, producing an eschar and resulting in a histologic pattern of coagulation necrosis. This process leads to edema, erythema, mucosal sloughing, ulceration, and necrosis of tissues. Dissociated anions of the acid ($Cl^-$, $SO_4^{2-}$, $PO_4^{3-}$) also act as reducing agents, further injuring tissue.

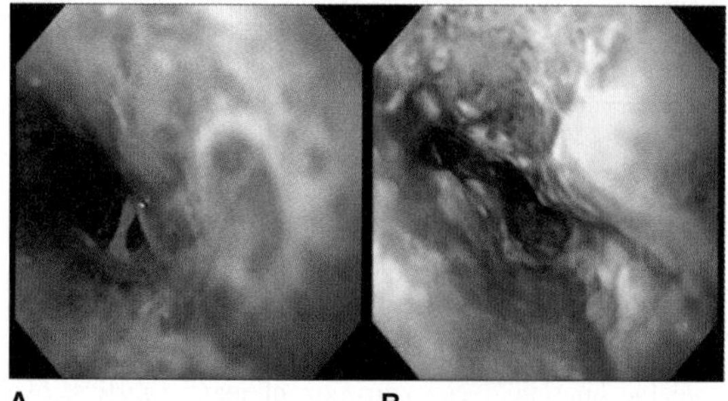

**FIGURE 76–2.** Endoscopic images of a 20-year-old man following ingestion of sodium hydroxide. (**A**) Grade IIa noncircumferential burn of the midesophagus. (**B**) Grade IIb circumferential burn of the distal esophagus. *(Used with permission from the Fellowship in Medical Toxicology, New York University Grossman School of Medicine, New York City Poison Center.)*

In most series, following an acid ingestion, both the gastric and esophageal mucosa are equally affected. On occasion, the esophagus is spared damage while severe injury is noted in the stomach (Fig. 76–3). This result tends to be a rarer finding than concomitant injury to both stomach and esophagus and is probably related to the rapid transit time of liquid acids through the upper gastrointestinal tract.

Chapters 68, 74, and 77 contain a more detailed discussion of mercury, phenol, and hydrofluoric acid, respectively, each a unique caustic.

### Classification and Progression of Caustic Injury

Esophageal and gastric burns are classified based on endoscopic visualization that employs a grading system similar to that used with dermal burns (Table 76–2).

## CLINICAL MANIFESTATIONS

The gastrointestinal tract, respiratory tract, eyes, and skin of the patient are potential sites of caustic injury. Caustics produce severe pain on contact with any of these tissues. By far, the majority of long-term morbidity and mortality from caustic exposure results from ingestion.

In general, patients who have ingested either alkalis or acids present and are managed in a similar manner. Oropharyngeal edema and burns lead to drooling and rapid airway compromise. Symptoms and findings of esophageal involvement include dysphagia and odynophagia, whereas epigastric pain and hematemesis are typical of gastric involvement. Respiratory tract damage occurs through direct inhalation or aspiration of vomitus, leading to the clinical manifestations of hoarseness, stridor, and respiratory distress. Injury results in epiglottitis, laryngeal edema and ulceration, pneumonitis, and impaired gas exchange. Tachypnea or hyperpnea results from either direct injury or as a compensatory response to a metabolic acidosis, which often is associated with elevated lactate concentrations from necrotic tissue or hemodynamic compromise.

**TABLE 76–2 Evaluation of Caustic Injuries and Their Management**

| *Grading of Injury by Endoscopic Visualization* | *Tissue Findings* | *Likelihood of Stricture Formation* | *Suggested Nutritional Support* | *Indication for Corticosteroids* | *Indications for Antibiotics* | *Indication for Stenting* |
|---|---|---|---|---|---|---|
| I | Hyperemia or edema of mucosa without ulcer formation | None | Resume diet as tolerated | None (unless airway edema mandates short course) | None | None<br>No stricture risk |
| IIa | Submucosal lesions, ulcers, exudates that are not circumferential | Low | Soft diet as tolerated or tube feeds (following nasogastric tube placement under direct visualization) | None (unless airway edema mandates short course) | Identified infection | None<br>No stricture risk |
| IIb | Submucosal lesions, ulcers, exudates that are near-circumferential | High, 75% | Because of risk of perforation, feeding via gastrostomy, jejunostomy, or total parenteral nutrition is recommended as rapidly as possible | Short course for alkaline ingestions only | Identified infection, or as part of a corticosteroid regimen | Intraluminal stents, nasogastric tubes are reasonable interventions to prevent strictures |
| III | Deep ulcers and necrosis into periesophageal tissues | High, near 100% | Because of risk of perforation, feeding via gastrostomy, jejunostomy, or total parenteral nutrition is recommended as rapidly as possible | Contraindicated (unless airway edema mandates short course) | Identified infection | Intraluminal stents, nasogastric tubes are reasonable interventions to prevent inevitable strictures |

Visual changes, eye pain, redness, burns, and ulceration of the eyes characterize ophthalmic exposure. Skin contact with caustics can result in pain, burns, and/or ulceration.

### Predictors of Injury

Various studies, mostly involving alkaline caustics, examine the predictive value of stridor, oropharyngeal burns, drooling, vomiting, and abdominal pain. In a landmark study, a combination of two or more of the signs (vomiting, drooling, stidor) was predictive of significant esophageal injury as visualized on endoscopy. This study has been validated by decades of clinical practice.

The abdominal examination is an unreliable indicator of the severity of injury. The presence of abdominal pain suggests tissue injury, but the absence of pain or findings on abdominal examination does not preclude life-threatening gastrointestinal damage. Esophageal perforations result in mediastinitis and are commonly associated with fever, dyspnea, chest pain, and subcutaneous emphysema of the neck and chest. Although indicative of viscus perforation, abdominal peritoneal signs are late findings.

Significant complications occur at various stages of wound recovery. Most importantly, these include airway compromise, hemodynamic instability secondary to hemorrhage from vascular erosion or septic shock, perforations of the gastrointestinal tract with the development of mediastinitis or peritonitis, and other overwhelming infections from bacteria residing in the oropharynx. A patient who survives acute injury with an acid or an alkali is at risk to subsequently develop stricture formation, gastric atony, decreased acid secretion, pseudodiverticula, and gastric outlet obstruction. Patients with strictures present with dysphagia and vomiting. Long-term survivors of moderate and severe caustic injury of the esophagus have a risk of esophageal carcinoma that is estimated to be 1,000 times higher than that of the general population and appears to present with a latency of up to 40 years.

## DIAGNOSTIC TESTING

### Laboratory

All patients with presumed serious caustic ingestion should have an evaluation of serum pH, blood type and crossmatch, complete blood count, coagulation parameters, and electrolytes. Absorption of nonionized acid from the stomach mucosa results in acidemia. Following ingestion of hydrochloric acid, hydrogen and chloride ions (both of which are accounted for in the measurement of the anion gap) dissociate in the serum, resulting in a hyperchloremic (normal anion gap) metabolic acidosis. Other acids, such as sulfuric acid, result in an elevated anion gap metabolic acidosis because the sulfate anion ($SO_4^{2-}$) is not measured in the calculation of the anion gap. Although alkalis are not absorbed systemically, significant necrosis of tissue results in a metabolic acidosis with an elevated lactate concentration.

### Radiology

Chest and abdominal radiographs are useful in the initial stages of assessment to detect gross signs of esophageal or gastric perforation. However, these studies have a limited sensitivity, and an absence of findings does not preclude perforation. Computed tomography (CT) scanning is considerably more sensitive than both radiography and ultrasound for detecting viscus perforation and is recommended for patients if endoscopy is unavailable or if the patient is critically ill. In addition, CT visualizes the esophagus and stomach distal to severe caustic burns that cannot be safely visualized using endoscopy and the serosal side of organs.

Another use of radiographic imaging is to noninvasively follow the patient after initial evaluation and stabilization. For example, contrast radiography is routinely used in the weeks or months following a caustic ingestion to detect esophageal narrowing representing stricture formation (Fig. 76–4).

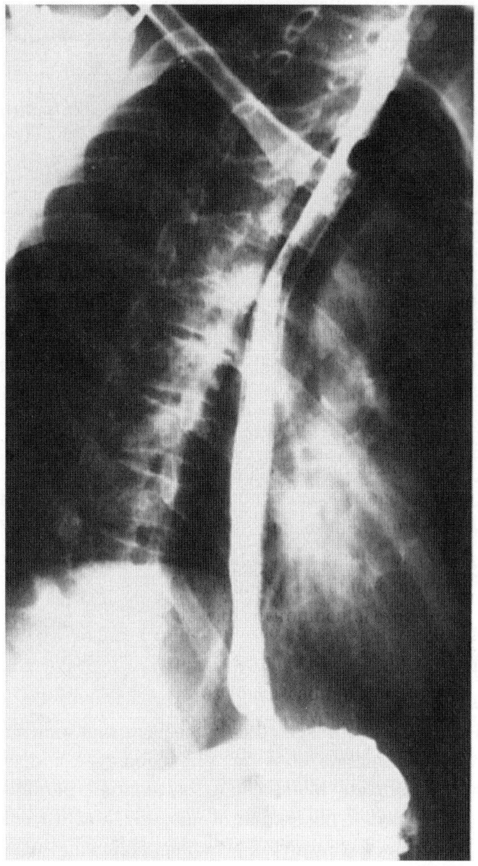



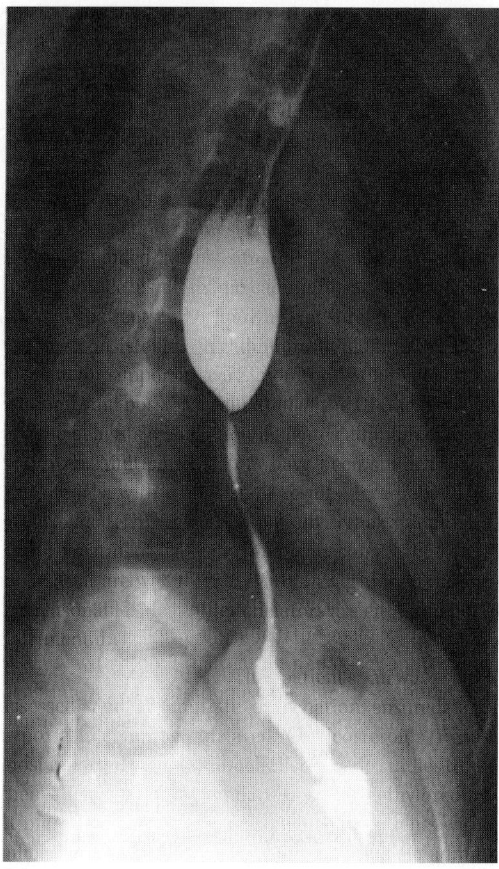



**FIGURE 76–4.** (**A**) Barium swallow several days after ingestion of liquid lye shows the esophagus to be atonic. There is poor coating of the esophagus, suggesting edema and intramural penetration. Note that the initial evaluation immediately following a caustic ingestion to assess the extent of injury is esophagoscopy, rather than a contrast esophagram. (**B**) Four months later, a repeat barium esophagram shows a severe stricture below the middle third of the esophagus. The barium barely passes the stricture, and the remainder of the esophagus is pencil thin. *(Used with permission from Emil J. Balthazar, MD, Professor of Radiology, New York University Langone Medical Center.)*

## Endoscopy

Endoscopy is recommended in: (1) all patients with intentional ingestions; (2) all acid ingestions regardless of symptoms (because of a lack of data); and (3) any patient with an unintentional ingestion of an alkaline caustic that has either stridor or both vomiting and drooling. Children with unintentional caustic ingestions who remain completely asymptomatic and tolerate liquids after a few hours of observation probably require no further medical care.

Early endoscopy serves multiple purposes. It offers a rapid means of obtaining diagnostic and prognostic information while shortening the period of time that patients forego nutritional support, permitting more precise treatment regimens. Patients found to have minimal or no evidence of gastroesophageal injury can be discharged or referred to psychiatry. A nasogastric tube may be passed under direct visualization in appropriate patients to facilitate caloric intake. Endoscopy is ideally performed within 12 hours and generally not later than 24 hours postingestion. We recommend against the use of endoscopic assessment after 24 hours and it should be avoided between 48 hours and 2 weeks postingestion; at this time, tissue strength is most compromised and the risk of perforation is greatest.

Most cases of perforation clearly linked to endoscopy have occurred when the endoscope was advanced through an esophagus with severe grade IIb or III lesions, which is a deviation from current endoscopic standards. In addition, perforations are also more likely to occur when rigid instruments are used in children or in uncooperative patients. Thus, the use of the flexible endoscope and adequate procedural sedation have decreased the complications from endoscopic evaluation. Some authors advocate the presence of a surgeon during endoscopy to assist in the assessment for potential surgical intervention.

Endoscopy permits limited evaluation of gastrointestinal injury. For example, the endoscopist is able to appreciate only the mucosal surface of tissues, not the serosal side. This is especially evident in stomach ulcerations, which often appear black and necrotic from a true burn through the layers of the stomach or from the effect of stomach acid on the blood exposed from a shallow lesion. As mentioned above, in these cases, endoscopic ultrasonography or CT scan improves assessment of injury depth. Often, however, only direct visualization of serosal and mucosal tissues with laparoscopy or laparotomy allows for definitive evaluation.

## MANAGEMENT

### Acute Management

The healthcare provider must first adhere to universal precautions using early decontamination. Decontamination should include removal of clothing and isolating it in a plastic bag for appropriate disposal and careful, copious irrigation of the patient's skin and eyes when indicated to remove any residual caustic and to prevent contamination of other patients, staff, and equipment. Concurrently, initial stabilization should include airway inspection and protection if indicated as well as basic resuscitation principles. Careful and constant attention to signs and symptoms of respiratory distress and airway edema, such as a change in voice, is essential and should prompt early endotracheal intubation as airway edema characteristically progresses rapidly over minutes to hours. Although not studied, dexamethasone 10 mg (intravenous) in adults and 0.6 mg/kg up to a total dose of 10 mg in children is reasonable for patients with these or other signs of caustic-induced airway compromise.

It is best to mobilize a team of the most skilled physicians early in case of unforeseen complications. Direct visual inspection of the vocal cords can be used to evaluate impending airway compromise when clinical signs and symptoms are unclear. However, a delay in prophylactic airway protection often makes subsequent attempts at intubation or bag–valve–mask ventilation difficult or impossible. Patients necessitating intubation are best served by direct visualization of the airway as perforation of edematous tissues is a grave complication that may occur during blind nasotracheal intubation attempts. Nonsurgical airway placement is recommended whenever possible as both cricothyrotomy and tracheostomy interfere with the surgical field if esophageal repair is required.

Following definitive airway management, large-bore intravenous access should be secured and volume resuscitation initiated. Both acid and alkali ingestions cause "third spacing" of intravascular fluid to the interstitial space, which can result in hypotension. Empiric volume resuscitation with clinical assessment should be used to guide individual fluid requirements. Serial physical examinations and constant monitoring of the vital signs, acid–base status, and urine output to assess the severity of the exposure and the progression in clinical status throughout the emergency department and/or hospital admission are imperative in patients with suspected serious caustic ingestion.

### Gastrointestinal Decontamination, Dilution, and Neutralization

Induced emesis is contraindicated, as it may cause reintroduction of the caustic to the upper gastrointestinal tract and airway. Activated charcoal is also not recommended, as it will interfere with tissue evaluation by endoscopy and preclude a subsequent management plan. Also, most caustics are not adsorbed to activated charcoal. Gastric emptying via cautious placement of a narrow nasogastric tube with direct visualization of the oropharynx and hypopharynx, followed by gentle suction is reasonable to remove the remaining acid in the stomach only in patients with large, life-threatening, intentional ingestions of acid who present within 30 minutes. Although this technique has never been studied and carries the risk of perforation, the outcome for this particular group of patients with massive exposure is often grave, and options for treatment are limited. In contrast, gastric emptying is contraindicated with alkaline and unknown caustic ingestions as blind passage of a nasogastric tube carries the risk of perforation of damaged tissues, a risk that outweighs the benefit.

The use of dilutional therapy was examined using in vitro, ex vivo, and in vivo models in an attempt to assess its efficacy in caustic ingestions. Data are limited, leading to weak recommendations. Dilutional therapy should be avoided in patients with nausea, drooling, stridor, or abdominal distention as it stimulates vomiting and results in reintroduction of the caustic into the upper gastrointestinal tract. Likewise, a child who refuses to swallow or take oral liquids should never be forced to do so. Thus, dilutional therapy with small volumes of water or milk is reasonable if it is limited to the first few minutes after ingestion in patients without airway signs or compromise and who are not complaining of significant pharyngeal, chest, or abdominal pain; are not vomiting; and are alert. Attempts at neutralization of ingested caustics are contraindicated.

### Surgical Management

The decision to perform surgery in patients with caustic ingestions is generally clear in the presence of either endoscopic or diagnostic imaging evidence of perforation, severe abdominal rigidity, or persistent hypotension. Many patients will not have an obvious indication for surgical intervention despite impending perforation, necrosis, sepsis, or delayed hemorrhage. Hypotension is a grave finding and often indicates perforation or significant blood loss. Also, patients with large ingestions (> 150 mL), shock, acidemia, or coagulation disorders tend to have severe findings on surgical exploration. It should be noted, again, that patients with severe acid injuries often lack abdominal pain, but generally have positive findings on diagnostic imaging. It is recommended to consult with a surgeon who is familiar with caustic ingestions for patients with grade IIb and III esophageal burns identified on endoscopy in case of progression of injury and surgery is required.

### Adjunctive Therapies

*Corticosteroids.* When required in these patients for other indications such as caustic-induced airway inflammation, short-term corticosteroids are recommended. For the prevention of limitations of strictures, corticosteroid therapy is contraindicated for grade I and IIa esophageal burns as the risk of strictures is mimimal. Similarly, while grade III burns often form strictures, they have a high risk of perforation, which is likely exacerbated by corticosteroids. Based on animal studies and one randomized prospective human trial, we currently recommend the use of corticosteroids in the treatment of grade

IIb lesions following alkaline ingestions. The regimen consists of a short course of methylprednisolone (1 g/1.73 $m^2$/day for 3 days), ranitidine, ceftriaxone, and total parenteral nutrition if needed based on confimed endoscopic findings in these patients. No data support the use of corticosteroids following acid ingestions.

***Antibiotics.*** No major outcome studies have investigated the use of antibiotics alone as prophylactic treatment for stricture prevention, and it is reasonable to reserve antibiotics for patients with an identified source of infection.

***$H_2$ Antagonists/Proton Pump Inhibitors.*** Histamine$_2$ antagonists or proton pump inhibitors theoretically help reduce acid production and injury after caustic ingestion and are thus reasonable as adjunctive therapy despite a lack of studies to demonstrate their efficacy.

***Stents and Feeding Tubes.*** A variety of other management strategies have been used in an attempt to prevent strictures and esophageal obstruction. Intraluminal stents and nasogastric tubes successfully maintain the patency of the esophageal lumen. Potential disadvantages of esophageal stents include mechanical trauma at the site and increased reflux, both of which may inhibit healing. Stents and feeding tubes provide the benefit of enteral nutrition and potential to prevent stricture formation and are reasonable on a case-by-case basis in discussion with surgery and gastroenterology consultants.

***Additional Considerations.*** Therapies with experimental support include β-amino propionitrile, penicillamine, *N*-acetylcysteine, halofuginone, vitamin E, sphingosylphosphorylcholine, colchicine, erythropoietin, mitomycin C, fibroblast growth factor, 5-fluorouracil, ibuprofen, and retinoic acid. These treatments are inadequately studied in humans and cannot be routinely recommended at this time.

## Disposition

The extent of tissue injury dictates the subsequent management and disposition of patients with caustic ingestions.

***Grade I Esophageal Injuries.*** Patients with isolated grade I injuries of the esophagus do not develop strictures and are not at increased risk of carcinoma. Their diet can be resumed as tolerated. No further therapy is required. These patients can be discharged from the emergency department as long as they are able to eat and drink and their psychiatric status is stable.

***Grade IIa Esophageal Injuries.*** If endoscopy reveals grade IIa lesions of the esophagus and sparing of the stomach, a soft diet can be resumed as tolerated or a nasogastric tube can be passed under direct visualization. If oral intake or feeding via a nasogastric tube is not feasible, feeding via gastrostomy, jejunostomy, or total parenteral nutrition is recommended as rapidly as possible. Providing interim enteral support is imperative as metabolic demands are increased in any patient with a significant caustic injury.

***Grades IIb and III Esophageal Injuries.*** Patients with grades IIb and III lesions must be followed for the complications of perforation, infection, and stricture development. Strictures are a debilitating complication that evolve over a period of weeks or months. In addition to stricture formation, patients with grade III burns are also at high risk for other complications, including fistula formation, infection, and perforation with associated mediastinitis and peritonitis.

## Chronic Treatment of Strictures

The mainstay of management of patients with esophageal strictures is endoscopic dilation. Measurement of maximal wall thickness is useful in determining long-term follow-up, type of nutritional support, and the potential need for surgical repair as an alternative to dilation. It also provides an indication for those who should undergo dilation under fluoroscopy to limit the risk of perforation. Patients with stricture formation require long-term endoscopic follow-up for the presence of neoplastic changes of the esophagus that may occur with a delay of several decades.

## Management of Ophthalmic Exposures

Ophthalmic exposures occur from splash injuries and malicious events as well as from the alkaline by-products of sodium azide released in automobile air bag deployment and rupture. The mainstay of therapy for these patients is immediate irrigation of each eye for a minimum of 15 minutes with 0.9% sodium chloride, lactated Ringer solution, or tap water. Several liters of irrigation fluid are recommended until a consistent normal pH (6.5 to 7.6) of ophthalmic secretions is achieved. A thorough eye examination should be completed, and ophthalmological follow-up should be arranged. Special Considerations: SC1 contains a more detailed description of the evaluation and management of caustic injuries of the eye.

# 77 HYDROFLUORIC ACID AND FLUORIDES

## HISTORY AND EPIDEMIOLOGY

Hydrofluoric acid has been known for centuries for its ability to dissolve silica. Today, hydrofluoric acid (HF) is widely used for glass etching, brick cleaning, etching microchips in the semiconductor industry, electroplating, leather tanning, rust removal, and the cleaning of porcelain. Exposures to HF often occur as unintentional occupational hazards. The hands are the commonest part of the body injured. In 1988, an oil refinery in Texas released a cloud of hydrogen fluoride gas that resulted in 939 people seeking hospital treatment with 94 of these patients requiring admission. Other fluoride salts are widely used in, for example, the steel industry, drinking water, toothpaste additives, electroplating, lumber treatment, and the glass and enamel industries.

## CHEMISTRY

Hydrofluoric acid is synthesized as the product of gaseous sulfuric acid and calcium fluoride, which is subsequently cooled to a liquid. Aqueous HF is a weak acid, with a pKa of 3.17. It is approximately 1,000 times less dissociated than equimolar hydrochloric acid. Hydrofluoric acid generally ranges in concentrations from 3% to 40%, for use in both industry and the home. Anhydrous HF is highly concentrated (> 70%) and used almost exclusively for industrial purposes.

Fluorine is the most electronegative element in the Periodic Table of the Elements owing to its relatively large number of protons in the nucleus compared to its molecular size, and the minimal amount of screening or shielding by inner electrons. Consequently, the corresponding anion of fluorine, the fluoride ion ($F^-$), is a weak base because it possesses only a limited ability to donate its electrons. Liberation of the fluoride ion is believed to be the major determinant of toxicity.

## PATHOPHYSIOLOGY

Exposures to HF occur via dermal, ophthalmic, inhalation, oral, and rectal routes. HF penetrates deeply into tissues prior to dissociating into hydrogen ions and highly electronegative fluoride ions. These fluoride ions avidly bind to extracellular and intracellular stores of calcium ($Ca^{2+}$) and magnesium ($Mg^{2+}$), depleting them, and ultimately leading to cellular dysfunction and cell death. The alteration in local calcium homeostasis causes neuroexcitation and accounts for the development of neuropathic pain. Furthermore, ischemia related to calcium dysregulation–mediated localized vasospasm is likely an additional contributory factor to the development of pain. Formation of insoluble salts of calcium and fluoride (most likely fluorapatite) is proposed as the etiology for the precipitous decrease in serum calcium. The anhydrous form of HF also produces a caustic burn similar to that caused by strong acids (Chap. 76). The minimal lethal oral dose in humans is approximately 5 to 10 g of NaF.

## CLINICAL EFFECTS

### Local Effects

***Dermal.*** The extent of tissue injury following dermal exposure is determined by the volume, concentration, and contact time with the tissues. High concentrations (> 20%) cause immediate pain with visible tissue damage. Exposure to household rust-removal products (6% and 12% HF) is often associated with a typical latency of several hours before pain develops. The initial site of injury typically appears relatively benign despite significant subjective complaints of pain. Over time, the tissue becomes hyperemic, with subsequent blanching and coagulative necrosis. As calcium complexes precipitate, a white discoloration of the affected area appears (Fig. 77–1). If more than 2.5% of the body surface area (BSA) is burned with highly concentrated HF, life-threatening systemic toxicity should be expected.

***Gastrointestinal.*** Intentional ingestion of concentrated HF (or other fluoride salts) causes significant gastritis yet often spares the remainder of the gastrointestinal tract. Patients promptly develop vomiting and abdominal pain. Systemic absorption is rapid and almost invariably fatal. Following HF ingestion, patients often present with altered mental status, that results from hemodynamic compromise, airway compromise, electrolyte abnormalities, or dysrhythmias.

***Ophthalmic.*** Hydrofluoric acid injury to the eye is usually more extensive than most other acids. Fluoride ions penetrate deeply to affect anterior chamber structures.

***Pulmonary.*** Patients with inhalational exposures present with a variety of signs and symptoms depending on the concentration and exposure time. Symptoms range from minor upper respiratory tract irritation and throat burning to shortness of breath, ulcers of the upper respiratory tract, stridor, hypoxemia, and hypocalcemia. Ophthalmic and dermal exposures are commonly associated with inhalational events.

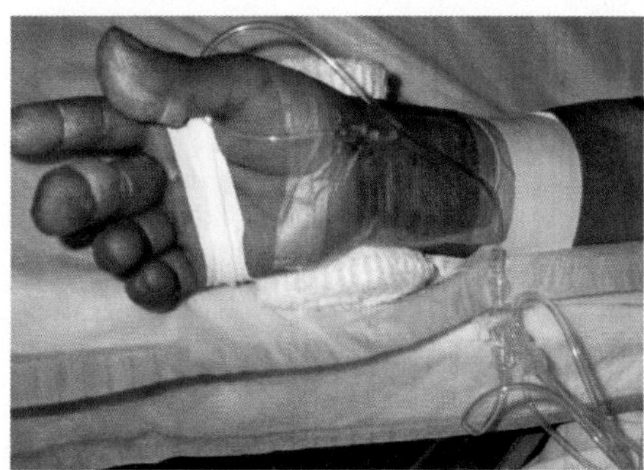

**FIGURE 77–1.** Severe injury to the fingers resulted from exposure to hydrofluoric acid. Note the arterial line in place for administration of calcium. *(Used with permission from the Fellowship in Medical Toxicology, New York Grossman University School of Medicine, New York City Poison Center.)*

## ASSESSING SEVERITY OF SYSTEMIC EFFECTS

Fatal exposures to HF by any route share the similar features of hypocalcemia, hypomagnesemia, and, in many cases, hyperkalemia as preterminal events. In some circumstances, the hypocalcemia severely disrupts the coagulation cascade, resulting in significant anticoagulation. Fatalities from HF occur as a result of either sudden-onset myocardial conduction failure or ventricular fibrillation.

Historical and clinical features of an HF exposure usually determine if the exposure is life-threatening. All oral and inhalational exposures are potentially fatal, as are burns of the face and neck, regardless of HF concentration. Inhalational exposure should be assumed for all patients with skin burns of greater than 5% BSA, any exposure to HF concentrations greater than 20%, and head and neck burns. Patients presenting with altered mental status directly related to HF are critically ill and necessitate rapid therapy. Hydrofluoric acid concentrations greater than 20% also have potential for significant toxicity in any patient, even if only a small surface area is exposed. As a general rule, patients who experience severe pain within minutes of contact are most likely exposed to a very high concentration of HF and their condition should be expected to rapidly deteriorate.

## DIAGNOSTIC TESTING

No monitoring or testing is required for uncomplicated small BSA exposures to low concentrations of HF. Diagnostic testing for systemic fluoride poisoning is currently based on monitoring of serum electrolytes. Calcium, magnesium, and potassium concentrations should be serially monitored. As systemic toxicity progresses, a metabolic acidosis will likely develop, necessitating a venous or arterial blood gas analysis. Serum fluoride concentrations are not readily available in a clinically relevant time frame. Electrocardiographic (ECG) findings of both hypocalcemia (prolonged QT interval) and hyperkalemia (eg, peaked T waves) are often reliable indicators of toxicity.

## MANAGEMENT

### General

For patients with more than localized exposure to low-concentration (< 20%) HF or any exposures to high-concentration (> 50%) HF, the mainstay of management is to prevent or limit systemic absorption, assess for systemic toxicity, and rapidly correct any electrolyte imbalances. Intravenous access should be obtained. An ECG should be obtained and examined for dysrhythmias and signs of hypocalcemia, hypomagnesemia, and hyperkalemia, and the patient should be attached to continuous cardiac monitoring. Rapid and serial determination of electrolytes is required. The airway should be assessed and protected early in patients with inhalation or ingestion, respiratory distress, ingestion with vomiting, or burns significant enough to cause a change in mental status or phonation. The most important therapy for skin exposures is the rapid removal of clothing and irrigation of the affected area with copious amounts of water or saline, whichever is more readily available.

### Dermal Toxicity

After irrigation, we recommend that a topical calcium gel be applied to the affected area. A commercial gel is available in the United States, but an acceptable substitute is reasonable and easily prepared. This is accomplished by mixing 3.5 g of calcium gluconate powder in 150 mL of sterile water-soluble lubricant, or 25 mL of 10% calcium gluconate in 75 mL of sterile water-soluble lubricant. This topical therapy for severe and non–life-threatening toxicity scavenges fluoride ions. Analgesics are recommended orally or parenterally as needed, but preferably not to the point of sedation, because local pain response is used to guide therapy. Digital nerve blocks with subcutaneous lidocaine or bupivacaine are also reasonable for patients with significant pain presenting 12 to 24 hours after the injury from a low concentration of HF and with no systemic signs of toxicity as calcium gluconate treatment is no longer necessary and and assessment of pain is not required to guide therapy.

Three other therapies have had variable success in human exposures: the application of calcium via intradermal, intravenous, and intraarterial routes. If topical gel therapy fails within the first few minutes of application, intradermal therapy with dilute calcium gluconate is a reasonable next step. Unfortunately, this treatment has limited usefulness and is not recommend in nondistensible spaces such as fingertips. The preferred method is to approach the wound from a distal point of injury and inject intradermally no more than 0.5 mL/cm$^2$ of 5% calcium gluconate. Effective pain relief is especially problematic for nailbed involvement, therefore other approaches are required. If the wound is large, under the nail, or on a section of the fingerpad or an area that is not amenable to intradermal injections, intraarterial calcium gluconate is the next most reasonable step. Placement should be ipsilateral and proximal to the affected area, usually in the radial or brachial artery. Cannulation must be confirmed to prevent extravasation. We recommend adding 10 mL of 10% calcium gluconate to either 40 mL of $D_5W$ (dextrose 5% in water) or 0.9% sodium chloride solution infused continuously over 4 hours. After the infusion is initiated, patients typically experience significant pain relief. Patients requiring an arterial line for treatment should be admitted to the hospital, as the majority will require more than one treatment.

Another reported therapy for localized HF poisoning is an intravenous Bier block technique that uses 25 mL of 2.5% calcium gluconate. In one case, the effects lasted 5 hours and there were no adverse events. Although the intravenous Bier block technique is not reported as being used in a substantial number of patients, it is reasonable, particularly when intraarterial infusion is problematic. Further data are required before this therapy is routinely recommended.

We routinely observe all patients with digital exposures to HF over 4 to 6 hours, as the pain often recurs and reapplication of the gel or an alternative therapy will be necessary. Even if successful pain control is achieved, the patient will require specialized follow-up and wound care.

### Inhalational Toxicity

Patients exposed to a low concentration of HF and treated with 4 mL of a 2.5% nebulized calcium gluconate solution demonstrated a subjective decrease in irritation with no adverse effects. Because nebulized calcium gluconate is a relatively benign therapy, we recommend that all patients with symptomatic inhalational exposures to any concentration of HF be administered a dilute solution of calcium gluconate.

### Ingestions

In patients with intentional ingestions of HF, gastrointestinal decontamination poses a dilemma. Gastric emptying via a nasogastric tube is reasonable in the absence of significant spontaneous emesis because these exposures are almost universally fatal. Healthcare providers should exercise extreme caution during this procedure because secondary dermal or inhalational exposures to the provider is possible in the absence of appropriate personal protective equipment. If there is a possibility of inhalation by the provider, the area should be well ventilated. Acceptable forms of hand protection include gloves made of nitrile, butyl rubber, polyvinyl chloride, or Neoprene.

We recommend a solution of a calcium or magnesium salt be administered orally as soon as possible to prevent HF penetration into the stomach and to provide an alternative source of cations for the damaging electronegative fluoride ions. Magnesium citrate in a standard cathartic dose, magnesium sulfate, or any of the calcium solutions can be administered orally to prevent absorption (Antidotes in Brief: A16). Based on limited research, calcium salts are preferred.

### Ophthalmic Toxicity

Patients with ophthalmic exposures should have each eye irrigated with 1 L of 0.9% sodium chloride solution, lactated Ringer solution, or water. Although there are limited data, repetitive or prolonged irrigation appears to worsen outcome. A complete ophthalmic examination should be performed after the patient is deemed stable, and an ophthalmology consultation should be obtained. The use of dilute calcium gluconate drops is not recommended at this time because of limited and conflicting evidence. Likewise, there is no role for gel therapy or ophthalmic injection.

### Systemic Toxicity

For systemic toxicity, the immediate intravenous administration of both calcium and magnesium salts is recommended. Calcium gluconate is preferred over calcium chloride because of the risks associated with extravasation (Antidotes in Brief: A32). Patients often require many grams of IV calcium salts to treat severe HF toxicity. We recommend that intravenous magnesium be administered to adults as 20 mL of a 20% magnesium sulfate solution (4 g) over 20 to 30 minutes. An approach that combines intravenous calcium or magnesium with local calcium or magnesium gels to limit absorption protects against life-threatening hypocalcemia and hyperkalemia. Urinary alkalinization is recommended to enhance the excretion of fluoride. Bicarbonate administration will also help address hyperkalemia when present. Although the use of quinidine, a potassium channel blocker, is protective in dogs, it has not been studied or used in humans, and at this time cannot be recommended prophylactically. However, in the presence of life-threatening ventricular dysrhythmias, quinidine (or any class III antidysrhythmic) is reasonable.

Hemodialysis is reasonable in patients with severe HF poisoning and acute kidney injury. There are several reported cases of successful clearance of fluoride ions via hemodialysis, with one case also using continuous venovenous hemodialysis. Because the reported clearance rate did not differ significantly from normally functioning kidneys, it is unclear whether hemodialysis alters outcome in patients with normal kidney function.

Antidotes in Brief

# A32 CALCIUM

## INTRODUCTION

Calcium is essential in maintaining the normal function of the heart, vascular smooth muscle, skeletal system, and nervous system. It is vital in enzymatic reactions, in neurohormonal transmission, and in the maintenance of cellular integrity. There are multiple toxicologic indications for calcium administration. Dosing and route vary based on these indications.

## HISTORY

Sidney Ringer performed controlled animal experiments in the 1880s demonstrating the importance of calcium in sustaining and resuscitating cardiac ventricular contraction. As the clinical use of calcium chloride antedated 1938, it was "grandfathered" under the United States (US) Food, Drug, and Cosmetic Act; calcium gluconate was approved in 1941.

## PHARMACOLOGY

### Chemistry/Preparation

For clinical use, calcium is prepared typically in combination with gluconate or chloride.

### Related Agents

Calcium acetate is used orally to treat hyperphosphatemia, particularly in patients with end-stage kidney disease. Other oral calcium salts such as calcium carbonate, citrate, lactate, glubionate, glycerophosphate, and polycarbophil are variously used as cariostatics, food additives, mineral supplements, and stool stabilizers.

### Pharmacokinetics

Calcium is the fifth most abundant element and the most abundant mineral in the body, and the third most common plasma cation after sodium and potassium. More than 99% of the 1 to 2 kg of calcium in the adult human is located in bone. Antidotal calcium is also variously reported as grams of the salt, mEq, or milimoles (mM) of calcium. One gram of calcium chloride contains 13.6 mEq (6.8 mM, 272.5 mg) of elemental calcium; 1 g of calcium gluconate contains 4.64 mEq (2.32 mM, 93 mg) of elemental calcium. In blood, the total calcium concentration is normally 8.5 to 10.6 mg/dL (2.13–2.65 mM, 4.25–5.3 mEq/L), of which approximately half is ionized and active. The remaining calcium is bound to negatively charged proteins (such as albumin and immunoglobulins) or loosely associated with anions such as phosphate, citrate, sulfate, lactate, and bicarbonate. Calcium concentrations are affected by pH, with increases in pH causing a decrease in ionized calcium and vice versa. Intracellular cytosolic free calcium concentrations are many orders of magnitude (~10,000-fold) lower than ionized calcium concentrations in the blood and extracellular fluid, creating a significant gradient. Calcium is excreted in feces as insoluble salts (80%) and renally (20%). Non–albumin-bound calcium is filterable at the glomerulus and is reabsorbed in the proximal tubule (60%–70%), in the thick ascending limb of Henle (20%–30%), and in the distal convoluted tubule (10%).

### Pharmacodynamics and Mechanisms of Action

Calcium is fundamental to neurotransmission, cardiovascular physiology, muscle performance, bone maintenance, coagulation, cellular exocytosis, and signaling. Cardiac excitation-contraction coupling is accomplished via sodium-triggered calcium influx through voltage-activated L-type calcium channels, which triggers ryanodine receptor type-2 calcium release, calcium binding to and activation of cardiac troponin C, and initiation of myofilament contraction.

## ROLE IN CALCIUM CHANNEL BLOCKER TOXICITY

Calcium enters cells in numerous ways. In cardiac and smooth muscles, the voltage-dependent L-type channels are inhibited by the calcium channel blockers (CCBs) available in the US. Patients with CCB overdose (Chap. 33) typically develop nausea, vomiting, hypotension, bradycardia, myocardial depression, sinus arrest, atrioventricular (AV) block, cardiovascular collapse, metabolic acidosis, hyperglycemia, shock, pulmonary edema, altered mental status, and seizures. Because CCBs do not alter either receptor-operated channels or the release of calcium from intracellular stores, the serum calcium concentration remains normal in overdose.

Pretreatment with calcium chloride or gluconate prevents hypotension associated with intravenous verapamil or diltiazem administered for supraventricular tachycardia. Intravenous administration of calcium to dogs poisoned with verapamil or diltiazem improved cardiac output secondary to increased inotropy. The heart rate and cardiac conduction were affected minimally, if at all. Case reports and reviews of the literature suggest variable responses to calcium in humans with CCB overdose.

As a relatively simple intervention, calcium is recommended as the initial therapy for symptomatic patients with CCB overdoses (Table A32–1). Several authors have successfully treated patients with much larger doses than recommended here, but without apparent adverse effects. However, following the use of large doses of calcium, hypercalcemia is expected, which is associated with potentially severe consequences including altered mental status, gut atony, myocardial depression, and intense vasoconstriction leading to multiorgan ischemia and death.

Because calcium chloride is extremely irritating to small vessels, subcutaneous tissue, and muscle, and causes necrosis following extravasation, it is usually only administered through a central venous line or intraosseously. Overwhelming clinical and experimental evidence supports the concept that

**TABLE A32–1 Calcium Salts for Intravenous Use**

| | *Calcium Gluconate*[a] | *Calcium Chloride* ($CaCl_2$)[a,b] |
|---|---|---|
| 10% solution | 10 mL = 1 g of $Ca^{2+}$ gluconate | 10 mL = 1 g of $CaCl_2$ |
| | 10 mL = 4.64 mEq = 93 mg = 2.32 mmol of elemental $Ca^{2+}$ | 10 mL = 13.6 mEq = 273 mg = 6.8 mmol of elemental $Ca^{2+}$ |
| | *or* | *or* |
| | 1 mL = 0.465 mEq = 9.3 mg = 0.23 mmol of elemental $Ca^{2+}$ | 1 mL = 1.36 mEq = 27.3 mg = 0.68 mmol of elemental $Ca^{2+}$ |
| Adult dose | 3 g (30 mL of 10% solution) over 10 minutes (unless in extremis—deliver over 60 seconds) | 1 g (10 mL of 10% solution) over 10 minutes (unless in extremis—deliver over 60 seconds) |
| | Repeat every 10–20 minutes up to 3–4 doses as necessary | Repeat every 10–20 minutes up to 3–4 doses as necessary |
| Pediatric dose (not to exceed the adult dose) | 60 mg/kg (0.6 mL/kg) of 10% solution infused over 5–10 minutes (unless in extremis—deliver over 60 seconds) | 20 mg/kg (0.2 mL/kg) infused over 5–10 minutes (unless in extremis—deliver over 60 seconds) |
| | Repeat every 10–20 minutes up to 3–4 doses as necessary | Repeat every 10–20 minutes up to 3–4 doses as necessary |

[a]Monitor calcium concentration after several doses. [b]Use of a central venous line is recommended to avoid extravasation.

simple dissociation of calcium from gluconate is responsible for releasing calcium, rather than hepatic metabolism.

The administration of calcium to a patient with toxicity from cardioactive steroids such as digoxin is potentially harmful. In the event of concurrent overdose with both a cardioactive steroid and a CCB, the early use of digoxin-specific antibody fragments (Antidotes in Brief: A22) will permit the subsequent safe use of calcium (Chap. 35).

## ROLE IN β-ADRENERGIC ANTAGONIST TOXICITY

The negative inotropic action of β-adrenergic antagonists is related to interference with both the forward and reverse transport of calcium in the sarcoplasmic reticulum and the inhibition of microsomal and mitochondrial calcium uptake (Chap. 32). In animals poisoned with β-adrenergic antagonists, calcium improved mean arterial pressure, the change in maximal left ventricular pressure over time, and peripheral vascular resistance, but it had no significant effect on bradycardia or QRS complex prolongation. Some case reports demonstrate a beneficial effect of intravenous calcium in β-adrenergic antagonist overdose. Because distinguishing an overdose of a CCB from that of a β-adrenergic antagonist is often clinically difficult and the two classes are sometimes ingested simultaneously, a trial of IV calcium is reasonable for an undifferentiated or mixed CCB and β-adrenergic antagonist overdose, if cardioactive steroid toxicity is excluded.

## ROLE IN HYPOCALCEMIA SECONDARY TO ETHYLENE GLYCOL

Following ethylene glycol poisoning (Chap. 79), metabolism of the parent molecule generates oxalic acid, which complexes with calcium and subsequently precipitates in the kidneys, brain, and elsewhere, and occasionally results in hypocalcemia. After exposure to ethylene glycol, it is reasonable to monitor the calcium concentration. Intravenous calcium is recommended in the doses in Table A32-1) to patients with signs or symptoms of hypocalcemia.

## ROLE IN HYPOCALCEMIA SECONDARY TO HYDROFLUORIC ACID AND FLUORIDE-RELEASING XENOBIOTICS

Hypocalcemia occurs in patients with life-threating burns from hydrofluoric acid (HF) or soluble salts of fluoride and bifluoride (Chap. 77). Patients should be treated with calcium in a manner similar to the hypocalcemia from other causes. For local HF toxicity, calcium gluconate is recommended topically and subcutaneously to manage minor to moderate cutaneous burns, and intraarterially to manage significant burns. A 2.5% topical calcium gluconate topical gel is marketed. In the event that the commercial preparation is unavailable, a topical calcium gel can be prepared by mixing 35 mL of a 10% calcium gluconate solution or 10 g of calcium carbonate tablets with 5 oz of water-soluble jelly. While the chloride salt is also acceptable for topical therapy, it should never be injected into tissues (subcutaneously or intramuscularly), because severe tissue necrosis can result. In patients with severe topical HF exposures, administration of regional IV calcium using a Bier block technique (10 mL of 10% calcium gluconate in a total volume of 40 mL) or intraarterial calcium (10 mL of 10% calcium gluconate in 50 mL in a total volume of 5% dextrose solution over 4 hours) is reasonable (Chap. 77). In patients with HF inhalation, nebulized 2.5% calcium gluconate (1.5 mL of 10% calcium gluconate solution with 4.5 mL of sterile water or 0.9% sodium chloride) is recommended in addition to systemic therapy.

## ROLE IN HYPERPHOSPHATEMIA

Inappropriate use of oral and rectal phosphates (eg, laxatives) can result in hypocalcemia, hyperphosphatemia, and hyperkalemia resulting in significant morbidity and mortality. Intravenous calcium is recommended for life-threatening hypocalcemia. However, because administration of calcium in the presence of hyperphosphatemia risks precipitation of calcium phosphate throughout the body, the risks and benefits of calcium administration versus hemodialysis and other therapies should be weighed in consultation with a nephrologist in non–life-threatening cases.

## ROLE IN HYPERMAGNESEMIA

Hypermagnesemia causes both direct and indirect depression of skeletal muscle function, resulting in neuromuscular blockade, loss of reflexes, and profound muscular paralysis. Intravenous calcium serves as a physiologic antagonist to these effects of magnesium and is recommended as in Table A32–1.

## ROLE IN HYPERKALEMIA

Calcium makes the membrane threshold potential less negative so that a larger stimulus is required to depolarize the cell. This stabilization antagonizes the hyperexcitability caused by modest hyperkalemia. However, when severe hyperkalemia exists, voltage-gated sodium channels are inactivated and cannot be depolarized, regardless of the strength of the impulse. Calcium transforms the voltage sensor of the sodium channel from inactive to closed, thus allowing the sodium channel to be opened with depolarization. The typical initial dose is 1 g of IV calcium gluconate. If hyperkalemia is secondary to the toxic effects of cardioactive steroids on the $Na^+,K^+$-adenosine triphosphatase (ATPase) pump, IV calcium can potentially exacerbate an already excessive intracellular calcium concentration, making IV calcium potentially harmful (Chap. 35). Digoxin-specific antibody fragments (Antidotes in Brief: A22) should be given for cardioactive steroid–induced hyperkalemia.

## ROLE IN CITRATE TOXICITY

Citrate binds calcium and other divalent cations. Blood products contain citrate to prevent coagulation. In massive transfusions, with citrate use in extracorporeal circuits, and in patients with liver disease (who metabolize citrate more slowly), excess citrate causes toxicity (hypocalcemia and, more rarely, hypomagnesemia). Calcium correction should be guided by clinical signs and ionized calcium determinations. Calcium should not be directly added to blood products, as this can cause clotting, but rather provided via a separate infusion line.

## ADVERSE EFFECTS AND SAFETY ISSUES

The adverse effects of hypercalcemia include nausea, vomiting, constipation, ileus, polyuria, polydipsia, nephrolithiasis, cognitive alterations, hyporeflexia, coma, vascular alterations, and dysrhythmias. Excessive calcium infusions led to death in a patient with CCB overdose. Neither calcium chloride nor calcium gluconate should be combined and administered intravenously with sodium bicarbonate or fluids containing phosphate. Calcium chloride is an acidifying salt, and it is extremely irritating to tissue. It is typically administered via central venous access and should never be given intramuscularly, subcutaneously, or perivascularly. The best reason for choosing calcium gluconate in almost all clinical situations is that the risk of tissue injury is far less. If extravasation occurs, subcutaneous injection of aliquots of hyaluronidase is reasonable to inject around the site to diminish tissue injury. (Special Considerations: SC7).

## PREGNANCY AND LACTATION

Calcium injection is US Food and Drug Administration Pregnancy Category C. Calcium is excreted as a natural component in human breast milk, but no definitive evaluations have been performed on potential adverse effects in the breastfed child following maternal intravenous calcium administration.

## DOSING AND ADMINISTRATION

Intravenous calcium must be administered slowly, at a rate not exceeding 0.7 to 1.8 mEq (14–36.1 mg) per minute, which equates to approximately one-half to one 10-mL vial of calcium chloride or one-and-one-half to three 10-mL vials of calcium gluconate over 10 minutes in adults, unless the patient is in extremis. More rapid administration can lead to vasodilation, hypotension, bradycardia, dysrhythmias, syncope, and cardiac arrest. In cases of life-threatening hypocalcemia or for a patient in extremis, a slow IV push is reasonable. Repeat doses are administered every 10 to 20 minutes for up to three to four doses as clinically indicated. Total and ionized calcium should be frequently monitored, particularly in light of the acid–base disturbances that occur in poisoned patients. Although intraosseous administration of calcium was used for vascular collapse, ensuring correct needle placement and the gluconate formulation are recommended, given the previous reports of limb ischemia.

## FORMULATION AND ACQUISITION

The two most commonly used formulations are calcium chloride (10%) and calcium gluconate (10%) (Table A32–1). A topical calcium gluconate gel (2.5%) 25 g is available. A commercially prepared emergency eyewash calcium gluconate 1% solution is available in 120-mL squirt bottles.

# 78 HYDROCARBONS

## HISTORY AND EPIDEMIOLOGY

The modern world could not exist without hydrocarbons. Crude oil processing involves heating to a set temperature within processors that separate (distill) hydrocarbon fractions by vapor (or boiling) point. Because of the relationship between boiling point and molecular weight, distillation roughly divides hydrocarbons into like-sized molecules. The most volatile fractions come off early as gases, and these are used primarily as heating fuels. The least volatile fractions (larger than about 10 or 12 carbons) are used chiefly for lubricants or as paraffins, petroleum jelly, or asphalt. The remaining midsized fractions (5 to 10 carbons) are those most commonly used in combustion fuels and as solvents. Petroleum distillates are also used as raw materials in the production of numerous finished products.

For decades in the United States (US), kerosene ingestion in children was a major public health concern. Only through public education, consumer product safety initiatives, and modernization of the use and distribution of cooking and heating fuels has this problem been largely eliminated. However, in resource-poor countries, these same challenges have yet to be resolved, with large numbers of children ingesting kerosene from poorly labeled and poorly secured containers.

Public attention and debate surround the hydrocarbon exposures following environmental spills. Even more controversial is the practice of "induced hydraulic fracturing" of rock or shale, commonly called "fracking." While the intent is to capture and collect trapped hydrocarbons, some escape into nearby aquifers, thereby entering water supplies or otherwise contaminating human environments. Hydrocarbon solvents are often volatile, making inhalation common in these exposures. The intentional misuse of volatile solvents by adolescents is discussed in more depth in Chap. 54.

Most commonly encountered hydrocarbons are mixtures of compounds, often obtained from a common petroleum distillation fraction. Table 78–1 lists frequently encountered hydrocarbons and their common uses. This chapter focuses principally on toxicity of hydrocarbons present in these commercially available mixtures. Individual hydrocarbons are discussed only when they are commonly available in purified form or when specific xenobiotics result in unique toxicologic concerns.

## CHEMISTRY

A *hydrocarbon* is an organic compound made up primarily of carbon and hydrogen atoms. This definition includes products derived from plants (terpenes such as pine oil and triglyceresin vegetable oil), animal fats (cod liver oil), natural gas, petroleum, or coal tar. There are two basic types of hydrocarbon molecules, *aliphatic* (straight or branched chains) and *cyclic* (closed ring), each with its own subclasses. An extensive discussion of organic chemistry is beyond the scope of this manual. When relevant, chemical properties will be highlighted in individual sections.

Physical properties of hydrocarbons vary by the number of carbon atoms and by molecular structure. Unsubstituted, aliphatic hydrocarbons that contain up to 4 carbons are gaseous at room temperature, 5- to 19-carbon molecules are liquids, and longer-chain molecules tend to be tars or solids. The various definitions of paraffin warrant discussion. In chemistry, *paraffin* is a general term for any saturated hydrocarbon (alkane). In North American common use, paraffin describes either medicinal paraffin or paraffin wax. *Medicinal paraffin* is the same as mineral oil, a viscous mixture of longer-chained alkanes (typically 15–50 carbon atoms per molecule) derived from a petroleum source. Outside North America, the term *paraffin* often refers to kerosene—a mixture of medium-chain alkanes typically used for lighting and heating. Halogenated hydrocarbons contain at least one halogen (eg, chlorine, fluorine, bromine) atom.

## PHARMACOLOGY

The effects of hydrocarbons on humans are chiefly related to interactions with lipid bilayers in cellular membranes. Acute central nervous system (CNS) toxicity from inhalational

**TABLE 78–1 Classification and Viscosity of Common Hydrocarbons**

| Compound | Common Uses | Viscosity (SUS)[a] |
|---|---|---|
| **Aliphatics** | | |
| Gasoline | Motor vehicle fuel | 30 |
| Naphtha | Charcoal lighter fluid | 29 |
| Kerosene | Heating fuel | 35 |
| Turpentine | Paint thinner | 33 |
| Mineral spirits | Paint and varnish thinner | 30–35 |
| Mineral seal oil | Furniture polish | 30–35 |
| Heavy fuel oil | Heating oil | > 450 |
| **Aromatics** | | |
| Benzene | Solvent, reagent, gasoline additive | 31 |
| Toluene | Solvent, spray paint solvent | 28 |
| Xylene | Solvent, paint thinner, reagent | 28 |
| **Halogenated** | | |
| Methylene chloride | Solvent, paint stripper, propellant | 27 |
| Carbon tetrachloride | Solvent, propellant, refrigerant | 30 |
| Trichloroethylene | Degreaser, spot remover | 27 |
| Tetrachloroethylene | Dry cleaning solvent, chemical intermediate | 28 |

[a]Direct values for kinematic viscosity in Saybolt universal seconds (SUS) were not available for the following compounds: naphtha, xylene, methylene chloride, carbon tetrachloride, trichloroethylene, perchloroethylene, and toluene. Saybolt universal seconds were calculated for these hydrocarbons by converting from available measurements in centipoise viscosity and/or centistokes viscosity using the following conversions: the value in centistokes is estimated by dividing centipoise by density at 68°F (20°C); SUS (Y) is approximated from centistokes (X) using $y = 3.2533x + 26.08$ ($R^2 = 0.9998$). Centipoise viscosity for naphtha was estimated from the value for butylbenzene. Centipoise viscosity for xylene is the average of *o*-, *m*-, and *p*-xylene.

occupational overexposure or recreational abuse parallels the effect of administering an inhaled general anesthetic. Inhaled solvent vapor produces unconsciousness in 50% of subjects, when the partial pressure in the lung reaches its median effective dose ($ED_{50}$). The $ED_{50}$ in occupational terms is effectively the same as the minimum alveolar concentration (MAC) in anesthesiology terms (Chap. 38). Numerous protein receptor interactions also occur. Toluene, trichloroethylene, perchloroethylene, and others inhibit neuronal calcium currents. The halogenated hydrocarbons increase the outward potassium rectifying current and decrease exocytosis of neuronal synaptic vesicles. Thus, no single mechanism fully explains the pharmacologic and toxicologic activity of volatile hydrocarbons on neuronal tissues.

## TOXICOKINETICS

Hydrocarbons are variably absorbed by ingestion, inhalation, or dermal routes. Human toxicokinetic data are lacking for most of these xenobiotics, therefore our understanding derives from in vitro studies and animal research. Partition coefficients are useful predictors of the rate and extent of the absorption and distribution of hydrocarbons into tissues. A partition coefficient for a given chemical species is the ratio of concentrations achieved between two different media at equilibrium. The blood-to-air, tissue-to-air, and tissue-to-blood coefficients directly relate to the pulmonary uptake and distribution of hydrocarbons. The tissue-to-blood partition coefficient is commonly derived by dividing the tissue-to-air coefficient by the blood-to-air coefficient. The higher the value, the greater the potential for distribution into tissue. Table 78–2 lists partition coefficients for commonly encountered hydrocarbons.

Inhalation is a major route of exposure for volatile hydrocarbons. Most cross the alveolar membrane by passive diffusion. Absorption of aliphatic hydrocarbons through the digestive tract is inversely related to molecular weight, ranging from complete absorption at lower molecular weights to approximately 60% for C-14 hydrocarbons, 5% for C-28 hydrocarbons, and essentially no absorption for aliphatic hydrocarbons with more than 32 carbons. Oral absorption of aromatic hydrocarbons with between 5 and 9 carbons ranges from 80% to 97%. Although the skin is a common area of contact with solvents, the dose of dermally absorbed hydrocarbons is small compared to other routes such as inhalation. However, with massive exposure (eg, whole-body immersion), dermal absorption contributes significantly to toxicity.

Once absorbed into the central compartment, hydrocarbons are distributed to target and storage organs based on their tissue-to-blood partition. During the onset of systemic exposure, hydrocarbons accumulate in tissues that have tissue-to-blood coefficients greater than 1 (eg, for toluene, the fat-to-blood partition coefficient is 60). Hydrocarbons can be eliminated from the body unchanged, for example, through expired air, or can be metabolized to more polar compounds, which are then excreted in urine or bile.

**TABLE 78–2 Kinetic Parameters of Selected Hydrocarbons**

| | *Partition Coefficients*[a] | | $t_{1/2}$ | | | |
|---|---|---|---|---|---|---|
| | ***Blood-to-Air*** | ***Fat-to-Air*** | $\alpha$ | $\beta$ | ***Elimination*** | ***Relevant Metabolites*** |
| **Aliphatics** | | | | | | |
| *n*-Hexane | 2 | 159 | 0.17 hours | 1.7 hours | 10%–20% exhaled; liver metabolism by CYP2E1 | 2-Hexanol, 2,5-Hexanedione, γ-valerolactone |
| Paraffin/tar | Not absorbed or metabolized | | — | | — | — |
| **Aromatics** | | | | | | |
| Benzene | 8.19 | 499 | 8 hours | 90 hours | 12% exhaled; liver metabolism to phenol | Phenol, catechol, hydroquinone, and conjugates |
| Toluene | 8–16 | 1,021 | 4–5 hours | 15–72 hours | Extensive liver extraction and metabolism | 80% metabolized to benzyl alcohol; 70% renally excreted as hippuric acid |
| *o*-Xylene | 34.9 | 1,877 | 0.5–1 hour | 20–30 hours | Liver CYP2E1 oxidation | Toluic acid, methyl hippuric acid |
| **Halogenated** | | | | | | |
| Methylene chloride | 5–10 | 120 | Apparent $t_{1/2}$ of COHb 13 hours | 0.7 hours | 92% exhaled unchanged<br>Low doses metabolized; high doses exhaled<br>Two liver metabolic pathways | (a) CYP2E1 to CO and $CO_2$ (b) Glutathione transferase to $CO_2$, formaldehyde, formic acid |
| Carbon tetrachloride | 1.6 | 359 | ~1.5 hours | 1.5–8 hours | Liver CYP2E1, some lung exhalation (dose-dependent) | Trichloromethyl radical, trichloromethyl peroxy radical, phosgene |
| Trichloroethylene | 9 | 554 | 3 hours | 30 hours | Liver CYP2E1—epoxide intermediate; trichloroethanol is glucuronidated and excreted | Chloral hydrate, trichloroethanol, trichloroacetic acid |
| 1,1,1-Trichloroethane | 1–3 | 263 | 0.7 hours | 53 hours | 91% exhaled; liver CYP2E1 | Trichloroacetic acid, trichloroethanol |
| Tetrachloroethylene | 10.3 | 1,638 | 2.7 hours | 33 hours | 80% exhaled; liver CYP2E1 | Trichloroacetic acid, trichloroethanol |

[a]Fat-to-blood partition coefficient is obtained by dividing the fat-to-air coefficient by the blood-to-air coefficient, as determined in rat models. All coefficients are determined at 98.6°F (37°C).

## PATHOPHYSIOLOGY AND CLINICAL FINDINGS

### Respiratory

Several factors are associated with pulmonary toxicity after hydrocarbon ingestion. These include specific physical properties of the xenobiotics ingested, the volume ingested, and the occurrence of vomiting. Physical properties of viscosity, surface tension, and volatility are primary determinants of aspiration potential.

*Dynamic (or absolute) viscosity* is the measurement of the ability of a fluid to resist flow. This property is measured with a rheometer and is typically given in units of pascal-seconds. More frequently, engineers work with *kinematic viscosity*, measured in square millimeters per second, or centistokes. An older system for measuring viscosity expresses kinematic viscosity in units of Saybolt universal seconds (SUS). Unfortunately, many policy statements were developed in an era when SUS units were popular, and many still describe viscosity in SUS units. Table 78–1 shows kinematic viscosity of common hydrocarbons, measured in SUS. An approximate unit conversion is given in the footnote of tables.

Hydrocarbons with low viscosities (< 60 SUS) have a higher tendency for aspiration. *Surface tension* is a cohesive force generated by attraction due to the Van der Waals forces between molecules. This influences adherence of a liquid along a surface ("its ability to creep"). The lower the surface tension, the more effectively the liquid will creep, leading to a higher aspiration risk. *Volatility* is the tendency for a liquid to become a gas. Hydrocarbons with high volatility tend to vaporize, displace oxygen, and potentially lead to transient hypoxia.

Aspiration is the main route of injury from ingested simple hydrocarbons. The mechanism of pulmonary injury, however, is not fully understood. Intratracheal instillation of 0.2 mL/kg of kerosene causes physiologic abnormalities in lung mechanics (decreased compliance and total lung capacity) and pathologic changes such as interstitial inflammation, polymorphonuclear exudates, intraalveolar edema and hemorrhage, hyperemia, bronchial and bronchiolar necrosis, and vascular thrombosis. These changes most likely reflect both direct toxicity to pulmonary tissue and disruption of the lipid surfactant layer.

Most patients who develop pulmonary toxicity following hydrocarbon ingestion will have an initial episode of coughing, gagging, or choking. This usually occurs within 30 minutes after ingestion and is presumptive evidence of aspiration. Pulmonary toxicity manifests as crackles, rhonchi, bronchospasm, tachypnea, hypoxemia, hemoptysis, acute respiratory distress syndrome, or respiratory distress. Clinical findings often worsen over the first several days but typically resolve within a week. Death is distinctly uncommon and typically occurs after a severe, progressive respiratory insult marked by hypoxia, ventilation–perfusion mismatch, and barotrauma.

Intravenous (IV), subcutaneous, and even intrapleural injection of hydrocarbons are reported. Severe hydrocarbon pneumonitis occurs following IV exposure. Animal experiments show that intravascular hydrocarbons injure the first capillary bed encountered. The clinical course after IV hydrocarbon injection is comparable to that of aspiration injury.

Radiographic evidence of pneumonitis develops in 40% to 88% of patients admitted following aspiration. Findings develop as early as 15 minutes or as late as 24 hours after exposure (Fig. 78–1). Chest radiographs performed immediately on initial presentation are not useful in predicting infiltrates in either symptomatic or asymptomatic patients. Ninety percent of patients who develop radiographic abnormalities do so by 4 hours postingestion. A small percentage (< 5%) of patients develop radiographic findings after a completely asymptomatic after a period of observation.

There are few reports of long-term follow-up on patients with hydrocarbon pneumonitis. Frequent respiratory tract infections are described after hydrocarbon pneumonitis, but these studies are not well controlled. Delayed formation of pneumatoceles occurs in isolated reports. Bronchiectasis and pulmonary fibrosis are reported but appear to be uncommon. In one study, 82% of patients examined 8 to 14 years after hydrocarbon-induced pneumonitis had asymptomatic minor pulmonary function abnormalities consistent with small-airway obstruction and loss of elastic recoil.

### Cardiac

The most concerning cardiac effect from hydrocarbon exposure is precipitation of dysrhythmias through myocardial sensitization. Cardiac sensitization is incompletely understood but likely results from alterations of sodium and potassium channels. Sensitization is also mediated by slowed conduction velocity through membrane gap junctions. All routes of exposure to hydrocarbons are potentially cardiotoxic. Malignant dysrhythmias are described with all classes of hydrocarbons, but halogenated compounds are most frequently implicated, followed by aromatic compounds. Atrial fibrillation, ventricular tachycardias, junctional rhythms, ventricular fibrillation, and cardiac arrest are reported. When this occurs in the context of inhalant abuse, it is termed the "sudden sniffing death syndrome." Prolongation of the QT interval in some cases raises additional concern for the development of torsade de pointes. Classically, sudden death follows an episode of sudden exertion, presumably associated with an endogenous catecholamine surge.

### Central Nervous System

Transient CNS excitation occurs after acute hydrocarbon inhalation or ingestion, but more commonly, CNS depression or general anesthesia occurs. In cases of aspiration, hypoxemia may contribute to CNS depression. Chronic occupational exposure or volatile substance use leads to a chronic neurobehavioral syndrome most notably described after toluene overexposure as toluene leukoencephalopathy, which also occurs after inhalational abuse. Clinical features include ataxia, spasticity, dysarthria, and dementia, consistent with leukoencephalopathy. Autopsy studies of the brains of patients chronically exposed to chronic toluene show atrophy and mottling of the white matter. Initial findings of white matter dementia include behavioral changes, impaired sense of smell, impaired concentration, and mild unsteadiness of hand movements and gait. Further exposure leads to slurred

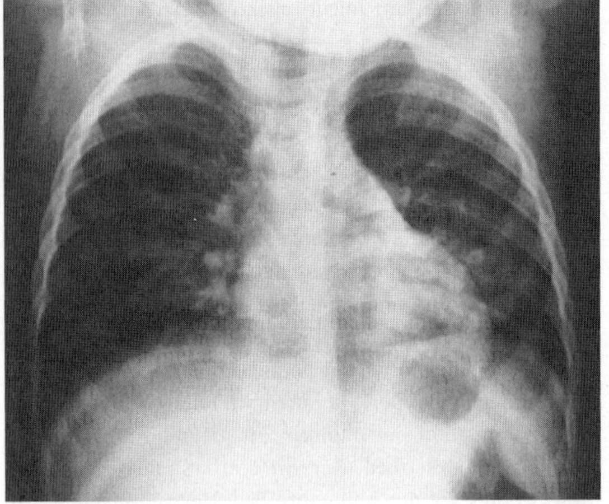

A

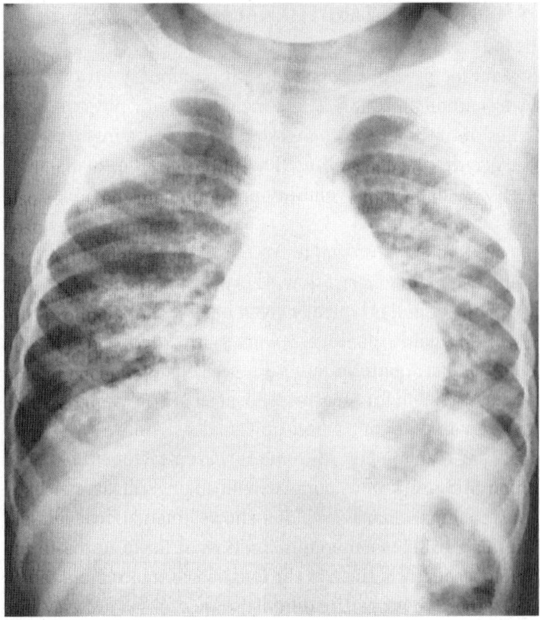

B

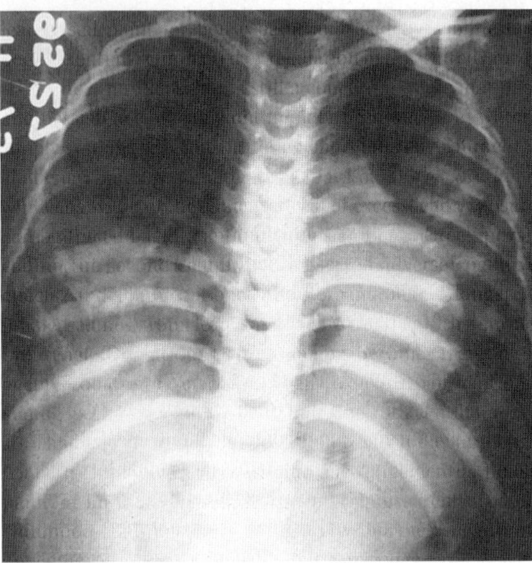

C

**FIGURE 78–1.** Three sequential radiographs of a young girl with severe hydrocarbon aspiration. (**A**) Initial: Patchy densities appear in the basilar areas of both lung fields with increased interstitial markings and peribronchial thickening. (**B**) Day 2: More extensive diffuse alveolar infiltrates are apparent. (**C**) Day 6: Dense consolidation and atelectasis are evident in the right lower lobe. *(Used with permission from Dr. Alexander Baxter, Department of Radiology, New York.)*

speech, nystagmus, head tremor, poor vision, deafness, stiff-legged and staggering gait, spasticity with hyperreflexia, plantar extension, and subsequent dementia.

### Peripheral Nervous System

Peripheral neuropathy is well described following occupational exposure to *n*-hexane or methyl-*n*-butyl ketone (MBK). This axonopathy results from a common metabolic intermediate, 2,5-hexanedione. The axonopathy typically begins in the distal extremities and progresses proximally (a classic, "dying-back" neuropathy). Cranial and peripheral neuropathies occur after acute and chronic exposure to trichloroethylene (TCE). Trichloroethylene exposure is also associated with trigeminal neuralgia.

### Gastrointestinal

Hydrocarbons irritate gastrointestinal mucous membranes. Nausea and vomiting are common after ingestion. As discussed earlier, vomiting increases the risk of pulmonary toxicity.

### Hepatic

The chlorinated hydrocarbons (Table 78–1) and their metabolites are hepatotoxic. In most cases, activation occurs via a phase I reaction to form a reactive intermediate. Carbon tetrachloride causes centrilobular necrosis after inhalational, oral, or dermal exposure. Hepatic injury, manifested as aminotransferase elevation and hepatomegaly, is usually reversible except in massive exposures. Vinyl chloride is a liver carcinogen.

### Renal

Acute kidney injury (AKI) and distal renal tubular acidosis occur in some painters and patients with volatile-substance use disorder. Toluene causes a renal tubular acidosis–like syndrome. Chronic hydrocarbon exposure is also associated with Goodpasture syndrome.

### Hematologic

Hemolysis is sporadically reported to occur following hydrocarbon ingestion. Benzene is a bone marrow suppressant and carcinogen.

### Immunologic

Hydrocarbons disturb the structural and functional integrity of membrane lipid bilayers by accumulating within the membrane and disrupting membrane lipopolysaccharides and proteins. This results in swelling and increased permeability to protons and other ions. Resultant toxicity directly destroys capillary endothelium. Additionally, there appears to be significant basement membrane dysfunction, and this is postulated to underlie both alveolar and glomerular toxicity of hydrocarbons. Immune mechanisms may account for basement membrane dysfunction in chronic exposures. Hydrocarbon exposure is suggested as one possible cause of the Goodpasture syndrome (immune dysfunction causing both pulmonary damage and glomerulonephritis).

### Dermatologic

Most hydrocarbon solvents cause nonspecific irritation of skin and mucous membranes. Repeated, prolonged contact can dry and crack the skin. The mechanism of dermal injury appears to be defatting of the lipid layer of the stratum corneum. Soft tissue injection of hydrocarbon is locally toxic, leading to necrosis. Particularly destructive lesions result from high-pressure injection gun injury. These injuries typically involve the extremities, with high-pressure injection of grease or paint into the fascial planes and tendon sheaths. Emergent surgical débridement is necessary in most of these cases.

## HYDROCARBONS WITH SPECIFIC AND UNIQUE TOXICITY

### *n*-Hexane

Hexane is a 6-carbon simple aliphatic hydrocarbon that is found in some brake-cleaning fluids, rubber cement, glues, spray paints, coatings, and silicones. Outbreaks of *n*-hexane–related neurotoxicity have occurred in printing plants, sandal shops, furniture factories, and automotive repair shops. Both *n*-hexane and MBK are well-known peripheral neurotoxins because of their common metabolic intermediate: 2,5-hexanedione. Similar 5- and 7-carbon species do not induce a comparable neurotoxicity, except those that are direct precursor intermediates in the metabolic pathway producing 2,5-hexanedione (Fig. 78–2).

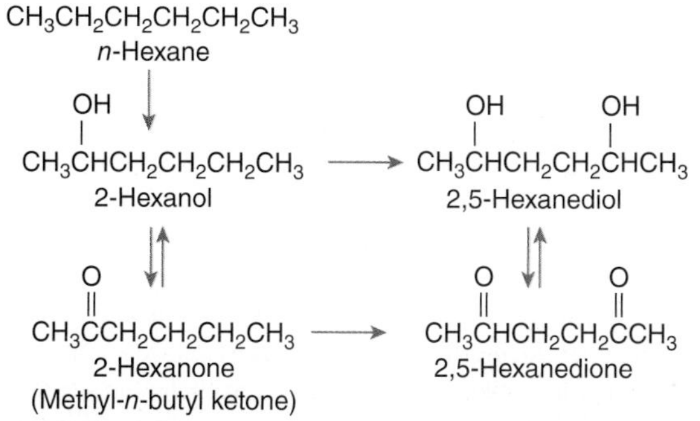

$CH_3CH_2CH_2CH_2CH_2CH_3$
*n*-Hexane
↓
OH on C2: $CH_3CHCH_2CH_2CH_2CH_3$ 2-Hexanol → OH, OH: $CH_3CHCH_2CH_2CHCH_3$ 2,5-Hexanediol
⇅ ⇅
O on C2: $CH_3CCH_2CH_2CH_2CH_3$ 2-Hexanone (Methyl-*n*-butyl ketone) → O, O: $CH_3CHCH_2CH_2CCH_3$ 2,5-Hexanedione

**FIGURE 78–2.** The metabolism of both organic solvents *n*-hexane and methyl-*n*-butyl ketone (MBK) produces the same common metabolite, 2,5-hexanedione.

### Methylene Chloride

Methylene chloride is commonly found in paint removers, cleansers, degreasers, and aerosol propellants. Like other halogenated hydrocarbons, it can rapidly induce general anesthesia by inhalation or ingestion. Unlike other hydrocarbons, methylene chloride and similar one-carbon halomethanes such as methylene dibromide are metabolized by CYP2E1 to carbon monoxide. Significant delayed and prolonged carboxyhemoglobinemia can occur (Table 78–2 and Chap. 95).

### Carbon Tetrachloride

Carbon tetrachloride ($CCl_4$), although not actually a hydrocarbon, has been used as an industrial solvent and reagent. Its use in the US declined dramatically since recognition of its toxicity caused the Environmental Protection Agency to restrict its commercial use. Absorption occurs by all routes, including dermal. Carbon tetrachloride is an irritant to skin and mucous membranes and gastric mucosa when ingested and can cause pneumonitis when aspirated and ventricular dysrhythmias once systemic absorption occurs. Carbon tetrachloride exposures are also hepatotoxic and nephrotoxic. Hepatotoxicity is typically manifested as reversible aminotransferase concentration elevations with or without hepatomegaly.

### Trichloroethylene

Trichloroethylene is a commonly used industrial solvent, cleanser, and degreaser. Systemically absorbed TCE competitively inhibits aldehyde dehydrogenase. Concomitant ethanol consumption results in a disulfiramlike reaction that is termed "degreaser's flush" (Chap. 51). Like other halogenated hydrocarbons, TCE is cardiotoxic, hepatotoxic, neurotoxic, and nephrotoxic.

### Benzene

Benzene is hematotoxic and associated with acute hemolysis or with the delayed development of aplastic anemia and acute myelogenous leukemia.

### Toluene

Chronic toluene abuse can also cause a syndrome that resembles transient distal renal tubular acidosis (RTA). Although the mechanism is incompletely understood, the acidosis results in great part from the urinary excretion of hippuric acid. Renal potassium loss results in symptomatic hypokalemia. Clinical findings are a hyperchloremic metabolic acidosis, hypokalemia, and aciduria.

### Pine Oil and Terpenes

Pine oil is an active ingredient in many household cleaning products. It is a mixture of unsaturated hydrocarbons composed of terpenes, camphenes, and pinenes. Patients who ingest pine oil often emit a strong pine odor. Wood distillates are readily absorbed from the gastrointestinal tract, and ingestion causes CNS and pulmonary toxicity without aspiration.

### Lipoid Pneumonia

Ingestion of low-viscosity hydrocarbons poses risk of pulmonary aspiration with subsequent acute pneumonitis. Conversely, viscous hydrocarbons rarely lead to pulmonary aspiration. However, inhalation of aerosolized oil droplets occurs in various occupational settings, resulting in lipoid pneumonia. The most common xenobiotics involved are mineral or vegetable oils. Initially, inhaled oil droplets are emulsified in the alveoli by surfactant, and then engulfed by alveolar macrophages. Unfortunately, macrophages are unable to readily process the internalized, exogenous oil. Symptoms of lipoid pneumonia are limited or even subclinical, but once they arise, illness may be prolonged from months to years. Ultimately, irreversible proliferative fibrosis may develop.

### Tar and Asphalt Injury

Asphalt workers are at risk for toxic gas exposure to hydrogen sulfide, carbon monoxide, propane, methane, and volatilized hydrocarbons. In addition, cutaneous exposure to these hot hydrocarbon mixtures causes severe burns. The material quickly hardens and is very difficult to remove. However, immediate cooling with cold water is important to limit further thermal injury. Complete removal is essential to ensure proper burn management and to limit infectious complications. Dissolving the material with mineral oil, petroleum jelly, or antibacterial ointments is met with variable success. Surface-active compounds combined with an ointment (De-Solv-it, Tween-80, Polysorbate 80) are more effective.

## DIAGNOSTIC TESTING

Laboratory and ancillary testing for hydrocarbon toxicity should be guided by available information regarding the specific xenobiotic, the route of exposure, and the best attempt at quantifying the exposure. The use of pulse oximetry and arterial blood gas testing in this group of patients is warranted for patients with respiratory symptoms. Early radiography is indicated in patients who are severely symptomatic; however, radiographs performed immediately after hydrocarbon ingestion have a poor predictive value for the occurrence of aspiration pneumonitis. In the asymptomatic patient, early radiography is not cost effective.

Specific diagnostic testing for hydrocarbon poisoning can be performed with bioassays for the specific hydrocarbon or its metabolites in blood, breath, or urine. These bioassays are not available in a clinically relevant time frame and should not be used to guide initial management of suspected hydrocarbon poisoning in the emergency setting. Patients with chronic exposures and CNS findings necessitate neuroimaging such as magnetic resonance imaging or positron emission tomography because computed tomography scan has limited utility except in those with severe disease.

## MANAGEMENT

Identification of the specific type, route, and amount of hydrocarbon exposure is rarely essential to achieve effective management. Decontamination is one of the cardinal principles of toxicology, with priority that is second only to stabilization of the cardiopulmonary status. Protection of rescuers with appropriate personal protective equipment and rescue protocols is paramount, especially in situations in which the victim has lost consciousness. Exposed clothing should be removed and safely discarded as further absorption or inhalation of hydrocarbons from grossly contaminated clothing can worsen systemic toxicity. Decontamination of the skin is a high priority in patients with massive hydrocarbon exposures, particularly those exposures involving highly toxic hydrocarbons. Soap and water should be the initial method of skin decontamination for the majority of hydrocarbons. The exception to this is phenol, for which water is often inadequate, and polyethylene glycol 400 (PEG 400) solution is recommended (Special Considerations: SC1).

Because of the high incidence of spontaneous emesis and the risk of aspiration in hydrocarbon ingestion, we recommend against routine attempts at gastric emptying. Activated charcoal (AC) has limited ability to decrease gastrointestinal absorption of hydrocarbons and may distend the stomach and predispose patients to vomiting and aspiration. Given the risk of spontaneous emesis and aspiration, we likewise recommend against the routine use of AC.

Since prophylactic antibiotics do not affect length of stay or otherwise impact the outcome of children with hydrocarbon aspiration, we recommend against routine antibiotic use in the management of patients with mild hydrocarbon pneumonitis. It is reasonable to administer antibiotics in patients with severe respiratory dysfunction. Similarly we recommend against the routine use of corticosteroids for hydrocarbon pulmonary toxicity, except in patients with bronchospasm or underlying reversible airways disease.

Patients with severe hydrocarbon toxicity pose unique problems for management. Respiratory distress requiring mechanical ventilation in this setting may be associated with a large ventilation–perfusion mismatch. The use of positive end-expiratory pressure (PEEP) in this setting is often beneficial. However, when very high levels of PEEP are required, there is an increased risk of barotrauma. High-frequency jet ventilation (HFJV), using very high respiratory rates (220–260) with small tidal volumes, has helped to decrease the need for PEEP. Patients who continue to have severe ventilation–perfusion mismatch despite PEEP and HFJV have benefited from extracorporeal membrane oxygenation (ECMO). Although there are case reports of clinical improvement of hydrocarbon pneumonitis with early administration of surfactant therapy, the evidence is poor and we do not recommend use of surfactant.

Hypotension in severe hydrocarbon toxicity raises additional concerns. The use of β-adrenergic agonists such as dopamine, epinephrine, isoproterenol, and norepinephrine should be avoided if possible, as certain hydrocarbons predispose to dysrhythmias. The recommended first-line treatments for hypotension is fluid resuscitation and minimizing PEEP, with phenylephrine used for refractory hypotension.

Management of dysrhythmias associated with hydrocarbon toxicity includes evaluation and correction of electrolyte and acid–base abnormalities such as hypokalemia and acidosis resulting from toluene, hypoxemia, hypotension, and hypothermia. Ventricular fibrillation poses a specific concern, as common resuscitation algorithms recommend epinephrine administration to treat this rhythm. If it is ascertained that the dysrhythmia emanates from myocardial sensitization by a hydrocarbon solvent, catecholamines should be avoided. In this setting, we recommend short-acting β-adrenergic antagonists such as esmolol as the treatment of choice for hydrocarbon-induced dysrhythmias.

We recommend hospitalization for those patients who have clinical evidence of toxicity and most individuals with intentional ingestions. Patients who do not have any initial symptoms, who have normal chest radiographs obtained at least 6 hours after ingestion, and who do not develop symptoms during the 6-hour observation period can be safely discharged. Patients who are asymptomatic on initial assessment but who have radiographic evidence of hydrocarbon pneumonitis can be safely discharged if they remain asymptomatic after a 6-hour observation period and are able to be reassessed with in 24 hours. Patients who have initial respiratory symptoms but quickly become asymptomatic during medical evaluation and remain so after a 6-hour observation period and who have a normal 6-hour chest radiograph can be discharged home. It is unclear how to manage asymptomatic patients who develop abnormal radiographic findings, but it is reasonable to observe them for and additional 12-24 hours for clinical illness.

# 79 TOXIC ALCOHOLS

## HISTORY AND EPIDEMIOLOGY

Methanol was a component of the embalming fluid used in ancient Egypt. Industrial production began in 1923, and today most methanol is used for the synthesis of other chemicals. Methanol-containing consumer products that are commonly encountered include model airplane and model car fuel, windshield washer fluid, solid cooking fuel for camping and chafing dishes, photocopying fluid, colognes and perfumes, and gas line antifreeze ("dry gas"). Methanol is also used as a solvent by itself or as an adulterant in "denatured" alcohol. There are sporadic epidemics of mass methanol poisoning, most commonly involving tainted fermented beverages.

Ethylene glycol was first synthesized in 1859 by Charles-Adolphe Wurtz and first widely produced as an engine coolant during World War II. Today its primary use remains as an engine coolant (antifreeze) in car radiators. Because of its sweet taste, it is often unintentionally consumed by animals and children.

Isopropanol is primarily available as rubbing alcohol. Typical household preparations contain 70% isopropanol. It is also a solvent used in many household, cosmetic, and topical pharmaceutical products. Perhaps because it is so ubiquitous, inexpensive, and with a common name that contains the word "alcohol," isopropanol ingestions are by far the most common toxic alcohol exposure reported to poison centers in the United States (US) every year.

## CHEMISTRY

Alcohols are hydrocarbons that contain a hydroxyl (–OH) group. The term "toxic alcohol" refers to alcohols other than ethanol that are not intended for ingestion. In a sense, this is arbitrary, since all alcohols are toxic, causing inebriation and end-organ effects. Primary alcohols, such as methanol and ethanol, contain a hydroxyl group on the end of the molecule (the terminal carbon), whereas secondary alcohols, such as isopropanol, contain hydroxyl groups bound to middle carbons. Ethylene glycol contains two hydroxyl groups; molecules with this characteristic are termed diols or glycols because of their sweet taste. Diethylene glycol is discussed in detail in Special Considerations: SC8.

## TOXICOKINETICS/TOXICODYNAMICS

### Absorption

***Ingestion.*** Alcohols are rapidly absorbed after ingestion but are not completely bioavailable because of metabolism by gastric alcohol dehydrogenase (ADH), as well as by first-pass hepatic metabolism. Ethylene glycol has an oral bioavailability of 92% to 100%.The bioavailabilities of methanol and isopropanol are not described, but are likely to be similar.

***Inhalation.*** Although methanol is absorbed in significant amounts by inhalation, poisoning by this route is uncommon. Cases of inhalational poisoning are reported with intentional inhalation of methanol as a drug of abuse, typically in the form of carburetor-cleaning fluid ("huffing") (Chap. 54), and with massive exposures of rescue workers responding to the scene of an overturned rail car filled with methanol. Ethylene glycol has low volatility and is not reported to cause poisoning by inhalation.

***Transdermal.*** Most alcohols have some dermal absorption, although isopropanol and methanol penetrate the skin much more effectively than ethylene glycol. Most reported cases of toxic alcohol poisoning by this route involve infants because of their greater body surface area–volume ratio and differences in permeability of infant skin compared to adults, and likely this also involved simultaneous inhalation. When transdermal methanol exposure is prolonged, severe toxicity is reported.

### Distribution

Once absorbed, alcohols are rapidly distributed to total body water. In human volunteers given an oral dose of methanol on an empty stomach, the measured volume of distribution was 0.77 L/kg, with a distribution half-life of about 8 minutes. This is only slightly longer than the absorption half-life, so serum concentrations often peak soon after ingestion and then decrease steadily. However, this is not necessarily the case in patients with large ingestions or with food in their stomachs prior to ingestion.

### Metabolism and Elimination

Without intervention, toxic alcohols are metabolized through successive oxidation by ADH and aldehyde dehydrogenase (ALDH), each of which is coupled to the reduction of $NAD^+$ to NADH.

Primary alcohols are metabolized first to aldehydes and then carboxylic acids (Figs. 79–1 and 79-2). Secondary alcohols are metabolized to ketones that cannot be further oxidized (Fig. 79–3).

In addition to their metabolites, methanol and ethylene glycol are also eliminated from the body as unchanged parent compounds. When kidney function is normal, ethylene glycol is cleared with a half-life of approximately 17 hours. In patients with renal impairment, the half-life is prolonged. Methanol does not have significant renal elimination and is cleared much more slowly than is ethylene glycol, presumably as a vapor in expired air (half-life 52 hours, with a longer half-life at very high concentrations).

## PATHOPHYSIOLOGY AND CLINICAL MANIFESTATIONS

### Acute Central Nervous System Effects

All alcohols cause inebriation, depending on the dose. Based on limited animal data, the higher-molecular-weight alcohols are more intoxicating than lower-molecular-weight alcohols. Therefore, isopropanol (MW 60.1) approximates ethylene glycol (MW 62.07), which is greater than ethanol (MW 46.07), which is greater than methanol (MW 32.04). However, the absence of apparent inebriation does not

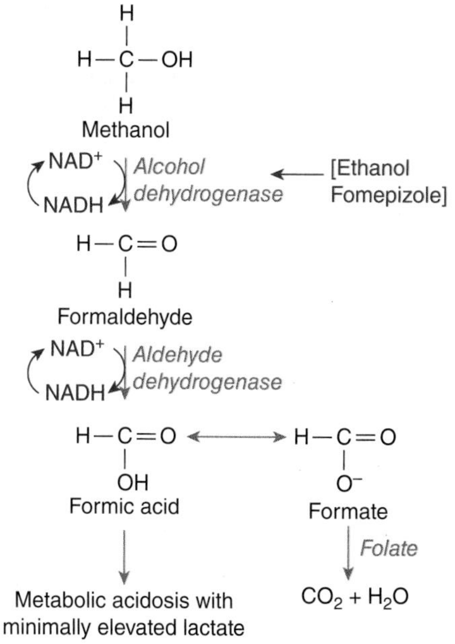

$H-C(H)(H)-OH$
Methanol
$NAD^+$ → NADH Alcohol dehydrogenase ← [Ethanol Fomepizole]
$H-C(H)=O$
Formaldehyde
$NAD^+$ → NADH Aldehyde dehydrogenase
$H-C(OH)=O$ ⟷ $H-C(O^-)=O$
Formic acid — Formate
↓ Metabolic acidosis with minimally elevated lactate
↓ Folate → $CO_2 + H_2O$

FIGURE 79–1. Major pathway of methanol metabolism.

exclude ingestion, particularly if the patient chronically drinks ethanol and is thereby tolerant to its central nervous system (CNS) effects. The CNS manifestations of toxic alcohol poisoning are incompletely understood. It is assumed by analogy that inebriation is similar to that of ethanol, in which effects are mediated through increased γ-aminobutyric acid (GABA) tone both directly and through inhibition of presynaptic GABA, $GABA_A$ receptors, as well as inhibition of the *N*-methyl-D-aspartate glutamate receptors.

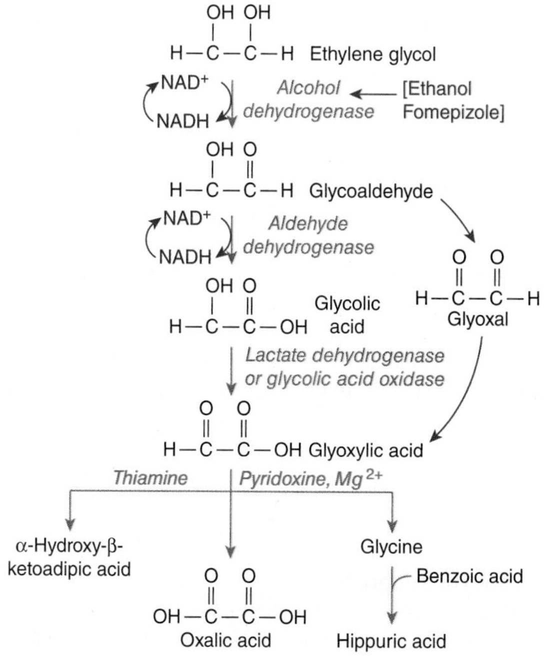

Ethylene glycol: $H-C(OH)-C(OH)-H$
$NAD^+$ → NADH Alcohol dehydrogenase ← [Ethanol Fomepizole]
Glycoaldehyde: $H-C(OH)-C(=O)-H$
$NAD^+$ → NADH Aldehyde dehydrogenase
Glycolic acid: $H-C(OH)-C(=O)-OH$
Glyoxal: $H-C(=O)-C(=O)-H$
Lactate dehydrogenase or glycolic acid oxidase
Glyoxylic acid: $H-C(=O)-C(=O)-OH$
Thiamine → α-Hydroxy-β-ketoadipic acid
Pyridoxine, $Mg^{2+}$ → Glycine; Glycine + Benzoic acid → Hippuric acid
Oxalic acid: $OH-C(=O)-C(=O)-OH$

FIGURE 79–2. Pathways of ethylene glycol metabolism. Thiamine and pyridoxine enhance formation of nontoxic metabolites.

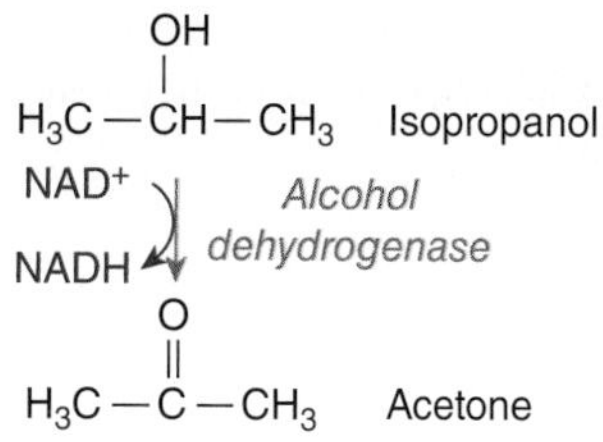

Isopropanol: $H_3C-CH(OH)-CH_3$
$NAD^+$ → NADH Alcohol dehydrogenase
Acetone: $H_3C-C(=O)-CH_3$

FIGURE 79–3. Isopropanol metabolism.

## Metabolic Acidosis

Metabolic acidosis with an elevated anion gap is a hallmark of toxic alcohol poisoning. This is a consequence of the metabolism of the alcohols to toxic organic acids. The acids have no rapid natural metabolic pathway of elimination, and therefore, they accumulate. In methanol poisoning, formic acid is responsible for the acidosis, whereas in ethylene glycol poisoning, glycolic acid is the primary acid responsible for the acidosis, with other metabolites making a minor contribution. Because acetone cannot be metabolized by ALDH, isopropanol has no organic acid metabolite and does not cause a metabolic acidosis.

## End-Organ Manifestations

Additional end-organ effects depend on which alcohol is involved. Methanol causes visual impairment, ranging from blurry or hazy vision or defects in color vision to "snowfield vision" or total blindness in severe poisoning. Formate is a mitochondrial toxin, inhibiting cytochrome oxidase, and it thereby interferes with oxidative phosphorylation. Although it is unclear why this results in ocular toxicity while other tissues are relatively spared, retinal pigmented epithelial cells and optic nerve cells appear to be uniquely susceptible. Interestingly, neurons in the basal ganglia appear to be similarly susceptible to this toxicity. Bilateral basal ganglia lesions and bilateral necrosis of the putamen (with or without hemorrhage), and less commonly, caudate nucleus are characteristic abnormalities visualized on cerebral computed tomography (CT) or magnetic resonance imaging (MRI) after methanol poisoning. Both retinal and neurologic toxicity in patients with methanol poisoning are often permanent.

Injury to other tissues also occurs. Both acute kidney injury (AKI) and pancreatitis are reported after methanol poisoning. Some of the AKI that results from methanol poisoning likely results from myoglobinuria. Patients with AKI were also more likely than a control group of patients to have severe poisoning, as manifested by low initial serum pH, high initial osmolality, and high peak formate concentration.

The most prominent end-organ effect of ethylene glycol is nephrotoxicity. The oxalic acid metabolite forms a complex with calcium to precipitate as calcium oxalate monohydrate crystals in the renal tubules, leading to AKI. In fact, the diagnosis of ethylene glycol poisoning is sometimes established following kidney biospy or at autopsy by demonstrating this abnormality. Ethylene glycol can also occasionally affect other organ systems. Uncommonly, in severe poisoning, the oxalic acid metabolite causes hypocalcemia by precipitation as calcium oxalate. Cranial nerve

(CN) abnormalities (CN VI, VII) are occasionally reported, possibly as a result of precipitation of calcium oxalate crystals in the brain.

## DIAGNOSTIC TESTING

### Toxic Alcohol and Metabolite Concentrations

Serum methanol, formate, ethylene glycol, oxalate, and isopropanol concentrations (as appropriate) would be the ideal tests to perform shortly after suspected toxic alcohol poisoning. However, these concentrations are most commonly measured by gas chromatography with or without mass spectrometry confirmation, methodologies that are not available in many hospital laboratories on a 24-hour basis, if at all. A newer dry chemistry "dipstick" technology for formate detection shows promise for rapid detection of cases of methanol poisoning with minimal equipment or skilled laboratory personnel. Patients with significant serum concentrations of ethanol generally do not have measurable formate concentrations even when there are significant serum concentrations of methanol, so serial testing of these patients would be necessary if methanol poisoning is suspected.

Patients presenting late after ingestion have already metabolized all parent compound to toxic metabolites and thus have low or no measurable toxic alcohol concentrations. Some authors actually advocate for routine testing for glycolic acid in addition to testing for the parent compound when ethylene glycol poisoning is suspected. Similarly, a formate concentration would be valuable when a patient presents late after methanol ingestion. Clearly, a low or undetectable toxic alcohol concentration must be interpreted within the context of the history and other clinical data, such as the presence of acidosis and end-organ toxicity, with glycolate and formate concentrations as potentially valuable additions.

Once alcohol concentrations are obtained, their interpretation represents a further point of controversy. Traditionally, a methanol or ethylene glycol concentration greater than 25 mg/dL was considered toxic, but the evidence supporting this as a threshold is often questioned. A systematic review found that 126 mg/dL was the lowest methanol concentration resulting in metabolic acidosis in a patient who arrived early after ingestion and met the inclusion criteria. The authors concluded that the available data are currently insufficient to apply a 25 mg/dL treatment threshold in a patient presenting early after ingestion without metabolic acidosis. However, until better data are available demonstrating the safe application of a higher concentration, it seems prudent to use a conservative concentration such as 25 mg/dL as a threshold for treatment.

Because of the problems with obtaining and interpreting actual serum concentrations, many surrogate markers are used to assess the patient with suspected toxic alcohol poisoning. The initial laboratory evaluation should include serum electrolytes, including calcium, blood urea nitrogen, serum creatinine concentrations, urinalysis, measured serum osmolality, and a serum ethanol concentration. Blood gas analysis with a lactate concentration is also helpful in the initial evaluation of ill-appearing patients.

### Anion Gap and Osmol Gap

As previously discussed, anion gap elevation is a hallmark of toxic alcohol poisoning. In fact, the possibility of methanol or ethylene glycol poisoning is often first considered when patients present with an anion gap metabolic acidosis of unknown etiology, frequently with no history of ingestion. Unless clinical information suggests otherwise, it is important to exclude metabolic acidosis with elevated lactate concentration and ketoacidosis, which are the most common causes of anion gap metabolic acidosis, before pursuing toxic alcohols in these patients. However, elevated lactate concentrations are often present in the setting of both methanol and ethylene glycol poisoning.

The unmeasured anions in patients with toxic alcohol poisoning are the dissociated organic acid metabolites discussed above. The metabolic acidosis takes time to develop, sometimes up to 16 to 24 hours for methanol. Thus, the absence of an anion gap elevation early after reported toxic alcohol ingestion does not exclude the diagnosis. If ethanol is present in the body, the development of metabolic acidosis will not begin to occur until enough ethanol has been metabolized such that it can no longer effectively inhibit ADH (see Ethanol Concentration, below).

A potential early surrogate marker of toxic alcohol poisoning is an elevated osmol gap. However, it is important to recognize that osmol gap elevation is neither sensitive nor specific for toxic alcohol poisoning. A low or normal osmol gap should not be used to definitively exclude a toxic alcohol ingestion. However, a markedly elevated osmol gap (> 50 mOsm/L) is difficult to explain by anything other than a toxic alcohol.

Further complicating matters, the anion gap and osmol gap have a reciprocal relationship over time. As the alcohols are metabolized to organic acid anions, the anion gap rises while the osmol gap falls. Thus, patients who present early after ingestion have a high osmol gap and normal anion gap, whereas those who present later have the reverse. Figure 79–4 depicts a more intuitive visual representation of this process.

### Ethanol Concentration

A serum ethanol concentration is an important part of the assessment of the patient with suspected toxic alcohol poisoning. The ethanol concentration is necessary to calculate osmolarity. In addition, because ethanol is the preferred substrate of ADH (4:1 over methanol and 8:1 over ethylene glycol on a molar basis), a significant concentration would be protective if coingested with a toxic alcohol. In fact, ethanol concentrations near 100 mg/dL (21.7 mmol/L) virtually preclude toxic alcohols as the cause of an unknown anion gap metabolic acidosis because the presence of such a concentration should have prevented metabolism to the organic acid. A possible exception would be ingestion of ethanol several hours after ingestion of a toxic alcohol.

### Lactate Concentration

Both methanol and ethylene glycol poisoning can result in elevated lactate concentrations, for different reasons. Formate, as an inhibitor of oxidative phosphorylation, leads to anaerobic metabolism and resultant lactate elevation. Additionally,

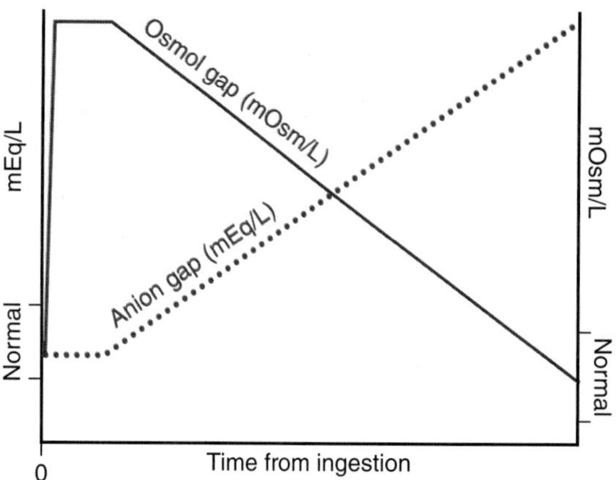


**FIGURE 79–4.** The reciprocal relationship of anion gap and osmol gap over time (hours). Note that patients presenting early may have a normal anion gap while patients who present late may have a normal osmol gap.

metabolism of all alcohols results in an increased NADH/$NAD^+$ ratio, which favors the conversion of pyruvate to lactate. Furthermore, hypotension and organ failure in severely poisoned patients also produces an elevated lactate concentration. However, lactate production by these mechanisms is rarely greater than 5 mmol/L.

In ethylene glycol poisoning, the glycolate metabolite also causes a false-positive lactate elevation when measured by some analyzers, particularly with whole blood arterial blood gas analyzers. In such cases, the degree of lactate elevation, which is often as high as 15 to 20 mmol/L, directly correlates with the concentration of glycolate present. This artifact can be exploited, using the presence of a "lactate gap" to diagnose ethylene glycol poisoning in hospitals where lactate assays are available with and without sensitivity to glycolate. Ingestion of propylene glycol also results in elevated lactate concentrations, but in this case, it is not a false-positive lactate but rather an accurate measurement of lactate, the principal metabolite of propylene glycol.

### Other Diagnostics

The urine provides some information in the assessment of the patient with suspected ethylene glycol poisoning. Calcium oxalate monohydrate (spindle-shaped) and dihydrate (envelope-shaped) crystals are often seen when the urine sediment is examined by microscopy, although this finding is neither sensitive nor specific. In fact, calcium oxalate crystals were only present in the urine of 63% of patients with proven ethylene glycol ingestion in one series.

Some brands of antifreeze contain fluorescein to facilitate the detection of radiator leaks. If one of these products is ingested and the urine is examined with a Wood lamp within the first 6 hours, there will often be urinary fluorescence. False-positive fluorescence also results from examining the urine in glass or plastic containers because of the inherent fluorescence of these materials, so if this test is performed, an aliquot of the urine should be poured onto a piece of white gauze or paper. Unfortunately, the utility of this test is quite limited.

The evaluation of patients with known or suspected ethylene glycol poisoning should also include serum calcium and creatinine concentrations. Depending on the clinical examination liver function tests, an electrocardiogram (ECG) and neuroimaging will be helpful.

### Diagnostic Testing and Risk Assessment

Many pediatric patients with toxic alcohol exposures have not actually ingested the product with which they are found. However, children who actually ingest toxic alcohols can be just as sick as adults, and smaller-volume ingestions are required to reach consequential serum concentrations, so risk assessment is particularly important for these patients.

If the ingested dose of a toxic alcohol is known, an estimate of the projected maximum serum concentration can be determined using the formula:

$$C = D/V_d$$

where C is the estimated blood concentration projected, D is the dose in grams, and $V_d$ is the volume of distribution (typically estimated at 0.6 L/kg) multiplied by the patient's weight in kilograms. Once the projected serum concentration is calculated, it can be compared to typical thresholds for treatment to decide whether the ingestion could potentially lead to a concerning serum concentration.

A review of reported toxic alcohol cases attempted to identify risk factors for mortality in adults with methanol or ethylene glycol poisoning. For methanol poisoning, no patient with an anion gap less than 30 mEq/L or an osmolar gap less than 49 mOsm/L died. A pH less than 7.22 was an even better predictor of mortality, as no patient with a pH greater than 7.22 died. For ethylene glycol, the tests were less useful. Other markers of poor outcomes in this study were initial creatinine higher than 1.65 mg/dL (146 μmol/L), seizure, and coma. Another retrospective study of risk factors for poor outcomes in methanol poisoning found that pH less than 7, coma, or a greater than 24-hour delay to presentation was associated with death. Formate, as discussed above, was a good predictor of outcome in one series, with concentrations less than 18 mg/dL associated with good outcomes and concentrations higher than 78.8 mg/dL associated with a 90% risk of mortality. In methanol-poisoned patients unlikely to die, the pH is of some use in predicting retinal toxicity. A retrospective study found a pH greater than 7.2 associated with a high likelihood of only transient visual sequelae.

## MANAGEMENT

As always, immediate resuscitation of critically ill patients starts with management of the airway, breathing, and circulation. Because alcohols cause respiratory depression and coma, intubation and mechanical ventilation are commonly necessary for patients with severe poisoning. Alcohol-induced vasodilation combined with vomiting often leads to hypotension, and many patients will require fluid resuscitation with intravenous crystalloid. Gastrointestinal decontamination is rarely, if ever, indicated for patients with toxic alcohols because of their rapid absorption and limited binding to activated charcoal. However, placement of a nasogastric tube and aspiration of any gastric contents are reasonable in intubated patients, as absorption is sometimes delayed after a large dose.

### Alcohol Dehydrogenase Inhibition

The most important part of the initial management of patients with known or suspected toxic alcohol poisoning (after initial resuscitation) is blockade of ADH. This allows time for the establishment of a definitive diagnosis and arrangement for hemodialysis while preventing the formation of toxic metabolites. Additionally, in some cases, ADH blockade will itself serve as definitive therapy.

Ethanol is the traditional method of ADH inhibition and is still the only option in most of the world, although it is rarely used in the US. Orally administered ethanol is effective and may be reasonable, particularly in rural areas where there is likely a significant delay in getting the patient to a hospital. Whether oral or IV, the goal is to rapidly reach and maintain a serum ethanol concentration of 100 mg/dL (21.7 mmol/L), which is challenging (Antidotes in Brief: A34).

Fomepizole is a competitive antagonist of ADH that has many advantages over ethanol. It reliably inhibits ADH when administered as an intravenous bolus, and concentrations do not need to be monitored as with an ethanol infusion. It does not cause inebriation and is associated with fewer adverse effects and fewer medication errors, so it does not require intensive care unit monitoring. For these reasons, it has become the preferred method of ADH blockade in the US, despite being significantly more expensive than ethanol. The dose of fomepizole is 15 mg/kg intravenously as an initial loading dose followed by 10 mg/kg every 12 hours. After 48 hours of therapy, fomepizole induces its own metabolism, so the dose must be increased to 15 mg/kg every 12 hours (Antidotes in Brief: A33).

Indications for fomepizole or ethanol therapy are based on the history or on laboratory data. It is reasonable to treat a patient with a history of methanol or ethylene glycol ingestion until concentrations are available because, as previously discussed, early signs and symptoms and laboratory markers other than serum concentrations are frequently absent. In addition, we recommend treating any patient with a life-threatening anion gap metabolic acidosis without another explanation or a markedly elevated osmol gap. Once concentrations are available, we recommend continuing therapy until the serum toxic alcohol concentration is predicted or measured to be below 25 mg/dL, although as discussed previously, this value is based more on consensus opinion than on data.

### Hemodialysis

The definitive therapy for symptomatic patients poisoned by toxic alcohols is hemodialysis. Hemodialysis clears both the alcohols and their toxic metabolites from the blood and corrects the acid–base disorder. The indications for hemodialysis have become more restricted with the advent of fomepizole because of its effectiveness combined with its low incidence of adverse effects. This is particularly true for ethylene glycol, which can generally be expected to be cleared within a few days once ADH is blocked, eliminating the need for hemodialysis as long as the glomerular filtration rate is normal. However, patients with end-organ toxicity or severe acidemia have significant amounts of toxic metabolites (a problem not addressed by ADH blockade), and acidemia is associated with poor prognosis.

The Extracorporeal Treatments in Poisoning (EXTRIP) group has published interdisciplinary consensus guidelines for dialysis in methanol poisoning (Table 79–1). The American Academy of Clinical Toxicology guidelines for ethylene glycol actually advise against hemodialysis for a concentration alone without clinical indications such as metabolic acidosis, AKI, end-organ effects, or worsening clinical status, and rates of hemodialysis for early ethylene glycol poisoning have declined in recent years.

Although hemodialysis effectively clears isopropanol and acetone from the blood, it is rarely if ever indicated for this purpose. Because isopropanol does not cause a metabolic acidosis and very rarely results in significant end-organ effects, the risks of hemodialysis likely outweigh the benefits.

Patients with high concentrations of toxic alcohols will require multiple courses of hemodialysis to clear the toxic alcohol and/or its metabolites, and reverse any metabolic acidemia that is present. If practicing in a setting where rapid determination of toxic alcohol concentrations is available, the need for further hemodialysis should be guided by the posthemodialysis concentration. Normalization of the osmol gap is another strategy to guide the required duration

**TABLE 79–1 EXTRIP Guidelines for Extracorporeal Treatment in Methanol Poisoning**

**Hemodialysis Recommended:**

1. Severe methanol poisoning
   a) coma
   b) seizures
   c) new vision deficit
   d) metabolic acidosis
      i) blood pH ≤ 7.15
      ii) persistent metabolic acidosis despite adequate support measures and antidotes
   e) serum anion gap ≥ 24 calculated by serum $[Na^+] - ([Cl^-] + [HCO_3^-])$
2. Serum methanol concentration
   a) > 70 mg/dL (21.8 mmol/L) in the context of fomepizole therapy
   b) > 60 mg/dL (18.7 mmol/L) in the context of ethanol treatment
   c) > 50 mg/dL (15.6 mmol/L) in the absence of an ADH antagonist
   d) in the absence of a serum methanol concentration, the osmol gap may be informative
3. In the context of impaired renal function

**To optimize the outcomes of extracorporeal treatment:**

4. Intermittent hemodialysis is the modality of choice in methanol poisoning. Continuous modalities are acceptable alternatives if intermittent hemodialysis is unavailable.
5. Alcohol dehydrogenase inhibitors and folic acid are to be continued during hemodialysis.
6. Extracorporeal treatment can be terminated when the methanol concentration is < 20 mg/dL (6.2 mmol/L) and a clinical improvement is observed.

Reproduced with permission from Roberts DM, Yates C, Megarbane B, et al. Recommendations for the role of extracorporeal treatments in the management of acute methanol poisoning: a systematic review and consensus statement. *Crit Care Med.* 2015;43(2):461-472.

of hemodialysis, and though not validated, seems reasonable. The important point with all of these strategies is that the duration of hemodialysis required is often much longer than a standard 4-hour course that would be used routinely in a patient with kidney failure, necessitating multiple or very long courses of hemodialysis. Regardless of how the duration of dialysis is determined, we recommend continuing ADH blockade during and after hemodialysis until a subsequent concentration of the toxic alcohol is below 20 mg/dL. Dosing recommendations for fomepizome and ethanol during hemodialys can be found in the two Antidotes in Brief (A33 and A34).

Continuous renal replacement therapy (CRRT) such as venovenous hemodiafiltration is used in some patients with toxic alcohol poisoning. Hemodialysis is much more efficient at clearing xenobiotics than CRRT and is the modality of choice if available. However, if there is a contraindication to hemodialysis or if hemodialysis is unavailable, continuous modalities are acceptable alternatives.

Because methanol poisoning is sometimes complicated by coagulopathy, anticoagulation during hemodialysis is at least a theoretical concern because of the potential risk of bleeding. In patients with laboratory evidence of coagulopathy, it is reasonable to perform hemodialysis or CRRT without systemic anticoagulation.

### Adjunctive Therapy

There are several therapeutic adjuncts to ADH blockade with or (especially) without hemodialysis that we recommend for these patients. Folate and leucovorin enhance the clearance of formate in animal models. Thiamine enhances the metabolism of ethylene glycol to ketoadipate, and pyridoxine enhances its metabolism to glycine and ultimately hippuric acid. Although all of these modalities offer theoretical advantages, they have yet to be proven to change outcome in humans. However, because of the safety of vitamin supplementation and the fact that many of these patients have alcohol use disorder and require folate and thiamine anyway, we recommend the use of folate, thiamine, and pyridoxine in patients with toxic alcohol poisoning (Antidotes in Brief: A12, A15, and A27).

Formate is much less toxic than undissociated formic acid, likely because formic acid has a much higher affinity for cytochrome oxidase in the mitochondria, the ultimate target site for toxicity. In addition, the undissociated form is better able to diffuse into target tissues. Alkalinization with a bicarbonate infusion shifts the equilibrium to favor the less toxic, dissociated form, in accordance with the Henderson-Hasselbalch equation. This also enhances formate clearance in the urine by ion trapping. In the absence of contraindications to a bicarbonate infusion (eg, hypokalemia, volume overload), alkalinization is reasonable in the patient with suspected methanol poisoning and a significant acidemia. A blood pH greater than 7.20 is a reasonable endpoint. Alkalinization is also reasonable for patients with ethylene glycol poisoning and life-threatening metabolic acidosis.

## POISONING EPIDEMICS

As discussed earlier, toxic alcohol poisoning epidemics can at times overwhelm local capacity to provide antidotal therapy and hemodialysis, necessitating triage decisions in allocating resources. Equally important is early recognition of an epidemic and effective communication with the population to try to identify affected people. Reaching patients before they become severely ill can potentially prevent bad outcomes. During an outbreak in Iran in 2013, multiple strategies were used, including text messaging, radio broadcasting, encouraging patients to find their drinking partners, and loudspeaker announcements near healthcare facilities, to encourage people to spread the word about contaminated alcoholic beverages, while emergency operation centers coordinated the medical response and distribution of patients to local dialysis centers. Another strategy to mitigate harm from methanol epidemics is empiric prehospital oral ethanol administration in patients with suspected methanol poisoning.

## OTHER ALCOHOLS

### Propylene Glycol

Propylene glycol is commonly used as an alternative to ethylene glycol in "environmentally safe" antifreeze. It is also used as a diluent for many pharmaceuticals (such as phenytoin and lorazepam). This alcohol is successively metabolized by ADH and ALDH to lactate, so a metabolic acidosis results. This can result in extremely high lactate concentrations that would typically be incompatible with life if generated by any disease process but are surprisingly well tolerated. Therapy is entirely supportive with cessation of the exposure if it relates to a pharmaceutical.

### Benzyl Alcohol

Benzyl alcohol is used as a preservative for intravenous solutions. Although it is no longer used in neonatal medicine, it was responsible for "neonatal gasping syndrome," involving multiorgan system dysfunction, metabolic acidosis, and death because of its metabolism to benzoic acid and hippuric acid (Chap. 19). Therapy is entirely supportive with cessation of the exposure if it relates to a pharmaceutical.

# A33 FOMEPIZOLE

Fomepizole is a potent competitive inhibitor of alcohol dehydrogenase (ADH) that prevents the formation of toxic metabolites from ethylene glycol and methanol. It also has a role in halting the disulfiram–ethanol reaction and in limiting the toxicity from a variety of xenobiotics that rely on alcohol dehydrogenase or CYP 2E1 for metabolism such as diethylene glycol.

## HISTORY

In 1963, Theorell described the inhibiting effect of pyrazole on horse ADH. The administration of pyrazole to animals poisoned with methanol and ethylene glycol improved survival but also had significant adverse effects. In 1969, Li and Theorell found that 4-methylpyrazole (fomepizole) inhibited ADH in human liver preparations and was relatively nontoxic. Subsequent studies of fomepizole in monkeys and humans poisoned with methanol and ethylene glycol confirmed both the inhibitory effect and relative safety of fomepizole.

## PHARMACOLOGY

### Mechanism of Action

Fomepizole is a potent competitive inhibitor of ADH with a very high affinity for ADH, thereby blocking the metabolism of methanol and ethylene glycol to their respective toxic metabolites. In human liver, the concentration of fomepizole needed to achieve inhibition is about 0.9 to 1 μm/L. Current dosing produces a serum fomepizole concentration of 100 to 300 μm/L to ensure a margin of safety.

## PHARMACOKINETICS

The volume of distribution of fomepizole is about 0.6 to 1 L/kg; it is metabolized to 4-carboxypyrazole, an inactive metabolite that accounts for 80% to 85% of the administered dose. Oral doses of fomepizole are rapidly absorbed, peak within 2 hours, and have an apparent half-life of 5.2 hours. When fomepizole is dosed every 12 hours, the elimination of fomepizole increases after 36 to 48 hours, most likely because of autoinduction requiring dosing adjustment (see below). Following a loading dose of 15 mg/kg of intravenous fomepizole, a mean peak concentration of 342 μm/L (28 mg/L) was achieved. The apparent half-life is 14.5 hours (in the presence of methanol or ethylene glycol), and 40 hours in the presence of ethanol, in addition to methanol or ethylene glycol. The hemodialysis clearance of fomepizole ranges from 50 to 137 mL/min.

## ROLE IN METHANOL TOXICITY

### In Vitro and Animal Studies

Studies using human livers demonstrate the inhibitory effect of fomepizole on ADH. Studies in monkeys, the animal species that most closely resembles humans in metabolizing methanol, also demonstrate the inhibitory effect of fomepizole in preventing the accumulation of formate (the toxic metabolite of methanol).

### Human Experience

In case series of patients given IV fomepizole, formate concentrations decreased, and the arterial pH increased. Case reports demonstrate similar findings.

### Effect on Methanol and Formate Concentrations

In humans treated with fomepizole, the apparent half-life of methanol was about 54 hours. Formate concentrations in patients with methanol poisoning treated with fomepizole decreased, with a half-life of 156 to 235 minutes in two studies.

## ROLE IN ETHYLENE GLYCOL TOXICITY

### In Vitro and Animal Studies

Monkeys given a uniformly lethal dose of ethylene glycol with fomepizole all survived.

### Human Experience

The first three patients treated with oral fomepizole improved clinically and tolerated the therapy. Subsequent case reports and case series using fomepizole orally or IV also demonstrated the effectiveness of fomepizole in preventing glycolate accumulation.

### Effect on Ethylene Glycol and Glycolate Concentrations in Humans

Kidney function is essential for the elimination of ethylene glycol. With normal kidney function, the half-life of ethylene glycol is about 8.6 hours. After fomepizole administration, the half-life of ethylene glycol is about 14 to 17 hours in patients with normal kidney function, and about 49 hours in patients with impaired kidney function defined as a serum creatinine greater than 1.2 mg/dL (106 μm/L). In a study where neither kidney function was defined nor the amount of glycolate excreted unchanged by the kidneys described, glycolate had a mean half-life of 10 ± 8 hours in patients treated with fomepizole before hemodialysis and a mean half-life of less than 3 hours during hemodialysis.

## ROLE IN TOXICITY FROM DIETHYLENE GLYCOL, DISULFIRAM, AND OTHER XENOBIOTICS

Fomepizole successfully terminated the adverse reactions resulting from the use of disulfiram administered to volunteers pretreated with a small dose of ethanol, in a person with alcohol use disorder surreptitiously given disulfiram by his wife, and in two patients who intentionally ingested ethanol in addition to an overdose of disulfiram.

Several animal studies and a few case reports suggest that fomepizole is effective in limiting the toxicity secondary to diethylene glycol (DEG), triethylene glycol, and 1,3-difluoro-2-propanol. Fomepizole blocks the metabolism of DEG to toxic metabolites and is recommended as early as possible after ingestion before metabolism of DEG occurs. Concomitant hemodialysis is also recommended. The role of fomepizole in overdoses secondary to 2-butoxyethanol (ethylene glycol monobutyl ether) is unclear, but fomepizole is reasonable for administration within several hours of ingestion and before rapid metabolism of butoxyethanol to butoxyacetic acid occurs.

## COMPARISON TO ETHANOL

Ethanol effectively and inexpensively inhibits the metabolism of methanol and ethylene glycol to their respective toxic metabolites and has been used for many years, but has many disadvantages compared to fomepizole. Ethanol causes central nervous system depression that is at least additive to that of the methanol or ethylene glycol, and dosing difficulties occur as a result of the rapid and often unpredictable rate of ethanol metabolism (Antidotes in Brief: A34). Fomepizole dosing is much easier and does not require therapeutic monitoring of its serum concentration. Ethanol is recommended for use only when fomepizole is not readily available. Ethanol might be preferred in a mass casualty situation until sufficient supplies of fomepizole can be procured.

## ADVERSE EFFECTS AND SAFETY ISSUES

The most common adverse effects of the use of fomepizole reported by the manufacturer (in a total of 78 patients and 63 volunteers) were headache (14%), nausea (11%), and dizziness, increased drowsiness, and dysgeusia or metallic taste (6%). Other less commonly observed adverse effects include phlebitis, rash, fever, and eosinophilia. The most common laboratory abnormality after fomepizole administration is a transient elevation of aminotransferase concentrations (never more than three times the upper limit of normal values), which was reported in 6 of 15 healthy volunteers.

## PREGNANCY AND LACTATION

Fomepizole is listed as Pregnancy Category C by the United States Food and Drug Administration. The risks of methanol and ethylene glycol poisoning are so severe (including neonatal death) that it is recommended that fomepizole be administered when toxicity is present or anticipated. There are no studies that have examined the amount of fomepizole in breast milk, although the low molecular weight suggests that it will be excreted into breast milk. It is recommended that breastfeeding be temporarily discontinued until fomepizole is predicted to be eliminated from the body (about 24 hours after the last dose) and the toxic alcohol has been eliminated.

## DOSING AND ADMINISTRATION

The loading dose of fomepizole is 15 mg/kg IV, followed in 12 hours by 10 mg/kg every 12 hours for four doses. If therapy is necessary beyond 48 hours, the dose is then increased to 15 mg/kg every 12 hours, for as long as necessary. Fomepizole must be diluted in 100 mL of NS (in adults) and infused over 30 min to avoid thrombophlebitis. Patients undergoing hemodialysis require additional doses of fomepizole to replace the amount removed during hemodialysis.

We recommend the administration of fomepizole at the beginning of hemodialysis if the last dose was given more than 6 hours earlier. At the completion of hemodialysis, we recommend the administration of the next scheduled dose if more than 3 hours have transpired, or one-half of the dose if 1 to 3 hours have passed. Following hemodialysis, dosing of fomepizole every 12 hours is reinstituted. A reasonable recommendation would be to administer the fomepizole every 8 hours during continuous kidney replacement therapy. Fomepizole therapy should be continued until the methanol or ethylene glycol is no longer present in sufficient concentrations to produce toxicity. We recommend continuing therapy until the serum toxic alcohol concentration is predicted or measured to be below 25 mg/dL in the absence of any acid–base disturbances.

## FORMULATION AND ACQUISITION

Fomepizole is marketed in branded and generic formulations in 1.5-mL vials of 1 g/mL.

# A34 ETHANOL

## INTRODUCTION AND HISTORY

Ethanol is used antidotally to limit the metabolism of xenobiotics metabolized by alcohol dehydrogenase (ADH). Ethanol has been used as an antidote for methanol poisoning since the 1940s and for ethylene glycol since the 1960s.

## PHARMACOLOGY

### Mechanism of Action

Ethanol is a competitive substrate for ADH, inhibiting the metabolism of xenobiotics such as methanol and ethylene glycol that employ this enzyme.

## AFFINITY FOR ALCOHOL DEHYDROGENASE

The molar affinity of ethanol for ADH is 67 times higher than its affinity for ethylene glycol and 15.5 times that of methanol. Using human ADH and a simulation model, the oxidation of 50 mM of methanol and ethylene glycol was inhibited by 20 mM (92 mg/dL) of ethanol and 50 μM (0.4 mg/dL) of fomepizole. Studies in methanol-poisoned monkeys revealed that when ethanol was administered at a molar ethanol-to-methanol ratio (E/M) of 1:4, the metabolism of methanol was reduced by 70%; at a 1:1 E/M ratio, metabolism was reduced by greater than 90%. When compared with methanol, smaller amounts of ethanol are required to block the metabolism of ethylene glycol, as the affinity of ethylene glycol for ADH is lesser than that of methanol.

## PHARMACOKINETICS

Ethanol can be given either orally or IV. The loading dose of ethanol must be followed by a maintenance dose, as metabolism is rapid. Concentrations of 20% to 30% (orally) and 5% to 10% IV are well tolerated. Intravenous administration has the advantage of complete absorption. Frequent serum ethanol determinations should be performed to ensure adequate dosing while also monitoring blood glucose and fluid and electrolyte status. Additionally, because ethanol is rapidly dialyzed, the maintenance dose should be tripled during hemodialysis and concentration must be checked every 1 to 2 hours to ensure that adequate protection is maintained.

## ROLE IN METHANOL AND ETHYLENE GLYCOL TOXICITY

When administered in a timely fashion after methanol and ethylene glycol ingestion and before the accumulation of the toxic metabolites, case reports and utilization in mass poisonings confirm the efficacy of ethanol in preventing sequelae. The half-life is approximately 40 hours (range 30.3–52.0 hours) for methanol-poisoned patients blocked with ethanol, which is quite similar to the 54 hours reported in patients treated with fomepizole. The half-life of ethylene glycol in patients with normal kidney function is about 17.5 hours, which was comparable with 17 hours in ethylene glycol–poisoned patients receiving fomepizole with normal kidney function.

## ADVERSE EFFECTS AND SAFETY ISSUES

Problems encountered with the administration of ethanol include further risk of central nervous system (CNS) depression, behavioral disturbances, or ethanol-related toxicity, such as nausea, emesis, hepatitis, pancreatitis, hypoglycemia, dehydration, various administration and monitoring errors resulting in fluctuating serum concentrations (subtherapeutic and supratherapeutic ethanol concentrations and premature discontinuation), and potential drug interactions resulting in disulfiramlike reactions.

## PREGNANCY AND LACTATION

Ethanol (injection) is United States (US) Food and Drug Administration Pregnancy Category C. Ethanol crosses the placenta and reaches the fetus. Ethanol is teratogenic, and the American Academy of Pediatrics (AAP) recommends that pregnant women abstain from all alcohol consumption. It is likely that the short duration of ethanol therapy, when used to compete with ADH, during the second or third trimester, has a minimal risk of inducing fetal alcohol syndrome. Ethanol should only be used following a risk-benefit analysis, particularly in the first trimester. Ethanol has been used to manage methanol poisoning in pregnancy when fomepizole was unavailable. Because of the potentially devastating maternal and fetal effects of methanol or ethylene glycol, if an antidote is required in a pregnant woman to treat an overdose and fomepizole is not available, then ethanol is recommended until fomepizole and/or hemodialysis can be performed. Ethanol crosses into breast milk and, depending on the dose of ethanol and the time since ingestion, causes CNS depression and ethanol toxicity in the breast-fed infant. We recommend that breastfeeding should be temporarily discontinued until the ethanol is eliminated as well as the toxic alcohol for which it is being used.

## DOSING AND ADMINISTRATION

Ethanol is given either orally or IV (Tables A34–1 and A34–2). We recommend either a serum ethanol concentration of 100 mg/dL, or at least a 1:4 molar ratio of ethanol to methanol or ethylene glycol, whichever is greater. Using this ratio, 100 mg/dL (approximately 22 mmol/L) of ethanol protects against 88 mmol/L (282 mg/dL) of methanol or 88 mmol/L (546 mg/dL) of ethylene glycol. After ADH is blocked with ethanol, renal, pulmonary, and extracorporeal routes of toxic alcohol removal become the sole mechanisms for elimination.

**TABLE A34–1 Intravenous Administration of 10% Ethanol**

| | Volume (mL)[b] (given over 1 hour as tolerated) | | | | | |
|---|---|---|---|---|---|---|
| *Loading Dose*[a] | *10 kg* | *15 kg* | *30 kg* | *50 kg* | *70 kg* | *100 kg* |
| 0.8 g/kg of 10% ethanol | 80 | 120 | 240 | 400 | 560 | 800 |
| | *mL/h for various weights*[d] | | | | | |
| *Maintenance Dose*[c] | *10 kg* | *15 kg* | *30 kg* | *50 kg* | *70 kg* | *100 kg* |
| *Ethanol naïve* | | | | | | |
| 80 mg/kg/h | 8 | 12 | 24 | 40 | 56 | 80 |
| 110 mg/kg/h | 11 | 16 | 33 | 55 | 77 | 110 |
| 130 mg/kg/h | 13 | 19 | 39 | 65 | 91 | 130 |
| *Ethanol tolerant* | | | | | | |
| 150 mg/kg/h | — | — | — | 75 | 105 | 150 |
| *During hemodialysis* | | | | | | |
| 250 mg/kg/h | 25 | 38 | 75 | 125 | 175 | 250 |
| 300 mg/kg/h | 30 | 45 | 90 | 150 | 210 | 300 |
| 350 mg/kg/h | 35 | 53 | 105 | 175 | 245 | 350 |

[a]A 10% V/V concentration yields approximately 100 mg/mL. [b]For a 5% concentration, multiply the amount by 2. [c]Infusion to be started immediately following the loading dose. Concentrations above 10% are recommended not to be used for intravenous administration. The dose schedule is based on the premise that the patient initially has a zero ethanol concentration. The aim of therapy is to maintain a serum ethanol concentration of 100 to 150 mg/dL, but frequent monitoring of the ethanol concentration is required because of wide variations in endogenous metabolic capacity. Ethanol will be removed by hemodialysis, and the infusion rate of ethanol must be increased during hemodialysis. Prolonged ethanol administration may lead to hypoglycemia. [d]Rounded to the nearest milliliter.

Adapted with permission from Roberts JR, Hedges J. *Clinical Procedures in Emergency Medicine*. Philadelphia, PA: WB Saunders; 1985.

## FORMULATION AND ACQUISITION

Commercial preparations of 5% ethanol in 5% dextrose are no longer available in the US for IV administration. Sterile ethanol USP can be added to 5% dextrose to make 10% ethanol concentration (55 mL of absolute ethanol is added to 500 mL of 5% dextrose to produce a total volume of 555 mL). In almost all circumstances (except in which the gastrointestinal tract cannot be used or mental status changes preclude oral administration), oral ethanol is recommended over the extemporaneous preparation of IV ethanol.

**TABLE A34–2 Oral Administration of 20% Ethanol**

| | Volume (mL) | | | | | |
|---|---|---|---|---|---|---|
| *Loading Dose*[a] | *10 kg* | *15 kg* | *30 kg* | *50 kg* | *70 kg* | *100 kg* |
| 0.8 g/kg of 20% ethanol, diluted in juice (administered orally or via nasogastric tube) | 40 | 60 | 120 | 200 | 280 | 400 |
| | *mL/h for various weights*[c,d] | | | | | |
| *Maintenance Dose*[b] | *10 kg* | *15 kg* | *30 kg* | *50 kg* | *70 kg* | *100 kg* |
| *Ethanol naïve* | | | | | | |
| 80 mg/kg/h | 4 | 6 | 12 | 20 | 28 | 40 |
| 110 mg/kg/h | 6 | 8 | 17 | 27 | 39 | 55 |
| 130 mg/kg/h | 7 | 10 | 20 | 33 | 46 | 66 |
| *Ethanol tolerant* | | | | | | |
| 150 mg/kg/h | — | — | — | 38 | 53 | 75 |
| *During hemodialysis* | | | | | | |
| 250 mg/kg/h | 13 | 19 | 38 | 63 | 88 | 125 |
| 300 mg/kg/h | 15 | 23 | 46 | 75 | 105 | 150 |
| 350 mg/kg/h | 18 | 26 | 53 | 88 | 123 | 175 |

[a]A 20% V/V concentration yields approximately 200 mg/mL. [b]Concentrations above 30% (60 proof) are not recommended for oral administration. The dose schedule is based on the premise that the patient initially has a zero ethanol concentration. The aim of therapy is to maintain a serum ethanol concentration of 100 to 150 mg/dL, but frequent monitoring of the ethanol concentration is required because of wide variations in endogenous metabolic capacity. Ethanol will be removed by hemodialysis, and the dose of ethanol must be increased during hemodialysis. Prolonged ethanol administration may lead to hypoglycemia. [c]Rounded to the nearest milliliter. [d]For a 30% concentration, multiply the amount by 0.66.

Adapted with permission from Roberts JR, Hedges J. *Clinical Procedures in Emergency Medicine*. Philadelphia, PA: WB Saunders; 1985.

## COMPARISON TO FOMEPIZOLE

Although the acquisition cost of fomepizole is greater than that for ethanol, the many advantages of fomepizole over ethanol make fomepizole the preferable antidote in most circumstances, and overall hospital costs including critical care resources, hemodialysis, and laboratory analyses are equivalent or less, depending on the healthcare and reimbursement system (Antidotes in Brief: A33 and Chap. 79). Ethanol is easier to deploy, particularly in the prehospital setting, in mass poisonings, or in resource-poor settings.

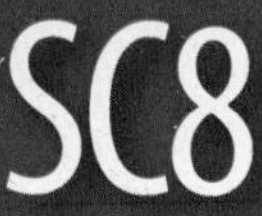

Special Considerations

# SC8 DIETHYLENE GLYCOL

## HISTORY AND EPIDEMIOLOGY

Diethylene glycol (DEG) is a solvent with physical and chemical properties similar to propylene glycol, a commonly used solvent for water-insoluble pharmaceuticals (Chap. 19). However, although it is only one carbon smaller than minimally toxic propylene glycol, DEG is a potent nephrotoxin and neurotoxin. Substitution of DEG for propylene glycol and other diluents in oral pharmaceutical elixirs has repeatedly caused epidemics of mass poisoning. In these recurring events, DEG was used instead of a safe and appropriate diluent such as glycerin or propylene glycol. Currently, DEG is also used as an antifreeze, as a finishing agent for wool, cotton, silk, and other fabrics, in dye manufacturing, and as a synthetic intermediate. In contrast to epidemics that result from adulterated pharmaceuticals, there are numerous isolated case reports of DEG poisoning from the consumption of DEG-containing products such as radiator fluid or antifreeze, brake fluid, solid cooking fuel, "fog solution," cleaning solutions, and wallpaper stripper.

## PHARMACOKINETICS/TOXICOKINETICS

### Absorption and Distribution

In rodents, DEG is highly (75%) and almost immediately absorbed after ingestion. The degree of protein binding and the volume of distribution (Vd) in humans is unknown, but the Vd in the rat is approximately 1 L/kg. In animal studies, diethylene glycol readily crosses the blood– brain barrier, and concentrations peak in brain tissue (cerebrospinal fluid concentration not reported) within 3 to 4 hours of exposure.

### Metabolism

Animal data demonstrate that as much as 40% of an ingested dose undergoes hepatic metabolism, with subsequent urinary elimination. Diethylene glycol is metabolized by alcohol dehydrogenase (ADH) to 2-hydroxyethoxyacetaldehyde, which is then further metabolized by aldehyde dehydrogenase (ALDH) to 2-hydroxyethoxyacetic acid (HEAA), which is then metabolized into diglycolic acid (DGA). The DEG ether bond linking the two ethylene glycol molecules is stable and is not hydrolyzed. Ingestion of DEG and subsequent metabolism do not therefore result in ethylene glycol release. However, a small amount of ethylene glycol is formed as an intermediate after formation of 2-hydroxyethoxyacetaldehyde (Fig. SC8–1). In rodents, HEAA concentrations peak approximately 4 hours following small DEG ingestions, but a delayed peak at 8 to 24 hours occurs with larger ingestions. Rats given large amounts of DEG with early administration of an ADH blocker such as ethanol or fomepizole do not accumulate DGA and do not develop nephrotoxicity.

### Elimination

Animal studies utilizing radiolabeled DEG report that more than 60% of a dose is eliminated within 24 hours of ingestion and more than 90% is eliminated within 72 hours. The majority of a DEG dose is eliminated unchanged in the urine (> 60%). Since elimination is largely renal, concentrations of DEG and both HEAA and DGA continue to rise in animals with impaired kidney function. Finally, small amounts DEG are eliminated in a dose-dependent fashion via fecal excretion (< 3%) and exhalation (< 7%). Diethylene glycol elimination undergoes zero-order kinetics for the first 9 to 18 hours following ingestion. First-order kinetics ensue thereafter, with apparent elimination half-lives that are dose-dependent and range from 3 to 13 hours. Apparent half-lives are prolonged to at least 13 hours in more substantial poisonings as kidney function becomes impaired.

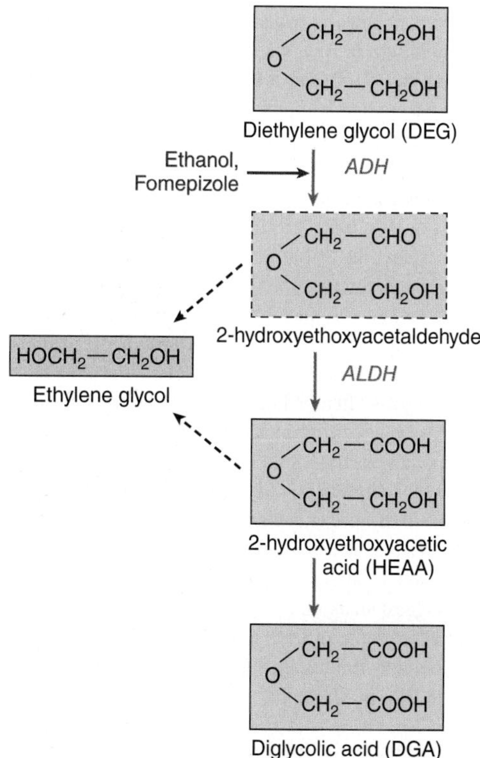


**FIGURE SC8–1.** Metabolic pathway for DEG based on animal studies and on the results presented in this chapter. Metabolites in solid boxes are observed following administration of DEG to animals; those in dashed boxes are theoretical intermediates. Because fomepizole reduced the amount of ethylene glycol in the urine, its origin is shown as coming from the aldehyde or acid intermediate, rather than from DEG itself. ALDH = aldehyde dehydrogenase. Diglycolic acid is also known as oxybisacetic acid. *(Used with permission of Oxford University Press, from Inhibition of metabolism of diethylene glycol prevents target organ toxicity in rats, Besenhofer LM, Adegboyega PA, et al; 117(1): 2010; permission conveyed through Copyright Clearance Center, Inc.)*

## TOXIC DOSE

Human data are limited, established primarily from the history of affected patients from mass poisonings, and usually represent an estimated cumulative exposure that occurred over a certain time period, rather than a single point of time. The median estimated toxic dose from the 1995 Haitian mass poisoning was approximately 1.5 g/kg (range, 0.25–4.94 g/kg) This estimation is similar to the doses reported for the DEG-contaminated elixir of sulfanilamide mass poisoning in the United States in the 1930s. Polyethylene glycol solutions with trace DEG concentrations yielding average total DEG exposures of 11 mg (range, 2–22 mg) administered for whole-bowel irrigation in adults do not cause adverse effects. Cumulative exposures at or above 250 mg/kg (the lower limit of the range reported in the Haiti mass poisoning) are potentially life threatening. The minimum toxic dose of DGA is unknown, but ingestion of 100 g in one adult was fatal.

## PATHOPHYSIOLOGY

Accumulation of HEAA and DGA in the blood causes a metabolic acidosis that can be prevented by early administration of an ADH inhibitor such as fomepizole. Although there are no published reports examining the efficacy of ethanol to block DEG metabolism, based on affinity studies with other toxic alcohols, it would also be expected to be efficacious. Inhibition of DEG metabolism with an ADH inhibitor prevents kidney and liver toxicity and decreases lethality in rodents. The parent compound (DEG) does not appear to be toxic based on these same studies. Diglycolic acid is likely to be the major if not sole cause of nephrotoxicity in DEG poisoning. Diglycolic acid is selectively taken up by renal tubule cells where it inhibits succinate dehydrogenase in the citric acid cycle. This results in interruption of mitochondrial respiration, leading to decreased energy production and proximal tubule cell necrosis. The histopathology of DEG-associated nephrotoxicity primarily involves the proximal convoluted tubules as expected and affects the renal cortex, in which necrosis, hemorrhage, and vacuolization develop. Elevations in hepatic aminotransferases also occur probably because of DEG, HEAA, and DGA accumulation in the liver. The neurotoxicity of DEG poisoning includes a severe peripheral neuropathy and encephalopathy of unclear mechanism. Limited results of cerebrospinal fluid samples taken from DEG-poisoned patients during the 2006 Panama mass poisoning suggest an association with DGA. The single reported human case of a pure DGA ingestion demonstrated clinical and pathologic findings, including severe neurotoxicity, very similar to DEG poisoning.

## CLINICAL MANIFESTATIONS

The signs, symptoms, and severity of DEG poisoning are dependent on various factors such as duration of exposure, dose, and other intrinsic host factors such as the presence of comorbidities. Following ingestion, symptoms typical of ethanol intoxication such as lethargy, confusion, "drunkenness," and altered mental status begin rapidly and last for several hours. Clinical signs and symptoms of a metabolic acidosis including tachypnea and hypernea are reported. Although nausea, vomiting, abdominal pain, diarrhea, headache, and confusion are reported in patients with DEG poisoning, nephrotoxicity (acute kidney injury {AKI}) remains the single consistent feature of all cases. This finding manifests over 1 to 3 days following ingestion as a progressive course of oliguria, anuria, or both. Some patients present with an AKI with profound metabolic acidosis and acidemia, while others present with vague gastrointestinal or respiratory symptoms and are found to have an AKI. This may be a manifestation of dose and duration of exposure. A bilateral cranial nerve VII (facial nerve) paralysis and peripheral extremity weakness often follow within several days. Some rapidly develop encephalopathy, coma, and death in the subsequent 24 to 48 hours.

Only those who develop some degree of AKI are at risk for developing neurotoxicity. Long-term outcomes among DEG poisoning survivors are not well characterized. Delayed-onset (beyond the typical initial course of acute DEG poisoning) renal and neurologic toxicity is unlikely to occur based on the single longitudinal study of DEG-poisoned survivors.

## DIAGNOSTIC TESTING

Although laboratory assays for DEG in whole blood, serum, plasma, and urine are commercially available at specialized toxicology testing laboratories, they are not available in most hospital laboratories and unlikely to return in a clinically meaningful time frame. The clinician will have to rely on a high index of suspicion, a good exposure history, and more commonly encountered "routine" testing methodologies including serum electrolytes, blood gas measurements, and kidney function studies upon initial presentation. While a high osmol gap (> 30 mOsm/L) is consistent with early poisoning, a low or normal gap should never be used to exclude that possibility (Chap. 79).

## TREATMENT

There is no evidence of clinical benefit or even reduced bioavailability of DEG following orogastric or nasogastric lavage or the administration of oral activated charcoal. Nevertheless, it is reasonable to perform nasogastric lavage for patients who presents recently (within 1–2 hours) only after ingestion of a large amount. It is also reasonable to administer a dose of activated charcoal if presentation is within 1 to 2 hours of ingestion. Because animal evidence suggests that the osmotic diuretic effect of DEG causes large urinary volume losses in the immediate postexposure period, adequate volume resuscitation should be performed as soon as possible. The patient should be closely monitored for decreases in urine output and fluid input and output recorded. Euvolemia should be maintained to assure a steady urine output. Careful attention to acid–base status is essential because acidemia enhances the toxicity of DGA. The use of intravenous sodium bicarbonate therapy for controlling metabolic acidosis is unstudied and therefore not routinely recommended at this time except for life-threatening acidemia.

Inhibition of ADH with fomepizole is recommended in suspected or known DEG poisoning to prevent nephrotoxicity, although most of the supporting evidence is from animal studies (Antidotes in Brief: A33). Because the dosing of fomepizole in humans with DEG poisoning is unstudied, it is reasonable to follow the regimen used for other toxic alcohols. Hemodialysis is recommended if clinical evidence of acidemia or end-organ toxicity is present. The endpoint of fomepizole therapy or need for additional rounds of dialysis is unclear. At this time, there are insufficient human data to conclude that fomepizole monotherapy (without hemodialysis) is completely protective in human DEG poisoning, therefore both therapies are recommended.

Because of the lack of rapid testing and limited information, all exposures to DEG present management dilemmas. Patients with a reliable history of a minimal ingestion, such as an unintentional sip of a low-concentration DEG-containing product, are unlikely to be at risk for toxicity. For those individuals, careful observation coupled with serial chemistries, venous blood gas measurements, and an initial osmol gap is reasonable. If any clinical evidence of nephrotoxicity or acidemia appears, then fomepizole is recommended in addition to hemodialysis. When the ingested dose exceeds 22 mg/kg and approaches 250 mg/kg, toxicity becomes likely and it is reasonable to proceed with at least fomepizole therapy and an attempt to obtain DEG-specific testing as well as the serial laboratory testing described earlier. Asymptomatic patients with ingestions beyond the "unintentional sip or taste" should be observed for at least 24 hours. Serial laboratory determinations to monitor acid–base status should be obtained and evaluated for at least 24 hours based on DEG toxicokinetics. For patients with signs or symptoms of alcohol intoxication who did not consume ethanol, a potentially life-threatening DEG dose should be suspected and both fomepizole and hemodialysis are recommended. The same approach is recommended for patients presenting to healthcare facilities with acidemia, oliguria, or anuria following DEG ingestion. Although there are no published reports examining the efficacy of ethanol to block DEG metabolism, it is expected to act similarly to fomepizole. Therefore, ethanol is a reasonable alternative therapy only if fomepizole is unavailable and a rapid transfer to another hospital is not possible.

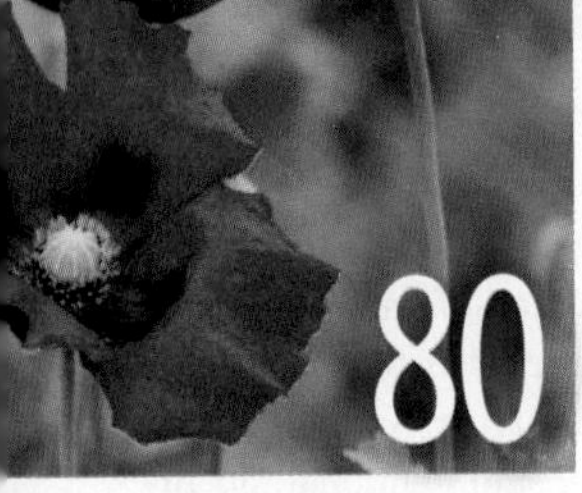



# 80 BARIUM

Normal serum concentration < 0.2 mg/L (1.46 μmol/L)

## HISTORY AND EPIDEMIOLOGY

Barium poisoning is reported following the intentional ingestion of soluble salts found in rodenticides, insecticides, or depilatories. Toxicity also occurs following occupational exposure to barium salts and explosions of the propellant barium styphnate. Despite barium sulfate being insoluble, rare cases of unintentional toxicity are reported as complications of administration of barium sulfate during radiographic procedures.

## CHEMISTRY

Elemental barium is not found in nature; it normally occurs in the salt form. Chemically, barium resembles calcium more than any other element. Barium salts are either water soluble or insoluble. The soluble salts (acetate, chloride, hydroxide, oxide, nitrate, and (poly)sulfide) are most commonly associated with toxicity. Barium (poly)sulfide produces toxicity through the formation of hydrogen sulfide when it combines with the acid normally present in the stomach. Barium carbonate is poorly water soluble at physiologic pH but increases significantly in an acid environment. In gastric acid, conversion to the highly soluble barium chloride occurs. Insoluble salts, such as arsenate, carbonate, chromate, fluoride, oxalate, and sulfate, are rarely associated with toxicity (Table 80–1).

## TOXICOKINETICS

Toxicity can occur from ingestion of as little as 200 mg of barium salt, although oral lethal doses are reported to range from 1 to 30 g barium salt. Following ingestion, 5% to 10% of soluble barium salts are absorbed, with the rate of absorption dependent on the water solubility of the salt. The time to peak serum concentrations is 2 hours, and the reported elimination half-life is between 18 and 85 hours. The predominant route of elimination is fecal, with renal elimination accounting for only 10% to 28% of total barium excretion. In symptomatic patients, serum barium concentrations range from 3.7 to 41.1 mg/L. Death is uncommon following ingestion but occurs most commonly in resource-poor locations.

Intravasation is a rare complication of radiologic studies in which barium sulfate is administered under pressure, such as a barium enema. Following a small perforation, barium sulfate leaks into the peritoneal cavity or portal venous system. Although sudden cardiovascular collapse occurs, it is unclear whether this is the result of venous occlusion (pulmonary embolism), overwhelming sepsis, or barium toxicity.

## PATHOPHYSIOLOGY

The hallmark of barium toxicity is hypokalemia, which results from redistribution of potassium from the extracellular to intracellular compartment. Barium inhibits calcium-activated potassium rectifier channels, reducing outward flow of potassium, and causes persistent $Na^+$,$K^+$-ATPase pump electrogenesis, leading to a shift of extracellular potassium into the cell. Intracellular potassium trapping leads to depolarization and paralysis. Additionally, the inhibition of potassium channels increases vascular resistance and reduces blood flow. There is also a possible direct effect of barium on either skeletal muscle or neuromuscular transmission.

## CLINICAL EFFECTS

Abdominal pain, nausea, vomiting, and diarrhea commonly occur within 1 hour of ingestion. Severe hypokalemia can occur within 2 hours and is associated with ventricular

**TABLE 80–1 Barium Salts: Solubility and Common Usages**

| *Barium Salt* | *Solubility (mg/L at 20°C)* | *Common Uses* |
|---|---|---|
| Acetate | 58.8 | Textile dyes |
| Carbonate | 0.02 increases in an acid pH; also, can be converted to barium chloride by gastric acid (HCl) | Rodenticide, welding fluxes, pigments, glass, ceramics, pyrotechnics, electronic devices, welding rods, ferrite magnet materials, optical glass, manufacture of caustic soda and other barium salts |
| Chloride | 375 | Textile dyes, pigments, boiler detergents, in purifying sugar, as mordant in dyeing and printing textiles, as water softener, in manufacture of caustic soda and chlorine, polymers, stabilizers |
| Fluoride | 1.2 | Welding fluxes |
| Nitrate | 87 | Optical glass, ceramic glazes, fireworks (green), explosives, antiseptic preparation |
| Oxide | 34.8 | In glass, ceramics, refining oils and sugar, as an additive in petroleum products and also as materials of plastics, pharmaceuticals, polymers, glass, and enamel industries |
| Styphnate | — | Propellant used in manufacture of explosive detonators |
| Sulfate | 0.002 | Radiopaque contrast solutions, manufacture of white pigments, paper making |
| Sulfide | Slightly soluble in $H_2O$ | Depilatories, manufacture of fluorescent tubes |

dysrhythmias, hypotension, profound flaccid muscle weakness, and respiratory failure. Hypertension is rarely noted and likely results from increased vascular resistance. Tissue injury results in metabolic acidosis with hyperlactatemia. Esophageal injury and hemorrhagic gastritis are also reported.

## DIAGNOSTIC STUDIES

Serum barium concentrations are not readily available, but values greater than 0.2 mg/L (1.46 μmol/L) are considered abnormal. Following acute exposures, patients should have serum electrolytes (particularly potassium and phosphate) measured hourly while performing continuous electrocardiogram monitoring. Acid–base status, kidney function, and creatine phosphokinase (CPK) should also be measured. A plain abdominal radiograph might demonstrate the presence of barium, but the sensitivity and specificity of radiography have never been determined.

## MANAGEMENT

Patients should be placed in a monitored setting with the capacity for respiratory support readily available. Toxicologic etiologies for flaccid paralysis such as hypermagnesemia, botulism, tick paralysis, and the administration of neuromuscular blockers should be evaluated while the serum potassium concentration is being determined. Once the hypokalemia is diagnosed, other causes of acute hypokalemia associated with paralysis such as periodic hypokalemic paralysis, toluene toxicity, and diuretic use should be evaluated if there is no history or laboratory confirmation of barium exposure. Patients who are asymptomatic at 6 hours with normal potassium concentrations can be discharged.

### Decontamination

Activated charcoal is unlikely to be effective because of poor adsorption. Orogastric lavage is reasonable in patients who present early after ingestion but is unlikely to provide extra benefit in patients who are already symptomatic or those who have had spontaneous emesis. Oral magnesium sulfate prevents absorption by precipitating unabsorbed barium ions to insoluble, nontoxic barium sulfate. The oral dose of magnesium sulfate is 250 mg/kg for children and 30 g for adults. Intravenous magnesium sulfate is not recommended as precipitation of barium in the renal tubules may cause acute kidney injury.

Patients in respiratory failure should receive assisted ventilation. Correction of hypokalemia is important to minimize the risk or to treat cardiac dysrhythmias. Large doses of potassium (for example 400 mEq in 24 hours) will be required to correct serum potassium but may still not improve muscle strength. As hypokalemia is caused by intracellular sequestration of potassium, potassium supplementation increases the total-body potassium load. In this situation, rebound hyperkalemia should be anticipated when barium is eliminated, especially in patients with impaired kidney function.

## ENHANCEMENT OF ELIMINATION

Hemodialysis and continuous renal replacement therapies increase barium elimination, stabilize potassium concentrations, and are reported to hasten clinical recovery. Either technique is reasonable in any severely symptomatic patient who does not respond to correction of hypokalemia.

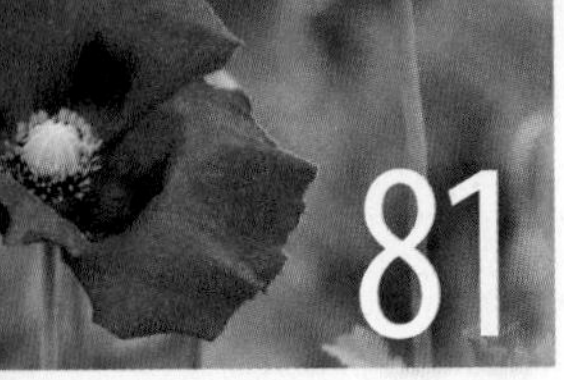

# 81 FUMIGANTS

## HISTORY AND EPIDEMIOLOGY

The proper use of pesticides has a beneficial role in human health by increasing the quality and quantity of crops. Alternatively, acute and chronic pesticide poisonings are significant causes of morbidity and mortality worldwide, especially in developing countries, making pesticide poisoning a global public health problem. Fumigants are nonspecific pesticides applied to kill and control rodents, nematodes, insects, weed seeds, and fungi anywhere in soil, in structures, and on crops, grains, and commodities. They represent a diverse group of pesticides that are dissimilar in their chemical structures, physical properties, and mechanisms of toxicity (Tables 81–1 and 81–2). Because fumigants exist as solids that release toxic gases on reacting with water (zinc phosphide, aluminum phosphide) or with acids (sodium or calcium cyanide), as liquids (ethylene dibromide, dibromochloropropane, formaldehyde) that can vaporize at ambient temperature, or as gases (methyl bromide, hydrogen cyanide, ethylene oxide), inhalation is the most common route of exposure. Their exposure risk is enhanced by their general lack of warning properties, non–species-selective effects, and high potency.

## METAL PHOSPHIDES AND PHOSPHINE

### Introduction

Metal phosphides are used to protect grain held in silos, in the holds of ships, and during transportation by rail. They are advantageous because of their low cost, high effectiveness in destroying harmful insects and rodents, freedom from toxic residue, and lack of adverse effects on seed viability. Following exposure to ambient moisture, the metal phosphides release phosphine gas ($PH_3$).

### History and Epidemiology

Unintentional poisoning as a result of negligence or ignorance is also reported. Also, aluminum phosphide (AlP) poisoning is one of the most common causes of poisoning both in adults and children in agricultural societies and resource-poor areas of countries, such as India, Sri Lanka, and Iran.

**TABLE 81–1 Physical Properties and Industrial Uses of Fumigants**

| *Fumigant* | *Color* | *State* | *Flammability* | *Odor* | *Use* |
|---|---|---|---|---|---|
| Phosphine | Colorless | Gas | High | Rotten fish<br>Garlic | Rodenticide |
| Methyl bromide | Colorless | Gas | No | None at low concentrations. Sweet chloroformlike at high concentrations | Soil<br>Structures<br>Crop |
| Dichloropropene | Yellow | Liquid | No | Garlic | Soil |
| Sulfuryl fluoride | Colorless | Gas | No | None | Structures |

### Physicochemical Properties

Commercially, AlP is most widely available as a greenish-gray tablet or pellet bag and granular form that has a garlic odor. The 3-g tablet usually contains AlP (56%), ammonium carbamate, and urea, which liberates $PH_3$ (up to 1 g), ammonia, and carbon dioxide. Zinc phosphide ($Zn_3P_2$) is available as a dark-gray powder or as quadrilateral crystals that have an odor of acetylene or rotten fish. Calcium phosphide ($Ca_3P_2$) is available as a reddish-brown crystal powder. Magnesium phosphide ($Mg_3P_2$) is a white crystalline solid.

In the presence of moisture or acid, metal phosphides are converted to $PH_3$. The release of $PH_3$ is even more vigorous after contact with an acid. In aqueous solutions, $PH_3$ produces phosphinic, phosphonic, and phosphoric acids, which are all caustic and produce exothermic reactions. Although $PH_3$ is colorless and odorless in pure form, the presence of substituted phosphines and diphosphines imparts a decaying fish or garlic odor that is detectable at very low concentrations.

### Toxicokinetics

Following ingestion, metal phosphides react with acidic fluid in the gastrointestinal (GI) tract to release $PH_3$, which is rapidly absorbed. Phosphine gas is also absorbed from respiratory tract mucosa if inhaled. Dermal absorption is insignificant. There are no data about distribution of $PH_3$ in humans, but a large volume of distribution is predicted. Its half-life ranges from 5 to 24 hours.

### Toxicodynamics

Phosphine gas is a protoplasmic toxin that blocks the electron transport chain and oxidative phosphorylation through noncompetitive inhibition of cytochrome-c oxidase. Phosphine gas decreases the activities of mitochondrial complexes I, II, IV, and V, which inhibits cellular respiration and ATP production and leads to the formation of highly reactive hydroxyl radicals that cause additional damage. Phosphine gas also inhibits catalase, induces superoxide dismutase, and reduces the glutathione (GSH) concentration. All of these effects combine to result in lipid peroxidation, protein denaturation of cell membranes, and DNA damage, leading to widespread cellular damage and ion channel dysfunction. Because $PH_3$ is caustic, it directly injures the alveolar capillary membrane in addition to producing oxidative injury, leading to an acute respiratory distress syndrome (ARDS).

### Toxic Dose

Ingestion of 1 g of zinc phosphide can cause toxicity in humans, and death is reported after ingestion of 4 g. Ingestion of 500 mg of AlP can be fatal.

### Clinical Manifestations

The smell of garlic or decaying fish on the breath is a common, but not universal finding, and results from oral or inhalational poisoning with metal phosphides and $PH_3$. After ingestion, the

**TABLE 81–2 Comparison of Clinical Effects of Fumigants**

| Fumigant | Mucous Membrane Irritation | Dermatitis | Burns (Frostbite) | Gastrointestinal: Nausea, Vomiting, Abdominal Pain | Hepatic Dysfunction | Chest Pain | Adult Respiratory Distress Syndrome | Nephrotoxicity | Hypotension | Dysrhythmias | Mental Status Changes |
|---|---|---|---|---|---|---|---|---|---|---|---|
| Phosphine | ++ | – | – | + | + | + | + | + | ++ | + | + |
| Methyl bromide | ± High concentration | + | + | + | + | + | + | + | + | + | + |
| Dichloropropene | + | + | – | + | + | + | + | + | + | + | + |
| Sulfuryl fluoride | ± High concentration | + | + | + | – | – | + | + | ++ | – | + |

– = Absent; + = Present; ++ = Very substantial; ± = Variable.

onset of toxicity usually is slightly more rapid for AlP (10–15 minutes) than for zinc phosphide (20–40 minutes). In patients with mild poisoning, nausea, repeated vomiting, thirst, diarrhea, abdominal discomfort or pain, especially epigastric pain, and tachycardia are common clinical manifestations. In those with moderate to severe effects, palpitations, tachypnea, GI manifestations, dysrhythmias, ARDS, hypotension, shock, and cardiovascular collapse occur rapidly. Restlessness, anxiety, dizziness, ataxia, numbness, paresthesias, and tremor are universally observed, but central nervous system (CNS) manifestations are not prominent until a secondary event, such as hypoxia, occurs. Late and severe neurologic findings include delirium, convulsions, ischemic/hemorrhagic stroke, and coma. Following limited $PH_3$ inhalational exposure, patients commonly have airway irritation and breathlessness. Other features include chest tightness, tachycardia, headache, nausea, vomiting, diarrhea, numbness, muscle weakness, and diplopia.

### Diagnostic Testing

Initial investigations should include electrocardiography (ECG) and continuous cardiac monitoring, chest radiograph, blood glucose, blood gases, serum electrolytes, complete blood count (CBC), and liver and kidney function studies. Hypokalemia is common after ingestion. Hypoglycemia as a result of impaired gluconeogenesis or glycogenolysis or possibly due to adrenal insufficiency is common and at times severe and persistent. Hyperglycemia and metabolic acidosis are also reported. Hemolysis, methemoglobinemia, leukopenia, and hyperbilirubinemia are unusual complications of metal phosphide poisonings. Echocardiography typically reveals cardiac dysfunction, dilation, and hypokinesia or akinesia of the left ventricle that typically resolves over several days. Chest radiography shows diffuse infiltration, pulmonary edema, ARDS, and atelectasis.

### Toxicologic Analyses

Chemical analysis for $PH_3$ in blood or urine is not recommended and is not typically helpful as $PH_3$ is rapidly oxidized to phosphite and hypophosphite. Both bedside and laboratory tests are available but unlikely to contribute to care.

### Prognosis

The mortality rate following ingestion of metal phosphides is reportedly 31% to 77%. Most of the deaths occur within 12 to 24 hours and are due to cardiovascular collapse. After 24 hours, most of the deaths are due to refractory shock, severe acidemia, and ARDS. Fulminant hepatic failure develops within 72 hours after poisoning and is another cause of delayed death. Metabolic acidosis with an elevated lactate concentration is an index of severity of AlP poisoning. A lactate concentration of 5.4 mmol/L at 4 hours and 2.8 mmol/L at 24 hours after ingestion was used to predict the likelihood of death in one study.

### Treatment

The victim should immediately be moved to fresh air, and supplemental oxygen should be provided as needed. Clinical staff and other healthcare professionals should use universal precautions (Special Considerations: SC1) with the understanding that particulate masks will not protect against $PH_3$. The patient's clothes should be removed sealed in plastic bags, and carefully discarded, and the skin and eyes decontaminated with water as early as possible. Following ingestion, gastric emptying is reasonable if it is done within a few hours and significant emesis has not already occurred. Oral administration of sodium bicarbonate, boric acid, or potassium permanganate are not recommended because of multiple associated risks and no proven benefit. Similarly, the routine use of activated charcoal is not recommended.

Standard supportive care to address ventilatory and vital sign abnormalities should be administered. If necessary, norepinephrine or phenylephrine are recommended. As there is no known specific antidote, intensive monitoring and supportive treatment are all that can be recommended. It is reasonable to correct severe acidemia with IV sodium bicarbonate. Based on one human trial, we recommend administering *N*-acetylcysteine (NAC) at a dose of 140 mg/kg IV infusion as a loading dose and 70 mg/kg IV infusion every 4 hours up to 17 doses. Also, administration of vitamin E (α-tocopherol) at a dose of 400 mg IM every 12 hours for 72 hours is reasonable as a free-radical scavenger in cases of life-threating toxicity. Because of the severe nature of this poisoning, many other pharmacotherapies have been tried, but there is insufficient evidence to recommend them at this time. When all other therapies are failing, extracorporeal life support is reasonable if available.

## METHYL BROMIDE

### History and Epidemiology

Today, methyl bromide ($CH_3Br$) is used widely as a fumigant for all types of dry food stuffs, in grain elevators, mills, ships, warehouses, greenhouses, and food-processing facilities for the control of nematodes, fungi, and weeds. It was also used as an insecticide, fire extinguisher, and refrigerant, although its domestic use was banned in 1987. Historically, poisonings involving the general public were mainly associated with the methyl bromide used in fire extinguishers. Other poisoning involved unauthorized entry into buildings being fumigated with methyl bromide.

Methyl bromide is a colorless gas at room temperature and standard pressure. It is 3 times heavier than air. It is odorless except at high concentrations, when it has a burning taste and sweet, chloroformlike smell. Commercially, it is available as a liquefied gas. Some formulations also contain chloropicrin or amyl acetate as a warning agent.

### Toxicokinetics

Inhalation is the primary route of exposure, although methyl bromide is rapidly absorbed through the dermal and oral routes. After absorption, methyl bromide or metabolites are rapidly distributed to many tissues, including the lungs, adrenals, kidneys, liver, brain, testis, and fat. The major organs of distribution observed immediately after exposure include fat, lungs, liver, adrenals, and kidneys.

Methyl bromide is partially converted to inorganic bromide, and bromide concentrations in blood and target organs increase after exposure to methyl bromide. It is metabolized to methyl glutathione by the enzyme glutathione *S*-transferase (GST) and is then converted into the neurotoxic metabolites of methanethiol and formaldehyde. Depending on the route of exposure, 16% to 40% is eliminated as metabolized methyl bromide in the urine and only 4% to 20% is eliminated in the expired air as parent compound. Biliary excretion accounts for about 46% of the elimination, generally within 24 hours following oral exposure.

### Toxicodynamics

Several mechanisms of toxicity are postulated, including the direct cytotoxic effect of the intact methyl bromide molecule or toxicity due to one of its metabolites. Methyl bromide is a potent alkylating agent with high affinity for sulfhydryl and amino groups. It irreversibly inhibits microsomal metabolism, interferes with protein synthesis, and may also alter by methylation many other cellular components such as GSH, proteins, DNA, and RNA.

### Clinical Manifestations

Inhalation of more than 10,000 ppm for more than a few minutes is sufficient to cause death. Severe poisoning produces tremor, convulsions, rapid loss of consciousness, dysrhythmias, and death. Convulsions generally occur in fatal cases, but ARDS, respiratory failure, and cardiovascular collapse are the leading causes of death. Pulmonary symptoms begin with cough or shortness of breath that rapidly progresses to bronchitis, pneumonitis, and ARDS. In contrast, following low-concentration exposure, there is a characteristic delay of up to 48 hours prior to the onset of clinical manifestations. Headache, dizziness, abdominal pain, nausea, vomiting, chest pain, and difficulty breathing are the manifestations of mild to moderate exposure. Some individuals initially manifest irritant symptoms of the eye, nasopharynx, and oropharynx, which are misdiagnosed as influenza or another viral illness. Visual disturbances such as blurred or double vision are also reported.

The neurologic effects of methyl bromide poisoning are the most consequential and often occur without antecedent irritant effects. Initial CNS signs and symptoms that manifest in the first few hours after exposure include headache, dizziness, numbness, drowsiness, euphoria, confusion, diplopia, dysmetria, dysarthria, agitation and mood disorders, or inappropriate affect. Those findings progress rapidly in the first day or manifest over several days including ataxia, intention tremor, fasciculation, myoclonus, delirium, seizures, and coma.

Methyl bromide also causes severe irritation, erythema, caustic skin injury, blisters, and vesicles predominantly in moist areas or pressure points such as the groin, axilla, and wrist. Liver and kidney damage is also described.

Most patients who develop seizures or coma will not survive, and in those who survive, recovery typically takes months. Permanent sequelae such as neuropsychiatric impairment, ataxia, muscular weakness, irritability, blurred vision, myoclonus, and electroencephalographic (EEG) disturbances are frequent.

### Diagnostic Testing

The standard laboratory evaluations, such as CBC, serum electrolytes, blood urea nitrogen (BUN), creatinine, ammonia concentration, blood gases, urinalysis, hepatic enzymes, chest radiography, and ECG, should be obtained after an acute exposure. Although a serum bromide concentration will help to confirm the diagnosis, it is not readily available in most laboratories. Bromide may falsely elevate chloride concentrations in some laboratories.

### Treatment

The poisoned or exposed individual should be immediately moved to fresh air. Rescue and decontamination should be performed only by personnel wearing personal protective equipment. In patients with respiratory and cardiac arrest, cardiopulmonary resuscitation should be initiated immediately when it is safe to perform. The clothing should be removed carefully, as methyl bromide adheres to clothing, including rubber and leather, and placed in plastic bags and disposed of appropriately. The affected skin should be washed with soap and water. Decontamination includes irrigation of the eyes with copious amounts of 0.9% sodium chloride solution or water. It is also reasonable to administer at least one dose of oral activated charcoal (AC) up to 1 to 2 hours following ingestion if the patient's airway is stable, although there is no supporting documentation for any benefit. Medical management should proceed as it would for any hazardous materials event (Chap. 101).

Management is primarily general and supportive care and often requires intensive care unit management of coma, seizures, ARDS, and hepatic and kidney failure. Seizures are common and difficult to control with traditional antiepileptics such as benzodiazepines. Pentobarbital, high-dose thiopental, and propofol are required in many cases. All exposed patients should be monitored for a minimum of 24 to 48 hours to detect delayed effects, especially ARDS.

## DICHLOROPROPENE

### History and Epidemiology

1,3-Dichloropropene is a volatile chlorinated aliphatic hydrocarbon that was introduced in 1945 and is primarily used as a soil fumigant for nematodes. Exposures are reported during production, application, and ingestion, most commonly in occupational settings where formulations are manufactured or applied.

### Toxicokinetics

Dichloropropene is rapidly absorbed by the oral, inhalational, and dermal routes. No human data describe systemic distribution. In humans, dichloropropene is metabolized in liver via oxidation in a phase I biotransformation, which is catalyzed by CYP2E enzymes and then glutathione-dependent biotransformation. Most of the glutathione-conjugated form of dichloropropene is eliminated by the kidneys, and smaller amounts are eliminated in the feces.

### Toxicodynamics

Human and animal health effects include damage to the liver, kidney, lung, CNS, myocardium, GI tract, skin, and mucous membranes. The exact mechanisms of toxicity are not clear, but glutathione depletion is documented in the rat model.

### Clinical Manifestations

Signs and symptoms of acute oral or inhalational exposure include nausea, vomiting, bloody diarrhea, pancreatitis, hepatotoxicity, tachycardia and hypotension, dyspnea, ARDS, CNS depression, acute kidney injury (acute tubular necrosis), and muscle pain and weakness. Coagulopathy and thrombocytopenia, hyperglycemia, severe metabolic acidosis, and intravascular fluid depletion secondary to hemorrhage are reported. Dermal manifestations include contact hypersensitivity, erythema, and profuse sweating. Mucous membrane irritation including erythema, edema, and irritation of the eyes, ears, nose, and throat occurs.

### Diagnostic Testing

Liver and kidney function should be monitored following acute poisoning. No additional or specific tests are recommended beyond those needed for supportive care.

### Treatment

Because of the volatility of dichloropropene, caution should be used to avoid continued inhalational and dermal exposure for both the patient and the healthcare professionals. Symptomatic and supportive care should be provided as for methyl bromide. Following ingestion, oral AC is reasonable, but there is no proven value. Orogastric lavage is also reasonable in a patient presenting shortly following ingestion. Exposed eyes should be irrigated with copious amounts of water or 0.9% sodium chloride solution for at least 15 minutes, and exposed skin should be similarly washed with soap. There are no data to support specific therapies beyond supportive care, although the use of antioxidant therapy and NAC warrants further study. The patients should be monitored for at least 24 hours after exposure.

## SULFURYL FLUORIDE

### History and Epidemiology

Sulfuryl fluoride has been used since 1957 as a structural fumigant insecticide to control wood-boring insects such as termites in homes. Structure or tent fumigation is performed by completely enclosing a house or other structure in plastic or a tarpaulin, and then sulfuryl fluoride is pumped in as a compressed gas. Chloropicrin is typically added as a warning agent.

### Toxicokinetics and Toxicodynamics

Sulfuryl fluoride gas is colorless, odorless, and heavier than air. Little is known about the toxicokinetics of sulfuryl fluoride in humans, and the exact mechanism of toxicity is not understood. The measurable fluoride concentrations in patients with sulfuryl fluoride poisoning and the development of fluorosis in models of chronic, low-concentration exposures suggest that the release of fluoride is of major pathophysiologic consequence.

### Clinical Manifestations

Case reports of sulfuryl fluoride exposure describe acute and subacute clinical courses that share many similarities to methyl bromide poisoning. Initial manifestations, especially in limited exposures, include nausea, vomiting, diarrhea, abdominal pain, cough, and dyspnea. Irritation of mucosal surfaces produces salivation and nasopharyngitis, lacrimation, and conjunctival injection. Central nervous system manifestations include paresthesias, irritability, agitation, tetany, refractory seizures, and coma. Finally, largely because of effects on calcium and magnesium, fluoride toxicity results in profound shock, cardiac dysrhythmias, wide QRS complexes, prolongation of the QT interval, torsade de pointes, hyperkalemia, and ARDS (Chap. 77).

### Diagnostic Testing

Patients with sulfuryl fluoride exposure require monitoring of serum calcium, magnesium, and potassium concentrations. Patients should have an ECG performed and be attached to continuous cardiac monitoring to observe for QRS complex widening, QT interval prolongation, and dysrhythmias. Serum fluoride concentrations, although not helpful for acute management, may help as a confirmatory diagnostic test.

### Treatment

Following inhalational exposure, patients should be disrobed to avoid further exposure to any liberated sulfuryl fluoride gas. In treating sulfuryl fluoride poisoning, aggressive treatment of hypocalcemia with calcium gluconate or calcium chloride should be expected (Antidotes in Brief: A32). Similar to the management of methyl bromide, intensive care is often required for seizures, dysrhythmias, bronchospasm, and ARDS. As the fluoride ion is excreted in the urine, fluid resuscitation is recommended to maintain a steady urine output.

## METHYL IODIDE

Iodomethane or methyl iodide is a monohalomethane and mainly used as a chemical reagent in the manufacturing of different pharmaceuticals and pesticides. It is proposed as a fumigant to replace methyl bromide. Human poisoning with methyl iodide is rare. There are reports of dermal exposure with severe burns, respiratory insufficiency, and delayed neuropsychiatric sequelae. Cerebellar and parkinsonian findings followed by the development of cognitive impairment and the late appearance of psychiatric disturbances (personality change) are reported.

There is no antidote for the treatment of methyl iodide poisoning. Successful treatment requires early diagnosis and cessation of exposure. It is difficult to distinguish the neurotoxic syndromes due to methyl iodide poisoning from other neurodegenerative conditions, infectious processes, and psychiatric disorders, especially when there is a lag time between exposure and onset of clinical manifestations.

# 82 HERBICIDES

## HISTORY, CLASSIFICATION, AND EPIDEMIOLOGY

Herbicides, defined as any chemical that regulates the growth of a plant, encompass a large number of xenobiotics of varying characteristics. Herbicides are used around the world for the destruction of plants in the home environment and also in agriculture in which weeds are particularly targeted. Poisoning follows acute (intentional or unintentional poisoning) or chronic (such as occupational) exposures. Depending on the herbicide and the characteristics of the exposure, this may lead to clinically significant poisoning, including death. This chapter focuses on the most widely used herbicides and also those associated with significant clinical toxicity.

Prior to the 1940s, the main method of weed control and field clearance was manual labor, which was time consuming and expensive. The first herbicide marketed was 2,4-dichlorphenoxyacetic acid (2,4-D) during the 1940s, followed by other phenoxy acid compounds. Paraquat was marketed in the early 1960s, followed by dicamba later that decade. Hundreds of xenobiotics are now classified as herbicides, and a much larger number of commercial preparations are marketed. Herbicides are the most widely sold pesticides in the world.

In well resourced countries, most acute herbicide exposures are unintentional and the majority of patients do not require admission to a hospital. Most deaths are due to paraquat and diquat, although recently, glyphosate and phenoxy acid compounds are more commonly implicated. Cases of severe poisoning that required hospitalization usually follow intentional self-poisoning. Significant toxicity including death also occurs with unintentional (eg, storage of an herbicide in food or drink containers) or criminal exposures.

### Classification

Table 82–1 lists the extensive range of herbicides in current use. By convention, they are subclassified according to their chemical class and their World Health Organization (WHO) hazard classification. Unfortunately, the utility of these (or any other) methods of classification to predict the hazard to humans with self-poisoning is not proven. The WHO categorizes pesticides by their median lethal dose ($LD_{50}$). This system does not consider morbidity or the effect of treatments.

### Contribution of Coformulations

Commercial herbicide formulations are identified by their active ingredients, but they almost always contain coformulants that often contribute to clinical toxicity. Hydrocarbon-based solvents and surfactants improve the contact of the herbicide with the plant and enhance penetration. Coformulants are generally considered "inactive" or "inert" because they lack herbicidal activity; however, increasingly their contribution to the human toxicity of a formulation is being appreciated. The most widely discussed example of a coformulant dominating the toxicity of an herbicide product is that of glyphosate-containing products, which is discussed below.

### Epidemiology

Herbicide poisoning is a major issue in resource-poor countries of the Asia-Pacific region where subsistence farming is common and herbicide use is relatively high. The incidence of poisoning with individual herbicides depends on their availability. Availability is associated with local marketing practices and is reflected in sales in the domestic sector. For example, paraquat poisonings are now comparatively rare in the United States (US), whereas the incidence of glyphosate poisoning has increased. Similarly, after paraquat was banned in Japan (late 1980s) and Korea (2012), there was an increase in the number of glufosinate poisonings.

### Regulatory Considerations

When properly used, most herbicide formulations have a low toxic potential for applicators because they are poorly absorbed across the skin and respiratory membranes. When inappropriately used, in particular when there is enteral (or rarely parenteral) exposure, toxicity is more pronounced. Regulatory bodies must evaluate not only the risk of toxicity, but also the cost and efficacy of herbicides and their fate in the environment. An ideal herbicide is one that is selective for the target plant and does not migrate far from the site of application. Selective targeting occurs when the herbicide is rapidly inactivated or binds strongly to soil components. For example, paraquat and glyphosate are inactivated when they contact soil, which is favorable because they remain in the region of application. By contrast, atrazine is more mobile, allowing it to leach into groundwater and migrate great distances.

## GENERAL COMMENTS FOR THE MANAGEMENT OF ACUTE HERBICIDE POISONING

### Diagnosis

Herbicide poisoning is diagnosed following a specific history or other evidence of exposure (such as an empty or partially used bottle) and associated clinical symptoms. A detailed history, including the type of herbicide, amount, time since poisoning, and symptoms, is essential. It is necessary to determine the actual brand in many cases because of variability in salts, concentrations, and coformulants. Depending on local laboratory resources, the diagnosis is confirmed using a specific assay, such as paraquat and glufosinate, but these are not usually available in a clinically meaningful time frame.

### Initial Management

An accurate risk assessment is necessary for the proper triage and subsequent management of patients with acute herbicide poisoning. Risk assessment involves an understanding of the dose ingested, time since ingestion, clinical features, patient factors, and availability of medical facilities. All intentional exposures should be assumed significant. If a patient presents to a facility that is unable to provide sufficient

**TABLE 82–1** Characteristics of the Major Herbicides Categorized by Chemical Class and WHO Hazard Classification

| *Chemical Class*[a] | *Applications, Usage Data, and Mechanism of Action in Plants, If Known*[b] | *WHO Hazard Class*[c] | *Compounds Included* | *Clinical Effects, Treatments, and Supportive Care* |
|---|---|---|---|---|
| Alcohol and aldehyde | Broad-spectrum contact herbicide | Ib | Allyl alcohol (prop-2-en-1-ol) and acrolein (the metabolite of allyl alcohol) | Local irritation, cardiotoxicity, pulmonary edema, and death. Administer *N*-acetylcysteine or mesna. |
| Amide | Selective for grasses pre- or postemergence<br>In 2012, acetochlor, propanil, metolachlor, and metolachlor-S were among the top herbicides used in the United States.<br>Multiple mechanisms of action, including inhibition of photosynthesis at photosystem II and/or inhibition of dihydropteroate synthase and/or inhibition of cell division through inhibition of the synthesis of very-long-chain fatty acids and/or inhibition of acetolactate synthase (interferes with branched amino acid synthesis) and/or inhibition of microtubule assembly.<br>Some compounds are also included in other chemical classes, including asulam (carbamate); oryzalin (dinitroaniline); clomeprop (phenoxy); diclosulam, flumetsulam, and metosulam (triazolopyrimidines). | III<br><br><br><br>U | *Anilide derivatives*: Acetochlor, alachlor, dimethachlor, flufenacet, mefluidide, metolachlor, propachlor, propanil (DCPA)<br>*Nonanilide derivatives*: Chlorthiamid, diphenamid<br>*Anilide derivatives*: Butachlor, clomeprop, diclosulam, flamprop, flumetsulam, metosulam, mefenacet, metazachlor, pentanochlor, pretilachlor<br>*Nonanilide derivatives*: Asulam, bromobutide, dimethenamid, isoxaben, napropamide, oryzalin, propyzamide, tebutam | See text for anilide derivatives. There are limited human data about the nonanilide derivatives. Lethargy or sedation preceded death in animals exposed to chlorthiamid. Behavioral changes, ataxia, and prostration were noted in animals exposed to diphenamid. Drowsiness and tachypnea were noted in goats following acute poisoning with napropamide. Oryzalin inhibits human carbonic anhydrase. Methemoglobinemia results, the treatment of which is methylene blue (Antidotes in Brief: A43). |
| Aromatic acid | In 2012, dicamba was the eighth most used herbicide in the domestic sector in the United States.<br>Dicamba is commonly coformulated with phenoxyacetic acid compounds.<br>Inhibits acetolactate synthase and/or inhibition of microtubule assembly and/or indole acetic acid–like (synthetic auxins). | III<br>U | Dicamba, 2,3,6-trichlorobenzoic acid (2,3,6-TBA)<br>Bispyribac, chloramben (amiben), chlorthal, clopyralid, pyriminobac, pyrithiobac, quinclorac, quinmerac | Bispyribac causes gastrointestinal irritation, sedation, and death (case fatality 1.8%; asystolic arrest reported). Minimal toxicity from dicamba, but some products are corrosive to the gut, and rhabdomyolysis and acute pancreatitis are reported. Human data are limited for the other compounds, particularly single-agent exposures. In animals, myotonia, dyspnea, and death are reported with dicamba and 2,3,6-TBA poisoning. |
| Arsenical | Unknown | III | Dimethylarsinic acid (cacodylic acid), methylarsonic acid (MAA or MSMA) | Chap. 59. |
| Benzothiazole | Indole acetic acid–like (synthetic auxins) and/or inhibits photosynthesis at photosystem II. | U | Benazolin, methabenzthiazuron | Limited human data. |
| Bipyridyl | Nonselective, postemergence, contact herbicide<br>Photosystem I electron diversion<br>These compounds are part of a larger group of quaternary ammonium herbicides, including difenzoquat, which is also a pyrazole compound (see below). | II | Paraquat, diquat | See text for paraquat and diquat. |
| Carbanilate | Inhibits photosynthesis at photosystem II and/or inhibits mitosis or microtubule organization. | U | Carbetamide, desmedipham, phenmedipham, propham | Limited human data. |
| Cyclohexane oxime | Postemergence, selective for grasses<br>Inhibits acetyl-CoA carboxylase (lipid biosynthesis inhibitors). | III<br>U | Butroxydim, sethoxydim, tralkoxydim<br>Alloxydim, cycloxydim, cyhalofop | Limited human data. |

| | | | | |
|---|---|---|---|---|
| Dinitroaniline | Preemergence, selective for grasses<br>In 2012, trifluralin and pendimethalin were among the top 20 herbicides used in the United States overall, while trifluralin and pendimethalin were among the top 10 used in the domestic sector.<br>Inhibits microtubule assembly. | III<br>U | Fluchloralin, pendimethalin<br>Benfluralin (benefin), butralin, dinitramine, ethalfluralin, oryzalin, prodiamine, trifluralin | Pendimethalin induces mild clinical toxicity in most cases, but gastroduodenal injury, sedation, seizures, hypotension, and death due to respiratory failure are reported, usually within 24 hours. Limited human data for the others.<br>Aniline metabolites are reported from trifluralin and oryzalin, which induce methemoglobinemia and hemolysis with prolonged exposures. For which methylene blue, blood transfusions and supportive care are recommended (Antidotes in Brief: A43). In rats, fluchloralin induces hyperexcitability, tremors, and convulsions prior to death. Agitation, trembling, and fatigue occur in rats following lethal doses of trifluralin. Many of these compounds are poorly absorbed and some are subject to enterohepatic recycling. |
| Dinitrophenol | Uncoupling (membrane disruption) | Ib | Dinoterb, DNOC (4,6-dinitro-*o*-cresol) | Limited human data; methemoglobinemia is reported in animals. Dinitrophenol uncouples oxidative phosphorylation. |
| Diphenylether | Postemergence (particularly broad leaves)<br>Contact herbicide, inhibits protoporphyrinogen oxidase, and/or inhibits carotenoid biosynthesis<br>Aclonifen is also an amine compound. | III<br>U | Acifluorfen, fluoroglycofen<br>Aclonifen, bifenox, chlomethoxyfen, oxyfluorfen | Limited human data. |
| Halogenated aliphatic | Inhibits lipid synthesis. | U | Dalapon, fluopropanate | Limited human data. |
| Imidazolinone | Inhibits acetolactate synthase, interfering with branched amino acid synthesis. | U | Imazamethabenz, imazapyr, imazaquin, imazethapyr | Limited human data. In a small case series, imazapyr induced sedation, respiratory distress, metabolic acidosis, hypotension, and hepatorenal dysfunction. |
| Inorganic | Nonselective | III<br>U | Sodium chlorate<br>Ammonium sulfamate | Nausea, vomiting, diarrhea, metabolic acidosis, kidney failure, hemolysis, methemoglobinemia, rhabdomyolysis, and disseminated intravascular coagulation. Treatment includes hemodialysis and erythrocyte and plasma transfusion. Methemoglobinemia is usually unresponsive to methylene blue (a single report suggested benefit when used within 6 hours of exposure).<br>Limited human data. |
| Nitrile | Preemergence, selective for grasses<br>Inhibits photosynthesis at photosystem II and/or inhibition of cell wall (cellulose) synthesis.<br>Commonly coformulated with phenoxyacetic acid compounds. | II<br>U | Bromoxynil, ioxynil<br>Dichlobenil | Limited human data of single-substance exposures. In animals, it uncouples oxidative phosphorylation and induces CNS toxicity. Similar clinical effects noted in humans. |
| Organic phosphorus | Bensulide: preemergence selective for grasses. Glyphosate and glufosinate are nonselective postemergence herbicides.<br>In 2012, glyphosate was the most used pesticide in the United States and the second most used in the domestic sector.<br>Bialaphos and glufosinate inhibit glutamine synthetase, bensulide inhibits lipid synthesis, and glyphosate inhibits EPSP synthase, which interferes with aromatic amino acid synthesis. | II<br>III<br>U | Butamifos, bialaphos (bilanafos), anilofos, bensulide, piperophos<br>Glufosinate<br>Fosamine, glyphosate | Limited human data. Bialaphos is metabolized to glufosinate in plants, but in humans, only the metabolite L-amino-4-hydroxymethyl-phosphonoyl-butyric acid has been found. Clinical effects of poisoning include apnea, amnesia, and metabolic acidosis. Anilofos and bensulide are shown to inhibit acetyl cholinesterase.<br>See text for glufosinate.<br>See text for glyphosate; limited human data for fosamine. |

(*Continued*)

**TABLE 82–1 Characteristics of the Major Herbicides Categorized by Chemical Class and WHO Hazard Classification (*Continued*)**

| *Chemical Class*[a] | *Applications, Usage Data, and Mechanism of Action in Plants, If Known*[b] | *WHO Hazard Class*[c] | *Compounds Included* | *Clinical Effects, Treatments, and Supportive Care* |
|---|---|---|---|---|
| Phenoxy | Postemergence, selective for grasses<br>In 2012, 2,4-D was the fifth most used herbicide in the United States but the most used in the domestic sector (mecoprop was third and MCPA ninth). | II | *Phenoxyacetic derivatives:* 2,4-D<br>*Nonphenoxyacetic derivatives:* haloxyfop, quizalofop-P | See text for phenoxyacetic derivatives; similar clinical features of toxicity are noted for the chlorinated nonphenoxyacetic acid compounds. Mild clinical toxicity from fenoxaprop-ethyl in acute overdose.<br>Limited human data on poisoning for others.<br>Fluazifop 0.07 mg/kg was safely administered to humans in a volunteer study. |
| | Inhibits acetyl-CoA carboxylase (lipid biosynthesis inhibitors; fops) or indole acetic acid-like (auxin growth regulators; chlorinated compounds). | III | *Phenoxyacetic derivatives:* MCPA, 2,4,5-T<br>*Nonphenoxyacetic derivatives:* Bromofenoxim, 2,4-DB, dichlorprop, diclofop, fluazifop, MCPB, mecoprop (MCPP), quizalofop, propaquizafop | |
| | Clomeprop is also an amide compound. | U | *Nonphenoxyacetic derivatives:* Clomeprop, fenoxaprop-ethyl | |
| Pyrazole | Inhibition of 4-hydroxyphenyl-pyruvate dioxygenase or photosystem I electron diversion (difenzoquat is also a quaternary ammonium compound) | II<br>III<br>U | Difenzoquat<br>Pyrazoxyfen, pyrazolynate<br>Azimsulfuron | Limited human data. |
| Pyridazine | Preemergence application. Inhibits photosynthesis at photosystem II. | III | Pyridate | Limited human data. |
| Pyridazinone | Inhibits photosynthesis at photosystem II or inhibits carotenoid biosynthesis at the phytoene desaturase step. | U | Chloridazon, norflurazon | Limited human data. In animals, chloridazon interferes with mitochondrial function. Respiratory distress, seizures, and paralysis precede death. |
| Pyridine | Inhibits carotenoid biosynthesis at the phytoene desaturase step and/or inhibits microtubule assembly and/or indole acetic acid–like (synthetic auxins). | III<br>U | Triclopyr<br>Diflufenican, dithiopyr, fluroxypyr, fluthiacet, picloram | Limited human data on poisoning, but triclopyr appears to be low toxicity, except for one case of acute poisoning with metabolic acidosis, coma, and cardiotoxicity; yet, recovery was complete. Triclopyr 0.5 mg/kg was safely administered to humans in a volunteer study. Picloram 5 mg/kg was safely administered to humans in a volunteer study. |
| Thiocarbamate | Preemergence, selective for grasses<br>Inhibits lipid synthesis. | II<br>III<br>U | EPTC, molinate, pebulate, prosulfocarb, thiobencarb, vernolate<br>Cycloate, esprocarb, triallate<br>Tiocarbazil | Molinate 5 mg was orally administered to volunteers. Limited human data, including effects on cholinesterase. Some compounds display variable inhibition of nicotinic receptors, esterases, and aldehyde dehydrogenase in animals. Cycloate induces neurotoxicity in rats. |
| Triazine | Mostly preemergence and nonselective<br>In 2007, atrazine was the second most used herbicide in the United States.<br>Inhibits photosynthesis at photosystem II. | II<br>III<br>U | Cyanazine, terbumeton<br>Ametryn, desmetryn, dimethametryn, simetryn<br>Atrazine, prometon, prometryn, propazine, simazine, terbuthylazine, terbutryn, trietazine | See text. |
| Triazinone | Inhibits photosynthesis at photosystem II. | II<br>III | Metribuzin, hexazinone<br>Metamitron | Limited human data. With hexazinone, rats and guinea pigs experience lethargy and ataxia, progressing to clonic seizures prior to death, while dogs were not particularly sensitive. Goats experience sedation, lethargy, and impaired respiration with metamitron poisoning. |
| Triazole | Postemergent, nonselective<br>Commonly coformulated with ammonium thiocyanate. Inhibits lycopene cyclase; chlorophyll or carotenoid pigment inhibitor. | U | Amitrole (aminotriazole) | Limited human data on single-agent exposures. Ingestion of 20 mg/kg in a human and > 4,000 mg/kg in rats did not induce symptoms. |

| Triazolone | Inhibits acetolactate synthase. | U | Flucarbazone | Limited human data. |
|---|---|---|---|---|
| Triazolopyrimidine | Inhibits acetolactate synthase. These herbicides are also amide compounds. | U | Diclosulam, flumetsulam, metosulam | Limited human data. Asthma is reported from occupational exposures to flumetsulam. |
| Uracil | Mostly preemergence. Inhibits photosynthesis at photosystem II. | U | Bromacil, lenacil, terbacil | Limited human data. |
| Urea | Both pre- and postemergence<br>Inhibits acetolactate synthase (interferes with branched amino acid synthesis) and/or inhibits photosynthesis at photosystem II and/or inhibition of carotenoid biosynthesis. | III<br>U | Isoproturon, isouron, tebuthiuron<br>Bensulfuron, chlorbromuron, chlorimuron, chlorotoluron, cinosulfuron, cyclosulfamuron, daimuron, dimefuron, diuron, fenuron, fluometuron, linuron, methyldymron, metobromuron, metoxuron, metsulfuron, monolinuron, neburon, nicosulfuron, primisulfuron, pyrazosulfuron, rimsulfuron, siduron, sulfometuron, thifensulfuron, triasulfuron, tribenuron, triflusulfuron | Limited human data. Some urea herbicides are metabolized to aniline compounds, which induce methemoglobinemia and hemolysis (similar to propanil, see text). Given the limited experience in treating poisonings with urea herbicides, it is reasonable to apply treatments described for amide herbicide poisoning (see text); success with methylene blue is reported. Wheezing is reported from occupational exposures to chlorimuron.<br>Animal studies suggest that isoproturon causes CNS depression and tebuthiuron causes lethargy, ataxia, and anorexia. |
| Miscellaneous | Clomazone: may be coformulated with propanil<br>Clomazone and fluridone: chlorophyll or carotenoid pigment inhibitor<br>Bentazone: pre- and postemergence for control of broadleaf plants. Inhibits photosynthesis.<br>Fluridone: chlorophyll or carotenoid pigment inhibitor | II<br>III<br>U | Clomazone, endothal<br>Bentazone, quinoclamine<br>Benfuresate, cinmethylin, ethofumesate, fluridone, flurochloridone, oxadiazon | Limited human data; in one case vomiting and gastric and pulmonary hemorrhage preceded death. Animal studies suggest that clomazone inhibits acetylcholinesterase and endothal induces lethargy, respiratory, and hepatic dysfunction. In vitro, clomazone induces oxidative stress and inhibits acetylecholinesterase.<br>Bentazone: gastrointestinal irritation, hepatic failure, acute kidney injury, dyspnea, muscle rigidity, confusion, death.<br>Limited human data. |

[a]Many of these classes can be further subclassified on the basis of chemical structure; however, the relationship between structure and clinical effects is not adequately described. The classification listed here is adapted from http://www.alanwood.net/pesticides/class_herbicides.html. Accessed December 9, 2012. [b]The mechanism by which a number of herbicides regulate plant growth is not fully described. The mechanisms listed here are adapted from http://www.plantprotection.org/HRAC/MOA.html (accessed December 9, 2012) and http://www.ces.purdue.edu/extmedia/WS/WS-23-W.html (accessed December 9, 2012). [c]WHO Hazard Classification scale for oral liquid exposures of the technical grade ingredient based on rat $LD_{50}$ (mg/kg body weight): Ia = "extremely hazardous," < 20 mg/kg; Ib = "highly hazardous," 20–200 mg/kg; II = "moderately hazardous," 200–2,000 mg/kg; III = "slightly hazardous," > 2,000 mg/kg; and U = "technical grade active ingredients of pesticides unlikely to present acute hazard in normal use."

CNS = central nervous system; WHO = World Health Organization.

medical and nursing care or does not have ready access to necessary antidotes, then arrangements should be made to rapidly and safely transport the patient to an appropriate healthcare facility.

For many herbicides, the initial management of an acute poisoning follows standard guidelines. All patients should receive prompt resuscitation emphasizing the airway, breathing, and circulation. Gastrointestinal toxicity, such as nausea, vomiting, and diarrhea, is common, leading to salt and water depletion that requires the administration of antiemetics and intravenous fluids.

Gastrointestinal decontamination decreases absorption of the herbicide from the gut, reducing systemic exposure. We generally recommend not to perform orogastric lavage in acute poisoning because patients usually present too late or have self-decontaminated from vomiting and diarrhea. However, gastric lavage with a small nasogastric tube is reasonable for patients presenting shortly after an ingestion of a liquid formulation for which treatment options are limited. Ingestion of a corrosive product is a relative contraindication. Oral activated charcoal is recommended if the patient presents within 1 to 2 hours of ingestion of an herbicide known to cause significant poisoning. In the case of herbicides with prolonged absorption (eg, propanil, MCPA), later administration of activated charcoal is reasonable. Dermal decontamination is recommended if the patient has incurred cutaneous exposure. The patient should be washed with soap and water, and contaminated clothes, shoes, and leather materials should be removed and safely discarded in sealed plastic bags.

Respiratory distress and hypoxia with focal respiratory crackles soon after presentation are likely to result from aspiration pneumonitis, which should be confirmed on chest radiography.

We recommend a minimum of 6 hours of observation for patients with a history of acute ingestion, unless otherwise stated below. For patients with a history of intentional ingestion and gastrointestinal symptoms, we recommend at least 24 hours of observation depending on the herbicide, given that clinical toxicity will progress or be delayed in some cases.

### Occupational and Secondary Exposures (Including Nosocomial Poisoning)

Concern has been expressed regarding the risk of nosocomial poisoning to staff and family members who are exposed to patients with acute herbicide poisoning. However, the risk to healthcare staff providing clinical care is low compared with other occupations, such as agricultural workers, in whom acute toxicity is rarely observed. Universal precautions using nitrile gloves are recommended to provide sufficient protection for staff members.

## AMIDE COMPOUNDS, PARTICULARLY ANILIDE DERIVATIVES

Anilide compounds are the most widely used amide herbicides, of which propanil (DCPA), alachlor, and butachlor are particularly common. Other amide herbicides and available toxicity data are listed in Table 82–1. Acute self-poisoning is reported, particularly in Asia where subsistence farming is common. The case fatality of propanil exceeds 10%, compared with a combined mortality of less than 3% for butachlor, metachlor, and alachlor.

### Pharmacology

Most of the clinical manifestations of propanil poisoning are mediated by its metabolites. 3,4-Dichlorophenylhydroxylamine is the most toxic metabolite and it directly induces methemoglobinemia and hemolysis in a dose-related manner. However, toxicity is not solely due to methemoglobinemia. Other possible toxicities from the metabolism of propanil include nephrotoxicity, lipid peroxidation, myelotoxicity, and immune dysfunction; the significance of these toxicities is poorly defined.

### Pharmacokinetics and Toxicokinetics

Absorption is rapid in animals, with a peak serum concentration expected 1 hour postingestion. The volume of distribution (Vd) of propanil is not defined but is expected to be large given that both propanil and 3,4-dichloroaniline are highly lipid soluble.

Anilide compounds undergo sequential metabolic reactions that produce toxic xenobiotics. *N*-Hydroxylation of 3,4-dichloroaniline produces the hydroxylamine compound that induces hemolysis and methemoglobinemia, which are the most obvious manifestations of propanil poisoning. These metabolic reactions are similar to those of dapsone, which are well characterized: the severity of methemoglobinemia relates to the amount of the dapsone hydroxylamine metabolite, which varies with dose, and cytochrome P450 activity (Chap. 97).

Propanil displays nonlinear toxicokinetics in humans with prolonged absorption continuing for approximately 10 hours following ingestion. The median apparent elimination half-life of propanil is 3.2 hours compared with 3,4-dichloroaniline, which has a highly variable elimination profile. In general, the concentration of 3,4-dichloroaniline exceeds that of propanil and remains elevated for a longer period. By 36 hours postingestion, the concentration of 3,4-dichloroaniline is low in survivors, so clinical toxicity is unlikely to increase beyond this time.

### Pathophysiology

The predominant clinical manifestation in acute poisoning is methemoglobinemia, which leads to end-organ dysfunction, including central nervous system depression, hypotension, and acidemia (Chap. 97). Sedation due to the direct effect of propanil or a hydrocarbon coformulant solvent causes hypoventilation, which contributes to cellular hypoxia.

### Clinical Manifestations

Methemoglobinemia, hemolysis and anemia, coma, and death are reported following acute propanil poisoning. These occur in the clinical context of cyanosis, acidemia, and progressive end-organ dysfunction. In one case series with a 10.7% fatality rate, the median time to death was 36 hours. Nausea, vomiting, diarrhea, tachycardia, dizziness, and confusion are also reported in patients who do not develop severe poisoning.

Alachlor, metachlor, and butachlor are less toxic than propanil, with a case fatality less than 3% with self-poisoning.

The manifestations of acute poisoning are usually mild, including gastrointestinal symptoms, agitation, dyspnea, and abnormal liver enzymes. Major symptoms include seizures, rhabdomyolysis, acidemia, kidney failure, and cardiac dysrhythmias; hypotension and coma preceded death. Methemoglobinemia is not reported.

### Diagnostic Testing

Patients with a history of propanil poisoning should be investigated for the presence of methemoglobinemia (Chap. 97). In the absence of co-oximetry, color charts can be used to support the diagnosis and severity of methemoglobinemia and to direct the use of antidotes at the bedside.

### Management

The minimum toxic dose has not been determined and the potential for severe poisoning and death is high, so all patients with amide herbicide ingestions should be treated as significant and monitored for a minimum of 12 hours. Patients with symptomatic ingestions should be treated cautiously, including continuous monitoring for 24 to 48 hours, preferably in an intensive care unit.

***Resuscitation and Supportive Care.*** Prompt resuscitation and close observation are required in all patients. Patients should be monitored clinically, including pulse oximetry, and receive supportive care, including supplemental oxygen, intravenous fluids, and ventilatory and hemodynamic support as required. In the absence of co-oximetry analysis, significant methemoglobinemia should be suspected when cyanosis does not correct with high-flow oxygen and ventilatory support. Hemoglobin concentrations should be monitored to detect hemolysis, and folate supplementation is recommended during the recovery phase if anemia is significant.

***Gastrointestinal Decontamination.*** Toxicokinetic studies of propanil demonstrate a prolonged absorption phase, so it is reasonable to administer activated charcoal to the patient as late as 2-4 hours postingestion.

***Extracorporeal Removal.*** Hemodialysis data are extremely limited, and based on a single report, it does not have a role in routine care.

***Antidotes.*** Methylene blue (Antidotes in Brief: A43) is the first-line treatment for methemoglobinemia. Methylene blue has a half-life of 5 hours, which is commonly shorter than that of 3,4-dichloroaniline, so rebound poisoning (ie, an increase in methemoglobin following an initial recovery postadministration of methylene blue) is anticipated and has been observed with a bolus regimen. Other potential treatments for methemoglobinemia from propanil include toluidine blue, *N*-acetylcysteine, ascorbic acid, and cimetidine, but no clinical studies have assessed the role of these potential antidotes in the management of propanil poisoning.

## BIPYRIDYL COMPOUNDS, PARAQUAT AND DIQUAT

Bipyridyl compounds are nonselective contact herbicides. The most widely used is paraquat but diquat is also commonly used. Paraquat is one of the most toxic pesticides available. Ingestion of as little as 10 to 20 mL of the 20% wt/vol solution is sufficient to cause death. Overall, the mortality rate varies between 50% and 90%; however, in cases of intentional self-poisoning with concentrated formulations, mortality approaches 100%. An increasing number of countries are banning the sale of paraquat in view of its high toxicity. Diquat is less toxic than paraquat, so it is frequently coformulated with paraquat (allowing a lower concentration of paraquat) or used as an alternative in countries where paraquat is severely restricted.

### Pharmacology

Paraquat and diquat formulations are highly irritating and often corrosive, causing direct injury. They induce intracellular toxicity by the generation of reactive oxygen species that nonspecifically damage the lipid membrane of cells, inducing cellular injury and death. Once paraquat enters the intracellular space, it is oxidized to the paraquat radical. This radical is subsequently reduced by diaphorase in the presence of nicotinamide adenine dinucleotide phosphate (NADPH) to re-form the parent paraquat compound and superoxide radical, a reactive oxygen species. This process is known as redox cycling (Fig. 82–1). The superoxide radical is susceptible to further reactions by other intracellular processes, leading to formation of other reactive oxygen species, including hydroxyl radicals and peroxynitrite. Reactive oxygen species are potent cytotoxics. Paraquat redox cycling continues if NADPH and oxygen are available. Depletion of NADPH prevents recycling of glutathione and interferes with other intracellular processes, including energy production and active transporters, exacerbating toxicity. Intracellular protective mechanisms, such as glutathione, superoxide dismutase, and catalase, are overwhelmed or depleted following large exposures. Taken together, these cytotoxic reactions induce cellular necrosis, which is followed by an influx of neutrophils and macrophages. The reactions contribute to the inflammatory response and promote fibrosis and destruction of normal tissue architecture over a number of days. Supplemental oxygen probably increases the generation of reactive oxygen species.

### Pharmacokinetics and Toxicokinetics

Absorption is limited following dermal and respiratory exposures. The oral bioavailability of paraquat in humans is estimated to be less than 5%. Absorption is rapid and the peak concentration occurs within 1 hour. Paraquat binds minimally to plasma proteins. Paraquat and diquat rapidly distribute to all tissues and then redistribute back to the central circulation. In humans, the distribution half-life is approximately 5 hours. Paraquat is taken up by alveolar cells through an active energy-dependent polyamine transporter. Paraquat accumulates in alveolar cells, peaking at around 6 hours postingestion in patients with normal kidney function, but later in the context of kidney impairment. Paraquat slowly redistributes from the lungs into the systemic circulation as the plasma concentration falls. By contrast, diquat uptake occurs to a limited extent.

Paraquat and diquat are not metabolized. Elimination is primarily renal, with more than 90% of a dose being excreted within the first 24 hours of poisoning if kidney function is maintained. Systemic clearance initially exceeds that of

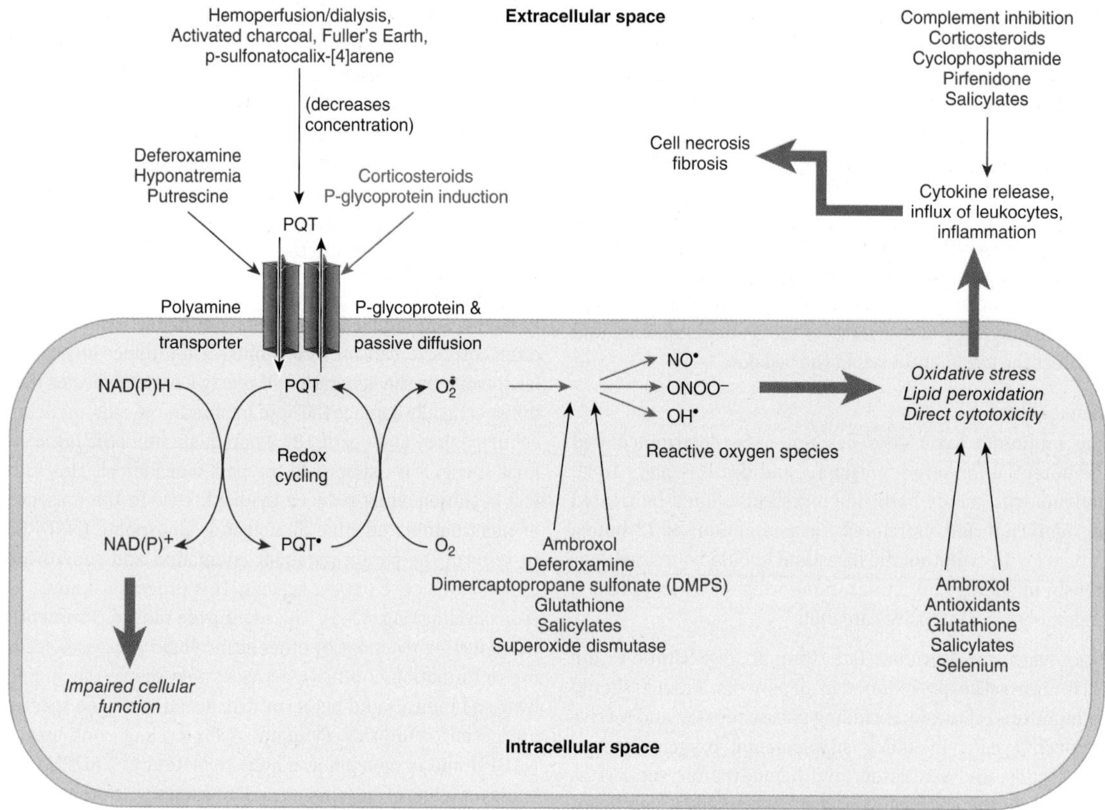


**FIGURE 82–1.** Toxicology of paraquat (PQT) and proposed mechanisms of action of potential treatments. Antioxidants include vitamins C and E and glutathione donors (particularly *N*-acetylcysteine, *S*-carboxymethylcysteine). PQT˙ = paraquat radical; NO˙ = nitric oxide; ONOO⁻ = peroxynitrite; OH˙ = hydroxyl radical.

glomerular filtration rate (GFR) because of active secretion. Impaired kidney function commonly occurs with paraquat and diquat poisoning, particularly beyond 24 to 48 hours postingestion, which decreases excretion and potentiates poisoning.

## Pathophysiology

Paraquat and diquat induce nonspecific cellular necrosis. Lung and kidney injuries are prominent in patients with acute paraquat poisoning because of the high concentrations found in these cells. Acute pneumonitis and hemorrhage, followed by ongoing inflammation and progressive pulmonary fibrosis, reduce oxygen diffusion and induce dyspnea and hypoxia, which interferes with normal cellular function. Paraquat induces acute tubular necrosis due to direct toxicity to the proximal tubule in particular and, to a lesser degree, distal structures. Varying degrees of oliguria, proteinuria, hematuria, and glycosuria are reported. Necrosis of the gastrointestinal tract limits absorption and causes fluid shifts that contribute to hypotension induced by direct vascular toxicity. Hypotension impairs tissue perfusion and, if uncorrected, progresses to irreversible shock.

## Clinical Manifestations

Topical exposures induce painful irritation to the eyes and skin, progressing to ulceration or desquamation. Intravenous administration induces severe poisoning from small amounts. Most ingestions of bipyridyl compounds induce poisoning. Ingestion of as little as 5 mL of paraquat 20% wt/vol causes death in more than 50% of cases.

Gastrointestinal toxicity occurs early, including nausea, vomiting, and abdominal and oral pain. Diarrhea, ileus, and pancreatitis are also reported. Necrosis of mucous membranes, occasionally referred to as pseudodiphtheria, and ulceration are prominent findings that occur within 12 hours. Dysphagia and odynophagia follow larger exposures and progress to esophageal rupture, pneumomediastinum and mediastinitis, subcutaneous emphysema, and pneumothorax, which are usually preterminal events.

Respiratory symptoms are prominent in patients with paraquat poisoning, including acute respiratory distress syndrome manifesting as dyspnea, hypoxia, and increased work of breathing. Ingestions of greater than 50 mL of 20% wt/vol formulation cause multiorgan dysfunction with rapid onset of death within days of ingestion in most patients. Features include hypotension, acute kidney and liver injury, severe diarrhea, and hemolytic anemia. By contrast, ARDS is less marked with diquat ingestion or following smaller exposures of paraquat (< 15–20 mL of 20% wt/vol formulations). In the case of paraquat, the acute respiratory impairment is often followed by progressive pulmonary fibrosis and death weeks or months postingestion. Diquat does not concentrate in the pneumocytes as readily as paraquat. Therefore, if the patient survives the multiorgan dysfunction, pulmonary fibrosis is less likely to occur.

Varying degrees of acute kidney injury and hepatic dysfunction occur. Acute kidney injury peaks around 5 days postingestion and resolves within 3 weeks in survivors. Seizures are reported with diquat poisoning and uncommonly with paraquat.

### Diagnostic Testing

The presence of a bipyridyl compound in blood confirms exposure, but availability of these assays is increasingly limited. The urinary dithionite test is a simple and quick method for confirming (or excluding) paraquat and diquat poisoning. A color change (blue for paraquat and green for diquat) confirms ingestion—the darker the color, the higher the concentration. If the test is negative on urine beyond 6 hours after ingestion, a large exposure is unlikely, but repeat testing should be conducted over 24 hours. When the dithionite test is conducted on plasma, a positive result is specific for death, but a negative test does not exclude severe poisoning or death.

Quantitative analysis of the concentration of paraquat in plasma is useful for prognostication, and a number of similar nomograms have been developed to assist with this process (eg, Fig. 82–2). The Severity Index of Paraquat Poisoning (SIPP) is also calculated with this information, by multiplying the plasma concentration (mg/L) by the time since ingestion (hours). Here, SIPP less than 10 predicts survival, SIPP 10 to 50 predicts death from lung fibrosis, and SIPP more than 50 predicts death from circulatory failure.

The rate of increase in creatinine concentration is a simple and practical test to predict prognosis. An increase less than 0.03 mg/dL/h (3 μmol/L/h) over 5 hours predicts survival, and an increase greater than 0.05 mg/dL/h (4.3 μmol/L/h) over 12 hours (sensitivity 100%, specificity 85%, likelihood ratio 7) predicts death. A similar relationship was noted for cystatin C, in which a rate of increase in cystatin C greater than 0.009 mg/L/h over 6 hours (sensitivity 100%, specificity 91%, likelihood ratio 11) predicted death. This method of prognostication is advantageous because it is determined irrespective of the time of poisoning.

### Management

Because death follows ingestion of as little as 5 mL of the 20% wt/vol paraquat, all exposures should be treated as potentially life threatening. Patients suspected of ingesting paraquat should be observed in hospital for at least 6 hours postingestion or until a urinary dithionite test is conducted. Many medical interventions are proposed for the treatment of patients with acute paraquat poisoning, but data supporting their efficacy are lacking. We have no evidence to recommend treatment with any of these regimens. The choice of which interventions should be administered to a patient is made on a case-by-case basis by the treating physician in consultation with relevant resources. In the context of the anticipated prognosis, detailed discussion with the patient and relatives early in the presentation is recommended to determine their preference for treatment. In general, a comprehensive treatment regimen is reasonable in patients who present very early (within 2 hours of poisoning) or those with a faintly positive dithionite urinary test. Here, treatments that reduce the exposure to paraquat by either reducing absorption or increasing clearance must be initiated promptly. In contrast, active treatment is not recommended in patients in whom this test is strongly positive, or those with hemodynamic compromise or evolving lung injury. Instead, palliation should be the priority, including supplemental oxygen for hypoxia and morphine for dyspnea and oropharyngeal and abdominal pain.

***Resuscitation and Supportive Care.*** Supplemental oxygen should only be administered to patients for palliation when there is confirmed hypoxia and/or prognosis is extremely poor. Although controlled hypoxia does not prevent the development of pulmonary injury, unnecessary supplemental oxygen theoretically hastens the progression of injury. In patients with established lung injury, ventilatory support is reasonable

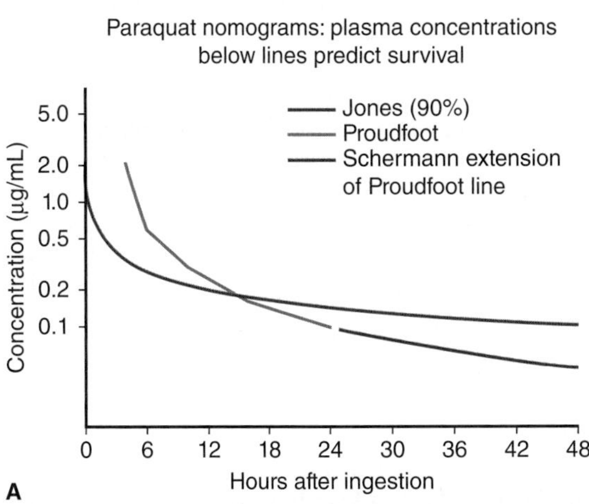


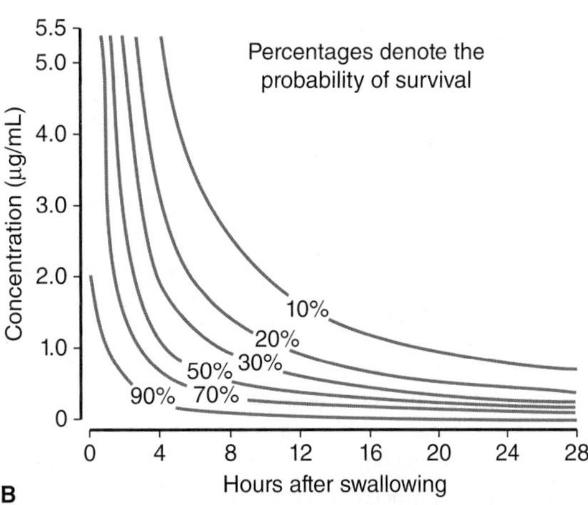


**FIGURE 82–2.** Nomograms for plasma paraquat concentrations. (**A**) Compilation of three nomograms proposed by Proudfoot et al, Scherrmann et al, and Jones et al. (**B**) Hart paraquat nomogram. In *A*, concentrations below lines predict survival. In *B*, lines link concentrations of equal probability of survival. *(Used with permission of Oxford University Press, from Prospects for treatment of paraquat-induced lung fibrosis with immunosuppressive drugs and the need for better prediction of outcome: a systematic review, Eddleston M, Wilks MF, Buckley NA, 96(11), 2003; permission conveyed through Copyright Clearance Center, Inc.)*

to improve oxygenation and reduce dyspnea. Intravenous fluids should be administered to patients who are volume depleted as this reduces the severity of acute kidney injury and promotes renal clearance of paraquat. Electrolyte abnormalities should be corrected as required. Analgesia for oral and abdominal pain should be administered as required. Plain radiographs or a computed tomography of the chest provides information on lung and esophageal injury, which may be prognostic, as noted above.

***Gastrointestinal Decontamination.*** Activated charcoal is recommended for all patients presumed to have ingested paraquat as soon as possible, within 2 hours of exposure. Paraquat is coformulated with an emetic so a degree of self-decontamination frequently occurs by the time of presentation to hospital. Fuller's Earth and activated charcoal decrease absorption of paraquat to a similar extent, but Fuller's Earth is in limited supply. Gastric lavage does not improve outcomes overall and is not recommended.

***Extracorporeal Removal.*** Hemoperfusion and hemodialysis increase the elimination of paraquat, which decreases the systemic exposure and potentially toxicity. Although published data regarding the efficacy of these treatments are contradictory or limited, extracorporeal treatments are recommended in cases of large exposures if the treatment can be initiated within a few hours of ingestion. Hemoperfusion is more efficient than hemodialysis, and elimination is maximized when treatment is initiated within the first couple of hours because the plasma concentration is high.

***Antidotes.*** A large number of potential antidotes are under study in the treatment of acute paraquat poisoning. The combination of antidotes (if any) that will improve outcomes is not known, so it is not possible to recommend specific antidotes or dosages in routine clinical care. Examples of specific potential antidotes are detailed here.

Immunosuppression with corticosteroids (dexamethasone or methylprednisolone) and cyclophosphamide are the most extensively studied antidotes in humans. Although nonrandomized studies support a potential benefit, this immunosuppressive regimen is not routinely recommended.

Generation of reactive oxygen species is an important step in the pathogenesis of paraquat poisoning. Administration of vitamin C (ascorbic acid), vitamin E (α-tocopherol), and glutathione and/or a glutathione donator (eg, *N*-acetylcysteine, *S*-carboxymethylcysteine, captopril) or other scavenging agents such as superoxide dismutase, amifostine, or deferoxamine is not routinely recommended because they are not proven to be beneficial, and potentially vitamin C might increase oxidative toxicity.

Salicylates are proposed to inhibit multiple steps in the pathogenesis of paraquat poisoning, including decreasing production of reactive oxygen species, inhibition of nuclear factor-κB, antithrombotic effects, and chelation of paraquat. A small pilot study noted a delayed time to death in patients receiving intravenous acetylsalicylic acid. However, it is premature to routinely recommend this therapy.

***Treatment Recommendations.*** In patients with a poor prognosis, active treatment, particularly with invasive modalities such as hemoperfusion/dialysis, will interfere with end-of-life care. Based on these principles, our recommendations favor intervention when there is a hope of recovery, while avoiding unfounded experimental technologies. The prognosis in patients presenting more than 12 hours after ingesting 50 mL or more of paraquat 20% wt/vol, those with a positive plasma dithionite test, or those with a SIPP greater than 50 is so poor that treatment should focus on symptom control and end-of-life support and palliation.

The prognosis in patients presenting within 6 hours of ingesting less than 50 mL of paraquat, those with a faint-positive dithionite test, or those with a SIPP less than 50 is also poor, but prompt multimodal treatment with volume resuscitation, oral activated charcoal (or Fuller's Earth), hemoperfusion or hemodialysis, intravenous corticosteroids, acetylsalicylate, *N*-acetylcysteine, deferoxamine, and vitamin E can be considered on a case-by-case basis. It cannot be overemphasized that potential benefits of these treatments (if any) is time-critical, so they must be commenced immediately. If any of these treatments are not available at the initial treatment center, it is reasonable to transfer the patient to a center that can provide them within the stated time frame. However, if resources are available and psychosocial or cultural factors support aggressive treatment, then the previously mentioned treatment regimen can be attempted (but a benefit is not anticipated).

## GLUFOSINATE

Glufosinate is a nonselective herbicide used predominantly in Japan and Korea. Commercial preparations contain 14% to 30% glufosinate as the ammonium or sodium salt, with anionic surfactants. Case fatalities between 6.1% and 17.7% are reported from glufosinate poisoning, and increasing age is a risk factor.

### Pharmacology

Glufosinate is neurotoxic, although the specific mechanism is incompletely described. Because it is structurally similar to glutamate, studies have explored whether it interferes with glutamate networks in the central nervous system. Studies in rats demonstrate both agonism and antagonism to glutamate receptors and no effect on other receptors in the brain. Glufosinate also interferes with glutamine synthetase activity, which induces hyperammonemia. The extent to which the surfactant contributes to clinical toxicity is not confirmed. Rat studies suggest that hemodynamic changes due to glufosinate ammonium formulations are entirely caused by the surfactant component rather than glufosinate itself.

### Pharmacokinetics and Toxicokinetics

The peak concentration is observed 1 hour postingestion in mice administered the formulated product, and less than 15% of a dose is absorbed by rats. Glufosinate does not appear to bind to plasma proteins to a significant extent. The Vd was calculated to be 1.44 L/kg in a case of acute poisoning. Glufosinate distributes into the central nervous system, but the rate of distribution to the cerebrospinal fluid has not been characterized. Glufosinate is subject to minimal metabolism, and the majority of the bioavailable dose of glufosinate is excreted unchanged in urine. Kinetic data in humans are limited to a small number of cases of acute intentional poisoning in which the elimination profile appeared biphasic with a distribution half-life of 2 to 4 hours and a terminal elimination of 10 to 18 hours.

### Pathophysiology

It is not known whether the manifestations of glufosinate poisoning represent a primary (toxic) or secondary (downstream) effect. The most important manifestations are neurologic, with respiratory impairment that reduces oxygen delivery and subsequently compromises cellular function. Hypotension also impairs tissue perfusion and, if uncorrected, progresses to shock. Failure to correct these abnormalities leads to irreversible cellular injury and death.

### Clinical Manifestations

Nausea and vomiting are early features of acute poisoning. An altered level of consciousness precedes severe neurotoxicity, which usually occurs within 24 hours, and includes seizures and central respiratory failure requiring ventilatory support. These toxicities often persist for a number of days. Other manifestations of acute poisoning include cardiac dysrhythmias, fever, amnesia, diabetes insipidus, and rhabdomyolysis.

### Diagnostic Testing

Glufosinate poisoning is diagnosed clinically in the context of a history of exposure. Glufosinate assays are available for clinical use in Japan, and a nomogram was developed for predicting clinical outcomes (Fig. 82–3). Clinical chemistry assays including kidney function, blood gases, electrolytes, creatine kinase, and ammonia concentrations support clinical management. Metabolic acidosis is more common with severe poisoning, and the ammonia concentration peaks 24 to 48 hours postingestion.

### Management

Toxicity is not consistently dose-dependent and severe symptoms are reported following unintentional ingestion, so all patients with oral exposures should be carefully monitored. Patients with confirmed exposures should be monitored for a minimum of 48 hours because the onset of clinical toxicity is often delayed.

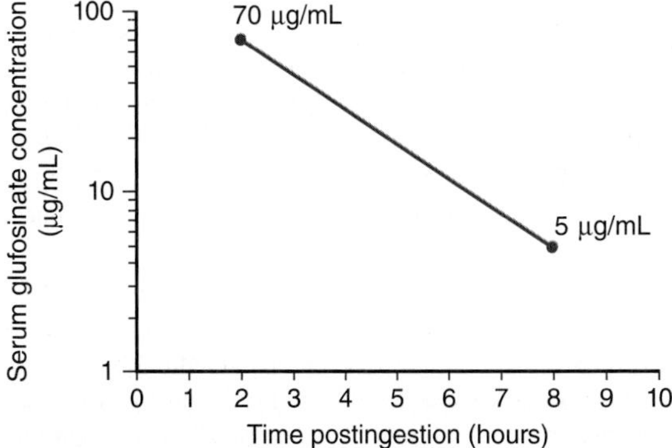


**FIGURE 82–3.** Glufosinate nomogram as described by Hori. Concentrations above the line are associated with more severe poisoning.

***Resuscitation and Supportive Care.*** Routine resuscitation, close observation, and supportive care are required. Careful monitoring for the onset of respiratory failure is necessary, and early intubation and ventilation are recommended in symptomatic patients. Given that glufosinate and metabolites are primarily renally cleared, intravenous fluids to maintain a consistent urine output are reasonable. Seizures should be treated in a standard manner initially with benzodiazepines as first-line therapy. Biochemical and acid–base abnormalities should be corrected as per usual care.

***Gastrointestinal Decontamination.*** In most reports of glufosinate poisoning, gastric lavage and activated charcoal were administered, but it is not possible to determine whether these interventions improved clinical outcomes. The high incidence of both seizures and respiratory failure from glufosinate poisoning are relative contraindications to the administration of activated charcoal to patients with an unprotected airway.

***Extracorporeal Removal.*** Although prompt hemodialysis in patients promotes a decrease in the concentration of glufosinate and probably ammonia, it is not known if this prevents the occurrence of neurotoxicity such as seizures, so its role in routine management is poorly defined. It is reasonable to administer these treatments in patients with severe poisoning and also in those with impaired kidney function.

***Antidotes.*** Specific antidotes are not available.

## GLYPHOSATE

Glyphosate is a nonselective postemergence herbicide. It is used extensively worldwide, most commonly as the isopropylamine salt but also a potassium salt. Glyphosate-containing herbicides are available in various formulations: 1% to 5% glyphosate (ready to use) or 30% to 50% (concentrate requiring dilution before use). In 2012, glyphosate was the most frequently used herbicide in the US and the second most commonly used herbicide in the domestic sector. Products containing glyphosate trimesium are less widely used and differ with respect to their toxicity profile. Glyphosate is banned in some countries because of data suggesting that it is a carcinogen. However, this topic is extensively debated, and in March 2017, the US Environmental Protection Agency concluded that glyphosate is not likely to be carcinogenic to humans.

### Pharmacology

Glyphosate inhibits 5-enolpyruvylshikimate-3-phosphate synthase in plants, which interferes with their aromatic amino acid synthesis; this enzyme is not present in humans. The mechanism of toxicity of glyphosate-containing herbicides to humans is not adequately described. The formulation is irritating and high concentrations are corrosive, causing direct injury to the gastrointestinal tract. Patients with severe poisoning manifest multisystem effects, suggesting that the formulation is either nonspecific in its action or that it interferes with a physiologic process common to a number of systems. Indeed, the mechanism of toxicity varies between different glyphosate salts. In two cases of glyphosate trimesium poisoning, cardiopulmonary arrest occurred within minutes of ingestion, which is not reported from glyphosate isopropylamine.

Experimentally, there is minimal (if any) mammalian toxicity from glyphosate itself. Surfactant coformulants are likely the more toxic component in glyphosate-containing herbicides. Systemic exposure to surfactants induces hypotension, which is primarily due to direct effects on the heart and blood vessels. Surfactants directly disrupt cellular and subcellular membranes, including those of mitochondria, which has the potential to lead to systemic symptoms.

### Pharmacokinetics and Toxicokinetics

The kinetics of the surfactant are not described. The relevance of the kinetics of glyphosate is questioned because its contribution to clinical toxicology is minimal. Glyphosate does not penetrate the skin to a significant extent. Up to 40% of an oral dose is absorbed in rats, although this could increase when ingested as a concentrated solution with injury to the gastrointestinal epithelium. The peak glyphosate plasma concentration occurs within 2 hours of ingestion and distribution appears to be limited. Glyphosate has an elimination half-life of less than 4 hours and is excreted unchanged in the urine.

### Pathophysiology

It is not known whether the manifestations of glyphosate poisoning represent a primary (toxic) or secondary (downstream) effect. Disruptions of oxidative phosphorylation globally impair normal cellular function as a result of limited energy supply. Hypotension and dysrhythmias impair tissue perfusion, and liver and kidney injuries induce metabolic disequilibria and acidemia, which impair normal physiologic processes. Pulmonary toxicity induces hypoxia, which further compromises normal cellular functioning.

### Clinical Manifestations

Abdominal pain with nausea, vomiting, and/or diarrhea are the most common manifestations of acute poisoning. Gastrointestinal burns and necrosis occur with high doses of concentrated formulations and are associated with hemorrhage. Severe poisoning manifests as multiorgan failure, including hypotension, cardiac dysrhythmias, kidney and liver dysfunction, hyperkalemia, pancreatitis, pulmonary edema or pneumonitis, altered level of consciousness including encephalopathy, seizures, and metabolic acidosis. Proposed risk factors for death include a large exposure, delayed presentation to hospital, elevated glyphosate concentration, and increasing age.

### Diagnostic Testing

Acute poisoning with a glyphosate-containing herbicide is diagnosed on the basis of a history of exposure and clinical findings. There are no readily available specific clinical investigations to guide management or estimate prognosis in acute poisoning. Although higher plasma glyphosate concentrations are associated with more severe poisoning, quantitative glyphosate assays are not routinely available for clinical use. Targeted laboratory and radiologic investigations should be conducted in patients demonstrating anything more than mild gastrointestinal symptoms. A typical assessment includes a complete blood count, electrolytes, kidney function, and a venous blood gas with lactate determination.

### Management

All patients except for those with trivial exposures should be observed for a minimum of 6 hours. If gastrointestinal symptoms are noted, then the patient should be observed for a minimum of 24 hours given that clinical toxicity may progress.

***Resuscitation and Supportive Care.*** All patients should receive prompt resuscitation, close observation, and routine supportive care; other treatments are largely empiric. The airway is usually maintained but respiratory distress and failure occur, which require supplemental oxygen and possibly mechanical ventilation. The optimal management of hypotension is complicated because its etiology is potentially related to hypovolemia, negative inotropy, and/or reduced vascular resistance. If the response to prompt administration of 20 to 30 mL/kg intravenous fluid to the patient is insufficient or there is increasing pulmonary congestion, then vasopressors are recommended.

Biochemical and acid–base abnormalities, such as hyperkalemia, should be corrected. Hemodialysis or hemofiltration should be administered to patients developing acute kidney injury per usual guidelines if active treatment is to be pursued. Survival is reported with severe glyphosate poisoning (respiratory failure, persistent ventricular tachycardia and shock refractory to inotropes, and acidemia) using extracorporeal membrane oxygenation therapy.

***Gastrointestinal Decontamination.*** No data exist to support the role of gastrointestinal decontamination in acute poisoning with glyphosate-containing herbicides.

***Extracorporeal Removal.*** The role of extracorporeal removal in routine care is not known, but we recommend using it in patients with severe poisoning.

***Antidotes.*** No specific antidotes are proposed or tested for the treatment of acute poisoning with glyphosate-containing herbicides, which relates in part to the unknown mechanism of toxicity.

## PHENOXY HERBICIDES (PHENOXYACETIC DERIVATIVES), INCLUDING 2,4-D AND MCPA

Phenoxy compounds are selective herbicides that are widely used globally. A large number of compounds are included in this category; however, the most commonly used are the phenoxyacetic derivatives. This includes 2,4-dichlorophenoxyacetic acid (2,4-D), 4-chloro-2-methylphenoxyacetic acid (MCPA), and mecoprop (MCPP). Other phenoxy herbicides and available toxicity data are listed in Table 82–1. In 2012, 2,4-D was the fifth most commonly used herbicide in the US but the most commonly used herbicide in the domestic sector.

Agent Orange, a defoliant popularly used by the US during the Vietnam War, was composed of an equal mixture of 2,4-D and 2,4,5-T. This product also contained contaminant dioxins, in particular 2,3,7,8-tetrachlorodibenzodioxin, which is a persistent organic pollutant that is alleged to induce chronic health conditions and cancer. This chapter discusses only the outcomes of acute exposures to phenoxy herbicides.

### Pharmacology

The formulation is irritating or caustic, causing direct injury to the gastrointestinal tract. Patients with severe poisoning manifest multisystem effects. Uncoupling of oxidative phosphorylation contributes to the development of severe clinical toxicity. Phenoxy acid compounds also inhibit the voltage-gated chloride channel (CLC-1) in skeletal muscles, which is thought to contribute to the neuromuscular toxicity of these compounds. Dysfunction of CLC-1 induces myotonia due to hyperpolarization of the cell membrane. Other possible mechanisms of toxicity relate to their similarity to acetic acid, interfering with the utilization of acetylcoenzyme A (acetyl-CoA), or action as a false messenger at cholinergic receptors.

### Pharmacokinetics and Toxicokinetics

Absorption is usually first order. However, the time to peak concentration is delayed with increasing doses, which suggests saturable absorption. In overdose, saturation of albumin binding occurs and the proportion of herbicide that is free (unbound) increases. This increases the Vd and prolongs the apparent plasma elimination half-life. Dose-dependent renal clearance is attributed to saturation of an active transport process or direct nephrotoxicity. Alterations in blood pH theoretically change tissue distribution because phenoxyacetic herbicides are weak acids (p*K*a approximately 3). Acidemia increases the proportion that is nonionized, and therefore lipophilic, which increases tissue binding and distribution. Experience with acute human poisonings noted a poor correlation between plasma concentrations and peak toxicity. This probably reflects a discordance between plasma (measured) and intracellular (eg, mitochondrial) concentrations.

### Pathophysiology

Direct injury to the gastrointestinal tract causes vomiting and diarrhea, which induces hypovolemia and electrolyte abnormalities. Uncoupling of oxidative phosphorylation disrupts mitochondrial function and causes inefficiency in energy production. There is an increase in heat production out of proportion to the generation of ATP. The initial physiologic response to uncoupling is to increase mitochondrial respiration to maintain the supply of ATP, which increases heat production and respiratory rate. As ATP depletion occurs, there is an increase in glycolysis, causing hypoglycemia and metabolic acidosis with an elevated lactate concentration. If the mitochondrial defect persists, then cell death occurs. Because mitochondria are the primary supplier of ATP for most physiologic systems, uncoupling of oxidative phosphorylation is expected to induce multisystem toxicity.

### Clinical Manifestations

Gastrointestinal toxicity, including nausea, vomiting, abdominal or throat pain, and diarrhea, is common. Other clinical features include neuromuscular findings (myalgia, rhabdomyolysis, weakness, myopathy, myotonia, and fasciculations), central nervous system effects (agitation, sedation, confusion, miosis), tachycardia, hypotension, acute kidney injury, and hypocalcemia.

Tachypnea with respiratory alkalosis occurs in patients with phenoxy herbicide poisoning, which is consistent with increased mitochondrial respiration from mild uncoupling. More severe poisoning is characterized by metabolic acidosis, hyperventilation, hyperthermia, elevated creatine kinase, generalized muscle rigidity, progressive hypotension, pulseless electrical activity, or asystole. The mortality from acute phenoxy herbicide poisoning is high. When death occurs, it is usually delayed by 24 to 48 hours postingestion and results from cardiorespiratory arrest.

### Diagnostic Testing

Commercial assays for the specific measurement of phenoxy herbicides are not available to assist in the diagnosis of acute poisoning. Further, their role in the management of acute poisoning is not confirmed because the relationship between plasma phenoxy herbicide concentration and clinical toxicity appears to be poor. Monitoring of electrolytes, kidney function, pulse oximetry, and blood gases is recommended to detect progression of organ toxicity. Hypoalbuminemia predisposes to severe poisoning. Creatine kinase should be determined because rhabdomyolysis is reported following acute poisoning. Urinalysis will identify myoglobinuria.

### Management

All patients with significant poisonings, particularly those with symptomatic oral ingestions, should be treated cautiously, including continuous monitoring for 24 to 48 hours preferably in an intensive care unit. Initial mild toxicity such as gastrointestinal symptoms with normal vital signs and level of consciousness does not preclude subsequent severe toxicity and death. Maintaining an adequate urine output (> 1 mL/kg/h) optimizes the renal excretion of phenoxy herbicides as well as decreases renal toxicity from rhabdomyolysis. Because signs consistent with uncoupling of oxidative phosphorylation are associated with a poor outcome, when present, more advanced treatments such as hemodialysis should be used. It is reasonable to correct electrolyte abnormalities and acidemia because acidemia promotes the distribution of weak acids and increases the intracellular concentration.

***Gastrointestinal Decontamination.*** Gastrointestinal decontamination is recommended to patients per the guidelines listed in Chap. 3. However, administration of activated charcoal beyond the usual time frame is reasonable given that absorption appears to be saturable.

***Extracorporeal Removal.*** Urgent hemodialysis is recommended in patients with severe poisoning. Because phenoxy compounds are small and water soluble and subject to saturable protein binding with large exposures (increasing the free concentration), they are likely to be cleared by extracorporeal techniques.

***Antidotes.*** There are no specific antidotes for phenoxy herbicides, but sodium bicarbonate or other alkalinizing agents favorably alter the kinetics of phenoxy herbicides. Plasma alkalinization theoretically limits the distribution of phenoxy compounds from the central circulation by "ion trapping." It is reasonable to alkalinize the urine to a pH greater than 7.5 in patients who are symptomatic, particularly if there are features of uncoupling of oxidative phosphorylation or metabolic acidosis. Alkalinization is rarely associated with adverse effects when administered to patients with care and close observation (Antidotes in Brief: A5).

## TRIAZINE COMPOUNDS, INCLUDING ATRAZINE

Triazine herbicides are widely used, and in 2012, atrazine was the second most used pesticide in the US. However, cases of acute poisoning are infrequent. Other herbicides included in this group are listed in Table 82–1. These selective herbicides are used pre- or post-emergence for weed control.

### Pharmacology

The mechanism of toxicity is not fully determined, although it might relate to uncoupling of oxidative phosphorylation. Atrazine is a direct arteriolar vasodilator.

### Pharmacokinetics and Toxicokinetics

Approximately 60% of an oral atrazine dose is absorbed in rats, and the concentration peaks beyond 3 hours. The absorption phase of triazine compounds appears to be prolonged in humans. Atrazine is rapidly dealkylated to a metabolite that binds strongly to hemoglobin and plasma proteins, allowing it to be detected in the blood for months. Metabolites are excreted in the urine, and around 25% of them are conjugated to glutathione. Dermal absorption of atrazine is incomplete but increases with exposure to the proprietary formulation.

### Clinical Manifestations

There are limited cases of triazine herbicide poisoning. Vomiting, depressed levels of consciousness, tachycardia, hypertension, acute kidney injury, and metabolic acidosis with an elevated lactate concentration were described in a patient with acute prometryn and ethanol poisoning. Similar clinical signs, in addition to hypotension with a low peripheral vascular resistance, were noted in a case of poisoning with atrazine, amitrole, ethylene glycol, and formaldehyde. This was followed by progressive multiorgan dysfunction and death due to refractory shock 3 days later.

### Diagnostic Testing

In a single case report, clinical toxicity did not directly relate to the concentration of prometryn, but the relationship to the concentration of metabolites was not determined. Routine biochemistry and blood gases are useful for monitoring for the development of systemic toxicity.

### Management

The limited number of publications of triazine herbicide poisoning is inadequate to guide specific management of patients with acute triazine poisoning. Routine resuscitation, close observation, and supportive care should be provided to all patients. Ventilatory support and correction of hypotension and metabolic disequilibria are appropriate.

***Gastrointestinal Decontamination.*** It is reasonable to administer activated charcoal to patients beyond 2 hours because of the slow absorption of these compounds.

***Extracorporeal Removal.*** Hemodialysis (HD) corrects the metabolic acidosis associated with poisoning but does not remove a substantial amount of xenobiotic. Therefore, the use of HD is only reasonable in cases of prometryn poisoning with refractory metabolic acidosis.

***Antidotes.*** No antidotes are available for the treatment of triazine herbicide poisoning.

# 83 INSECTICIDES: ORGANIC PHOSPHORUS COMPOUNDS AND CARBAMATES

## INTRODUCTION

Pesticide poisoning kills approximately 150,000 people each year, with anticholinesterase compounds responsible for about two-thirds of these deaths. Most deaths occur in rural Asia where intentional self-harm is common and where highly toxic organic phosphorus (OP) insecticides are still widely used. Severe occupational or unintentional poisoning also happens where these highly toxic insecticides are used, but deaths are generally less common. A further threat is the terrorist use of OP insecticides such as parathion to poison a water supply or flour used in bread baking.

## HISTORY AND EPIDEMIOLOGY

The first potent organic phosphorus (OP) anticholinesterase was synthesized by Clermont in 1854. In 1932, Lange and Krueger wrote of choking and blurred vision following inhalation of dimethyl and diethyl phosphorofluoridates. Their account inspired Schrader in Germany to begin investigating these compounds, initially as pesticides, and later as warfare agents (Chap. 98). Carbamates were first identified by Western scientists in the 19th century when the use of the Calabar bean (*Physostigma venenosum*) was recognized in tribal cultural practice in West Africa.

Although the term *organophosphate* is often used in both clinical practice and literature to refer to all phosphorus-containing pesticides that inhibit cholinesterase, phosphates are compounds in which the phosphorus atom is surrounded by four oxygen atoms, which is not the case for most OP compounds. Some chemicals, such as parathion, contain thioesters, whereas others are vinyl esters. Those cholinesterase-inhibiting (anticholinesterase) insecticides that contain phosphorus are collectively termed *organic phosphorus* compounds in this chapter. Those that contain the OC=ON linkage are termed carbamates. Anticholinesterase pesticides are broadly grouped according to their toxicity by the World Health Organization (WHO) (Table 83–1).

The case fatality for OP and carbamate poisoning varies according to the insecticides used in local agriculture (and therefore taken for self-harm) and the healthcare services available. Where fast-acting, highly toxic pesticides are used for self-harm, deaths will occur before patients present to hospital. Hospital-based data therefore will have a falsely low case fatality, although often still high at 10% to 30%. Although still a major clinical problem in resource-poor regions of the world, the current annual estimate of at least 100,000 deaths is substantially less than previous estimate from the 1990s to 2000s of 200,000 per year. As the most toxic WHO Toxicity Class 1a and 1b insecticides are gradually being withdrawn from agriculture across the world, the case fatality for OP and carbamate pesticide poisoning is declining.

**TABLE 83–1 WHO Classification of Pesticide Toxicity**

| | | $LD_{50}$ for the rat (mg/kg body weight) | | | |
|---|---|---|---|---|---|
| | | Oral | | Dermal | |
| | Class | Solids | Liquids | Solids | Liquids |
| Ia | Extremely hazardous | ≤ 5 | ≤ 20 | ≤ 10 | ≤ 40 |
| Ib | Highly hazardous | 5–50 | 20–200 | 10–100 | 40–400 |
| II | Moderately hazardous | 50–500 | 200–2,000 | 100–1,000 | 400–4,000 |
| III | Slightly hazardous | > 500 | > 2,000 | > 1,000 | > 4,000 |

## PHARMACOLOGY

### Organic Phosphorus Compounds

Organic phosphorus compound poisoning results in a rise in the concentration of acetylcholine (ACh) at muscarinic and nicotinic cholinergic synapses, which, in turn, leads to the syndrome of cholinergic excess. Figure 83–1 shows the basic formula for cholinesterase-inhibiting OP compounds. The "X" or "leaving group" provides a means of classifying OP insecticides into four main groups (Table 83–2). Direct-acting OP compounds (oxons) inhibit acetylcholinesterase (AChE) without needing to be metabolized in the body. However, many pesticides, such as parathion and malathion, are indirect inhibitors (prodrugs or thions) requiring partial metabolism (to paraoxon and malaoxon, respectively) within the body to become active. Desulfuration to the oxon occurs in the intestinal mucosa and liver following absorption.

The OPs bind to a hydroxyl group at the active site deep inside a cleft in the AChE enzyme. As the leaving group of the OP insecticide is split off by AChE, a stable but reversible bond results between the remaining substituted phosphorus of the OP and AChE, effectively inactivating the enzyme (Figs. 83–2 and 83–3).

### Carbamates

Carbamate insecticides are *N*-methyl carbamates derived from carbamic acid (Fig. 83–4). When exposed to carbamates, AChE undergoes carbamylation in a manner similar to phosphorylation by OP compounds, allowing ACh to accumulate in synapses. However, aging does not occur, and the carbamate–AChE bond hydrolyzes spontaneously, reactivating the enzyme. As such, the duration of cholinergic symptoms in carbamate poisoning is generally less than 24 hours.

$$R_2-\overset{\overset{R_1}{|}}{\underset{\underset{X}{|}}{P}}=O \text{ (or S)}$$

FIGURE 83–1. General structure of organic phosphorus compounds. X represents the leaving group. $R_1$ and $R_2$ may be aromatic or aliphatic groups that can be identical.

**TABLE 83–2** The Classification of Organic Phosphorus Compounds by Groups, Showing Leaving Groups and Examples of Each Group

| Classification | Example |
|---|---|
| Group 1–phosphorylcholines<br>Leaving group: substituted quaternary nitrogen<br>Echothiophate iodide | 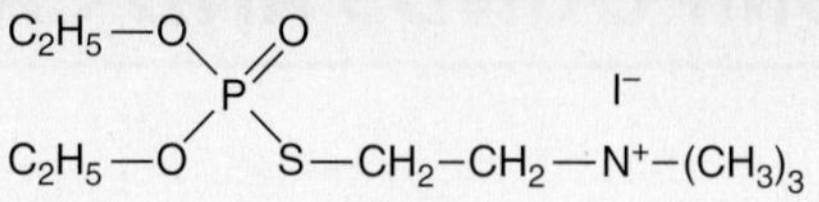 Echothiophate iodide: $(C_2H_5-O)_2P(=O)-S-CH_2-CH_2-N^+-(CH_3)_3\ I^-$ |
| Group 2–fluorophosphates<br>Leaving group: fluoride<br>Dimefox, sarin, mipafox | 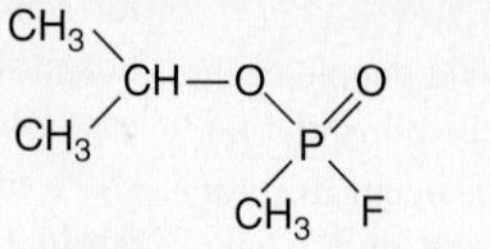 Sarin: $(CH_3)_2CH-O-P(=O)(CH_3)F$ |
| Group 3–cyanophosphates, other halophosphates<br>Leaving group: CN, SCN, OCN, halogen other than fluoride<br>Tabun | 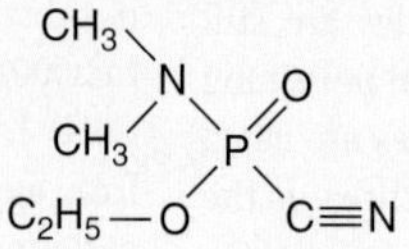 Tabun: $(CH_3)_2N-P(=O)(O-C_2H_5)C{\equiv}N$ |
| Group 4–multiple constituents<br>Leaving group:<br>Dimethoxy<br>Azinphos-menthyl, bromophos, chlorothion, crotoxyphos, dicapthon, dichlorvos, dicrotophos, dimethoate, fenthion, malathion, mevinphos, parathion-methyl, phosphamidon, temephos, trichlorfon<br>Diethoxy<br>Carbophenothion, chlorfenvinphos, chlorpyriphos, coumaphos, demeton, diazinon, dioxathion, disulfoton, ethion, methosfolan, parathion, phorate, phosfolan, TEPP<br>Other dialkoxy<br>Isopropyl paraoxon, isopropyl parathion<br>Diamino<br>Schradan<br>Chlorinated and other substituted dialkoxy<br>Haloxon<br>Trithioalkyl<br>Merphos<br>Triphenyl and substituted triphenyl<br>Triorthocresyl phosphate (TOCP)<br>Mixed substituent<br>Crufomate, cyanofenphos | Parathion: $(C_2H_5-O)_2P(=S)-O-C_6H_4-NO_2$<br>Triorthocresyl phosphate: $O=P(O-C_6H_4-CH_3)_3$ |

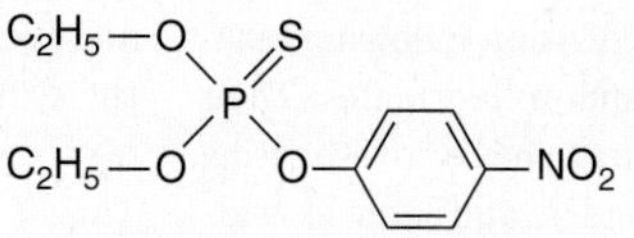

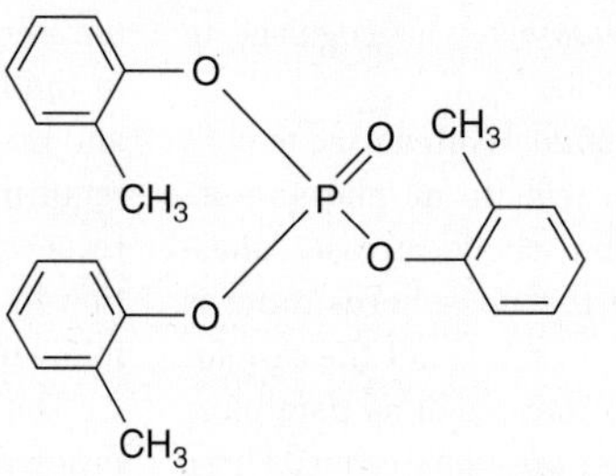

## PHARMACOKINETICS AND TOXICOKINETICS

### Organic Phosphorus Compounds

Organic phosphorus compounds are well absorbed from the lungs, gastrointestinal tract, mucous membranes, and conjunctiva following inhalation, ingestion, or topical contact. Although absorption through intact skin appears to be relatively low, percutaneous exposure to highly toxic compounds can cause severe toxicity. The presence of broken skin, dermatitis, and higher environmental temperatures further enhances cutaneous absorption.

The time to peak plasma concentration (Cmax) after self-poisoning is unknown. Human volunteer studies, using very low doses of chlorpyrifos, found Cmax to be around 6 hours after ingestion. However, patients ingesting large amounts of oxon or fast-acting thion OPs often become symptomatic within minutes, suggesting that absorption is rapid. In addition, the chlorpyrifos study was performed with pure chlorpyrifos, not the formulated agricultural pesticide with

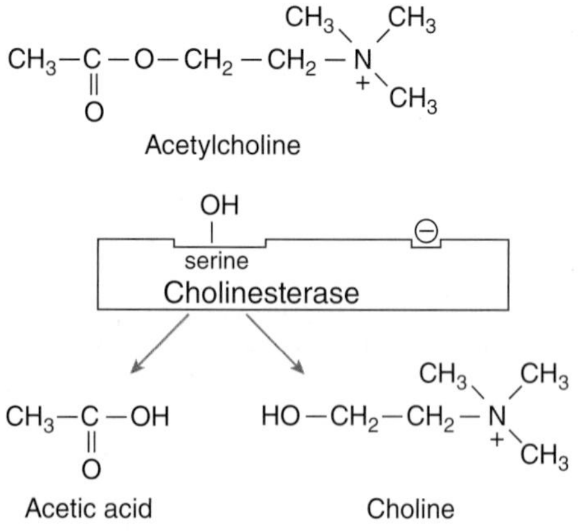

**FIGURE 83–2.** Normal metabolism of acetylcholine by acetylcholinesterase to choline and acetic acid.

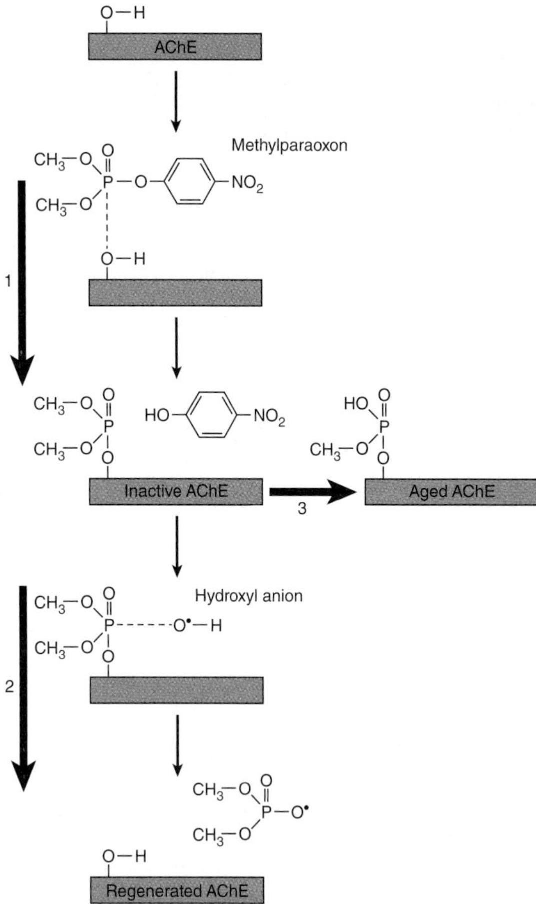


**FIGURE 83–3.** Mechanism of inhibition of acetylcholinesterase by an organic phosphorus compound. A dimethylated organic phosphorus pesticide (eg, methylparaoxon) inhibits AChE function by phosphorylating the serine hydroxyl group at the active site of the enzyme (reaction 1). This reaction occurs very quickly. Active AChE is subsequently regenerated by a hydroxyl ion attacking the acetylated serine residue, removing the phosphate moiety, and releasing active enzyme (reaction 2). This regenerative process, however, is much slower than inhibition, requiring hours to days to occur (spontaneous reactivation $t_{1/2}$ ~0.7 hours for dimethyl and 30 hours for diethyl compounds). While in the inactive state, the enzyme is prone to "aging" (reaction 3) in which one alkyl side chain of the phosphoryl moiety is removed nonenzymatically, leaving a hydroxyl group in its place. Aged AChE can no longer react with water and regeneration no longer occurs. This reaction occurs considerably faster with enzymes that are inhibited by dimethylated pesticides ($t_{1/2}$ ~3.3 hours) than those inhibited by diethylated pesticides ($t_{1/2}$ ~30 hours). The slower the regenerative process, the greater the quantity of inactive AChE available for aging. Pralidoxime catalyzes the regeneration of active acetylcholinesterase by exerting a nucleophilic attack on the phosphoryl group, transferring it from the enzyme to itself. By speeding up reaction 2, it reduces the quantity of inactive AChE available for aging. However, because aging occurs more rapidly with dimethylated OP compounds, pralidoxime is only useful before about 12 hours with dimethylated enzyme. *(Reproduced with permission from Eddleston M, Szinicz L, Eyer P, et al. Oximes in acute organophosphorus pesticide poisoning: a systematic review of clinical trials. QJM. 2002;95(5):275-283.)*

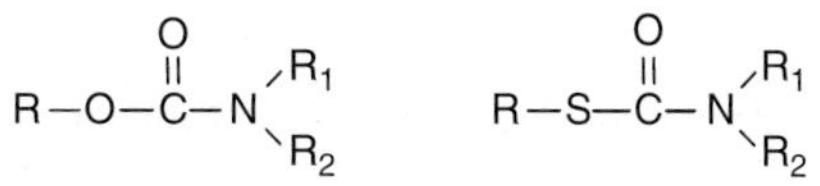

$R{-}O{-}C({=}O){-}N(R_1)(R_2)$    $R{-}S{-}C({=}O){-}N(R_1)(R_2)$

**FIGURE 83–4.** General structure of carbamate insecticides.

solvents and surfactants that would be ingested for self-harm. These solvents potentially change the toxicokinetics of the OP compound. Most OP compounds are lipophilic, with a large volume of distribution, and therefore rapidly distribute into tissue and fat, where they are protected from metabolism. Redistribution from these stores allows measurement of circulating OP compound concentrations for up to 48 days after ingestion.

Thion OPs are activated by cytochrome P450 enzymes in the liver and intestinal mucosa. Studies indicate that the activity of the human plasma enzyme paraoxonase (PON) is related to susceptibility to some acute and chronic effects of OP poisoning. Paraoxonase is an A-esterase that can hydrolyze the active (oxon) metabolites of some but not all OP insecticides. Some authors propose that genetic polymorphisms in human PON activity lead to variations in interindividual susceptibility to some OP compounds. However, the clinical relevance of these polymorphisms after poisoning is unclear.

### Carbamates

Carbamate insecticides are absorbed across skin and mucous membranes and by inhalation and ingestion. Peak cholinesterase inhibition occurred within 30 minutes of oral administration in rats. Most carbamates undergo hydrolysis, hydroxylation, and conjugation in the liver and intestinal wall, with 90% excreted in the urine within 3 to 4 days.

## PATHOPHYSIOLOGY

### Cholinesterase Inhibition

Acetylcholine is a neurotransmitter found throughout the nervous system (Fig. 83–5). Organic phosphorus and carbamate compounds are inhibitors of carboxylic ester hydrolases within the body, including acetylcholinesterase (AChE, EC 3.1.1.7), butyrylcholinesterase (plasma or pseudocholinesterase, BuChE, EC 3.1.1.8), plasma and hepatic carboxylesterases (aliesterases), paraoxonases (A-esterases), chymotrypsin, and other nonspecific proteases.

Under normal circumstances, virtually all ACh released by the axon is hydrolyzed rapidly, with choline undergoing reuptake into the presynaptic terminal where it is reused to synthesize ACh. Acetylcholinesterase is found in human nervous tissue and skeletal muscle, and on erythrocyte (ie, red blood cell {RBC}) cell membranes. Inhibition of AChE at synapses is generally thought to account for all, or the majority, of clinical features of both OP and carbamate compound poisoning.

### Effect of Coformulants and Alcohol

Patients who drink agricultural pesticides in self-harm actually ingest formulated pesticides rather than the pure anticholinesterase "active ingredient" (AI). Organic phosphorus compounds sold for agricultural use are typically emulsifiable concentrates (EC) in which the AI (eg, dimethoate) is mixed with an organic solvent such as xylene or cyclohexanone and a surfactant/emulsifier. These compounds used for coformulation are highly variable, and as a result, coformulants often differ between the same OP produced by two companies, and for different OPs produced by one company. The clinical

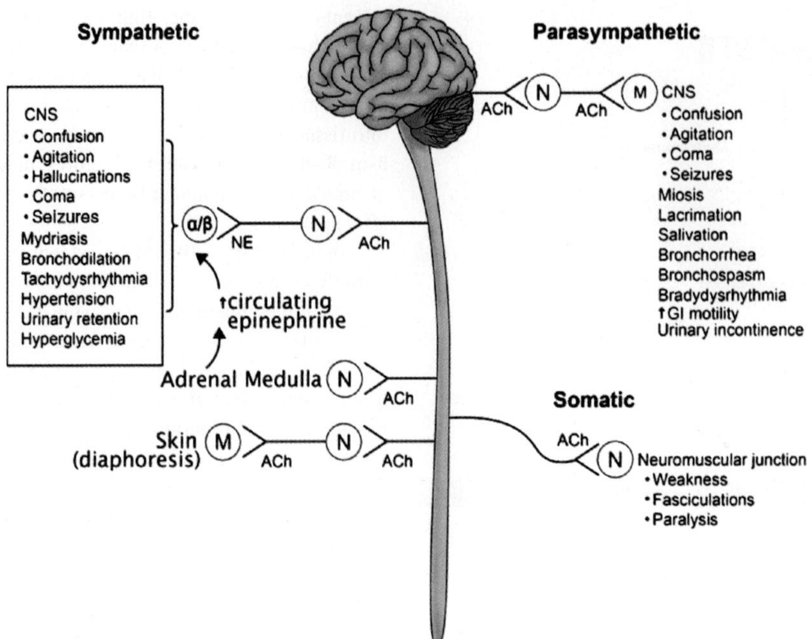


**FIGURE 83–5.** Pathophysiology of cholinergic syndrome as it affects the autonomic and somatic nervous systems.

effect of self-poisoning with these coformulants, in addition to the carbamate or OP AI, is not yet clear. One major effect of the solvent/surfactant occurs after aspiration. Ingestion of large quantities of OPs or carbamates causes rapid loss of consciousness and respiratory arrest, increasing the risk of aspiration with pesticide AI, solvent, surfactant, and gastric contents.

Pesticides are frequently coingested with ethanol, raising questions about the effect of the alcohol on outcome after OP poisoning. In one study, high ethanol blood concentrations were associated with high dimethoate concentrations, suggesting that inebriation caused people to drink larger amounts of pesticide, worsening outcome due to the direct toxic effects of the pesticide rather than a complication of ethanol.

## CLINICAL MANIFESTATIONS

Clinical manifestations vary according to the particular OP insecticide involved, the dose and route of exposure, and the time since exposure. Features are classified as acute (usually less than 24 hours), delayed (from 24 hours to 2 weeks), and late (after 2 weeks).

### Acute Toxicity—Organic Phosphorus Compounds

Clinical findings of acute toxicity from OPs derive from excessive stimulation of muscarinic and nicotinic cholinergic receptors by ACh in the central and autonomic nervous systems and at skeletal neuromuscular junctions (Fig. 83–5). The typical patient with severe OP poisoning is one who is unresponsive, with pinpoint pupils, muscle fasciculations, diaphoresis, emesis, diarrhea, salivation, lacrimation, urinary incontinence, and (after self-poisoning) an odor of garlic or solvents.

***Timing of Clinical Features.*** The timing of onset of symptoms varies according to the route, the degree of exposure, and the particular OP involved. This is important because more rapid onset of poisoning will reduce the likelihood of the patient reaching health care safely, before onset of respiratory failure or of complications such as aspiration. Out-of-hospital cardiorespiratory arrest in most parts of the world will result in the patient's death. Some patients ingesting large quantities of concentrated agricultural formulations become symptomatic as soon as 5 minutes following ingestion. Most patients with acute poisoning become symptomatic within a few hours of exposure, and practically all who will become ill show some features within 24 hours. In contrast, patients ingesting thions that are slowly converted to active oxons (such as fenthion) often do not show symptoms for hours.

Symptoms following OP exposure last for variable lengths of time, again based on the compound and the circumstances of the poisoning. For example, highly lipophilic compounds, such as dichlofenthion or fenthion, cause recurrent cholinergic effects for many days in some patients following oral ingestion as they are released from fat stores.

***Clinical Features.*** Patients usually present awake and alert, complaining of anxiety, restlessness, insomnia, headache, dizziness, blurred vision, depression, tremors, and/or other nonspecific symptoms. In moderate-severe poisoning, the level of consciousness then deteriorates rapidly to confusion, lethargy, and coma. Where careful observational studies have been done, convulsions appear to be uncommon in adult OP pesticide poisoning compared to OP nerve agent poisoning. The convulsions are likely due to hypoxia.

The effects of excessive ACh on the autonomic nervous system are variable because cholinergic receptors are found in both the sympathetic and parasympathetic nervous systems. Excessive muscarinic activity is characterized by several mnemonics, including "SLUDGE" (salivation, lacrimation, urination, defecation, gastric cramps, emesis) and "DUMBELS" (defecation, urination, miosis, bronchospasm or bronchorrhea, emesis, lacrimation, salivation). Of these, miosis is the most consistently encountered sign. Profuse bronchorrhea mimics pulmonary edema. Excessive fluid loss results in salt and water depletion. Body temperature is often low acutely, rising to normal or higher with treatment and time. Although muscarinic findings are emphasized in these mnemonics, muscarinic signs are not always clinically dramatic or initially predominant. Parasympathetic effects can be offset by excessive autonomic activity from stimulation of nicotinic adrenal receptors (resulting in catecholamine release) and postganglionic sympathetic fibers. Mydriasis, bronchodilation, and urinary retention can occur as a result of sympathetic activity.

Cardiovascular manifestations reflect mixed effects on the autonomic nervous system (including increased sympathetic tone), together with the consequences of OP-induced hypoxia and hypovolemia. Admission heart rate is usually normal, with relatively few patients showing a tachycardia greater than 100 beats/min or bradycardia less than 60 beats/min. Patients who receive atropine before admission are infrequently tachycardic. The literature is filled with reports of QT interval prolongation and ventricular dysrhythmias. However, these reports are complicated by the fact that many patients had their electrocardiogram (ECG) done before they received any atropine or were so ill that atropine was ineffective. In a case series of oxygenated and atropinized OP-poisoned patients in intensive care, QT interval prolongation was noted in nine (27.3%) of 33 patients, but in only five was the corrected QT (QTc) interval greater than 500 ms. However, bradycardia and torsade de pointes occurred after stopping atropine in five patients, suggesting that atropine had been treating a potential complication of OP poisoning.

Hypotension occurs because of stimulation of vascular receptors by excessive circulating ACh, severe volume loss, or myocardial dysfunction. Acute respiratory complications of OP poisoning (Figs. 83–6 and 83–7) include the direct pulmonary effects of bronchorrhea and bronchoconstriction, neuromuscular junction (NMJ) failure in the diaphragm and intercostal muscles, and loss of central respiratory drive. Both bronchorrhea and bronchoconstriction respond to adequate atropine therapy. Unfortunately, neither NMJ failure nor loss of central respiratory drive responds to atropine, and patients must be ventilated until respiratory function recovers. An additional early respiratory complication is hydrocarbon aspiration that may occur after ingestion of commercially formulated pesticides.

Acetylcholine stimulation of nicotinic receptors also governs skeletal muscle activity. The effects of excessive cholinergic stimulation at the NMJ are similar to those of a depolarizing neuromuscular blocker (succinylcholine) and initially result in fasciculations or weakness. Severe poisoning results in paralysis.

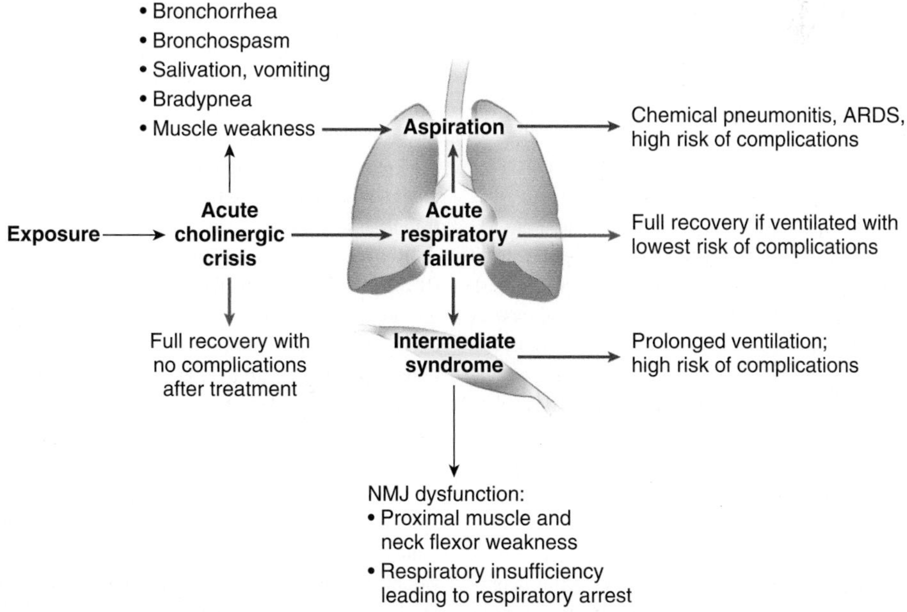


**FIGURE 83–6.** Respiratory system toxicity secondary to organic phosphorus compound poisoning. ARDS = acute respiratory distress syndrome; NMJ = neuromuscular junction.

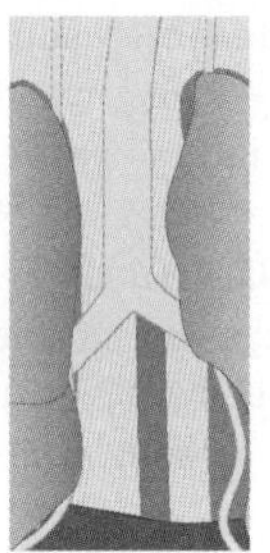


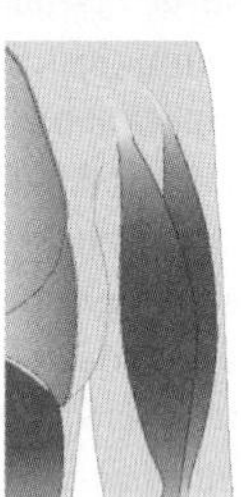


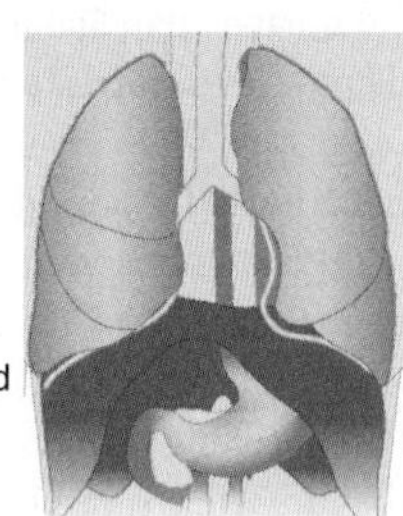


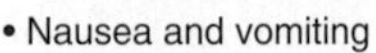


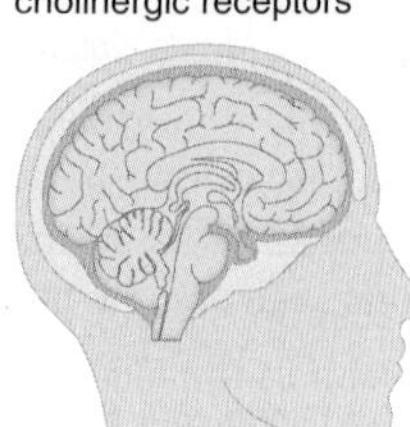


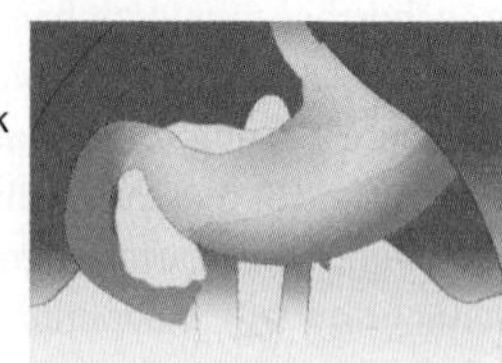


**FIGURE 83–7.** Pulmonary complications of organic phosphorus poisoning. Exposure to organic phosphorus compounds causes the acute cholinergic syndrome characterized by reduction in central respiratory drive, bronchospasm, and hypoxia due to bronchorrhea and alveolar edema, and depolarizing neuromuscular junction (NMJ) block. This can resolve or progress to acute respiratory failure. Reduced consciousness and loss of airway control increase the risk of aspiration, resulting in chemical pneumonitis that will worsen oxygenation and progress to acute respiratory distress syndrome (ARDS).

## Acute Toxicity—Carbamates

The acute effects of poisoning from carbamate insecticides are similar to those of OP insecticides. Cholinergic features tend to last for shorter durations after poisoning, often for a matter of hours, rather than days.

## Delayed Syndromes

***Neuromuscular Junction Dysfunction (Intermediate Syndrome).*** A syndrome of delayed muscle weakness without cholinergic features or fasciculations resulting in respiratory failure is called the intermediate syndrome. The syndrome is defined as occurring 24 to 96 hours after acute OP poisoning and after resolution of the cholinergic crisis. Patients develop proximal muscle weakness, especially of the neck flexors, and cranial nerve palsies, and progress to respiratory failure that lasts for up to several weeks. Consciousness is preserved unless complicated by hypoxia. The first sign is often weakness of neck flexion such that patients cannot lift their head off the bed. Although the exact pathophysiology of the syndrome is unknown, it is clearly due to NMJ dysfunction, with respiratory failure resulting from weakness affecting the diaphragm and intercostal muscles. Solvents may have a contributory role. Preservation of consciousness suggests that the central respiratory drive is not involved.

Clinical examination for proximal muscle weakness remains the most reliable means of identifying the occurrence of intermediate syndrome. Electromyograms often show tetanic fade and suggest both pre- and postsynaptic involvement. The majority of patients developing weakness do not progress to respiratory failure, indicating that intermediate syndrome is a spectrum disorder.

***Organic Phosphorus Compound–Induced Delayed Neuropathy.*** Peripheral neuropathies occur days to weeks following acute exposures, due to phosphorylation and inhibition of the enzyme neuropathy target esterase (NTE, now identified as a lysophospholipase). This enzyme catalyzes breakdown of endoplasmic reticulum-membrane phosphatidylcholine, the major phospholipid of eukaryotic cell membranes. Neuropathic OPs (such as chlorpyrifos, dichlorvos, isofenphos, methamidophos) cause a transient loss of NTE activity, putatively disrupting membrane phospholipid homeostasis, axonal transport, and glial–axonal interactions. Delayed neuropathies are not usually associated with carbamate insecticides.

Neuropathies even sometimes result from exposure to OPs that do not inhibit RBC cholinesterase or produce clinical cholinergic toxicity. The more commonly implicated chemicals include triaryl phosphates, such as triorthocresyl phosphate (TOCP), and dialkyl phosphates, such as mephosfolan, mipafox, and chlorpyrifos. Pathologic findings demonstrate effects primarily on large distal neurons, with axonal degeneration preceding demyelination.

Contaminated foods and beverages were responsible for epidemics of OP compound–induced delayed polyneuropathies and encephalopathy. In the 1930s, thousands of individuals in the United States became weak or paralyzed after drinking an illegal alcohol supplement containing TOCP—an outbreak nicknamed "Ginger Jake paralysis." Vague distal muscle weakness and pain are often the presenting symptoms and progress to paralysis. The administration of atropine or pralidoxime does not alter the onset and clinical course of these symptoms. Recovery of these patients is variable and occurs over months to years, with residual deficits common.

### Behavioral Toxicity

Behavioral changes also occur after acute or chronic exposure to OP compounds. Signs and symptoms include confusion, psychosis, anxiety, drowsiness, depression, fatigue, and irritability. Electroencephalographic changes last for weeks in some cases. Although multiple small studies have shown some effect, thus far there is no clear evidence for neuropsychiatric deficits resulting from subclinical exposure to OPs.

### Chronic Toxicity

Chronic exposure most commonly occurs in workers who have regular contact with OPs, but also occurs in individuals who have repeated contact with insecticides in their living environment. Studies link the onset of Parkinson disease with chronic exposure to pesticides including OP compounds. Overall, the studies have been retrospective in nature and confounded by recall bias. However, one case–control study using a geographic information system–based exposure assessment tool to estimate ambient exposure to OPs in central California found an adjusted odds ratio of 2.24 (95% confidence interval, 1.58–3.19).

## DIAGNOSTIC TESTING

### Organic Phosphorus Compounds

When faced with a patient in cholinergic crisis who presents with a history of acute exposure to an OP cholinesterase inhibitor insecticide, the diagnosis is straightforward. Although there are a variety of clinical signs for the cholinergic crisis (eg, DUMBELS, SLUD), most patients with significant poisoning are simply identified by the presence of pinpoint pupils, excessive sweat, and breathing difficulty. However, when the history is unreliable or does not suggest poisoning, the clinician must turn to other means to confirm the diagnosis of OP or carbamate poisoning. However, treatment of an ill patient with a cholinergic syndrome should not await confirmation of the diagnosis.

The most appropriate laboratory tests for confirming cholinesterase inhibition by insecticides are tests that measure (1) specific insecticides and active metabolites in biologic tissues and (2) cholinesterase activity in plasma or blood. Unfortunately, although urine and serum assays for OP compounds and their metabolites are available, such testing is rarely obtainable within hours. Moreover, toxic concentrations are not established for most compounds. Currently, therefore, verifying cholinesterase inhibitor poisoning relies on measurement of cholinesterase activity.

*Cholinesterase Activity.* The two cholinesterases commonly measured are butyrylcholinesterase (BuChE, plasma cholinesterase, EC 3.1.1.8) and RBC acetylcholinesterase (AChE, EC 3.1.1.7). The former is produced by the liver and then secreted into the blood, where it metabolizes xenobiotics, such as succinylcholine and cocaine. Red blood cell AChE is expressed from the same gene as the enzyme found in neuronal synapses. The main difference is in their mechanism of membrane attachment. Inhibition of either RBC AChE or BuChE only serves as a marker for cholinesterase inhibitor poisoning, because inhibition of these enzymes specifically does not contribute to signs and symptoms of poisoning. After a significant exposure, BuChE activity usually decreases first, followed by a decrease in RBC AChE activity. The sequence is highly variable, but by the time patients present with acute symptoms, activities of both cholinesterases have usually decreased well below baseline values.

*Butyrylcholinesterase.* Butyrylcholinesterase activity usually recovers before RBC AChE activity, returning to normal within a few days after a mild exposure. The wide normal range of BuChE activity allows for patients with high-normal values to suffer significant decreases in activity, yet still register near normal BuChE activity on assay. Additionally, day-to-day variation in the activity of this enzyme in healthy individuals may be as high as 20%. Furthermore, because BuChE inhibition varies between OPs and does not cause clinical effects, an admission value by itself is of little value in predicting outcome.

*Red Blood Cell Acetylcholinesterase.* Red blood cell AChE activity is thought to more accurately reflect nervous tissue AChE activity than plasma BuChE, with greater than 50% required for clinical features. Acutely, for some OPs, RBC AChE activity correlates closely with nervous system AChE activity, with NMJ dysfunction associated with greater than 70% inhibition. However, this is not always the case. After poisoning, and in the absence of oximes, RBC AChE takes many weeks to recover because erythrocytes in circulation at the time of OP exposure must be replaced. An average of 66 days is necessary for RBC AChE activity to recover following severe inhibition, and activity may take up to 100 days to return to normal. Decreased RBC AChE activity also results from exposures or conditions other than OP or carbamate poisoning, for example, pernicious anemia and during therapy with antimalarial or antidepressant medicines (Table 83–3).

### Carbamates

Carbamates inhibit neuronal AChE, RBC AChE, and BuChE. The relative ease with which spontaneous decarbamylation of AChE takes place results in the measurement of relatively normal RBC AChE activity despite severe cholinergic symptoms if the assay is not performed within several hours of sampling.

### Atropine Challenge

An atropine challenge (administration of 0.6–1 mg of atropine to test for cholinergic features responsive to atropine) was once commonly recommended. However, there are no studies of the sensitivity and specificity of the test or of its predictive values. Patients with substantial poisoning will show no response to the small dose of atropine; in contrast, patients with either mild poisoning or no poisoning will develop antimuscarinic features. In the light of this lack of clarity on usefulness, we recommend against this approach to diagnosis.

### Differential Diagnosis

The differential diagnosis for cholinergic poisoning includes three main categories (Table 83–4).

**TABLE 83–3 Interpreting Cholinesterase Activity Values**

| | *Red Blood Cell Acetylcholinesterase* | *Butyrylcholinesterase* |
|---|---|---|
| Advantage | Better reflection of synaptic inhibition | Easier to assay, declines faster |
| Site | RBC | CNS white matter, plasma, liver, pancreas, heart |
| Regeneration (untreated) | 1% per day | 25%–30% in the first 7–10 days |
| Normalization (untreated with oxime) | 35–100 days | 28–42 days |
| Use | Unsuspected prior exposure with normal butyrylcholinesterase | Acute exposure |
| Clinical false depression | Pernicious anemia, hemoglobinopathies, antimalarial treatment, oxalate blood tubes | Liver dysfunction, malnutrition, hypersensitivity reactions, drugs (succinylcholine, codeine, morphine), pregnancy or deficiency |

CNS = central nervous system; RBC = red blood cell.

## MANAGEMENT

### Organic Phosphorus Compounds

The primary cause of death after anticholinesterase poisoning is respiratory failure and hypoxemia. This results from muscarinic effects on the cardiovascular and pulmonary systems (bronchospasm, bronchorrhea, aspiration, bradydysrhythmias, or hypotension), nicotinic effects on skeletal muscles (weakness and paralysis), loss of central respiratory drive, and rarely seizures (Figs. 83–6 and 83–7). Therefore, initial treatment for a patient exposed to OP compounds should be directed at ensuring an adequate airway and ventilation and at stabilizing cardiorespiratory function by reversing excessive muscarinic effects. Seizures not secondary to hypoxemia should be treated with a standard benzodiazepine antiepileptic.

**TABLE 83–4 Categories of Cholinergic Poisoning**

- Cholinesterase inhibitors
  - Organic phosphorus insecticides
  - Organic phosphorus ophthalmic medications
  - Carbamate insecticides
  - Carbamate medications
- Cholinomimetics
  - Pilocarpine
  - Carbachol
  - Aceclidine
  - Methacholine
  - Bethanechol
  - Muscarine-containing mushrooms
- Nicotine alkaloids
  - Coniine
  - Lobeline
  - Nicotine

Maintenance of the patient's airway should be ensured by early endotracheal intubation and positive-pressure ventilation in patients who are comatose, have significant weakness, or are unable to handle copious secretions. Only a neuromuscular blocker that is not primarily metabolized by cholinesterases should be used to induce pharmacologic paralysis if needed. The duration of action of succinylcholine and mivacurium will be prolonged in the presence of low BuChE activity, causing paralysis lasting for several hours.

***Antimuscarinic Therapy.*** Excessive muscarinic activity should be controlled at the same time as resuscitation to aid respiration and oxygenation. The muscarinic antagonist atropine competitively blocks ACh at muscarinic receptors to reverse excessive secretions, miosis, bronchospasm, vomiting, diarrhea, diaphoresis, and urinary incontinence. For adolescents and adults, an intravenous loading bolus of between 1 and 2 mg (depending on the severity of symptoms) is recommended; doses for children should start at 0.05 mg/kg up to adult doses. Doses should be titrated against effect, individualizing therapy for the patient. The most rapid method of controlling excessive cholinergic activity is to give doubling doses every 3 to 5 minutes if the response to the previous dose is inadequate. Atropine dosing should aim to reverse bronchorrhea and bronchospasm and to provide adequate blood pressure and heart rate for tissue oxygenation (eg, systolic blood pressure > 90 mm Hg and heart rate > 80 beats/min). All variables are easily and rapidly assessed. Once atropinization occurs, an infusion of atropine is recommended initially giving 10% to 20% of the total loading dose per hour (usually maximum 2 mg/h). Regular checks for signs of under- or overatropinization should guide the use of further boluses followed by changes in the infusion rate or discontinuation of the infusion.

The presence of marked tachycardia (> 120–140 beats/min in a well-hydrated patient not withdrawing from alcohol), mydriasis, absent bowel sounds, and urinary retention after atropine administration indicates over-atropinization or atropine toxicity. This is unnecessary and possibly dangerous because of associated hyperthermia, confusion, and agitation. However, tachycardia is not an absolute contraindication to atropine therapy because it can result from hypoxia, hypovolemia, aspiration pneumonitis, or agitation.

Atropine does not reverse nicotinic effects. Therefore, patients who improve after receiving atropine should be closely monitored in a critical care setting for impending respiratory failure from delayed NMJ dysfunction (Antidotes in Brief: A35).

### Oximes

Phosphorylated AChE undergoes hydrolytic regeneration at a very slow rate. However, this process can be enhanced by using an oxime such as pralidoxime chloride (2-PAM) or obidoxime (Fig. 83–3). Regeneration of AChE lowers ACh concentrations, improving both muscarinic and nicotinic effects. An immediate rise in RBC AChE activity, hopefully paralleling a rise in neuronal AChE activity, occurs after effective administration of oximes. Since phosphorylated AChE becomes aged, and therefore unresponsive to oximes, therapy is recommended early, within 3 to 4 hours of exposure, after dimethoxy OP poisoning. In contrast, oximes can still be highly efficacious 48 hours after diethoxy OP poisoning, with some effect even when given several days after exposure. We recommend an intravenous loading dose of pralidoxime chloride of 30 mg/kg (up to 2 g) over 15 to 30 minutes. This is followed by a maintenance infusion of 8 to 10 mg/kg/h (up to 650 mg/h) in adults and 10 to 20 mg/kg/h (up to 650 mg/h) in children (Antidotes in Brief: A36).

### Benzodiazepines

Animal studies demonstrate that administering benzodiazepines along with oximes in the treatment of poisoning with OP nerve agents or the insecticide dichlorvos increases survival and decreases the incidence of seizures and neuropathy. However, seizures are uncommon in large case series of patients poisoned by OP insecticides, and no clinical studies have been performed yet to determine whether benzodiazepines offer benefit to humans. In the absence of this evidence, benzodiazepines should be used to treat OP-related seizures and agitation and to aid intubation, but should not be given routinely to all cases.

### Other Drug Treatments

The therapies discussed above affect only limited mechanisms involved in OP poisoning. Multiple additional therapies have been tested in animals, but none have been shown to be beneficial in large clinical trials and none are used widely in clinical practice. Treatments that have been proposed include magnesium or clonidine to reduce presynaptic acetylcholine release, fresh-frozen plasma as a source of BuChE for scavenging OP pesticides, and sodium bicarbonate. Lipid emulsions have also been suggested because of the high lipid solubility of most OP insecticides and their solvents; however, an in vitro study suggested that the lipid actually stabilizes the OP from degradation. More definitive studies are required; none of these therapies are currently recommended for anticholinesterase poisoning.

### Decontamination

Cutaneous absorption of OP pesticides and carbamates requires removal of all clothing as soon as possible after resuscitation and administration of atropine and oxygen. Medical personnel should avoid self-contamination by wearing neoprene or nitrile gloves. Skin should be triple-washed with water, soap, and water, and rinsed again with water. Cutaneous absorption also results from contact with OP and carbamate compounds in vomitus and diarrhea if the initial exposure was by ingestion. Exposed leather clothing or products should be discarded because decontamination is very difficult once impregnation has occurred.

In potentially life-threatening acute ingestions, if emesis has not occurred, the patient presents within 2 hours, and the airway can be protected, the stomach contents should be evacuated by lavage using a nasogastric tube. Although there are data suggesting that activated charcoal adsorbs some OP insecticides, a study of Sri Lankan patients with OP or carbamate poisoning found no clear benefit from the use of multiple-dose activated charcoal. For patients with anticholinesterase poisoning in whom the airway can be protected, we recommend a single dose of 1 g/kg activated charcoal.

Healthcare providers must always maintain caution when coming into contact with stomach contents or other body fluids when managing these cases. Bystanders were poisoned by providing mouth-to-mouth resuscitation to a victim of an intentional ingestion of diazinon. Clinical experience from South Asia suggests that nosocomial poisoning with OP pesticides is unlikely as long as standard universal precautions are followed.

### Extracorporeal Elimination

Hemodialysis and/or hemoperfusion are sometimes recommended for OP and carbamate insecticide–poisoned patients, particularly in East Asia. However, at present, there are insufficient data to recommend extracorporeal purification for anticholinesterase insecticide poisoning.

### Disposition

After atropinization, patients with cholinesterase inhibitor poisoning should be carefully and frequently observed for evidence of (1) deteriorating neurologic function and potential paralysis and (2) need for an increase or reduction in atropine dosing. Cholinesterase activities can be measured to monitor their recovery. However, clinical assessment is a more reliable marker of recovery because cholinesterase activities are often substantially reduced for many days after poisoning. We do not recommend using cholinesterase activities to make decisions on discharge. It is reasonable to discharge a patient who becomes asymptomatic and has not required atropine for 1 to 2 days. Although recurrent cholinergic crises and/or respiratory failure can occur after several days, such patients have usually previously shown clinical signs of toxicity. Patients should not be allowed to go home wearing clothing that was worn when the poisoning occurred.

### Carbamates

The treatment of patients with carbamate insecticide poisoning is similar to treatment of patients with OP poisoning. Urgent resuscitation and titrated dosing of atropine should be performed for all patients. The efficacy of oximes for carbamate poisoning is unclear. Fortunately, because of the rapid hydrolysis of the carbamate-AChE complex (see above), symptoms, including weakness and paralysis, usually resolve within 24 to 48 hours without oxime therapy. We do not recommend the routine administration of oximes to patients poisoned by carbamate insecticides. However, administering pralidoxime to a poisoned patient in a cholinergic crisis is appropriate when it is not known whether the patient is suffering from OP or carbamate pesticide poisoning.

# A35 ATROPINE

## INTRODUCTION

Atropine is a competitive antagonist at both central and peripheral muscarinic receptors that is used to treat patients with signs and symptoms from muscarinic agonists and acetylcholinesterase inhibitors such as organic phosphorus pesticides.

## HISTORY

Many plants such as *Atropa belladonna* contain the tropane alkaloids atropine and/or scopolamine. In the early 1800s, atropine was isolated and purified from these plants. In the 1860s, Fraser experimented with the dose–response relationship between atropine and physostigmine in various organs such as the heart and the eye. Experiments in the 1940s with cholinesterase inhibitors demonstrated that atropine reversed many of the effects of physostigmine and protected animals against doses 2 to 3 times the dose necessary to kill 50% of the animals ($LD_{50}$).

## PHARMACOLOGY

### Chemistry

Atropine (DL-hyoscyamine), like scopolamine (L-hyoscine), is a tropane alkaloid with a tertiary amine structure that allows central nervous system (CNS) penetration. Quaternary amine antimuscarinic agents, such as glycopyrrolate, and ipratropium do not cross the blood–brain barrier into the CNS.

### Mechanism of Action

Cholinergic receptors consist of muscarinic and nicotinic subtypes. Muscarinic receptors are widely distributed throughout the peripheral and central nervous systems. Cholinesterase inhibitors prevent the breakdown of acetylcholine by acetylcholinesterase, thereby increasing the amount of acetylcholine available to stimulate cholinergic receptors at both muscarinic and nicotinic subtypes, although the degree of effect varies widely among the class. Atropine is a competitive antagonist of acetylcholine only at muscarinic receptors and not nicotinic receptors.

### Pharmacokinetics and Pharmacodynamics

Atropine is absorbed rapidly from most routes of administration, including inhalation, oral, and intramuscular (IM). Ingestion of 1 mg of atropine produces maximal effects on heart rate and on salivary secretions at 1 and 3 hours, respectively, and lasts from 12 to 24 hours. The apparent volume of distribution ($V_d$) is about 2 to 2.6 L/kg. The serum concentrations of atropine are similar at 1 hour following either 1 mg intravenously (IV) or IM in adults. The elimination half-life is 6.5 hours. One investigation of the oral bioavailability of atropine eye drops in healthy adults revealed, on average, 65% systemic absorption, but with a wide individual variability. The time to maximum serum concentration was 30 minutes and the elimination half-life was 2.5 hours. Given the short supply of parenteral atropine during a mass casualty event, atropine eye drops may prove to be a useful substitute. Following inhalation, the time to peak atropine concentration of atropine averaged 1.3 hours, and thus inhaled atropine is not recommended for poisoning emergencies.

## ROLE IN ORGANIC PHOSPHORUS AND CARBAMATE TOXICITY

Atropine is recommended as the first line in therapy for the muscarinic effects of organic phosphorus and carbamate toxicity, which prevents patients from drowning in their own secretions. The benefits of adding pralidoxime to atropine were noted in the 1950s, and in the 1960s, pralidoxime was established as a standard antidote in addition to atropine for these xenobiotics (Antidotes in Brief: A36).

## ADVERSE EFFECTS AND SAFETY ISSUES

When too much atropine is administered, the patient demonstrates classic signs of peripheral antimuscarinic toxicity: hot, dry, flushed skin, urinary retention, absent bowel sounds, tachycardia, mydriasis, and central antimuscarinic activity, including restlessness, confusion, and hallucinations or CNS depression. In the absence of a cholinergic agent, these adverse effects begin at 0.5 mg IV in the adult. However, in the presence of a muscarinic agonist or an anticholinesterase agent, the effects may not occur until many milligrams of atropine are administered. In adults, low doses (0.5 mg) of atropine sometimes cause a paradoxical bradycardia of about 4 to 8 beats/min, which does not occur with rapid IV administration.

## USE IN PREGNANCY

Atropine is classified by the United States Food and Drug Administration as Pregnancy Category C. Atropine crosses the placenta and may cause tachycardia in the near-term fetus. The American Academy of Pediatrics classifies atropine as compatible with breast feeding.

## DOSAGE AND ADMINISTRATION

The ideal dosage regimen of atropine for organic phosphorous pesticide poisoning in adults has never been studied in a randomized controlled trial. However, experience suggests that atropine should be initiated in adults in doses of 1 to 2 mg IV for mild to moderate poisoning and 3 to 5 mg IV for severe poisoning with unconsciousness. We recommend that this dose be doubled every 3 to 5 minutes as needed. The most important end point for adequate atropinization is clear lungs and the reversal of the muscarinic toxic syndrome. Once this end point has been achieved, a maintenance dose of atropine may be needed. We recommend administering 10% to 20% of the loading dose as an IV infusion every hour as a starting point with meticulous, frequent reevaluation and titration to achieve desired clinical end points while monitoring for signs of anticholinergic toxicity from excess atropine.

The IV or intraosseous starting dose of atropine in children is 0.05 mg/kg up to the adult dose. Although a minimum dose of 0.1 mg has been advocated, this dose would be toxic to infants less than 5 kg and is not recommended.

### Dosing for Chemical Weapons Nerve Agents

In a conscious adult with cholinergic effects, 2 mg of atropine IV or IM should be administered every 5 to 10 minutes until shortness of breath improves and drying of secretions occurs. Based on a limited amount of information, total doses of 2 to 4 mg of atropine are usually sufficient, which is much lower than the dose for most organic phosphorus compound exposures. Patients who are unconscious or apneic require higher total doses, usually on the order of 5 to 15 mg.

The appropriate total "Mark I Nerve Agent Antidote Kit" (NAAK) autoinjector doses of atropine for children depend on age and weight. For ages 3 to 7 (13–25 kg), one autoinjector (2 mg) of atropine is recommended; for ages 8 to 14 years, two autoinjectors (4 mg) are recommended, and for patients older than 14 years, three autoinjectors (6 mg) of atropine are recommended. In an emergency for children younger than 3 years of age, a risk-to-benefit analysis would suggest injecting one autoinjector of atropine (2 mg). We recommend that children younger than 1 year be administered one pediatric atropine autoinjector (0.5 mg if available) and children older than 1 year be administered the NAAK autoinjector as described above.

## FORMULATION AND ACQUISITION

Atropine sulfate injection (USP) is available in many different strengths, with the following concentrations in each 1-mL vial or ampule: 50 μg, 300 μg, 400 μg, 500 μg, 800 μg, and 1 mg. Atropine is also available in prefilled 5- or 10-mL syringes with a concentration of 0.1 mg/mL for adults and in 5-mL syringes with a concentration of 0.05 mg/mL for children.

The AtroPen Auto-Injector is a prefilled syringe designed for IM injection by an autoinjector into the outer thigh. It is available in four strengths: 0.25 mg, 0.5 mg (Blue Label), 1 mg (Dark Red Label), and 2 mg (Green Label). Atropine is also packaged in a kit with a second autoinjector containing 600 mg of pralidoxime in 2 mL of sterile water for injection with 40 mg of benzyl alcohol and 22.5 mg of glycine. The atropine autoinjector contains 2.1 mg of atropine. This particular combination kit is called a "Mark I NAAK" and is designed for IM use in case of a nerve agent attack. The Mark I NAAK was replaced by the DuoDote Autoinjector System and the analogous, military-designated Antidote Treatment Nerve Agent Autoinjector (ATNAA), which sequentially administers 2.1 mg of atropine in 0.7 mL followed by 600 mg of pralidoxime chloride in 2 mL IM through the same syringe. Other sources of atropine to consider in an emergency during a shortage would be atropine eye drops, which come as a 1% concentration (10 mg/mL).

# A36 PRALIDOXIME

## INTRODUCTION

Pralidoxime is the only cholinesterase-reactivating agent currently available in the United States (US). It is used concomitantly with atropine in the management of patients poisoned by organic phosphorus (OP) and carbamate pesticides. Administration should be initiated as soon as possible because of the aging associated with the organic phosphorus–cholinesterase bond, but pralidoxime may remain effective for days after an exposure depending on the speed of aging. Continuous infusion is preferable to intermittent administration for patients with serious toxicity, and a prolonged therapeutic course of several days is often required.

## HISTORY

Identification of an anionic site on acetylcholinesterase (AChE) led to the theory that a compound could be developed that would bind to this site and remove the phosphate ester, thereby reactivating AChE. In 1951, Wilson demonstrated the key concept that cholinesterases inhibited by organic phosphorus compounds could be reactivated using hydroxylamine. Several hydroxylamine derivatives were studied and led to the design of pralidoxime (2-PAM), which American and British scientists independently synthesized in 1955.

## PHARMACOLOGY

### Chemistry

Pralidoxime chloride is a quaternary pyridinium oxime with a molecular weight of 173 Da. Pralidoxime iodide has a molecular weight of 264 Da and is less water soluble than the chloride salt.

### Related Medications

Obidoxime (Toxogonin, LuH-6) is an oxime used outside the US that contains two active sites per molecule. On a molar basis, obidoxime is approximately 10 to 20 times more effective in reactivating AChE than pralidoxime. The H series of oximes (named after Hagedorn; HI-6, HIo-7) were developed to act against the chemical warfare nerve agents (Chap. 98). These oximes have superior effectiveness against sarin, VX, and certain types of newer pesticides (eg, methylfluorophosphonylcholines). Unfortunately, they are less efficacious for traditional OP insecticide poisoning, and their toxicity profile is less defined.

### Mechanism of Action

Organic phosphorus compounds are powerful inhibitors of acetylcholinesterase (AChE; true cholinesterase, found in red blood cells, nervous tissue, and skeletal muscle) and plasma cholinesterase or butyrylcholinesterase (BuChE) (found in plasma, liver, heart, pancreas, and brain). The OP binds and inactivates the esteratic site on the enzyme (Fig. 83–3). This reaction results in the accumulation of acetylcholine at muscarinic and nicotinic synapses in the peripheral and central nervous systems, leading to the clinical manifestations of OP poisoning. Following phosphorylation, the enzyme is inactivated and can undergo one of three processes; endogenous hydrolysis, reactivation by a xenobiotic such as pralidoxime, or aging, which renders it incapable of reactivation.

Pralidoxime binds to the phosphate on the OP, successfully releasing it from the AChE enzyme, and restoring enzymatic function. Pralidoxime is important at nicotinic sites where atropine is ineffective, most often typically improving muscle strength within 10 to 40 minutes after administration. Pralidoxime is also synergistic with atropine; it liberates cholinesterase enzyme so that additional acetylcholine can be metabolized, while atropine inhibits the effects of acetylcholine directly at cholinergic receptors.

## PHARMACOKINETICS AND PHARMACODYNAMICS

In volunteers, the $V_d$ is about 0.8 L/kg and the $t_{1/2}$ is 75 minutes. Pralidoxime is renally excreted, and within 12 hours, 80% of the dose is recovered unchanged in the urine. A dose of 10 mg/kg (IM or IV) to volunteers results in peak plasma concentrations of 6 μg/mL (reached 5–15 minutes after IM injection) and a plasma half-life of approximately 75 minutes. In a human volunteer study, an intravenous loading dose of 4 mg/kg over 15 minutes followed by 3.2 mg/kg/h for a total of 4 hours maintained pralidoxime serum concentrations greater than 4 μg/mL for 4 hours.

In poisoned patients receiving continuous infusions of pralidoxime, the $V_d$ was 2.77 L/kg and the $t_{1/2}$ was 3.44 hours. In poisoned children and adolescents, the $V_d$ varied with severity of poisoning from 8.8 L/kg in the severely poisoned patients to 2.8 L/kg in moderately poisoned patients. The $t_{1/2}$ was 3.6 hours.

Autoinjector administration of 600 mg of pralidoxime chloride in an adult man (9 mg/kg) produced a concentration above 4 μg/mL at 7 to 16 minutes, a maximum plasma concentration of 6.5 μg/mL at about 28 minutes, and a half-life of 2 hours. Kinetics with other autoinjectors are similar.

## ROLE IN ORGANIC PHOSPHORUS COMPOUND TOXICITY: EFFICACY RELATED TO TIME OF ADMINISTRATION AFTER POISONING

The sooner after exposure to an OP, the more likely pralidoxime is to be effective because of the reduced likelihood of aging. However, there is no absolute time limitation on reactivation function, as long as the patient remains symptomatic. Experimental studies produced wide variations in results depending on the OP tested and other variables.

## ROLE IN ORGANIC PHOSPHORUS COMPOUND TOXICITY: HUMAN TRIALS

There are four randomized clinical trials examining the efficacy of pralidoxime for the management of OP poisoning. Two trials used doses of pralidoxime now considered to be insufficient, and neither study demonstrated a benefit for pralidoxime. The third clinical trial included patients who were moderately to severely poisoned with an OP and received a 2-g loading dose of pralidoxime iodide over 30 minutes before being randomized to receive 1 g over 1 hour every 4 hours for 48 hours or a continuous infusion of 1 g/h for 48 hours. In the continuous pralidoxime infusion arm, there was a significant reduction in atropine requirements, a smaller number of patients required intubation, fewer days of intubation were needed, and a reduction in mortality was noted from 8% to 1%. A fourth trial was unable to demonstrate a beneficial effect of patients given pralidoxime versus placebo. In comparison to the third study, these patients arrived much later to care facilities (4.4 vs 2 hours) and received less concomitant supportive care interventions. These differences are likely the result of varied methodologies.

## ROLE IN CARBAMATE TOXICITY

Acetylcholinesterases inactivated by most carbamates spontaneously reactivate with half-lives of 1 to 2 hours, and typical clinical recovery occurs in several hours. However, in severe cases, cholinergic findings may persist for 24 hours. Pralidoxime is rarely indicated for patients with carbamate poisoning, but it is not contraindicated as was once suggested. In fact, there are cases reports, particularly with aldicarb, in which pralidoxime appears to improve outcome. Pralidoxime should not be withheld in a seriously poisoned patient out of concern that a cholinergic xenobiotic is a carbamate. Pralidoxime should almost always be used in conjunction with atropine. Rarely, pralidoxime has been used as the sole therapy in OP or carbamate poisoning when only nicotinic findings were present.

## ADVERSE EFFECTS AND SAFETY ISSUES

At therapeutic doses of pralidoxime in humans, adverse effects are minimal and include transient dizziness, blurred vision, and elevations in diastolic blood pressure. Rapid IV bolus administration has produced sudden cardiac and respiratory arrest as a result of laryngospasm and muscle rigidity. An important safety issue is inadvertent provider or patient contact with the "active" needle end of autoinjectors or autoinjector systems, triggering unintended administration, self-administration, needle injury, or delivery to an unintended site.

## PREGNANCY AND LACTATION

Pralidoxime is US Food and Drug Administration Pregnancy Risk Category C. The use of pralidoxime should not be withheld because of pregnancy. It is unknown whether pralidoxime is excreted into breast milk.

## DOSING AND ADMINISTRATION

The optimal dosage regimen for pralidoxime is unknown. We recommend a loading dose of pralidoxime chloride of 30 mg/kg (up to 2 g) over 15 to 30 minutes followed by a maintenance infusion of 8 to 10 mg/kg/h for adults (up to 650 mg/h) and 10 to 20 mg/kg/h for children (up to 650 mg/h). Although IV administration is preferred, IM administration is acceptable until IV access is secured. Reconstitute a 1-g vial of pralidoxime with 3 mL of sterile water or 0.9% sodium chloride for injection for IM use. Intraosseous administration is likely to be as effective or superior to IM delivery and was demonstrated to achieve excellent serum concentrations in a swine model.

For nerve agent and mass casualty exposures, one to three injections with a pair of autoinjectors containing 2.1 mg of atropine followed by 600 mg of pralidoxime chloride or one to three injections of a DuoDote autoinjector should be administered into the outer thigh and held in place for 10 seconds. The number of autoinjector doses administered to a child depends on the age and weight of the child. For children aged 3 to 7 years (13–25 kg), one autoinjector of atropine and one autoinjector of pralidoxime are recommended for administration. For children aged 8 to 14 years, two autoinjectors of atropine and two autoinjectors of pralidoxime are recommended for administration. For children older than 14 years, the adult dose is recommended. For children younger than 3 years, during an emergency, one autoinjector of atropine and one of pralidoxime may be administered in accordance with a risk-to-benefit analysis.

## DURATION OF TREATMENT

It is a reasonable approach to discontinue pralidoxime when the patient has improved and no longer requires atropine. The patient must be observed carefully for recrudescence of toxicity from a fat-soluble long-acting OP. If symptoms return, therapy with pralidoxime and atropine should be continued for at least an additional 24 hours.

## FORMULATION AND ACQUISITION

Pralidoxime chloride (Protopam) is supplied in 20-mL vials containing 1 g of powder for reconstitution. Pralidoxime chloride is also available for IM administration by an autoinjector containing 600 mg of pralidoxime and is packaged with an autoinjector containing 2.1 mg of atropine as a "Mark I Nerve Agent Antidote Kit (NAAK)." The Mark I NAAK was replaced by the DuoDote Autoinjector System and the analogous, military-designated Antidote Treatment Nerve Agent Autoinjector (ATNAA), which sequentially administers 2.1 mg of atropine followed by 600 mg of pralidoxime chloride IM through the same syringe. Pralidoxime is maintained as part of the Strategic National Stockpile (SNS) formulary in repositories in numerous locations throughout the US.

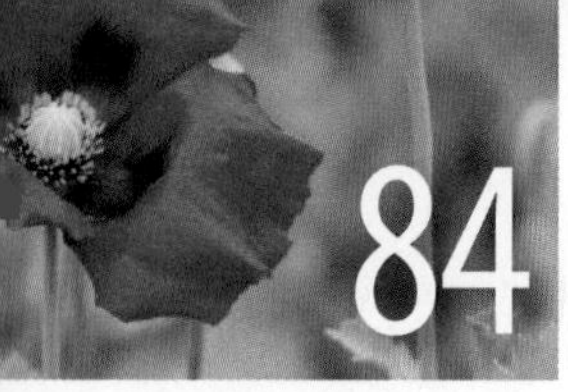

# 84 INSECTICIDES: ORGANIC CHLORINES, PYRETHRINS/PYRETHROIDS, AND INSECT REPELLENTS

## ORGANIC CHLORINE PESTICIDES

### History and Epidemiology

Paul Müller demonstrated the insecticidal properties of dichlorodiphenyltrichloroethane (DDT) in the early 1940s, and in doing so introduced the new class of organic chlorine insecticides. These insecticides were inexpensive to produce, nonvolatile, environmentally stable, and had relatively low acute toxicity when compared to previous insecticides. Most organic chlorines have a negative temperature coefficient, making them more insecticidal at lower temperatures and less toxic to warm-blooded organisms. Their widespread use from the 1940s until the mid-1970s revolutionized modern agriculture. Because of their stability, organic chlorines were used extensively in structural protection (termites, carpenter ants) and soil treatments. Medical and public health applications of DDT and its analogs were also found in the control of typhus body louse and eradication of malaria in many countries by eliminating the mosquito vector. By 1953, DDT alone was credited for saving an estimated 50 million lives and with averting one billion cases of human disease, and is credited with eliminating malaria from the United States (US) and Europe.

However, the properties that made these chemicals such effective insecticides were suspected as posing environmental hazards: they are slowly metabolized, lipid soluble, chemically stable, and environmentally persistent. Rachel Carson, a biologist with the US Fish and Wildlife Service, claimed that since organic chlorines are bioconcentrated and biomagnified up the food chain, this persistence could eventually lead to increases in cancer in the future, as well as having adverse effects on wildlife. The controversy arose when scientific opinions suggested that organic chlorine residues caused eggshell thinning and decreased reproductive success in predatory birds. Hearings before the Environmental Protection Agency (EPA) regarding DDT registration focused also on the unproven fear of placing future generations at risk of cancer. This, and the demonstration of persistent DDT residues in all humans, even those living in areas where DDT was never utilized, led to the severe restriction or total ban of DDT and most other organic chlorines in North America and Europe.

There is considerable evidence that since DDT was banned, less-effective replacements have placed many more millions at risk for malaria, and this is at least in part responsible for millions of preventable deaths from this disease. For these reasons, the World Health Organization (WHO) exempted DDT from its list of banned pesticides, and it is still widely used for malaria control programs in many countries because alternatives are more expensive and must be applied more frequently.

The organic chlorine pesticides are grouped into four categories based on their chemical structures and similar toxicities (Table 84–1).

### Toxicokinetics

***Absorption.*** All of the organic chlorine pesticides are well absorbed orally and by inhalation; transdermal absorption is variable (Table 84–1).

***Distribution.*** All organic chlorines are lipophilic, a property that allows penetration to their sites of action in insects and mammals. The fat-to-serum ratios at equilibrium are high, in the range of 660:1 for chlordane; 220:1 for lindane; and 150:1 for dieldrin. Central nervous system (CNS) redistribution of the organic chlorines to the blood and then to fat most likely accounts for the apparent rapid CNS recovery despite the persistent substantial total-body burden.

***Metabolism.*** The high lipid solubility and very slow metabolic disposition of DDT, DDE (dichlorodiphenyl dichloroethylene, the primary metabolite of DDT), dieldrin, heptachlor, chlordane, mirex, and chlordecone cause significant adipose tissue storage and increasing body burdens in chronically exposed populations. Organic chlorines that are rapidly metabolized and eliminated, such as endrin (an isomer of dieldrin), endosulfan, lindane, methoxychlor, dienochlor, chlorobenzilate, dicofol, and toxaphene tend to have less persistence in body tissues, despite being highly lipid soluble.

Most organic chlorines are metabolized by the hepatic microsomal enzyme systems by dechlorination and oxidation, with subsequent conjugation. However, for some insecticides, metabolism results in the production of a metabolite with more toxicity than the parent compound, such as heptachlor to heptachlor epoxide, chlordane to oxychlordane, and aldrin to dieldrin.

***Elimination.*** The half-lives of fat-stored compounds and poorly metabolized organic chlorines such as DDT and chlordecone are measured in months or years, compared to the elimination half-life of lindane, which is 21 hours in adults. The primary route of excretion of the organic chlorines is in the bile, but most also produce detectable urinary metabolites. However, as with other compounds excreted in bile, most of the organic chlorines, such as mirex and chlordecone, have significant enterohepatic or enteroenteric recirculation.

### Mechanisms of Toxicity

Organic chlorine insecticides affect the membranes of excitable cells by interfering with repolarization, by prolonging depolarization (both are $Na^+$ channel effects), or by impairing the maintenance of the polarized state of the neuron (γ-aminobutyric acid {$GABA_A$} chloride ionophore effects). The end result is hyperexcitability of the nervous system and repetitive neuronal discharges with subsequent inhibition of further depolarization (Fig. 84–1).

This occurs primarily in the peripheral nervous system, DDT and its analogs preferentially bind to the $Na^+$ channel when the M gate is open, allowing prolonged inward sodium

**TABLE 84–1 Classification of Organic Chlorine Pesticides**

| *Classes of Organic Chlorines* | *Specific Organic Chlorine* | *Current EPA Registration (US)* | *Acute Oral Toxicity (Man)* | *Dermal Absorption* | *Lipid Solubility* | *Specific Characteristics* |
|---|---|---|---|---|---|---|
| Hexachlorocyclohexanes | Lindane ($\gamma$ isomer) | Topical scabicide; agricultural use canceled 2006 | Moderate | High | Low | Seizures, CNS excitation; musty odor |
| DDT and analogs | DDT—Dichlorodiphenyltrichloroethane | Banned 1972 | Slightly to moderately | Low | Highest | Tremors, CNS excitation; odorless |
| | Methoxychlor | Banned 2003 | Slightly | Low | Moderate | Less toxic DDT substitute |
| | Dicofol | Residential use banned 1998; cotton, citrus, apple industries | Slightly | Low | Low | |
| | Chlorobenzilate | Banned 1983 | Slightly | Low | Low | Much less environmental persistence than DDT |
| Cyclodienes and related compounds | Aldrin | Banned 1974 | Highly | High | High | Rapidly metabolized to dieldrin; mild "chemical" odor |
| | Dieldrin | Banned 1974 | Highly | High | High | Stereoisomer of endrin; early and late seizures; odorless |
| | Endrin | Banned 1974 | Very Highly | High | None | Most toxic organic chlorine; rapid-onset seizures, status epilepticus |
| | Chlordane | Banned 1988 | Moderately | High | High | Early and late seizures occur |
| | Endosulfan | RED 2002 | Highly | High | Low | Strong sulfur odor |
| | Heptachlor | Restricted: fire ant control, soil treatment | Moderately | High | High | Toxic metabolite heptachlor epoxide; odor of camphor |
| | Isobenzan | Never registered | Highly | Moderate | High | Also inhibits $Mg^{2+}$-ATPase; mild "chemical" odor |
| | Dienochlor | Banned | NA | Low | Low | Toxic metabolite binds to glutathione |
| | Toxaphene (polychlorinated camphene) | Banned 1982 | Moderately to highly | Low | Low | Seizures; turpentinelike odor, often mixed with parathion |
| Chlordecone and Mirex | Chlordecone | Banned 1977 | Moderately | High | High | "Kepone shakes"; seizures not seen, structurally similar to mirex |
| | Mirex | Banned 1976 | Slightly | High | High | (?) Converted to chlordecone, toxicity identical |

CNS = central nervous system; RED = re-registration eligibility decision: EPA = Environmental Protection Agency: US = United States: CNS = central nervous system.

conductance, repetitive action potentials, and extended tail currents. Dichlorodiphenyltrichloroethane also inhibits $Ca^{2+}$-ATPase, located on the external cell membrane. Inhibition of this pump likely contributes to membrane instability and repetitive discharges due to a reduction in external calcium concentrations.

The cyclodienes and lindane act as GABA antagonists. They inhibit GABA binding at the $GABA_A$-receptor-chloride ionophore complex in the CNS, by interacting at the picrotoxin binding site (Fig. 84–2). Although the mechanisms of action of mirex and chlordecone are completely understood, they inhibit $Na^+$,$K^+$-ATPase, and $Ca^{2+}$-ATPase.

## Drug Interactions

There are theoretical consequences of hepatic enzyme induction, such as enhanced metabolism of therapeutic drugs and/or reduced efficacy. A large group of workers poisoned by chlordecone over many months had some increased hepatic microsomal activity but no evidence of drug interactions or adverse clinical effects. There are no definitive reports of enhanced metabolism of therapeutic drugs or adverse reactions because of microsomal enzyme induction in man.

## Clinical Manifestations

***Acute Exposure.*** In sufficient doses, organic chlorines lower the seizure threshold (DDT and related $Na^+$-channel xenobiotics) or remove inhibitory influences (antagonism to GABA effects) and produce peripheral and CNS stimulation, with resultant tremors, seizures, respiratory failure, and death. After DDT exposure, tremor is often the only initial manifestation, except following extensive exposure. Nausea, vomiting, hyperesthesia of the mouth and face, paresthesias of the face, tongue, and extremities, headache, dizziness, myoclonus, leg weakness, agitation, and confusion can follow large exposures. Seizures only occur after very high exposures, usually following large intentional ingestions. However, with lindane, the cyclodienes, and toxaphene, there typically are no prodromal signs or symptoms, and more often than not, the first manifestation of toxicity is a generalized seizure, usually within 1 to 2 hours of ingestion. The seizures are often

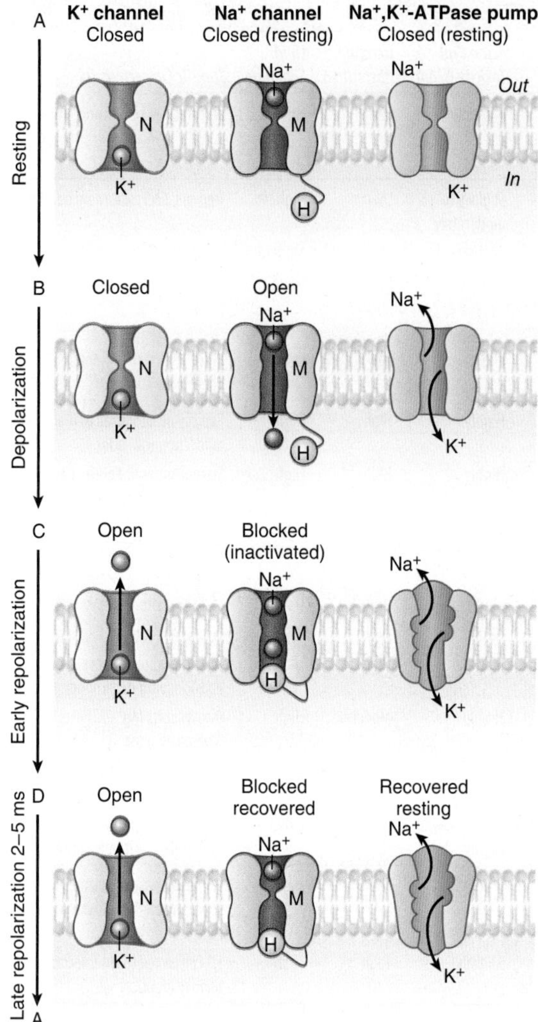


**FIGURE 84–1.** Sodium channel. Schematic drawing of voltage-gated neuronal $Na^+$ channel: demonstrating four phases of activation: (1) Closed, resting state: M gate closed, H gate open, cell is at normal polarized state, ready for activation. (2) Stimulus resulting in depolarization causes voltage-dependent M gate to open, allowing rapid $Na^+$ flow intracellularly, depolarizing the cell (H gate is open). (3) Inactivated (blocked) state: M gate still open, but depolarization causes a conformational change in the channel, and causes H gate to rapidly close (voltage independent), inactivating intracellular $Na^+$ flow. $K^+$ channels open to assist in repolarization (4) As repolarization is accomplished by $Na^+,K^+$-ATPase and $K^+$ channels, the voltage-dependent M gate closes again, conformational change reverts back to a recovered/resting position, and the H gate reopens. When the $K^+$ channel and $Na^+,K^+$-ATPase have completed repolarization, the resting state (1) will be restored.

self-limited, but recurrent seizures and even status epilepticus are reported. In contrast, the cyclodienes are also notable for their propensity to cause seizures that often recur for several days following an acute exposure. If the seizures are brief and hypoxia has not occurred, recovery is usually complete. Hyperthermia secondary to central mechanisms, increased muscle activity, and/or aspiration pneumonia is common. Status epilepticus is a common occurrence in patients with intentional endosulfan ingestions.

***Lindane: Specific Risks.*** Patients are at risk for developing CNS toxicity from improper topical therapeutic use, such as excessive amounts used, or applications to abraided or inflammed skin, or after baths or under occlusive dressings; young children (< 2 years) and the elderly appear to be at greatest risk. Toxicity also occurs after unintentional oral ingestion of topical preparations. In 2009, the American Academy of Pediatrics (AAP) recommended stopping the use of lindane for the treatment of lice or scabies, even as second-line therapy.

***Chronic Exposure.*** Chlordecone (Kepone), unlike the other organic chlorines, produces an insidious picture of chronic toxicity related to its extremely long persistence in the body. Because of poor industrial hygiene practices in a makeshift chlordecone factory in Hopewell, Virginia, 133 workers were heavily exposed for 17 months in 1974–1975. They developed a clinical syndrome consisting of a prominent tremor of the hands, a fine tremor of the head, and trembling of the entire body, known as the "Kepone Shakes." Other findings included

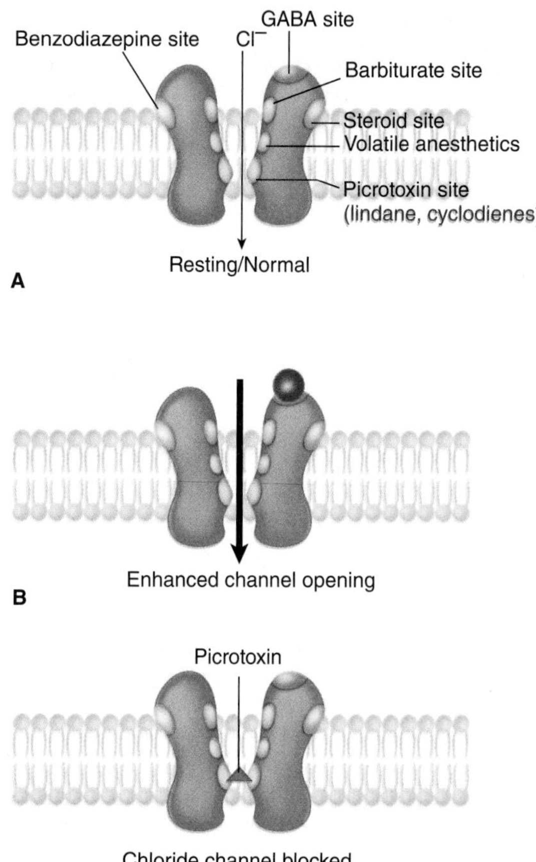


**FIGURE 84–2.** GABA chloride channel. (**A**) Under resting conditions, a tonic influx of chloride maintains the nerve cell in a polarized state. (**B**) Binding of GABA or an indirect-acting GABA agonist (eg, barbiturate, volatile anesthetic) opens the chloride channel. The subsequent chloride influx hyperpolarizes the cell membrane, making the neuron less likely to propagate an action potential in response to a stimulus. (**C**) GABA antagonists, such as picrotoxin, block the chloride channel, reducing chloride influx. The resulting decreased membrane polarity causes the neuron to become hyperexcitable to even those stimuli that are normally subthreshold in nature.

weakness, opsoclonus (rapid, irregular, dysrhythmic ocular movements), ataxia, altered mental status, rash, weight loss, and elevated liver enzymes.

***DDT and Breast Cancer.*** Dichlorodiphenyltrichloroethane and other organic chlorine insecticides have estrogenic effects. Because breast cancer incidence rates in the US have steadily climbed 1% per year since the 1940s, coinciding with the worldwide use of DDT, it is postulated that women who have higher concentrations of estrogenic organic chlorine compounds (eg, DDT, polychlorinated biphenyls {PCBs}) are at risk for developing breast cancer. A meta-analysis of 22 studies found strong evidence to discard the putative relationship between *p,p'*-DDE concentrations and breast cancer risk; two more recent meta-analyses also confirmed the lack of any increased risk for breast cancer associated with DDT or DDE.

### Diagnostic Information

The history of exposure to an organic chlorine pesticide is the most critical piece of information, because exposure is otherwise rare. Following ingestion, abdominal radiographs often reveal the presence of a radiopaque chlorinated pesticide, because chlorine increases the radiopacity of the xenobiotics (Chap. 5). A large number of other xenobiotics lead to seizures as the first manifestation of toxicity and must be in the differential of an unknown exposure.

### Laboratory Testing

Gas chromatography can detect organic chlorine pesticides in serum, adipose tissue, and urine. If the patient's history and toxidrome are obvious, then laboratory evaluation is unnecessary, as this determination will not alter the course of management, and these blood tests are not available on an emergent basis. At present, there are no data correlating health effects and serum or tissue concentrations.

### Management

As with any patient who presents with an altered mental status, dextrose and thiamine should be administered as clinically indicated. Skin decontamination is essential. Clothing should be removed and placed in a plastic bag and disposed of appropriately as a biohazardous waste, and the skin washed with soap and water. Healthcare providers should be protected with rubber gloves and aprons. Because these pesticides are almost invariably liquids, a nasogastric tube is reasonable for suction and lavage of gastric contents, if the ingestion was recent (Chap. 3). The benefit of activated charcoal (AC) is limited, and therefore, AC is not routinely recommended. Standard seizure control with benzodiazepines and barbiturates is recommended as needed, and additional medications such as propofol may also be necessary, due to the risk of recurrent seizures and status epilepticus. The use of cholestyramine, a nonabsorbable bile acid–binding anion exchange resin that was successfully used in chlordecone poisonings in humans (see below), showed a statistically significant benefit on decreasing seizure incidence and mortality in a murine experimental model. There is some evidence that sucrose polyester (ie, olestra, a nonabsorbed synthetic dietary oil substitute) increases excretion of a wide variety of fat-soluble organic chlorine chemicals, especially those undergoing enterohepatic recirculation, by fecal elimination. Sucrose polyester is a reasonable, inexpensive, and more palatable alternative to cholestyramine to increase excretion in patients with chronic organic chlorine toxicity. Cholestyramine or sucrose polyester resin is recommended for all patients symptomatic from chlordecone, and other organic chlorines. Chlordecone undergoes both enterohepatic and enteroenteric recirculation, which can be interrupted by cholestyramine at a dosage of 16 g/day. Cholestyramine increased the fecal elimination of chlordecone 3- to 18-fold in industrial workers exposed during the Hopewell epidemic, resulting in clinical improvement. Sucrose polyester is a reasonable adjunct for enhancing excretion.

### Chlorfenapyr

Chlorfenapyr is a member of a newer class of pesticides known as pyrroles. Chlorfenapyr itself is a pro-insecticide and requires CYP enzyme metabolic activation producing the free pyrrole, which is a lipophilic weak acid with very strong insecticidal activity. Pyrrole interferes with ATP production by uncoupling mitochondrial oxidative phosphorylation. Acute ingestions have a high case-fatality rate. A unique, consistent, yet disturbing feature of these poisonings is a long latency (lasting several days to 2 weeks) between ingestion and onset of toxic effects. Symptoms begin with nausea, fever, and diaphoresis, which is usually followed by CNS manifestations and complete cardiovascular collapse and death. Some cases had relatively mild clinical effects of intermittent fever, thirst, and diaphoresis for a few days as the only abnormality prior to rapid collapse and death. No specific therapy is known to be beneficial.

## PYRETHRINS AND PYRETHROIDS

The natural pyrethrins are the active extracts from the flower *Chrysanthemum cinerariaefolium.* These insecticides are important historically, having been used in China since the first century A.D., and developed for commercial application by the 1800s. Pyrethrins and pyrethroids (synthetic pyrethrin derivatives) are found in more than 2,000 commercially available products. These insecticides are highly effective contact poisons, and their lipophilic nature allows them to readily penetrate insect chitin (exoskeleton). They have a rapid paralytic effect ("knock down") on insects that results from paralysis of the nervous system through interactions at the voltage-dependent $Na^+$ channel. When applied properly, they have essentially no systemic mammalian toxicity because of their rapid hydrolysis. Pyrethrins break down rapidly in light and in water, and therefore have no environmental persistence or bioaccumulation. This fact makes the pyrethrins extremely safe after human exposures but unsuitable for commercial agriculture, because the constant reapplication would be cost prohibitive.

The pyrethroids are the synthetic derivatives of the natural pyrethrins (Table 84–2). They were developed in an effort to produce more environmentally stable products for use in agriculture. The predominant classification scheme used

**TABLE 84–2 Synthetic Pyrethroids in Common Use**

| *Pyrethroid Class* | *Generic Name* | *Generation of Pyrethroid, Dates Introduced (If Available)* |
|---|---|---|
| Type I | Allethrin | 1st generation; first synthetic pyrethroid, 1949 |
| | Bioallethrin | 2nd generation, 1969; trans isomer of allethrin |
| | Dimethrin | Not available |
| | Phenothrin | 2nd generation, 1973 |
| | Resmethrin | 2nd generation, 1967; 20× strength of pyrethrum |
| | Bioresmethrin | 2nd generation, 1967; 50× strength of pyrethrum, isomer of resmethrin |
| | Tetramethrin | 2nd generation, 1965 |
| | Permethrin | 3rd generation, 1972; effective topical scabicide and miticide, low toxicity |
| | Bifenthrin | 4th generation |
| | Prallethrin | 4th generation |
| | Imiprothrin | 3rd generation, 1998 |
| Type II | Fenvalerate | 3rd generation, 1973 |
| | Acrinathrin | 4th generation |
| | Cyfluthrin | 4th generation |
| | Cyhalothrin | 4th generation |
| | Cypermethrin | 4th generation |
| | Deltamethrin | 4th generation |
| | Esfenvalerate | 4th generation |
| | Fenpropathrin | 4th generation, 1989 |
| | Flucythrinate 70124-77-5 | 4th generation |
| | Fluvalinate 102851-06-9 | 4th generation |
| | Imiprothrin 72963-72-5 | 4th generation, 1998 |
| | Tefluthrin 79538-32-2 | 4th generation |
| | Tralomethrin 66841-25-6 | 4th generation |

today is based on the structure of the pyrethroid, its clinical manifestations in mammalian poisoning, its actions on insect nerve preparations, and its insecticidal activity. Type I pyrethroids have a simple ester bond at the central linkage without a cyano group. Commonly used type I pyrethroids include permethrin, allethrin, tetramethrin, and phenothrin. The type II pyrethroids have a cyano group at the carbon of this ester linkage. Type II pyrethroids in common use include cypermethrin, deltamethrin, fenpropathrin, fluvalinate, and fenvalerate. The cyano group greatly enhances neurotoxicity of the type II pyrethroids in both mammals and insects. The development of the pyrethroids can also be divided into "generations," based on efficacy and dates of introduction.

## Toxicokinetics

***Absorption.*** Pyrethrins are well absorbed orally and via inhalation, but skin absorption is poor. The oral toxicity of pyrethrins in mammals is extremely low, because they are so readily hydrolyzed into inactive compounds. Their dermal toxicity is even lower, owing to their slow penetration and rapid metabolism. The pyrethroids are more stable than the natural pyrethrins, and significant systemic toxicity occurs following large ingestions. An average of 35% (range 27%–57%) of orally administered cypermethrin is absorbed in human volunteers. In the same volunteer study, a mean of 1.2% (range 0.85%–1.8%) of dermally applied cypermethrin in soybean oil vehicle was absorbed systemically.

***Distribution.*** The pyrethroids and pyrethrins are lipophilic and, as such, are rapidly distributed to the CNS. Because they are rapidly metabolized, there is no storage or bioaccumulation, which limits chronic toxicity.

***Metabolism.*** Natural pyrethrins are readily metabolized by mammalian microsomal enzymes, and hence are essentially nontoxic to humans. The synthetic pyrethroids are readily metabolized in animals and man by hydrolases and the CYP microsomal system to metabolites of lower toxicity than the parent compounds. Piperonyl butoxide, a CYP enzyme inhibitor in insects, enhances the potency of pyrethrins and pyrethroids 10- to 300-fold to target insects. Testing of piperonyl butoxide on CYP metabolism in humans revealed no effect.

***Elimination.*** There is no evidence that the pyrethroids undergo enterohepatic recirculation. Parent compounds, and metabolites of the pyrethroids, are found in the urine.

## Pathophysiology

Pyrethrins and pyrethroids prolong the activation of the voltage-dependent $Na^+$ channel by binding to it in the open state, causing a prolonged depolarization. Although DDT affects primarily the insect peripheral nervous system (PNS), the pyrethroids affect the insect CNS as well as the PNS. The mammalian voltage-dependent $Na^+$ channel, unlike the insect, has many isoforms, which helps explain the relative resistance in mammalian species (> 1,000-fold less susceptible). Different pyrethroids have varied effects on these mammalian $Na^+$ channels.

Pyrethroids also have activity at certain isoforms of the voltage-sensitive $Ca^{2+}$ channel, which would explain the neurotransmitter release that occurs in pyrethroid poisoning. Additionally, pyrethroids block voltage-sensitive $Cl^-$ channels in test animals, producing the salivation. Some studies show some interference of the type II pyrethroids with the $GABA_A$-mediated inhibitory $Cl^-$ channels in high concentrations, which probably contributes to the seizures following severe poisoning by type II pyrethyroids.

## Clinical Manifestations

Pyrethrum probably has an $LD_{50}$ of well over 1 g/kg in man, as extrapolated from animal data. Most cases of toxicity associated with the pyrethrins are the result of allergic reactions. The synthetic pyrethroids can cause histamine release in vitro, but generally do not induce IgE-mediated allergic reactions. Excluding the rare possibility of skin irritation or allergy, the type I pyrethroids are unlikely to cause systemic toxicity in humans. Poisoning with type II pyrethroids causes paresthesias, salivation, nausea, vomiting, dizziness, fasciculations, altered mental status, coma, seizures, and acute respiratory distress syndrome. A review of more than 500 cases of acute pyrethroid poisoning from China highlights some similar manifestations between a massive acute type II pyrethroid overdose and an organic phosphorus compound overdose (salivation, vomiting, seizures). However, serious atropine toxicity and death have resulted when poisoning from a type II pyrethroid was mistaken for an organic phosphorus compound, and treatment was directed at these seemingly muscarinic signs. Although the type II pyrethroids contain a cyanide moiety, cyanide poisoning does not occur, and cyanide antidotal therapy is not indicated. Because the pyrethroids are rapidly metabolized and are not biopersistent compounds, they are shown not to cause cumulative toxicity.

### Treatment

Initial treatment should be directed toward skin decontamination, as most poisonings occur from exposures by this route. For patients with intentional ingestions of a type II pyrethroid, we recommend a single standard dose of AC, provided the diluent of the pyrethroid does not contain a petroleum solvent because of concerns for an increased risk of aspiration. Contact dermatitis and acute systemic allergic reactions should be treated with antihistamines, corticosteroids, and inhalational β-adrenergic agonists as clinically indicated.

Treatment of systemic toxicity is entirely supportive and symptomatic, because no specific antidote exists. Benzodiazepines should be used for tremor and seizures. Topical vitamin E oil (D,L-α-tocopherol) is especially effective in preventing and treating the cutaneous paresthesias due to topical pyrethroid exposures.

## ARTHROPOD REPELLENTS

Mosquitoes transmit more diseases to humans than any other biting insect. Worldwide, more than 700 million people are infected yearly by mosquito bites that transmit diseases such as malaria, viral encephalitis, yellow fever, dengue fever, West Nile, Zika, bancroftian filariasis, and epidemic polyarthritis.

*N,N*-Diethyl-3-methylbenzamide (DEET) has been the time-tested primary weapon for the past 5 decades. However, much controversy continues to surround DEET despite a remarkable safety profile with over a half-century of global use by billions of people. A growing trend in the US and many Western cultures is a chemophobia against synthetic products like DEET. Many people favor plant-based "natural" or "organic" repellents, paralleling the increasing consumer preference for natural or organic foods. Several xenobiotics are proposed, but thus far, few have been shown by objective blinded studies to even approach the efficacy of DEET, much less surpass it. Numerous comprehensive reviews of the subject demonstrated the superiority of DEET in most cases, and it remains the insect repellent standard by which all others are measured (Table 84–3).

### DEET

The topical insect repellent DEET was patented by the US Army in 1946 and has been commercially marketed in the US since 1956. Currently, it is used worldwide by more than 200 million persons annually. The EPA estimates that 38% of the US population uses DEET each year. Formulations of DEET can be purchased without prescription in concentrations ranging from 5% to 100%, and in multiple formulations of solutions, creams, lotions, gels, and aerosol sprays. Mosquitoes are attracted to their hosts by temperature and chemical attractants, principally $CO_2$ and lactate. While it was once thought that DEET repels insects due to interference with the chemoreceptors that detect lactic acid and $CO_2$, novel work demonstrated that DEET itself is actually detected by the olfactory receptors of mosquitoes and repels them independently of whether the normal physical or chemical attractants are present.

***Toxicokinetics.*** DEET is extensively absorbed via the gastrointestinal tract. Skin absorption is significant, depending on the vehicle and the concentration. DEET is lipophilic, and skin absorption usually occurs within 2 hours. The volume of distribution is large, in the range of 2.7 to 6.2 L/kg in animal studies. DEET is extensively metabolized by oxidation

**TABLE 84–3 Comparative Efficacy and Toxicity of Commonly Available Insect Repellents**

| *Insect Repellent* | *EPA Approval* | *EPA Toxicity Rating*[a] | *Efficacy in Lab and Field Studies*[b] | *Notes* |
|---|---|---|---|---|
| DEET | 1957 (1980) | III | Most efficacious in lab and field studies; proven protection against ticks and mosquitoes | > 50 years of experience, billions of users<br>10%–30% solution: safe, effective when used as directed |
| Picaridin (Bayrepel) | 2001 | IV | 20% solution:<br>Lab: Equivalent to DEET<br>Field: Essentially equivalent to DEET | All studies done on 20% picaridin; no studies done with 7% US formula<br>Recommended by CDC as a DEET alternative |
| IR3535 (substituted β amino acid) | 1999 | IV | Lab: Inferior to DEET<br>Field: None available | Recommended by CDC as a DEET alternative |
| Oil of lemon eucalyptus (*p*-menthane diol) | 2000 | IV (I, ocular) | Equivalent to DEET for mosquitoes; not tested for tick bite prevention | Recommended by CDC as a DEET alternative |
| BioUD (2-undecanone) | 2007 | IV | Lab: Equivalent to 7% DEET<br>Field: Equal to 25% and 30% DEET | Studies performed by patent holders and developers of IR, no impartial evidence |
| Citronella oil | 1948 | IV | Lab study: Ineffective | Candles only provide some repellency when within 1 meter |

EPA: Environmental Protection Agency; CDC: Centers for Disease Control and Prevention. [a]EPA Acute Toxicity Ratings: Category I = very highly or highly toxic; Category II = moderately toxic; Category III = slightly toxic; Category IV = practically nontoxic (see Table 84-4 for definitions). [b]Lab tests: arm-in-cage studies for mosquito repellency; field studies: actual biting or tick attachment assays in natural conditions.

and hydroxylation by the hepatic microsomal enzymes, primarily by the isozymes CYP2B6, 3A4, 2C19, and 2A6. DEET is excreted in the urine within 12 hours, mainly as metabolites, with 15% or less appearing as the parent compound.

***Pathophysiology.*** The exact mechanism of DEET toxicity is unknown.

***Clinical Manifestations.*** Most calls to poison centers regarding DEET exposures involve minor or no symptoms, and symptomatic exposures occur primarily when DEET is sprayed in the eyes or inhaled. A single case report of severe poisoning developed in a man with extreme exposure. He used 30% DEET on his entire body several times daily for a prolonged time period, with an entire bottle used the day prior to admission. He developed weakness and nausea that progressed to confusion and shortness of breath. Metabolic acidosis, with an elevated lactate concentration, acute kidney injury requiring hemodialysis, and worsening weakness requiring mechanical ventilation developed. His blood DEET concentration was 130 ppb (μg/L). No seizures developed, and he experienced a full neurologic recovery after a prolonged hospitalization. When toxicity data and the few cases of encephalopathy and death allegedly related to DEET use are closely analyzed, the actual role of DEET remains purely speculative.

***Treatment.*** Patients with DEET exposures are treated with supportive care aimed at the primarily neurologic symptoms. In cases of dermal exposures, skin decontamination with soap and water should be a priority to prevent further absorption. For patients with intentional oral ingestions, it is reasonable to give a single dose of AC if it has been less than 2 hours after ingestion and there are no contraindications such as seizures, decreased mental status, or vomiting.

## LEGAL STANDARDS FOR AN INSECTICIDE LABEL

The Federal Insecticide, Fungicide, and Rodenticide Act of 1962 established criteria for a "signal word" on an insecticide label, which implies the degree of toxicity based on an oral $LD_{50}$. Also, the label on the original container of these products is usually instructive and should always be brought to the medical facility (Table 84–4).

**TABLE 84–4 United States Environmental Protection Agency Toxicity Classification of Pesticides**

| *Category and Signal Word* | *Oral $LD_{50}$ (mg/kg)* | *Dermal $LD_{50}$ (mg/kg)* | *Inhalation $LC_{50}$ (mg/L)* | *Eye Irritation* | *Skin Irritation* |
|---|---|---|---|---|---|
| I Danger | 0–50 | 0–200 | 0–0.05 | Corrosive: corneal opacity not reversible within 21 days | Corrosive |
| II Warning | 50–500 | 200–2,000 | 0.05–0.5 | Corneal opacity reversible within 8–21 days; irritation persisting for 7 days | Severe irritation at 72 hours |
| III Caution | 500–5,000 | 2,000–20,000 | 0.5–5.0 | Corneal opacity; irritation reversible within 7 days | Moderate irritation at 72 hours |
| IV None | > 5,000 | > 20,000 | > 5.0 | Irritation cleared within 24 hours | Mild or slight irritation at 72 hours |

$LD_{50}$: The dose that is lethal to 50% of test animals; $LC_{50}$: The concentration in air that is lethal to 50% of test animals.

# 85 PHOSPHORUS

Normal Concentration

| | |
|---|---|
| Serum | 3–4.5 mg/dL (1–1.4 mmol/L) as phosphate |

## HISTORY AND EPIDEMIOLOGY

The word *phosphorus* comes from the ancient Greek *phos*, which means light, and *phorus*, which means bringing. White phosphorus gained public notoriety as the main ingredient in strike-anywhere matches. Workplace exposure to phosphorus produced "phossy jaw," or mandibular necrosis, that was first documented in 1838. Because of the fire hazard presented by strike-anywhere matches, their use was discontinued. Most current matches use red phosphorus in the striking pad on the matchbook. White phosphorus is used to manufacture insecticides and fertilizer, as an incendiary, and in fireworks.

## CHEMISTRY AND PHARMACOLOGY

Elemental phosphorus exists in three allotropes: black phosphorus, a nontoxic compound that does not ignite spontaneously; red phosphorus, a fairly innocuous phosphorus intermediate in reactivity between black and white phosphorus; and white phosphorus, a highly reactive and dangerous element. White phosphorus is a tetramer, $P_4$, which is a waxy paste, and is insoluble in water. The presence of impurities in white phosphorus accounts for the general description of white phosphorus as yellow phosphorus. White phosphorus undergoes rapid oxidation upon contact with oxygen, with the resultant liberation of heat, light, and dense white smoke. Phosphorus pentoxide generates phosphoric acid when dissolved in water. Following explosion, white phosphorus is broadly disseminated in a dense cloud of white smoke with a garlic odor. The smoke is phosphoric acid, which can produce pulmonary, ophthalmic, and dermal irritation.

Red phosphorus differs from the white allotrope by its crystalline form, its lack of phosphorescence, and its markedly reduced reactivity with oxygen. Red phosphorus will slowly degrade to highly toxic phosphine gas ($PH_3$) and phosphorous acid.

## PHARMOCOKINETICS AND TOXICOKINETICS

White phosphorus is rapidly absorbed from the intestinal tract and subsequently taken up primarily by the tissues of the liver, renal cortex, bowel mucosa, epidermis, hair follicles, pancreas, and adrenal cortex. Within several hours of ingestion 69% to 73% of the total ingested dose is identified concentrated in the liver. Because phosphorus is highly lipid soluble, significant absorption can also occur after skin or mucosal exposure. Penetrating wounds and dermal burns enhance the systemic absorption of phosphorus. The lethal dose is reported to be 1 mg/kg.

## PATHOPHYSIOLOGY

Externally, white phosphorus reacts with oxygen (ie, burns) to form phosphorus pentoxide and other phosphorus oxides. Phosphorus pentoxide readily reacts with water in an exothermic reaction, producing corrosive phosphoric acid. A resurgence of injury related to red phosphorus results from methamphetamine production. Red phosphorus is used in conjunction with elemental iodine to produce hydroiodic acid, the ultimate reducing agent required to convert ephedrine to methamphetamine. In this situation, red phosphorus causes fire because of its unintentional conversion to highly flammable white phosphorus. Toxicity occurs because during heating, the reaction products of iodine and red phosphorus often generate phosphine ($PH_3$), a pulmonary irritant (Chap. 81). Otherwise, red phosphorus has limited direct toxicologic significance. All further references to phosphorus in this chapter refer to white phosphorus.

## CLINICAL MANIFESTATIONS

### General

The clinical manifestations of oral phosphorus poisoning are classically described in three stages. The initial effects are delayed for a few hours, and the degree of delay partially depends on the dose. During the first phase, patients experience vomiting, hematemesis, and abdominal pain, with hypotension and death occurring within 24 hours after large ingestions. During the second stage, there is transient resolution of the toxic effects. During the third stage, the patient develops hepatic injury with coagulopathy, jaundice, and acute kidney injury with oliguria and uremia. However, clinical experience demonstrates that three distinct phases are the exception rather than the rule, with significant overlap or absence of the "quiescent" second stage and death potentially occurring within hours of ingestion.

### Gastrointestinal

Initial symptoms after ingestion include nausea, vomiting, and abdominal pain. Both diarrhea and constipation are reported but are much less common. The breath and vomitus are sometimes described as having a garlic or musty sweet odor. The vomitus and diarrhea are sometimes luminescent and smoking, but this specific finding occurs infrequently. Phosphorus causes an inflammatory injury to the gastrointestinal (GI) tract characterized by local hemorrhage and hematemesis, but generally perforation does not occur. Massive GI bleeding occurs later in the clinical course, particularly when hepatic failure and coagulopathy are present.

### Renal/Electrolytes

In humans, acute kidney injury from phosphorus is most likely acute tubular necrosis resulting from hypotension, salt and water depletion, and a direct toxic effect. Significant electrolyte disturbances result from both ingestion and dermal absorption of phosphorus. Hypocalcemia is common, but hypercalcemia is also occasionally reported. Hyperphosphatemia reportedly accompanies the hypocalcemia but is not universal and can occur at any time in the clinical course. Hyperkalemia is occasionally reported and may be secondary to tissue injury and acute kidney injury. These electrolyte disturbances are likely a leading cause of early mortality from phosphorus.

### Cardiovascular

When death occurs within 24 hours of the ingestion, it is likely the result of cardiovascular collapse. Electrocardiographic (ECG) abnormalities include abnormal T waves, QT interval prolongation, ST segment changes, and dysrhythmias. Autopsies of poisoned patients demonstrated fatty degeneration of the myocardium and vacuolated cytoplasm many hours postingestion.

### Hepatic

Phosphorus increases oxygen consumption in the hepatocyte. Uncoupling of oxidative phosphorylation is the likely mechanism, and there is a decrease in intrahepatocyte adenosine triphosphate (ATP) concentrations. Massive hepatic steatosis is a hallmark of white phosphorus toxicity, with a rise in hepatic triglycerides beginning within 2 hours and peaking in 36 hours. Hepatic necrosis may be prominent, particularly in zone 1, in distinction to most other classic hepatotoxins, such as acetaminophen, which produce zone 3 necrosis. Early elevation of the aspartate aminotransferase, coagulopathy, and jaundice are poor prognostic markers.

### Nervous System

Central nervous system effects include headache, altered mental status, coma, and rarely seizures. Patients with initial alterations in mental status or coma have an increased mortality rate independent of the presence of any electrolyte abnormalities.

### Dermal/Mucous Membranes

Dermal phosphorus exposure causes extensive burns, and this occurs most frequently in the military setting. The burns are described as emitting a garlic odor and displaying a yellow color that fluoresces under ultraviolet light. The smoke produced by burning white phosphorus contains phosphorus pentoxide and is irritating to the conjunctiva and mucosa of the oropharynx and lungs. Following a large burn, systemic illness manifested by electrolyte, cardiovascular, and hepatic abnormalities results from absorbed phosphorus. Healing time from phosphorus burns is prolonged when compared with thermal burns.

## DIAGNOSTIC TESTING

Serum elemental phosphorus concentrations are not clinically available, and a serum phosphate concentration while potentially elevated does not reflect the serum elemental phosphorus concentration or any body burden of elemental phosphorus. The diagnosis of phosphorus poisoning must rely on the history and physical examination. However, for optimal supportive care of the patient, many laboratory factors must be monitored, such as ECG, electrolytes, serum pH, hepatic function, glucose, kidney function, and coagulation parameters.

## MANAGEMENT

### Protection of Healthcare Workers

Care must be taken to prevent exposure of healthcare personnel. Phosphorus contained in vomitus or stool can be hazardous. Personnel should wear protective equipment to prevent direct contact with phosphorus.

### General

Life-support measures, such as airway protection and fluid resuscitation, should be provided. A complete blood count, hepatic enzymes, coagulation parameters, basic metabolic panel, serum phosphate, and serum calcium should be measured. Electrolytes, in particular, should be assayed frequently. Hypocalcemia, hyperphosphatemia, and hyperkalemia should be expeditiously treated using standard modalities. Frequent measurement of vital signs and continuous cardiac monitoring are essential. Kidney function, as well as urine output, must be evaluated. Ophthalmic irrigation should be performed if eye irritation is present.

### Dermal Exposure

The patient with a cutaneous exposure should be immediately washed with or immersed in water. Irrigation is the only treatment shown to decrease burn size, length of hospital stay, and mortality. Any areas where white phosphorus remains must be kept wet at all times, as the substance may reignite if it is exposed to ambient oxygen.

Careful debridement is the next critical step as wounds that have not undergone adequate decontamination heal poorly, requiring additional debridement. Fragments of phosphorus from the wound should be placed under water to prevent a fire hazard. Particles of phosphorus can be visualized by using a Woods lamp as the chemical burns have a yellowish fluorescence. Because of the increased solubility of phosphorus in hydrophobic solvents, it is important not to use ointments until the wound is completely decontaminated. Copper sulfate reacts with phosphorus to produce copper phosphide, a dark compound that is more easily visualized in the tissues. This dark material coats the particle and decreases the reaction of phosphorus with oxygen for a limited time. It is reasonable to utilize dilute copper sulfate solutions (0.5%–1.0%) applied once to the wound and then rinsed off with water. The copper phosphide–coated particles must be removed as they still react slowly.

Silver nitrate (1%–2% solution) is suggested by some as a potential solution to replace the use of copper sulfate. However, since there are no human data, it is not recommended at this time. Patients with significant burns should be admitted to a burn intensive care unit for close monitoring of cardiovascular, kidney, and electrolyte status for several days at the minimum.

### Gastrointestinal Exposure

There is no good evidence that GI decontamination or antidotal therapy is efficacious following phosphorus ingestion. However, despite the lack of data of efficacy, given the poor outcome of patients with large ingestions of phosphorus, gastric decontamination is recommended, even if vomiting has occurred. Either an orogastric (OG) or nasogastric (NG) tube should be used, with the OG tube being preferred (Chap. 3). Because of the risk of fire and explosion, it would be reasonable to keep the free end of the OG tube under water while inserting and instilling small amounts of water (not air) to check for proper placement, although this is only supported by one case report. Hepatic injury is more likely with ingested phosphorus than following dermal exposure. *N*-Acetylcysteine (NAC) would be reasonable as a potential adjunct in the treatment of phosphorus toxicity because of its antioxidant effects. A standard intravenous NAC regimen is recommended (see Antidotes in Brief: A3).

# 86 SODIUM MONOFLUOROACETATE AND FLUOROACETAMIDE

## HISTORY AND EPIDEMIOLOGY

Sodium monofluoroacetate (SMFA, 1080) is synthesized by plants such as gifblaar (*Dichapetalum cymosum*), which is native to Brazil, Australia, and South and West Africa and developed as a rodenticide. Fluoroacetamide (1081) is a similar compound. Use of either was banned in the United States in 1972 except in the form of collars intended to protect sheep and cattle from coyotes. Currently, SMFA is used in New Zealand and Australia as a vertebrate pesticide.

## TOXICOKINETICS AND TOXICODYNAMICS

Sodium monofluoroacetate is an odorless, tasteless white powder with the consistency of flour. SMFA and fluoroacetamide are well absorbed orally, and poisoning has also occurred from inhalation. Detailed toxicokinetic data are lacking in humans. The serum half-life is estimated to be 6.6 to 13.3 hours in sheep, and the estimated lethal dose in humans is 2 to 10 mg/kg.

## PATHOPHYSIOLOGY

Sodium monofluoroacetate and fluoroacetamide are structural analogs of acetic acid. Monofluoroacetic acid enters the mitochondria where it is converted to monofluoroacetyl-coenzyme A (CoA) by acetate thiokinase. Next, citrate synthase joins the monofluoroacetyl-CoA complex with oxaloacetate to form fluorocitrate. Finally, fluorocitrate covalently binds aconitase, irreversibly inhibiting all citric acid cycle activity.

Inhibition of aconitase impairs energy production, leading to metabolic acidosis with an elevated lactate concentration. Glutamate depletion leads to urea cycle disruption and ammonia accumulation. Increased citrate chelates divalent cations, causing hypocalcemia.

## CLINICAL MANIFESTATIONS

Most patients will develop symptoms within 6 hours following ingestion. The most common symptoms recorded at the time of emergency department presentation are nausea and vomiting (74%), diarrhea (29%), agitation (29%), and abdominal pain (26%). Low systemic vascular resistance, seizures, and QT interval prolongation are also reported. Respiratory distress, hypotension, and seizures are prognostic of death, which typically occurs within 72 hours of hospitalization.

## DIAGNOSTIC TESTING

Although SMFA and fluoroacetamide can be confirmed with gas chromatography-mass spectrometry and thin-layer chromatography, neither of these studies can be performed in a clinically relevant time period. A combination of history, signs, symptoms, and common laboratory tests can assist with the diagnosis. A complete blood cell count revealing leukocytosis, electrolytes, and arterial blood gas demonstrating hypokalemia, hypocalcemia, and an acidemia are supportive.

The electrocardiogram findings will be consistent with the electrolyte abnormalities and include a prolonged QT interval. Atrial fibrillation with a rapid ventricular response, ventricular tachycardia, and other dysrhythmias are all described.

## TREATMENT

Initial decontamination should include removal of clothes and cleansing of skin with soap and water. Since there is no antidote for SMFA or fluoroacetamide poisoning, orogastric lavage is reasonable for patients who present to the emergency department prior to significant emesis. For patients who present within 1 to 2 hours of ingestion, we recommend oral activated charcoal.

In animal models, ethanol and glycerol monoacetate (monoacetin) improve survival presumably by acting as acetate donors for incorporation into the citric acid cycle. Both are converted to acetyl-CoA and compete for binding of citrate synthase with monofluoroacetyl-CoA. Ethanol has been used in human cases, and a reasonable therapeutic dose is one that would achieve and maintain an ethanol serum concentration of 100 mg/dL (Antidotes in Brief: A34).

In a mouse model, the combination of calcium, sodium succinate, and α-ketoglutarate improved survival, presumably by providing citric acid cycle intermediates distal to the inhibited aconitase. These antidotes were not effective unless calcium was coadministered, emphasizing the importance of replenishing electrolytes. Access to α-ketoglutarate or sodium succinate for a human case would be limited and its use is reasonable as long as accompanied by electrolyte replacement.

Hypotension and shock should be treated with intravenous fluids followed by a vasopressor such as norepinephrine. Supportive care, correction of electrolyte abnormalities (calcium and potassium), ethanol infusion, and monitoring for dysrhythmias and seizures are the mainstays of treatment.

# 87 STRYCHNINE

## HISTORY AND EPIDEMIOLOGY

Strychnine occurs naturally in *Strychnos nux vomica*, a tree native to tropical Asia and North Australia. It is also found in South Asian *Strychnos ignatii* and *Strychnos tiente* trees. The alkaloid is an odorless, colorless, crystalline powder with a bitter taste. Strychnine was introduced as a rodenticide in 1540 and subsequently used medically as a cardiac, respiratory, and digestive stimulant, an analeptic, and an antidote for barbiturate and opioid overdoses. By 1982, 172 commercial products contained strychnine, including 77 rodenticides, 25 veterinary products, and 41 products for human use. Currently, strychnine is restricted to nonhuman use and is mainly used as an insecticide, pesticide, and rodenticide.

Strychnine poisoning was once common, killing more than three American children per week in the 1920s. Currently, although strychnine poisoning is uncommon in the United States, deaths are still reported worldwide. Exposures result from suicidal and homicidal attempts, unintentional poisoning from a Chinese herbal medicine (Maqianzi), a Cambodian traditional remedy (slang nut), and adulteration of street drugs.

## TOXICOKINETICS

While the lethal dose of strychnine is commonly quoted at 50 to 100 mg (1–2 mg/kg), deaths from doses as low as 5 to 10 mg are reported. Some of this variation can be attributed to the route of administration, with parenteral being more toxic than oral.

Strychnine is rapidly absorbed from the gastrointestinal tract and mucous membranes, and there is at least one report of dermal poisoning. There is minimal protein binding and a large volume of distribution (13 L/kg). In postmortem samples, the highest concentrations of strychnine are found in the liver, bile, blood, and gastric contents.

Between 1% and 30% of strychnine is excreted unchanged in urine. Strychnine is metabolized primarily by CYP3A4 to produce the major metabolite strychnine-*N*-oxide, which has about one-tenth the toxicity of strychnine. Several other urinary metabolites are identified. In humans, elimination follows first-order kinetics with a half-life of 10 to 16 hours.

### Pathophysiology

Strychnine is a postsynaptic, competitive, glycine-receptor antagonist. With the loss of the glycine inhibition to the motor neurons in the ventral horn, there is an increased impulse transmission to the muscles, resulting in generalized muscular contraction. Tetanus toxin causes similar muscular contractions by preventing the release of glycine from the presynaptic neuron. In dogs, strychnine has positive chronotropic and inotropic effects on the heart, but this effect is unlikely to be consequential in human poisoning.

### Clinical Manifestations

Symptoms usually begin about 15 to 60 minutes following ingestion and occur sooner with parenteral or nasal administration. Delayed presentations are rarely reported, with a 10-hour delay in one case. The hallmark of strychnine toxicity is generalized involuntary muscular contractions resulting in neck, back, and limb pain. The contractions are easily triggered by trivial stimuli and usually last for 30 seconds to 2 minutes in each episode, repeatedly for a duration of 12 to 24 hours. These unopposed contractions result in the classical signs of opisthotonos, trismus, and risus sardonicus, with flexion of the upper limbs and extension of lower limbs. Hyperreflexia, clonus, and nystagmus also occur. Because strychnine affects glycine inhibition mainly in the spinal cord, the patient retains a normal level of consciousness until metabolic complications become severe. These characteristics often result in descriptions such as "conscious seizure" or "spinal seizure" being used to describe strychnine poisoning.

Hypotension and hypertension, as well as bradycardia and tachycardia, are all reported. Hyperthermia results from the increased muscular activity, and severe hyperthermia should be expected. Other nonspecific signs and symptoms include dizziness, vomiting, and chest and abdominal pain.

Death results mainly from hypoxia and hypoventilation secondary to muscle contractions. Later life-threatening complications include rhabdomyolysis with subsequent myoglobinuria and acute kidney failure, hyperthermia with multiorgan failure, pancreatitis, aspiration pneumonia, anoxic brain injury, and adult respiratory distress syndrome. Rarely, local neuromuscular sequelae such as weakness, myalgias and compartment syndrome are reported.

### Differential Diagnosis

The diagnosis of strychnine poisoning is mainly established on clinical grounds, although several etiologies need to be considered. Tetanus presents with similar muscular hyperactivity, but the clinical course is more gradual in onset and more protracted. Generalized seizures can be differentiated by the normal sensorium, at least in the initial phase, and by an electroencephalogram (EEG) if necessary. A lumbar puncture is helpful to exclude meningitis or encephalitis. Hypocalcemia, hyperventilation, and myoclonus secondary to kidney or liver failure are evaluated by relevant routine laboratory testing. Although a drug-induced dystonic reaction should be considered when there is relevant drug use history, dystonic reactions are usually static, and strychnine poisoning results in dynamic muscular events. Serotonin toxicity, malignant hyperthermia, neuroleptic malignant syndrome, and stimulant-associated toxicity all resemble late phases of strychnine poisoning, but other features of the history or physical examination usually help distinguish them from either strychnine poisoning or tetanus.

### Diagnostic Testing

Most laboratory abnormalities associated with strychnine poisoning are a result of the intense muscle contractions. Metabolic acidosis and respiratory acidosis result from hypoventilation and from diaphragmatic and respiratory muscle failure. Survival in patients with serum pHs in the range of 6.5 to 6.6 is common. Other laboratory abnormalities include hyperlactatemia, hyperkalemia, acute kidney injury, markers of muscle injury, a stress-induced leukocytosis, elevated liver enzymes, hypocalcemia, hypernatremia, and hypokalemia.

Strychnine can be detected by various analytical methods. However, with the exception of the bedside colorimetric reaction, none of these tests are routinely available in a timeframe to assist clinical decision making.

### Management

Orogastric lavage is reasonable, and activated charcoal binds strychnine effectively and should be given at a dose of 1 g/kg body weight. Because patients rapidly suffer airway compromise, endotracheal intubation is indicated before attempting gastrointestinal decontamination. Forced diuresis, peritoneal dialysis, hemodialysis, and hemoperfusion are not indicated.

Supportive treatment remains the most important aspect of care, and the objective is to rapidly terminate muscle hyperactivity. Unnecessary stimuli and manipulation of the patient should be avoided as these trigger muscle contractions. Rapidly acting parenteral benzodiazepines such as midazolam or diazepam remain the first-line treatment. The initial dose of benzodiazepine should be the standard dose used for agitation and hyperactivity, although doses greater than 1 mg/kg diazepam or its equivalent may be needed. Dosing should be repeated at appropriate intervals until the patient becomes relaxed. Barbiturates or neuromuscular blockade is recommended if benzodiazepines do not produce rapid control. It is important to remember that strychnine has no direct effects on consciousness, so that sedation must always accompany neuromuscular blockade. Therapy is recommended for 24 hours and then the patient can be weaned from the respirator as tolerated.

Hyperthermia should be treated by active cooling with ice water immersion. Metabolic acidosis rapidly subsides when muscular activity is controlled. Treatment for rhabdomyolysis includes adequate fluid administration to ensure good urine output (> 1 mL/kg/h), and urinary alkalinization is reasonable to prevent myoglobin precipitation in renal tubules. The management in the first few hours of strychnine poisoning is crucial for survival.

For patients unintentionally exposed to strychnine who remain without symptoms, an observation period of 12 hours is sufficient to exclude a significant risk.

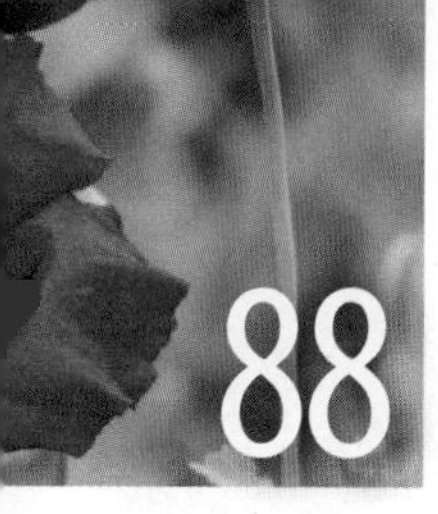



# 88 ARTHROPODS

## TAXONOMY

*Arthropoda* means "joint-footed" in Latin and describes the jointed bodies and legs connected to a chitinous exoskeleton of arthropods. The majority of arthropods are benign to humans and environmentally beneficial. However, some spiders have toxic venoms that produce dangerous, painful lesions or significant systemic effects. Important clinical syndromes are produced by bites or stings from animals in the phylum Arthropoda, specifically the classes Arachnida (spiders, scorpions, and ticks) and Insecta (bees, wasps, hornets, and ants) (Table 88–1). Infectious diseases transmitted by arthropods are not discussed in this chapter.

Arthropoda comprises the largest phylum in the animal kingdom. It includes more species than all other phyla combined (Fig. 88–1). "Bites" are different from "stings." Bites are defined as creating a wound using the oral pole while "stings" occur from a modified ovipositor at the aboral pole.

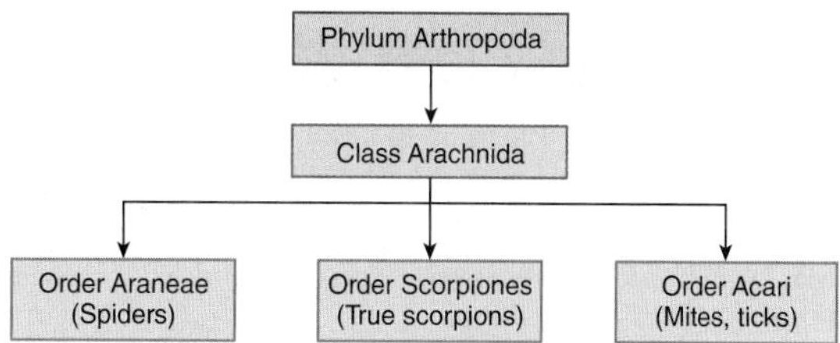


**FIGURE 88–1.** Taxonomy of the phylum Arthropoda.

## HISTORY AND EPIDEMIOLOGY

Since the time of Aristotle, spiders and their webs were used for medicinal purposes. One *Latrodectus* species has an infamous history of medical concern, hence the name *mactans*, which means "murderer" in Latin. Hysteria regarding spider bites peaked during the 17th century in the Taranto region of Italy. The syndrome tarantism, which is characterized by lethargy, stupor, and a restless compulsion to walk or dance, was blamed on *Lycosa tarantula*, a spider that pounces on its prey like a wolf. Deaths were associated with these outbreaks. Dancing the rapid tarantella to music was the presumed remedy. Approximately 200 species of spiders are associated with envenomations. Eighteen genera of North American spiders produce poisonings that require clinical intervention (Table 88–2).

## BLACK WIDOW SPIDER (*LATRODECTUS MACTANS*; HOURGLASS SPIDER)

Five species of widow spiders are found in the United States (US): *Latrodectus mactans* (black widow; Fig. 88–2A), *Latrodectus hesperus* (Western black widow), *Latrodectus variolus* (found in New England, Canada, south to Florida, and west

**TABLE 88–1 North American Insects and Other Arthropods That Bite, Sting, or Nettle Humans**

| *Arthropod* | *Description* |
|---|---|
| Honeybee (*Apis mellifera*) | Hairy, yellowish brown with black markings |
| Bumblebee and carpenter bee (*Bombus* spp and *Xylocopa* spp) | Hairy, larger than honeybees and colored black and yellow |
| Vespids (yellow jackets, hornets, paper wasps) | Short-waisted, robust, black and yellow or white combination |
| Schecoids (thread-waisted wasps) | Threadlike waist |
| Nettling caterpillars (browntail, Io, hag, and buck moths, saddleback and puss caterpillars) | Caterpillar shaped |
| Southern fire ant (*Solenopsis* spp) | Ant shaped |
| Spiders (Arachnida) black widow, brown recluse | Body with 2 regions: cephalothorax and abdomen; 8 legs |
| Scorpions (*Centruroides* spp.) | Eight-legged, crablike, stinger at the tip of the abdomen; pedipalps (pincers) highly developed (not a true insect) |
| Centipedes (Chilopoda) | Elongated, wormlike, with many jointed segments and legs; one pair of poison fangs behind head |

**TABLE 88–2 North American Spiders of Medical Importance**

| *Genus* | *Common Name* |
|---|---|
| *Araneus* spp | Orb weaver |
| *Argiope* spp | Orange argiope |
| *Bothriocyrtum* spp | Trap door spider |
| *Chiracanthium* spp | Running spider |
| *Drassodes* spp | Gnaphosid spider |
| *Heteropoda* spp | Huntsman spider |
| *Latrodectus* spp | Widow spider |
| *Liocranoides* spp | Running spider |
| *Loxosceles* spp | Brown, violin, or recluse spider |
| *Lycosa* spp | Wolf spider |
| *Misumenoides* spp | Crab spider |
| *Neoscona* spp | Orb weaver |
| *Peucetia* spp | Green lynx spider |
| *Phiddipus* spp | Jumping spider |
| *Rheostica (Aphonopelma)* spp | Tarantula |
| *Steatoda grossa* | False black widow spider |
| *Eratigena* spp | Hobo spider |
| *Ummidia* spp | Trap door spider |

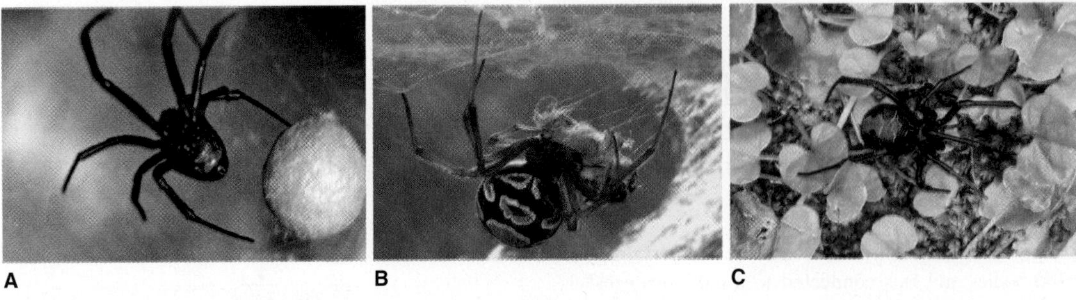


**FIGURE 88–2.** Widow spiders. **(A)** A black widow spider, Latrodectus mactans. Though spiders are mostly harmless to man, two genera, Latrodectus, and Loxosceles, which includes the brown recluse spider, Loxosceles reclusa, inflict bites that are poisonous to humans. *(Used with permission from Public Health Image Library, CDC.)* **(B)** Close-up of an upside down female Brown Widow (Latrodectus geometricus) eating an insect and clinging to a web. *(Used with permission from NHPA/James Carmichael, Jr.)* **(C)** A venomous female Redback spider, Latrodectus hasselti. *(Used with permission from cbstockfoto/Alamy Stock Photo.)*

to eastern Texas, Oklahoma, and Kansas), *Latrodectus bishopi* (red widow of the South), and *Latrodectus geometricus* (brown widow or brown button spider; Fig. 88–2B). Dangerous widow spiders in other parts of the world include *L. geometricus* and *Latrodectus tredecimguttatus* (European widow spider found in southern Europe), *Latrodectus hasselti* (red back widow spider found in Australia, Japan, and India; Fig. 88–2C), and *Latrodectus cinctus* (found in South Africa). These spiders live in temperate and tropical latitudes in places such as stone walls, crevices, wood piles, outhouses, barns, stables, and rubbish piles.

The female *L. mactans* is shiny, jet-black, and large (8–10 mm), with a rounded abdomen and a red hourglass mark on its ventral surface. Her larger size and ability of her fangs to penetrate human skin make her more venomous and toxic than the male spider, which resembles the immature spider in earlier stages of development and is smaller, lighter in color, and has a more elongated abdomen and fangs that usually are too short to envenomate humans.

## Pathophysiology

The venom is more potent on a volume-per-volume basis than the venom of a pit viper and contains a number of toxins, the most important of which for humans is α-latrotoxin. α-Latrotoxin binds to the specific presynaptic receptors and triggers a cascade of events that ultimately causes exocytosis of norepinephrine, dopamine, neuropeptides, acetylcholine, glutamate, and γ-aminobutyric acid (GABA). This massive release of neurotransmitters is what causes the clinical envenomation syndrome known as latrodectism.

## Clinical Manifestations

A sharp pain typically described as a pinprick occurs as the victim is bitten. A pair of red spots often evolve at the site, although the bite is commonly unnoticed. The bite mark itself tends to be limited to a small puncture wound or wheal and flare reaction that often is associated with a halo. One grading system divides the severity of the envenomation into three categories. Grade 1 envenomations range from no symptoms to local pain at the envenomation site with normal vital signs. Grade 2 envenomations involve muscular pain at the site with migration of the pain to the trunk, diaphoresis at the bite site, and normal vital signs. Grade 3 envenomations include the grade 2 findings with abnormal vital signs; diaphoresis distant from the bite site; generalized myalgias to back, chest, and abdomen; and nausea, vomiting, and headache.

The myopathic syndrome of latrodectism involves muscle cramps that usually begin 15 to 60 minutes after the bite. The muscle cramps initially occur at the site of the bite, but later involve rigidity of other skeletal muscles, particularly muscles of the chest, abdomen, and face. Large muscle groups are affected first. Additional clinical findings include "facies latrodectismica," which consists of sweating, contorted, grimaced face associated with blepharitis, conjunctivitis, rhinitis, cheilitis, and trismus of the masseters. Nausea, vomiting, sweating, tachycardia, hypertension, muscle cramping, restlessness, compartment syndrome at the site of the bite, and, rarely, priapism are also reported. Recovery usually ensues within 24 to 48 hours, but clinical findings are reported to last several days with more severe envenomations. Life-threatening complications include severe hypertension, respiratory distress, myocardial infarction, cardiovascular failure, and gangrene. Death with modern care is distinctly uncommon.

## Diagnostic Testing

Laboratory data generally are not helpful in management or predicting outcome. Currently, no specific laboratory assay is capable of confirming latrodectism.

## Management

Treatment involves establishing an airway and supporting respiration and circulation, if indicated. Wound evaluation and local wound care, including tetanus prophylaxis, are essential.

The routine use of antibiotics is not recommended. Pain management is a substantial component of patient care and depends on the clinical findings. Using the grading system, grade 1 envenomations require only cold packs and orally administered nonsteroidal antiinflammatory drugs. For grade 2 and 3 envenomations, intravenous (IV) opioids and benzodiazepines are often reasonable for pain control and muscle spasm.

*Latrodectus* antivenom (Merck) is rapidly effective and curative. In the US, the antivenom formulation is effective for all species but is available as a crude hyperimmune horse serum that is reported to cause anaphylaxis and serum sickness. The morbidity of latrodectism is high, with pain, cramping, and autonomic disturbances, but mortality is low. Hence controversy exists over when to administer the black widow antivenom (BW-AV). We recommend BW-AV for severe reactions (eg, hypertensive crisis or intractable pain), to high-risk patients (eg, pregnant women), or for treatment of priapism (Antidotes in Brief: A37).

## BROWN RECLUSE SPIDER (*LOXOSCELES RECLUSA*; VIOLIN OR FIDDLEBACK SPIDER)

*Loxosceles reclusa* has a brown violin-shaped mark on the dorsum of the cephalothorax, three dyads of eyes arranged in a semicircle on top of the head, and legs that are five times as long as the body. It is small (6–20 mm long) and gray to orange or reddish brown (Fig. 88–3). Spiders in the genus *Loxosceles* have a worldwide distribution. In the US, other species of this genus, which include *L. rufescens*, *L. deserta*, *L. devia*, and *L. arizonica*, are prominent in the Southeast and Southwest. *L. rufescens* was inadvertently introduced in several buildings in New York City. The peak time for envenomation is from spring to autumn, and most victims are bitten in the morning. Because in a majority of patients the spider is unavailable for inspection, the diagnosis of spider bite is frequently misused, and a diagnosis of a dermatonecrotic wound of uncertain etiology would be more accurate.

### Pathophysiology

The venom is cytotoxic. The two main constituent enzymes of the venom are sphingomyelinase D and hyaluronidase, though other subcomponents include deoxyribonuclease, ribonuclease, collagenase, esterase, proteases, alkaline phosphatase, and lipase. Hyaluronidase is a spreading factor that facilitates the penetration of the venom into tissue but does not induce lesion development. Sphingomyelinase D causes dermato necrosis and red blood cell hemolysis and also causes platelets to release serotonin. Sphingomyelinase also reacts with sphingomyelin in the red blood cell membrane to release choline and *N*-acylsphingosine phosphate, which triggers a chain reaction, releasing inflammatory mediators, such as thromboxanes, leukotrienes, prostaglandins, and neutrophils, leading to vessel thrombosis, tissue ischemia, and skin loss. Early perivascular collections of polymorphonuclear leukocytes with hemorrhage and edema progress to intravascular clotting. Coagulation and vascular occlusion of the microcirculation occur, ultimately leading to necrosis.

### Clinical Manifestations

The clinical spectrum of loxoscelism is divided into three major categories. The first category includes bites in which very little, if any, venom is injected. A small erythematous papule appears, which then becomes firm before healing and is associated with a localized urticarial response. In the second category, the bite undergoes a cytotoxic reaction. The bite initially is reported to be painless or have a stinging sensation, followed by blistering, bleeding, and ulceration 2 to 8 hours later. The lesion then increases in diameter, with demarcation of central hemorrhagic vesiculation, then ulceration, the development of violaceous necrosis surrounded by ischemic blanching of skin and outer erythema, and, finally, induration over 1 to 3 days. This is also known as the "red, white, and blue" reaction (Fig. 88–3). Necrosis of the central blister occurs in 3 to 4 days, with eschar formation between 5 and 7 days. After 7 to 14 days, the wound becomes indurated and the eschar falls off, leaving an ulceration that heals by secondary intention. The third category consists of systemic loxoscelism, which is not predicted by the extent of cutaneous reaction, and occurs 24 to 72 hours after the bite. The young are particularly susceptible. The clinical manifestations of systemic loxoscelism include fever, chills, weakness, edema, nausea, vomiting, arthralgias, petechial eruptions, rhabdomyolysis, disseminated intravascular coagulation, hemolysis that is reported to progress to

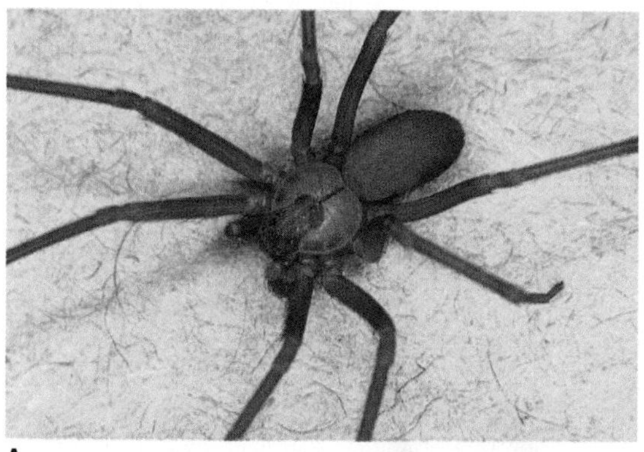

A

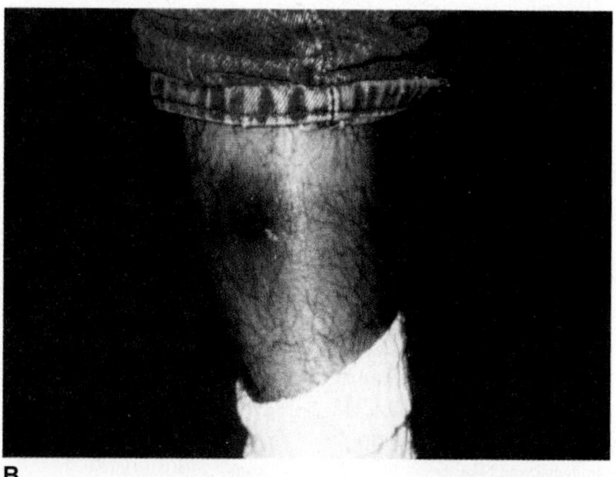

B

**FIGURE 88–3.** Brown recluse spider. (**A**) *Loxosceles reclusa*. Note the image of the violin, which gives the spider its common name, "the fiddleback spider." *(Used with permission from CDC/Margaret Parsons.)* (**B**) A typical envenomation from the brown recluse spider. *(Used with permission from the Fellowship in Medical Toxicology, New York University Grossman School of Medicine, New York City Poison Center.)*

hemoglobinuria, acute kidney injury, and death. However, in North America, the incidence of systemic illness and mortality is rare.

### Diagnostic Testing

Bites from other spiders, such as *Cheiracanthium* (sac spider), *Phidippus* (jumping spider), and *Argiope* (orb weaver), also produce necrotic wounds. These spiders are often the actual culprits when the brown recluse is mistakenly blamed. Definitive diagnosis is achieved only when the biting spider is positively identified. No routine laboratory test for loxoscelism is available for clinical application, but several techniques are presently used for research purposes.

Clinical laboratory data include the findings of hemolysis, hemoglobinuria, and hematuria. Coagulopathy is often present, with laboratory data significant for elevated fibrin split products, decreased fibrinogen concentrations, and a positive D-dimer assay. Other tests include increased prothrombin time (PT) and partial thromboplastin time (PTT), leukocytosis, spherocytosis, Coombs-positive hemolytic anemia, thrombocytopenia, or abnormal kidney and liver function tests.

### Treatment

Optimal local treatment of the lesion is controversial. The most prudent management of the dermatonecrotic lesion is wound care, immobilization, tetanus prophylaxis, analgesics, and antipruritics as warranted (Table 88–3). Early use of dapsone (in patients who develop a central purplish bleb or vesicle within the first 6–8 hours) is reported to inhibit local infiltration of the wound by polymorphonuclear leukocytes. However, there is not enough information to recommend the use of dapsone in the management of *Loxosceles* envenomation at this time. Hepatitis, methemoglobinemia (Chap. 97), and hemolysis are associated with dapsone use.

Patients manifesting systemic loxoscelism or those with expanding necrotic lesions should be admitted to the hospital. All patients should be monitored for evidence of hemolysis, acute kidney injury, or coagulopathy. If hemoglobinuria ensues, increased IV fluids and urinary alkalinization can be used in an attempt to prevent acute kidney injury. Hemolysis, if significant, can be treated with transfusions. Patients with coagulopathy should be monitored with serial complete blood cell counts, platelet counts, PT, PTT, fibrin split products, and fibrinogen. Disseminated intravascular coagulopathy requires treatment, based on severity.

**TABLE 88–3 Management of Brown Recluse Spider Bite**

| *General Wound Care* | *Local Wound Care* | *Systemic* |
|---|---|---|
| Clean | Serial observations | Antipruritic/antianxiety and/or analgesics |
| Tetanus prophylaxis as indicated | Natural healing by granulation | Antibiotics for secondary bacterial infection |
| Immobilize and elevate bitten extremity | Delayed primary closure | Antivenom (experimental) |
| Apply cool compresses; avoid local heat | Delayed secondary closure with skin graft | |
| | Gauze packing, if applicable | |

## HOBO SPIDER (*ERATIGENA AGRESTIS*, NORTHWESTERN BROWN SPIDER, WALCKENAER SPIDER)

Formerly known as *Tegenaria agrestis*, the hobo spider is native to Europe and was introduced to the northwestern US (Washington, Oregon, Idaho) in the 1920s or 1930s. There is only one confirmed hobo spider bite resulting in a necrotic lesion. The other cases implicating Hobo spiders as a cause for dermatonecrotic injuries are based on proximity of the Hobo spider or other large brown spiders that are unidentified.

### Pathophysiology

The toxin was fractionated, with three peptides identified as having potent insecticidal activity and no discernible effects in mammalian in vivo assays. Insects envenomated with *E. agrestis* venom and the insecticidal toxins purified from the venom developed a slowly evolving spastic paralysis. Currently, little is known about the toxin and its mechanism of action in humans.

### Clinical Manifestations

The toxicity of hobo spider venom is questionable; however, it occasionally causes dermatonecrosis secondary to infection. Other causes of dermatonecrotic lesions should be excluded. The most common symptom associated with the spider bite is a headache that persists for up to 1 week. Other manifestations, including nausea, vomiting, fatigue, memory loss, visual impairment, weakness, and lethargy, are reported.

### Diagnostic Testing

No specific laboratory assay confirms envenomation with *E. agrestis* spider.

### Treatment

Treatment emphasizes local wound care and tetanus prophylaxis, although systemic corticosteroids are reasonable for hematologic complications.

## TARANTULAS

Tarantulas are primitive mygalomorph spiders that belong to the family Theraphosidae, a subgroup of Mygalomorphae (Greek word *mygale* for field mouse) (Fig. 88–4). Because of

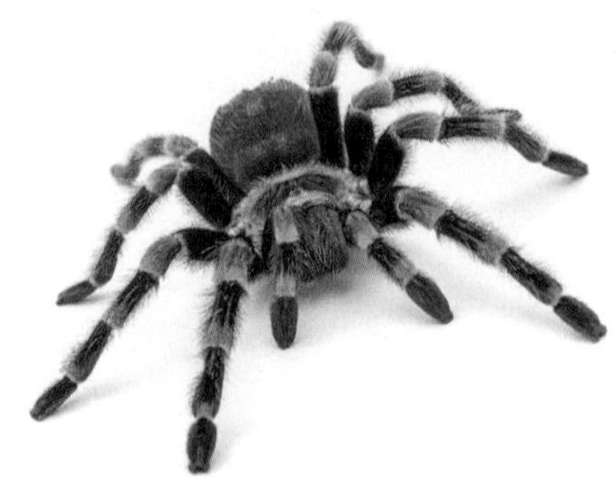

**FIGURE 88–4.** The Mexican redknee tarantula, *Brachypelma smithi*. *(Used with permission from Pets in Frames/Shutterstock.)*

their great size and reputation, tarantulas are often feared. They have poor eyesight and usually detect their victims by touch and vibrations. Their defense lies in either their painful bite with erect fangs or by barraging their victim with urticating hairs that are released on provocation. Only the New World tarantulas (tarantulas indigenous to the Americas) have and use the urticating hairs to defend themselves.

Tarantulas bite when provoked or roughly handled. Based on the few case reports, their venom has relatively minor effects in humans but can be deadly for canines and other small animals, such as rats, mice, cats, and birds. At least four genera of tarantulas (*Lasiodora*, *Grammostola*, *Acanthoscurria*, and *Brachypelma*) possess urticating hairs that are released in self-defense when the tarantulas rub their hind legs against their abdomen rapidly to create a small cloud. Urticarial hairs or setae are composed of chitin, lipoproteins, and mucopolysaccharides, which are recognized as foreign bodies triggering a humoral response in the mammalian immune system. Besides cell-mediated inflammation, spider setae also trigger IgE-mediated hypersensitivity.

### Pathophysiology

Tarantula venom contains hyaluronidase, nucleotides (adenosine triphosphate, adenosine diphosphate, and adenosine monophosphate), and polyamines (spermine, spermidine, putrescine, and cadaverine) that are essential to prey. Venom causes skeletal muscle necrosis when injected intraperitoneally in mice. The primary injury results in rupture of the plasma membrane, followed by the inability of mitochondria and sarcoplasmic reticulum to maintain normal concentrations of calcium in the cytoplasm leading to cell death.

### Clinical Manifestations

Although relatively infrequent in occurrence, bites present with puncture or fang marks. They range from being painless to a deep throbbing pain that is reported to last several hours without any inflammatory component. Fever occurs in the absence of infection, suggesting a direct pyrexic action of the venom. Rarely, bites create a local histamine response with resultant itching, and hypersensitive individuals can have more severe reactions and, less commonly, mild systemic effects such as nausea and vomiting. Contact reactions from the urticating hairs are more likely to be the health hazard than the spider bite. The urticating hairs provoke local histamine reactions in humans and are especially irritating to the eyes, skin, and respiratory tract. Tarantula urticating hairs cause intense inflammation that often remains pruritic for weeks.

### Treatment

Treatment is largely supportive. Cool compresses and analgesics should be given as needed. All bites should receive local wound care, including tetanus prophylaxis if necessary. If the hairs are barbed, as in some species, they can be removed by using adhesive such as duct tape or cellophane tape followed by compresses or irrigation with 0.9% sodium chloride solution. Urticarial reactions should be treated with oral antihistamines and topical or systemic corticosteroids. If the hairs are located in the eye, then surgical removal will be required, followed by medical management of inflammation.

## FUNNEL WEB SPIDERS

Australian funnel web spiders cause a severe neurotoxic envenomation syndrome in humans. The fang positions of funnel web spiders are vertical relative to their body, which requires the spider to rear back and lift the body to attack. The length of fangs reaches up to 5 mm. This spider bites tenaciously and occasionally requires extraction from the victim. *Atrax robustus*, also called the Sydney funnel web spider, is the best known and is located around the center of Sydney, Australia. The Sydney funnel web spider is considered one of the most poisonous spiders. It was responsible for 14 deaths between 1927 and 1980, at which time an antivenom was introduced.

### Pathophysiology

Originally called robustotoxin from *A. robustus* spider and versutoxin from the *Hadronyche versuta* spider, the single toxin, which is now referred to as atracotoxin or atraxin, is the lethal protein component of *A. robustus* venom. Atracotoxin targets mammals by increasing the ion conductance at voltage-gated sodium channels via trapping the channel in an inward conformational change, preventing the closure of the ion channel, thereby evoking a fulminant neurotransmitter release at the autonomic and/or somatic synapses. Hence atracotoxin produces an autonomic storm, releasing acetylcholine, noradrenaline, and adrenaline.

### Clinical Manifestations

A biphasic envenomation syndrome is described in humans. Phase 1 consists of localized pain at the bite site, perioral tingling, piloerection, and regional fasciculations (most prominent in the face, tongue, and intercostal muscles). Fasciculations progress to more overt muscle spasm; masseter and laryngeal involvement may threaten the airway. Other features include tachycardia, hypertension, cardiac dysrhythmias, nausea, vomiting, abdominal pain, diaphoresis, lacrimation, salivation, and acute respiratory distress syndrome (ARDS), which often is the cause of death in phase 1. Phase 2 consists of resolution of the overt cholinergic and adrenergic crisis; secretions dry up, and fasciculations, spasms, and hypertension resolve. This apparent improvement is occasionally followed by the gradual onset of refractory hypotension, apnea, and cardiac arrest.

### Treatment

Pressure immobilization using crepe bandage to limit lymphatic flow and immobilization of the bitten extremity are reported to inactivate the venom and are recommended to be applied if symptoms of envenomation are present. Funnel web venom is one of the few animal toxins known to undergo local inactivation. The patient should be transferred to the nearest hospital with the bandage in place and then stabilized and placed in a resuscitation facility with adequate ampules of antivenom readily available before the bandage is removed; otherwise, a precipitous envenomation will potentially occur during the removal of the pressure bandage. A purified IgG antivenom protective against *Atrax* envenomations was developed in rabbits. The starting dose is two ampules if systemic signs of envenomations are present and four ampules if the patient develops ARDS or decreased mental status. Doses are repeated every 15 minutes until

**TABLE 88–4 Scorpions of Toxicologic Importance**

| |
|---|
| Australia: *Lychas marmoreus, Lychas* spp, *Isometrus* spp, *Cercophonius squama, Urodacus* spp |
| India: *Buthus tamulus* |
| Mexico: *Centruroides* spp |
| Middle East: *Androctonus crassicauda, Androctonus australis, Buthus minax, Androctonus australis, Buthus occitanus, Leiurus quinquestriatus* |
| Spain: *Buthus occitanus* |
| South Africa: *Androctonus crassicauda* |
| South America: *Tityus serrulatus* |
| United States: *Centruroides exilicauda* |

clinical improvement occurs. That being said, the efficacy of antivenom is debated. Serum sickness is rare after funnel web antivenom administration.

## SCORPIONS

Scorpions are invertebrate arthropods that have existed for more than 400 million years. Of the 650 known living species, most of the lethal species are in the family Buthidae (Table 88–4). Their five-segmented metasoma ("tail") contains a terminal bulbous segment called the *telson* that contains the venom apparatus (Fig. 88–5). More than 100,000 medically significant stings likely occur annually worldwide, predominantly in the tropics and North Africa.

### Pathophysiology

Components of scorpion venom are complex and species specific. Four neurotoxins, designated toxins I to IV, were isolated from *C. exilicauda*. Some of the toxins target excitable membranes, especially at the neuromuscular junction, by opening sodium channels. The results are repetitive depolarization of nerves in both sympathetic and parasympathetic nervous systems causing catecholamine and acetylcholine release, respectively.

### Clinical Manifestations

A three-category classification system for scorpion envenomations worldwide is used. Category 1 is "mild" and involves local manifestations such as erythema, edema, sweating, numbness, and fasciculations. Category 2 is "moderate" and involves abdominal pain, vomiting, generalized diaphoresis, tachypnea, tachycardia or bradycardia, hypertension, agitation, hypersalivation, dysphagia, fever, and/or hyperglycemia. Category 3 is "severe" and indicates patients who present with cardiovascular complications such as congestive heart failure, dilated cardiomyopathy, cardiogenic shock, dysrhythmias, or severe hypertension. Severe envenomation also includes pulmonary manifestations such as pulmonary edema and ARDS; gastrointestinal findings such as acute pancreatitis or peptic ulceration; as well as neurologic manifestations such as hypertensive encephalopathy, coma, or seizures. The presence of diarrhea is associated with increased incidence of respiratory failure, neurologic failure, liver failure, and death. This system has been adapted for US envenomations, where symptoms begin almost immediately and reach maximum severity in about 5 hours (Table 88–5).

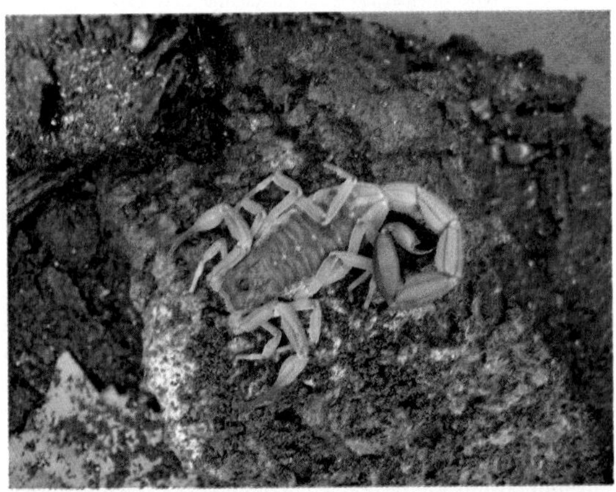

**FIGURE 88–5.** The Brazilian scorpion, *Tityus serrulatus*, shown here to demonstrate the typical features of scorpions. Note the telson (stinger) located on the tail. *(Used with permission from Dr. Michael Seiter, University of Vienna, Austria.)*

**TABLE 88–5 Envenomation Gradation for *Centruroides exilicauda* (Bark Scorpion)**

| Grade | Signs and Symptoms |
|---|---|
| I | Site of envenomation<br>Pain and/or paresthesias<br>Positive tap test (severe pain increases with touch or percussion) |
| II | Grade I in addition to<br>Pain and paresthesias remote from sting site (eg, paresthesias moving up an extremity, perioral "numbness") |
| III | One of the following:<br>Somatic skeletal neuromuscular dysfunction: jerking of extremity(ies), restlessness, severe involuntary shaking and jerking, which may be mistaken for seizures<br>Cranial nerve dysfunction: blurred vision, roving eye movements (opsoclonus) hypersalivation, dysphagia, tongue fasciculation, upper airway dysfunction, slurred speech |
| IV | Both cranial nerve dysfunction and somatic skeletal neuromuscular dysfunction |

### Treatment

Because most envenomations do not produce severe effects, local wound care, including tetanus prophylaxis and pain management, usually is all that is warranted. In young children or patients who manifest severe toxicity, hospitalization is recommended. Treatment emphasizes support of the airway, breathing, and circulation. However, children rarely require respiratory support. Continuous intravenous midazolam infusion is often used for *C. exilicauda* scorpion envenomation until resolution of the abnormal motor activity and agitation occurs. An equine-derived F(ab′)2 product for *Centruroides* spp. envenomation was approved in the US in 2011 (Antidotes in Brief: A38). Indications include neurotoxicity, which primarily occurs in children younger than 10 years, and intractable pain in adults.

## TICKS

In 1912, Todd described a progressive ascending flaccid paralysis after bites from ticks. Three families of ticks are recognized: (1) Ixodidae (hard ticks), (2) Argasidae (soft ticks), and (3) Nuttalliellidae (a group that has characteristics of both hard and soft ticks and not thought to be parasitic compared to ixodids and argasids). The terms *hard* and *soft* refer to a dorsal scutum or "plate" that is present in the Ixodidae but absent in the Argasidae. The paralytic syndrome is induced following envenomation during the larva, nymph, and adult stages and is related to the tick obtaining a blood meal. The following discussion focuses only on tick paralysis (TP) or tick toxicosis and not on any of the infectious diseases associated with tick bites. In North America, *Dermacentor andersoni* (Rocky Mountain wood tick), *Dermacentor variabilis* (American dog tick), and *Amblyomma americanum* (Lone Star tick) are the most commonly implicated causes of TP. Typically, tick toxicosis occurs in the Southeast, Rocky Mountain, and Pacific Northwest regions of the US, but cases are also reported in the Northeast. In Australia, the *Ixodes holocyclus* or Australian marsupial tick is the most common offender.

### Pathophysiology

Venom secreted from the salivary glands during the blood meal is absorbed by the host and systemically distributed. The neurotoxin "ixobotoxin", inhibits the release of acetylcholine at the neuromuscular junction and autonomic ganglia, very similar to botulinum toxin.

### Clinical Manifestations

Usually the tick must remain on the person for at least 3 days in order to result in systemic effects. Several days must pass before tick salivary glands begin to secrete significant quantities of toxin. Once secreted, the toxin does not act immediately and undergoes binding and internalization, in a similar sequence to botulinum toxin. Children appear listless, weak, ataxic, and irritable for several days before they develop an ascending paralysis that begins in the lower limbs. Fever usually is absent. Other manifestations include sensory symptoms such as paresthesias, numbness, and mild diarrhea. These symptoms are followed by absent or decreased deep-tendon reflexes and an ascending generalized weakness that can progress to bulbar structures involving speech, swallowing, and facial expression within 24 to 48 hours, as well as fixed, dilated pupils and disturbances of extraocular movements. Unlike the *Dermacentor* spp of North America, removal of the *I. holocyclus* tick does not result in dramatic improvement for several days to weeks.

The differential diagnosis is extensive and includes Guillain-Barré syndrome (GBS), the Miller-Fisher variant of Guillain-Barré, poliomyelitis, botulism, transverse myelitis, myasthenia gravis, periodic paralysis, elapid snakebites, marine neurotoxin poisoning, acute cerebellar ataxia, and spinal cord lesions (Chap. 11). The cerebrospinal fluid remains normal, and the rate of progression is rapid, unlike GBS and poliomyelitis. The edrophonium test to assess for myasthenia gravis is negative. Nerve conduction studies in patients with TP frequently resemble those of patients with early stages of GBS.

### Treatment

Other than removal of the entire tick, which is curative, treatment is entirely supportive. Proper removal of the tick is very important; otherwise, infection or incomplete tick removal can result. The tick should be grasped as close to the skin surface as possible with blunt curved forceps, tweezers, or gloved hands and pulled straight up. Steady pressure without crushing the body should be employed. After tick removal, the site should be disinfected. Since *I. holocyclus* of Australia is considerably more toxic and patients are more likely to deteriorate before they improve, close observation is required for several days until improvement is certain.

## HYMENOPTERA: BEES, WASPS, HORNETS, YELLOW JACKETS, AND ANTS

Within the order Hymenoptera are three families of clinical significance: Apidae (honeybees and bumblebees), Vespidae (yellow jackets, hornets, and wasps), and Formicidae (ants, specifically fire ants). These insects (Fig. 88–6) are of great medical importance because their stings are the most commonly reported and can cause acute toxic and fatal allergic reactions. Honeybee workers only sting once. Their stinger is a modified ovipositor that resides in the abdomen and its shaft is barbed and has a venom sac attached. Once the stinger embeds into the skin, the stinger disembowels the bee. Bumblebees, however, can sting multiple times. Vespids are more aggressive and able to sting multiple times.

### Pathophysiology

Several allergens (Table 88–6) and pharmacologically active compounds are found in honeybee venom. Melittin is the principal component of honeybee venom. It acts as a detergent to disrupt the cell membrane and liberate potassium and biogenic amines. Histamine release by bee venom is largely mediated by mast cell degranulation peptide. Apamin is a neurotoxin that acts on the spinal cord. Apamin binds to the $Ca^{+2}$-triggered $K^{+}$ channel and depresses delayed hyperpolarization. Phospholipase $A_2$ and hyaluronidase are the chief enzymes in bee venom.

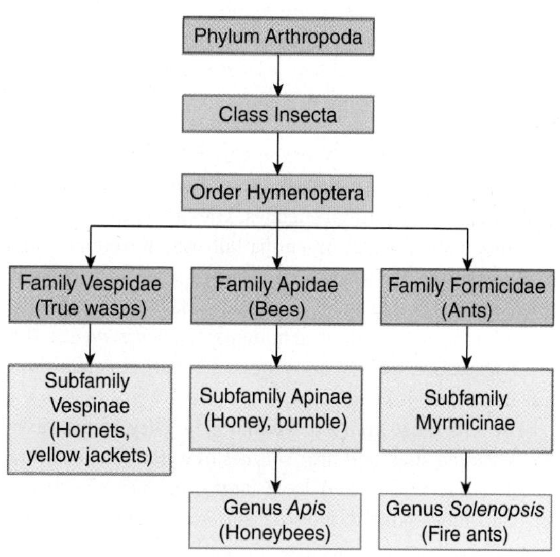


**FIGURE 88–6.** Taxonomy of the order Hymenoptera.

TABLE 88–6 Composition of Hymenoptera Venom

| *Vespid (Wasps, Hornets, Yellow Jackets)* | *Apids (Honeybees)* | *Formicids (Fire Ants)* |
|---|---|---|
| Biogenic amines (diverse) | Biogenic amines (diverse) | Biogenic amines (diverse) |
| Phospholipase A | Phospholipase A | Phospholipase $A_2$ |
| Phospholipase B | Phospholipase B | Hyaluronidase |
| Hyaluronidase | Hyaluronidase | Piperidines |
| Acid phosphatase | Acid phosphatase | |
| Mast cell–degranulating peptide | Minimine | |
| Kinin | Mellitin | |
| | Apamin | |
| | Mast cell–degranulating peptide | |

### Clinical Manifestations

Normally, the honeybee sting results in immediate pain, a wheal-and-flare reaction, and localized edema without a systemic reaction. Vomiting, diarrhea, and syncope occur with a higher dose of venom resulting from multiple stings. Toxic reactions occur with multiple stings (more than 500 stings are described as possibly fatal) and occur with Africanized honeybees and include gastrointestinal (GI) effects, headache, fever, syncope and, rarely, rhabdomyolysis, acute kidney injury, and seizures. This type of toxic reaction differs from the hypersensitivity reactions or anaphylactic reactions because it is not an IgE-mediated response, but rather a direct effect from the venom itself.

### Treatment

Application of ice at the site usually is sufficient to halt discomfort. Stingers from honeybees should be removed by scraping with a credit card or scalpel, as opposed to pulling, which potentially releases additional retained venom. Since the stinger in other bee species typically stays within the insect, this removal technique will not be necessary if other bee species are involved. Therapy is aimed at supportive care that includes standard therapy for anaphylaxis with epinephrine, diphenhydramine, and corticosteroids when indicated.

## FIRE ANTS

There are native fire ants in the US, but the imported fire ants *Solenopsis invicta* and *Solenopsis richteri* are significant pests that have no natural enemies. They are native to Brazil, Paraguay, Uruguay, and Argentina but were introduced into Alabama in the 1930s. They have spread rapidly throughout the southern US, damaging crops, reducing biologic diversity, and inflicting severe stings to humans. *Solenopsis invicta*, the most aggressive species, now infests 13 southern states and was introduced into Australia.

Fire ants range from 2 to 6 mm in size. They live in grassy areas, garden sites, and near sources of water. The nests are largely subterranean and have large, conspicuous, dome-shaped, above-ground mounds (up to 45 cm above the ground), with many openings for traffic. The mounds can contain 80,000 to 250,000 workers and one or more queens that live for 2 to 6 years and produce 1,500 eggs daily. Fire ants are named for the burning pain inflicted after exposure, and necrosis can result at the site. The imported fire ant attacks with little warning. By firmly grasping the skin with their mandibles, both the fire ant and the jumper ant can repeatedly inject venom from a retractile stinger at the end of the abdomen. Pivoting at the head, the fire ant injects an average of seven or eight stings in a circular pattern.

### Pathophysiology

The venom inhibits $Na^+,K^+$-ATPases, reduces mitochondrial respiration, uncouples oxidative phosphorylation, adversely affects neutrophil and platelet function, inhibits nitric oxide synthetase, and perhaps activates coagulation. There is also some in vivo evidence that the venom inhibits nitric oxide synthetase activity and has direct cardiotoxic, convulsant, and respiratory depressant activities.

### Clinical Manifestations

In the US, residents of healthcare facilities who are immobile or cognitively impaired are at risk for fire ant attacks, especially when the facility lacks pest control techniques for fire ants. Three categories are suggested based on the reactions to the imported fire ant: local, large local, and systemic. *Local reactions* occur in nonallergic individuals. *Large local reactions* are defined as painful, pruritic swelling at least 5 cm in diameter and contiguous with the sting site. *Systemic reactions* involve signs and symptoms remote from the sting site. The sting initially forms a wheal that is described as a burning itch at the site, followed by the development of sterile pustules. In 24 hours, the pustules umbilicate on an erythematous base. Pustules last 1 to 2 weeks. Large reactions lead to tissue edema sufficient to compromise blood flow to an extremity. Anaphylaxis occurs in 0.6% to 6% of persons who have been stung. The majority of individuals who die after fire ant attacks succumb to heart failure possibly as a result of the direct myocardial toxicity of the venom.

### Diagnosis

Clinical clues such as pustule development at the sting site after 24 hours, species identification, and history help to identify fire ant exposure. No laboratory assays to determine exposure are available.

### Treatment

Local reactions require cold compresses and cleansing with soap and water. We recommend topical or injected lidocaine with or without 1:100,000 epinephrine, and topical vinegar and salt mixtures to decrease pain at the site of the bite and sting. Large local reactions should be treated with oral corticosteroids, antihistamines, and analgesics. Secondary infections should be treated with antibiotics. It is reasonable for systemic reactions to be treated with intramuscular or intravenous epinephrine.

## BUTTERFLIES, MOTHS, AND CATERPILLARS

Butterflies and moths are insects of the order Lepidoptera. Caterpillar species from about 12 families of moths and rarely butterflies worldwide can inflict serious human injuries, including urticarial dermatitis, allergic reactions, consumptive coagulopathy, acute kidney injury, intracerebral hemorrhage, arthritis, joint deformity, and even altered mental status, ataxia, and dysarthria. *Lepidopterism* is a general term that describes the systemic adverse effects, and *erucism* is the term used for isolated cutaneous effects.

### Pathophysiology

The composition of the venom varies according to the different caterpillar species. The pathophysiology is not well understood, but the venom contains formaldehyde and several uncharacterized histamine analogs that cause both acute allergic reactions and chronic effects on bone, joints, and cartilage that are thought to be autoimmune mediated. A protein called lonomin isolated from the *Lonomia achelous* caterpillar causes coagulopathy.

### Clinical Manifestations

The pathophysiologic effects of venomous caterpillar exposures are classified into seven distinct clinical syndromes to guide clinicians in making earlier, more species-specific diagnoses to direct therapies.

1. Erucism is the preferred term for caterpillar dermatitis caused by contact with caterpillar urticating hairs, spines, or toxic hemolymph.
2. Lepidopterism is a systemic illness caused by a constellation of adverse effects resulting from direct or aerosol contact with caterpillar, cocoon, or moth urticating hairs, spines, or body fluids and is characterized by generalized urticaria, headache, conjunctivitis, pharyngitis, nausea, vomiting, bronchospasm, wheezing, and, rarely, dyspnea.
3. Dendrolimiasis is a chronic form of lepidopterism caused by direct contact with urticating hairs, spines, or hemolymph of living or dead central Asian pine-tree lappet moth caterpillars or their cocoons and is characterized by urticating maculopapular dermatitis, migratory inflammatory polyarthritis, migratory inflammatory polychondritis, chronic osteoarthritis, and, rarely, acute scleritis.
4. Ophthalmia nodosa is a chronic ocular condition characterized by initial conjunctivitis with subsequent panuveitis caused by corneal penetration and subsequent intraocular migration of urticating hairs from lymantriid caterpillars and moths and therapsid spiders (tarantulas).
5. Consumptive coagulopathy results from exposure to the South American *Lonomia saturniid* moth caterpillars. High fatality rates result from venom-induced, intracerebral hemorrhage, and acute kidney injury, possibly due to a combination of venom nephrotoxicity and microcirculatory fibrin deposition. The hemorrhagic syndrome presents as a disseminating intravascular coagulopathy and as a secondary fibrinolysis with skin, mucosal, and visceral bleeding, acute kidney injury, and intracerebral hemorrhage.
6. Seasonal ataxia is a syndrome of unsteady gait and dysarthria, which occurs after the ingestion of the caterpillar of *Anaphe venata.* This occurs in areas of Nigeria where the caterpillars are a source of protein. Ingestion of the roasted larvae causes nausea and vomiting and progresses to dizziness, ataxia, and unsteady gait in more than 90% of victims. These findings may take weeks to months for resolution. Dysarthria and impaired consciousness are also reported. The pathogenesis is related to thiamine deficiency induced by thiaminases contained in the larvae (Antidote in Brief: A27).
7. Pararamose is similar to dendrolimiasis with pruritic or painful dermatitis associated with arthritis and joint deformity, arising from contact with the caterpillar of *Premolis semirufa,* which are found in the Brazilian Amazon rain forests.

### Treatment

Management for most dermal caterpillar envenomations is entirely supportive and includes washing the area with soap and water; "no touch" drying of the sting site with a hair dryer; gentle stripping of the bite site with cellophane or adhesive duct tape; and application of ice packs with cooling enhanced by initial topical swabbing with isopropyl alcohol. Rings should be removed in anticipation for potential swelling of the extremity, and tetanus prophylaxis should be updated accordingly. Treatment of ophthalmic lesions depends upon the exposure classification and should be managed by an ophthalmologist.

Opioids are recommended if minor analgesics do not provide relief. If muscle cramps develop, benzodiazepines are reasonable. Topical corticosteroids are reasonable to decrease local inflammation. Antihistamines such as diphenhydramine (25–50 mg for adults and 1 mg/kg, maximum 50 mg, in children) are recommended to relieve pruritus and urticaria. Nebulized β-agonists and epinephrine administered intramuscularly should be used for more severe respiratory symptoms and anaphylactoid/anaphylactic-type reactions.

For hemorrhagic syndrome resulting from exposure to *L. obliqua* caterpillar, besides restoration of clotting factors, platelet, and cryoprecipitate infusions, an antidote called the antilonomic serum is available and is used for treatment of the hemorrhagic syndrome in Brazil. It is important to involve an experienced hematologist for suspected *Lonomia* envenomation and very important to distinguish *Lonomia obliqua* from *Lonomia achelous* because the cryoprecipitate, purified fibrinogen, and antifibrinolytic drugs, such as aprotinin and ε-aminocaproic acid, were used successfully in *Lonomia achelous* but exacerbated the hemorrhagic effects in *Lonomia obliqua* with fatal consequences. Patients exposed to either species should receive neither whole blood nor fresh plasma, which aggravates the clinical effects. Treatment for the seasonal ataxia includes supportive care with the administration of thiamine 100 mg orally every 8 hours, which reversed symptoms within 48 hours without long-term sequelae in a double-blinded placebo-controlled trial (Antidote in Brief: A27).

## BLISTER BEETLES

Blister beetles are plant-eating insects that exude the blistering irritant cantharidin as a presumed defense mechanism. They are found in the eastern US, southern Europe, Africa, and Asia. Most are from the order Coleoptera, family

Meloidae. When the beetles sense danger, they exude cantharidin by filling their breathing tubes with air, closing their breathing pores, and building up body fluid pressure until fluid is pushed out through one or more leg joints. Cantharidin, also known popularly as *Spanish fly*, takes its name from the Mediterranean beetle *Cantharis vesicatoria.* It has been ingested as a sexual stimulant for millennia. The aphrodisiac properties are related to the ability of cantharidin to cause vascular engorgement and inflammation of the genitourinary tract upon elimination, hence the reports of priapism and pelvic organ engorgement. Cantharidin poisoning is reported by cutaneous exposure, unintentional inoculation, and inadvertent ingestion of the beetle itself.

## Pathophysiology

Although the mechanism of action of cantharidin has not been elucidated, one study suggests that cantharidin inhibits the activity of protein phosphatases type 1 and 2A. This inhibition alters endothelial permeability by enhancing the phosphorylation state of endothelial regulatory proteins and results in elevated albumin flux and dysfunction of the barrier. Enhanced permeability of albumin is thought to be responsible for the systemic effects of cantharidin.

## Clinical Manifestations

Cantharidin causes an urticarial dermatitis that is manifested several hours after exposure by burns, blisters, or vesiculobullae. In addition to the local effects, cantharidin can be absorbed through the epidermis and cause systemic toxicity, with diaphoresis, tachycardia, hematuria, and oliguria from extensive dermal exposure. Ophthalmic findings from direct contact with the beetle or hand contamination include decreased vision, pain, lacrimation, corneal ulcerations, filamentary keratitis, and anterior uveitis.

When cantharidin is ingested, severe GI disturbances and hematuria occur. Initial patient complaints typically include burning of the oropharynx, dysphagia, abdominal cramping, vomiting, hematemesis followed by lower GI tract hematochezia, and tenesmus. Genitourinary effects include dysuria, urinary frequency, hematuria, proteinuria, and acute kidney injury impairment. Most symptoms resolve over several weeks.

## Diagnostic Testing

Although methods exist to identify cantharidin, they are not routinely available in a clinically relevant time frame.

## Treatment

Treatment is largely supportive. Wound care and tetanus status should be assessed. For keratoconjunctivitis, an ophthalmologist should be consulted early in the clinical course and the patient should be treated with topical corticosteroids (prednisolone 0.125%), mydriatics (cyclopentolate 1%), and antibiotics (ciprofloxacin 0.3%).

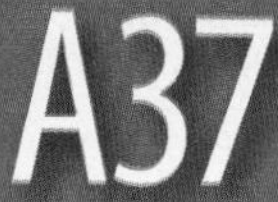

# A37 ANTIVENOM: SPIDER

## INTRODUCTION

The terms *antivenom* and *antivenin* are often used interchangeably. Except when it refers to a specific brand name, the term *antivenom* is used in this Antidotes in Brief. Antivenom for spiders is prepared by immunizing animals with venom and then collecting the immune serum for administration (Table A37–1).

## HISTORY

The two most notable genera of spiders of medical importance in the United States (US) are *Latrodectus* and *Loxosceles.* There is no commercially available antivenom for treatment of *Loxosceles* spp. envenomation at this time and only one commercially available *Latrodectus* spp. antivenom in the US. Black Widow Spider Antivenin (Merck & Co, Inc) (Merck BW-AV) The use of BW-AV is controversial, as mortality from bites is low and complications including death following BW-AV are rarely reported. An $F(ab')_2$ antivenom will likely be safer, but has not been approved for use by the US Food and Drug Administration (FDA) at the time of this writing.

## PHARMACOLOGY

### Chemistry, Preparation, and Mechanism of Action

Antivenom for spiders is prepared by immunizing animals with nontoxic amounts of venom. The majority of antivenom manufacturers use horses, since they are relatively easy to maintain, and large volumes of serum can be obtained at one time without harming the animal. During

**TABLE A37–1 Worldwide Availability of Spider Antivenom**

| *Species Name* | *Country* | *Name* | *Manufacturer* |
|---|---|---|---|
| ***Atrax, Hadronyche (Funnel web Spider)*** | | | |
| | Argentina | Anti Latrodectus Antinvenom | Instituto Nacional de Produccion de Biologicos (Equine IgG) |
| | Australia | Funnel Web Spider Antivenom | CSL Ltd (Rabbit IgG) |
| ***Latrodectus (Black widow, Redback)*** | | | |
| | Australia | Red Back Spider Antivenom | CSL Ltd (Equine $F(ab')_2$) |
| | Croatia | Antilatrodectus mactans/Tredecimguttatus Serum | Institute of Immunology (Equine IgG) |
| | Mexico | Aracmyn | Instituto Bioclon (Equine $F(ab')_2$) |
| | South Africa | SAIMR Spider Antivenom | SAIMR (Equine IgG) |
| | USA | Antivenom Latrodectus Mactans | Merck & Company (Equine IgG) |
| ***Loxosceles (Brown spiders)*** | | | |
| | Brazil | Antiloxosceles Serum | Centro de Producao e Pesquisas de Immunbiologicos (Equine IgG) |
| | Brazil | Soro Antiarachnidico | Instituto Butantan (contains *Loxosceles* spp, *Tityus* spp, and *Phoneutria* spp Antivenom) (Equine IgG) |
| | Peru | Antiloxosceles Serum | Instituto Nacional de Salud, Centro Nacional de Production de Biologicos (Equine IgG) |

antivenom production, efforts are made to remove animal proteins such as albumin.

The antivenom exists as either whole IgG, Fab, or $F(ab')_2$. Whole IgG antivenom is the easiest and least expensive to manufacture. Because of its size, it is the least filterable at the glomerulus, has the smallest volume of distribution, and has a longer elimination half-life than either Fab or $F(ab')_2$. $F(ab')_2$ antivenom has an intermediate size and elimination half-life and a lower risk of anaphylaxis compared to whole IgG. The Fab antivenom is the smallest molecule in size, has the largest volume of distribution, and is eliminated by the kidneys. Antivenoms target, bind, neutralize, and promote elimination or redistribution of toxins from body tissues.

### Pharmacokinetics and Pharmacodynamics

There is no published intravenous pharmacokinetic or pharmacodynamic information available on Merck BW-AV. Animal studies demonstrated that intramuscular administration of $F(ab')_2$ and IgG antivenom had poor bioavailability (36%–42%) and a delayed time to peak concentrations (48–96 hours) and produced very low serum venom concentrations. Redback spider (*L. hasseltii)* antivenom (RBS-AV) is available in Australia. Following intramuscular administration, studies demonstrate no circulating RBS-AV in serum up to 5 hours, compared to detection within 30 minutes following intravenous administration.

## ROLE IN *LATRODECTUS* SPECIES (*L. BISHOPI, L. GEOMETRICUS, L. HESPERUS, L. INDISTINCTUS, L. MACTANS, L. VARIOLUS*)

The administration of the BW-AV is controversial. Although black widow envenomation is associated with severe muscle pain, cramping, and autonomic disturbances, mortality is low. Symptomatic treatment can almost always be accomplished with muscle relaxants and opioids, individually or in combination.

Some authors believe that because of anaphylaxis, BW-AV has too high a risk-to-benefit ratio to justify its use. In selected patients, however, the use of antivenom reduces pain and suffering, shortens the course of the envenomation, and reduces or eliminates the need for hospitalization. We believe that indications for antivenom administration include severe muscle cramping, hypertension, diaphoresis, nausea, vomiting, and respiratory difficulty that is unresponsive to other therapy. A shortage of Merck BW-AV prompted the finding that RBS-AV also neutralizes the venom of *L. mactans* in a mouse model. Anawidow, a polyvalent $F(ab')_2$, is an equine-derived antivenom created for *L. mactans* in both Argentina and Mexico and is undergoing the US FDA approval process at this time.

## ROLE IN FUNNEL WEB SPECIES (*ATRAX* AND *HADRONYCHE*)

A rabbit IgG–based funnel web spider (*Atrax robustus* and others) antivenom is available in Australia. Since the introduction of the antivenom, no deaths have been reported. Complete response following administration of antivenom was reported in 97% of envenomations in one series.

## ROLE IN *LOXOSCELES* SPECIES (*L. RECLUSA, L. LAETA, L. RUFESCENS, L. ARIZONICA, L. UNICOLOR*)

Envenomation by the brown recluse spider *Loxosceles reclusa* is associated with low but significant morbidity, particularly in the midwest and southeast US. Experimental anti-*Loxosceles* Fab blocked dermatonecrosis in a rabbit model, but only if provided within 24 to 48 hours of envenomation. National laboratories in Brazil and Argentina produce antivenoms for *L. reclusa, L. boneti,* and *L. rufescens.*

## ADVERSE EFFECTS AND SAFETY ISSUES

Death from bronchospasm and anaphylaxis is a rarely reported complication of whole IgG BW-AV administration, as is serum sickness. Serum sickness is dose-dependent and is less likely when a dose of one to two vials is administered.

Because Australian RBS-AV is an $F(ab')_2$, it has a lower reported incidence of early allergic reactions (0.5%–0.8%), and a review of the US National Poison Data System reported a 3.4% rate of adverse drug reactions following administration of the BW-AV and a reported incidence of serum sickness of less than 5%. No serious adverse effects or deaths occurred in a randomized controlled Analatro trial.

## PREGNANCY AND LACTATION

Black widow envenomations during pregnancy are relatively rare. Merck BW-AV is Pregnancy Category C. It is not known whether antivenom is excreted in human milk.

## DOSING AND ADMINISTRATION

The recommended dose of the BW-AV is one vial reconstituted with 2.5 mL of sterile water for injection and then diluted in 50 mL of saline for intravenous administration over 15 minutes. Intramuscular administration is not routinely recommended. The initial dose of antivenom in funnel web spider envenomation is two vials in patients with any signs or symptoms of envenomation and four vials for patients with acute respiratory distress syndrome or decreased consciousness. The dosage for children is the same as for adults.

## FORMULATION AND ACQUISITION

Merck BW-AV is supplied as a powder along with a 2.5-mL vial of sterile diluent for reconstitution. The antivenin must be stored and shipped at 2°C to 8°C (36°F–46°F) but should never be frozen. The reconstituted antivenin color ranges from light straw to very dark iced tea, but color has no effect on potency. Although a 1-mL vial of horse serum (1:10 dilution) for sensitivity testing is also included, we recommend against its use. Because *Latrodectus* venoms are virtually identical by immunologic and electrophoretic mechanisms, the RBS-AV created for *L. mactans* is presumed to be effective in other species of *Latrodectus* as well. The Antivenom Index maintained by the Association of Zoos and Aquariums (https://www.aza.org/antivenom-index/) (Phone: 301-562-0777) is accessible at US Poison Centers and also serves as a resource.

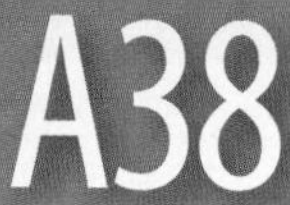

# A38 ANTIVENOM: SCORPION

## INTRODUCTION

*Centruroides exilicauda* (formerly known as *Centruroides sculpturatus*) is the only scorpion of medical importance in the United States (US). It is indigenous to the deserts of Arizona, but also can be found in Texas, New Mexico, California, and Nevada. Occasionally, envenomations occur in nonindigenous areas of the country from "stowaway" scorpions in travelers' luggage.

## HISTORY

Antivenom for the *Centruroides* spp was first produced in horses in Mexico in the 1930s. In 1947, antivenom was produced from rabbits and cats. The Antivenom Production Laboratory at Arizona State University (APL-ASU) began producing antivenom to *C. sculpturatus* in goats in 1965. This antivenom was used for treatment of scorpion stings in Arizona until 2004. In June 2000, Silanes Laboratory received orphan drug status for a *Centruroides* scorpion antivenom, an equine $F(ab')_2$ derived from *C. limpidus*, *C. noxius*, *C. suffusus*, and *C. meisei* manufactured by Instituto Bioclon of Mexico, and sold as Centruroides (Scorpion) Immune $F(ab')_2$ (Equine) Injection (Anascorp). In August 2011, Centruroides (Scorpion) Immune $F(ab')_2$ (Equine) Injection was approved by the US Food and Drug Administration (FDA) for the treatment of *C. exilicauda* envenomations.

## PHARMACOLOGY

Antivenom for scorpions is prepared in the same manner as other antivenom products (Antidotes in Brief: A37 and A39).

### Pharmacokinetics and Pharmacodynamics

Measured pharmacokinetic parameters (mean ± standard deviation) for Centruroides (Scorpion) Immune $F(ab')_2$ (Equine) Injection in adult humans are: clearance, 83.5 ± 38.4 mL/h; half-life, 159 ± 57 hours; and steady-state volume of distribution (Vdss), 13.6 ± 5.4 L.

## ROLE IN *CENTRUROIDES* SPECIES

The safety and efficacy of Centruroides (Scorpion) Immune $F(ab')_2$ (Equine) Injection are documented in both animals and humans. A prospective, randomized, double-blinded, controlled trial demonstrated a clear benefit in reduction of signs and symptoms of scorpion envenomation by 4 hours post-administration in greater than 95% of patients, and a reduction in quantity of sedative administered (mean midazolam dose of 0.1 mg/kg {0.0–0.2 mg/kg}) in treated patients versus 4.6 mg/kg (0.1–16.7 mg/kg) in controls. Because of the high cost of Centruroides (Scorpion) Immune $F(ab')_2$ (Equine) Injection, some hospitals have adopted guidelines advocating for a single-vial initial dose rather than the US FDA-approved three-vial initial dose.

## ADVERSE EFFECTS AND SAFETY ISSUES

Adverse effects reported from cumulative clinical trial data revealed that 2.2% of patients experienced severe adverse reactions (respiratory distress, aspiration, hypoxia, ataxia, pneumonia, and eye swelling) following Centruroides (Scorpion) Immune $F(ab')_2$ (Equine) Injection administration. However, these symptoms occurred in the setting of acute *Centruroides* envenomation, limiting the direct attribution of symptoms to antivenom administration alone. The most common adverse effects reported included vomiting (4.7%), pyrexia (4.1%), rash (2.7%), nausea (2.1%), and pruritus (2%). No deaths were reported in clinical trials of Centruroides (Scorpion) Immune $F(ab')_2$ (Equine) Injection. Patients with known equine protein allergies or previous exposure to Centruroides (Scorpion) Immune $F(ab')_2$ (Equine) Injection or other equine-derived antivenoms or antitoxins may also be at increased risk because of previous sensitization.

## PREGNANCY AND LACTATION

Centruroides (Scorpion) Immune $F(ab')_2$ (Equine) Injection is Pregnancy Category C. Anascorp should only be administered in pregnant women if clearly needed for alleviation of symptoms and after other therapies have been utilized. It is unknown whether Anascorp is excreted in human breast milk.

## DOSING AND ADMINISTRATION

Centruroides (Scorpion) Immune $F(ab')_2$ (Equine) Injection should be reconstituted (5 mL sterile 0.9% sodium chloride solution/vial) and diluted to a total volume of 50 mL. The recommended dose is three vials intravenously over 10 minutes. Thereafter, administer one additional vial at a time at 30- to 60-minute intervals as needed for symptom control. Although antivenom is highly effective, concerns about its cost persist.

## FORMULATION AND ACQUISITION

Centruroides (Scorpion) Immune $F(ab')_2$ (Equine) Injection is supplied as a sterile lyophilized preparation in a single-use vial that should be stored at room temperature up to 25°C (77°F). The Antivenom Index, maintained by the Association of Zoos and Aquariums (https://www.aza.org/antivenom-index/), which is accessible to the America's Poison Centers, may serve as a resource in the event of difficulty obtaining antivenom. The World Health Organization's World Directory of Poison Control Centres (http://www.who.int/gho/phe/chemical_safety/poisons_centres/en/) might assist those outside of the US to source more exotic antivenoms.

**TABLE A38–1 Worldwide Scorpion Antivenoms**

| *Species* | *Country* | *Name* | *Manufacturer* | *Antibody Type* |
|---|---|---|---|---|
| ***Centruroides* species *(elegans, exilicauda, gertschi, limpidus, noxius, suffusus)*** | Mexico | Suero Antialacran Alacramyn | Instituto Bioclon | Equine $F(ab')_2$ |
| | United States | Anascorp Centruroides (Scorpion) Immune $F(ab')_2$ | Instituto Bioclon | Equine $F(ab')_2$ |
| ***Androctonus* species** | | | | |
| | Algeria | Antiscorpion Serum | Institut Pasteur d'Algerie | Equine $F(ab')_2$ |
| | Egypt | Purified Polyvalent Antiscorpion Serum | Egyptian Organization for Biological Products and Vaccines (VACSERA) | Equine $F(ab')_2$ |
| | France | ScorpiFAV | Aventis Pasteur | Equine $F(ab')_2$ |
| | Germany | Scorpion Antivenom | Twyford | Equine $F(ab')_2$ |
| | Iran | Polyvalent Scorpion Antivenom | Razi Vaccine and Serum Research Institute | Equine $F(ab')_2$ |
| | Tunisia | Scorpion Antivenom | Institut Pasteur de Tunis | Equine $F(ab')_2$ |
| | Turkey | Scorpion Antivenom | Refik Saydam Hygiene Center | Equine $F(ab')_2$ |
| ***Buthus* species** | | | | |
| | Algeria | Antiscorpion Serum | Institut Pasteur d'Algerie | Equine $F(ab')_2$ |
| | Egypt | Purified Polyvalent Antiscorpion Serum | VACSERA | Equine $F(ab')_2$ |
| | France | ScorpiFAV | Aventis Pasteur | Equine $F(ab')_2$ |
| | Germany | Scorpion Antivenom | Twyford | Equine $F(ab')_2$ |
| | India | Scorpion Venom | Haffkine Biopharmaceutical | Equine $F(ab')_2$ |
| | Saudi Arabia | Polyvalent Scorpion Antivenom | National Antivenom and Vaccine Production Center (NAVPC) | Equine $F(ab')_2$ |
| | Tunisia | Scorpion Antivenom | Institut Pasteur de Tunis | Equine $F(ab')_2$ |
| ***Leiurus* species** | | | | |
| | Egypt | Purified Polyvalent Antiscorpion Serum | VACSERA | Equine $F(ab')_2$ |
| | France | ScorpiFAV | Aventis Pasteur | Equine $F(ab')_2$ |
| | Saudi Arabia | Polyvalent Scorpion | NAVPC | Equine $F(ab')_2$ |
| | Tunisia | Scorpion Antivenom | Institut Pasteur de Tunis | Equine $F(ab')_2$ |
| | Turkey | Scorpion Antivenom | Refik Saydam Hygiene Center | Equine $F(ab')_2$ |
| ***Mesobuthus* species** | | | | |
| | India | Monovalent Scorpion Antivenom | Central Research Institute | Equine $F(ab')_2$ |
| | Iran | Polyvalent Scorpion Antivenom | Razi Vaccine and Serum Research Institute | Equine $F(ab')_2$ |
| ***Odontobuthus doriae*** | | | | |
| | Iran | Polyvalent Scorpion Antivenom | Razi Vaccine and Serum Research Institute | Equine $F(ab')_2$ |
| ***Palamnaeus* species** | | | | |
| | India | Monovalent Scorpion Antivenom | Central Research Institute | Equine $F(ab')_2$ |
| ***Parabuthus* species** | | | | |
| | South Africa | SAIMR Scorpion Antivenom | South African Vaccine Producers | Equine $F(ab')_2$ |
| ***Scorpio maurus*** | | | | |
| | Egypt | Purified Polyvalent Antiscorpion Serum | VACSERA | Equine $F(ab')_2$ |
| | France | ScorpiFAV | Aventis Pasteur | Equine $F(ab')_2$ |
| | Iran | Polyvalent Scorpion Antivenom | Razi Vaccine and Serum Research Institute | Equine $F(ab')_2$ |
| | Turkey | Scorpion Antivenom | Refik Saydam Hygiene Center | Equine $F(ab')_2$ |
| ***Tityus* species** | | | | |
| | Argentina | Scorpion Antivenom | Instituto Nacional | Equine Fab |
| | Brazil | Soro Antiscorpionico | Instituto Butantan | Equine Sera |
| | Brazil | Soro Antiarachnidico | Instituto Butantan, | Equine IgG |
| | Brazil | Antiscorpion Serum IVB | Instituto Vital Brazil S.A. | Equine IgG |
| | Brazil | Antiescopionico | Fundacao Ezequiel Dias | Equine $F(ab')_2$ |

## SCORPIONS NOT NATIVE TO NORTH AMERICA

### *Leiurus* Species

The *Leiurus quinquestriatus* scorpion is indigenous to Africa, Asia, and the Middle East, including Egypt, Israel, Jordan, Kuwait, Lebanon, Oman, Qatar, Saudi Arabia, Syria, and Turkey. Antivenom to *L. quinquestriatus* is currently made in France, Germany, Israel, Saudi Arabia, Egypt, Tunisia, and Turkey (Table A38–1). In observational studies, an intravenous infusion of 5 to 20 mL of *Leiurus* antivenom was needed to control venom effects, and only patients given antivenom within the first several hours demonstrated significant benefit. The rate of allergic reactions for the Turkish antiscorpion antivenom is reported to be 1.6% to 6.6%. The recommended dose of the Israeli *L. quinquestriatus* antivenom is 5 to 15 mL for intravenous use, although several authors report lack of clinical efficacy of this particular antivenom.

### *Tityus* Species

*Tityus* species of scorpions are endemic to South America, particularly Brazil. An F(ab′) antivenom is available from Fundaç-ão Ezequiel Dias (FUNED), in Belo Horizonte, Brazil. The usual dose of the antivenom is 20 mL as an intravenous infusion. In a series of 18 patients with *T. serrulatus* envenomation treated with antivenom, vomiting and local pain decreased within 1 hour, and cardiorespiratory manifestations disappeared within 6 to 24 hours in all patients except the two presenting with acute respiratory distress syndrome.

### Other Species

Scorpion antivenom in South Africa is an equine-derived antivenom available from the South African Vaccine Producers. Scorpi-FAV, produced by Aventis Pasteur, is produced for treatment of *Androctonus* spp, *Buthus occitanus*, and *L. quinquestriatus*.

*Buthus tamulus* monovalent red scorpion antivenom serum produced by Central Research Institute of India is an equine-derived lyophilized antivenom for the venom of *Mesobuthus tamulus*. The manufacturer recommends a dosage of one vial, although a dose of five vials significantly decreased mortality in one study.

In Pakistan, the treatment of scorpion stings was modified in 1991 to include the administration of five vials of antivenom. A retrospective case series of 950 patients treated with and without antivenom was compared to 968 cases treated after the five-vial protocol was initiated. A statistically significant decrease in mortality was demonstrated.

*Parabuthus* spp. antivenom from South African Vaccine Producers is an equine-derived antivenom to *Parabuthus* spp. In one study, antivenom was unavailable for a period of time allowing for a unique design of matched pair of patients. Patients who received antivenom had a significant decrease in hospital stay after receiving one (5-mL) vial. Pain, hypersalivation, fasciculations, tremor, and bladder distension responded best to antivenom, whereas dysphagia, ptosis, and local swelling were more resistant.

# 89 MARINE ENVENOMATIONS

Human contact with venomous marine creatures is common, with serious harm resulting from biological toxins or mechanical injury inflicted by the stinging apparatus. Venomous invertebrates include the phylum Cnidaria (jellyfish, anemones), Mollusca (snails, octopods), and Echinodermata (sea stars, sea urchins). Sea snakes and spiny fish are the common venomous vertebrates.

## INVERTEBRATES

### Cnidaria

The phylum Cnidaria (formerly Coelenterata) includes more than 9,000 species, of which approximately 100 are known to injure humans. Commonly referred to as jellyfish, their phylogenetic designations separate "true jellyfish" and other organisms into distinct classes (Table 89–1; Fig. 89–1A, B). All species possess microscopic cnidae (the Greek *knide* means nettle), which are highly specialized organelles consisting of an encapsulated hollow barbed thread bathed in venom. Thousands of these stinging organelles, called nematocysts (*or* cnidocysts), are distributed along tentacles. A trigger mechanism called a cnidocil regulates nematocyst discharge. Pressure from contact with a victim's skin, or chemical triggers such as osmotic change, stimulates discharge of the thread and toxin from its casing (Fig. 89–2). Although all Cnidaria feature cnidae, only those whose barbed thread can penetrate the human epidermis for intradermal venom delivery inflict injury. Among these are members of the subphylum Cubozoa (sea wasp, Irukandji jellyfish), Hydrozoa (Portuguese man-of-war, bluebottle), Scyphozoa (sea nettle, mauve stinger), and a class of Anthozoa (anemones).

Locations with documented Cnidaria-related deaths include the United States (US) (Florida, North Carolina, Texas), Australia, the Indo-Pacific region (Malaysia, Langkawi Islands, Philippines, Solomon Islands, Papua New Guinea), and the coast of China. Since 1884, approximately 70 deaths in Australia have been attributed to *C. fleckeri*. Approximately 20 to 40 deaths are reported yearly in the Philippines from unidentified species of the Chirodropidae family.

***Cubozoa.*** Members of Cubozoa are not true jellyfish. Animals of this subphylum have a cube-shaped bell with four corners, each supporting between 1 and 15 tentacles. Cubozoa species produce the greatest morbidity and mortality of all Cnidaria. The subphylum comprises two main families of toxicologic importance: Chirodropidae and Carybdeidae.

The Chirodropidae family is well known for the sea wasp (*Chironex fleckeri*, Greek *cheiro* means hand, Latin *nex* means death; therefore, "assassin's hand"). When full grown, the bell of the sea wasp, a type of box jellyfish, measures 25 to 30 cm in diameter, and 15 tentacles are attached at each "corner" of the bell. These tentacles extend up to 3 m in length. The Carybdeidae family is most notable for the Irukandji jellyfish (*Carukia barnesi*). Its small size, with a bell diameter of only 2.5 cm, limits detection in open waters.

***Hydrozoa.*** Members of the Hydrozoa class are also not true jellyfish. The order Siphonophorae (Physaliidae family) includes two unusual creatures of toxicologic concern: *Physalia physalis*, the Portuguese man-of-war, and its smaller counterpart, *Physalia utriculus*, the bluebottle. They are pelagic (floating) colonial Hydrozoa, meaning one "jellyfish" is actually a colony

**TABLE 89–1 Characteristics of Common Cnidaria**

| Latin Name | Common Name | Common Habitat (Coastal Waters) |
|---|---|---|
| Cubozoa class | | |
| *Chironex fleckeri*[a] | Sea wasp | Tropical Pacific Ocean, Indian Ocean, Gulf of Oman |
| *Carukia barnesi*[a] | Irukandji jellyfish | North Australian |
| *Chiropsalmus spp*[a] | Sea wasp or fire medusa | North Australian, Philippines, Japan, Indian Ocean, Gulf of Mexico, Caribbean |
| *Chiropsalmus quadrigatus*, *C. quadrumanus* | Box jellyfish | Western Atlantic, Gulf of Mexico, Pacific |
| *Carybdea alata* | Hawaiian box jellyfish | Hawaii |
| *Carybdea rastoni* | Jimble | Australia |
| Hydrozoa class | | |
| *Physalia physalis*[a] | Portuguese man-of-war | Eastern US from Florida to North Carolina, Gulf of Mexico, Australia (rare reports) |
| *Physalia utriculus* | Bluebottle | Tropical Pacific Ocean, particularly Australia |
| *Millepora alcicornis* | Fire coral | Widespread in tropical waters, including Caribbean |
| Scyphozoa class | | |
| *Chrysaora quinquecirrha* | Sea nettle | Chesapeake Bay, widely distributed in temperate and tropical waters |
| *Stomolophus meleagris* | Cabbage head or cannonball jellyfish | Gulf of Mexico, Caribbean |
| *Stomolophus nomurai*[a] | Lion's mane | Yellow Sea between China and South Korea |
| *Cyanea capillata* | Lion's mane or hair jellyfish | Northwest US to Arctic Sea, Norway and Great Britain, Australia |
| *Pelagia noctiluca* | Mauve stinger or purple-striped jellyfish | Wide distribution in tropical zones |
| *Linuche unguiculata* | Thimble jellyfish | Florida, Mexico, and Caribbean |
| Anthozoa class | | |
| *Anemonia sulcata* | European stinging anemone | Eastern Atlantic, Mediterranean, Adriatic Sea |
| *Actinodendron plumosum* | Hell's fire anemone | South Pacific |
| *Actinia equina* | Beadlet anemone | Great Britain, Ireland |

[a]Well-documented human fatalities.

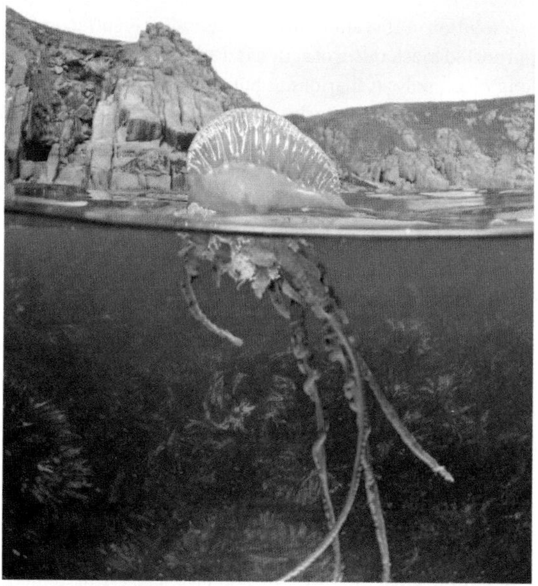


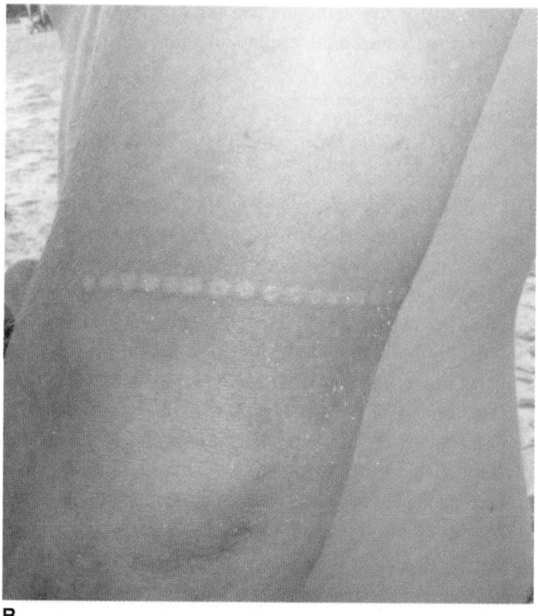


**FIGURE 89–1.** (**A**) North Atlantic Portuguese man-of-war *Physalia physalis* with multiple tentacles dangling in the water. The tentacles filled with venomous nematocysts extend several meters in length. *(Used with permission from NHPA/Charles Hood/Photoshot.)* (**B**) Linear vesicular eruption from contact with an unidentified jellyfish in the South Atlantic Ocean. *(Used with permission from David Goldfarb.)*

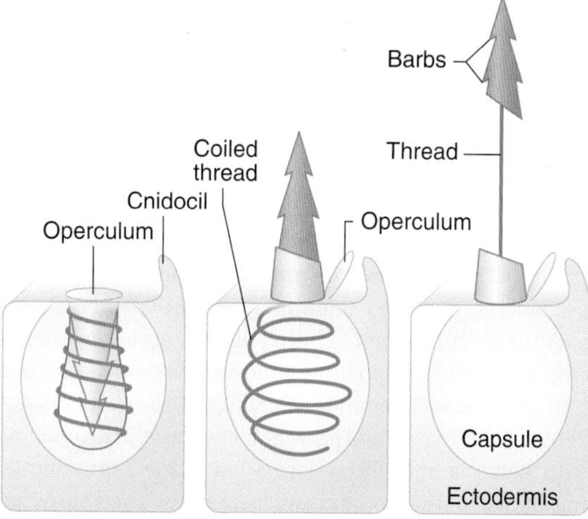


**FIGURE 89–2.** The structure and function of the nematocyst of the jellyfish (Cnidaria). The barbed thread rests inverted and spring-loaded in the nematocyst, which measures approximately 10 to 20 μm. Upon mechanical or osmotic stimulation of the trigger mechanism (called the cnidocil), the hinged operculum places the barb in its upright position and the thread uncoils, propelling itself outward. Venom stored in the capsule flows through the thread into the victim's tissue.

of multiple specialized animals (zooids) in a formed mass. The easily recognizable pneumatophore (blue sail) that floats above the surface of the water is filled with up to 13% carbon monoxide, 15% to 20% oxygen, and nitrogen for the remaining partial pressure. Tentacles of *P. physalis* reach lengths exceeding 30 m and contain more than 750,000 nematocysts in each of its numerous tentacles (up to 40). *Physalia utriculus* has only one tentacle that measures up to 15 m.

The Anthomedusae order includes the sessile *Millepora alcicornis* (fire coral) that exists as a fixed colony of hydroids. It appears much like true coral and has a white to yellow-green lime carbonate exoskeleton. Small nematocyst-containing tentacles protrude through minute surface gastropores. The overall structure ranges from 10 cm to 2 m.

***Scyphozoa.*** True jellyfish belong to the class Scyphozoa and are extremely diverse in size, shape, and color. Common varieties known to envenomate humans are *Cyanea capillata* (lion's mane or hair jelly), *Chrysaora quinquecirrha* (sea nettle), and *Pelagia noctiluca* (mauve stinger). The mauve stinger is easily recognized; it appears pink in daylight and phosphorescent at night. Larvae of *Linuche unguiculata* cause seabather's eruption (SBE).

***Anthozoa.*** The Anthozoa class of Cnidaria does not feature a medusa ("jellyfish") stage in its life cycle and is thus marked by sessility. Its diverse membership includes true corals, soft corals, and anemones. Only the anemones are of toxicologic importance. They are common inhabitants of reefs and tide pools and attach themselves to rock or coral. Armed with modified nematocysts known as *sporocysts* and *basitrichous isorhiza* located on their tentacles, they produce stings similar to those of organisms from other Cnidaria classes.

## Cnidaria Dermatitis

***Epidemiology.*** Stings from Cnidaria and subsequent dermal eruptions represent the overwhelming majority of marine envenomations. In Australia, approximately 10,000 stings per year are recorded from *Physalia* spp alone. Stings occur with greatest frequency on hotter than average days with low winds, particularly during times of low precipitation. Related to changes in ocean pH and temperature as a result of climate change, the size of jellyfish blooms and the subsequent incidence of Cnidaria envenomation have increased. In addition, the geographical distribution of venomous jellyfish is expanding.

***Pathophysiology.*** Dermal eruptions after *Cnidaria* envenomation occur due to both toxin and immune system–mediated mechanisms. The exact composition varies by class, but in general, toxins are subdivided into four types: enzymes (phospholipase $A_2$, metalloproteases), pore-forming toxins, neurotoxins, and nonprotein bioactive components (serotonin, histamine). Phospholipase $A_2$ enzymatically cleaves glycerophospholipids into arachidonic acid and thus induces inflammation. Metalloproteases break down extracellular matrix and prevent hemostasis. Tissue edema with necrosis and blister formation ensues. Intradermal injection of both serotonin and histamine causes vasodilation and pain. Two myotoxins from *C. fleckeri* cause powerful sustained muscle contractions in isolated muscle fibers. An immune-mediated response to venom further explains some sting-related symptoms.

***Clinical Manifestations.*** Most patients with stings are treated beachside and never require hospitalization. The vast majority of patients who seek medical care do so because of severe pain without evidence of systemic poisoning. Envenomation by *C. fleckeri* inflicts the most severe pain and is frequently associated with systemic toxicity. An erythematous whiplike linear rash with a "frosted ladder" appearance develops. The pain often is excruciating and requires parenteral analgesia.

*Millepora alcicornis* (fire coral) is a common cause of stings in southern US and Caribbean waters. Although a member of the same phylogenetic class as *P. physalis*, it produces far less significant injuries. It is a nuisance to divers who touch the coral and suffer moderate burning pain for hours. Untreated pain generally lessens within 90 minutes, with skin wheals flattening at 24 hours and resolving within 1 week. Hyperpigmentation persists for up to 8 weeks. Following stings from sea anemones, victims develop either immediate or delayed pain. Skin findings range from mild erythema and itching to ulceration.

***Diagnosis.*** The diagnosis is clinical. Following severe stings from a variety of *Cnidaria*, urinalysis, complete blood count (CBC), and serum creatinine measurements serve to detect the presence of hemolysis and subsequent risk of kidney injury.

***Management.*** Initial interventions after *Cnidaria* envenomation are directed toward stabilization of cardiopulmonary abnormalities in cases of severe envenomation. Secondary measures are directed toward the prevention of further nematocyst discharge, which could intensify pain and enhance toxicity. Vinegar is a common first-line treatment for topical application following *Cnidaria* stings. In vitro trials with *C. fleckeri* tentacles demonstrate complete irreversible inhibition of nematocyst discharge following a 30-second application. Similar experiments demonstrate that vinegar is effective for Morbakka (large Cubozoan in Australia), *Carybdea rastoni*, and *C. barnesi*. Unfortunately, vinegar causes nematocyst discharge when applied to *C. capillata*, *C. quinquecirrha*, and *P. physalis*. Hence, therapy must be guided by geographic location. Stingose is an aqueous solution of 20% aluminum sulfate and 1.1% surfactant. Its purported mechanism of action is denaturing of proteins and long-chain polysaccharides. A human volunteer trial involving stings from live tentacles of *C. fleckeri* demonstrated pain relief within 5 seconds of Stingose application. Similar results were achieved following treatment of stings from *C. quinquecirrha*. A small randomized controlled trial found Stingose superior to saltwater irrigation after Physalia envenomation.

Ice packs provided rapid, effective relief for patients with mild to moderate pain from *Cnidaria* stings in Australia. In contrast, hot water immersion (HWI) at 45°C for 20 minutes provided pain relief to 87% of victims of bluebottle (*P. utriculus*) stings in a randomized controlled trial. In vitro data support thermal denaturing of *C. fleckeri* cardiotoxin. No human randomized controlled trials exist to assess the efficacy of HWI in *C. fleckeri* envenomation.

Pressure immobilization bandaging is a technique that applies sufficient pressure to a wound to impede lymphatic drainage and prevent the entrance of venom into systemic circulation. Given the lack of evidence suggesting benefit, coupled with clear in vitro evidence of increased venom delivery with this technique, we recommend against the use of pressure immobilization bandaging for treatment of Cnidaria stings.

### Cnidaria Cardiotoxicity

***Epidemiology.*** The majority of victims do not present to healthcare facilities following *Cnidaria* envenomation. Although older reports suggest a 15% to 20% fatality rate following *C. fleckeri* envenomation, a prospective study of stings from Cubozoa over 1 year in Australia revealed no dysrhythmias, pulmonary edema, or death. No patient received antivenom, and analgesia was the only pharmacotherapy implemented. Although most victims suffer only local severe pain, serious systemic toxicity occurs rarely, and may include vertigo, ataxia, paralysis, delirium, syncope, respiratory distress, cardiogenic pulmonary edema, hypotension, and dysrhythmias. In a series of 10 reported deaths from *C. fleckeri*, all occurred in children, suggesting vulnerability due to lower body mass and thinner dermis.

***Pathophysiology.*** Cnidaria venoms contain a variety of components that induce cardiotoxicity. The cardiotoxin of *C. fleckeri* has not yet been fully identified but is believed to be a pore-forming toxin that increases $Na^+$ permeability in cardiac tissue. Cardiovascular collapse results from osmotic dysregulation of endothelial and cardiac tissues. Cardiac effects in animals include negative inotropy, conduction delays, ventricular tachycardia, and coronary artery vasoconstriction. Cardiotoxicity also results from blockade of voltage-gated $Na^+$ and $K^+$ channels. *Physalia* spp venom inhibits $Ca^{2+}$ entry into the sarcoplasmic reticulum. Similar mechanisms are proposed for *Chrysaora*, *Chiropsalmus*, and *Stomolophus*. *Chrysaora quinquecirrha* venom induces atrioventricular block and produces myocardial ischemia, hypertension, dysrhythmias, and nerve conduction block, as well as hepatic and renal necrosis.

***Clinical Manifestations.*** Fatality is documented to occur with only 4 m of tentacle markings. Death is rapid, preventing many victims from reaching medical care, or even the shore. Survival is possible with immediate cardiopulmonary resuscitation (CPR).

***Diagnosis.*** *Cnidaria* cardiotoxicity should be suspected in all drowning victims with linear skin lesions. Patients not in cardiac arrest present with hypotension and cardiac conduction abnormalities. An electrocardiogram is prudent to identify treatable dysrhythmias. Envenomation impairs coronary perfusion, and serial troponin assays are recommended.

***Management.*** Rescuer efforts should focus on immediate nematocyst inactivation, tentacle removal, and basic life support. Box jellyfish whole IgG antivenom is effective in animal models and in vitro experiments. However, distance from medical care limits the ability to obtain antivenom in a timely fashion. Although box jellyfish antivenom can be administered by paramedics via intramuscular (IM) injection, poor IM absorption and incomplete venom neutralization with antivenoms, as well as delayed peak serum concentrations, limit the utility of this approach. The manufacturer recommends treating initially with one vial intravenously (IV) diluted 1:10 with saline or three undiluted vials (1.5–4 mL each) IM at three separate sites, if IV access is unavailable. Although available in Australia since 1970, to this date, no survival is attributable to the administration of antivenom, and there are multiple fatalities despite its use. If available, antivenom administration is recommended but does not replace supportive care.

Although successfully utilized for the treatment of pain associated with *C. fleckeri* stings, HWI is unlikely to demonstrate benefit in the treatment of cardiotoxicity. Immersion in hot water is impractical for the critically ill patient, and penetrance of heat is limited to superficial tissues and will not denature circulating cardiotoxins.

### Irukandji Syndrome

***Epidemiology.*** Stings from the Portuguese man-of-war (*Physalia physalis*) and the Irukandji jellyfish (*Carukia barnesi*) are associated with the development of Irukandji syndrome. However, an unidentified species produced three cases of an Irukandjilike syndrome in the Florida Keys, and six cases were reported off the coast of Hawaii. This suggests a more diverse geographical distribution and possibly multiple responsible organisms.

***Pathophysiology.*** *Carukia barnesi*, the Irukandji jellyfish, likely induces its dramatic vasopressor effects via catecholamine release. Porcine studies with intravenous *C. barnesi* venom administration show a 4,000- and 1,000-fold increase in norepinephrine and epinephrine, respectively.

***Clinical Manifestations.*** Individuals afflicted often notice a mild sting while they are in the water; however, skin findings typically are absent. Severe systemic symptoms develop after a latent period of 5 to 40 minutes and mimic a catecholamine surge including tachycardia, hypertension, piloerection, hyperpnea, headache, pallor, restlessness, apprehension, sweating, and a sense of impending doom. A prominent feature is severe diffuse muscle spasms that come in waves and preferentially affect the back. Spasms are described as unbearable and frequently require parenteral analgesia. Symptoms generally abate over several hours but can last up to 2 days. Hypertension is universal, severe, and can result in intracranial hemorrhage. Hypotension frequently follows, requiring vasopressor support. Pulmonary edema can develop within hours. Echocardiograms consistently reveal global ventricular dysfunction.

***Diagnosis.*** Irukandji syndrome is a clinical diagnosis. Electrocardiogram, serial cardiac biomarkers, and echocardiography are recommended to screen for myocardial damage and Takotsubo (stress) cardiomyopathy.

***Management.*** Vinegar irrigation, or HWI, prevents further envenomation as discussed above and is recommended early in the course of treatment. Further treatment for Irukandji syndrome should focus on analgesia and blood pressure control. Several modalities for control of severe hypertension are reasonable and include phentolamine, nitroglycerin, and IV magnesium sulfate. Because hypotension occurs in late stages of toxicity, clinicians should only administer a short-acting titratable antihypertensive such as nicardipine for control of initial hypertension.

### Seabather's Eruption

***Epidemiology.*** Cases of Seabather's eruption (SBE) occur in clusters. Variation in intensity and frequency occurs from year to year as exemplified by a 25-year hiatus during which no cases were reported in Florida, followed by more than 10,000 cases in 1992.

***Pathophysiology.*** Seabather's eruption is the result of envenomation by the larvae of *Linuche unguiculata* and *Edwardsiella lineata*. The larvae appear as pin-sized (0.5 mm) brown to green-brown spheres in the upper 2 inches of the water and are typically unnoticed. The eruption displays a characteristic delay in onset of symptoms and is effectively treated with steroids, suggesting a primary immune-mediated process.

***Clinical Manifestation.*** The pruritic papular eruption occurs mostly in areas covered by a bathing suit as a result of larvae trapped under the garments. Only 50% of people reported a stinging sensation while they were in the water, and 25% reported itching upon exiting the water. The remainder of patients developed symptoms within 11 hours. Skin lesions develop within hours of itching and appear as discrete, closely spaced papules, with pustules, vesicles, and urticaria. Itching often is severe and prevents sleep. New lesions typically continue to develop over 72 hours. The average duration of symptoms is just under 2 weeks. Systemic symptoms such as chills, headache, nausea, vomiting, and malaise occur occasionally.

***Diagnosis.*** The diagnosis of SBE is based on history and physical examination.

***Management.*** Topical application of vinegar is known to deactivate nematocysts of *Linuche unguiculata*. Antihistamines and topical corticosteroids are also reasonable therapies.

## MOLLUSCA

The phylum Mollusca comprises Cephalopoda (octopus, squid, and cuttlefish) and Gastropoda (cone snails). Cephalopod species of toxicologic concern are limited to the blue-ringed octopus *Hapalochlaena maculosa* and the greater blue-ringed

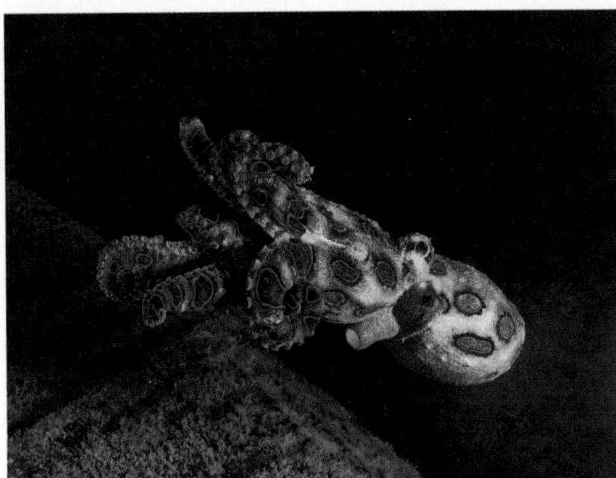

**FIGURE 89–3.** The blue-ringed octopus, *Hapalochlaena maculosa*. *(Used with permission from Yusran Abdul Rahman/Shutterstock.)*

octopus *Hapalochlaena lunulata*. The blue-ringed and greater blue-ringed octopods are found in the Indo-Pacific region, primarily in Australian waters (Fig. 89–3). Of the 400 species of cone snails that belong to the genus *Conus*, 18 are implicated in human envenomations.

## Cephalopoda

***Epidemiology.*** The blue-ringed octopus is a relatively small (12–20 cm) animal that lives camouflaged in crevices and rock piles around Australia, the Indo-Pacific region, and Japan. It normally displays a yellow-brown color, but flashes iridescent blue rings to warn and repel predators. The species is not aggressive and only bites humans when handled, and evenomations and deaths are rarely reported. Poisoning also occurs when the blue-ringed octopus is consumed as tetrodotoxin (TTX) is also highly concentrated in its integument.

***Pathophysiology.*** Symbiotic bacteria in the salivary glands of the blue-ringed octopus produce tetrodotoxin (TTX). The parrotlike beak of the octopus creates small punctures in human skin through which venom is introduced. Tetrodotoxin blocks $Na^+$ conductance in neurons. Other venom components such as serotonin (5-HT), hyaluronidase, tyramine, histamine, tryptamine, octopine, taurine, acetylcholine, and dopamine lead to profound hypotension and subsequent global ischemia.

***Clinical Manifestations.*** The blue-ringed octopus creates one or two puncture wounds with its jaws, inflicting only minor discomfort. A wheal typically develops with erythema, tenderness, and pruritus as a result of the histamine content of the venom. Tetrodotoxin exerts a curarelike effect characterized by paralysis without depressing mental status. Symptoms include perioral and intraoral paresthesias, diplopia, aphonia, dysphagia, ataxia, weakness, nausea, vomiting, flaccid muscle paralysis, respiratory failure, and death. Detailed case reports describe rapid onset of symptoms within minutes. If cardiac and pulmonary support are adequate, near-complete recovery of neuromuscular function occurs within 24 to 48 hours.

***Diagnostic Testing.*** An assay can detect TTX in the urine or serum, but it is unlikely to yield results prior to death or resolution of symptoms.

***Management.*** Patients with compromised respiratory effort require basic airway management and ventilator support. Norepinephrine or phenylephrine is recommended based on animal data that indicate they successfully raise blood pressure to physiologic levels. Epinephrine and dopamine lacked efficacy in these same models.

## Gastropoda

***Epidemiology.*** Cone snails predominantly inhabit the Indo-Pacific, including all parts of Australia, New Guinea, Solomon Islands, and the Philippines. Estimates suggest only 16 human deaths have occurred worldwide. *Conus geographicus* (fish hunting cone) is the most common species implicated, and fatality is estimated in up to 25% of envenomations.

***Pathophysiology.*** Cone snails have a hollow proboscis that contains a disposable radular tooth bathed in venom. Similar to a harpoon, the barbed tooth is fired from the proboscis to hunt or in defense. Human envenomations occur when the shells are handled. *Conus* species contain approximately 100 peptides or *conotoxins* in their venom along with hyaluronidases, proteases, and lipases that aid in local tissue breakdown and diffusion of venom (Table 89–2).

***Clinical Manifestations.*** Localized symptoms range from a slight sting to excruciating pain, tissue ischemia, cyanosis, and numbness. Systemic symptoms include weakness, diaphoresis, diplopia, blurred vision, aphonia, dysphagia, generalized muscle paralysis, respiratory failure, cardiovascular collapse, and coma. Systemic symptoms occur within 30 minutes of envenomation; respiratory arrest occurs shortly thereafter. Death is rapid and occurs within an hour.

***Diagnostic Testing.*** Whereas most venomous marine animals leave a visible injury, hypodermal injection by the radula toothlike structure produces minimal tissue injury easily overlooked on physical examination. Surrounding discoloration and local edema provide clues of envenomation. Because of the risk for dysrhythmias, an electrocardiogram should be performed in addition to continuous cardiac monitoring.

**TABLE 89–2 Conus Peptide Targets**

| *Peptide* | *Receptor Type* | *Mechanism* |
|---|---|---|
| *Ligand-gated ion channels* | | |
| Conantokins | NMDA | Inhibits conductance |
| α-Conotoxin | Nicotinic | Competitive antagonism |
| σ-Conotoxin | $5\text{-}HT_3$ | Noncompetitive antagonism |
| M1 | | Neuromuscular junction |
| M2 | | Neuronal receptors |
| *Voltage-gated ion channels* | | |
| δ-Conotoxin | | Delayed channel activation |
| κ-Conotoxin | $K^+$ | Channel blockade |
| μ-Conotoxin | $Na^+$ | Channel blockade |
| ω-Conotoxin | $Ca^{2+}$ | Channel blockade |
| *G-protein linked* | | |
| Conopressin-G | Vasopressin receptor | Receptor agonism |
| Contulakin-G | Neurotensin receptor | Receptor agonism |

***Management.*** Primary interventions include maintenance of airway, breathing, and circulation. Global flaccid paralysis requires short-term mechanical ventilation, but usually resolves within 24 hours. Cardiac dysrhythmias require electrical cardioversion. Antidysrhythmics that block $Na^+$ channels could theoretically worsen the patient's dysrhythmia and should be avoided. Hypotension should be treated with intravenous fluids and norepinephrine as appropriate.

### Echinodermata, Annelida, and Porifera

The Echinodermata phylum includes sea stars, brittle stars, sea urchins, sand dollars, and sea cucumbers. Annelida are segmented worms that include the Polychaetae family of bristle worms. Sponges are classified in the Porifera phylum. One feature that all three phyla share is the passive envenomation of people who mistakenly handle or step on them. Most stings are mild.

***Epidemiology.*** Echinoderms, annelids, and sponges are ubiquitous ocean inhabitants. The crown-of-thorns sea star (*Acanthaster planci*) is found in the warmest waters of Polynesia to the Red Sea and is a particularly venomous species because of its sharp spines that easily puncture human skin. Sea urchins inhabit all oceans of the world. They are nonaggressive, slow moving bottom dwellers, and human envenomation typically results from stepping on or handling the animal. The most venomous are species of *Diadema*, *Echinothrix*, and *Asthenosoma*. Bristle worms such as *Hermodice caruncula*ta typically inhabit tropical waters such as those of Florida and the Caribbean. However, some species thrive in the frigid waters of Antarctica. The fire sponge *Tedania ignis* is a brilliant yellow-orange sponge identified in large numbers off the coast of Hawaii and in the Florida Keys. Other common American sponges are *Neofibularia nolitangere* (poison-bun sponge or touch-me-not sponge) and *Microciona prolifera* (red sponge). *Neofibularia mordens* (Australian stinging sponge) is a common Southern Australian variety. In the Mediterranean, sponges are often colonized with sea anemones that inflict severe stings.

***Pathophysiology.*** Venom contained within the spines of sea urchins consists of steroid glycosides, 5-HT, hemolysin, protease, acetylcholinelike substances, and bradykininlike substances. Some species harbor neurotoxins. Sea stars contain toxic saponins (plancitoxin I and II) with hemolytic and anticoagulant effects as well as histaminelike substances. Sea cucumbers excrete holothurin, a sulfated triterpenoid oligoglycoside, from the anus (organs of Cuvier) as a defense. The toxin inhibits neural conduction in fish, leading to paralysis. Some sea cucumbers eat Cnidaria and subsequently secrete their venom. Sponges have toxins that include halitoxin, odadaic acid, and subcritine, the nature of which is uncertain. Dried sponges are nontoxic; however, on rewetting, they produce toxicity even after several years.

***Clinical Manifestations.*** Sea urchin envenomation presents as intense burning with local tissue reaction, including edema and erythema. Reports of other manifestations including death are not well substantiated. The Pacific urchin *Tripneustes* produces a neurotoxin with a predilection for cranial nerves. Retention of sea urchin spine fragments predisposes the patient to development of painful granulomata. Spine penetration of a joint induces synovitis. Small cuts on the skin from handling sea stars allow venom to penetrate, leading to contact dermatitis. The crown-of-thorns sea star causes severe pain, nausea, vomiting, and muscular paralysis. Massive hemolysis and hepatic necrosis were reported after a single-stinger envenomation. Cutaneous, scleral, or corneal exposure to sea cucumbers triggers contact dermatitis, intense corneal inflammation, and even blindness. Bristle worms are shrouded with bristles that produce a reddened urticarial rash. Symptoms typically are mild and resolve over several hours to days. Contact with the fire sponge, poison-bun sponge, or red-moss sponge causes erythema, papules, vesicles, and bullae that generally subside within 3 to 7 days. Some victims develop fever, chills, and muscle cramps. Skin desquamation occurs at 10 days to 2 months, with chronic skin changes lasting several months.

***Diagnosis.*** Radiographic or ultrasonographic imaging of the affected body part is recommended to assess for the presence of remnant foreign bodies. Following crown-of-thorns envenomation, a complete blood count and liver function tests are reasonable given the risk for hemolysis and hepatotoxicity.

***Management.*** The primary objective following envenomation from sea urchins and crown-of-thorns starfish is analgesia. Submersion of the affected extremity in hot water (105°–115°F; 40.6°–46.1°C) and administration of oral analgesics often are sufficient as several components of the venom are thermolabile. Spines frequently crumble with attempted extraction and often require surgical exploration of the tract for complete removal. Antibiotic prophylaxis is recommended for patients with immune compromise risk factors such as diabetes or other comorbidities. Although most infections likely are secondary to human skin flora, marine flora such as *Mycobacterium marinum* and *Vibrio parahaemolyticus* are potential wound contaminants, and *M. marinum* is associated with the formation of granulomata after sea urchin envenomation. Treatment of sponge exposures usually requires only removal of spicules using adhesive tape or the edge of a credit card. Antihistamines and topical corticosteroids often provide no relief from stinging sponges.

## VERTEBRATES

### Snakes

Sea snakes are elapids and are divided into two subfamilies: Hydrophiinae and Laticaudinae. Distinction from eels is made by the presence of scales and the absence of fins and gills. All 52 species of sea snakes are venomous and at least six species are implicated in human fatalities. The most common species cited in human envenomation are *Enhydrina schistosa*, the beaked sea snake, and *Pelamis platurus*, the yellow-bellied sea snake.

***Epidemiology.*** Sea snakes are common to the tropical and temperate Indian and Pacific Oceans, but they are also found along the eastern Pacific Coast of Central and South America and the Gulf of California. There are no venomous sea snakes in the Atlantic Ocean or Mediterranean. The majority of envenomations occur along the coasts of Southeast Asia, the Persian Gulf, and the Malay Archipelago (Malaysia). Workers of the fishing industry are at greatest risk as snakes frequently get trapped in fishing nets. Sea snakes generally are docile, except when provoked, or during the mating season. Two species, the Stokes' sea snake (*Astoria stokesii*) and beaked sea snake (*Enhydrina schistosa*), are known for aggression. The true incidence of sea snake envenomation is unknown because many bites are not recorded. Worldwide, the number of deaths per year approaches 150, with an overall mortality rate estimated between 3.2% and 30%.

***Pathophysiology.*** All sea snakes have small front fangs. Their venom is neurotoxic, myotoxic, nephrotoxic, and hemolytic. Known components of the venom include acetylcholinesterase, hyaluronidase, leucine aminopeptidase, 5′-nucleotidase, phosphodiesterase, and phospholipase A. The neurotoxin is similar to that of cobra and krait venom and targets postsynaptic acetylcholine (ACh) receptors, creating a blockade at the neuromuscular junction. Presynaptic effects include initial enhanced ACh release and subsequent inhibition of ACh release.

***Clinical Manifestations.*** Bites typically are painless or inflict minimal discomfort initially despite significant envenomation as venom contains few inflammatory or necrotic factors. Between one and four fang marks are common. The diagnosis often is obscured because victims do not associate the slight prick following the bite with later onset of ascending paralysis. Symptoms progress within minutes, although a delay of up to 6 hours is possible. Painful muscular rigidity and myoglobinuria are hallmarks of sea snake myotoxicity. Myoglobinuria develops between 30 minutes and 8 hours after the bite. This is followed by ascending paralysis from acetylcholine receptor blockade by the neurotoxic venom fraction and muscle destruction from myotoxic fraction. Massive potassium release from damaged muscle tissue coupled with impaired kidney function from myoglobin nephropathy predisposes to fatal dysrhythmias. Other classic symptoms include dysphagia, trismus, ptosis, aphonia, nausea, vomiting, fasciculations, and ultimately respiratory insufficiency, seizures, and coma.

***Diagnostic Testing.*** Laboratory diagnostics are directed toward identifying hemolysis, myonecrosis, hyperkalemia, and acute kidney injury. Serum electrolytes, creatinine, and creatine phosphokinase, as well as a CBC and urinalysis, should be obtained. Elevated concentrations of hepatic enzymes indicate severe envenomation. Serial measurement of these parameters is recommended.

***Management.*** Prehospital management of sea snakebites mirrors treatment of terrestrial snakebites (Chap. 92) and includes immobilization of the extremity. A pressure immobilization bandage is reasonable to impede lymphatic drainage, but tourniquets that impede venous or arterial flow are not recommended. Airway and respiratory effort require close monitoring because paralysis develops rapidly.

Currently, only one equine Fab antivenom specific to sea snake bites is available (Table 89–3). No controlled human trials have evaluated the efficacy of sea snake antivenom, although case reports suggest improved outcomes and more rapid recovery with its use. In the event that sea snake antivenom is not available, Thai neuro polyvalent antivenom (NPAV) and tiger snake antivenom are reasonable alternatives. Epinephrine and antihistamines should be readily available.

**TABLE 89–3 Antivenom, Initial Dosing by Route**

| Organism | Intravenous Dosing | Intramuscular Dosing |
|---|---|---|
| *Box jellyfish* | | |
| *C. fleckeri* | 1 vial as 1:10 dilution[a] | 3 vials (undiluted) |
| *Sea snake* | | |
| *E. schistose* (beaked sea snake) | 1–3 vials as 1:10 dilution,[a] up to 10 vials in severe cases | Not recommended |
| *N. scutatus* (terrestrial tiger snake) | 1 vial as 1:10 dilution[a] | Not recommended |
| *Stonefish* | | |
| *S. trachynis* | 1 vial as 1:10 dilution,[a] high risk of anaphylactoid reaction | 1 vial (undiluted) for every 2 punctures |

[a]Dilution in pediatric patients: 1:5 to avoid volume overload.

## Fish

Several fish utilize defensive venoms. Stingrays and spiny fish are known to pose a threat to humans. Although rare, death is typically the result of mechanical trauma rather than toxicological effects of venom. Stingrays are members of the class Chondrichthyes (order Rajiformes: skates and rays). Families include Dasyatidae (whip ray or sting ray), Urolophidae (round ray), Myliobatidae (batfish or eagle ray), Gymnuridae (butterfly ray), and Potamotrygonidae (river ray, freshwater). Spiny fish of the family Scorpaenidae include a variety of venomous creatures (Table 89–4). Stonefish display a mottled color and are covered in mucus that allows for growth of algae, making them well camouflaged among rocks and reefs (Fig. 89–4).

***Epidemiology.*** There are 11 different species of stingrays in US coastal waters. Most envenomations occur when the animal is inadvertently stepped on. In one review, a total of 17 fatalities resulting from trunk wounds, hemorrhage, or tetanus were identified worldwide. Three populations are at highest risk for spiny fish envenomation: fishermen sorting the catch from nets, waders, and aquarium enthusiasts. Only five deaths from Scorpaenidae have been reported; all resulted from stonefish and are poorly documented. In the US, Scorpaenidae stings occur in the Florida Keys, in the Gulf of Mexico, off the coast of California, and in Hawaii. Lionfish (genus *Pterois*) (Fig. 89–5) are common to home aquariums and account for most poison center calls involving spiny fish envenomation in the US. Weeverfish inhabit shallow temperate waters with sandy or muddy bottoms in the eastern Atlantic and Mediterranean, including the European Coast extending to the southern tip of Norway.

***Pathophysiology.*** Tapered, bilaterally retroserrated spines covered by an integumentary sheath emanate from the stingray tail. The ventrolateral groove contains venom glands that saturate the spine with venom and mucus. Puncture of the victim

**TABLE 89–4 Spiny Fish**

| *Latin Name* | *Common Name* | *Habitat (Coastal Waters)* |
|---|---|---|
| Scorpaenidae family | | |
| *Pterois* | | |
| *P. volitans* | Lionfish (also zebrafish, turkeyfish, or red firefish) | Indo-Pacific region, Florida to North Carolina (nonnative to US coast) |
| *P. lunulata* | Lionfish or butterfly cod | |
| *Synanceja* | | |
| *S. trachynis* | Australian estuarine stonefish | Indo-Pacific region (Pacific and Indian Oceans) |
| *S. horrida* | Indian stonefish | |
| *S. verrucosa* | Reef stonefish | |
| *Scorpaena* | | |
| *S. cardinalis* | Red rock cod, scorpionfish | Australia |
| *S. guttata* | California sculpin, scorpionfish | California |
| *Notesthes robusta* | Bullrout | Australia |
| *Gymnapistes marmoratus* | Cobbler | Australia |
| Trachinidae family | | |
| *Trachinus* | | |
| *T. vipera* | Lesser weeverfish | Great Britain to Northwest Africa, throughout |
| *T. draco* | Greater weeverfish (also adderpike, stingfish, or seacat) | Mediterranean and Black Seas |

disrupts the integrity of the integument overlying the stinger. This releases the venom, which contains several amino acids, serotonin, 5′-nucleotidase, and phosphodiesterase.

Scorpaenidae have 12 to 13 dorsal, 2 pelvic, and 3 anal spines that are covered with an integumentary sheath. Glands at the base contain 5 to 10 mg of venom each; the amount of venom released is proportional to the pressure applied to the spine. Ornate pectoral fins are not venomous. Venom can remain stable for 24 to 48 hours after the fish dies. Three main toxins are isolated from various species of stonefish: stonustoxin (SNTX), verrucotoxin (VTX), and trachynilysin (TLY). SNTX induces formation of hydrophilic pores in cell membranes leading to cell destruction. Verrucotoxin, isolated from *S. verrucosa*, shares homology with SNTX in that both block cardiac $Ca^{2+}$ channels. Trachynilysin forms pores in cell membranes that allow $Ca^{2+}$ entry and causes release of ACh from nerve endings at motor end plates and increased catecholamine release. *Synanceja trachynis* venom causes endothelium-dependent vasodilation and cardiovascular collapse in rats, which appears to be mediated by muscarinic and adrenergic receptors. Stonefish venom also contains a powerful hyaluronidase inducing local tissue destruction and systemic absorption of venom. Other venoms of Scorpaenidae include proteinase, phosphodiesterase, alkaline phosphomonoesterase, arginine esterase, arginine amidinase, 5′-nucleotidase, acetylcholinesterase, and biogenic amines.

***Clinical Manifestations.*** Stingray wounds cause intense pain out of proportion to the appearance of the wound. Symptoms peak 30 to 90 minutes after injury and may persist for 48 hours. Local edema, cyanosis and ischemia due to vasospasm, erythema, and petechiae follow rapidly. Tissue hypoperfusion results in necrosis and ulceration. Symptoms include weakness, nausea, vomiting, diarrhea, vertigo, headache, syncope, seizures, muscle cramps, fasciculations, hypotension, and dysrhythmias. Chest and abdominal wounds, as well as tetanus, have caused death.

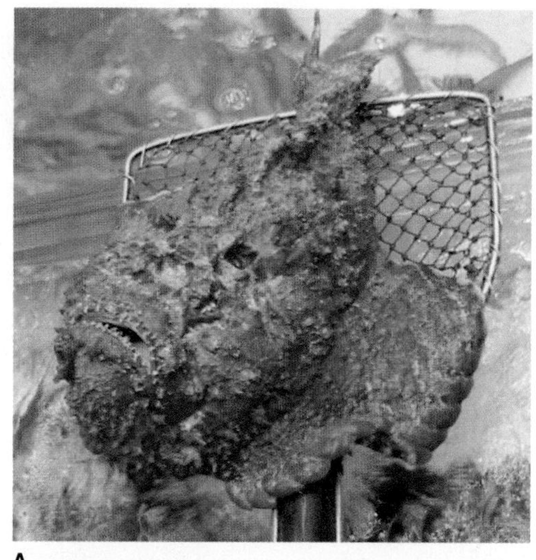

A

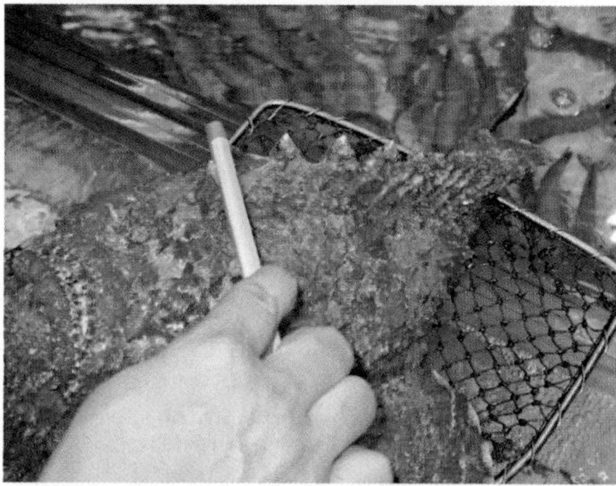

B

**FIGURE 89–4.** The stonefish, *Synanceja* spp. Note the stinging spines on the close-up. *(Used with permission from the Fellowship in Medical Toxicology, New York University Grossman School of Medicine, New York City Poison Center.)*

Stings from stonefish produce immediate, severe pain with rapid wound cyanosis and edema that progresses up the injured extremity. Pain reaches a maximum after 30 to 90 minutes and usually resolves over 6 to 12 hours, although some patients experience pain for days. Headache, vomiting, abdominal pain, delirium, seizures, limb paralysis, hypertension, respiratory distress, dysrhythmias, congestive heart failure, and hypotension characterize systemic toxicity. Wound healing requires months. Symptoms of *P. volitans* envenomation include pain, swelling, nausea, numbness, joint pain, anxiety, headache, dizziness, and cellulitis.

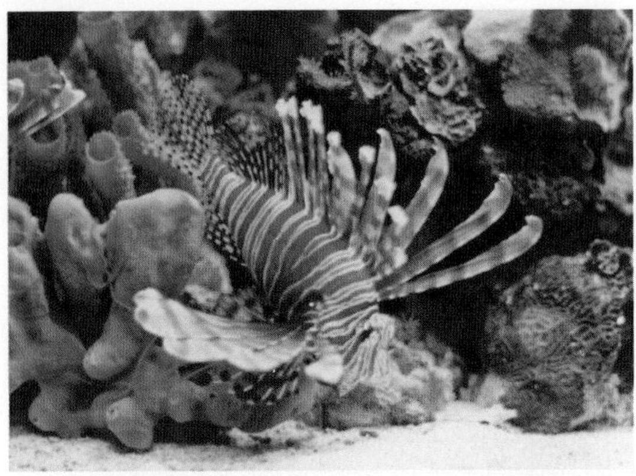

A

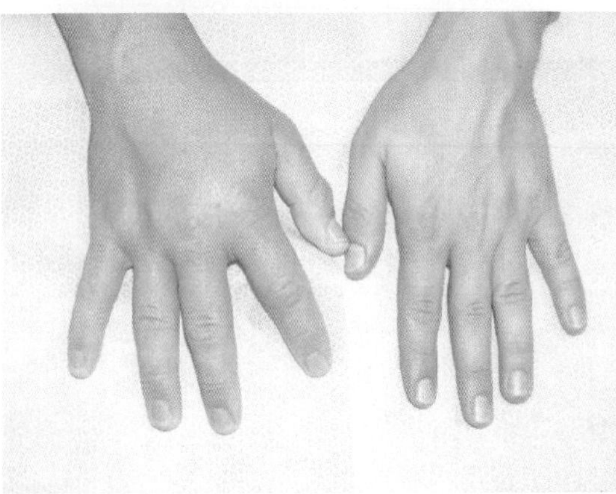

B

**FIGURE 89–5.** (**A**) The lionfish, *Pterois volitans*. (**B**) This patient's hand was envenomated by his pet lionfish while cleaning his aquarium. *(Used with permission from the Fellowship in Medical Toxicology, New York University Grossman School of Medicine, New York City Poison Center.)*

***Diagnosis.*** The most commonly affected area is the lower extremities. Imaging of the affected body part is indicated because of the potential of retained foreign bodies. Stingray spines are denser than human tissue and easily identified on radiographs. However, if only the sheath of the spine remains in the wound, radiography is unlikely to reveal this foreign body. Ultrasonography is recommended for patients with a negative radiography. Stings from stone fish are associated with compartment syndrome. Compartment pressures should be evaluated for a patient with significant pain, pallor, poikilothermia, paresthesias, or loss of distal pulses.

***Management.*** Wounds inflicted by stingrays and spiny fish should be carefully examined for imbedded foreign material. Stingray wounds have the potential to be extensive and require surgical attention for vascular or tendinous disruption. Tetanus immune status should be addressed. Prophylactic antibiotics decrease rates of wound infection; a quinolone and cefazolin are the recommended therapy. In a series of 576 stings from stingrays off the Californian coast, 69% of patients reported significant relief of local pain with HWI. In a human volunteer study in which subjects received a subcutaneous injection of stingray venom, severe pain developed immediately and was alleviated with water heated to 122°F (50°C). Pain increased with application of cold water. In patients undergoing HWI due to stonefish envenomation, antibiotics should be administered early due to the theoretical increased rate of growth of *Vibrio vulnificus* and subsequent necrotizing fasciitis. Although patients occasionally required a single dose of oral or parenteral analgesia, clinicians rarely prescribed analgesics on discharge. Severe vasospasm can generate limb-threatening ischemia.

Stonefish antivenom is an equine-derived IgG Fab raised against the venom of *S. trachynis*. Anecdotal reports suggest it provides effective relief from pain without acute adverse effects. Rash and serum sickness can develop several days postinjection. The manufacturer recommends IM administration of stonefish antivenom and advises against IV administration because of increased risk of anaphylactoid reaction. Administration is indicated for systemic toxicity or refractory pain. The number of puncture wounds guides therapy: one vial for one to two punctures, two vials for three to four punctures, and three vials for five or more punctures. Epinephrine and diphenhydramine should be readily available for treatment of airway emergencies and anaphylactic reactions.

# 90 MUSHROOMS

The diversity of mushroom species is evident in our grocery stores, our restaurant menus, and our environment. The enhanced culinary interest in mushrooms has led to experimentation by young and old residents and our newest immigrants and their young children reaching for what might become an innocuous (common) or a serious (rare) ingestion. This chapter offers general information on the most consequential toxicologic groups of mushrooms and emphasizes clinical diagnosis over mushroom identification. Additional mushroom syndromes are discussed in Table 90–1.

## EPIDEMIOLOGY

Unintentional ingestions of mushrooms, particularly in children, represent a small but relatively constant percentage of consultations requested from poison centers. Although the methods of codification of patients with mushroom exposure have changed over the past 35 years, cumulative American Association of Poison Control Centers (AAPCC) data consistently demonstrate the relative benignity of the vast majority of exposures. The inability of most healthcare providers to correctly identify the ingested mushroom and the rarity of lethal outcomes are also demonstrated by the accumulated data. In 75% to 95% of exposures, the exact species was unidentified. More than 50% of exposed individuals had no symptoms. Most patients were treated at home and rarely had major toxicity. During the 35 years covered by the AAPCC data, fewer than 100 patients died of their mushroom ingestion. Most deaths were associated with *Amanita* spp.

## CLASSIFICATION AND MANAGEMENT

This chapter does not address molds, mildews, and yeasts, which in addition to mushrooms are all categorized as fungi. The unifying principle for fungi is the lack of the photosynthetic capacity to produce nutrition. Survival is achieved by the enzymatic capacity of these organisms to integrate into living materials and digest them. Because mushroom species vary widely with regard to the xenobiotics they contain, and because identifying them with certainty is difficult, a system of classification based on clinical effects is more useful than one based on taxonomy. In many cases, management and prognosis can be determined with a high degree of confidence from the history and the geographic origin of the mushroom, the initial signs and symptoms, the organ system or systems involved, and coexistent factors or conditions. Most unintentional ingestions in small children involve at the most tasting common backyard mushrooms, which almost invariably results in no symptoms and no risks. Identification of the mushroom by photography will permit enhancement of the toxicologist's efforts at reassurance.

## GROUP I: CYCLOPEPTIDE-CONTAINING MUSHROOMS

Worldwide, most mushroom fatalities are associated with cyclopeptide (amatoxin) containing species. Approximately 50 to 100 cases are reported annually in Western Europe with fewer in Asia, Australia, Africa, and North and South America. In North America, there are two distinct ranges of cyclopeptide-containing species along the West Coast (California to British Columbia) and along the East Coast (Maryland to Maine). These mushrooms include a number of *Amanita* species, including *A. verna*, *A. virosa*, and *A. phalloides*; *Galerina* spp, including *G. autumnalis*, *G. marginata*, and *G. venenata*; and *Lepiota* species, including *L. helveola*, *L. josserandi*, and *L. brunneoincarnata* (Fig. 90–1). Early differentiation of cyclopeptide poisonings from other types of mushroom poisoning is difficult (Fig. 90–2).

*A. phalloides* contains 15 to 20 cyclopeptides, each with an approximate weight of 900 Da. The amatoxins (cyclic octapeptides), phallotoxins (cyclic heptapeptides), and virotoxins (cyclic heptapeptides) are the best studied. There is no evidence for the toxicity of virotoxins in humans. Of these three chemically similar cyclopeptide molecules, phalloidin (the principal phallotoxin) appears to be rapid-acting, whereas amanitin tends to cause more delayed manifestations. The amatoxins are the most toxic of the cyclopeptides, leading to liver, kidney, and central nervous system (CNS) damage. These polypeptides are heat stable. α-Amanitin is the principal amatoxin responsible for human toxicity following ingestion. Approximately 1.5 to 2.5 mg of amanitin can be obtained from 1 g of dry *A. phalloides*, and as much as 3.5 mg/g can be obtained from some *Lepiota* spp. A 20-g mushroom contains well in excess of the 0.1 mg/kg amanitin considered lethal for humans.

The amanitins are highly bioavailable and rapidly absorbed from the gastrointestinal (GI) tract. Amatoxins show limited protein binding and are present in the plasma at low concentrations for 24 to 48 hours. Hepatocellular entry of α-amanitin is facilitated by a sodium-dependent bile acid transporter. Several studies demonstrate that a member of the organic anion–transporter (OAT) polypeptide family localized in the sinusoidal membranes of human hepatocytes facilitates hepatocellular α-amanitin uptake. Once inside the cells, the cytotoxicity of amanitin results from its interference with RNA polymerase II, preventing the transcription of DNA and thereby suppressing protein synthesis resulting in cell death. α-Amanitin is enterohepatically recirculated. Target organs are those with the highest rate of cell turnover, including the GI tract epithelium, hepatocytes, and kidneys. Amatoxins do not cross the placenta, as demonstrated by the absence of fetal toxicity in severely poisoned pregnant women.

In an intravenous radiolabeled amatoxin study in dogs, 85% of the amatoxin was recovered in the urine within the first 6 hours, whereas less than 1% was found in the blood at that time. The extreme variabilities of the type and quantity of amanitin ingested, the host, the delay from the time of ingestion to collection, and the management make interpretations of amatoxin concentrations exceedingly difficult.

Several variable techniques for quantitative and qualitative evaluation of amatoxins are utilized. Amatoxins can be detected

**TABLE 90–1** Mushroom Toxicity Overview

| *Representative Genus/Species* | *Xenobiotic* | *Time of Onset of Symptoms* | *Primary Site of Toxicity* | *Clinical Findings* | *Mortality* | *Specific Therapy*[a] |
|---|---|---|---|---|---|---|
| I | | | | | | |
| *Amanita phalloides, A. tenuifolia, A. virosa*<br>*Galerina autumnalis, G. marginata, G. venenata*<br>*Lepiota josserandi, L. helveola* | Cyclopeptides<br>Amatoxins<br>Phallotoxins | 5–24 h | Liver | Phase I: GI toxicity—N/V/D<br>Phase II: Quiescent<br>Phase III: N/V/D, jaundice, ↑ AST, ↑ ALT, ↑ Bilirubin, hepatic failure | 30% | Potential benefit early of activated charcoal<br>Hemoperfusion/hemodialysis<br>Silibinin<br>Polymyxin B<br>Potential benefit late for *N*-acetylcysteine |
| II | | | | | | |
| *Gyromitra ambigua, G. esculenta, G. infula* | Gyromitrin (metabolite: monomethylhydrazine) | 5–10 h | CNS | Seizures, abdominal pain, N/V, weakness, hepatorenal failure | Rare | Benzodiazepines, pyridoxine 70 mg/kg IV (max 5 g) |
| III | | | | | | |
| *Clitocybe dealbata, Omphalotus olearius,* most *Inocybe* spp, *Boletus eastwoodiae* | Muscarine | 0.5–2 h | Autonomic nervous system | Peripheral muscarinic effects—salivation, bradycardia, lacrimation, urination, defecation, diaphoresis | Rare | Atropine—Adults: 1–2 mg<br>Children: 0.02 mg/kg with a minimum of 0.1 mg |
| IV | | | | | | |
| *Coprinopsis atramentaria, C. insignis* | Coprine (metabolite: 1-aminocyclopropanol) | 0.5–2 h | Aldehyde dehydrogenase | Disulfiramlike effect with ethanol, tachycardia, N/V, flushing | Rare | Antiemetics<br>Fluid resuscitation<br>Fomepizole for refractory toxicity |
| V | | | | | | |
| *Amanita gemmata, A. muscaria, A. pantherina, Tricholoma muscarium* | Ibotenic acid, muscimol | 0.5–2 h | CNS | GABAergic effects, rare delirium, hallucinations, dizziness, ataxia | Rare | Benzodiazepines during excitatory phase |
| VI | | | | | | |
| *Psilocybe cyanescens, P. cubensis,*<br>*Gymnopilus spectabilis,*<br>*Psathyrella foenisecii* | Psilocybin, psilocin | 0.5–1 h | CNS | Ataxia, N/V, hyperkinesis, hallucinations, illusions | Rare | Benzodiazepines for agitation |
| VII | | | | | | |
| *Clitocybe nebularis,*<br>*Chlorophyllum molybdites,*<br>*C. esculentum, Lactarius* spp, *Paxillus involutus* | Various<br>GI irritants | 0.3–3 h | GI | Malaise, N/V/D | Rare | Symptomatic care |
| VIII | | | | | | |
| *Cortinarius orellanus, C. rubellus, C. gentilis* | Orellanine, orellinine | > 1 day–weeks | Kidney | Phase I: N/V<br>Phase II: Oliguria, acute kidney injury | Rare | Hemodialysis for acute kidney injury |
| IX | | | | | | |
| *Amanita smithiana,*<br>*A. proxima, A. pseudoporphyria* | Allenic norleucine | 0.5–12 h | Kidney | Phase I: N/V<br>Phase II: Oliguria, acute kidney injury | None | Hemodialysis for acute kidney injury |
| X | | | | | | |
| *Tricholoma equestre* (Europe),<br>*Russula subnigricans* (Japan, China) | Cycloprop-2-enecarboxylic acid | 24–72 h<br>0.5–2 h | Muscle (skeletal and cardiac) | Fatigue, N/V, muscle weakness, myalgias, ↑ CK, facial erythema, diaphoresis, myocarditis | 10% | Sodium bicarbonate, hemodialysis for acute kidney injury |
| XI | | | | | | |
| *Trogia venenata,*<br>*Amanita franchetti,*<br>*Ramaria rufescens* | 2*R*-amino-4,5-hydroxy-5-hexynoic acid | 1–5 days<br>2–15 h<br>2–15 h | Cardiac and skeletal muscle | Tachycardia, GI symptoms, myalgias, tremor, seizures, dizziness, weakness, syncope, palpitations, ventricular fibrillation | High? | Intensive care monitoring |

*(Continued)*

**TABLE 90–1 Mushroom Toxicity Overview (*Continued*)**

| *Representative Genus/Species* | *Xenobiotic* | *Time of Onset of Symptoms* | *Primary Site of Toxicity* | *Clinical Findings* | *Mortality* | *Specific Therapy*[a] |
|---|---|---|---|---|---|---|
| XII | | | | | | |
| *Clitocybe acromelalga, C. amoenolens* | Acromelic acids | 24 h | Peripheral nervous system | Erythromelalgia, paresthesias—hands and feet, dysesthesias, erythema, edema | None | Symptomatic care |
| XIII | | | | | | |
| *Pleurocybella porrigens* | Unknown | 1–31 days | CNS | Encephalopathy, convulsions, myoclonus in patients with chronic kidney failure | High (30%) | Hemodialysis |
| *Hapalopilus rutilans* | Polyporic acid | > 12 h | GI, CNS | N/V, abdominal pain, vertigo, ataxia, drowsiness, encephalopathy | None | Symptomatic care |
| XIV | | | | | | |
| *Paxillus involutus, Clitocybe claviceps? Boletus luridus?* | Involutin | Following repeated exposure 0.5–3 h | Red blood cell, kidney | Hemolytic anemia, acute kidney injury | Rare | Hemodialysis |
| XV | | | | | | |
| *Lycoperdon perlatum, L. pyriforme, L. gemmatum* | Spores | Hours | Pulmonary, GI | Cough, shortness of breath, fever, nausea, vomiting | None | Corticosteroids |

[a]Supportive care (fluids, electrolytes, and antiemetics) as indicated.
AST/ALT = aspartate- and alanine aminotransferase; CK = creatine phosphokinase; CNS = central nervous system; D = diarrhea; GI = gastrointestinal; N = nausea; V = vomiting.

by high-performance liquid chromatography, thin-layer chromatography, ion trap mass spectrometry, and radioimmunoassay in gastroduodenal fluid, serum, urine, stool, and liver and kidney biopsies for several days following an ingestion.

## Clinical

Phase I of cyclopeptide poisoning resembles severe gastroenteritis, with profuse watery diarrhea that is delayed until 5 to 24 hours after ingestion. Early onset of GI distress before 5 hours is strong support for another non-*Amanita* species or an etiology other than mushroom ingestion. Transient improvement occurs during phase II from 12 and 36 hours after ingestion, although hepatic injury begins during this phase. Gastrointestinal manifestations including nausea, vomiting, abdominal pain, and diarrhea may persist during the entirety of the clinical course. Although many patients recover, some progress to phase III, which is manifested by hepatic and renal toxicity and even death 2 to 6 days after ingestion. Although hepatotoxicity begins within the second phase of toxicity, clinical hepatotoxicity with elevated concentrations of bilirubin, aspartate aminotransferase (AST), and alanine aminotransferase (ALT), hypoglycemia, jaundice, and hepatic coma are not manifest until 2 to 3 days after ingestion.

## Treatment

Survival rates in case series of variable numbers of patients poisoned by *A. phalloides* who received supportive care, fluid and electrolyte repletion, high-dose penicillin G, dexamethasone, or other therapies are between 70% and 100%. Many of these case series have excellent survival rates with extremely

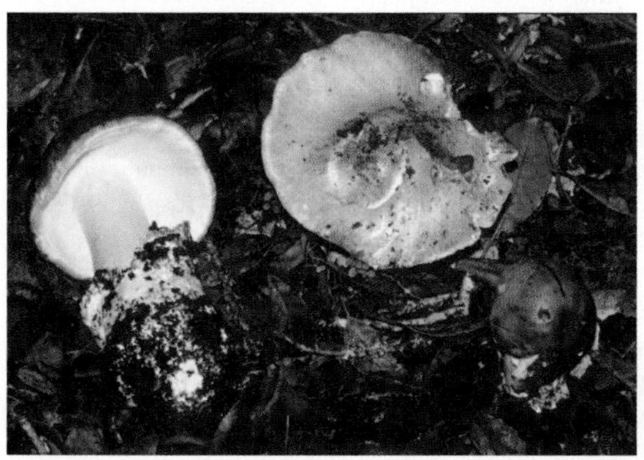
A

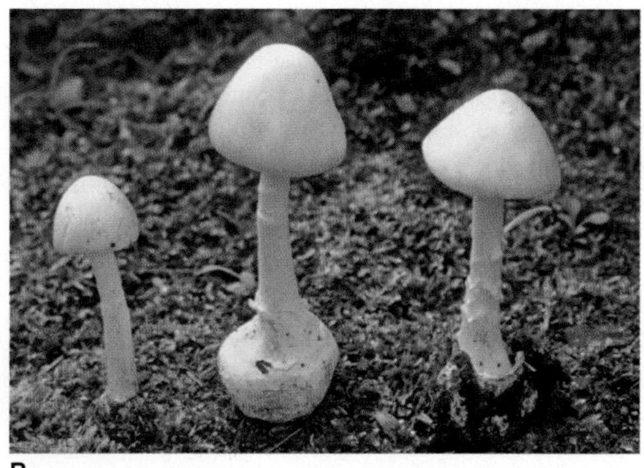
B

**FIGURE 90–1.** Group I: Cyclopeptide-containing mushrooms. (**A**) *Amanita phalloides* and (**B**) *Amanita virosa*. *(Used with permission from John Plischke III.)*

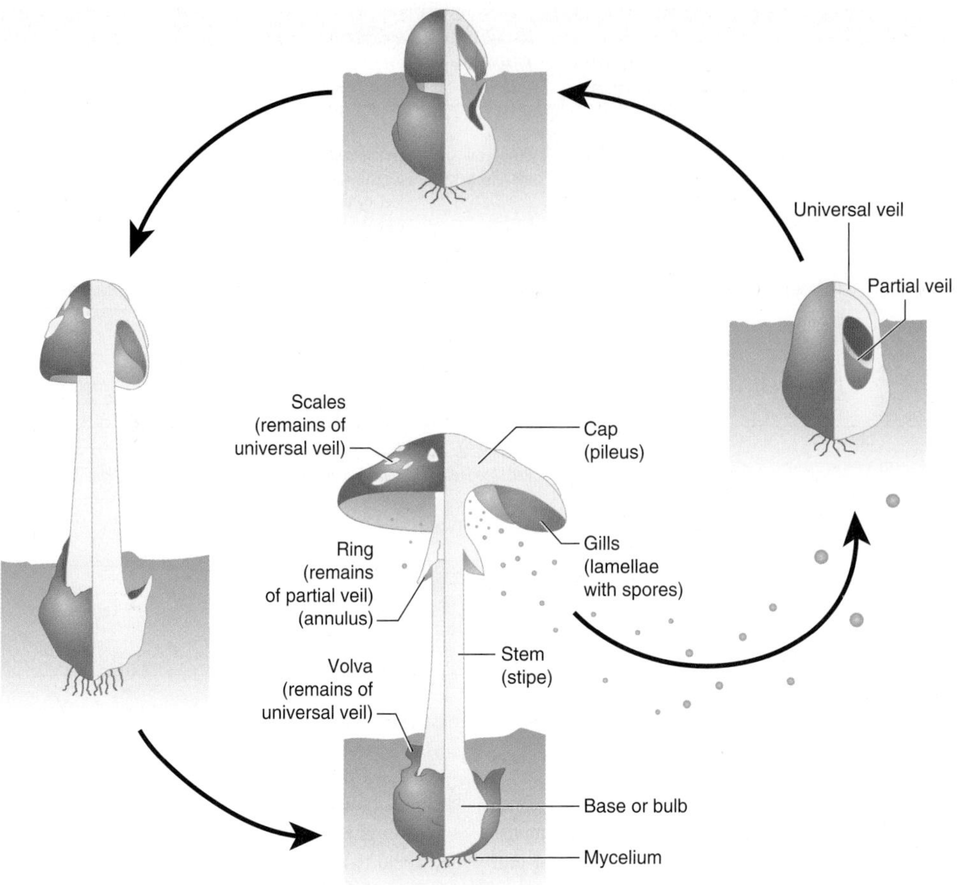


**FIGURE 90–2.** In the more highly specialized mushrooms, such as the *Amanita* species shown here, two veils of tissue cover the fruiting body and its constituent parts during its development. The outer enclosing bag, known as the universal veil ruptures as the fruiting body expands to leave a volva at the base and fragments on the cap. The inner partial veil that covers the developing gills is pulled away as the cap opens to leave a ring on the stem.

variable therapeutic interventions, limiting the capacity to determine the need for, or efficacy of, most of the standard conservative therapeutic regimens. Fluid and electrolyte repletion and treatment of hepatic compromise are essential. Intravenous 0.9% sodium chloride solution and electrolytes usually are necessary because of substantial fluid losses due to vomiting and diarrhea. Dextrose repletion titrating to serum glucose concentration (> 100 mg/dL) is reasonable because of nutritional compromise, hepatic failure, or glycogen depletion. Orogastric lavage is not necessary unless the patient presents within several hours after the ingestion because any substantial quantity of ingested toxin almost invariably induces emesis and catharsis.

Activated charcoal both adsorbs the amatoxins and improves survival in laboratory animals. Activated charcoal is safe, logical, and a valuable therapeutic strategy at least during the first 12 to 24 hours following mushroom ingestion. Although the clinical presentation often is delayed, 1 g/kg body weight of activated charcoal is reasonable for oral administration every 2 to 4 hours (if the patient is vomiting, an antiemetic is indicated) or by continuous nasogastric infusion. Data are insufficient to recommend either continuous nasogastric duodenal aspiration or biliary drainage.

Despite some experimental and clinical support, we no longer recommend thioctic (α-lipoic) acid, cimetidine, or penicillin G. *N*-Acetylcysteine is reasonable in patients with liver injury. The optimal dosing is unknown, but we typically recommend the standard acetaminophen regimen (Antidotes in Brief: A3).

The active complex of milk thistle (*Silybum marianum*) is silymarin, which is a lipophilic extract composed of three isomeric flavonolignans: silibinin, silychristin, and silydianin. Silibinin competitively inhibits the organic anion transporter (OATP1B3) that is responsible for the uptake and enterohepatic recycling of α-amanitin. Although some in vitro and animal experiments support the use of silibinin, there are no controlled human trials. A 20-year retrospective review of European and American case reports of more than 2,000 hospitalized patients with amatoxin-induced mushroom poisoning concluded that silibinin alone or in combination with *N*-acetylcysteine showed the most promise as hepatoprotective therapies. Silibinin is routinely available as a nonprescription supplement in most pharmacies and appears to be safe and well tolerated in patients with chronic liver disease. A dose of silibinin 20 to 50 mg/kg/day is reasonable in humans, even though it is not approved as a therapeutic for hepatic disease by the Food and Drug Administration (FDA) in the United States (US).

In a response to the continuing quest for a successful antidote for α-amanitin poisoning, a group of investigators with computer modeling and simulation screened clinical drugs sharing bioisosterism with α-amanitin. They subsequently found in an in silico study that polymyxin B had significant chemical similarities and molecular dynamics that successfully competed at the same interface and displaced α-amanitin from binding sites with RNA polymerase II. Polymyxin B was then used in vivo to demonstrate that all mice given a specified dose of α-amanitin died, whereas when polymyxin B was given simultaneously, all mice survived. In the absence of any proven antidote, polymyxin B at a dose of at least 7,500 Units/kg every 12 hours for 1 to 2 days is reasonable to administer as a life-saving gesture when there is certainty that a cyclopeptide-containing species was ingested.

Forced diuresis, hemodialysis, plasmapheresis, hemofiltration, and hemoperfusion are often considered shortly after ingestion, but most studies offer neither clinical evidence of benefit nor supportive pharmacokinetic data for any of these therapies. These therapies are not routinely recommended. Because of the absence of prospective, controlled studies of exposure to amatoxins, in addition to the extreme variability of success with many regimens, multiple-dose activated charcoal and supportive care remain the standard therapy.

Extracorporeal albumin dialysis, molecular adsorbent recirculating system, and fractionated plasma separation and adsorption system are detoxification techniques used in patients with fulminant hepatic failure to remove water-soluble and albumin-bound xenobiotics while providing renal support. None of the available studies of these bridging systems are randomized or controlled. The clinical experience is solely in the care of patients with grave hepatotoxicity at a delayed stage limiting any potential for significant conclusions. These two techniques permit time for hepatic regeneration or sufficient bridging time to orthotopic liver transplantation.

The criteria and timing for liver transplantation following amatoxin poisoning are far less established than for fulminant viral hepatitis, in which grade III or IV hepatic encephalopathy, marked hyperbilirubinemia, increased international normalized ratio (INR) and azotemia are the well-established criteria for transplantation. From 1998 to 2014, the US Acute Liver Failure Study group of 2,224 patients had only 18 patients (five with acute liver injury and 13 with acute liver failure) who were suggested to have had severe hepatotoxicity secondary to an amatoxin. Many survived acute liver failure without transplant, and all those with liver transplant survived. The grim prognosis associated with hepatic coma secondary to *Amanita* spp poisoning has led several transplant groups to consider hepatic transplantation for encephalopathic patients with prolonged INRs (> 6), persistent hypoglycemia, metabolic acidosis, increased concentrations of serum ammonia and AST, and hypofibrinogenemia. Because there are no definitive transplant criteria for amatoxin-associated acute liver injury and acute liver failure, the judgment of a transplant team is essential. It is our belief that rapid transfer to a regional liver transplantation center offers the safest site for high-quality care and for decision making with regard to timing for liver transplantation in the face of advancing liver failure.

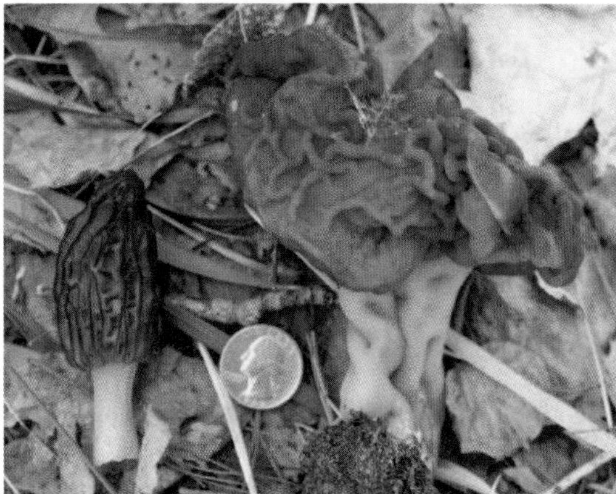

**FIGURE 90–3.** Group II: Gyromitrin-containing mushrooms. A true morel (*Morchella* spp) on the left is compared to a false morel (*Gyromitra esculenta*) on the right. *(Used with permission from John Trestrail.)*

## GROUP II: GYROMITRIN-CONTAINING MUSHROOMS

Members of the gyromitrin group include *Gyromitra esculenta*, *G. ambigua*, and *G. infula*. *G. esculenta* enjoy a reputation of being edible in the western US but of being toxic in other areas. The most common error occurs in the spring, when an individual seeking the nongilled, brainlike *Morchella esculenta* (morel) finds the similar *G. esculenta* (false morel) (Fig. 90–3).

These mushrooms are found commonly in the spring under conifers and are easily recognized by their brainlike appearance. Poisonings with these mushrooms are exceptionally uncommon in the US, representing less than 1% of all recognized events, whereas these poisonings are considered more common in Europe. *Gyromitra* mushrooms contain the nonvolatile insoluble gyromitrin. The metabolism of gyromitrin is shown in Figure 90–4.

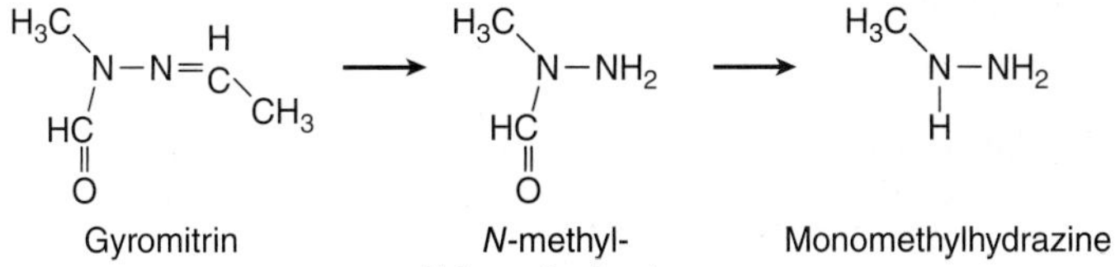

Gyromitrin → *N*-methyl-*N*-formylhydrazine → Monomethylhydrazine

**FIGURE 90–4.** *Gyromitra* mushrooms contain gyromitrin, which undergoes hydrolysis to yield a family of *N*-methyl-formylhydrazines. These molecules on subsequent hydrolysis yield *N*-methyl-*N*-formylhydrazine and monomethylhydrazine.

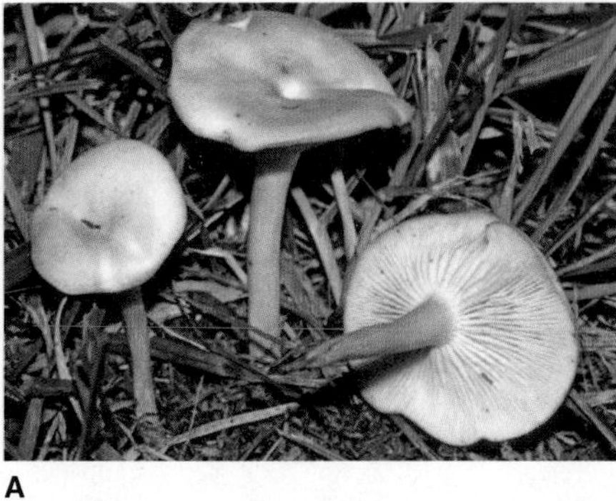
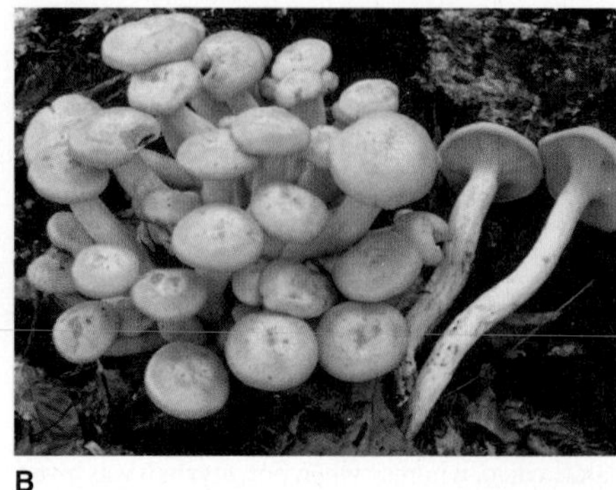

**FIGURE 90–5.** Group III: Muscarine-containing mushrooms. (**A**) *Clitocybe dealbata*. (**B**) *Omphalotus olearius*. *(Used with permission from John Plischke III.)*

The hydrazine moiety reacts with pyridoxine, resulting in inhibition of pyridoxal phosphate–related enzymatic reactions. This impairs the production of the inhibitory neurotransmitter γ-aminobutyric acid (GABA).

The initial signs and symptoms of toxicity from these mushrooms occur 5 to 10 hours after ingestion and include nausea, vomiting, diarrhea, and abdominal pain. Patients manifest headaches, weakness, and diffuse muscle cramping. Rarely in the first 12 to 48 hours, patients develop nystagmus, ataxia, delirium, stupor, convulsions, and coma. Most patients improve dramatically and return to normal function within several days.

Activated charcoal 1 g/kg body weight is recommended for administration. Benzodiazepines are appropriate for initial management of seizures. Under most circumstances, supportive care is adequate treatment. Pyridoxine (vitamin $B_6$) in doses of 70 mg/kg IV up to 5 g is recommended to limit seizures and other neurologic symptoms (Antidotes in Brief: A15).

## GROUP III: MUSCARINE-CONTAINING MUSHROOMS

Mushrooms that contain muscarine include numerous members of the *Clitocybe* species, such as *C. dealbata* (the sweater) and *C. illudens* (*Omphalotus olearius*), and the *Inocybe* species, which include *I. iacera*, *I. lanuginosa*, and *I. geophylla* (Fig. 90–5).

Clinical manifestations usually develop within 0.25 to 2 hours and typically last several additional hours with complete resolution within 24 hours. Muscarine and acetylcholine are similar structurally and have comparable clinical effects at the muscarinic receptors. Peripheral manifestations include bradycardia, miosis, salivation, lacrimation, vomiting, diarrhea, bronchospasm, bronchorrhea, and micturition. Central muscarinic manifestations do not occur because muscarine, a quaternary ammonium compound, does not cross the blood–brain barrier. No nicotinic manifestations such as diaphoresis or tremor occur. Significant toxicity is uncommon, limiting the need for more than supportive care. Rarely, atropine (1–2 mg given IV slowly for adults or 0.02 mg/kg IV for children) is reasonable when titrated and repeated as frequently as indicated to reverse symptomatology.

## GROUP IV: COPRINE-CONTAINING MUSHROOMS

*Coprinus* mushrooms, particularly *C. atramentarius* (*Coprinopsis atramentaria*), contain the toxin coprine (Fig. 90–6). These mushrooms grow abundantly in temperate climates in grassy or woodland fields. They are known as "inky caps" because the gills that contain a peptidase autodigest into an inky liquid shortly after picking. The edible member of this group, *Coprinus comatus* (shaggy mane), is nontoxic, and probably its misidentification results in collectors' errors. Coprine metabolites have a disulfiramlike effect. Inhibition of acetaldehyde dehydrogenase results in accumulation of acetaldehyde and its associated adverse effects, which take at least 0.5 to 2 hours to manifest if the patient ingests alcohol concomitantly or subsequent to

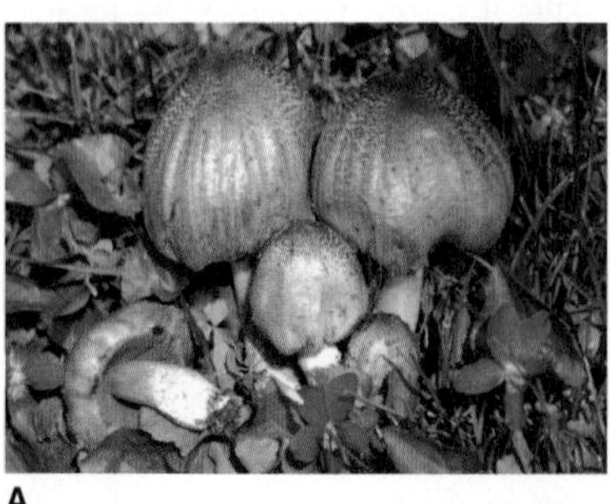
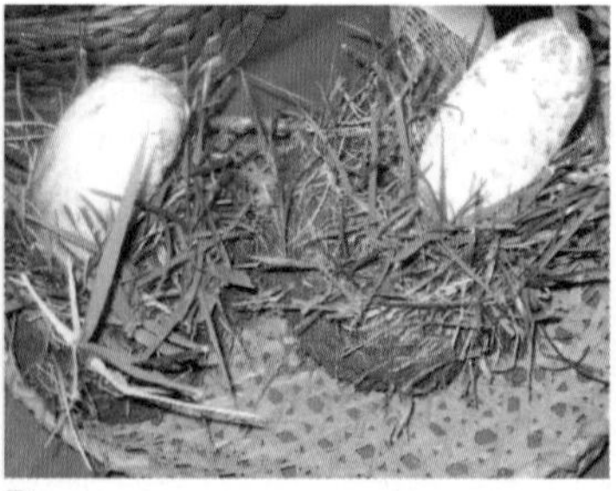
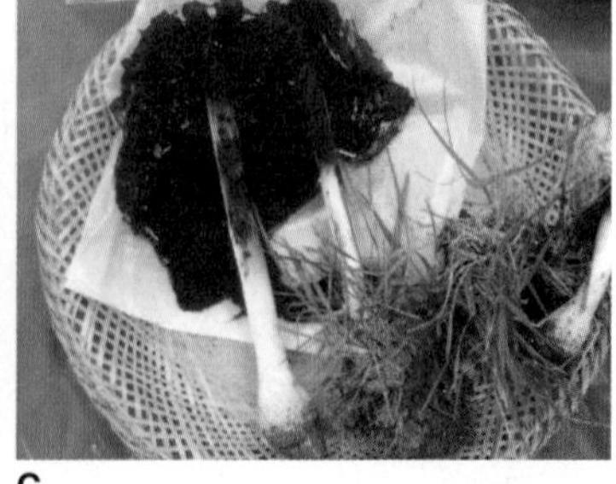

**FIGURE 90–6.** Group IV: Coprine-containing mushrooms. (**A**) *Coprinopsis atramentaria*; (**B**) and (**C**) show *Coprinus comatus* (shaggy mane). Image B shows an early form, which later is self-digested, demonstrating the gill liquefaction in image C. *(Image A used with permission from John Plischke III, and images B and C used with permission from Lewis Nelson.)*

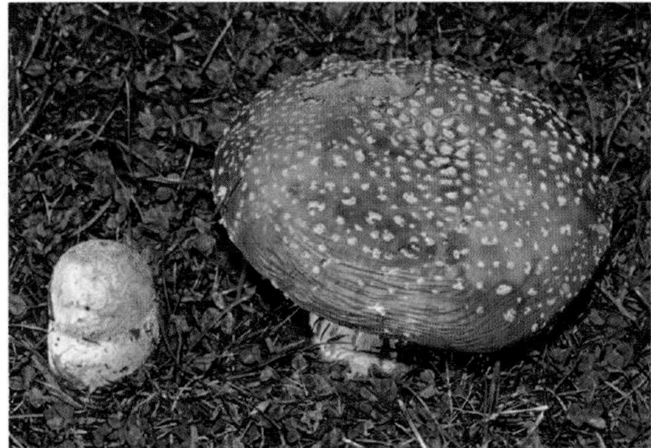

**FIGURE 90–7.** Group V: Muscimol-containing mushrooms. This image of *Amanita muscaria* highlights different development forms and colors. *(Used with permission from John Plischke III.)*

eating a coprine-containing mushroom. For the subsequent 48 to 72 hours following coprine-containing mushroom ingestion, if ethanol ingestion occurs, toxicity ensues. Within 0.5 to 2 hours of ethanol ingestion, tachycardia, flushing, nausea, and vomiting occur. Treatment is symptomatic with fluid repletion and antiemetics such as metoclopramide or ondansetron, although clinical manifestations usually are mild and resolve within several hours. Prophylactic use of fomepizole (Antidotes in Brief: A33) immediately following ingestion of ethanol and coprine-containing mushrooms would be reasonable, and therapeutic use would be appropriate if persistent toxicity occurs associated with an elevated ethanol concentration, although no case reports or studies are published.

## GROUP V: IBOTENIC ACID– AND MUSCIMOL-CONTAINING MUSHROOMS

Most of the mushrooms in this class are primarily in the *Amanita* species, which includes *A. muscaria* (fly agaric), *A. pantherina*, and *A. gemmate* (Fig. 90–7). They exist singly scattered throughout the US woodlands. The brilliant red or tan cap (pileus) is that of the mushroom commonly depicted in children's books and is easily recognized in the fields during summer and fall. Small variable quantities of ibotenic acid and its decarboxylated metabolite muscimol are found in these mushrooms. Ibotenic acid is an amino acid that acts as a glutamate agonist at *N*-methyl-D-aspartate (NMDA) receptors. Muscimol acts as a γ-aminobutyric acid type A ($GABA_A$) agonist.

Most patients who develop symptoms have intentionally ingested large quantities of these mushrooms while seeking a hallucinatory experience. Within 0.5 to 2 hours of ingestion, these mushrooms produce somnolence, dizziness, auditory and visual hallucinations, dysphoria, seizures, and agitated delirium in adults and the excitatory glutamatergic manifestations of myoclonic movements. Seizures and other neurologic findings predominate in children. Treatment is invariably supportive. Most symptoms respond solely to supportive care, although a benzodiazepine is recommended for excitatory CNS manifestations.

## GROUP VI: PSILOCYBIN-CONTAINING MUSHROOMS

Psilocybin-containing mushrooms include *Psilocybe cyanescens, Psilocybe cubensis, Conocybe cyanopus, Panaeolus cyanescens, Gymnopilus spectabilis*, and *Psathyrella foenisecii* (Fig. 90–8). These mushrooms have been used for native North and South American religious ceremonies for thousands of years. They grow abundantly in warm, moist areas of the US. They are readily available through drug culture magazines and the Internet.

Psilocybin is rapidly and completely hydrolyzed to psilocin in vivo. Serotonin, psilocin, psilocybin, bufotenine, dimethyltryptamine, and lysergic acid diethylamide (LSD) are very similar structurally and presumably act at the $5\text{-HT}_2$ receptor site. The effects of psilocybin as a serotonin agonist and antagonist are discussed in Chap. 52.

The psilocybin and psilocin rapidly (within 1 hour of ingestion) produce CNS effects, including ataxia, hyperkinesis, visual illusions, and hallucinations. Some patients manifest GI distress, tachycardia, mydriasis, anxiety, lightheadedness, tremor, and agitation. Most pateints return to normal within 6 to 12 hours. Treatment for hallucinations usually is supportive, although administering a benzodiazepine is reasonable when reassurance proves inadequate.

## GROUP VII: GASTROINTESTINAL TOXIN–CONTAINING MUSHROOMS

By far the largest group of mushrooms is a diverse group that contains a variety of ill-defined GI toxins. Many of the hundreds of mushrooms in this group fall into the "little brown mushroom" category. Some *Boletus* spp, *Lactarius* spp, *O. olearius, Rhodophyllus* spp, *Tricholoma* spp, *Chlorophyllum*

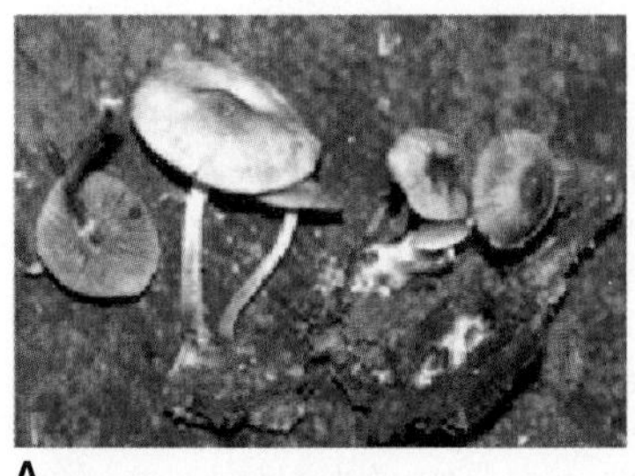

A

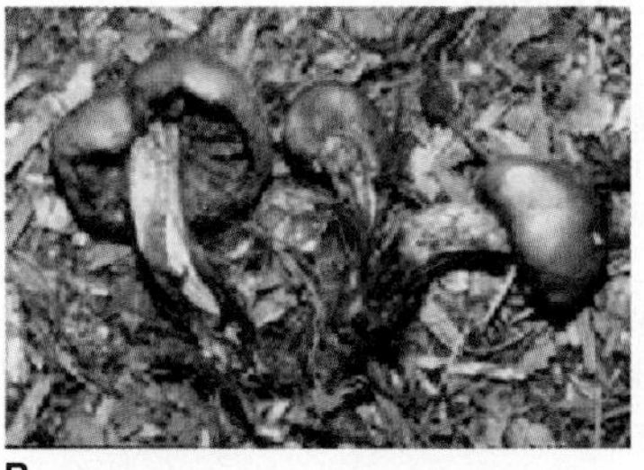

B

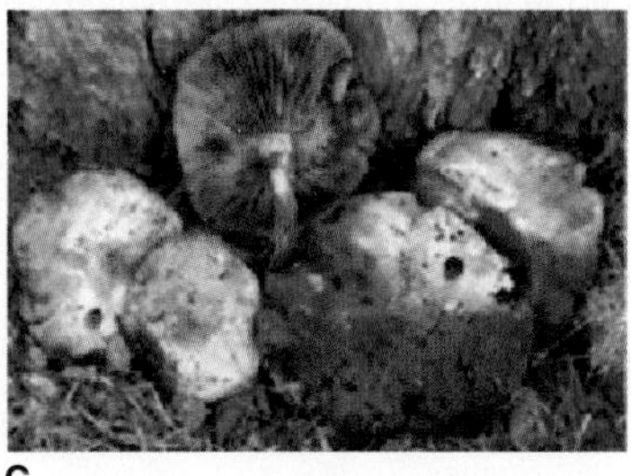

C

**FIGURE 90–8.** Group VI: Psilocybin-containing mushrooms. Three examples of hallucinogenic mushrooms: (**A**) *Psilocybe cyanescens*, (**B**) *Psilocybe caerulipes*, and (**C**) *Gymnopilus spectabilis*. *(Used with permission from John Plischke III.)*

**TABLE 90–2 Mushroom Toxicity: Correlation Between Organ System Affected, Time of Onset of Toxic Manifestations, and Mushroom Xenobiotic Responsible**

| | Time of Onset | | |
|---|---|---|---|
| *Organ System* | *Early: < 5 h* | *Middle: 5–24 h* | *Late: > 24 h* |
| Cardiac muscle | | | 2*R*-amino-4, 5-hexynoic acid, Group XI |
| Gastrointestinal | Allenic norleucine<br>2*R*-amino-4, 5-hexynoic acid<br>Coprine<br>Group VII<br>Psilocybin<br>Muscarine | Allenic norleucine<br>Amatoxin<br>Gyromitrin | Orellanine and orellinine |
| Liver | | | Amatoxin |
| Immunologic | Involutin<br>Spores | | |
| Nervous | Ibotenic acid and muscimol<br>Psilocybin | Gyromitrin | Acromelic acid<br>Gyromitrin<br>Polyporic acid |
| Kidney | | | Allenic norleucine<br>Orellanine and orellinine |
| Skeletal muscle | Cycloprop-2-enecarboxylic acid, Group X | | |

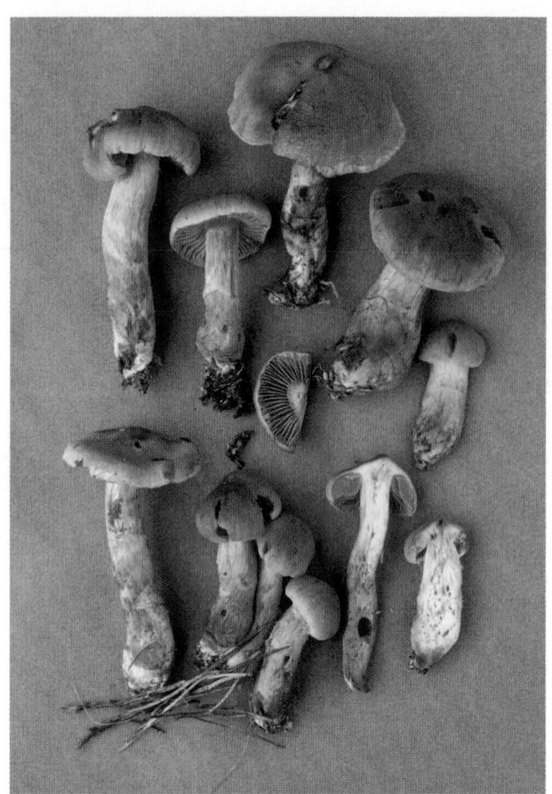

**FIGURE 90–9.** Group VIII: Orellanine- and orellinine-containing mushrooms: *Cortinarius rubellus*. *(Used with permission from Roger Phillips/Alamy Stock Photo.)*

*molybdites*, and *Chlorophyllum esculentum* are mistaken for edible or hallucinogenic species. A frequently reported error is the confusion of the jack-o'-lantern (*Omphalotus olearius*) with the edible species of chanterelle (*Cantharellus cibarius*).

The toxins associated with this group are not identified. Gastrointestinal toxicity occurs 0.3 to 3 hours after ingestion when epigastric distress, malaise, nausea, vomiting, and diarrhea are evident. Treatment includes fluid resuscitation with control of vomiting and diarrhea. The clinical course is brief and the prognosis excellent. Those mushroom ingestions resulting in GI toxicity more than 5 hours after ingestion are considered in Table 90–2. When symptoms seem to persist, the clinician must consider a mixed ingestion of another potentially toxic mushroom group.

## GROUP VIII: ORELLANINE- AND ORELLININE-CONTAINING MUSHROOMS

*Cortinarius* mushrooms, such as *C. rubellus* and *C. orellanus*, are commonly found throughout North America and Europe Figure 90–9. The *C. orellanus* toxin orellanine is reduced by photochemical degradation to orellinine, which is further reduced to the nontoxic orelline. The toxic compound orellanine is similar to paraquat and diquat and may have comparable mechanisms of action, although precise knowledge is limited (Chap. 82). Other nephrotoxins are isolated from certain *Cortinarius* spp and result in tubular damage, interstitial nephritis, and tubulointerstitial fibrosis.

Orellanine is rapidly removed from the plasma within 48 to 72 hours and concentrated in the urine in a soluble form. Initial manifestations occur 24 to 72 hours after ingestion and initially include headache, nausea, vomiting, and diarrhea followed by chills, polydipsia, anorexia, oliguria, and flank and abdominal pain. Oliguric kidney failure develops several days to weeks after initial symptoms. The only initial laboratory abnormalities include hematuria, pyuria, and proteinuria. Nephrotoxicity is characterized by interstitial nephritis with tubular damage and early fibrosis of injured tubules with relative glomerular sparing. Hepatotoxicity is rarely reported.

Hemodialysis and renal transplantation are used for the treatment of acute kidney failure. No evidence suggests that secondary detoxification by plasmapheresis or hemoperfusion is of any benefit in preventing chronic kidney failure even when initiated in the first 48 hours.

## GROUP IX: ALLENIC NORLEUCINE–CONTAINING MUSHROOMS

*Amanita smithiana* poisoning is reported in the Pacific Northwest and the Mediterranean area. Because the mature specimen often lacks any evidence of a partial or universal veil, these mushrooms are not recognized as *Amanita* species. It appears that all of the poisoned individuals were seeking the edible pine mushroom matsutake (*Tricholoma magnivelare*), a highly desirable lookalike (Fig. 90–10). The *A. smithiana*, *A. proxima*, *A. abrupta*, and *A. pseudoporphyria* possess two amino acid toxins: allenic norleucine (2-amino-4,5-hexadienoic acid) and possibly 1,2-amino-4-pentynoic acid.

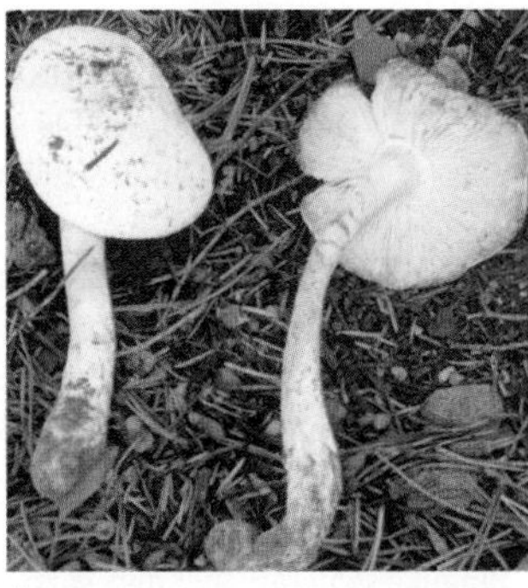
A

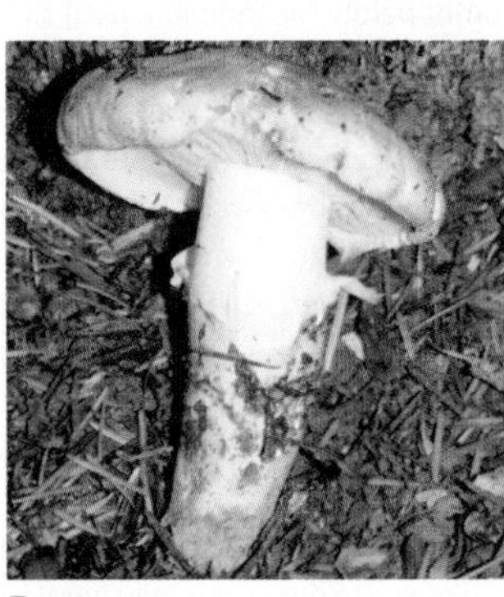
B

**FIGURE 90–10.** Group IX: Allenic norleucine-containing mushrooms: (**A**) *Amanita smithiana* compared to (**B**) *Tricholoma magnivelare* (matsutake, the mushroom with which it has been mistaken). *(Used with permission from John Plischke III.)*

Initial effects were noted from 0.5 to 12 hours following ingestion of either raw or cooked specimens. Gastrointestinal manifestations, including anorexia, nausea, vomiting, abdominal pain, and diarrhea, occurred frequently, accompanied by malaise, sweating, and dizziness. In some cases, vomiting and diarrhea persist for several days. The patients typically presented for care 3 to 6 days after ingestion, at which time they were oliguric or anuric. Acute kidney injury manifested 4 to 6 days following ingestion, with marked elevation of blood urea nitrogen and creatinine. Lactate dehydrogenase and ALT concentrations frequently were elevated, whereas amylase, AST, alkaline phosphatase, and bilirubin were only infrequently abnormal.

There is no known antidote for these nephrotoxins. Activated charcoal, although of no proven benefit, is reasonable in standard doses when a patient in the northwest US presents with early GI manifestations after mushroom ingestions. In view of the substantial morbidity associated with *A. smithiana* ingestions, historic, clinical, and/or temporal evidence of this ingestion would be a reasonable indication for charcoal hemoperfusion or hemodialysis when the patient presents in the early phase (12–24 hours) of exposure. When a patient presents with renal compromise several days, as opposed to weeks, following mushroom ingestion and with a history of early, as opposed to delayed, GI manifestations, the clinician may be able to suggest *A. smithiana* as the etiology compared to *Cortinarius* spp exposure.

## GROUP X: CYCLOPROP-2-ENECARBOXYLIC ACID–CONTAINING MUSHROOMS

There are several reports of *Tricholoma equestre* (*Tricholoma flavovirens*) ingestions in Poland and France, where although this mushroom is considered edible it has resulted in significant severe myotoxicity. In the first report, 12 patients who ingested *T. equestre* mushrooms for three consecutive days developed severe rhabdomyolysis. All patients developed fatigue, muscle weakness, and myalgias 24 to 72 hours following the last mushroom meal. The individuals also developed facial erythema, nausea without vomiting, and profuse sweating. Some patients had maximal creatine phosphokinase (CK) concentrations greater than 500,000 U/L. Electromyography and biopsies showed myofibrillar injury and edema consistent with an acute myopathy. Dyspnea, muscle weakness, acute myocarditis, dysrhythmias, congestive heart failure, and death ensued in three patients. Autopsy demonstrated myocardial lesions identical to those found in the peripheral muscles.

Similar clinical presentations are reported in China, Taiwan, and Japan associated with the ingestion of *Russula subnigricans*. Patients also manifest nausea, vomiting, diarrhea, malaise, fatigue, muscle weakness, dark urine, and oliguria. In these reports, rhabdomyolysis (CK in 100s–10,000s U/L) and oliguric kidney failure necessitating hemodialysis occurred in several patients with rare deaths. A toxin—cycloprop-2-ene carboxylic acid extracted from *R. subnigricans*—caused severe myotoxicity in mice, but a mechanism is not defined and there are other proposed myotoxins also recognized in this species.

## GENERAL MANAGEMENT ISSUES

Because ingestion of certain mushrooms may lead to toxicity with substantial morbidity or mortality, patients with suspected mushroom ingestions require a rigorous approach. Precise identification of the genus and species involved will make assessment, management, and follow-up easier and more logical. Unintentional ingestions in children in their yards are usually limited exposures to nontoxic mushrooms resulting in no symptoms necessitating solely reassurance by the certified specialist in Poison Information. For patients with intentional ingestions of potentially toxic mushrooms, it is recommended that activated charcoal be administered. If nausea and vomiting persist, an antiemetic is recommended to ensure that the patient can retain activated charcoal. Appropriate life support measures are recommended as necessary. Fluids, electrolytes, and dextrose repletion, as needed, are essential.

The clinical course for *A. smithiana* poisoning has led us to suggest an alteration in the initial approach to include patients in the northwest US who have early onset (0.5–5 hours) of GI distress following mushroom ingestion as potentially at risk, as *A. smithiana* has a significant association with kidney failure. Prior to the recognition of this mushroom poisoning, all patients who had early onset of nausea, vomiting, diarrhea, and abdominal cramps were presumed to be poisoned by a member of the groups containing either the GI toxins or muscarine. The more we learn, the more it is obvious that these clinical time courses as described in Table 90–2 are rough estimates and the clinician should recognize that the quality of our understanding of mushroom toxicology is improving, but speciation, time course, actual mycologic chemistry, and management are based on limited evidence.

## DISPOSITION

It is important to remember that many patients with mushroom ingestions present with mixed and incomplete signs and symptoms. Whereas some ingestions produce "purer" symptom complexes than others, some ingestions, such as those of *A. muscaria*, produce GI and CNS effects, and still other ingestions, such as those of *Cortinarius* spp, have acute GI and delayed kidney manifestations. Treatment or partial treatment may further confound the assessment. Because the clinical course of mushroom poisoning can be deceptive, all patients who manifest early GI symptoms (< 5 hours) and remain symptomatic for several hours despite supportive care (Tables 90–1 and 90–2) should be admitted to the hospital. Patients whose delayed initial presentation (≥ 5 hours) is suggestive of amatoxin exposure should be hospitalized, as should any patient postingestion who cannot be followed safely or reliably as an outpatient. All patients with symptoms following unknown ingestions require subsequent follow-up.

## IDENTIFICATION

Visualizing and analyzing the gross, microscopic, or chemical characteristics of the ingested mushroom remain vital strategies that are infrequently used. When the whole mushroom or parts are unavailable, the diagnosis must be based on the clinical presentation. Most often, no rapidly available studies in emergency departments or clinical chemistry laboratories are available to assist with identification. In Italy and Japan, real-time polymerase chain reaction (PCR) technology has been developed for multiple species for evaluations of cooked mushrooms and gastric aspirates. Future development of this technique may prove clinically useful.

Although mushroom identification is a difficult task, this section may be helpful to the clinician dealing with a suspected case of mushroom toxicity. However, it is generally best to rely on symptomats, not mushroom appearances, to confirm a diagnosis. As a general rule, positive identification of the mushroom should be left to the mycologist or toxicologist. The most important anatomic features of both edible and poisonous mushrooms are their pileus, stipe, lamellae or gills, and volva (Fig. 90–2).

- Pileus: Broad, caplike structure from which hang the gills (lamellae), tubes, or teeth.
- Stipe: Long stalk or stem that supports the cap; the stipe is not present in some species.
- Lamellae: Platelike or gilllike structures on the undersurface of the pileus that radiate out like the spokes of a wheel. The spores are found on the lamellae. Some mushrooms have pores or toothlike structures on their pili, which contain the spores. The mode of attachment of the lamellae to the stipe is noteworthy in making an identification.
- Volva: Partial remnant of the veil found around the base of the stipe in some species.
- Veil: Membrane that may completely or partially cover the lamellae, depending on the stage of development. The "universal" veil covers the underside, the spore-bearing surface of the pileus.
- Annulus: Ringlike structure that may surround the stipe at some point below the junction, with the cap that is a remnant of the partial veil.
- Spores: Microscopic reproductive structures that are resistant to extremes in temperature and dryness, produced in the millions on the spore-bearing surface (see Lamellae). Of all the characteristics of a particular mushroom species, spores are the least variable, although many mushrooms have similar-appearing spores. A spore print is helpful in establishing an identification. A spore print viewed microscopically is comparable to a bacterial Gram stain. Spore colors range from white to black and include shades of pink, salmon, buff, brown, and purple. Spore color in general is constant for a species.

## THE UNKNOWN MUSHROOM

1. The most important determinant is whether the ingested mushroom is one of the high-morbidity varieties, especially *Amanita* spp.
2. An attempt should be made to obtain either the collected mushrooms, a photograph, or a detailed description of their features. Arrange for transport of the mushroom in a dry paper bag (not plastic). Ensure that the mushroom is neither moistened nor refrigerated, either of which will alter its structure. Remember that gastric contents may contain spores that are very difficult to find but can be crucial for analysis.
3. If the mushroom cap is available, make a spore print by placing the pileus spore-bearing surface side down on a piece of paper for at least 4 to 6 hours in a windless area. The spores that collect on the paper can be analyzed for color. White spore prints can be visualized more easily on white paper by tilting the paper and looking at it from an angle.
4. Concomitant with step 3, contact a mycologist and use the best resources available for identification. A botanical garden usually has expert mycologists on staff, or a local mycology club can locate a mycologist. A regional poison control center almost always can provide this expertise or locate an expert.

# 91 PLANTS

Approximately 5% of all human exposures reported to poison centers involve plants. The large number of exposures probably occur because plants are so accessible and attractive to youngsters. Approximately 80% of these cases involve individuals younger than 6 years. More than 80% of patients reported to the American Association of Poison Control Centers (AAPCC) as being exposed were asymptomatic, less than 20% had minor to moderate symptomats, and less than 7% necessitated a healthcare visit. The benignity of these exposures in the United States (US), largely due to the unintentional nature of the event, is represented by a fatality rate of less than 0.001%. However, in other parts of the world, plant exposures, particularly those taken for self-harm and where healthcare is less accessible, carry a significant risk and public health burden. This chapter addresses the toxicologic principles associated with the most potentially dangerous plants.

## HISTORY AND CLASSIFICATION OF PLANT XENOBIOTICS

Aconitine, from monkshood, is believed by the Greeks to be the first poison—"lycoctonum"—created by the goddess Hecate from the foam of the mouth of Cerebrus. The science of pharmacognosy, which is the science of medicines derived from natural sources developed from a system of classification outlined here.

1. Alkaloids: Molecules that react as bases and contain nitrogen. Alkaloids typically have strong pharmacologic activity that defines many major toxidromes.
2. Glycosides: Organic compounds that yield a sugar or sugar derivative (the glycone) and a nonsugar moiety (the aglycone) upon hydrolysis.
3. Terpenes and resins: Assemblages of 5-carbon units (isoprene unit) with many types of functional groups (eg, alcohols, phenols, ketones, and esters) attached. This is the largest group of secondary metabolites, of which approximately 20,000 are identified.
4. Proteins, peptides, and lectins: Proteins consist of amino acid units with various side chains, and peptides consist of linkages among amino acids. Lectins are glycoproteins classified according to the number of protein chains linked by disulfide bonds and by binding affinity for specific carbohydrate ligands, particularly galactosamines.
5. Phenols and phenylpropanoids: Phenols contain phenyl rings and have one or more hydroxyl groups attached to the ring. Phenylpropanoids consist of a phenyl ring attached to a propane side chain.

Plant chemistry is complex. The simplified presentation of one xenobiotic per plant per symptom group used in Table 91–1 deemphasizes the fact that plants contain multiple xenobiotics that work independently or in concert. Our focus is on exposures to flowering plants (angiosperms) related to foraging, dietary, or occupational contact, except for some gymnosperms or algae and, rarely, medicinal contact (Chap. 16). Uncertainty is compounded by the fact that plants themselves are inherently variable, and potency and type of xenobiotic depend on the season, geography, growing environment, plant part, and methods of processing.

## IDENTIFICATION OF PLANTS

Positive identification of the plant species should be attempted whenever possible, especially when the patient becomes symptomatic. Communication with an expert botanist, medical toxicologist, or poison center is highly recommended and can be facilitated by transmission of digital images. Provisionally, simple comparison of the species in question with pictures or descriptions from a field guide of flora may help exclude the identity of the plant from among the most life-threatening.

## APPROACH TO THE EXPOSED PATIENT AND UNDERSTANDING RISK

Identified plant species most frequently reported to poison centers are indicated in Table 91–1. In most cases, these species provide reassurance because most exposures result in benign outcomes, and only a few among these are regularly life threatening depending on the circumstances of the exposure. The difficult task in human plant toxicology is the lack of adequate data to determine risk. Typically, evaluations of risk are based on poison center data and usually cite the numerous calls without clinical consequence as a part of the risk equation. Basic decontamination and supportive care should be instituted as appropriate for the clinical situation, with poison center consultation.

## TOXIC CONSTITUENTS IN PLANTS, TAXONOMIC ASSOCIATIONS, AND SELECTED SYMPTOMS

### Alkaloids

Alkaloids figure prominently in the history of human–plant interactions, ranging from epidemics of poisoning caused by ergot-infected rye bread in the Middle Ages to dependency on cocaine, heroin, and nicotine in contemporary time. Numerous examples of toxic constituents of these families are given in the following discussion, which begins with a description of the major toxidromes that involves alkaloids

***Anticholinergic: Belladonna Alkaloids*** (Fig. 91–1). The belladonna alkaloids are from the family Solanaceae and the plants are identified as members of this family by their characteristic flowers (most familiar from nightshade, potato, or tomato flowers). The belladonna alkaloids have potent antimuscarinic effects, manifested by tachycardia, hyperthermia, dry skin and mucous membranes, skin flushing, diminished bowel sounds, urinary retention, agitation, disorientation,

**TABLE 91–1 Primary Toxicity of Common Important Plant Species**

| *Plant Species (Family)* | *Typical Common Names* | *Primary Toxicity* | *Xenobiotic(s)* | *Class of Xenobiotic* |
|---|---|---|---|---|
| *Abrus precatorius* (Euphorbiaceae)[a] | Prayer beans, rosary pea, Indian bean, crab's eye, Buddhist's rosary bead, jequirity pea | Gastrointestinal | Abrin | Protein, lectin, peptide, amino acid |
| *Aconitum napellus* and other *Aconitum* spp (Ranunculaceae)[a] | Monkshood<br>Friar's cap<br>Wolfsbane | Cardiac, neurologic | Aconitine and related compounds | Alkaloid |
| *Acorus calamus* (Araliaceae) | Sweet flag, rat root, flag root, calamus | Gastrointestinal | Asarin | Phenol or phenylpropanoid |
| *Aesculus hippocastanum* (Hippocastanaceae) | Horse chestnut | Hematologic | Esculoside (6-β-D-glucopyranosyloxy-7-hydroxycoumarin) | Phenol or phenylpropanoid |
| *Agave lecheguilla* (Amaryllidaceae) | Agave | Dermatitis | Aglycones, smilagenin, sarsasapogenin | Saponin glycoside |
| *Aloe barbadensis, Aloe vera,* others (Liliaceae/Amaryllidaceae) | Aloagave | Gastrointestinal | Barbaloin, iso-barbaloin, aloinosides | Anthraquinone glycoside |
| *Anabaena and Aphanizomenon*[a] | Blue-green algae | Neurologic | Saxitoxinlike | Guanidinium |
| *Anacardium occidentale*, many others (Anacardiaceae) | Cashew, many others | Contact dermatitis | Urushiol oleoresins | Terpenoid |
| *Anthoxanthum odoratum* (Poaceae) | Sweet vernal grass | Hematologic | Coumarin | Phenol or phenylpropanoid |
| *Areca catechu* (Arecaceae) | Betel nut | Cholinergic | Arecoline | Alkaloid |
| *Argemone mexicana* (Papaveraceae) | Mexican pricklepoppy | Gastrointestinal | Sanguinarine | Alkaloid |
| *Argyreia nervosa* | Hawaiian baby woodrose seeds | Neurologic | Lysergic acid amide | Alkaloid |
| *Argyreia* spp (Convolvulaceae) | Morning glory | Neurologic | Lysergic acid derivatives | Alkaloid |
| *Aristolochia reticulata, Aristolochia* spp (Aristolochiaceae)[a] | Texan or Red River snake root | Renal, carcinogenic | Aristolochic acid | Alkaloid relative as derivative of isothebaine |
| *Artemisia absinthium* (Compositae/Asteraceae)[a] | Absinthe | Neurologic | Thujone | Terpenoid |
| *Asclepias* spp (Asclepiadaceae)[a] | Milk weed | Cardiac | Asclepin and related cardenolides | Cardioactive steroid |
| *Astragalus* spp (Fabaceae)[a] | Locoweed | Metabolic, neurologic | Swainsonine | Alkaloid |
| *Atractylis gummifera* (Compositae)[a] | Thistle | Hepatic | Atractyloside, gummiferine | Glycoside |
| *Atropa belladonna* (Solanaceae)[a] | Belladonna | Anticholinergic | Belladonna alkaloids | Alkaloid |
| *Azalea* spp (Ericaceae)[a,b] | Azalea | Cardiac, neurologic | Grayanotoxin | Terpenoid |
| *Berberis* spp (Ranunculaceae) | Barberry | Oxytocic, cardiovascular | Berberine | Alkaloid |
| *Blighia sapida* (Sapindaceae)[a] | Ackee fruit | Metabolic, gastrointestinal, neurotoxic | Hypoglycin | Protein, lectin, peptide, amino acid |
| *Borago officinalis* (Boraginaceae)[a] | Borage | Hepatic (venoocclusive disease) | Pyrrolizidine alkaloids | Alkaloid |
| *Brassaia* spp[b] | Umbrella tree | Dermatitis, mechanical and cytotoxic | Oxalate raphides | Carboxylic acid |
| *Brassica nigra* (Brassicaceae) | Black mustard | Dermatitis, irritant | Sinigrin | Glucosinolate (isothiocyanate glycoside) |
| *Brassica oleracea* var. capitata | Cabbage | Metabolic (precursor to goitrin, antithyroid compound) | Progoitrin | Isothiocyanate glycoside |
| *Cactus* spp[b] | Cactus | Dermatitis, mechanical | Nontoxic | None |
| *Caladium* spp (Araceae)[b] | Caladium | Dermatitis, mechanical and cytotoxic | Oxalate raphides | Carboxylic acid |
| *Calotropis* spp (Asclepiadaceae)[a] | Crown flower | Cardiac | Asclepin and related cardenolides | Cardioactive steroid |
| *Camellia sinensis* (Theaceae) | Tea, green tea | Cardiac, neurologic | Theophylline, caffeine | Alkaloid |

(*Continued*)

**TABLE 91–1 Primary Toxicity of Common Important Plant Species (*Continued*)**

| *Plant Species (Family)* | *Typical Common Names* | *Primary Toxicity* | *Xenobiotic(s)* | *Class of Xenobiotic* |
|---|---|---|---|---|
| *Cannabis sativa* | Cannabis, marijuana, Indian hemp, hashish, pot | Neurologic | Tetrahydrocannabinol | Terpenoid, resin, oleoresin |
| *Capsicum frutescens, Capsicum annuum, Capsicum* spp (Solanaceae)[b] | Capsicum, cayenne pepper | Dermatitis, irritant | Capsaicin | Phenol or phenylpropanoid |
| *Cascara sagrada, Rhamnus purshiana, Rhamnus cathartica* (Rhamnaceae) | Cascara, sacred bark, chittern bark, common buckthorn | Gastrointestinal | Cascarosides, *O*-glycosides, emodin | Anthraquinone glycoside |
| *Cassia senna, Cassia angustifolia* (Fabaceae) | Senna | Gastrointestinal | Sennosides | Anthraquinone glycoside |
| *Catha edulis* (Celastraceae) | Khat | Cardiac, neurologic | Cathinone | Alkaloid |
| *Catharanthus roseus* (formerly *Vinca rosea*) (Apocynaceae) | Catharanthus, vinca, madagascar periwinkle | Gastrointestinal | Vincristine | Alkaloid |
| *Caulophyllum thalictroides* (Berberidaceae) | Blue cohosh | Nicotinic | *N*-Methylcytisine and related compounds | Alkaloid |
| *Cephaelis ipecacuanha, Cephaelis acuminata* (Rubiaceae)[a] | Syrup of ipecac | Gastrointestinal, cardiac | Emetine/cephaline | Alkaloid |
| *Chlorophytum comosum*[b] | Spider plant | Dermatitis, contact and allergic | Urushiol oleoresins | Terpenoid |
| *Chondrodendron* spp, *Curarea* spp, *Strychnos* spp[a] | Tubocurare, curare | Neurologic | Tubocurarine | Alkaloid |
| *Chrysanthemum* spp, *Taraxacum officinale*, other Compositae (Asteraceae)[b] | Chrysanthemum, dandelion, other Compositaceae | Contact dermatitis | Sesquiterpene lactones | Terpenoid |
| *Cicuta maculata* (Apiaceae/Umbelliferae)[a] | Water hemlock | Neurologic | Cicutoxin | Alcohol |
| *Cinchona* spp (Rubiaceae)[a] | Cinchona | Cardiac, cinchonism | Quinidine | Alkaloid |
| *Citrus aurantium* (Rutaceae)[a] | Bitter orange | Cardiac, neurologic | Synephrine | Alkaloid |
| *Citrus paradisi* (Rutaceae) | Grapefruit | Drug interactions | Bergamottin, naringenin, or naringen | Phenol or phenylpropanoid |
| *Claviceps purpurea, Claviceps paspali* (Claviceptacea = fungus)[a] | Ergot | Cardiac, neurologic, oxytocic | Ergotamine and related compounds | Alkaloid |
| *Coffea arabica* (Rubiaceae) | Coffee | Cardiac, neurologic | Caffeine | Alkaloid |
| *Cola nitida, Cola* spp (Sterculiaceae) | Kola nut | Cardiac, neurologic | Caffeine | Alkaloid |
| *Colchicum autumnale* (Liliaceae)[a] | Autumn crocus | Multisystem | Colchicine | Alkaloid |
| *Conium maculatum* (Apiaceae/Umbelliferae)[a] | Poison hemlock | Nicotinic, neurologic, respiratory, renal | Coniine | Alkaloid |
| *Convallaria majalis*[a] | Lily of the valley | Cardiac | Convallatoxin, strophanthin (~40 others) | Cardioactive steroid |
| *Coptis* spp (Ranunculaceae) | Goldenthread | Oxytocic, cardiovascular | Berberine | Alkaloid |
| *Crassula* spp[b] | Jade plant | Gastrointestinal | Nontoxic | None |
| *Crotalaria* spp (Fabaceae)[a] | Rattlebox | Hepatic (venoocclusive disease) | Pyrrolizidine alkaloids | Alkaloid |
| *Croton tiglium* and *Croton* spp (Euphorbiaceae) | Croton | Carcinogen, gastrointestinal | Croton oil | Lipid and fixed oil, also contains tropane alkaloid and diterpene |
| *Cycas circinalis*[a] | Queen sago, indu, cycad | Neurologic | Cycasin | Glycosides |
| *Cytisus scoparius* (Fabaceae)[a] | Broom, Scotch broom | Nicotinic, oxytocic | Sparteine | Alkaloid |
| *Datura stramonium* (Solanaceae)[a] | Jimson weed, stramonium, locoweed | Anticholinergic | Belladonna alkaloids | Alkaloid |

(*Continued*)

**TABLE 91–1 Primary Toxicity of Common Important Plant Species (*Continued*)**

| *Plant Species (Family)* | *Typical Common Names* | *Primary Toxicity* | *Xenobiotic(s)* | *Class of Xenobiotic* |
|---|---|---|---|---|
| *Delphinium* spp (Ranunculaceae)[a] | Larkspur | Cardiac, neurologic | Methyllycaconitine | Alkaloid-related xenobiotic |
| *Dieffenbachia* spp (Araceae)[b] | Dieffenbachia | Dermatitis, mechanical and cytotoxic | Oxalate raphides | Carboxylic acid |
| *Digitalis lanata*[a] | Grecian foxglove | Cardiac | Digoxin, lanatosides A–E (contains ~70 cardiac glycosides) | Cardioactive steroid |
| *Digitalis purpurea*[a] | Purple foxglove | Cardiac | Digitoxin | Cardioactive steroid |
| *Dipteryx odorata, Dipteryx oppositifolia* (Fabaceae) | Tonka beans | Hematologic | Coumarin | Phenol or phenylpropanoid |
| *Ephedra* spp, especially *sinensis* (Ephedraceae/Gnetaceae = Gymnosperm)[a] | Ephedra, Ma-huang | Cardiac, neurologic | Ephedrine and related compounds | Alkaloid |
| *Epipremnum aureum* (Araceae)[b] | Pothos | Dermatitis, mechanical and cytotoxic | Oxalate raphides | Carboxylic acid |
| *Erythroxylum coca* | Coca | Neurologic, cardiac | Cocaine | Alkaloid |
| *Eucalyptus globus* or spp[b] | Eucalyptus | Dermatitis, contact and allergic | Eucalyptol | Terpenoid |
| *Euphorbia pulcherrima, Euphorbia* spp (Eurphorbiaceae)[b] | Poinsettia | Dermatitis, contact and allergic | Phorbol esters | Terpenoid |
| *Galium triflorum* (Rubiaceae) | Sweet-scented bedstraw | Hematologic | Coumarin | Phenol or phenylpropanoid |
| *Ginkgo biloba* (Ginkgoaceae) | Ginkgo | Dermatitis, contact and allergic<br>Hematologic<br>Neurologic | Urushiol oleoresins<br>Ginkgolides A–C, M<br>4-Methoxypyridoxine in seeds only | Terpenoid<br>Terpenoid<br>Alkaloid, pyridine |
| *Gloriosa superba* (Liliaceae)[a] | Meadow saffron | Multisystem | Colchicine | Alkaloid |
| *Glycyrrhiza glabra*[a] | Licorice | Metabolic, renal | Glycyrrhizin | Saponin glycoside |
| *Gossypium* spp | Cotton, cottonseed oil | Metabolic | Gossypol | Terpenoid |
| *Hedeoma pulegioides* (Lamiaceae)[a] | Pennyroyal | Hepatic, neurologic, oxytoxic | Pulegone | Terpenoid |
| *Hedera helix* (Araliaceae)[b] | Common ivy | Not absorbed | Hederacoside C, α-hederin, hederagenin | Cardioactive steroid |
| *Hedysarium alpinum* (Fabaceae) | Wild potato | Metabolic, neurologic | Swainsonine | Alkaloid |
| *Heliotropium* spp (Compositae/Asteraceae)[a] | Ragwort | Hepatic (venoocclusive disease) | Pyrrolizidine alkaloids | Alkaloid |
| *Helleborus niger*[a] | Black hellebore, Christmas rose | Cardiac | Hellebrin | Cardioactive steroid |
| *Hydrastis canadensis* (Ranunculaceae)[a] | Goldenseal | Neurologic, oxytocic, cardiovascular, respiratory | Hydrastine, berberine | Alkaloid |
| *Hyoscyamus niger* (Solanaceae)[a] | Henbane, hyoscyamus | Anticholinergic | Belladonna alkaloids | Alkaloid |
| *Hypericum perforatum* (Clusiaceae) | St John's wort | Dermatitis, photosensitivity, neurologic, xenobiotic interactions | Hyperforin, hypericin | Terpenoid |
| *Ilex paraguariensis* (Aquifoliaceae) | Maté, Yerba Maté, Paraguay tea | Cardiac, neurologic | Caffeine | Alkaloid |
| *Ilex* spp berries (Aquifoliaceae)[b] | Holly | Gastrointestinal | Mixture. Alkaloids, polyphenols, saponins, steroids, triterpenoids | Unidentified |
| *Illicium anisatum* (Illiciaceae)[a] | Japanese Star anise | Neurologic | Anasatin | Terpenoid |
| *Ipomoea tricolor* and other *Ipomoea* spp (Convolvulaceae) | Morning glory | Neurologic | Lysergic acid derivatives | Alkaloid |
| *Jatropha curcas* (Euphorbiaceae) | Black vomit nut, physic nut, purging nut | Gastrointestinal | Curcin | Protein, lectin, peptide, amino acid |
| *Karwinskia humboldtiana*[a] | Buckthorn, wild cherry, tullidora, coyotillo, capulincillo, others | Neurologic, respiratory | Toxin T-514 | Phenol or phenylpropanoid |

(*Continued*)

TABLE 91–1 Primary Toxicity of Common Important Plant Species (*Continued*)

| *Plant Species (Family)* | *Typical Common Names* | *Primary Toxicity* | *Xenobiotic(s)* | *Class of Xenobiotic* |
|---|---|---|---|---|
| *Laburnum anagyroides* (syn. *Cytisus laburnum*; Fabaceae)[a] | Golden chain, laburnum | Nicotinic | Cytisine | Alkaloid |
| *Lantana camara* (Verbenaceae) | Lantana | Dermatitis, photosensitivity | Lantadene A and B, phylloerythrin | Terpenoid |
| *Lathyrus sativus*[a] | Grass pea | Neurologic, skeletal | β-*N*-Oxalylamino-L-alanine (BOAA); β-aminopropionitrile (BAPN) | Protein, lectin, peptide, amino acid |
| *Lobelia inflata* (Campanulaceae) | Indian tobacco | Nicotinic | Lobeline | Alkaloid |
| *Lophophora williamsii* | Peyote or mescal buttons | Neurologic | Mescaline | Alkaloid |
| *Lupinus latifolius* and other *Lupinus* spp (Fabaceae) | Lupine | Nicotinic | Anagyrine | Alkaloid |
| *Lycopersicon* spp (Solanaceae)[a] | Tomato (green) | Gastrointestinal, neurologic, anticholinergic | Tomatine, tomatidine | Glycoalkaloid |
| *Mahonia* spp (Ranunculaceae) | Oregon grape | Oxytocic, cardiovascular | Berberine | Alkaloid |
| *Mandragora officinarum* (Solanaceae)[a] | European or true mandrake | Anticholinergic | Belladonna alkaloids | Alkaloid |
| *Manihot esculentus* (Euphorbiaceae)[a] | Cassava, manihot, tapioca | Metabolic, neurotoxic, spastic paresis, and visual disturbances | Linamarin | Cyanogenic glycoside |
| *Melilotus* spp (Fabaceae/Legumaceae) | Sweet clover (spoiled moldy) | Hematologic | Dicumarol | Phenol or phenylpropanoid |
| *Mentha pulegium* (Lamiaceae)[a] | Pennyroyal | Hepatic, neurologic, oxytocic | Pulegone | Terpenoid |
| *Microcystis* and *Anabaena* spp | Blue-green algae (cyanobacteria) | Hepatotoxic, dermatitis, photosensitivity | Microcystin | Protein, lectin, peptide, amino acid |
| *Myristica fragrans* | Nutmeg, pericarp = mace | Neurologic (hallucinations) | Myristicin, elemicin | Terpenoid |
| *Narcissus* spp and other (Amaryllidaceae, Liliaceae) | Narcissus | Dermatitis, mechanical and cytotoxic | Lycorine, homolycorin | Alkaloid |
| *Nerium oleander*[a] | Oleander | Cardiac | Oleandrin | Cardioactive steroid |
| *Nicotiana tabacum, Nicotiana* spp (Solanaceae)[a] | Tobacco | Nicotinic | Nicotine | Alkaloid |
| *Oxytropis* spp (Fabaceae) | Locoweed | Metabolic, neurologic | Swainsonine | Alkaloid |
| *Papaver somniferum* | Poppy | Neurologic | Morphine/other opium derivatives | Alkaloid |
| *Paullinia cupana* (Sapindaceae) | Guarana | Cardiac, neurologic | Caffeine | Alkaloid |
| *Pausinystalia yohimbe* (Rubiaceae)[a] | Yohimbe | Cardiac, cholinergic | Yohimbine | Alkaloid |
| *Philodendron* spp (Araceae)[b] | Philodendron | Dermatitis, mechanical and cytotoxic | Oxalate raphides | Carboxylic acid |
| *Phoradendron* spp (Loranthaceae or Viscaceae) | American mistletoe | Gastrointestinal | Phoratoxin, ligatoxin | Protein, lectin, peptide, amino acid |
| *Physostigma venenosum* (Fabaceae)[a] | Calabar bean, ordeal bean | Cholinergic | Physostigmine | Alkaloid |
| *Phytolacca americana* (Phytolaccaceae)[a] | Pokeweed, poke | Gastrointestinal | Phytolaccotoxin | Protein, lectin, peptide, amino acid |
| *Pilocarpus jaborandi, Pilocarpus pinnatifolius* (Rutaceae)[a] | Pilocarpus, jaborandi | Cholinergic effects | Pilocarpine | Alkaloid |
| *Piper methysticum*[a] | Kava kava | Hepatic, neurologic | Kawain, methysticine, yangonin, other kava lactones | Terpenoid, resin, oleoresin |
| *Plantago* spp | Plantago (seed husks) | Gastrointestinal | Psyllium | Carbohydrate |
| *Podophyllum emodi* (Berberidaceae)[a] | Wild mandrake | Gastrointestinal and neurologic effects | Podophyllin (lignan) | Phenol or phenylpropanoid |

(*Continued*)

**TABLE 91–1 Primary Toxicity of Common Important Plant Species (*Continued*)**

| *Plant Species (Family)* | *Typical Common Names* | *Primary Toxicity* | *Xenobiotic(s)* | *Class of Xenobiotic* |
|---|---|---|---|---|
| *Podophyllum peltatum* (Berberidaceae)[a] | Mayapple | Gastrointestinal and neurologic effects | Podophyllin (lignan) | Phenol or phenylpropanoid |
| *Populus* spp (Salicaceae) | Poplar species | Salicylism | Salicin | Glycoside |
| *Primula obconica* (Primulaceae) | Primrose | Dermatitis, contact and allergic | Primin | Phenol or phenylpropanoid |
| *Prunus armeniaca, Prunus* spp, *Malus* spp (Rosaceae)[a] | Apricot seed pits, wild cherry, peach, plum, pear, almond, apple, and other seed kernels | Metabolic acidosis, respiratory failure, coma, death | Amygdalin, emulsin | Cyanogenic glycoside |
| *Pteridium* spp (Polypodiaceae) | Bracken fern | Carcinogen, thiaminase | Ptaquiloside | Terpenoid |
| *Pulsatilla* spp (Ranunculaceae) | Pulsatilla | Dermatitis, contact | Ranunculin, protoanemonin | Glycoside |
| *Quercus* spp | Oak | Metabolic, livestock toxicity | Tannic acid | Phenol or phenylpropanoid |
| *Ranunculus* spp (Ranunculaceae) | Buttercups | Dermatitis, contact | Ranunculin, protoanemonin | Glycoside |
| *Rauwolfia serpentine* (Apocynaceae) | Indian snakeroot | Cardiac, neurologic | Reserpine | Alkaloid |
| *Remijia pedunculata* (Rubiaceae)[a] | Cuprea bark | Cardiac, cinchonism | Quinidine | Alkaloid |
| *Rhamnus frangula* (Rhamnaceae) | Frangula bark, alder buckthorn | Gastrointestinal | Frangulins | Anthraquinone glycoside |
| *Rheum officinale, Rheum* spp (Polygonaceae) | Rhubarb | Gastrointestinal<br>Metabolic | Rhein anthrones<br>Oxalic acid (soluble) | Anthraquinone glycoside<br>Carboxylic acid |
| *Rheum* spp (Polygonaceae) | Rhubarb species | Urologic | Oxalates | Carboxylic acid |
| *Rhododendron* spp (Ericaceae)[a] | Rhododendron | Cardiac, neurologic | Grayanotoxins | Terpenoid including resin and oleoresin |
| *Ricinus communis* (Euphorbiaceae)[a] | Castor or rosary seeds, purging nuts, physic nut, tick seeds | Gastrointestinal | Ricin, curcin | Protein, lectin, peptide, amino acid |
| *Robinia pseudoacacia* (Fabaceae)[a] | Black locust | Gastrointestinal | Robin (robinia lectin) | Protein, lectin, peptide, amino acid |
| *Rumex* spp (Polygonaceae) | Dock species | Urologic | Oxalates | Carboxylic acid |
| *Salix* spp (Salicaceae) | Willow species | Salicylism | Salicin | Glycosides, other |
| *Sambucus* spp (Caprifoliaceae) | Elderberry | Metabolic | Anthracyanins | Cyanogenic glycoside |
| *Sanguinaria canadensis* (Papaveraceae) | Sanguinaria, bloodroot | Gastrointestinal | Sanguinarine | Alkaloid |
| *Schefflera* spp (Araceae)[b] | Umbrella tree | Dermatitis, mechanical and cytotoxic | Oxalate raphides | Carboxylic acid |
| *Schlumbergera bridgesii*[b] | Christmas cactus | Dermatitis, mechanical | Nontoxic | None |
| *Senecio* spp (Compositae/Asteraceae)[a] | Groundsel | Hepatic (venoocclusive disease) | Pyrrolizidine alkaloids | Alkaloid |
| *Sida carpinifolia* (Malvaceae) | Locoweed | Metabolic, neurologic | Swainsonine | Alkaloid |
| *Sida cordifolia* (Malvaceae)[a] | Bala | Cardiac, neurologic | Ephedrine and related compounds | Alkaloid |
| *Solanum americanum* (Solanaceae)[a] | American nightshade | Gastrointestinal, neurologic, anticholinergic | Solasodine, soladulcidine, solanine, chaconine | Glycoalkaloid |
| *Solanum dulcamara* (Solanaceae)[a,b] | Bittersweet woody nightshade | Gastrointestinal, neurologic, anticholinergic | Solanine, chaconine, belladonna alkaloids | Alkaloid |
| *Solanum nigrum* (Solanaceae)[a] | Black nightshade, common nightshade | Gastrointestinal, neurologic, anticholinergic | Solanine, chaconine, belladonna alkaloids | Alkaloid |
| *Solanum tuberosum* (Solanaceae)[a] | Potato (green), leaves | Gastrointestinal, neurologic, anticholinergic | Solanine, chaconine | Alkaloid |
| *Spathiphyllum* spp (Araceae)[b] | Peace lily | Dermatitis, mechanical and cytotoxic | Oxalate raphides | Carboxylic acid |
| *Spinacia oleracea* (Chenopodiaceae) | Spinach, others | Urologic | Oxalates | Carboxylic acid |

(*Continued*)

**TABLE 91–1 Primary Toxicity of Common Important Plant Species (*Continued*)**

| *Plant Species (Family)* | *Typical Common Names* | *Primary Toxicity* | *Xenobiotic(s)* | *Class of Xenobiotic* |
|---|---|---|---|---|
| *Strychnos nux-vomica, Strychnos ignatia* (Loganiaceae)[a] | Nux vomica, Ignatia, St Ignatius bean, vomit button | Neurologic | Strychnine, brucine | Alkaloid |
| *Swainsonia* spp (Fabaceae) | Locoweed | Metabolic, neurologic | Swainsonine | Alkaloid |
| *Symphytum* spp (Boraginaceae)[a] | Comfrey | Hepatic (venoocclusive disease) | Pyrrolizidine alkaloids | Alkaloid |
| *Tanacetum vulgare* (= *Chrysanthemum vulgare*; Compositae/Asteraceae)[a] | Tansy | Neurologic | Thujone | Terpenoid |
| *Taxus baccata, Taxus brevifolia*, other *Taxus* spp (Taxaceae)[a] | English yew, Pacific yew | Cardiac | Taxine | Alkaloid |
| *Theobroma cacao* (Sterculiaceae) | Cocoa | Cardiac, neurologic | Theobromine | Alkaloid |
| *Thevetia peruviana*[a] | Yellow oleander | Cardiac | Thevetin | Cardioactive steroid |
| *Toxicodendron radicans, Toxicodendron toxicarium, Toxicodendron diversilobum, Toxicodendron vernix, Toxicodendron* spp, many others (Anacardaceae)[b] | Poison ivy, poison oak, poison sumac | Dermatitis, contact and allergic | Urushiol oleoresins | Terpenoid |
| *Tribulus terrestris* (Fabaceae) | Caltrop, puncture vine | Dermatitis, photosensitivity in animals | Steroidal saponins (aglycones, diosgenin, yamogenin) | Saponin glycoside |
| *Trifolium pratense* and other (Fabaceae/Legumaceae) | Red clover | Phytoestrogen, hematologic | Formononetin, Biochanin A, coumarin | Phenol (isoflavone) |
| *Tussilago farfara* (Compositae/Asteraceae)[a] | Coltsfoot | Hepatic (venoocclusive disease) | Pyrrolizidine alkaloids | Alkaloid |
| *Urginea maritima, Urginea indica*[a] | Red, or Mediterranean squill, Indian squill, sea onion | Cardiac | Scillaren A, B | Cardioactive steroid |
| *Veratrum viride, Veratrum album, Veratrum californicum* (Liliaceae)[a] | False hellebore, Indian poke, California hellebore | Cardiac | Veratridine | Alkaloid |
| *Vicia fava, Vicia sativa* (Fabaceae) | Fava bean, vetch | Hematologic | Vicine, convicine | Glycoside |
| *Viscum album* (Loranthaceae or Viscaceae) | European mistletoe | Gastrointestinal | Viscumin | Protein, lectin, peptide, amino acid, lignan, polypeptide |
| *Wisteria floribunda* (Fabaceae) | Wisteria | Gastrointestinal | Cystatin | Protein, lectin, peptide, amino acid |

[a]Reports of life-threatening effects from plant use. [b]Plants reported commonly among calls to poison centers.

and hallucinations (Chap. 1). The onset of symptoms typically occurs 1 to 4 hours postingestion, and more rapidly if the plants are smoked or consumed as a brewed tea. When used appropriately, physostigmine limits the duration of delirium and prevents unnessary medical testing (Antidotes in Brief: A11).

***Nicotine and Nicotinelike Alkaloids: Nicotine, Anabasine, Lobeline, Sparteine, N-Methylcytisine, Cytisine, and Coniine.*** Nicotine toxicity (other than from inhaled sources) occurs via ingestion of leaves of *Nicotiana tabacum*, cigarettes and their remains, e-cigarette refill, organic insecticidal products, and transdermally among farm workers harvesting tobacco (green tobacco sickness) (Chap. 55). A dose of nicotine as small as 1 mg/kg of body weight can be lethal, although it is more likely with doses greater than 4 mg/kg. Overstimulation of the nicotinic receptors by high doses of the alkaloid produces nicotinism, a toxidrome that progresses from gastrointestinal (GI) symptoms to diaphoresis, mydriasis, fasciculations, tachycardia, hypertension, hyperthermia, seizures, respiratory depression, and death (Chap. 55).

These manifestations are also produced by alkaloids other than nicotine such as lobeline (found in all parts of *Lobelia inflata*), sparteine from broom (*Cytisus scoparius*) and *N*-methylcytisine from blue cohosh (*Caulophyllum thalictroides*), and cytisine from laburnum or golden chain (*Cytisus laburnum*).

The most famous description of the end stages of nicotinic toxicity dates from approximately 2,400 years ago by an observer of Socrates' fatal ingestion of a decoction of poison hemlock (*Conium maculatum*).

> *the person who had administered the poison went up to him and examined for some little time his feet and legs, and then squeezing his foot strongly asked whether he felt him. Socrates replied that he did not and said to us when the effect of the poison reached his heart, Socrates would depart.*

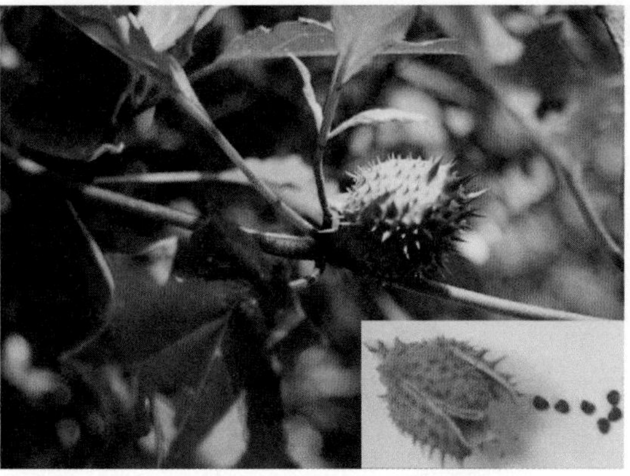

**FIGURE 91–1.** Jimsonweed (*Datura stramonium*) initially has a showy white tubular flower that becomes a prickly fruit (pod) following maturation. Inset: The pod (inset) of jimsonweed holds multiple small seeds containing atropine and scopolamine. *(Used with permission from the Fellowship in Medical Toxicology, New York University Grossman School of Medicine, New York City Poison Center.)*

Birds do not experience coniine toxicity but provide a vector for poisoning. This is especially well documented in Italy, where the toxic alkaloid coniine was detected in bird meat, as well as in the blood, urine, and tissue of some poisoned individuals. Of 17 poisoned Italian patients, all had elevated hepatic aminotransferases and myoglobin concentrations, and five had acute tubular necrosis. Death developed 1 to 16 days following ingestion.

***Cholinergic Alkaloids: Arecoline, Physostigmine, and Pilocarpine.*** Betel chewing has been a habitual practice in the tropical Pacific, Asia, and East Africa. The "quid" consists of betel nut (*Areca catechu*) and other ingredients. The effects of acute exposure to arecoline, the major alkaloid, include sweating, salivation, hyperthermia, and rarely death. Physostigmine is an alkaloid derived from the Calabar bean (*Physostigma venenosum*), where it is present in concentrations of 0.15% (Antidotes in Brief: A11). Pilocarpine is derived from *Pilocarpus jaborandi* from South America. Reversal of toxicity can be achieved by atropine.

***Psychotropic Alkaloids: Lysergic Acid and Mescaline.*** Hallucinations from the direct serotonin effects of lysergic acid diethylamide (LSD) and its derivatives and from the amphetaminelike serotoninergic effects of the mescaline alkaloids are reported following ingestion of morning glory seeds (*Ipomoea* spp) and peyote cactus (*Lophophora williamsii*), respectively (Chap. 52).

***Alkaloidal Central Nervous System Stimulants and Depressants: Ephedrine, Synephrine, Cathinone, and Opioids.*** The use of ephedrine-containing *Ephedra* spp in herbal dietary supplement products was banned by the US Food and Drug Administration (FDA) in 2004 because of the associated cardiovascular toxicity and deaths. Synephrine, a xenobiotic structurally related to ephedrine, occurs in bitter orange (*Citrus aurantium*), which is ingested as a plant, in foods such as marmalades, as a dietary supplement, or as a traditional medicine. Although illegal in the US, another plant ingested for its CNS-stimulant activity is khat (*Catha edulis*). The plant contains cathinone (α-aminopropiophenone) and cathine ((+)-norpseudoephedrine). In addition, opioids derived from the poppy plant (*Papaver* spp) are prototypic CNS depressants and analgesics (Chap. 9).

***Pyrrolizidine Alkaloids.*** Approximately half of the 350 different pyrrolizidine alkaloids characterized to date are toxic when ingested. Chronic exposures stimulate the proliferation of the intima of hepatic vasculature and result in hepatic venoocclusive disease (HVOD). Acute hepatocellular toxicity can occur following ingestion of 10 to 20 mg of pyrrolizidine alkaloid and is probably caused by an oxidant effect producing hepatic necrosis. An estimated 20% of patients with acute pyrrolizidine alkaloid poisoning die, 50% recover completely, and the rest develop subacute or chronic manifestations of HVOD.

***Isoquinoline Alkaloids: Sanguinarine, Berberine, and Hydrastine.*** Adverse effects on human health due to consumption of edible mustard oil adulterated with argemone oil are reported. Sanguinarine was detected in 26 family members who consumed a mustard oil contaminated with seeds of Mexican pricklypoppy (*Argemone mexicana*). All patients suffered GI distress followed by peripheral edema, skin darkening, erythema, skin lesions, perianal itching, anemia, and hepatomegaly. Ascites developed in 12%, and myocarditis and congestive heart failure occurred in approximately a third of affected individuals. Berberine is structurally similar to sanguinarine and also has cardiac depressant effects.

***Other Alkaloids: Emetine/Cephaline, Strychnine/Curare, and Swainsonine.*** Emetine and cephaline are derived from *Cephaelis ipecacuanha*. They are the principal active constituents in syrup of ipecac, which produces emesis. Chronic use of syrup of ipecac, typically by patients with eating disorders or medical child abuse, causes cardiomyopathy, smooth muscle dysfunction, myopathies, electrolyte and acid–base disturbances related to excessive vomiting, and death. Poisoning in patients ingesting plant material is not reported. The convulsant alkaloids strychnine and brucine are found in various members of the genus *Strychnos* (Chap. 87).

Curare is an extract of the bark of *Chondrodendron tomentosum* and certain members of the genus *Strychnos*. The physiologically active xenobiotic is D-tubocurarine chloride, a competitive antagonist of acetylcholine at nicotinic receptors in the neuromuscular junction. Curare is the molecule from which most nondepolarizing neuromuscular blockers are derived (Chap. 39).

Swainsonine is isolated from *Swainsonia canescens*, *Astragalus lentiginosis* (spotted locoweed), as well as several species in the genera *Oxytropis* and *Ipomoea*, and several fungi. After subsisting on seeds containing swainsonine for nearly 4 months, a naturalist forager manifested profound muscular weakness and died in the wilderness. Swainsonine inhibits the glycosylation of glycoproteins by α-mannosidase II of the Golgi apparatus, resulting in a lysosomal storage disease. Adverse effects include hepatic, pancreatic, and respiratory manifestations, as well as lethargy and nausea.

## Glycosides

***Saponin Glycosides: Cardiac Glycosides, Glycyrrhizin, Ilex Saponins*** (Fig. 91–2). Poisoning by virtually all cardioactive steroidal glycosides is clinically indistinguishable from poisoning by

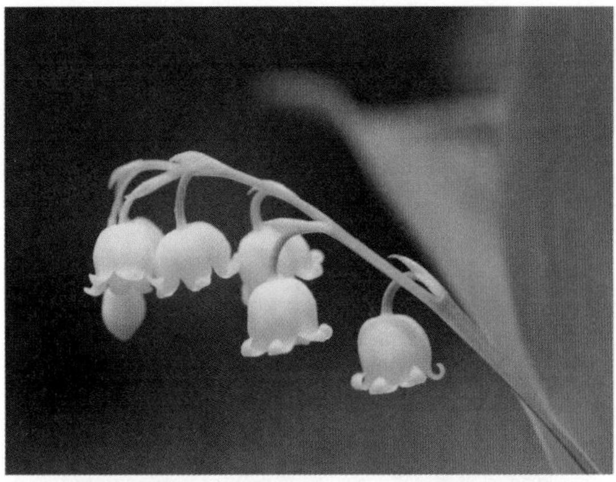

A

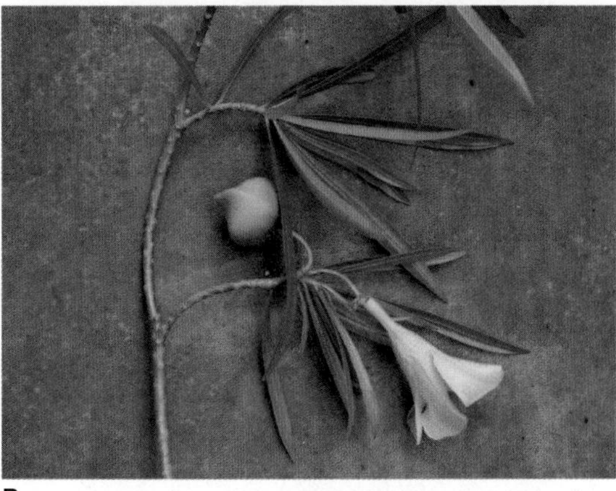

B

**FIGURE 91–2.** Saponin-glycoside containing plants: (**A**) Lily of the valley (*Convallaria majalis*) contains the cardioactive steroid convallatoxin. (*Used with permission from Imagemore/SuperStock.*) (**B**) Yellow oleander (*Thevetia peruviana*) contains a cardioactive steroid, thevetin. (*Used with permission from Darren Roberts, MD.*)

digoxin (Chap. 35), which itself is a cardioactive steroid derived from *Digitalis lanata*. However, compared with toxicity from pharmaceutical digoxin, toxicity resulting from the cardioactive steroidal glycosides found in plants has markedly different pharmacokinetic characteristics. For example, digitoxin in *Digitalis* spp has a plasma half-life as long as 192 hours (average 168 hours). Poisonings by oleander and yellow oleander occur predominantly in the Mediterranean and in the Near and Far East. These two plants are popular attractive ornamentals and commonly result in poisoning in the US and Europe.

Activated charcoal was beneficial in preventing death after suicide attempts with yellow oleander in Sri Lanka and its use should not be delayed in the face of uncertain plant identity. In addition, various cardioactive steroids respond differently to therapeutic use of digoxin-specific antibody fragments. Use of very large doses of digoxin-specific antibody may be necessary to capitalize on the therapeutic cross-reactivity between digoxin-specific antibody and the nondigoxin cardioactive steroids, such as oleander (Antidotes in Brief: A22).

***Glycyrrhizin.*** Glycyrrhizin is a saponin glycoside derived from *Glycyrrhiza glabra* (licorice) and other *Glycyrrhiza* spp. Glycyrrhizin inhibits 11-β-hydroxysteroid dehydrogenase, an enzyme that converts cortisol to cortisone. When large amounts of licorice root are consumed chronically, cortisol concentrations rise, resulting in pseudo-hyperaldosteronism because of its affinity for renal mineralocorticoid receptors. Chronic use eventually leads to hypokalemia with muscle weakness, sodium and water retention, hypertension, and dysrhythmias.

***Ilex Species.*** Holly berries from more than 300 *Ilex* spp are commonly ingested by children, especially during winter holidays. The saponin glycosides appear to be responsible for GI symptoms such as nausea, vomiting, diarrhea, and abdominal cramping that result from ingestion of the berries.

***Cyanogenic Glycosides: (S)-Sambunigrin, Amygdalin, Linamarin, and Cycasin.*** Cyanogenic glycosides yield hydrogen cyanide on complete hydrolysis. The species that are most important to humans are cassava (*Manihot esculenta*), which contains linamarin, and *Prunus* spp, which contain amygdalin. The fleshy fruit of *Prunus* spp in the Rosaceae are nontoxic (apricots, peaches, pears, apples, and plums), but the leaves, bark, and seed kernels contain amygdalin, which is metabolized to cyanide. Amygdalin was the active ingredient of Laetrile, an apricot pit extract promoted in the 1970s for its supposed selective toxicity to tumor cells. Its sale was restricted in the US because it lacked efficacy and safety. However, patients went to other countries for Laetrile therapy, which was marketed as "vitamin B-17," and available through alternative medicine providers. The manifestations of cyanide poisoning and treatment involving use of hydroxocobalamin and the cyanide antidote kit are detailed elsewhere (Chap. 96 and Antidotes in Brief: A41 and A42).

Chronic manifestations include visual disturbances (amblyopia), upper motor neuron disease with spastic paraparesis, and hypothyroidism. These findings are associated with thiocyanate accumulation, which may lead to degeneration of the α-amino-3-hydroxy-5-methyl-isoxazole-4-propionic acid (AMPA)–containing neurons that are first stimulated and then destroyed in neurolathyrism. Similarly, seeds of cycads contain cycasin and neocycasin, which belong to the family of cyanogenic glycosides, as well as neurotoxins. On the island of Guam, indigenous peoples develop a devastating amyotrophic lateral sclerosis–parkinsonism dementia complex (ALS-PDC) that appears associated with ingestion of *Cycas circinalis* seeds or the flying foxes that feed extensively upon the cycads.

***Anthraquinone Glycosides: Sennoside and Others.*** Anthraquinone laxatives are regulated both as nonprescription pharmaceuticals and as dietary supplements. These glycosides stimulate colonic motility, probably by inhibiting $Na^+,K^+$-adenosine triphosphatase (ATPase) in the intestine, which promotes accumulation of water and electrolytes in the gut lumen.

***Other Glycosides: Salicin, Atractyloside, Carboxyatractyloside, Vicine, and Convicine.*** Salicin is an inactive glycoside until it is hydrolyzed to produce salicylic acid (Chap. 10). *Atractylis gummifera* was a favorite agent for homicide during the reign of the Borgias. Atractyloside, the toxic xenobiotic, primarily inhibits oxidative phosphorylation in the liver by inhibiting the ADP/ATP antiporter blocking influx of adenosine diphosphate (ADP) into hepatic mitochondria and outflow of ATP to the rest of the cell. Death or severe illness as a result of liver failure or hepatorenal disease following ingestion is reported.

Favism is a potentially fatal disorder brought about by eating fava beans or vetch seeds (*Vicia faba, Vicia sativa*, respectively). These seeds contain the pyrimidine glycosides vicine and convicine (divicine is the aglycone of vicine). Consumption of these compounds by individuals with an inborn error of metabolism (glucose-6-phosphate dehydrogenase deficiency) can cause acute hemolytic crisis.

### Terpenoids and Resins: Ginkgolides, Kava Lactones, Thujone, Anisatin, Ptaquiloside/Thiaminase, and Gossypol

Ginkgolides in *Ginkgo biloba* result in antiplatelet aggregation effects. Reports of spontaneous bleeding are associated with ingestion of Ginkgo leaf products. Another xenobiotic found only in the seed, 4-methoxypyridoxine (pyridine alkaloid), is associated with seizures. A mechanism similar to isoniazid-induced seizures is plausible, suggesting treatment with pyridoxine phosphate (Chap. 29 and Antidotes in Brief: A15).

Kava lactones are found in kava (*Piper methysticum*) and cause central and peripheral nervous system effects. Proposed mechanisms include effects at γ-aminobutyric acid type A ($GABA_A$) and $GABA_B$ receptors or local anesthetic effects. Acute effects following ingestion include peripheral numbness, weakness, and sedation. More than 70 cases of hepatotoxicity, several requiring liver transplantation, are associated with both acute and chronic effects of kava extracts on cytochrome oxygenases or other yet-to-be-defined etiologies.

Thujone is one of many terpenes associated with seizures. It is found in the wormwood plant (*Artemisia absinthium*), in absinthe (the liquor flavored with *A. absinthium*), and in some strains of tansy (*Tanacetum vulgare*). The α- and β-isomers of thujone likely work similarly to camphor to produce CNS depression and seizures. Absinthism is characterized by seizures and hallucinations, permanent cognitive impairment, and personality changes. Acute and chronic absinthism led to a worldwide ban of the alcoholic beverage absinthe, which contained thujone, in the early 1900s. Symptoms were more likely related to the alcohol use.

Anisatin is found in *Illicium* spp. This terpenoid produces seizures as a noncompetitive GABA antagonist. The Chinese star anise (*Illicium verum*) is sometimes used in teas and occasionally is confused or contaminated with other species of *Illicium*, particularly Japanese star anise *Illicium anisatum*. These contaminations caused small epidemics of tonic–clonic seizures, particularly, but not exclusively, in infants after use of the tea to treat their infantile colic. At least 40 individuals who consumed teas brewed from "star anise" experienced seizures, motor disturbances, other neurologic effects, and vomiting. These cases include at least 15 infants treated for infantile colic with this home remedy. This trend prompted the US FDA to issue an advisory regarding the health risk from remedies sharing the common name "star anise."

### Proteins, Peptides, and Lectins: Ricin and Ricinlike, Pokeweed, Mistletoe, Hypoglycin, Lathyrins, and Microcystins (Fig. 91–3)

Toxalbumins such as ricin and abrin are lectins that are such potent cytotoxins that they are used as biologic weapons. Ricin, extracted from the castor bean (*Ricinus communis*), exerts its cytotoxicity by inhibiting the 60S ribosome. In addition to the GI manifestations of vomiting, diarrhea, and

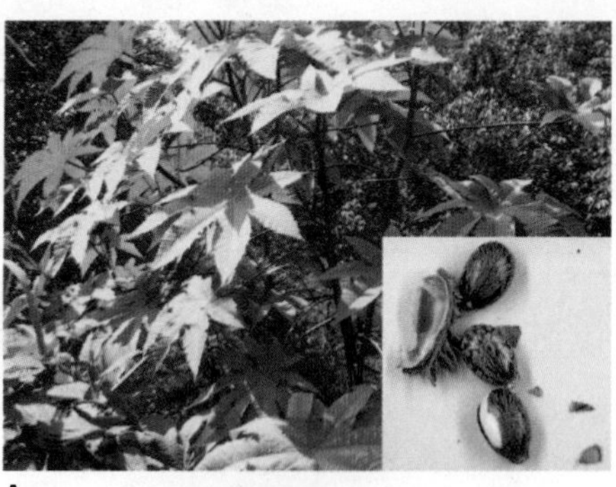

A

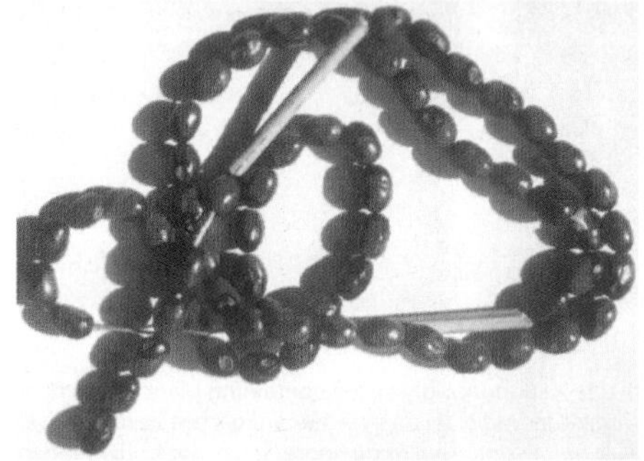

B

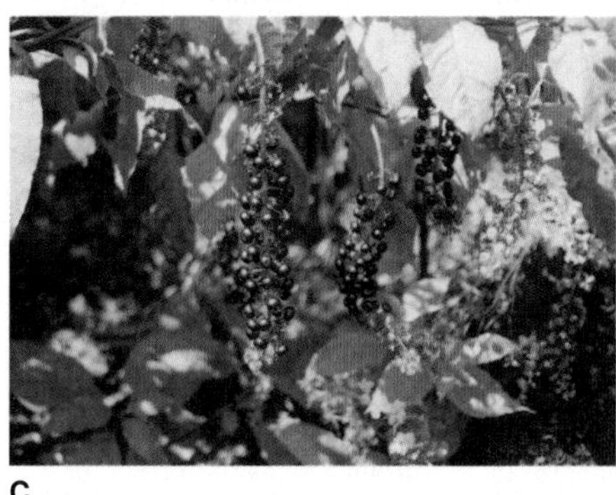

C

**FIGURE 91–3.** Protein-, peptide-, and lectin-containing plants: (**A**) The castor bean plant. The seedpods come in bunches, two of which appear near the center of the image. Each seedpod typically contains three seeds. Inset: Castor beans (*Ricinus communis*), which contain the toxalbumin ricin. By interfering with protein synthesis, ricin may cause multiorgan system failure when administered parenterally. However, its oral absorption is poor, and most oral poisonings cause gastroenteritis. (**B**) Rosary pea (*Abrus precatorius*) containing abrin, a toxalbumin that inhibits protein synthesis. The peas are shown strung together as a rosary. (**C**) Pokeweed (*Phytolacca americana*) has a large rootstock. The unripe berries contain phytolaccatoxin, which produces gastroenteritis, but the mature, purple berries are often consumed. *(Used with permission from the Fellowship in Medical Toxicology, New York University Grossman School of Medicine, New York City Poison Center.)*

dehydration, ricin can cause cardiac, hematologic, hepatic, and renal toxicity. All contribute to death in humans and animals. Despite the obvious toxicity of this compound, death probably can be prevented by early and aggressive fluid and electrolyte replacement after ingestion (but not injection or inhalation; Chap. 99). Although chewing of one seed by a child liberates enough ricin to produce death, this outcome (or even serious toxicity) is uncommon, even if the seeds are chewed, probably because GI absorption of the ricin is poor and supportive care is effective. Activated charcoal should be administered promptly following ingestion. Other ricin-like lectins are found in *Abrus precatorius* (jequirity pea, rosary pea), *Jatropha* spp, *Trichosanthes* spp (eg, *T. kirilowii* or Chinese cucumber), *Robinia pseudoacacia* (black locust), *Phoradendron* spp (American mistletoe), *Viscum album* (European mistletoe), and *Wisteria* spp (wisteria).

The most commonly ingested toxic plant lectins in the US are from pokeweed (*Phytolacca americana*), which is eaten as a vegetable but rarely causes toxicity or death. Pokeweed leaves are consumed after boiling without toxic effect if the water is changed between the first and second boiling (parboiling). When this detoxification technique is not followed, violent GI effects can ensue 0.5 to 6 hours after ingestion. Nausea, vomiting, abdominal cramping, diarrhea, hemorrhagic gastritis, and death may occur. In addition, bradycardia and hypotension, perhaps induced by an increase in vagal tone, may be associated with nausea and vomiting. Phytolaccatoxin and pokeweed mitogen are found in all plant parts and produce a lymphocytosis 2 to 4 days after ingestion that may last for 10 days, but this is without clinical consequence.

Hypoglycin A and hypoglycin B are found in the unripe fruit and seeds of *Blighia sapida* (Euphorbiaceae), or ackee. The tree is native to Africa but was imported to Jamaica in 1778. Epidemics of illness (Jamaican vomiting sickness) associated with consumption of the unripe ackee fruit (raw and cooked) occur in Africa but are more common in Jamaica, where ackee is the national dish. Cases of hypoglycin A poisoning are also associated with canned ackee fruit and recently with epidemic poisonings from litchi fruit in India. Hypoglycin A is metabolized to methylene cyclopropyl acetic acid, which competitively inhibits the carnitine–acyl coenzyme (CoA) transferase system. This prevents importation of long-chain fatty acids into the mitochondria, preventing their β-oxidation to precursors of gluconeogenesis. In addition, increased concentrations of glutaric acid may inhibit glutamic acid decarboxylase, which produces GABA from glutamic acid. This not only depletes GABA but also increases concentrations of excitatory glutamate, which produces seizures. Insulin concentrations remain unaffected by hypoglycin and metabolites. Convulsions, coma, and death can ensue, with death occurring approximately 12 hours following consumption. Laboratory findings are notable for profound hepatic aminotransferase and bilirubin abnormalities and aciduria and acidemia without ketonemia. Autopsy reveals fatty degeneration of liver, particularly microvesicular steatosis, and other organs with depletion of glycogen stores. Left untreated, patient mortality reaches 80%, with 85% of the fatal cases suffering seizures. Treatment with dextrose and fluid replacement is essential. Benzodiazepines control seizures but may fail if the seizures are related to depletion of GABA. In this situation, an alternative anticonvulsant, such as a barbiturate or propofol, should be utilized. L-Carnitine therapy may exert a theoretical therapeutic role similar to that noted with valproic acid toxicity (Chap. 21 and Antidotes in Brief: A10). Its use, however, in this situation is not studied.

The lathyrins β-*N*-oxalylamino-L-alanine (BOAA) and β-aminopropionitrile (BAPN) are peptides from the grass pea (*Lathyrus sativus*) found in the seeds and leaves, respectively. β-*N*-Oxalylamino-L-alanine produces neurolathyrism and BAPN produces osteolathyrism in individuals with a dietary dependence on this plant. Neurolathyrism is nearly indistinguishable from spastic paresis associated with consumption of improperly prepared cassava (see section Cyanogenic Glycosides). Thiol oxidation with depletion of nicotinamide adenine dinucleotide (NADH) dehydrogenase in neuronal mitochondria (ie, excitatory AMPA receptors) may be the common etiology. β-Aminopropionitrile affects bone matrix and leads to bone pain and skeletal deformities that develop in adulthood. These diseases occur in areas where the plants are endemic, the food is consumed for 2 months or more, and when diets are otherwise poor in protein and possibly in zinc.

Microcystins are found in several cyanobacteria (blue-green algae) belonging to various species of the genera *Microcystis*, *Anabaena*, *Nodularia*, *Nostoc*, and *Oscillatoria*. They elaborate a series of peptides called microcystins and nodularins (*Nodularia spumigena*). These compounds produce hepatotoxicity by inhibiting phosphatases and causing deterioration of the microfilament function in hepatocytes, leading to cell shrinkage and bleeding into the hepatic sinusoids. Although most cases of untoward effects from blue-green algae occur in animals, the potential for harm was demonstrated by use of microcystin-contaminated water in a dialysis unit in Brazil. Unfiltered water was identified as the risk factor for liver disease in 100 patients who attended the dialysis center (Chap. 4). Fifty of these patients died of acute liver failure following early signs of nausea, vomiting, and visual disturbances.

### Phenols and Phenylpropanoids: Coumarins, Capsaicin, Karwinskia Toxins, Naringenin and Bergamottin, Asarin, Nordihydroguaiaretic Acid, Podophyllin, Psoralen, and Esculoside

Phenols and phenylpropanoids represent one of the largest groups of plant secondary metabolites. Coumarins and their isomers are phenylpropanoids that are discussed in Chap. 31. Capsaicin is derived from *Capsicum annuum* or other species of chili or cayenne peppers. Capsaicin causes release of the neuropeptide substance P from sensory C-type nerve fibers resulting in immediate intense local pain. Skin irrigation, dermal aloe gel, analgesics, and oral antacids are therapeutic agents that may be helpful as appropriate. Irritated eyes should be treated with irrigation and, if severe, topical analgesia, but the pain generally resolves without sequelae within 24 hours.

Karwinskia toxins are found in plants commonly named buckthorn, coyotillo, tullidora, wild cherry, or capulincillo (*Karwinskia humboldtiana*). Uncoupling of oxidative phosphorylation or dysfunction of peroxisome assembly and integrity is described as the mechanism of action of T-514 on Schwann cells. Within a few days of ingestion, a symmetric motor neuropathy ascends from the lower extremities to produce a bulbar paralysis that may lead to death. Deep-tendon reflexes are abolished in affected areas, but cranial nerve findings are absent. Treatment is supportive, with mechanical ventilation as needed, and recovery typically is slow.

Naringin, naringenin, and bergamottin inhibit CYP3A4 and P-glycoprotein. Grapefruit juice consumption can increase circulating concentrations of drugs reliant on these mechanisms for metabolic elimination. Comedication with St John's wort (*Hypericum perforatum*) resulted in decreased plasma concentrations of a number of xenobiotics. Hyperforin is found in St John's wort and is associated with plant–xenobiotic interactions through strong induction of CYP3A4-mediated drug metabolism as well as induction of P-glycoprotein.

### Carboxylic Acids: Aristolochic Acids, Oxalic Acid, and Oxalate Raphides

Aristolochic acids are present in most members of the genus *Aristolochia*. Consumption of these compounds can cause aristolochic acid nephropathy (AAN), a progressive renal interstitial fibrosis frequently associated with urothelial malignancies (Chap. 16).

Certain plant families, such as the Araceae, Chenopodiaceae, Polygonaceae, and Amaranthaceae, and several of the grass families are rich in oxalates. Human dietary sources include rhubarb, spinach, strawberries, chocolate, tea, and nuts. Human consumption of soluble oxalate-rich foods correlates with kidney stone formation.

The insoluble calcium oxalate raphides that are present in certain plants, usually in the Araceae family, are found in conjunction with a protein toxin that increases the painful irritation to skin or mucous membranes.

### Alcohols: Cicutoxin

Cicutoxin is found in *Cicuta maculata* (water hemlock), *Cicuta douglasii* (western water hemlock), and *Oenanthe crocata* (hemlock water dropwort). Ingestion of any part of these plants constitutes the most common form of lethal plant ingestion in the US. These ingestions usually involve adults who incorrectly identify the plant as wild parsnip, turnip, parsley, or ginseng. Although the mechanism is not fully understood, cicutoxin may noncompetitively inhibit GABA receptors or block potassium channels. Clinical findings of mild or early poisonings consist of GI symptoms (nausea, vomiting, epigastric discomfort) and begin as early as 15 minutes after ingestion. Diaphoresis, flushing, dizziness, excessive salivation, bradycardia, hypotension, bronchial secretions with respiratory distress, and cyanosis occur and rapidly progress to violent seizures and status epilepticus. Immediate gastric lavage is recommended if practical, and benzodiazepines should be administered for seizures.

## EFFECTS SHARED AMONG DIFFERENT CLASSES OF XENOBIOTICS

### Plant–Xenobiotic Interactions

Examples of CYP3A4 induction and inhibition are listed above. Excessive intake of broccoli provides enough vitamin K to competitively inhibit the effects of warfarin on vitamin K activation.

### Sodium Channel Effects: Aconitine, Veratridine, Zygacine, Taxine, and Grayanotoxins

Several unrelated plants produce xenobiotics that affect the flow of sodium at the sodium channel. The mechanism of action depends on the individual alkaloid. For instance, aconitine and veratrum alkaloids tend to open the channels to influx of sodium, whereas others (eg, taxine) tend to block the flow, and grayanotoxins both increase and block sodium flow. The sodium channel opener aconitine from *Aconitum* spp or *Delphinium* spp has the most persistent toxicity and the lowest therapeutic index among the many active alkaloid ingredients of these toxic plants called aconite. Aconitine opens the voltage-dependent sodium channel, initially increasing cellular excitability. By prolonging sodium current influx, neuronal and cardiac repolarization eventually slows.

Approximately one teaspoon (2–5 g) of the root may cause death. The aconitine alkaloids are rapidly absorbed from the GI tract, and the calculated half-life of aconitine is 3 hours. Central nervous system effects typically progress from paresthesias to CNS depression, respiratory muscle depression, paralysis, and seizures. Nausea, vomiting, diarrhea, and abdominal cramping occur. Cardiotoxicity progresses from bradycardia with atrioventricular conduction blockade to increased ventricular automaticity resulting in diverse tachydysrhythmias. Antidysrhythmic success with lidocaine is limited, and amiodarone and flecainide are currently the antidysrhythmics of choice. Orogastric lavage and/or administration of activated charcoal should be performed for any patient displaying signs or symptoms consistent with poisoning from this category of plants, or in those who are believed to have a potentially toxic exposures. Given the potential for rapid cardiovascular deterioration, equipment and staff for cardiac pacing, and extracorporeal membrane oxygenation (ECMO) should be prepared and used for conventional indications.

Ingestion of veratridine and other veratrum alkaloids (from *Veratrum viride* and other *Veratrum* spp) generally results from foraging errors where the root appears similar to leeks (*Allium porrum*) and above-ground parts appear similar to gentian (*Gentiana lutea*) used for teas and wines in Europe. Symptoms develop within an hour of ingestion and include headache followed by nausea, vomiting, and less frequently bradycardia and diarrhea. Zygacine from *Zigadenus* spp (death camas) and other members of the lily family produces the same toxic effects as veratridine alkaloids (vomiting, hypotension, and bradycardia).

Taxine, derived from the yew, is another alkaloid mixture of sodium channel effectors that tend to close the channel (*Taxus baccata*) (Fig. 91–4). Toxic alkaloids are contained within the bark, leaves, and hard central seed but not in the surrounding fleshy red aril, which partly explains the low

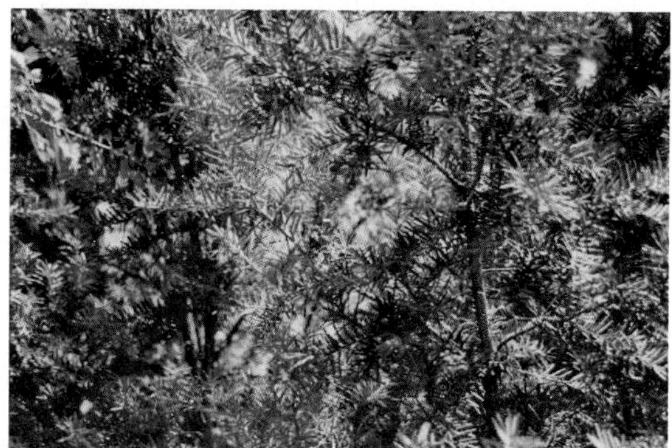

**FIGURE 91–4.** The yew (*Taxus* spp.) is a common garden shrub that produces taxine, a cardiotoxin. Though the fleshy red aril is nontoxic, the hard seed it contains is toxic. *(Used with permission from the Fellowship in Medical Toxicology, New York University Grossman School of Medicine, New York City Poison Center.)*

rate of toxicity in reported cases of unintentional exposure. Clinical manifestations of yew poisoning include dizziness, nausea, vomiting, diffuse abdominal pain, tachycardia (initially), and convulsions followed by bradycardia, respiratory paralysis, and death.

Grayanotoxins (formerly termed andromedotoxins) are present in leaves of various species of *Rhododendron*, *Azalea*, *Kalmia* (Fig. 91–5), and *Leucothoe* (Ericaceae). They exert their toxic effects via sodium channels, which they open or close, depending on the toxin. Grayanotoxins are concentrated in honey made in areas with densely populated grayanotoxin-containing plants, mainly in the Mediterranean. Bradycardia, hypotension, GI manifestations, mental status changes ("mad honey"), and seizures are described in patients suffering grayanotoxin toxicity.

### Antimitotic Alkaloids and Resins: Colchicine, Vincristine, and Podophyllum

Consumption of colchicine from plant sources such as autumn crocus (*Colchicum autumnale*) produces a spectrum of effects, including nausea, vomiting, watery diarrhea, hypotension, bradycardia, electrocardiographic abnormalities, diaphoresis,

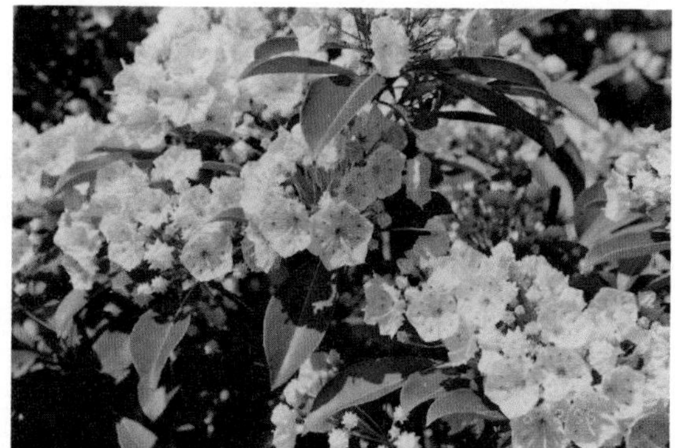

**FIGURE 91–5.** Mountain laurel (*Kalmia latifolia*), an evergreen shrub, contains the sodium channel opener grayanotoxin, which produces dysrhythmias. *(Used with permission from the Fellowship in Medical Toxicology, New York University Grossman School of Medicine, New York City Poison Center.)*

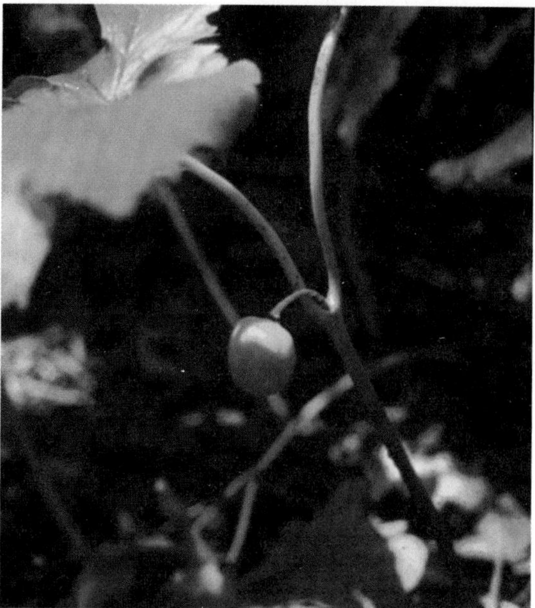

**FIGURE 91–6.** The mayapple (*Podophyllum peltatum*) develops from an initial nodding flower that grows from the stem of this low-lying ground cover plant. The whole plant contains podophyllotoxin (podophyllin), though the apple is generally considered the least toxic part. *(Used with permission from the Fellowship in Medical Toxicology, New York University Grossman School of Medicine, New York City Poison Center.)*

alopecia, bone marrow depression, acute kidney injury, hepatic necrosis, hemorrhagic lung injury, convulsions, and death. The mechanism of toxicity is disruption of microtubule formation in mitotic cells. Vincristine and vinblastine are two other alkaloids used as chemotherapeutics and are both isolated from the Madagascar periwinkle (*Catharanthus roseus*). No reports of poisoning by these alkaloids following ingestion of the plant could be found. Podophyllum resin is the dry, alcoholic extract of the rhizomes and roots of mayapple (*Podophyllum peltatum*) (Fig. 91–6). The dry resin consists of up to 20% podophyllotoxin, α- and β-peltatin, desoxypodophyllotoxin, and dehydropodophyllotoxin. Podophyllotoxins make up 20% of the resin from the roots of mayapple (*P. peltatum*). As a group, they disrupt tubulin formation, producing multisystem organ failure (Chap. 7).

### Plant-Induced Dermatitis

A large number of plants result in undesirable dermal, mucous membrane, and ocular effects, and they represent the most common adverse effects reported to US poison centers and occupational health centers. Plant-induced dermal disorders are readily categorized into four mechanistic groups, that is, dermatis that results from (1) mechanical injury, (2) irritant molecules that penetrate the skin, (3) allergy, or (4) photosensitivity (direct and hepatogenous).

Exposures to commonly available household plants such as dumbcane (*Dieffenbachia* spp), *Philodendron* spp, and *Narcissus* bulbs can lead to mechanical injury and painful microtrauma produced by bundles of tiny needlelike calcium oxalate crystals called raphides. Packages of hundreds of raphides called idioblasts contain proteolytic enzymes.

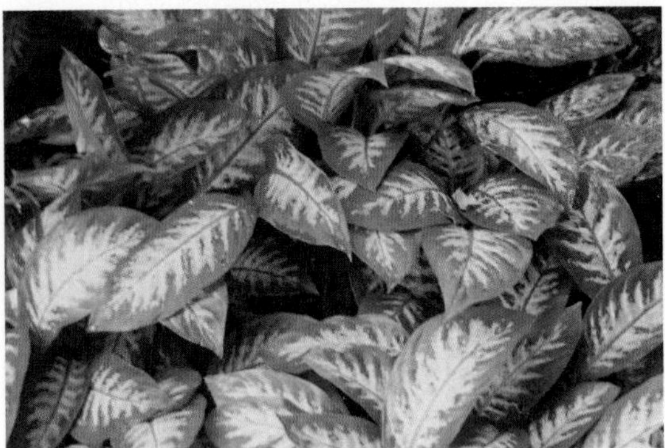

**FIGURE 91–7.** This dumbcane (*Dieffenbachia* sp) plant is representative of the Arum family, which typically have variegated, waxy leaves. Many contain insoluble crystals of calcium oxalate arranged in idioblasts, which may be ejected following trauma to the leaf. *(Used with permission from the Fellowship in Medical Toxicology, New York University Grossman School of Medicine, New York City Poison Center.)*

*Dieffenbachia* (more than 30 species) (Fig. 91–7) exposures are commonly reported household or malicious plant exposures, although such exposures are rarely serious. When the leaves are chewed, immediate oropharyngeal pain and swelling occur. Severe oral exposures can be excruciating and progress to profuse salivation, dysphagia, and loss of speech. Soothing liquids, ice, parenteral opioids, corticosteroids, and airway protection may be indicated, but antihistamines provide little relief. The edema and pain typically begin to subside after 4 to 8 days. Ocular exposure to the sap may produce chemical conjunctivitis, corneal abrasions, and, rarely, permanent corneal opacifications. Similar exposures to oxalate raphide-containing household plants in the same family (*Philodendron, Brassaia, Epipremnum aureum, Spathiphyllum,* and *Scheflera* spp) are not as painful as those to dumbcane, presumably because the crystals are packaged differently and do not simultaneously deliver proteolytic enzymes.

Irritant dermatitis results from low-molecular-weight xenobiotics such as phorbol esters (from Euphorbiaceae) that directly penetrate the skin without antecedent mechanical injury. Phorbol esters found in spurges (Euphorbiaceae) are contained in milky sap that is capable of producing erythema, desquamation, and bullae. Allergic contact dermatitis results from type IV hypersensitivity response and, unlike irritant dermatitis, requires prior exposures to the xenobiotic before symptoms manifest. The most infamous of these xenobiotics are the urushiol oleoresins derived from catechols that are found in *G. biloba* (Ginkgoaceae) and members of the Proteaceae (eg, *Macadamia integrifolia*) and the Anacardaceae. The latter family is notable for inclusion of poison ivy (*Toxicodendron radicans*), poison oak (*Toxicodendron toxicarium, Toxicodendron diver-silobum*), and poison sumac (*Toxicodendron vernix*), as well as mango (*Mangifera indica*), pistachio (*Pistacia vera*), cashew (*Anacardium occidentale*), and Indian marking nut "Bhilawanol" (*Semecarpus anacardium*). Upon first exposure, urushiol resins penetrate the skin and react with proteins to form antigens to which the body forms antibodies. Upon reexposure to urushiol resins, inflammatory mediators are released, leading to urticaria, itching, swelling, and pain. In extreme cases, these reactions can progress to type I hypersensitivity. Therapy includes washing with soap and water, application of topical corticosteroids, and for those at risk for frequent exposure (eg, forestry workers), desensitization. Allergic contact dermatitis is the most common plant-induced occupational injury. In the US, 33% of 462 floral shops surveyed reported that at least one employee had developed contact dermatitis.

Direct photosensitivity dermatitis is produced when compounds such as psoralens or other linear furocoumarins come into direct contact with the skin or are digested and become bloodborne to dermal capillary beds, where they interact with sunlight. These photosensitizing agents are activated by ultraviolet A radiation (320–400 nm), producing singlet oxygen and DNA adducts. More than 200 of these xenobiotics have been identified in at least 15 plant families, including food sources, such as Apiaceae (anise, caraway, carrot, celery, chervil, dill, fennel, parsley, and parsnip), Rutaceae (grapefruit, lemon, lime, bergamot, and orange), Solanaceae (potato), and Moraceae (figs) family.

# 92 NATIVE (US) VENOMOUS SNAKES AND LIZARDS

## EPIDEMIOLOGY

### Snakes

More than 3,000 species of snakes are identified worldwide, with nearly 800 species considered venomous. All venomous species are classified taxonomically into one of four general groups. These include the families Viperidae, Elapidae, and Colubridae, as well as the Atractaspidinae, a subfamily of the Lamprophiidae family. The United States (US) is home to nearly 30 species and subspecies of venomous snakes (Table 92–1). All belong to either the Crotalinae subfamily of Viperidae or the Elapidae family.

The majority of snake species in North America are rear-fanged, nonvenomous members of the Colubridae family. Venomous snakes are found throughout most of the US. They are much more common in the southern and western states than in the northern states. The true number of bites that occur each year is not accurately known, but an average of 5,000 native venomous snakebites are reported to US poison centers annually. Mortality is rare in the US, with fewer than 10 deaths per year reported. The majority of snakebites in the US occur between April and September, with the peak number reported in July. Men comprise 75% of snakebite victims and children represent about 10% to 15% of reported cases. Most victims are bitten on an extremity because bites often occur when an individual is purposely handling a known venomous snake.

Snake enthusiasts often keep nonnative (exotic) species as pets. Approximately 30 to 50 bites from a large variety of exotic venomous snakes are reported to poison control centers each year.

**TABLE 92–1 Medically Important Snakes of the United States**

| Genus | Species | Common Name |
|---|---|---|
| Crotalinae | | |
| *Crotalus* | *adamanteus* | Eastern diamondback rattlesnake |
| | *atrox* | Western diamondback rattlesnake |
| | *cerastes* | Sidewinder[a] |
| | *cerberus* | Arizona black rattlesnake |
| | *horridus* | Timber rattlesnake |
| | *lepidus* | Rock rattlesnake[a] |
| | *mitchellii* | Speckled rattlesnake[a] |
| | *molossus* | Black-tailed rattlesnake[a] |
| | *oreganus* | Western rattlesnake[a] |
| | *pricei* | Twin-spotted rattlesnake[a] |
| | *ruber* | Red diamond rattlesnake[a] |
| | *scutulatus* | Mojave rattlesnake[a] |
| | *stephensi* | Panamint rattlesnake |
| | *tigris* | Tiger rattlesnake |
| | *viridis* | Prairie rattlesnake[a] |
| | *willardi* | Ridgenose rattlesnake[a] |
| *Sistrurus* | *catenatus* | Massasauga[a] |
| | *miliarius* | Pygmy rattlesnake[a] |
| *Agkistrodon* | *contortrix* | Copperhead[a] |
| | *piscivorus* | Cottonmouth[a] |
| Elapidae | | |
| *Micrurus* | *fulvius* | Eastern coral snake |
| *Micrurus* | *tener* | Texas coral snake[a] |

[a]Subspecies identified for this species.

***Pit Vipers.*** The majority of native venomous snakes are members of the Crotalinae subfamily of Viperidae. These crotaline species are variably referred to as crotalids, New World vipers, or pit vipers. The term "pit viper" describes the presence of a pitlike depression behind the nostril that contains a heat-sensing organ used to locate prey (Figs. 92–1 and 92–2). Crotalinae have front, mobile fangs that are paired, needlelike structures that can retract on a hingelike mechanism into the roof of the mouth. Rattlesnakes have the longest fangs, reaching 3 to 4 cm. Of crotalid bites for which the type of snake is reported, about half are rattlesnake species, and the remainder are copperheads and cottonmouths. Deaths following snakebite are almost always due to rattlesnakes, although rare deaths are reported from copperhead bites.

***Coral Snakes.*** Coral snakes (genera *Micrurus* and *Micruroides*) represent the Elapidae family in North America. These brightly colored snakes typically have easily identifiable red, yellow, and black bands along the length of their bodies. In the US, coral snakes and the similarly colored nonvenomous scarlet king snake are often confused. Coral and king snakes can be distinguished by their color patterns. Whereas coral snakes have black snouts, king snakes have red snouts. Both species have red, yellow, and black rings, but in different sequences: the red and yellow rings touch in the coral snake

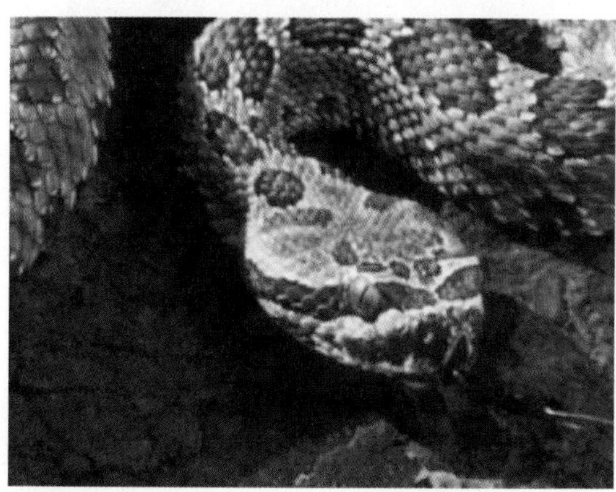

**FIGURE 92–1.** Pit vipers have a triangular-shaped head, vertically elliptical pupils, and heat-sensing pits behind the nostril.

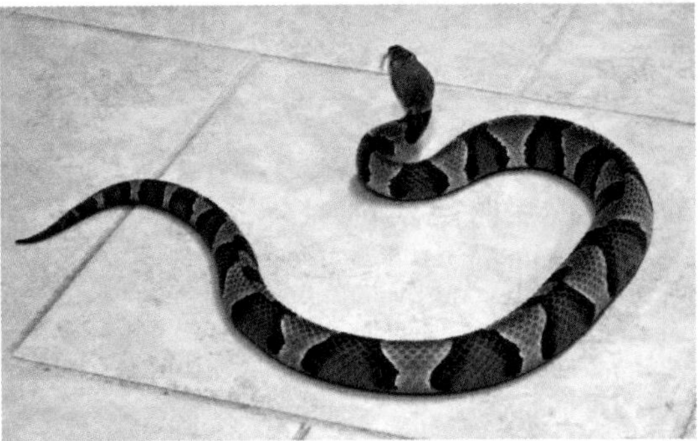

**FIGURE 92–2.** Copperhead (*Agkistrodon contortrix*). *(Used with the permission from Michelle Ruha, MD.)*

but are separated by black rings in king snakes ("Red on yellow kills a fellow; red on black, venom lack") (Fig. 92–3).

Elapids possess front-fixed fangs. The fangs of coral snakes are small, and discrete fang marks may not be obvious after envenomation. Coral snakes often latch on to a victim or "chew" for a few seconds in an attempt to deliver venom. A history of this activity may help identify a coral snakebite when the offending reptile cannot be located.

Coral snakes are responsible for approximately 2% of bites reported to US poison centers, of which *Micrurus fulvius* (the Eastern coral snake) is responsible for the greatest morbidity and mortality.

### Lizards

There are two species of lizard that are known to produce envenomation in humans. These are the Gila monster (*Heloderma suspectum*), which is native to the desert southwestern US, and the beaded lizard (*H. horridum*), which is found in Mexico. Both species are members of the Helodermatidae family (Fig. 92–4). Bites by the Gila monster and beaded lizard are extremely uncommon, even in areas where the lizards are endemic. Gila monsters are known for their forceful bites. They can hang on and "chew" for as long as 15 minutes, and they may be difficult to disengage.

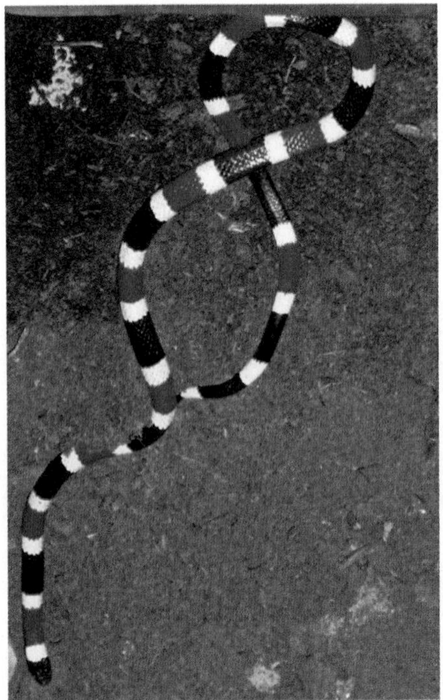

**FIGURE 92–3.** Coral snake with characteristic black snout and red bands bordered by yellow bands. *(Used with permission from Banner Good Samaritan Medical Center Department of Medical Toxicology.)*

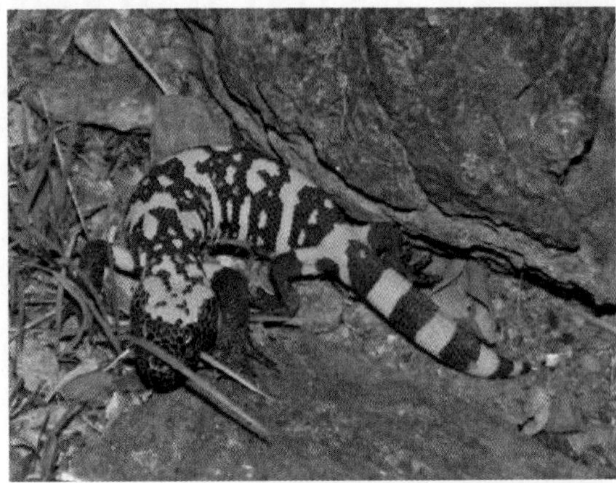

A

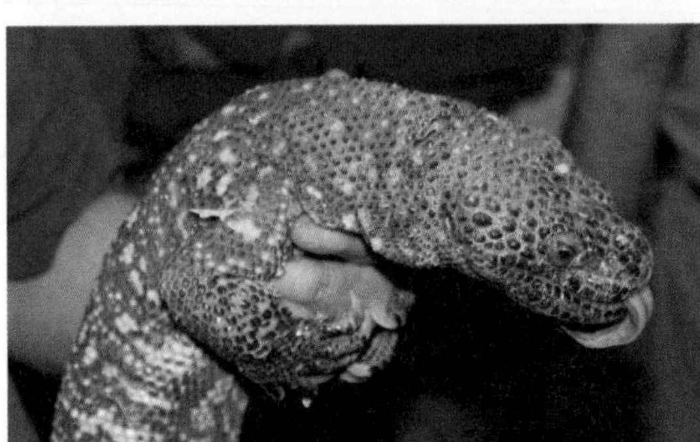

B

**FIGURE 92–4.** (**A**) Young Gila monster (*Heloderma suspectum*). *(Used with the permission from Steven Curry, MD.)* (**B**) Beaded lizard (*Heloderma horridum*). *(Used with the permission from Michelle Ruha, MD.)*

The helodermatid lizards have a less effective venom delivery system than venomous snake species. The lizards possess paired venom glands that are located on either side of the anterior lower mandible. Venom ducts carry the venom from the glands to the base of grooved teeth. When a tooth produces a puncture wound, the venom travels by capillary action into the grooves and then into the wound.

## PHARMACOLOGY

### Snakes

Snake venom is a complex mixture of proteins, peptides, lipids, carbohydrates, and metal ions. The content and potency of venom in any given snake vary depending on age, diet, and geography. Thus, an adult snake may have significantly different venom composition than a young snake of the same species. The actions of only a fraction of snake venom components are fully understood.

### Lizards

Helodermatid venom contains a complex mixture of components similar to those of snake venoms. Nonenzymatic components include helospectins and helodermin, which are vasoactive peptides that activate adenylate cyclase, and exendin-3 and exendin-4, which stimulate glucose-dependent insulin secretion. Discovery of exendins in *Heloderma* venom lead to development of exenatide a glucagonlike peptide-1 (GLP-1) receptor agonist used in the management of diabetes.

## PHARMACOKINETICS AND TOXICOKINETICS

### Snakes

Very few pharmacokinetic studies of snake venom exist, and much remains unknown regarding absorption, distribution, and elimination of venom following a bite. When a snake bites, venom is usually deposited subcutaneously. In some cases, fangs reach muscle or even directly access vasculature. Systemic absorption of venom usually occurs via the lymphatic system. Available human and animal data suggest that venom antigens are absorbed into blood within minutes of envenomation, with peak concentrations detected within 4 hours. Venom antigens are also detected in urine as early as 30 minutes after envenomation. The elimination half-life of snake venom appears to be long.

### Lizards

Pharmacokinetic studies of helodermatid venom are not available.

## PATHOPHYSIOLOGY

### Snakes

***Pit Vipers.*** Crotaline venom has the potential to simultaneously damage tissue, affect blood vessels and blood, and alter transmission at the neuromuscular junction. It is difficult to attribute specific pathology or pathophysiology to any particular component of snake venom. In fact, clinical effects often occur as the result of several venom components (Table 92–2).

**TABLE 92–2 Major Venom Components of Crotalinae Snakes**

| *General Clinical Effect* | *Responsible Venom Components* |
|---|---|
| Local tissue damage | Metalloproteinases<br>Phospholipases $A_2$<br>Hyaluronidase |
| Coagulation effects[a] | C-type lectinlike proteins<br>Metalloproteinases[b]<br>Serine proteases[b]<br>Phospholipases $A_2$ |
| Platelet effects[c] | Disintegrins<br>C-type lectinlike proteins<br>Metalloproteinases<br>Phospholipases $A_2$ |
| Neurotoxic effects | Phospholipases $A_2$ |

[a]Venom contains both pro- and anticoagulants, with anticoagulant effects predominating in North American crotaline envenomation. [b]Include thrombinlike enzymes as well as fibrinogenolytic enzymes. [c]Venom may contain factors that inhibit, activate, or affect aggregation of platelets.

***Coral Snakes.*** Coral snake venom contains neurotoxins that produce systemic neurotoxicity. Unlike crotaline venom, coral snake venom does not cause local tissue injury. Similar to neurotoxins present in other elapid species, coral snake neurotoxins bind and competitively block postsynaptic acetylcholine receptors at the neuromuscular junction, leading to weakness and paralysis.

### Lizards

The pathophysiology of helodermatid venom is poorly understood. It is suggested that hyaluronidase contributes to spreading of venom throughout tissue. Gilatoxin is believed to produce hypotension and other findings such as angioedema by increasing bradykinin concentrations.

## CLINICAL MANIFESTATIONS

### Snakes

The clinical presentation of North American snake envenomation is highly variable and depends upon many factors, including the species of snake, the amount and potency of venom deposited, the location of the bite, and patient factors, such as comorbidities. For bites by nonnative species, it is important to identify the species so that specific antivenom can be sought.

***Pit Vipers.*** Envenomation by North American pit vipers is characterized by local swelling and cytotoxic effects. Hematologic effects are common, and there is the potential for development of systemic illness and neurotoxicity. Most patients exhibit only a subset of possible effects of envenomation. In addition, some of the signs and symptoms in a given individual, such as nausea or tachycardia, may be related to fear rather than to envenomation.

The clinical presentation following a pit viper bite can range from benign to life threatening (Table 92–3). One finding common to nearly all victims is the presence of an identifiable disruption of skin integrity. Most commonly, one or two distinct punctures are present, though occasionally, patients exhibit multiple punctures, small lacerations, or scratches (Fig. 92–5). Because pit viper bites result in injection of venom only about 75% of the time, approximately 25% of bites do not result in envenomation and are considered "dry bites." Unfortunately, it is impossible to diagnose a dry bite without an extended period of observation, because some patients have delayed onset of findings for as much as 8 to 10 hours following the bite and some subsequently develop serious illness.

Rarely, patients bitten by crotalids experience classic anaphylaxis from the venom itself, which complicates evaluation or mimics a severe systemic reaction to venom. Previous sensitization to venom results in development of IgE antibodies to venom in these patients. This is thought to occur more frequently in patients who have previously experienced a snakebite but is also observed in snake handlers who are thought to be sensitized to snake proteins through inhalation or skin contact. The presence of pruritus and urticaria or wheezing, uncommon with envenomation, should suggest anaphylaxis.

***Coral Snakes.*** Coral snake fangs are small and nonmobile, and as a result, bites are less likely than pit viper bites to

**TABLE 92–3 Evaluation and Treatment of Crotaline Envenomation**

| *Extent of Envenomation* | *Clinical Observations* | *Antivenom Recommended*[a] | *Other Treatment* | *Disposition* |
|---|---|---|---|---|
| None ("dry bite") | Fang marks are present, but no local or systemic effects after 8–12 hours | No | Local wound care<br>Tetanus prophylaxis | Discharge after 8–12 hours of observation |
| Minimal | Minor, nonprogressing, local swelling and discomfort without systemic effects or hematologic abnormalities | No | Local wound care<br>Tetanus prophylaxis | Admit to monitored unit for 24-hour observation |
| Moderate | Progression of swelling beyond area of bite with or without local tissue destruction, hematologic abnormalities, or non–life-threatening systemic effects | Yes | Intravenous fluids<br>Cardiac monitoring<br>Analgesics<br>Follow laboratory parameters<br>Tetanus prophylaxis | Admit to intensive care unit |
| Severe | Marked progressive swelling, pain with or without local tissue destruction<br>Systemic effects such as diarrhea, weakness, shock, or angioedema, and/or pronounced thrombocytopenia or coagulopathy | Yes | Intravenous fluids<br>Cardiac monitoring<br>Analgesics<br>Follow laboratory parameters<br>Oxygen<br>Vasopressors<br>Tetanus prophylaxis | Admit to intensive care unit |

[a]See Antidotes in Brief: A39 for dosing recommendations.

lead to envenomation. An estimated 40% of patients bitten by a coral snake are subsequently determined to be envenomated, with rates for the Eastern coral snake species possibly higher. Coral snake fangs do not always produce easily identifiable puncture wounds. In addition to the absence of a discernable wound in some victims, coral snake envenomations are characterized by potentially serious neurotoxicity without impressive local symptoms. The effects of envenomation are characteristically delayed for a number of hours. Neurologic abnormalities reported with coral snake envenomation include paresthesias, slurred speech, ptosis, diplopia, dysphagia, stridor, muscle weakness, fasciculations, and paralysis. The major cause of death is respiratory failure secondary to neuromuscular weakness. Muscle weakness takes weeks to months to resolve completely. With respiratory support, however, paralysis is completely reversible. Pulmonary aspiration is a common sequela in the subacute phase.

### Lizards

The rate of envenomation following Gila monster bites is not known, but one case series reported 40% dry bites. Pain is immediate following a bite, and local soft tissue edema often develops within minutes. Swelling extends from the puncture site, though not as commonly or dramatically as occurs following pit viper envenomation. Helodermatid venom does not produce local tissue necrosis, but erythema at the wound site and extension of erythema to an entire extremity are well described. Lymphangitic streaking is also reported. Nausea, vomiting, and diaphoresis are reported following helodermatid envenomation. Patients are often tachycardic and hypotensive. There are numerous reports of upper airway angioedema developing after bites by both Gila monsters and beaded lizards.

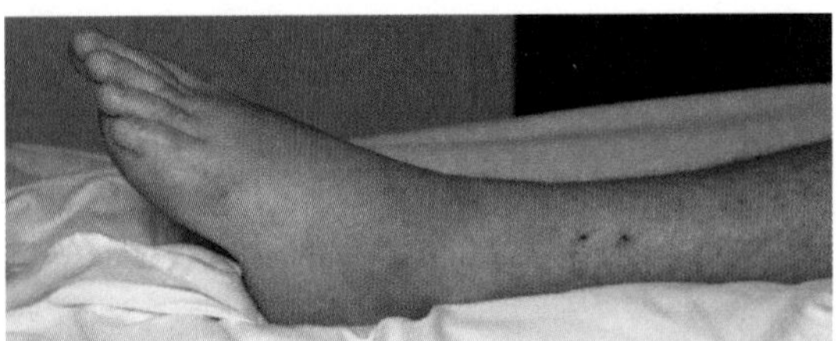

**FIGURE 92–5.** Rattlesnake bite to the lower leg, with characteristic edema and bluish discoloration of the foot due to ecchymosis. *(Used with the permission from Michelle Ruha, MD.)*

## DIAGNOSTIC TESTING

### Snakes

Diagnosis of North American snake envenomation is based on a history of a snakebite and presence of clinical signs of envenomation. There are no available laboratory assays for detection of venom in a wound. Platelet counts, fibrinogen concentrations, and prothrombin times (PTs) are useful in the diagnosis of pit viper envenomation if they are abnormal. However, normal results do not exclude envenomation because thrombocytopenia and coagulopathy do not develop in all patients with pit viper envenomation.

### Lizards

The diagnosis of helodermatid envenomation is based on the history of a bite and presence of physical examination findings consistent with envenomation. There are no laboratory studies that are available to confirm or exclude the diagnosis, but a complete blood count may reveal leukocytosis.

## MANAGEMENT

### Snakes

When a patient with a snake bite presents for care, the initial objectives are to determine the presence or absence of envenomation, provide basic supportive therapy, treat the local and systemic effects of envenomation, and limit tissue loss or functional disability (Table 92–3). A combination of medical therapy (mainly supportive care and, often, antivenom) and in some cases conservative surgical treatment (mainly debridement of devitalized tissue), individualized for each patient, will provide the best results. In general, the more rapidly treatment is instituted, the shorter the period of disability.

**Pit Vipers.** *Prehospital care.* No first aid measure or specific field treatment has been proven to positively affect outcome following a crotaline envenomation. Prehospital care should generally be limited to immobilization of the affected limb, placement of an intravenous catheter, treatment of life-threatening clinical findings, and rapid transport to a medical facility. If transport time is long and pain is severe, administration of analgesics is recommended. Patients who are volume depleted, vomiting, or experiencing systemic effects such as diarrhea should be given an intravenous fluid bolus. Hypotension that does not quickly respond to a fluid bolus should be treated with epinephrine, since early hypotension is most likely due to anaphylaxis, anaphylactoid reaction to venom, or venom-induced vasodilation.

*Hospital care.* When a patient presents to the hospital with history of crotaline snakebite, it is important to first determine whether an envenomation has occurred. Although most patients show early evidence of envenomation, absence of symptoms at presentation is not uncommon, and not all asymptomatic patients ultimately have "dry" bites. Patients who present with puncture wounds but without swelling or other evidence of envenomation must be observed for delayed onset of symptoms. An observation period of 8 hours for *Agkistrodon* bites and 12 hours for rattlesnake bites is recommended. If no swelling develops and laboratory study samples drawn at least 8 hours from the time of the bite remain normal and unchanged, the bite is likely "dry" and the patient is safe for discharge from medical care with instructions to return if new pain or swelling develops.

*Supportive.* The initial in-hospital assessment of North American crotaline envenomation should focus on airway, breathing, and circulation. Patients with evidence of angioedema or with bites to the face or tongue need to be observed closely for signs of airway compromise and intubated early, before swelling progresses to the point of airway obstruction. All patients, regardless of presenting symptoms, should have an intravenous catheter placed in an unaffected extremity and an IV fluid bolus is recommended. Patients presenting with cardiovascular collapse should receive large volumes of fluid. An epinephrine continuous infusion, starting at 0.1 μg/kg/min and titrating as needed, is the authors' vasopressor of choice for signs of shock following envenomation.

Immobilization of the affected extremity in a padded splint in near-full extension and elevation above the level of the heart to avoid dependent edema are recommended. Marking the leading edge of swelling with a pen or sequentially measuring extremity circumference will help to identify progression of edema. A baseline complete blood count, PT, and fibrinogen concentration should be obtained initially and repeated in 4 to 6 hours. Patients who are systemically ill should also have electrolytes, creatinine phosphokinase, creatinine, glucose, and urinalysis checked. Pain should be treated with opioid analgesics as needed, and tetanus prophylaxis should be addressed. The patient should be reassessed frequently with repeat physical examinations, specifically noting any progression of swelling. Prophylactic antibiotics should not be given.

*Antivenom.* Patients with dry bites or mild envenomations, such as those who present with only localized swelling that fails to progress, do not meet criteria for antivenom (Table 92–3). Patients who present with progressive swelling, thrombocytopenia, coagulopathy, neurotoxicity, or significant systemic toxicity are candidates for antivenom therapy. Antivenom given in a timely manner can reverse coagulopathy and thrombocytopenia and halt progression of local swelling. Antivenom also reduces compartment pressure and limits venom-induced decreases in perfusion pressure, potentially preventing the need for fasciotomy.

Two available US Food and Drug Administration (FDA)-approved antivenoms for North American pit viper envenomation currently exist. Crotalidae polyvalent immune Fab is administered IV in an initial dose of four to six vials reconstituted in 0.9% sodium chloride solution. The recommended starting dose for patients who present with cardiovascular collapse or serious active bleeding is 8 to 12 vials. Details on dosing and administration can be found in Antidotes in Brief: A39. Pregnant patients and children who meet criteria for treatment should also receive antivenom.

An alternative antivenom for the treatment of North American rattlesnake envenomation is US. Crotalidae equine immune $F(ab')_2$, which is made using venoms of *Bothrops asper* and *Crotalus simus*. The initial dose of Crotalidae equine immune $F(ab')_2$ is 10 vials. Details on dosing and administration can be found in Antidotes in Brief: A39.

*Surgery.* Surgery is not routinely indicated following snakebites. An extensive review of the literature failed to identify any evidence to support the use of fasciotomy in the treatment of snakebites. When compartment syndrome is suspected, intracompartmental pressures should be measured. It is reasonable to attempt to treat moderately elevated compartment pressures with antivenom initially. If compartment pressures are rising despite administration of antivenom or if the patient develops evidence of limb ischemia, fasciotomy is recommended.

Patients with bites to the digit sometimes present with evidence of ischemia. The compromised finger appears cyanotic or pale, tense, and lacks sensation. The small diameter of the digit and limited ability of the skin to expand essentially create a small compartment. In such cases, it is recommended to perform a digital dermotomy, in which a longitudinal incision is made through the skin on the medial or lateral aspect of the digit in order to decompress the neurovascular structures. Dermotomy should not be performed prophylactically in cases of digital envenomation, as most patients have good outcome without any surgical intervention. Debridement of hemorrhagic blebs and blisters is often performed to evaluate underlying tissue and relieve discomfort. Some patients require surgical debridement of necrotic tissue or even amputation of a digit 1 to 2 weeks after the bite. Referral to a hand surgeon is appropriate for patients with evidence of extensive tissue necrosis.

*Blood Products.* Immeasurably low fibrinogen concentrations, PTs greater than 100 seconds, and platelet counts less than 20,000/mm$^3$ are routinely encountered after rattlesnake envenomation. Such abnormal laboratory results alone should not prompt the clinician to treat with blood products in the absence of clinically significant bleeding. The mainstay of treatment for crotaline envenomation–induced hematopathology is antivenom, not blood products. Rarely, a patient will have clinically significant bleeding, and antivenom alone will not correct the platelets and fibrinogen. In such cases, fresh frozen plasma, cryoprecipitate, packed red blood cells, or platelet transfusions are recommended to replace losses.

In some cases, thrombocytopenia is difficult, or impossible, to correct with even large amounts of antivenom. The Timber rattlesnake, for example, is known for producing thrombocytopenia resistant to antivenom. In the absence of bleeding, thrombocytopenia is a benign, self-limiting disorder, resolving within 2 to 3 weeks of envenomation. It is best to closely follow patients with resistant thrombocytopenia who are not bleeding, rather than attempt further platelet transfusions or antivenom administration.

*Follow-Up Care.* Hospital stays for patients with uncomplicated pit viper envenomations are typically short, lasting approximately 1 to 2 days. Upon discharge from the hospital, patients often have residual swelling and functional disability. Some will have continued progression of hemorrhagic bullae with underlying necrosis. Patients should have an out-patient follow-up evaluation to ensure wounds are healing appropriately and extremity function is returning. If joint mobility does not return to baseline as swelling resolves, the patient should be referred for physical and occupational therapy.

In a significant proportion of rattlesnake bite patients treated with Crotalidae polyvalent immune Fab antivenom, a return of swelling, coagulopathy, or thrombocytopenia is noted days to weeks after initial resolution with effective antivenom treatment. This is termed "recurrence" of venom effect and is attributed to the interrelated kinetics and dynamics of venom and antivenom. Simply stated, Fab antivenom has a clinical half-life shorter than that of venom. The most reasonable way to address possible late hematologic effects of crotaline envenomation is careful outpatient follow-up after hospital discharge. Provide careful discharge instructions and consider all patients who have been treated with Crotalidae polyvalent immune Fab antivenom to be at risk for late hematologic toxicity. Patients must be warned not to undergo dental or surgical procedures for up to 3 weeks unless platelet and coagulation studies are documented to be normal immediately prior to the procedure. High-risk activities, such as contact sports, should be avoided. All patients with rattlesnake bites should have platelets and coagulation studies measured 2 to 3 days, and again 5 to 7 days, after the last antivenom treatment. If values are abnormal or trending in the wrong direction, the studies should be repeated every few days until normal and stable. Because copperhead envenomation is much less likely to produce severe hemotoxicity, one set of follow-up laboratory studies to screen for late thrombocytopenia or coagulopathy is reasonable in this population. We recommend retreatment for any patient with evidence of bleeding, as well as patients with severe isolated thrombocytopenia (platelets < 25,000/mm$^3$) or moderate thrombocytopenia (platelets 25,000–50,000/mm$^3$) in combination with severe coagulopathy (fibrinogen < 80 mg/dL). When the decision is made to retreat a patient with late hemotoxicity with antivenom, an initial starting dose of two vials is recommended. Based on anecdotal experience, if platelet counts do not increase after two to three doses of antivenom, additional antivenom is unlikely to be effective. Response to platelet transfusions is also often poor.

***Coral Snakes.*** As with North American pit viper bites, patients who are bitten by North American coral snakes should be taken to a hospital for definitive medical care as soon as possible. There are no field treatments that have been shown to affect outcome in these patients, although use of a pressure immobilization bandage (PIB) is reasonable if transport to a hospital will be prolonged or delayed. Patients who present for care after a PIB has been placed should have the dressing left in place until resuscitative equipment and personnel are present and, ideally, antivenom is available. The PIB should be checked to ensure it is not functioning as a tourniquet.

Patients with a history concerning for possible Eastern or Texas coral snakebite should be observed for 24 hours in a monitored unit where resuscitative measures, including endotracheal intubation, can be performed. Because neuromuscular weakness and respiratory paralysis can develop quickly, endotracheal intubation is reasonable at the first sign of bulbar paralysis. In the past, treatment with Antivenin (*Micrurus fulvius*) (equine origin) North American Coral Snake Antivenin was recommended for all patients in whom there is strong suspicion of coral snakebite, even in the absence of signs of envenomation. We recommend a conservative approach, defined as waiting for symptoms to develop before administering antivenom.

If a patient is symptomatic following a coral snake envenomation, antivenom, if available, is indicated. If antivenom is unavailable, supportive care including mechanical ventilation may be necessary for many weeks. Additionally, a trial of neostigmine to reverse the neurotoxic effects of venom is reasonable.

### Lizards

Management of helodermatid envenomation consists of supportive care. There is no antivenom available against lizard venom. Routine wound care should be performed, and the clinician should look for the presence of teeth in the wound. There is no evidence to guide clinicians when deciding whether to administer antibiotics to patients with erythema surrounding and extending from the bite site. Most case reports describing patients with erythema also report empiric use of antibiotics. There are no reports of confirmed infections following these bites.

Patients who are symptomatic following a bite should be attached to a cardiac monitor and have an intravenous catheter inserted. Although serious morbidity from lizard bites is unusual, life-threatening manifestations of envenomation are reported. Angioedema, other evidence of respiratory compromise, or airway obstruction should prompt endotracheal intubation. Hypotension should be treated with intravenous fluid boluses as well as vasopressors such as epinephrine. Epinephrine, corticosteroids, and antihistamines are recommended for the treatment of anaphylactoid reactions.

Antidotes in Brief

# A39 ANTIVENOM FOR NORTH AMERICAN VENOMOUS SNAKES (CROTALINE AND ELAPID)

## INTRODUCTION

The focus of treatment for the snakebite victim is a careful assessment, supportive care, evaluating for signs of envenomation, and ultimately, determining the need for antivenom.

## HISTORY

### Crotalidae Polyvalent Immune Fab (Ovine)

Historically, Wyeth (Marietta, PA) manufactured Antivenin Crotalidae Polyvalent (ACP) for treatment of crotaline snakebites in the United States (US). It was a poorly purified whole IgG product derived from horse serum with significant risk for acute and delayed allergic reactions. In October 2000, the US Food and Drug Administration (FDA) approved Crotalidae polyvalent immune Fab (Fab antivenom) marketed as CroFab. This antivenom is derived from sheep serum and digested to remove extraneous proteins as well as the Fc portion of the antibody. Fab antivenom is a less allergenic alternative to the previously manufactured horse serum product from Wyeth (Table A39–1). Equine-derived Crotalidae immune $F(ab')_2$ (Anavip; $F(ab')_2$ antivenom) was more recently approved by the US FDA as an alternative treatment for North American Crotalidae. Unlike the Fab antivenom, this $F(ab')_2$ product keeps the Fab fragments joined to form a larger antibody complex and, as such, is expected to prolong the duration of action (Fig. A39–1).

### North American Coral Snake Antivenin (Equine)

For decades, Wyeth Laboratories manufactured Antivenin (*Micrurus fulvius*) (Equine), which is more commonly known as North American Coral Snake Antivenin (NACSA), for treatment of envenomations by the eastern coral snake (*Micrurus fulvius*) and Texas coral snake (*Micrurus tener*). Although production was temporarily discontinued, at the time of writing, the manufacturer will only provide the antivenom on an "as-needed basis."

## PHARMACOLOGY

### Mechanism of Action

In general, the mechanism of action of antivenoms remains the same regardless of the preparation. The antibody fragments bind and neutralize venom components.

### Crotalidae Polyvalent Immune Fab (Ovine)

***Chemistry/Preparation.*** Crotalidae polyvalent immune Fab (Fab antivenom) is produced by inoculating sheep with the venom of one of the following crotaline snake species: the Eastern diamondback rattlesnake (*Crotalus adamanteus*), Western diamondback rattlesnake (*Crotalus atrox*), cottonmouth (*Agkistrodon piscivorus*), and Mojave rattlesnake (*Crotalus scutulatus*). The species-specific antivenom is then prepared by isolating the antibodies from the sheep serum and digesting the IgG antibodies with papain. This refining process eliminates most of the Fc portion of the immunoglobulin and other potentially immunogenic sheep proteins. All four species-specific antivenoms are then combined to form the final polyvalent product.

***Pharmacokinetics.*** The pharmacokinetics of Fab antivenom are poorly studied. The half-life is estimated between 12 and 23 hours. Although a similarly prepared and sized ovine Fab product yielded a volume of distribution of 0.3 L/kg, a clearance of 32 mL/min, and an elimination half-life of approximately 15 hours, these parameters are not necessarily applicable to Fab antivenom.

### Crotalidae Immune $F(ab')_2$ (Equine)

***Chemistry/Preparation.*** Crotalidae immune $F(ab')_2$ ($F(ab')_2$ antivenom) is manufactured by immunizing horses with the venom of the fer-de-lance (*Bothrops asper*) and the Central American rattlesnake (*Crotalus durissus*). The horse serum is then prepared by pepsin digestion to remove the Fc portion of the antibody creating an $F(ab')_2$ product.

***Pharmacokinetics.*** The pharmacokinetics of $F(ab')_2$ antivenom provide a much longer duration of action than its Fab

**TABLE A39–1 Comparison of Crotalid and Elapid Antivenoms**

| *Antivenom* | *Snake Species Used in Production* | *Digestion* | *Origin* | *Recommended Dosing*[a] |
|---|---|---|---|---|
| Crotalidae Polyvalent Immune Fab | *Crotalus atrox*<br>*Crotalus adamenteus*<br>*Crotalus scutulatus*<br>*Agkistrodon piscivorus* | Papain | Ovine | 4–6 vials repeated as needed to achieve control; then 2 vials every 6 h × 3 doses |
| Crotalidae Immune $F(ab')_2$ | *Bothrops asper*<br>*Crotalus durissus* | Pepsin | Equine | 10 vials repeated as needed to achieve control |
| North American Coral Snake Antivenin | *Micrurus fulvius* | None | Equine | 3–5 vials repeated as needed for clinical improvement |

[a]As recommended by respective package inserts.

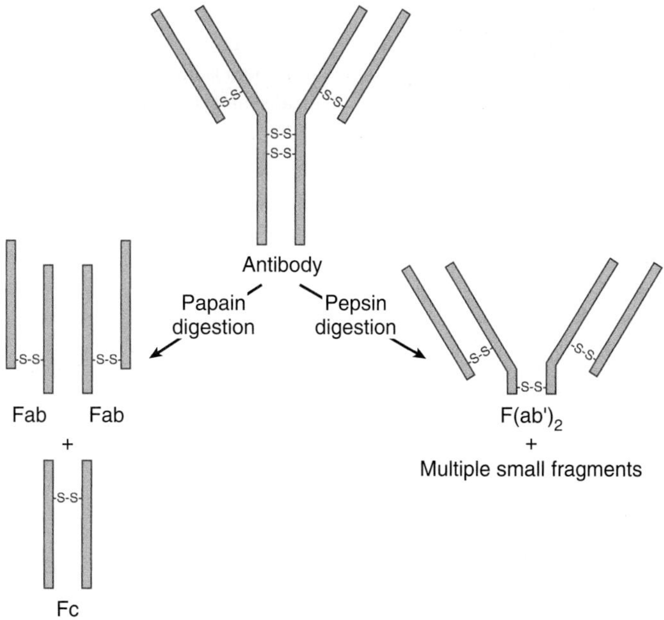


**FIGURE A39–1.** Antibody fragments produced from various digestion treatments during the production of antivenoms.

counterpart. The mean elimination half-life is 133 hours. The volume of distribution is 0.2 L/kg, and the clearance is 1.6 mL/min.

### North American Coral Snake Antivenin IgG (Equine)

***Chemistry/Preparation.*** North American Coral Snake Antivenin (NACSA) is manufactured by immunizing healthy horses with venom from the Eastern coral snake (*Micrurus fulvius*). The horse serum is then purified and concentrated before it is lyophilized for storage as a whole IgG product.

***Pharmacokinetics.*** The pharmacokinetics of NACSA are unknown and unstudied.

## CLINICAL USE

### Crotalidae Polyvalent Immune Fab (Ovine)

Although crotalidae polyvalent immune Fab (Fab antivenom) is designed using the venoms of four North American crotalids, murine lethality studies demonstrate activity against the venom of six other crotaline snake species (*Crotalus viridis helleri*, *C. molossus molossus*, *C. horridus horridus*, *C. horridus atricaudatus*, *Agkistrodon contortrix contortrix*, and *Sistrurus miliarus barbouri*). In addition to these 10 crotalid species, numerous case reports document benefit after envenomation by many other North American crotalids.

Following an envenomation, the major indications for Fab antivenom administration are (1) progression of swelling, (2) significant coagulopathy or thrombocytopenia, (3) neuromuscular toxicity, or (4) hemodynamic compromise. Furthermore, antivenom is also recommended when patients demonstrate muscle fasciculations, weakness, or shock. When indications are met, antivenom should be administered as soon as possible. We recommend against giving antivenom prophylactically to individuals without evidence of envenomation or for localized tissue swelling when other signs of envenomation are absent. This is interpreted as swelling localized to only the bite site or swelling that does not cross a major joint (Chap. 92).

### Crotalidae Immune $F(ab')_2$ (Equine)

Although Crotalidae Immune $F(ab')_2$ ($F(ab')_2$ antivenom) is derived from the venoms of two snake species less commonly encountered in North America, $F(ab')_2$ antivenom effectively neutralizes the venom from 15 different North American snakes. However, as compared to the Fab ovine counterpart, the dose required for neutralization was higher in nearly every case. Clinical indications for use are the same as for Fab antivenom.

### North American Coral Snake Antivenin IgG (Equine)

North American Coral Snake Antivenin (NACSA) is the recommended treatment for envenomation by the eastern coral snake (*Micrurus fulvius*) and Texas coral snake (*Micrurus tener*). This antivenom does not treat envenomations from coral snakes found in Mexico, Central America, or South America. Furthermore, bites by the less virulent Arizona coral snake (Sonoran, *Micruroides euryoxanthus*) do not produce significant envenomation requiring treatment with antivenom. Indications for NACSA administration include the development of any signs or symptoms consistent with coral snake envenomation such as paresthesias, slurred speech, ptosis, diplopia, dysphagia, stridor, muscle weakness, fasciculations, and paralysis.

In the absence of antivenom, the mainstay of treatment consists of supportive care. In particular, if respiratory failure results from muscle weakness, prolonged mechanical ventilation is often necessary until neurologic recovery. Paralysis is completely reversible; however, it typically takes weeks to months to resolve completely.

## ADVERSE EFFECTS AND SAFETY ISSUES

### Crotalidae Polyvalent Immune Fab (Ovine)

Acute hypersensitivity reactions are the most significant safety concerns when administering antivenom to patients. Urticaria, rash, bronchospasm, pruritus, angioedema, anaphylaxis, and delayed serum sickness are all associated with use of Fab ovine antivenom. The reported incidence of acute reactions is approximately 5% to 6%.

When antivenom is administered too rapidly, nonimmunogenically mediated anaphylactoid reactions also occur. If the patient requires rapid administration of antivenom because of the severity of the envenomation, $H_1$ histamine receptor antagonists and an epinephrine infusion should be readily available in case symptoms develop.

For acute anaphylactic reactions, the antivenom is stopped, and supportive and pharmacologic therapy begun. Intravenous epinephrine at 2 to 4 μg/min (0.03–0.06 μg/kg/min for children) should be initiated and then titrated to effect. After the symptoms of hypersensitivity resolve, the antivenom is restarted only in patients at high risk for significant morbidity or mortality from envenomation. In such cases, the diluted antivenom infusion is restarted at 1 to 2 mL/h, while the epinephrine infusion is continued. The antivenom infusion rate is slowly increased as tolerated. If anaphylaxis recurs, the antivenom is stopped and the epinephrine infusion increased until symptoms resolve.

In addition to acute allergic reactions, delayed hypersensitivity reactions including serum sickness are reported to occur in 16% of patients. Most episodes of serum sickness are mild and include urticaria, pruritus, and malaise. Arthralgias, lymphadenopathy, and fever also develop. In rare severe cases, glomerulonephritis, vasculitis, myocarditis, and neuritis occur. We recommend that patients with serum sickness symptoms receive treatment with 2 mg/kg (a maximum dose of 60 mg per day for adults) of oral prednisone and tapered over 2 to 3 weeks. Oral $H_1$ receptor antagonists are reasonable for immediate symptomatic treatment as well. The vast majority of patients are managed as outpatients, and most respond favorably to this regimen.

### Crotalidae Immune F(ab′)$_2$ (Equine)

Although its use in the US is limited, adverse effects and safety issues remain the same for F(ab′)$_2$ as for Fab antivenoms. Monitoring for and treatment of acute and delayed adverse reactions is the same as described for Fab antivenom.

### North American Coral Snake Antivenin IgG (Equine)

Acute and delayed hypersensitivity reactions are the most significant safety concerns when providing antivenom products to patients. The risk of acute hypersensitivity reactions with NACSA is approximately 20%. Patients with a known horse serum allergy or who have been treated with equine-derived antivenoms previously should only receive treatment with NACSA if there is a significant risk of severe morbidity or mortality and appropriate management for anaphylactic reactions is readily available. For these patients we recommend using an intravenous epinephrine infusion (2–4 μg/min for adults) prior to antivenom administration. The antivenom is then started at a very low rate of infusion, and if tolerated, the rate is increased. If an acute allergic reaction develops, the antivenom is immediately stopped and the epinephrine drip titrated for symptoms.

## PREGNANCY AND LACTATION

### Crotalidae Polyvalent Immune Fab (Ovine)

Pregnant patients who meet criteria for treatment should also receive antivenom, which is currently listed as Category C by the US FDA. Continuous fetal monitoring is important. It is unknown if Fab antivenom is excreted in breast milk.

### Crotalidae Immune F(ab′)$_2$ (Equine)

Pregnant patients who meet criteria for treatment should also receive antivenom, which is currently listed as Category C by the US FDA. No evidence exists concerning use during pregnancy. Continuous fetal monitoring is important. It is unknown if F(ab)$_2$ antivenom is excreted in breast milk.

### North American Coral Snake Antivenin (Equine)

Currently NACSA does not have a US FDA pregnancy listing. Considering the severe morbidity associated with coral snake envenomation, we recommend that pregnant patients who meet criteria for treatment receive antivenom. Continuous fetal monitoring is important. It is unknown if NACSA is excreted in breast milk.

## DOSING AND ADMINISTRATION

### Crotalidae Polyvalent Immune Fab (Ovine)

According to the manufacturer, the only contraindication is an allergy to papaya or papain. Antivenom should be administered in a monitored setting in which resuscitation can be performed and airway supplies are readily available. Antivenom is packaged in vials as a lyophilized powder, which must be reconstituted and diluted as described in the package insert. The initial recommended dose is at least four to six vials based on clinical experience or consultation with an expert. The vials are mixed in 250 mL 0.9% sodium chloride solution and administered over 1 hour. For patients who present with cardiovascular collapse or life-threatening toxicity, we recommend a starting dose of 8 to 12 vials of Fab antivenom.

In order to avoid serious adverse reactions, the first dose of antivenom is administered cautiously at an initial rate of 10 mL/h. If after 5 minutes no adverse reactions occur, then the rate is doubled every few minutes, as tolerated by the patient, with the goal of infusing the first dose over 1 hour. If the patient tolerates the initial dose, subsequent doses can be given at a rate of 250 mL/h without a need for rate titration. The total dose of antivenom required to control an envenomation varies widely. We define control as improvement in hemodynamic parameters as normalization is not always possible. After achieving control, maintenance doses of two vials every 6 hours for three doses are recommended. An algorithm for Fab antivenom administration for moderate to severe crotaline envenomation is shown in Fig. A39–2. Some patients will demonstrate recurrence of swelling during their maintenance infusions. For this reason, close monitoring of extremity swelling is recommended for 18 to

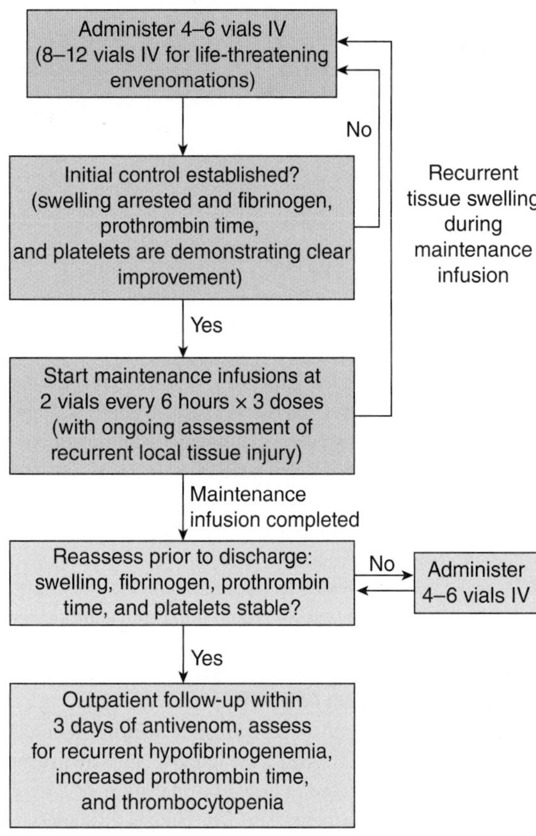


**FIGURE A39–2.** Algorithm for Crotalidae Polyvalent Immune Fab administration for treatment of moderate-to-severe Crotaline envenomation.

24 hours after control has been achieved. Despite successful completion of maintenance antivenom doses, some patients also develop a recurrence of coagulopathy and/or thrombocytopenia. Therefore, we recommend repeat prothrombin time, fibrinogen, and platelet counts be performed 2 to 3 days and again 5 to 7 days in all patients after hospital discharge to ensure late recurrent hematologic effects have not developed.

### Crotalidae Immune F(ab′)$_2$ (Equine)

Prior to administration, the same preparation should occur for F(ab′)$_2$ administration as for Fab antivenoms. However, there are no contraindications listed on the F(ab′)$_2$ package insert. Antivenom is packaged in vials as a lyophilized powder, which must be reconstituted and diluted as specified in the package insert.

The initial recommended dose of F(ab′)$_2$ is 10 vials, which are mixed in 250 mL 0.9% sodium chloride solution and administered over 1 hour. For the first 10 minutes, the infusion rate is 25 to 50 mL/h, which is then increased to the full 250-mL/h rate until completion if no allergic reactions develop. Repeat doses of 10 vials are recommended until control is achieved. Clinical trials suggest maintenance dosing is not needed. However, the package insert recommends four vials adminstered over one hour as needed for recurrent venom effects and at least 18 hours of monitoring after obtaining control. The caveats for Fab antivenom administration (infusion rate and treatment of allergic reactions) apply to F(ab′)$_2$ antivenom. Recurrent venom effects still occur in 5% to 10% of case. After hospital discharge, outpatient monitoring is still recommended as experience with this antivenom is limited.

### North American Coral Snake Antivenin IgG (Equine)

Prior to administration, the same preparation should occur for NACSA administration as for the other antivenoms. Antivenom is packaged in vials as a lyophilized powder, which must be reconstituted and diluted as specified in the package insert. The initial recommended dose of NACSA is three to five vials based on availability and clinical experience. The vials are mixed in 250 mL 0.9% sodium chloride solution and administered over 1 hour. Additional antivenom doses are indicated for the evolution of any neurologic abnormalities including, but not limited to, paresthesias, slurred speech, ptosis, diplopia, dysphagia, stridor, muscle weakness, fasciculations, and paralysis. The caveats for crotaline antivenom administration (infusion rate and treatment of allergic reactions) apply to coral snake antivenom, except less antivenom is usually required for coral snakes.

## FORMULATION AND ACQUISITION

### Crotalidae Polyvalent Immune Fab (Ovine) and Crotalidae Immune F(ab′)$_2$ (Equine)

Hospitals with native crotaline species within their region should maintain Fab antivenoms at all times. Because the timely administration is the cornerstone of treatment, attempting to obtain antivenom at the time of an emergency will likely introduce a significant delay to treatment and exacerbate morbidity.

### North American Coral Snake Antivenin IgG (Equine)

In order to obtain NASCA, contact the local poison center or Pfizer, which currently holds the rights to this antivenom. Poison centers have access to the online Antivenom Index, which is useful when attempting to locate coral snake antivenom. Otherwise, Pfizer will provide the antivenom on an as-needed basis.

Special Considerations

# SC9 EXOTIC NONNATIVE SNAKE ENVENOMATIONS

## HISTORY AND EPIDEMIOLOGY

Current estimates place the worldwide annual incidence of snakebites as high as 5.5 million, of which roughly 50% are thought to be from venomous snakes. Estimated annual complications include 400,000 amputations and approximately 100,000 deaths. Snakes, although feared by many, are popular around the world as pets. This Special Consideration will discuss the evaluation and management of patients envenomated in the United States (US) by nonnative snakes (also known as exotic snakes). A review from 2005 through 2011 of the National Poison Data System (NPDS), maintained by the American Association of Poison Control Centers (AAPCC), confirmed 258 exotic snakebites reports, of which 218 were identified by genus and species, from a total of 71 different varieties. Forty-three percent of these bites were from Viperidae, with the top four species being gaboon viper (*Bitis gabonica*), bush master (*Lachesis mutus*), the sharpnosed viper (*Deinagkistrodon acutus*), and the hognosed viper (*Bothrops ophroyomegas*). Thirty-nine percent of these bites were from Elapidaes, most commonly the monocellate cobra (*Naja naja kaouthia*), black necked spitting cobra (*Naja nigricollis*), and the black mamba (*Dendroaspis polylepis*).

## TAXONOMY

The naming of snakes has evolved, and the renaming currently continues at a rapid pace as a result of advances in DNA testing and research. There are approximately 2,700 snake species in the world, of which 20% are known to be venomous to humans. Venomous snakes are divided into four major families as shown in Table SC9–1.

## ANTIVENOM INDEX

The Antivenom Index (AI), created as a joint effort of the Association of Zoos and Aquariums (AZA) and the AAPCC, is a database that contains the location of all nonnative snake antivenoms stored throughout the zoos in the US. The AI can be searched by the common name or the scientific name of the venomous snake and results in a list of possible snakes that match the searched term. A list of antivenoms active against each genus and species is displayed, including which zoos stock them and how many vials are available. Additional information includes antivenom package inserts (many of which are translated into English), which include the expiration dates, and additional information such as links to various recommendations on the housing, stocking, and administration of antivenoms. Access to the AI is limited to the AZA and the AAPCC (all US poison centers have access and can be reached at 1-800-222-1222).

## VENOM TOXICITY

Common venom components from the Elapidae and Viperidae families are classified as neurotoxic, hemotoxic, and/or myotoxic. Elapidae venom commonly causes neurotoxic effects such as blurred vision, paresthesias, ptosis, paralysis of facial muscles, difficulty swallowing, respiratory paralysis, and generalized flaccid paralysis. In contrast, Viperidae venom commonly causes hemotoxicity and myotoxicity, although some species also have neurotoxic effects. The hematologic effects include petechiae, purpura, ecchymosis, bleeding, and changes in platelets and coagulation parameters. Myotoxic effects include swelling, necrosis, and skin blebs and are accompanied by elevations of creatine kinase and aminotransferases with possible impairment of kidney function.

## CLINICAL PRESENTATION AND INITIAL MANAGEMENT

It is useful to consult with an expert to help identify the snake and determine specific signs, symptoms, and treatment options. Experts are found at local poison centers or a local zoological society or serpentarium. The clinical presentation of patients with exotic snake envenomation is extremely variable as mentioned in the above section. Several basic

**TABLE SC9–1 Taxonomy of Venomous Snakes**

| *Family* | *Subfamily* | *Representative Species* |
|---|---|---|
| Elapidae | Elipinae | Cobras (*Naja* spp.) |
| | | King cobras (*Ophiophagus hannah*) |
| | | Mambas (*Dendroaspis* spp.) |
| | | Kraits (*Bungarus* spp.) |
| | | Coral snakes (*Micrurus* spp. and *Micruroides* spp.) |
| | Hydrophiinae | Various sea snakes |
| | Laticaudinae | Sea kraits |
| Viperidae | Azemiopinae | Fea's viper (*Azemiops feae*) |
| | Viperinae (Old World vipers) | Russell's viper (*Vipera russelii*) |
| | | Gaboon viper (*Bitis gabonica*) |
| | | Saw-scaled viper (*Echis carinatus*) |
| | | Death adders (*Acanthophis* spp.) |
| | Crotalinae (pit vipers) | Rattlesnakes (*Crotalus* and *Sistrurus* spp.) |
| | | Copperheads (*Agkistrodon* spp.) |
| Atractaspididae | | Stiletto snakes (*Atractaspis* spp.) |
| Colubridae | | African boomslang (*Dispholidus typus*) |
| | | Twig snake (*Thelotornis* spp.) |

| TABLE SC9–2 General Approach to a Patient With an Exotic Snake Envenomation |
|---|
| Immobilize the bitten limb in a dependent position and rapidly transport the patient to a medical facility. Initiate irrigation with water if the eyes are exposed. |
| Determine the time and location of bite, and mark the borders. Follow and mark the progression over time. |
| Determine the species responsible for the bite. If the bite occurred at a zoo, the zoo may have a written plan for management of the specific species ready to accompany the patient (often a zoo employee) that includes the name of species, appropriate first aid, other management guidelines, and any antivenom that is available. Patients who own exotic snakes may know the identity but often use misleading or inaccurate common names, in which case, it is necessary to contact a local herpetologist, who often can be found through the poison center or a local zoo, to help identify the snake. |
| Standard resuscitation techniques are indicated for cardiovascular or respiratory failure. |
| Initiate volume repletion if there is massive hemorrhage or hypotension. |
| Physical examination should include evaluation of signs of local envenomation (pain, swelling, bleeding, and bruising), painful and tender enlargement of lymph nodes, hypotension, spontaneous bleeding, ptosis, muscle tone, cranial nerve function, myalgias, and a complete neurotoxic assessment. Laboratory assessment should include a complete blood count, coagulation profile, electrolytes and kidney function, creatine kinase, aminotransferase, urinalysis for blood and myoglobin, and an electrocardiogram. |
| Begin the process of locating, obtaining, and receiving permission to administer antivenom, even if it is unclear that foreign antivenom will be available or required. |
| Prepare for the treatment of anaphylaxis if foreign antivenom is to be administered. |
| Because of uncertainties in prediction of clinical evolution and severity of symptom presentation, close monitoring in an intensive care unit is preferred for all patients with exotic envenomations. This will allow for appropriate clinical and laboratory monitoring specific to the needs of the patient. A minimum of 24 hours of hospital observation is recommended to assess delayed evolution of signs or symptoms. Follow-up for serum sickness is reasonable. |

steps are recommended for the initial management of these patients as outlined in Table SC9–2.

## Zoological and Exotic Antivenoms

Hospitals in the US are not permitted to stock antivenoms for exotic snakes that have not been produced for the US market and submitted to the Food and Drug Administration (FDA) process for drug sale and administration. Zoos are permitted to stock antivenoms for the species of snakes locally housed for the purpose of treating an unintentional exposure, but importation requires permits from the US Department of Agriculture.

## Hospital Use of Exotic Antivenoms

To administer foreign antivenoms to patients, the antivenom must have an Investigational New Drug (IND) Application filed with the US FDA. This can either be done ahead of time or with emergency approval by the US FDA. Because delays to care are inevitable, it is important to have a detailed plan that includes hospital personnel and relevant outside consultants. Challenges should be expected with locating the correct antivenom and transporting it to the hospital. Once brought to the facility, the treating physician should contact the US FDA to obtain approval to administer the antivenom as an IND under emergency use. Contact numbers are found at http://www.fda.gov/RegulatoryInformation/Guidances/ucm126491.htm. In addition, informed consent from the patient is required, and both the Institutional Review Board (IRB) and Drug and Formulary Committee must be notified and provide approval. Many IRBs have emergency processes to expedite such a request. If such approval cannot be obtained in a clinically relevant time, the IRB must be notified of the emergency treatment within five working days of the administration. The physician must also complete the appropriate IND paperwork (Form FDA 1571) and submit a comprehensive case report. The pharmacy department should also be notified as soon as possible to allow the staff time to begin investigating preparation and administration instructions. Having knowledge of these required procedures will expedite the administration of the antivenom.

## Other Therapies

Because of some homology across snake venoms, it is possible to use antivenom derived against specific snakes in the treatment of envenomation from other snakes with related venoms. US FDA–approved coral snake antivenom was used in an experimental model of nonnative elapid envenomation. Similarly, US FDA–approved crotalid antivenom demonstrated efficacy against mice treated with venom from *Crotalus durissus terrificus*, *Bothrops atrox*, and *Bitis gabonica*. In fact, a single case report demonstrates utilization of this principle of cross-reactivity when a patient envenomated by *C. durissus terrificus* was successfully treated with US FDA–approved Crotalidae Polyvalent Immune Fab. Such cross-reactivity should never be assumed based on common or taxonomic identification. The manufacturer of Crotalidae Polyvalent Immune Fab lists experimental cross-reactivity with a number of species in the AI (Table SC9–3). The decision to use Crotalidae Polyvalent Immune Fab for a patient envenomated by a non-US species of snake with known experimental cross-reactivity should be based on the severity of envenomation, the availability of species-specific antivenom, and the risks associated with administration of species-specific antivenom versus the risks of Crotalidae Polyvalent Immune Fab (Antidotes in Brief: A39).

The venom of many neurotoxic snakes interferes with neuromuscular transmission similar to neuromuscular blockers used in clinical medicine (Chap. 39). Neostigmine increases the $LD_{50}$ of animals treated with *Naja haje haje* venom. Clinical data suggest improvement in neurologic deficits and respiratory failure after neostigmine is given to humans suffering neurotoxic snake envenomation. Patients typically received 0.5 to 1 mg of neostigmine IV immediately following pretreatment with 0.5 to 0.6 mg of atropine IV, repeated every 10 to 30 minutes based on response. Because the complications of atropine and neostigmine at these doses are small, administration is reasonable if antivenom is unavailable or delayed.

It is important to remember that there is a wide variation in the standards for preparation of antivenoms around the world. Although many products are highly purified antibody

**TABLE SC9–3 Experimental Cross-Reactivity Between Crotalidae Polyvalent Immune Fab and Nonnative Snakes Is Suggested for These Species[a]**

| Genus | Species and Subspecies | Common Name | Natural Habitat |
|---|---|---|---|
| *Agkistrodon* | *bilineatus bilineatus* | Cantil, common cantil, Mexican moccasin, tropical moccasin, Mexican cantil | Mexico and Central America |
| | *bilineatus howardgloydi* | Castellana | Honduras, Nicaragua, and Costa Rica |
| | *bilineatus lemosespinali* | Cantil, Mexican moccasin | Mexico and Central America |
| | *bilineatus russeolus* | Cantil, common cantil, Mexican moccasin | Mexico and Central America |
| | *bilineatus taylori* | Taylor's cantil, ornate cantil | Mexico |
| *Bothriechis* | *aurifer* | Yellow-blotched palm pit viper, Guatemalan palm viper | Mexico and Guatemala |
| | *bicolor* | Guatemalan palm pit viper, Guatemalan tree viper | Mexico, Guatemala, and Honduras |
| | *rowleyi* | Mexican palm pit viper | Mexico |
| | *schlegelii* | Eyelash viper | Central and South America |
| *Bothrops* | *asper* | Fer-de-lance | Mexico and South America |
| | *moojeni* | Brazilian lancehead | Brazil |
| *Crotalus* | *basiliscus* | Mexican west coast rattlesnake, Mexican green rattler | Mexico |
| | *cerastes cerastes* | Sidewinder, horned rattlesnake, sidewinder rattlesnake | US and northwestern Mexico |
| | *cerastes cercobombus* | Sonoran Desert sidewinder, Sonoran sidewinder | US and northwestern Mexico |
| | *durissus durissus* | South American rattlesnake, tropical rattlesnake | South America |
| | *durissus totonacus* | Totonacan rattlesnake | Northern Mexico |
| | *durissus tzabcan* | Middle American rattlesnake, Central American rattlesnake, tzabcan | Mexico and Central America |
| | *enyo enyo* | Baja California rattlesnake, Lower California rattlesnake | US and northwestern Mexico |
| | *exsul (Ruber)* | Red diamond rattlesnake, red rattlesnake, red diamond snake | Baja California, Mexico |
| | *exsul exsul (Ruber)* | Red diamond rattlesnake, red rattlesnake, red diamond snake | Baja California, Mexico |
| | *intermedius gloydi* | Oaxacan small-headed rattlesnake | Mexico |
| | *lannomi* | Autlán rattlesnake | Mexico |
| | *lepidus castaneus* | Rock rattlesnake | US and Mexico |
| | *lepidus klauberi* | Banded rock rattlesnake, green rattlesnake, green rock rattlesnake | US and Mexico |
| | *lepidus lepidus* | Rock rattlesnake, green rattlesnake, blue rattlesnake | US and Mexico |
| | *lepidus maculosus* | Durango rock rattlesnake | Mexico |
| | *lepidus morulus* | Rock rattlesnake | Mexico |
| | *mitchelli angelensis* | Angel de la Guarda Island speckled rattlesnake | Angel de la Guarda Island, Mexico |
| | *mitchelli mitchelli* | Speckled rattlesnake, Mitchell's rattlesnake, white rattlesnake | US and Mexico |
| | *mitchelli muertensis* | El Muerto Island speckled rattlesnake | El Muerto Island, Mexico |
| | *mitchelli pyrrhus* | Southwestern speckled rattlesnake, Mitchell's rattlesnake | US and Mexico |
| | *molossus estabanensis* | San Esteban Island rattlesnake | San Esteban Island, Mexico |
| | *molossus molossus* | Northern black-tailed rattlesnake, green rattler | US and Mexico |
| | *molossus nigrescens* | Mexican black-tailed rattlesnake | US and Mexico |
| | *molossus oaxacus* | Oaxacan black-tailed rattlesnake | Mexico |
| | *polystictus* | Mexican lance-headed rattlesnake, lance-headed rattlesnake | Mexico |
| | *pricei miquihuanus* | Eastern twin-spotted rattlesnake | Mexico |
| | *pricei pricei* | Western twin-spotted rattlesnake | Mexico |
| | *pusillus* | Tancitaran dusky rattlesnake | Mexico |
| | *ruber lorenzoensis* | San Lorenzo Island rattlesnake | San Lorenzo Island, Mexico |
| | *ruber lucasensis* | San Lucan diamond rattlesnake | Mexico |
| | *ruber ruber* | Red diamond rattlesnake | US and Mexico |
| | *scutulatus salvini* | Huamantlan rattlesnake | Mexico |
| | *scutulatus scutulatus* | Mojave rattlesnake | US and Mexico |
| | *stejnegeri* | Long-tailed rattlesnake | Mexico |
| | *tigris* | Tiger rattlesnake, tiger rattler | US and Mexico |
| | *tortugensis* | Tortuga Island diamond rattlesnake, Tortuga Island rattlesnake | Tortuga Island, Mexico |
| | *transversus* | Cross-banded mountain rattlesnake | Mexico |
| | *triseriatus aquilus* | Querétaro dusky rattlesnake, Queretaran dusky rattlesnake | Mexico |
| | *triseriatus armstrongi* | Western dusky rattlesnake | Mexico |
| | *triseriatus triseriatus* | Dusky rattlesnake | Mexico |
| | *viridis caliginus* | Coronado Island rattlesnake | Coronado Island, Mexico |

(*Continued*)

**TABLE SC9–3 Experimental Cross-Reactivity Between Crotalidae Polyvalent Immune Fab and Nonnative Snakes Is Suggested for These Species[a] (*Continued*)**

| *Genus* | *Species and Subspecies* | *Common Name* | *Natural Habitat* |
|---|---|---|---|
| | *willardi amabilis* | Del Nido ridge-nosed rattlesnake | Mexico |
| | *willardi meridionalis* | Southern ridge-nosed rattlesnake | Mexico |
| | *willardi obscurus* | Animas ridge-nosed rattlesnake | US and Mexico |
| | *willardi silus* | Chihuahuan ridge-nosed rattlesnake | Mexico |
| | *willardi willardi* | Arizona ridge-nosed rattlesnake | US and Mexico |
| *Ophryacus* | *undulatus* | Mexican horned pit viper, undulated pit viper | Mexico |
| *Porthidium* | *dunni* | Dunn's hognosed pit viper | Mexico |
| | *godmani* | Godman's montane pit viper, Godman's pit viper | Mexico and Central America |
| | *hespere* | Colima hognosed pit viper | Mexico |
| | *nasutum* | Rainforest hognosed pit viper, horned hog-nosed viper | Mexico, Central America, and South America |
| | *yucatanicum* | Yucatán hognosed pit viper | Mexico |
| *Sistrurus* | *ravus* | Mexican pigmy rattlesnake, Mexican pygmy rattlesnake | Mexico |

[a]"Cross-reactivity" defined here as experimental evidence supplied by the manufacturer to the Antivenom Index. Although clinical evidence of benefit is lacking, use of Crotalidae Polyvalent Immune Fab is reasonable in these envenomations based on a risk-to-benefit analysis when species-specific antivenom is lacking, delayed, or contraindicated (due to allergy), and the envenomation is a risk to life or limb.

fragments, some continue to use whole immunoglobulins that have a sufficient risk for anaphylaxis. Prior to antivenom administration, preparations must be made to treat anaphylaxis. The appropriate level of nursing care and monitoring should be available, IV access should be secured, and standard drugs (epinephrine, corticosteroids, antihistamines) and airway management equipment should be immediately available.

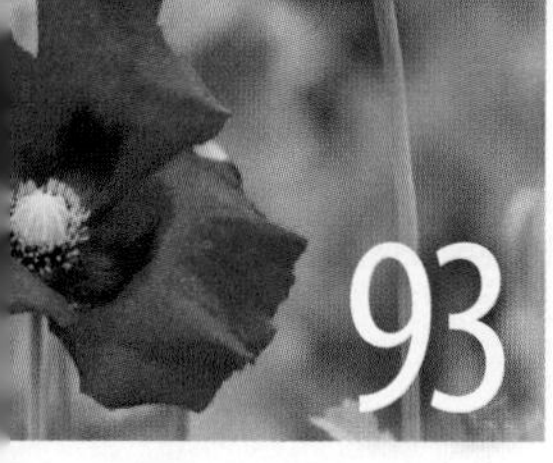



# 93 SMOKE INHALATION

## HISTORY AND EPIDEMIOLOGY

Smoke is generated as the result of thermal degradation of a material. It is a complex mixture of heated air containing suspended solid and liquid particles (aerosols), gases, and vapors. The complex and ever-growing variety of materials used in our environment contributes to the broad spectrum of xenobiotics present in typical smoke (Table 93–1).

Smoke inhalation is a complex medical syndrome involving diverse toxicologic injuries, making care of smoke-injured patients very challenging. These injuries occur both locally within the respiratory tract and systemically. It is, in fact, smoke inhalation—not thermal burns—that is the leading cause of death from fires. An estimated 50% to 80% of fire-related deaths result from smoke inhalation rather than dermal burns or trauma, and deaths related to smoke inhalation occur much more prevalently in an enclosed-space environment. Compared with other industrialized countries, the United States has one of the highest rates of fire-related deaths in the world. Disastrous enclosed-space fires are a frequent reminder of the role of inhalation injury in fire deaths. Despite improved firefighting resources, mass casualties from smoke inhalation are common.

**TABLE 93–1 Common Materials and Their Thermal Degradation Products**

| *Materials* | *Thermal Degradation Products* |
|---|---|
| Wool | Ammonia, carbon monoxide, chlorine, cyanide, hydrogen chloride, phosgene |
| Silk | Ammonia, cyanide, hydrogen sulfide, sulfur dioxide |
| Nylon | Ammonia, cyanide |
| Wood, cotton, paper | Acetaldehyde, acetic acid, acrolein, carbon monoxide, formic acid, formaldehyde, methane |
| Petroleum materials | Acetic acid, acrolein, carbon monoxide, formic acid |
| Polystyrene | Styrene |
| Acrylic | Acrolein, carbon monoxide, hydrogen chloride |
| Plastics | Aldehydes, ammonia, chlorine, cyanide, hydrogen chloride, nitrogen oxides, phosgene, |
| Polyvinyl chloride | Carbon monoxide, chlorine, hydrogen chloride, phosgene |
| Polyurethane | Cyanide, isocyanates |
| Melamine resins | Ammonia, cyanide |
| Rubber | Hydrogen sulfide, sulfur dioxide |
| Sulfur-containing materials | Sulfur dioxide |
| Nitrogen-containing materials | Cyanide, isocyanates, oxides of nitrogen |
| Fluorinated resins | Hydrogen fluoride |
| Fire retardant materials | Hydrogen bromide, hydrogen chloride |

## PATHOPHYSIOLOGY

Toxic thermal degradation products are classified into three categories: simple asphyxiants, irritant gases, and chemical asphyxiants (Table 93–2). Simple asphyxiants, such as carbon dioxide, exert their toxicity by displacing oxygen, resulting in an oxygen-deprived environment, thereby decreasing the amount of oxygen available for absorption. Irritant gases are chemically reactive compounds that exert a local effect on the respiratory tract (Chap. 94). For irritant gases, the degree of water solubility is the most important chemical characteristic in determining the timing and anatomic location of respiratory tract injury. Highly water-soluble xenobiotics, such as ammonia and hydrogen chloride, primarily injure the upper airway by rapidly combining with mucosal water, leaving little of the parent compound to travel further down the airway. These xenobiotics quickly damage mucosal cells, which subsequently release mediators of inflammation or reactive oxygen species (ROS). Xenobiotics with low water solubility, such as phosgene and oxides of nitrogen, react with the upper respiratory mucosa and eyes more slowly and do not elicit the irritation and aversion stimului that prompt an escape response. These xenobiotics more typically reach the distal lung parenchyma, where they react slowly to create delayed toxic effects. Xenobiotics with intermediate water solubility, such as chlorine and isocyanates, are more likely to result in damage to both the upper and lower respiratory tracts.

Damage to the tracheobronchial tree is mediated by inhaled particulates and toxic gases, which result in deposition of corrosives and oxidants. Direct thermal injury is less likely to occur as a result of the efficient cooling ability of the upper airways. Direct injury to the tracheobronchial tree and an intense inflammatory response lead to an increase in airway resistance from mucosal edema, bronchoconstriction, and accumulation of intraluminal debris and airway secretions.

**TABLE 93–2 Toxic Thermal Degradation Products**

| *Asphyxiants* | *Irritants* |
|---|---|
| **Simple** | **High Water Solubility (Upper Airway Injury)** |
| Carbon dioxide | Ammonia |
| **Chemical** | Hydrogen chloride |
| Carbon monoxide | Sulfur dioxide |
| Hydrogen cyanide | **Intermediate Water Solubility (Upper and Lower Respiratory Tract Injury)** |
| Hydrogen sulfide | Chlorine |
| Oxides of nitrogen | Isocyanates |
| | **Low Water Solubility (Pulmonary Parenchymal Injury)** |
| | Oxides of nitrogen |
| | Phosgene |

Irritant xenobiotics that reach the alveoli injure the lung parenchyma. Pathophysiologic changes of acute respiratory distress syndrome (ARDS) decrease lung compliance and bacterial defenses and lead to ventilation–perfusion mismatch with intrapulmonary shunting, increased extravascular lung water, and microvascular permeability. Lung compliance is further decreased by atelectasis when xenobiotics inactivate pulmonary surfactant. In addition, ventilation–perfusion mismatch occurs when pulmonary blood flow is diverted both by hypoxia and vasoactive mediators of inflammation. Xenobiotics cause additional injury by impairing clearance by the mucociliary apparatus, altering alveolar macrophage function, and impairing phagocytosis of bacteria, all of which predispose to pulmonary infections and sepsis. The combination of the delayed toxic effects of some inhaled xenobiotics and the slowly developing inflammatory response helps explain the progression of parenchymal injury during the first 24 hours after smoke exposure.

Thermal degradation of organic material produces finely divided carbonaceous particulate matter (soot) suspended in hot gases. These carbonaceous particles adsorb other combustion products from the environment and then adhere to the mucosa of the airways, allowing adsorbed irritant xenobiotics to desorb and react with the mucosal surface moisture. The deposition of these particles in the respiratory tract depends on their size, with particles of 1 to 3 μm reaching the alveoli.

Chemical asphyxiants considered are primarily carbon monoxide (CO), hydrogen sulfide, and cyanide. These chemical asphyxiants impair extrapulmonary oxygen delivery or utilization, with the route of exposure being commonly smoke inhalation, without much, if any, direct pulmonary toxicity, per se (Chaps. 95 and 96). Combustion of nitrogen-containing materials also generates oxides of nitrogen, which are irritants and rarely induces the formation of methemoglobin (Chap. 97).

## CLINICAL MANIFESTATIONS

The primary clinical problem in smoke inhalation is respiratory compromise; therefore, clinical evaluation should specifically address this issue. Additionally, systemic toxicity from inhaled chemicals, such as CO and cyanide, can lead to cardiovascular dysfunction and hypotension and can directly and indirectly impair mental status. Clinical symptoms suggestive of significant smoke exposure include eye, mouth, and throat irritation. Cough, chest tightness, and complaints of dyspnea are common.

On examination, burns to the face or singed hairs of the head, face, or nasal passages are associated with an increased risk of inhalational injury but are not present in all patients with significant inhalational injury. Soot around the mouth or nares is also indicative of an increased risk. Changes in voice and difficulty managing airway secretions (drooling or hypersalvation) are important signs of progressive airway edema. Ophthalmic examination should occur in all patients who either complain of ocular symptoms or whose symptoms are unable to be obtained because of unresponsiveness. Rhonchi, crackles, and wheezing on chest auscultation are suggestive of inhalational injury, but these finding are often delayed by 24 to 36 hours and are a poor prognostic indicator if present on initial patient presentation. Tachycardia and tachypnea occur secondary to hypoxemia and systemic xenobiotic toxicity. Hypotension occurs secondary to hypoxemia and systemic toxicity and presents with faint or absent peripheral pulses. Altered mental status, including agitation, confusion, or coma, is most often attributable to hypoxia from either pulmonary compromise or cellular hypoxia, but altered consciousness also results from direct effects of systemic xenobiotics, such as CO, or from concomitant trauma or drug or alcohol intoxication.

## DIAGNOSTIC TESTING

Diagnostic studies should focus on assessing for airway and pulmonary injury as well as the ability of the patient to oxygenate and ventilate. Analysis of either an arterial blood gas (ABG) or a venous blood gas (VBG), cooximetry and chest radiography (CXR) should be obtained initially in all patients with smoke inhalation. Healthcare professionals should obtain a rapid lactate concentration in all seriously ill patients with smoke inhalation to aid in evaluation of possible cyanide toxicity.

An ABG analysis assesses both pulmonary function (gas exchange) and blood pH. Measurement of oxygen saturation by transcutaneous pulse oximetry is unreliable in patients with smoke inhalation because of the potential presence of dyshemoglobinemias. Cooximetry measures both carboxyhemoglobin and methemoglobin levels and is recommended in those with significant exposure or signs or symptoms of smoke inhalation. Blood pH and lactate concentration are more useful tools in acutely assessing for cyanide exposure. A blood lactate concentration of 10 mmol/L or greater suggests cyanide poisoning and supports the administration of empiric antidotal treatment to critically ill fire-exposed patients.

Chest radiography is recommended early in the assessment of patients with smoke inhalation but is an insensitive indicator of pulmonary injury. The most frequent abnormal findings on initial CXR are diffuse alveolar and interstitial changes, found in up to 34% of patients. Serial CXRs after a baseline study are generally more helpful in detecting evolving pulmonary injury after smoke inhalation (Fig. 93–1). Computed tomography (CT) of the lungs is a more sensitive modality than plain radiography for detecting early pulmonary injury after smoke inhalation. However, since there are no data to support improved patient outcomes when using CT, we recommend against the routine use of CT scanning in all patients with smoke inhalation.

In intubated patients, diagnostic fiberoptic bronchoscopy remains the standard in assessing smoke inhalational injury. Bronchoscopy allows for direct visualization of the upper airways, allows for grading of the injury, and helps to determine those at risk for developing inhalational injury. Early diagnostic bronchoscopy has yet to show an improvement in patient outcome, but because it aids in diagnosis and helps assess the severity of injury, it is reasonable to perform in intubated patients with suspicion of inhalation injury.

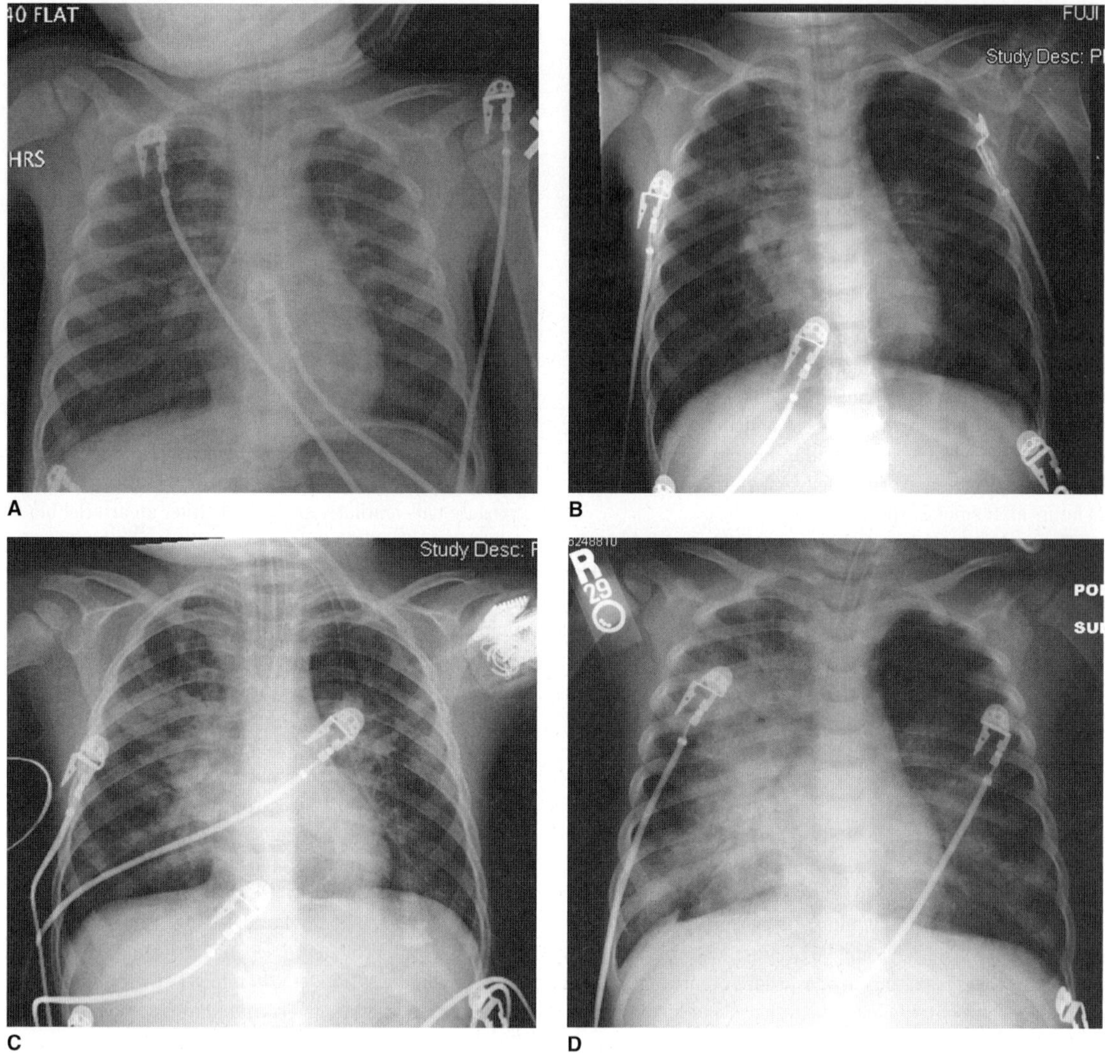


**FIGURE 93–1.** (**A**) Initial chest radiograph of a 3-year-old boy involved in a structural fire (approximately 60 minutes after the event). (**B**) Chest radiograph approximately 3 hours after exposure demonstrating the appearance of right upper lobe and perihilar infiltrates. (**C**) Evolution of chest radiograph findings approximately 17 hours after initial exposure demonstrating evolution of the right upper and perihilar infiltrates. (**D**) Approximately 60 hours after exposure demonstrating diffuse alveolar and interstitial infiltrates representative of inhalation-induced acute respiratory distress syndrome. *(Used with permission from The University of Virginia Medical Toxicology Fellowship Program.)*

## MANAGEMENT

From oxygen acquisition to cellular utilization, the final common pathophysiologic effect from smoke injury is hypoxia. Basic critical care strategies that optimize oxygen delivery and utilization are of primary importance in treatment. In critically ill patients, insert two large-bore intravenous (IV) lines and provide appropriate fluid resuscitation as clinically warranted to optimize perfusion and aid in oxygen delivery. The clinical effects of smoke exposure and their appropriate treatment are described in Fig. 93–2.

Critical airway compromise is often present upon initial hospital presentation or develops in the ensuing hours. A major pitfall in the management of patients with smoke inhalation is failing to appreciate the possibility of rapid deterioration. For signs of current or impending airway compromise, upper airway patency must be rapidly established. When obvious oropharyngeal burns are observed, upper airway injury almost certainly is present. Direct evaluation of the upper airway, preferably with fiberoptic endoscopy, is essential for assessing patients at high risk for inhalation airway injury. Other indications for early intubation include coma, stridor, and full-thickness circumferential neck burns. Patients requiring transfer to other institutions or those who require prolonged imaging studies are often candidates for prophylactic intubation.

Even if overt injuries are not visualized, distal injury is often present and underestimated. Pathophysiologic changes in the lung result in progressive hypoxia over hours to days. Basic treatment of progressive respiratory failure includes continuous positive airway pressure, mechanical ventilation using lung protective strategies, positive end-expiratory pressure (PEEP), and vigorous clearing of pulmonary secretions.

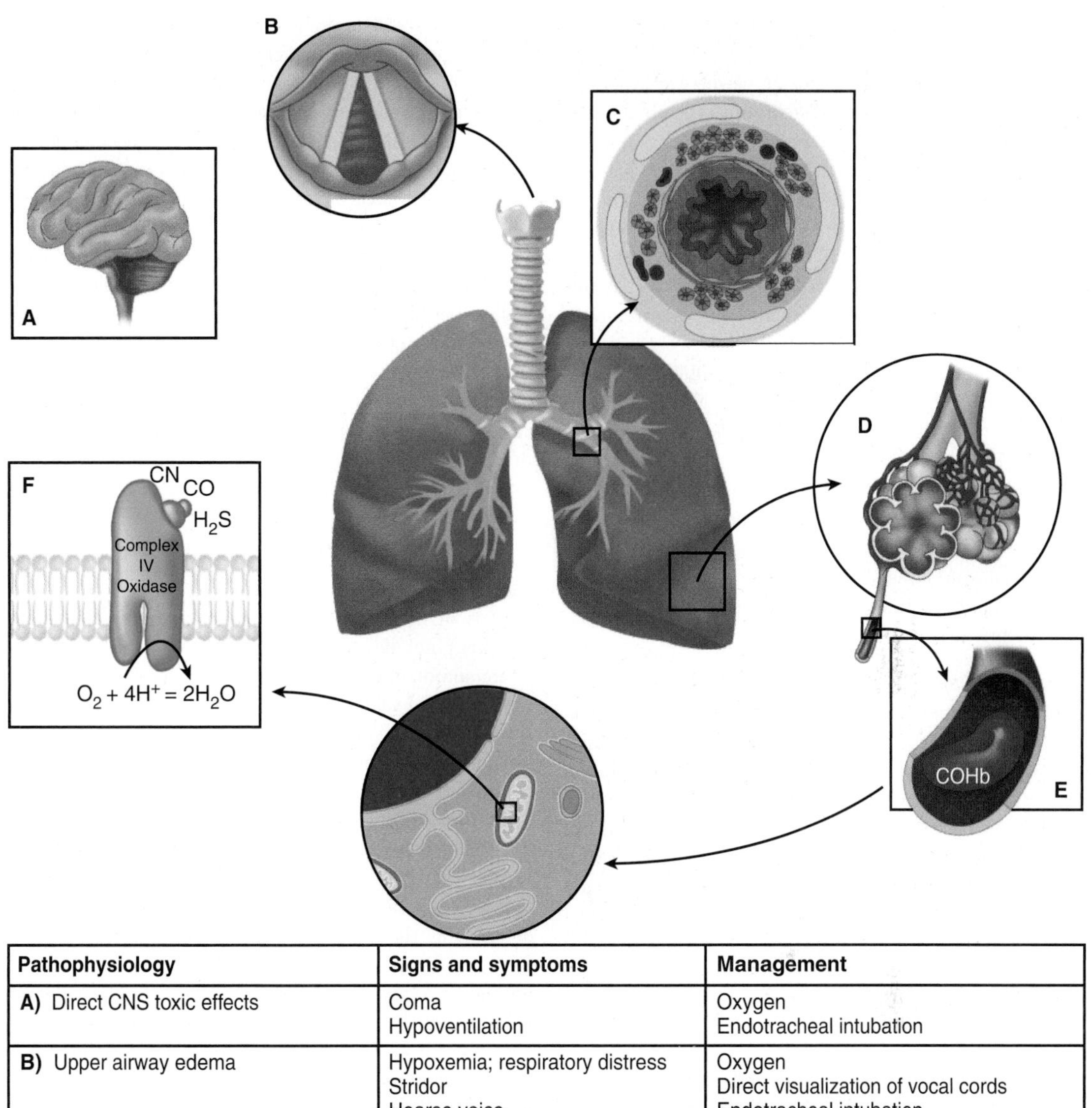


| Pathophysiology | Signs and symptoms | Management |
|---|---|---|
| **A)** Direct CNS toxic effects | Coma<br>Hypoventilation | Oxygen<br>Endotracheal intubation |
| **B)** Upper airway edema | Hypoxemia; respiratory distress<br>Stridor<br>Hoarse voice | Oxygen<br>Direct visualization of vocal cords<br>Endotracheal intubation |
| **C)** Bronchiolar airway obstruction<br>Mucosal edema<br>Intraluminal debris and casts<br>Inspissated secretions<br>Bronchospasm | Respiratory distress<br>Hypoxemia<br>Wheezes<br>Cough<br>Increased peak airway pressures | Oxygen<br>Removal of debris and secretions<br>Chest physiotherapy<br>Frequent airway suctioning<br>Therapeutic bronchoscopy<br>Inhaled β-adrenergic agonists |
| **D)** Atelectasis<br>Surfactant destruction<br>Acute respiratory distress syndrome (ARDS) | Respiratory distress<br>Hypoxemia<br>Crackles<br>Chest radiographic changes | Oxygen<br>Continuous positive airway pressure<br>Mechanical ventilation<br>Lung protective ventilation |
| **E)** Impaired oxygen-carrying capacity and delivery (carbon monoxide or methemoglobinemia) | CNS depression or seizures<br>Myocardial ischemia<br>Dysrhythmias<br>Metabolic acidosis | Oxygen<br>Hyperbaric oxygen as clinically indicated<br>Methylene blue as clinically indicated |
| **F)** Impaired oxygen use at tissues (cyanide, hydrogen sulfide, and/or carbon monoxide) | CNS depression or seizures<br>Myocardial ischemia<br>Dysrhythmias<br>Metabolic acidosis | Oxygen<br>Ensure adequate tissue perfusion<br>Treat suspected cyanide toxicity with cyanide antidote<br>Hyperbaric oxygen as clinically indicated |

**FIGURE 93–2.** The final common pathway from all pathophysiologic changes that occur in smoke inhalation is hypoxia. All treatments should be focused on improving oxygen delivery and oxygen utilization. CNS = central nervous system.

Recommendations for limiting barotrauma in mechanically ventilated patients include using a low tidal volume (6–8 mL/kg) and PEEP and allowing permissive hypercapnia as necessary. The role of extracorporeal membrane oxygenation (ECMO) in victims of smoke inhalation is unclear. Although multiple case reports document its use in patients with inhalational injury, there is limited evidence and no high-quality studies to support its use in smoke inhalation injury. However, as expertise in the use of ECMO has greatly progressed in recent years, it seems reasonable to use this modality as a rescue therapy in patients failing more conventional ventilation strategies.

A significant amount of pulmonary injury after smoke inhalation is attributable to free radical damage. Although human data are currently limited, with only animal studies and human retrospective data available, it would be reasonable to use nebulized unfractionated heparin (typically either 10,000 U of heparin nebulized every 4 hours) and *N*-acetylcysteine for the treatment of intubated patients with bronchoscopy-confirmed smoke inhalation and associated ARDS. Care should be taken to monitor for pneumonia, which, in one study, had a higher incidence in treated patients.

### Carbon Monoxide

The initial treatment strategy for patients with CO poisoning should focus on optimizing oxygen delivery to the tissues. Optimal timing of hyperbaric oxygen (HBO) administration is often during the same period when intensive resuscitative efforts and focused ventilator management are required and could limit attention to these important therapies. The decision to treat a patient with smoke inhalation with HBO should take into account risks and other clinical requirements when determining the appropriate therapy because the therapeutic priority is meticulous supportive care and high-flow oxygen therapy (Chap. 95 and Antidotes in Brief: A40).

### Cyanide

Cyanide is a common product of combustion, with toxic concentrations often measured in fire victims. Because rapid determination of blood cyanide concentrations is not readily available in the prehospital setting or in the emergency department, surrogate markers must be used to help establish the diagnosis. Cyanide poisoning should be suspected in patients involved in enclosed-space fires with evidence of smoke inhalation, particularly in the presence of altered mental status, hemodynamic instability, or metabolic acidosis with an elevated lactate concentration. A blood lactate concentration of 10 mmol/L is a sensitive indicator of cyanide toxicity. For patients with suspected cyanide poisoning, specific treatment of cyanide toxicity should be implemented while other life support measures are instituted. Systematic reviews of various cyanide antidotes conclude that it is possible to survive even cardiorespiratory arrest caused by cyanide poisoning if the patient is provided optimal supportive care and an appropriate antidote (Chap. 96 and Antidotes in Brief: A41). In the prehospital setting or if unable to obtain a rapid lactate concentration, the presence of altered mental status or hemodynamic instability is a reasonable indication to administer hydroxocobalamin.

### Associated Injuries

Victims of fires have respiratory compromise and other pathology not directly related to smoke inhalation, such as trauma or other underlying medical problems. Trauma from falls or explosions must be suspected and treatment started simultaneously with treatment of burns and inhalation injury. Comatose patients should be evaluated for other causes of their status and should receive naloxone, thiamine, and hypertonic dextrose as indicated.

Xenobiotics often injure the skin or mucous membranes in addition to the respiratory mucosa. The duration of contact of a xenobiotic with tissue is an important factor in determining the extent of chemical injury to the skin and eyes. Rapid removal of soot from the skin or eyes helps to prevent continued injury. The eyes should be evaluated for corneal burns caused by thermal or irritant chemical injury. Patients with signs of ophthalmic irritation should have their eyes irrigated, and dermal decontamination should be performed as necessary to prevent burns from toxin-laden soot adherent to the skin (Special Considerations: SC1).

# 94 SIMPLE ASPHYXIANTS AND PULMONARY IRRITANTS

In a 24-hour period, an average adult human at rest will be exposed to 11,500 L of air. There are a number of protective mechanisms within the respiratory system to prevent exposure to xenobiotics, but these mechanisms can be overwhelmed. Diverse xenobiotics act at unique points in the respiratory system to limit or impair tissue oxygenation and are discussed in many chapters of this book. Two mechanistically distinct groups of xenobiotics are capable of interfering with gas exchange to produce hypoxia: simple asphyxiants and pulmonary irritants.

## HISTORY AND EPIDEMIOLOGY

Unlike most xenobiotic exposures, simple asphyxiant and pulmonary irritant poisonings frequently occur on a mass scale due to the magnitude of these exposures. For example, the large-scale emission of carbon dioxide ($CO_2$) from Lake Nyos, a carbonated volcanic crater lake in Cameroon, resulted in nearly 2,000 human deaths and many more livestock deaths. Chlorine and phosgene were used in battle during World War I, resulting in thousands of Allied deaths (Chap. 98). Unexpected release of other irritant inhalants leads to large-scale poisoning. In 1984, an inadvertent release of methyl isocyanate (MIC) in Bhopal, India, resulted in immediate and persistent respiratory symptoms in approximately 200,000 local inhabitants, with approximately 2,500 deaths.

Isolated exposures to individuals occur as well, often in workplaces, and more frequently in contained spaces (eg, indoors). Simple asphyxiation is also a painless and relatively undetectable method for committing suicide.

## SIMPLE ASPHYXIANTS

Simple asphyxiants work primarily by displacing oxygen from ambient air, unlike chemical asphyxiants, which cause cellular hypoxia and are discussed in Chaps. 95 to 97. Virtually every gas, excluding oxygen, is capable of acting as a simple asphyxiant.

### Pathophysiology

Simple asphyxiants displace oxygen from ambient air, thereby reducing the fraction of inspired oxygen ($FiO_2$) in air to below 21%, and result in a decrease in the partial pressure of oxygen. Simple asphyxiants have no pharmacologic activity. For this reason, exceedingly high ambient concentrations of these gases are necessary to produce asphyxia. Asphyxiation typically occurs in confined spaces or with rapid release of large volumes of simple asphyxiants.

### Clinical Manifestations

A patient exposed to any simple asphyxiant gas will develop characteristic clinical findings of hypoxia (Table 94–1). Exposure to simple asphyxiants does not impair $CO_2$ exchange, and hypercapnia does not occur. Because dyspnea develops more rapidly from hypercapnia than hypoxemia, the breathlessness associated with physical or simple chemical asphyxiation does not develop until severe hypoxemia intervenes. In these circumstances, victims frequently succumb to hypoxemia without ever developing the expected warning symptoms. In the case of $CO_2$ inhalation, hypercapnia occurs very rapidly, which itself produces acute cognitive impairment.

### Specific Xenobiotics

***Noble Gases: Helium, Neon, Argon, and Xenon.*** Helium has the lowest molecular weight and is the smallest member of the noble gas family of elements. Helium is used by divers to replace nitrogen to prevent nitrogen narcosis at depth (see Nitrogen). Even using gas mixtures of 50% helium, divers have no adverse effects as long as a normal partial pressure of oxygen is maintained by the mixture at depth. At depth, the quantity (molar quantity, not volume) of air inspired per breath is several-fold greater than at sea level. The lower density of helium than nitrogen results in a lower viscosity of the inhaled air, with a marked decrease in flow resistance. This property of helium is the basis for its use in patients with increased airway resistance (heliox mixture).

All noble gases, when compressed, form cryogenic liquids, which expand rapidly to their gas phase on decompression. Liberation of these gases in closed spaces results in either asphyxiation or freezing injuries, or both. Xenon, unlike the other noble gases, has unique anesthetic properties because of its high lipid solubility and inhibition of *N*-methyl-D-aspartic acid (NMDA) receptors.

***Short-Chain Aliphatic Hydrocarbon Gases: Methane, Ethane, Propane, and Butane.*** The short-chain aliphatic hydrocarbon gases are primarily used in the compressed form as fuel. Methane ($CH_4$) has no known direct toxicity. Methane, also known as "natural gas" and "swamp gas," is present in high ambient concentrations in bogs of decaying organic matter. Methane exposure is an occupational hazard for miners who historically carried canaries into their workplace as an "early warning" sign for the presence of toxic gases or oxygen deficiency. Methane is odorless and undetectable without sophisticated equipment. For this

**TABLE 94–1 Clinical Findings Associated with Reduction of Inspired Oxygen**

| *$FiO_2$* [a] | *Signs and Symptoms* |
|---|---|
| 21 | None |
| 12–16 | Tachypnea, hyperpnea, (resultant hypocapnia), tachycardia, reduced attention and alertness, euphoria, headache, mild incoordination |
| 10–14 | Altered judgment, incoordination, muscular fatigue, cyanosis |
| 6–10 | Nausea, vomiting, lethargy, air hunger, severe incoordination, coma |
| < 6 | Gasping respiration, seizure, coma, death |

[a]At sea level, barometric pressure; appropriate adjustments must be made for altitude and depth exposures.

$FiO_2$ = fraction of inspired oxygen.

reason, natural gas is intentionally adulterated with a small concentration of ethyl mercaptan, a stenching agent, which is responsible for the well-recognized sulfur odor of natural gas.

Ethane ($C_2H_6$) is an odorless component of natural gas and is used as a refrigerant. It has characteristics similar to methane and is occasionally implicated as a simple asphyxiant. Propane ($C_3H_8$) is widely used in its compressed, liquefied form both as an industrial and domestic fuel and as an industrial solvent. Butane ($C_4H_{10}$) is a common fuel and solvent. Deliberate butane inhalation from cigarette lighters or air fresheners for recreational purposes is associated with cardiovascular dysfunction and cerebral damage (Chap. 54).

***Carbon Dioxide.*** Although not a simple asphyxiant gas by definition because it produces physiologic effects, $CO_2$ closely resembles simple asphyxiants from a toxicologic viewpoint. Dry ice, the frozen form of $CO_2$, is extremely cold (−141.3°F; −78.5°C) and undergoes conversion from solid to gas without liquefaction, a process known as sublimation. Poisoning occurs when dry ice is allowed to sublimate in a closed space, such as the cabin of a car or in a cold storage room. Furthermore, inadvertent connection of respirable gas hoses to $CO_2$ is reported in both industrial and medical settings, with resultant worker and patient fatalities.

**Pharmacology and Pathophysiology.** Carbon dioxide, an end product of normal human metabolism, dissolves in the plasma and is in equilibrium with carbonic acid ($H_2CO_3$). The pH at the central chemoreceptors, reflective of the dissolved carbon dioxide ($PCO_2$), is responsible for our respiratory drive, and $PCO_2$ is tightly controlled by the central nervous system (CNS) through regulation of breathing. When ambient concentrations increase, uptake of $CO_2$ occurs, which further stimulates respiration, thereby further increasing the uptake of ambient $CO_2$.

**Clinical Manifestations.** Subacute poisoning occurs during hypoventilation when a patient fails to eliminate endogenous $CO_2$, develops hypercapnia, and typically presents with gradual somnolence. This is linked to respiratory failure, as in the case of emphysema or opioid poisoning. In experimental models in which a normal $FiO_2$ is maintained, massive $CO_2$ inhalation produces CNS and respiratory system manifestations within seconds.

***Nitrogen Gas.*** Although nitrogen, like $CO_2$, produces clinical effects independently of hypoxemia, most poisonings are characterized by the manifestations of a simple asphyxiant. Poisoning by nitrogen gas is uncommon but occurs after rapid evaporation of the supercooled liquid.

**Pharmacology and Pathophysiology.** Nitrogen is a colorless, odorless, and tasteless gas that makes up 78% by volume of air. Under standard conditions, it is inert and has no direct physiologic toxicity.

**Clinical Manifestations.** Inadvertent connection of air-line respirator hoses to nitrogen results in acute asphyxiation, with unconsciousness occurring in approximately 12 seconds and death shortly thereafter. More indolent inhalational poisoning by nitrogen is characterized by impairment of intellectual function and judgment, giddiness, and euphoria, which is qualitatively similar to ethanol intoxication. More severely poisoned patients manifest the spectrum of depressed mental status. Nitrogen poisoning, also known as *nitrogen narcosis*, occurs in underwater divers while they are breathing air that contains 70% nitrogen and causes many deaths in the subaquatic environment. The underlying mechanism of nitrogen narcosis is unknown, but the simple structure and relatively high lipophilicity of nitrogen suggest a mechanism similar to that of the anesthetic gases.

Dermal exposure to liquid nitrogen produces frostbite because liquid nitrogen is extremely cold and ingestion of liquid nitrogen similarly produces a freezing injury of the gastrointestinal (GI) tract.

### Treatment

Treatment of all individuals poisoned by simple asphyxiants begins with immediate removal of the persons from exposure and provision of ventilatory assistance. Provision of supplemental oxygen is preferable, but room air usually suffices. Restoration of oxygenation through spontaneous or mechanical ventilation occurs after only several breaths. Support of vital functions is the mainstay of therapy but is generally unnecessary after a brief exposure.

## PULMONARY IRRITANTS

The irritant gases are a heterogeneous group of chemicals that produce toxic effects via a final common pathway: destruction of the integrity of the mucosal barrier of the respiratory tract (Table 94–2).

### Pathophysiology

In the lung, irritant chemicals damage both the type I pneumocytes and the surfactant-producing type II pneumocytes. Neutrophil influx, recruited in response to macrophage-derived inflammatory cytokines such as tumor necrosis factor (TNF)-α, releases toxic mediators that disrupt the integrity of the capillary endothelial cells. This host defense response results in accumulation of cellular debris and plasma exudate in the alveolar sacs, producing the characteristic clinical findings of the acute respiratory distress syndrome (ARDS). The specific mechanisms by which the irritant gases damage the pulmonary endothelial and epithelial cells vary. Many irritant gases require dissolution in lung water to liberate their ultimate toxicant, which often is an acid. Experimental models assessing the water solubility of a gas to predict the location of its associated lesions generally agree with the clinical data.

### Clinical Manifestations

Regardless of the mechanism by which the mucosa is damaged, the clinical presentations of patients exposed to irritant gases are similar. Those exposed to gases that result in irritation within seconds generally develop mucosal injury limited to the upper respiratory tract. The rapid onset of symptoms is usually a sufficient signal to the patient to escape the exposure. Patients present with nasal or oropharyngeal pain in addition to drooling, mucosal edema, cough, or stridor. Chemosis and skin irritation are often noted because concomitant ocular and cutaneous exposure to the gases usually

**TABLE 94–2 Characteristics of Common Respiratory Irritants**

| *Gas* | *Source or Exposure* | *Solubility (g%)*[a] | *Detection Threshold (ppm)* | *Regulatory Standard (ppm)*[b] | *IDLH*[c] *(ppm)* | *STEL (ppm)* |
|---|---|---|---|---|---|---|
| Ammonia | Fertilizer, refrigeration, synthetic fiber synthesis | H | 5 | 50 | 300 | 35 |
| Cadmium oxide fumes | Welding | I | Odorless | 0.005 mg/m$^3$ | 9 mg/m$^3$ (as Cd) | NA |
| Carbon dioxide | Exhaust, dry ice sublimation, environmental disasters | P | Odorless | 5000 | 40,000 | 30,000 |
| Chloramine | Bleach plus ammonia | H | NA | NR | NR | NR |
| Chlorine | Water disinfection, pulp, and paper industry | I | 0.3 | 0.5 | 10 | 1 |
| Copper oxide fumes | Welding | I | NA | 0.1 mg/m$^3$ | 100 mg/m$^3$ (as Cu) | NA |
| Ethylene oxide | Sterilant | H | 500 | 1 | 800 | 5 |
| Formaldehyde | Chemical disinfection | H | 0.8 | 0.016 | 20 | 2 |
| Hydrogen chloride | Chemical reactions | H | 1–5 | 5 | 50 | 5 |
| Hydrogen fluoride | Glass etching, semiconductor industry | H | 0.042 | 3 (as F) | 30 (as F) | 6 |
| Hydrogen sulfide | Petroleum industry, sewer, manure pits | P | 0.025 | | 100 | 50 |
| Mercury vapor | Electrical equipment, thermometers, catalyst, dental fillings, metal extraction, heating or vacuuming elemental mercury | I | Odorless | 0.1 mg/m$^3$ | 10 mg/m$^3$ | 0.05 |
| Methane | Natural heating gas, swamp gas | M | Odorless | NR | NR | NR |
| Methyl bromide | Fumigant | M | 20 | 20 | 250 | NA |
| Nickel carbonyl | Nickel purification, nickel coating, catalyst | P | 1–3 | 0.001 | 2 (as Ni) | 0.1 |
| Nitrogen | Cryotherapy | P | Odorless | NR | NR | NR |
| Nitrogen dioxide | Chemical synthesis, combustion emission | P | 0.12 | 3 | 20 | 5 |
| Nitrous oxide | Anesthetic gas, whipping cream dispensers (abuse), racing fuel additive | P | 2 | 25 | 100 | NA |
| Ozone | Disinfectant, produced by high-voltage electrical equipment | P | 0.05 | 0.1 | 5 | 0.1 |
| Phosgene | Chemical synthesis, combustion of chlorinated compounds | P | 0.5 | 0.1 | 2 | 0.1 |
| Phosphine | Fumigant, semiconductor industry | P | 2 | 0.3 | 50 | 1 |
| Propane | Liquified propane gas | P | Odorless | 1000 | 2100 | NR |
| Sulfur dioxide | Environmental exhaust | H | 1 | 2 | 100 | 5 |
| Zinc chloride fumes | Artificial smoke (no longer in use) | H | NA | 1 mg/m$^3$ | 50 mg/m$^3$ | 2 mg/m$^3$ |
| Zinc oxide | Welding | P | Odorless | 5 mg/m$^3$ | 500 mg/m$^3$ | 10 mg/m$^3$ |

[a]g% = grams of gas per 100 mL water; if applicable. Solubility: I = insoluble; P = poor; M = medium; H = high. [b]Standards are either threshold limit value-time weighted average (TLV-TWA) set by the American Conference of Governmental Industrial Hygienists (ACGIH) or permissible exposure limits (PELs) set by the Occupational Safety and Health Administration (OSHA). [c]Immediately dangerous to life and health (IDLH): National Institute for Occupational Safety and Health (NIOSH), revised 1994. (Documentation for each IDLH is available at http://www.cdc.gov/niosh/idlh/idlhintr.html.)

F = fluorine; NA = not available; NR = no regulatory standard; STEL = short-term exposure limit (15-minute average not to be exceeded).

is unavoidable. Gases that are less rapidly irritating do not typically provide an adequate signal of their presence and therefore do not prompt expeditious escape by the exposed individual. In this case, prolonged breathing allows entry of the toxic gas farther into the bronchopulmonary system, where delayed toxic effects are subsequently noted. Tracheobronchitis, bronchiolitis, bronchospasm, and ARDS are typical inflammatory responses of the airway and represent the spectrum of acute lower respiratory tract injury.

The most characteristic and serious clinical manifestation of irritant gas exposure is ARDS. Acute respiratory distress syndrome is a nonspecific syndrome that consists of the clinical, radiographic, and physiologic abnormalities caused by pulmonary inflammation and alveolar filling that must be both acute in onset and not attributable solely to pulmonary capillary hypertension as occurs in patients with congestive heart failure. Patients with ARDS present with dyspnea, chest tightness, chest pain, cough, frothy sputum, wheezing or crackles, and arterial hypoxemia. Typical radiographic abnormalities include bilateral pulmonary infiltrates with an alveolar filling pattern and a normal cardiac silhouette that differentiates this syndrome from congestive heart failure.

## Specific Xenobiotics

### *Acid- or Base-Forming Gases Highly Water-Soluble Xenobiotics*

**Ammonia ($NH_3$).** Ammonia is a common industrial and household chemical whose odor and irritancy are

**A.** $3\ NaOCl + 2\ NH_3 \rightarrow NH_2Cl + NHCl_2 + 3\ NaOH$

**B.** $NH_2Cl + H_2O \rightarrow HOCl + NH_3$

$HOCl \rightarrow HCl + \{O\}$

**FIGURE 94–1.** Chloramine chemistry. (**A**) Sodium hypochlorite (bleach) plus ammonia form monochloramine and dichloramine. (**B**) Chloramine dissolves in water to liberate hypochlorous acid, hydrochloric acid, ammonia, and nascent oxygen {O}, an oxidant.

characteristic and serve as an effective warning signal of exposure. Dissolution of $NH_3$ in water to form the base ammonium hydroxide ($NH_4OH$) rapidly produces severe upper airway irritation. Patients with exposures to highly concentrated $NH_3$ or exposures for prolonged periods develop tracheobronchial or pulmonary inflammation.

**Chloramines.** This series of chlorinated nitrogenous compounds (Fig. 94–1) includes monochloramine ($NH_2Cl$), dichloramine ($NHCl_2$), and trichloramine ($NCl_3$). The chloramines are most commonly generated by the admixture of ammonia with sodium hypochlorite (NaOCl) bleach, often in an effort to potentiate their individual cleansing powers. On dissolution of the chloramines in the epithelial lining fluid, hypochlorous acid (HOCl), ammonia, and oxygen radicals are generated, all of which act as irritants. Although less water soluble than ammonia, the chloramines typically promptly produce symptoms. Because these initial symptoms are often mild, however, they often do not prompt immediate escape, resulting in prolonged or recurrent exposure with pulmonary and ocular symptoms predominating.

**Hydrogen Chloride (HCl).** Dissolution of HCl gas in lung water after inhalation similarly produces hydrochloric acid.

**Hydrogen Fluoride (HF).** Hydrogen fluoride gas dissolves in epithelial lining fluid to form the weak acid hydrofluoric acid. The intact HF molecule is the predominant form in solution, and few free hydronium ions ($H_3O^+$) are liberated. Low-dose inhalational exposures result in irritant symptoms, and large exposures cause bronchial and pulmonary parenchymal destruction. Inhalation results in ARDS, but death usually is related to systemic fluoride poisoning (Chap. 77).

**Sulfur Dioxide and Sulfuric Acid ($SO_2$ and $H_2SO_4$).** Sulfur dioxide is highly water soluble and has a characteristic pungent odor that provides warning of its presence at concentrations well below those that are irritating. In the presence of catalytic metals (Fe, Mn), environmental sulfur dioxide is readily converted to sulfurous acid ($H_2SO_3$) within water droplets. Sulfurous acid is a major environmental concern and the cause of "acid rain." Exposure to atmospheric sulfur dioxide results in a roughly dose-related bronchospasm, which is most pronounced and difficult to treat in patients with asthma. Inhalation of sulfurous acid or dissolution of sulfur dioxide in epithelial lining fluid produces typical pathologic and clinical findings associated with ARDS. Large acute exposures produce the expected acute irritant response of both the upper and lower respiratory tracts, and pulmonary dysfunction (see Asthma and Reactive Airways Dysfunction Syndrome) in some persists for several years.

**A.** $HCl + HOCl \rightarrow Cl_2 + H_2O$

**B.** $Cl_2 + H_2O \rightarrow 2\ HCl + \{O\}$

$Cl_2 + H_2O \rightarrow HCl + HOCl$

**FIGURE 94–2.** Chlorine chemistry. (**A**) Formation of chlorine gas from the acidification of hypochlorous acid. (**B**) Dissolution of chlorine in mucosal water to generate both hydrochloric and hypochlorous acids (hydrogen chloride {HCl} and hypochlorous acid {HOCl}) and nascent oxygen {O}, an oxidant.

### *Intermediate Water-Soluble Xenobiotics*

**Chlorine ($Cl_2$).** Although chlorine gas is not generally available for use in the home, domestic exposure to chlorine gas is common. The admixture of an acid to bleach liberates chlorine gas (Fig. 94–2). Chlorine gas is also generated when aging swimming pool chlorination tablets, such as calcium hypochlorite {$Ca(OCl)_2$} or trichloro-*s*-triazinetrione (TST) decompose. Inadvertent mixture of $Ca(OCl)_2$ and TST results in excessive chlorine gas generation, which is also explosive.

The odor threshold for chlorine is low, but distinguishing toxic from permissible air concentrations is difficult until toxicity manifests. The intermediate solubility characteristics of chlorine result in only mild initial symptoms after moderate exposure and allow a substantial time delay, typically several hours, before clinical symptoms develop. Chlorine dissolution in lung water generates HCl and hypochlorous (HOCl) acids. Hypochlorous acid rapidly decomposes into HCl and nascent oxygen (O). The unpaired nascent oxygen atom produces additional pulmonary damage by initiating a free radical oxidative cascade. Although the majority of life-threatening chlorine poisonings occur after acute large exposures, patients with chronic, low-concentration or recurrent exposures and patients with exposure to moderate concentrations often manifest increased bronchial responsiveness (see Asthma and Reactive Airways Dysfunction Syndrome).

### *Poorly Water-Soluble Xenobiotics*

**Hydrogen Sulfide ($H_2S$).** Hydrogen Sulfide exposures occur most frequently in the waste management, petroleum, and natural gas industries. Hydrogen sulfide exposure also rarely occurs in hospital workers using acid cleaners to unblock drains clogged with plaster of Paris sludge. The generation of $H_2S$ by mixing household chemicals in a closed automobile, a trend referred to as "detergent suicide," produces a potential threat to the responders. Hydrogen sulfide inhibits mitochondrial respiration in a fashion similar to that of cyanide (Chap. 96).

Hydrogen sulfide has the distinctive odor of "rotten eggs," which, although helpful in diagnosis, is not specific. Despite a sensitive odor threshold of several parts per billion, rapid olfactory fatigue ensues, providing a misperception that the exposure and its attendant risk have diminished. At low and moderate concentrations ($\leq$ 500 ppm), upper respiratory tract mucosal irritation occurs and is the principal toxicity. The rapidity of death in patients exposed to high $H_2S$ concentrations makes it difficult to conclude whether simple asphyxiation or cytochrome oxidase inhibition is causal in most cases.

**Phosgene ($COCl_2$).** During World War I, phosgene was an important chemical weapon that produced countless deaths (Chap. 98). Exposure to phosgene initially produces limited manifestations but results in acute mucosal irritation after intense exposure. In fact, the pleasant odor of fresh hay, rather than prompting escape, disturbingly promotes prolonged breathing of the toxic gas. The most consequential clinical effect related to phosgene exposure is delayed ARDS. Because the onset is typically delayed up to 24 hours, prolonged observation of patients thought to be phosgene-poisoned is warranted.

***Oxidant Gases.*** Rather than acidic or alkaline metabolites, free radicals mediate the pulmonary toxicity of certain irritant gases. Many of the chemicals discussed participate in both acid–base and oxidant types of injury. However, the clinical distinction between acid- or alkali-forming irritants and oxidants is difficult but is therapeutically relevant.

**Oxygen ($O_2$).** Oxygen toxicity is uncommon in the workplace but, ironically, is common in hospitalized patients. Although prolonged, high-concentration exposures to $O_2$ produce CNS and retinal toxicity, pulmonary damage is more common. Humans can tolerate 100% $O_2$ at sea level for up to 48 hours without significant acute pulmonary damage. Under hyperbaric conditions (2.0 atmospheres absolute), oxygen toxicity develops within 3 to 6 hours. Acute respiratory distress syndrome occurs in approximately 5% of patients administered hyperbaric oxygen for therapeutic purposes. Delayed pulmonary fibrosis, presumably from healing of subclinical injury, develops in patients breathing lower concentrations of $O_2$ at sea level for shorter periods.

Generation of reactive oxygen species (ROS), including superoxide ($O_2^{-\cdot}$), hydroxyl radical (OH·), hydrogen peroxide (HOOH), singlet oxygen (O·), and nitric oxide (NO), produces cellular necrosis, increases pulmonary capillary permeability, and induces apoptosis. Current techniques for preventing pulmonary oxygen toxicity emphasize reduction of the inspired oxygen concentration by use of positive end-expiratory pressure (PEEP) ventilation.

**Oxides of Nitrogen (NOx).** The most important substances included in this series are the stable free radicals nitrogen dioxide ($NO_2$) and NO, as well as nitrogen tetroxide (dinitrogen tetroxide {$N_2O_4$}), nitrogen trioxide ($N_2O_3$), and nitrous oxide ($N_2O$). Oxides of nitrogen are products of combustion and decomposition. In the absence of ventilation, high concentrations of $NO_2$ accumulate in silos such that an individual entering the silo is rapidly asphyxiated from the depletion of oxygen. Additionally, substantial quantities of $NO_2$ remaining after incomplete ventilation are associated with delayed-onset pulmonary toxicity characteristic of silo filler's disease.

The various oxides of nitrogen directly oxidize respiratory tract cellular membranes but more typically generate reactive nitrogen intermediates, or radicals, such as $ONOO^-$, which subsequently damage the pulmonary epithelial cells. In addition, dissolution in respiratory tract water generates nitric acid ($HNO_3$) and NO, which produce injury consistent with other inhaled acids.

**Ozone ($O_3$).** Ozone is abundant in the stratospheric region found between 5 and 31 miles above the planet. Ozone is formed by the action of ultraviolet light on oxygen molecules and is an important component of photochemical smog. As such, it contributes to chronic lung disease. Because of its high electronegativity, ozone is one of the most potent oxidizers available.

The pulmonary toxicity associated with ozone primarily results from its high reactivity toward unsaturated fatty acids and amino acids with sulfhydryl functional groups. Ozonation and free radical damage to the lipid component of the membrane initiate an inflammatory cascade. Increased permeability of the pulmonary epithelium results in alveolar filling from the transudation of proteins and fluids characteristic of ARDS.

***Miscellaneous Pulmonary Irritants.***

**Methyl Isocyanate.** Methyl isocyanate (MIC) is one of a series of compounds sharing a similar isocyanate (N=C=O) moiety. Toluene diisocyanate (TDI) and diphenyl-methane diisocyanate (MDI) are important chemicals in the polymer industry. In those exposed to MIC in Bhopal, ARDS was evident both clinically and radiographically. Methyl isocyanate is a significantly more potent respiratory irritant than the other regularly used isocyanate derivatives such as TDI.

**Riot Control Agents: Capsaicin, Chlorobenzylidene Malononitrile, and Chloroacetophenone.** Historically, riot control agents consisted primarily of chloroacetophenone (military designation, CN) or chlorobenzylidene malononitrile (military designation, CS). Both are white solids that are dispersed as aerosols. After low-concentration exposure, ocular discomfort and lacrimation alone are expected, accounting for the common appellation *tear gas*. The effects are transient, and complete recovery within 30 minutes is typical, although long-lasting pulmonary effects are described (see Asthma and Reactive Airways Dysfunction Syndrome). Closed-space exposure is associated with significant ocular toxicity, dermal burns, laryngospasm, ARDS, or death. Because of their high potential for severe toxicity, CN and CS were replaced for civilian use by oleoresin capsicum (OC), also known as *pepper spray* or *pepper mace*.

Capsaicin interacts with the transient receptor potential vanilloid-1 (TRPV1). Stimulation of this receptor invokes the release of substance P, a neuropeptide involved with transmission of pain impulses. Substance P also induces neurogenic inflammation, which, in the lung, results in ARDS and bronchoconstriction (see Asthma and Reactive Airways Dysfunction Syndrome).

**Metal Pneumonitis.** Acute inhalational exposures to certain metal compounds produce clinical effects identical to those of the chemical irritants. For example, exposure to zinc chloride fumes for just a few minutes is associated with ARDS and death (Chap. 73). Other metals are discussed in their respective chapters (Chaps. 61, 68, and 69). The mechanism of toxicity typically relates to overwhelming oxidant stress with a pronounced inflammatory response as measured by serum cytokine (eg, TNF-$\alpha$) concentrations, consistent with the role of metals in redox reactions. Patients with metal-induced pneumonitis present with chest tightness, cough, fever, and signs consistent with ARDS. In particular, metal pneumonitis should be differentiated from the more common and substantially less consequential metal fume fever, discussed later in this chapter. In addition to standard supportive measures, patients with acute metal-induced pneumonitis should be hospitalized, and it is reasonable to administer corticosteroids. Chelation therapy has no documented benefit for treatment of patients with ARDS but is indicated based on conventional indications.

## MANAGEMENT

### Standard and Supportive Measures

Management of patients with acute respiratory tract injury begins with meticulous support of airway patency by limiting bronchial and pulmonary secretions and maintaining oxygenation. Supplemental oxygen, bronchodilators, and airway suctioning should be used for standard indications. Corticosteroid therapy use is reasonable whether inhaled or intravenous, and based largely on institutional practices for the management of patients with ARDS. Prone positioning during ventilation; PEEP; early neuromuscular blockade; and low-volume, low-pressure, lung-protective strategies are successful in enhancing the oxygenation of patients with ARDS of various causes but are not necessarily successful in improving outcome. Lower tidal volume mechanical ventilation using 6 mL/kg and plateau pressures of 30 cm $H_2O$ attenuated the inflammatory response and resulted in a lower mortality rate and less need for mechanical ventilation than traditional volume ventilation with 12 mL/kg. It is recommended to reduce the inspired concentration of oxygen to below 50% as rapidly as possible because patients poisoned by irritant gases have enhanced susceptibility to oxygen toxicity as a result of depletion of endogenous antioxidant barriers.

### Neutralization Therapy

A therapy unique to several of the acid- or base-forming irritant gases is chemical neutralization. Although contraindicated in acid or alkali ingestion because of concern of an exothermic reaction in the process of neutralization, the large surface area of the lung and the relatively small amount of xenobiotic present allow dissipation of the heat and gas generated during neutralization. Case studies suggest that nebulized 2% sodium bicarbonate is beneficial in patients poisoned by acid-forming irritant gases. The vast majority of these cases involve chlorine gas exposure, and most patients received other symptomatic therapies as well. Although there appears to be no specific benefit for patients exposed to chloramine, nebulized bicarbonate therapy appears to be safe and is reasonable to administer. The sodium bicarbonate solution should be used in a sufficiently dilute form to prevent irritation. Typically, 1 mL of 7.5% or 8.4% sodium bicarbonate solution is added to 3 mL sterile water (resulting in an ~2% solution for nebulization) (Antidotes in Brief: A5). Patients receiving nebulized bicarbonate therapy require observation beyond the time of symptom resolution. Because administration of neutralizing acids for alkaline irritants, such as ammonia, has not been attempted, we recommend against their use at this time.

### Antioxidants

Antioxidants include reducing agents such as ascorbic acid, *N*-acetylcysteine, free radical scavengers such as vitamin E, and enzymes such as superoxide dismutase. Although the concept of treating pulmonary oxidant stress with antioxidants or free radical scavengers is intriguing, most currently available evidence suggests that these xenobiotics offer negligible benefit in humans.

### Xenobiotic-Directed Therapy

Patients with inhalational exposure to hydrogen fluoride should undergo frequent electrocardiographic evaluations and correction of serum electrolytes. Administration of nebulized 2.5% calcium gluconate, prepared as 1.5 mL 10% calcium gluconate plus 4.5 mL 0.9% sodium chloride solution or sterile water, is recommended to limit systemic fluoride absorption and is reasonable to administer. Systemic calcium salts should be administered as needed to correct hypocalcemia (Chap. 77 and Antidotes in Brief: A32).

## OTHER INHALED PULMONARY XENOBIOTICS

A particulate, or dust, is a solid dispersed in a gas. Dust is a substantial source of occupational particulate exposure and is an important cause of acute pulmonary toxic syndromes. A respirable particulate must have an appropriately small size (generally < 10 microns) and aerodynamic properties to enter the terminal respiratory tree. Nonrespirable particulates, also called *nuisance dusts*, are trapped by the upper airways and are not generally thought to cause pulmonary damage. In distinction from the irritant gases, there is no unifying toxic mechanism among the respirable particulates. Many of the particulate diseases, such as asbestos exposure and its sequelae, are chronic in nature; only the acute and subacute syndromes are discussed here.

### Inorganic Dust Exposure

Silicosis results from inhalation of crystalline silica ($SiO_2$). Exposure-related effects include cough, asthma, chronic obstructive pulmonary disease, and sarcoidlike lung changes. Although typically a chronic occupational disease, intense subacute silica dust exposure produces acute silicosis in a few weeks and even death within 2 years. The mechanism of toxicity relates to the relentless inflammatory response generated by the pulmonary macrophages. These cells engulf the indigestible particles and are destroyed, releasing their lytic enzymes and oxidative products locally within the pulmonary parenchyma. Patients present with dyspnea, cor pulmonale, restrictive lung findings, and classic radiographic findings. Treatment is limited and includes steroids and supportive care.

### Organic Dusts

Inhalation of dusts from cotton or similar natural fibers, usually during the refinement of cotton fibers (byssinosis), produces chest tightness, dyspnea, and fever that typically begin within 3 to 4 hours of exposure. Similar reactions occur after inhalation of hay, silage, grain, hemp, or compost dust. Symptoms often resolve during the workweek but return after a weekend hiatus. Byssinosis is caused by an endotoxin present on the cotton and is not immunologic in nature. "Grain fever" is caused by a respirable compound associated with grain dust, as occurs during harvesting, milling, and transporting.

### Hypersensitivity Pneumonitis

Hypersensitivity pneumonitis, also known as extrinsic allergic alveolitis, is the final common pathway for many different organic dust exposures. The name attached to the individual syndrome typically identifies the associated occupation or substrate. For example, *bagassosis* is the term associated with sugar cane (bagasse), and *farmer's lung* is the term associated with moldy hay, although both conditions are caused by thermophilic *Actinomycetes* spp. When associated with puffball mushroom spores (*Lycoperdon* spp), the syndrome is called *lycoperdonosis*; when caused by bird droppings, it is called *bird fancier's lung*. The implicated allergen is capable of depositing in the pulmonary parenchyma and eliciting a cell-mediated (type IV) immunologic response. Clinical findings include fever, chills, and dyspnea beginning 4 to 8 hours after exposure. The chest radiograph is typically normal but also reveals diffuse or discrete infiltrates. Progressive disease is associated with a honeycombing pattern on the radiograph and a restrictive lung disease pattern on formal pulmonary function testing. It is reasonable to administer corticosteroids and recommended to avoid the antigen.

## Metal Fume Fever and Polymer Fume Fever

Metal fume fever is a recurrent influenzalike syndrome that develops several hours after exposure to metal oxide fumes generated during welding, galvanizing, or smelting. In addition to dyspnea, cough, chest pain, and fever, patients experience headache, a metallic taste, myalgias, and chills. Direct pulmonary toxicity does not occur, and patients with metal fume fever generally have normal chest radiographs. Many metal oxides are capable of eliciting this syndrome, but it is noted most frequently in patients who weld galvanized steel, which contains zinc. Antigen release with immunologic response appears to be responsible for the induction of symptoms. On subsequent exposure, proinflammatory cytokines, such as TNF-$\alpha$, and various interleukins are detected in bronchoalveolar lavage fluid. However, because symptoms often occur with the first exposure to fumes, a direct toxic effect on the respiratory mucosa presumably exists.

The management of patients with metal fume fever is supportive and includes analgesics and antipyretics. There is no specific antidote, and we recommend against chelation therapy unless otherwise indicated. The natural course of metal fume fever involves spontaneous resolution within 48 hours. Persistent symptoms are rare and should prompt investigation of other etiologies.

A remarkably similar syndrome occurs subsequent to inhaling pyrolysis products of fluorinated polymers (eg, Teflon), which is aptly termed *polymer fume fever*. As with metal fumes, very large exposures to polymer fumes result in direct pulmonary toxicity. Supportive care is the therapy of choice.

## Asthma and Reactive Airways Dysfunction Syndrome

Asthma, or *reversible airways disease*, is a clinical syndrome that includes intermittent episodes of dyspnea, cough, chest pain or tightness, wheezes on auscultation, and measurable variations in expiratory airflow. Episodes typically are triggered by a xenobiotic or physical stimulus and resolve over several hours with appropriate therapy. The underlying process is immunologic in most cases, with allergen-triggered release of inflammatory mediators causing bronchiolar smooth muscle contraction and subsequent inflammation. Because asthma affects 5% to 10% of the world's population and the triggers often are nonspecific, it is not surprising that work-aggravated asthma is extremely common.

**TABLE 94–3 Common Xenobiotic Sensitizers Producing Occupational Asthma**

| *Molecular Weight* | *Example* | *Primary Risk Occupations* |
|---|---|---|
| **High** | | |
| Proteins | Crab shell protein | Seafood processors |
| **Low** | | |
| Acrylate | Plastics | Adhesives, plastics |
| Glutaraldehyde | Sterilant | Healthcare workers |
| Isocyanates | Toluene diisocyanate | Polyurethane foam, automobile painters |
| Metals | Nickel sulfate | Nickel platers |
| Trimellitic anhydride | Curing agent for epoxy and paint | Chemical workers |
| Wood dust | Western red cedar (*Thuja plicata*) | Foresters, carpenters |

Occupational asthma, or asthma occasioned by a workplace exposure to a sensitizing xenobiotic, accounts for perhaps up to 25% of all newly diagnosed asthma in adults. Exposure to one of the 250 or more known sensitizers (Table 94–3) is usually associated with a latency period of weeks or months of exposure before symptom onset. After symptoms begin, however, they recur consistently after reexposure to the inciting trigger agent. Because contact with a trigger is difficult to avoid, reassignment or an outright occupational change is occasionally required. Treatment for exacerbations is comparable to standard asthma therapy and should include bronchodilators and corticosteroids as appropriate.

Acute exposure to irritant gas results in the development of a persistent asthmalike syndrome also termed *reactive airways dysfunction syndrome* (RADS), *irritant-induced asthma*, or *occupational asthma without latency*. Virtually every irritative xenobiotic is reported to cause this syndrome. In comparison with patients who develop occupational asthma, patients who develop RADS have a lower incidence of atopy and are exposed to xenobiotics not typically considered to be immunologically sensitizing. In addition, the airflow improvement with $\beta_2$-adrenergic agonist therapy is significantly better in patients with occupational asthma. Bronchial biopsy performed in patients with RADS generally reveals a chronic inflammatory response. The role of corticosteroids is undefined, but animal models suggest an antiinflammatory benefit, and they are recommended as for any other patient with acute bronchospasm. Recovery often takes months, with the delay related to either ongoing low-level exposures or persistent irritation of impaired tissue.

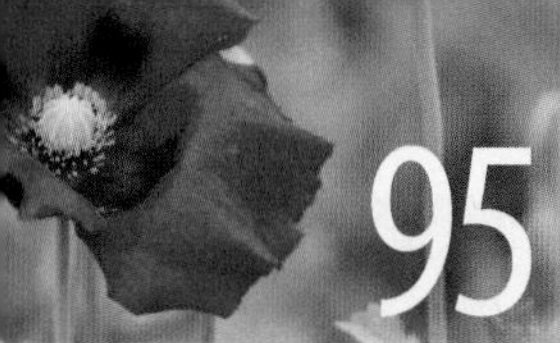

# 95 CARBON MONOXIDE

| **Carbon Monoxide (CO)** | | |
|---|---|---|
| Gas density | = | 0.968 (air = 1.0) |
| Blood carboxyhemoglobin level | | |
| Nonsmokers | = | 1%–2% |
| Smokers | = | 5%–10% |
| Action level | > | 10% |
| TLV–TWA | = | 50 ppm |

## HISTORY AND EPIDEMIOLOGY

Carbon monoxide (CO) is formed during the incomplete combustion of virtually any carbon-containing compound. Because it is an odorless, colorless, and tasteless gas, it is remarkably difficult to detect in the environment even when present at high ambient concentrations and is a leading cause of poisoning morbidity and mortality in the United States. Although fires are the most commonly recognized reason for exposure, many clusters of CO poisoning are associated with power failures during catastrophic weather, such as ice storms, blizzards, and hurricanes. Potential sources of CO abound in our society (Table 95–1). Despite catalytic converters and other emission controls, many unintentional CO deaths are still caused by motor vehicle exhaust.

While fatality is a concern, the larger problem with CO poisoning is the associated morbidity that survivors risk even after acute treatment. The most serious complication is persistent or delayed neurologic sequelae (DNS) or delayed neurocognitive sequelae, which occur in up to 50% of patients with symptomatic acute poisonings.

## TOXICOKINETICS

Carbon monoxide is readily absorbed after inhalation. After its absorption, CO is carried in the blood, primarily bound to hemoglobin. The Haldane ratio states that hemoglobin has approximately 200 to 250 times greater affinity for CO than for oxygen. Therefore, CO is primarily confined to the blood compartment, but eventually up to 15% of total CO body content is taken up by tissue, primarily bound to myoglobin. The elimination half-life of CO is dependent on the $PO_2$ (see Management section below).

**TABLE 95–1 Sources of Carbon Monoxide Implicated in Poisonings**

| |
|---|
| Anesthetic absorbents |
| Banked blood |
| Camp stoves and lanterns |
| Charcoal grills |
| Coffee roasting |
| Fires |
| Formic acid decomposition mixed in sulfuric acid |
| Gasoline-powered equipment (eg, generators, power washers) |
| Ice-resurfacing machines (propane powered) |
| Internal combustion engine (boat, car, truck) |
| Methylene bromide |
| Methylene chloride |
| Natural gas combustion furnaces (water heaters, ranges, and ovens) |
| Propane powered forklifts |
| Underground mine explosions |
| Wood pellet storage |

Methylene chloride, a paint stripper, is another source of CO. It is readily absorbed through the skin or by ingestion or inhalation and is metabolized in the liver to CO. Carboxyhemoglobin (COHb) levels typically peak 8 to 12 hours later and range from 10% to 50%.

## PATHOPHYSIOLOGY

The most obvious deleterious effect of CO is binding to hemoglobin, rendering it incapable of delivering oxygen to the cells. Therefore, despite adequate partial pressures of oxygen in blood ($PO_2$), there is decreased arterial oxygen content. Further insult occurs because CO causes a leftward shift of the oxyhemoglobin dissociation curve, thus decreasing the offloading of oxygen from hemoglobin to tissue. The net effect of all these processes is the decreased ability of oxygen to be delivered to tissue. Carbon monoxide toxicity cannot be attributed solely to COHb-mediated hypoxia. For CO to reach tissue, it has to be dissolved in the plasma rather than bound to hemoglobin. Carbon monoxide interferes with cellular respiration by binding to mitochondrial cytochrome oxidase.

In vitro rat models demonstrate that this oxidative stress causes mitochondrial damage with protein oxidation and lipid peroxidation, particularly in the hippocampus and corpus striatum. Although no comparable brain studies exist in humans, the peripheral lymphocytes and monocytes of CO-poisoned patients show cytochrome oxidase inhibition accompanied by increased lipid peroxidation. Inactivation of cytochrome oxidase is only an initial part of the cascade of inflammatory events that results in ischemic reperfusion injury to the brain after CO poisoning (Fig. A40–1). Simultaneously, with all this perivascular oxidative stress in the brain, there is activation of excitatory amino acids, which ultimately is responsible for the subsequent neuronal cell loss.

Myoglobin, another heme protein, binds CO with an affinity about 60 times greater than it binds oxygen. About 10% to 15% of the total-body store of CO is extravascular, primarily binding to myoglobin. This binding partially explains the myocardial impairment that occurs in both animal studies and low-level exposures in patients with ischemic heart disease. The combination of COHb formation, which decreases oxygen-carrying capacity, and carboxy-myoglobin in the heart, which decreases oxygen extraction, contributes to the preterminal dysrhythmias that occurs in poisoned animals.

Several studies suggest that CO effects on the cardiovascular system are necessary for ischemic reperfusion injury of the brain. Hypotension is an essential component and results from a combination of myocardial depression and vasodilation. Carbon monoxide, perhaps because of its similarity to nitric oxide (NO), activates guanylate cyclase, which in turn relaxes vascular smooth muscle. Also, CO further displaces NO from platelets, resulting in additional vasodilation. These factors contribute to the hypotension that occurs in animal experiments with exposure to high concentrations of CO. Such an episode of hypotension leads to syncope, portending a worse clinical outcome.

## CLINICAL MANIFESTATIONS

### Acute Exposure

The earliest symptoms associated with CO poisoning are often nonspecific and readily confused with other illnesses, typically a viral syndrome. The initial symptoms are typically headache, dizziness, and nausea. Carbon monoxide poisoning is also frequently misdiagnosed as food poisoning, gastroenteritis, and even colic in infants.

The central nervous system (CNS) is the organ system that is most sensitive to CO poisoning. Acutely, otherwise healthy patients may manifest headache, dizziness, and ataxia at COHb levels as low as 15% to 20%, with higher levels or longer exposures causing syncope, seizures, or coma. Within 1 day of exposures that result in coma, many patients show decreased density in the central white matter and globus pallidus on computed tomography (CT) (Fig. 95–1) or magnetic resonance imaging (MRI). Autopsies show involvement of other areas, including the cerebral cortex, hippocampus, cerebellum, and substantia nigra.

Continued exposure to CO leads to symptoms attributable to cardiac and cerebral oxygen deficiency. Tachycardia is followed by angina, premature ventricular contractions, myocardial infarctions, ventricular dysrhythmias, and cardiac dysfunction. Troponin elevations often occur even in the absence of any coronary artery disease or electrocardiographic (ECG) or echocardiographic changes.

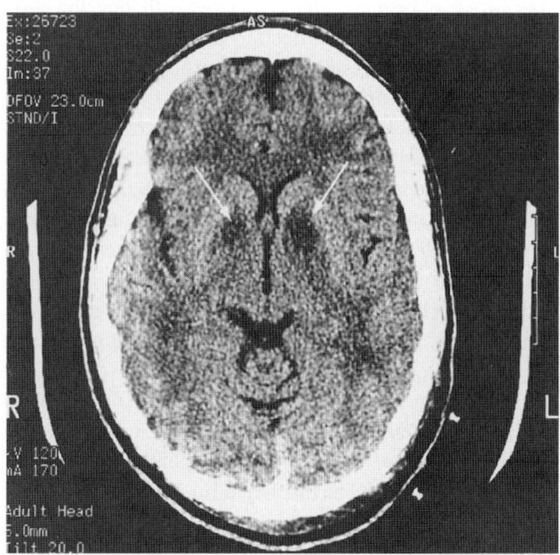


**FIGURE 95–1.** Computed tomography scan of the brain showing bilateral lesions of the globus pallidus (arrows) in a patient with poor recovery from severe carbon monoxide poisoning. *(Used with permission from the Fellowship in Medical Toxicology, New York University Grossman School of Medicine, New York City Poison Center.)*

Metabolic changes reflect the toxic effects of CO better than any particular COHb level. Patients with mild CO poisoning develop respiratory alkalosis in an attempt to compensate for the reduction in oxygen-carrying capacity and delivery. More substantial exposures result in metabolic acidosis with lactate production that accompanies tissue hypoxia. The importance of metabolic acidosis was highlighted in a retrospective series of CO-poisoned patients, in whom hydrogen ion concentration was a better predictor of poor recovery during initial hospitalization than was COHb level.

Although the brain and heart are the most sensitive, other organs also manifest the effects of CO poisoning. Pulmonary edema and ARDS are common, although smoke inhalation may be causative or contributory. Myonecrosis and even compartment syndromes occur and can lead to acute kidney injury (AKI). Retinal hemorrhages occur with exposures longer than 12 hours. Cherry-red skin coloration occurs only after lethal or near-lethal exposure and represents a combination of CO-induced vasodilation, concomitant tissue ischemia, and failure to extract oxygen from arterial blood. Another classic but uncommon phenomenon is the development of cutaneous bullae after severe exposures. These bullae are thought to be caused by a combination of pressure necrosis and possibly direct CO effects in the epidermis.

## NEUROCOGNITIVE SEQUELAE

The persistent or delayed effects of CO poisoning are varied and include dementia, amnestic syndromes, psychosis, parkinsonism, paralysis, chorea, cortical blindness, apraxia and agnosia, peripheral neuropathy, and incontinence. Neurocognitive sequelae involve lesions of the cerebral white matter. If not diagnosed at initial poisoning, neurologic deterioration is delayed and preceded by a lucid period of 2 to 40 days after the initial poisoning. Most cases of delayed neurocognitive sequelae are associated with loss of consciousness (LOC) during the acute phase of toxicity.

## CHRONIC EXPOSURE

Often, patients complain of persistent headaches and cognitive problems after long-term exposure to low concentrations of CO. Unfortunately, to date, there have been no controlled studies demonstrating that in the absence of a severe acute poisoning episode, this type of exposure results in any long-term sequelae.

## DIAGNOSTIC TESTING

The most useful diagnostic test obtainable in a suspected CO poisoning is a COHb level. Of note, in blood samples from neonates, falsely high COHb levels up to 8% can occur because of interference of fetal hemoglobin with spectroscopy. The usual method for measuring COHb is with a cooximeter, a device that spectrophotometrically reads the percentage of total hemoglobin saturated with CO. Traditionally, arterial blood was used for this determination; however, venous blood levels are accurate because there is little CO extraction from hemoglobin across the capillary bed. Refrigerated heparinized samples yield accurate COHb levels for months and at room temperature for 28 days, making retrospective clinical and postmortem evaluations reliable. The prior administration of hydroxocobalamin, interferes with COHb levels leading to falsely low levels on selected cooximeters, which could result in misdiagnosis.

Because of the similarities in extinction coefficients, COHb is misinterpreted as oxyhemoglobin on most types of pulse oximetry. Early models of a commercial bedside pulse cooximeter showed very poor agreement, mischaracterizing half the patients with levels over 15% as lower. Subsequently, two other cohorts of emergency department (ED) patients, using a later model of the same device, found that it measured COHb well, with a bias of 0.6% to 3% and precision of 3.3%. Because the pulse cooximeter is noninvasive, it can be used for initial screening of ED patients for occult CO poisoning who present with nonspecific symptoms and for field screening of mass casualties.

Additional laboratory tests are useful in severe poisoning cases. Metabolic acidosis with elevated lactate concentration is a more reliable index of severity than a measurement of the COHb level. Unfortunately, even arterial pH does not correlate well with either initial neurologic examination or the COHb level, making it a poor criterion for deciding the need for hyperbaric oxygen (HBO) treatment. Specificity of lactate is low in smoke inhalation victims, in whom it is used to indicate concomitant cyanide poisoning (Chap. 96). Continuous cardiac monitoring and a 12-lead ECG are essential to identify ischemia or dysrhythmias in symptomatic patients with preexisting coronary artery disease or severe exposure. Creatine phosphokinase is useful for diffuse myonecrosis, whereas troponin elevations are indicative of cardiac involvement.

The problem with using COHb levels to base treatment is that there is a wide variation in clinical manifestations across patients with identical COHb levels. Furthermore, particular COHb levels are not predictive of symptoms or final outcome. Admission COHb levels are also inaccurate predictors of peak levels, and the use of nomograms to extrapolate to earlier levels is not validated.

## NEUROPSYCHOLOGICAL TESTING

The extent of neurologic insult from CO can be assessed with a variety of tests. The most basic is documentation of the normal neurologic examination, including a quick mini mental status examination. A more sensitive indicator of the acute effects of CO on cortical function is a detailed neuropsychological test battery developed specifically for CO patients. The advantages of such testing, which usually takes about 30 minutes, are that it can reliably distinguish 79% of the time between CO-poisoned patients and control participants, and it shows improvement with appropriate HBO treatment. Unfortunately, such testing shows a sensitivity of only 77% and a specificity of 80% for CO poisoning.

## NEUROIMAGING

Acute changes on CT scans of the brain often occur within 12 hours of CO exposure that resulted in LOC. Symmetric low-density areas in the region of the globus pallidus, putamen, and caudate nuclei are frequently noted. Changes in the globus pallidus and subcortical white matter early within the first day after poisoning are associated with poor outcomes (Fig. 95–1). Magnetic resonance imaging is superior to CT in detecting cerebral white matter basal ganglia lesions after CO poisoning. One study found a much higher incidence of periventricular white matter changes on MRIs done within the first day after exposure. However, such changes had no correlation with COHb level or cognitive sequelae. Single-photon emission CT (SPECT) and positron emission tomography (PET) show promise but are not widely available.

Electroencephalograms (EEGs) complement perfusion studies in the evaluation of CO-poisoned patients. Although initial studies demonstrate that many patients have regional EEG abnormalities after poisoning, it is unknown if these are predictive of persistent or delayed neurologic problems.

## MANAGEMENT

The mainstay of treatment is initial attention to the airway. One hundred percent oxygen should be provided as soon as possible by either nonrebreather face mask or endotracheal tube. Although concerns have been raised regarding toxicity from excess oxygen, patients poisoned with CO can still have cellular hypoxia despite normal oxygen saturation. It is important to remember that a nonrebreathing mask only delivers 70% to 90% oxygen; a positive-pressure mask or an endotracheal tube is necessary to achieve higher oxygen concentrations. High-flow nasal cannula also effectively lowers COHb levels. The immediate effect of oxygen is to enhance the dissociation of COHb. In volunteers, the half-life of COHb is reduced from a mean of 5 hours (range, 2–7 hours) when breathing room air (21% oxygen) to approximately 1 hour (range, 36–137 minutes) when breathing 100% oxygen at normal atmospheric pressure. Actual poisoned patients show a range in half-lives of 36 to 137 minutes (mean, 85 minutes) when breathing 100% oxygen; the longer elimination half-lives appear to be most often associated with long, low-level exposures. The duration of treatment is unclear, with a valid end point being the resolution of symptoms, usually accompanied by a COHb below 5%.

Continuous cardiac monitoring and intravenous (IV) access are necessary in any patient with systemic toxicity from CO poisoning. Hypotension should initially be treated with IV fluids, with the addition of inotropes for persistent myocardial depression. Standard advanced cardiac life support protocols should be followed for the treatment of patients with life-threatening dysrhythmias. Patients with a depressed mental status should have a rapid blood glucose checked. We recommend not giving sodium bicarbonate for correction of any acidemia unless the acidemia is profound (usually pH < 7.0 or a serum bicarbonate concentration < 5 mEq/L) because it will cause left shift of the oxyhemoglobin dissociation curve, further impairing tissue oxygenation.

### Hyperbaric Oxygen

Hyperbaric oxygen (HBO) therapy is the treatment of choice for patients with significant CO exposures. But its most obvious effect is not the most important. One hundred percent oxygen at ambient pressure reduces the half-life of COHb from about 320 minutes to 85 minutes; at 2.5 atmospheres absolute (ATA), it is reduced to 20 minutes. Actual CO-poisoned victims treated with HBO have COHb half-lives ranging from 4 to 86 minutes. Hyperbaric oxygen also increases the amount of dissolved oxygen by about 10 times, which is sufficient alone to supply metabolic needs in the absence of hemoglobin. This is rarely an important clinical issue because most patients are already stabilized and have appreciably decreased COHb with ambient oxygen before preparation for an HBO treatment.

Therefore, HBO is more than just a modality to clear COHb more quickly than ambient oxygen (Antidotes in Brief: A40). More importantly, in multiple animal models of CO exposure, hyperbaric, but not normobaric, oxygen therapy prevents brain lipid peroxidation. This effect persists with clinically relevant delays to HBO therapy. Clinical studies of the effectiveness of HBO in preventing neurologic damage from CO are not as convincing as basic science studies would suggest. In uncontrolled human clinical series, the incidence of persistent neuropsychiatric symptoms, including memory impairment, ranged from 12% to 43% in patients treated with 100% oxygen and was as low as 0% to 4% in patients treated with HBO. Additionally, several controlled clinical trials evaluated the efficacy of HBO in CO poisoning with varied results.

Based on the strong animal and basic science experience, positive human studies, and few adverse effects, it is not surprising that the Underwater and Hyperbaric Medical Society (UHMS) recommends HBO for all CO patients with signs of serious toxicity. We believe that HBO is safe and indicated for serious CO poisoning, even though there is still substantial disagreement in the interpretation of the existing evidence regarding its usefulness.

***Indications for Hyperbaric Oxygen Therapy.*** Although the specific recommendations for HBO after acute CO poisoning are listed (Table 95–2), they are not prospectively evaluated. There are no completely reliable predictors for screening out patients who will do well without HBO treatment. Some authors recommend a more selective use of HBO because of cost and difficulties in transport if the primary facility lacks a chamber. However, complications that make such transfers and treatment unsafe are rare.

| TABLE 95–2 Recommended Indications for Hyperbaric Oxygen[a] |
|---|
| Syncope (transient loss of consciousness) |
| Coma |
| Seizure |
| Altered mental status (Glasgow Coma Scale score < 15) or confusion |
| Carboxyhemoglobin > 25%; independent of signs or symptoms |
| Abnormal cerebellar function |
| Pregnancy with a carboxyhemoglobin ≥ 15% |
| Fetal distress in pregnancy |
| Equivocal cases with age > 35 years and prolonged exposure (≥ 24 h) |

[a]Patients with these risk factors for cognitive sequelae have the highest potential to benefit from hyperbaric oxygen treatment.

***Delayed Administration of Hyperbaric Oxygen.*** The optimal timing and number of HBO treatments for CO poisoning are unclear. Patients treated later than 6 hours after exposure tend to have worse outcomes in terms of delayed sequelae (30% versus 19%) and mortality (30% versus 14%). However, patients benefit even if treated later. In the most recent randomized clinical trial showing beneficial effects of HBO, although all patients were treated within 24 hours of exposure, 38% of patients were treated later than 6 hours after exposure. Improvement in neurologic function was noted in this group. Therefore, it is reasonable to perform HBO, contingent on transport limitations, if the patient can receive HBO within 24 hours of removal from exposure.

***Repeat Treatment with Hyperbaric Oxygen.*** A randomized clinical trial demonstrated that three HBO treatments within the first 24 hours improved cognitive outcome. Unfortunately, there was no group treated with only one or two HBO sessions in that study. Regardless, it is reasonable to give up to three treatments for patients with persistent symptoms, particularly coma, who do not resolve after their first HBO session. With the lack of prospective studies comparing single versus multiple courses of HBO therapy, multiple treatments are not recommended as a routine at this time.

### Treatment of Pregnant Patients

The management of CO exposure in the pregnant patient is difficult because of the potential adverse effects of both CO and HBO. A literature review of all CO exposures during pregnancy revealed a high incidence of fetal CNS damage and stillbirth after severe maternal poisonings. Traditionally, it was thought that fetal hemoglobin had a high affinity for CO. Pregnant ewe studies show a delayed but substantive increase in COHb levels in fetuses, exceeding the level and duration of those in the mothers. Thus, it appeared that fetuses were a sink for CO and could be poisoned at concentrations lower than mothers. However, such data do not apply to humans because in vitro evidence demonstrates that as opposed to sheep, human fetal hemoglobin actually has less affinity for CO than maternal hemoglobin. The more important issue with maternal CO exposure is the precipitous decrease in fetal arterial oxygen content that occurs following CO poisoning.

The approach to treatment of seriously symptomatic CO-poisoned pregnant patients is problematic. All patients should receive 100% oxygen by face mask, at least until the mother is asymptomatic. However, CO absorption and elimination are slower in the fetal circulation than in the maternal circulation. Unfortunately, pregnant patients were excluded from all prospective trials documenting the efficacy of HBO. However, treatment of pregnant patients with HBO is not without theoretical risk. Animal studies show conflicting results on the effects of HBO on fetal development. This is in marked contrast to the extensive Russian experience, in which hundreds of pregnant women were treated with HBO, apparently without significant perinatal complications and with improvement in fetal and maternal status for their underlying conditions of toxemia, anemia, and diabetes. Thus, it appears that HBO should be safe and have the same efficacy for pregnant patients as in nonpregnant patients. There currently is no scientific validation for an absolute level at which to provide HBO therapy for a pregnant patient with CO exposure. Somewhat arbitrarily, we recommend a threshold for HBO in pregnant patients as a COHb level, regardless of symptoms, of greater than or equal to 15%. Pregnant patients should not be treated any differently if they meet the criteria for HBO described above (Table 95–2). Additional criteria include any signs of fetal distress, such as abnormal fetal heart rate.

### Treatment of Children

It is suggested that children are more sensitive to the effects of CO because of their increased respiratory and metabolic rates. Epidemiologic studies suggest that children become symptomatic at COHb levels lower than commonly expected in adults. The other problem is that these younger patients have unusual presentations. Although most children manifest nausea, headache, or lethargy, an isolated seizure or vomiting is sometimes the only manifestation of CO toxicity in an infant or child. When interpreting COHb levels in infants, clinicians must be aware of two confounding factors. First, many older cooximeters give falsely elevated COHb levels in proportion to the amount of fetal hemoglobin present. Second, CO is produced during breakdown of protoporphyrin to bilirubin. Therefore, infants normally have higher levels of COHb, which are even higher in the presence of kernicterus.

There are alternative clinical markers better than COHb for gauging toxicity in children. An elevated lactate concentration was found in 90.1% of 674 pediatric patients admitted for CO poisoning. Many children with elevated troponin concentrations after CO poisoning had normal ECGs or just subtle transitory T-wave changes from repolarization abnormalities. The echocardiogram is abnormal in approximately 50% of patients found to have an elevated troponin concentration, usually showing a temporary decrease in left ventricular function and ejection fraction.

Although children are likely more susceptible to acute toxicity with CO, their long-term outcomes appear to be more favorable than for adults. A low incidence of DNS in patients treated only with 100% oxygen at normal pressures is used as an argument to avoid HBO. Often, children exposed to CO under similar circumstances with a parent, although appearing well, are treated simultaneously with the sick parent, especially if a multiplace chamber is available.

### Novel Neuroprotective Treatments

A variety of neuroprotective therapeutics were tested in animal models. They are targeted primarily at preventing the delayed neurologic sequelae associated with serious CO poisoning. One of the simplest treatments tested is insulin. In CO poisoning of rodents, hyperglycemia is associated with worse neurologic outcome. However, insulin, independent of its glucose-lowering effect, is protective after ischemic insults. In rodent studies, improved neurologic outcome, as measured by locomotor activity, occurs in those with CO poisoning treated with insulin. In light of these findings, it is reasonable to treat documented hyperglycemia with insulin in patients with serious CO poisoning.

Although there are experimental data in support of dizocilpine, ketamine, dimethyl sulfoxide, disulfiram, 3-*N*-butylphtalide (a celery seed extract), dexamethasone, allopurinol, and erythropoietin, data are insufficient to recommend their use at this time.

## PREVENTION

Early diagnosis prevents much of the morbidity and mortality associated with CO poisoning, especially in unintentional exposures. The increased quality of home CO-detecting devices allows personal intervention in the prevention of exposure. If a patient presents complaining that his or her CO alarm sounded, it is important to realize that the threshold limit concentration for the alarm is set roughly to approximate a COHb level of 10% at worst. Alarms are not designed to activate for prolonged low-level exposures to prevent epidemic alarming during winter thermal inversions in large cities.

Routine laboratory screening of ED patients during the winter is not very efficacious in diagnosing unsuspected CO poisoning; the yield is less than 1% for patients tested in whom the diagnosis of CO exposure was already excluded by history. Instead, selecting patients with CO-related complaints, such as headache, dizziness, or nausea, increases the yield to 5% to 11%. During the winter, risk factors such as gas heating or symptomatic cohabitants in patients with influenzalike symptoms such as headache, dizziness, or nausea, particularly in the absence of fever, are the most useful method for deciding when to obtain COHb levels for potential patients.

The issue of symptomatic cohabitants is especially important from a preventive standpoint. Alerting other cohabitants to this danger and effecting evacuation prevents needless morbidity and mortality. This is especially critical for multifamily domiciles, such as hotels, that have resulted in dramatic collective exposures and even deaths. Most communities have multiple resources for on-site evaluation. Usually the local fire department or utility company can either check home appliances or measure ambient CO concentrations with portable monitoring equipment.

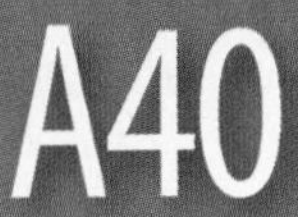


# HYPERBARIC OXYGEN

## INTRODUCTION

Hyperbaric oxygen (HBO) is used therapeutically in poisoning by carbon monoxide (CO), methylene chloride, hydrogen sulfide ($H_2S$), and carbon tetrachloride ($CCl_4$). It is also a recognized therapy for air or gas embolism and for functional anemia that arises from oxidants that induce methemoglobinemia.

## HISTORY

Hyperbaric medicine became established as a clinical discipline in the latter half of the 20th century with a focus on treatment of decompression sickness. The first hyperbaric chamber was built in New York by Corning in 1891. The first case reports of HBO for documented CO poisoning appeared in 1960.

## PHARMACOLOGY

### Chemistry and Preparation

Pressures applied while patients are in the hyperbaric chamber usually are 2 to 3 atmospheres absolute (ATA). Treatments generally last for 1.5 to 8 hours and are performed one to three times daily. Monoplace (single-person) chambers usually are compressed with pure oxygen. Multiplace (2–14 patients treated simultaneously) chambers are pressurized with air, and patients breathe pure oxygen through a tight-fitting face mask, a head tent, or an endotracheal tube.

### Mechanisms of Action

During treatment, the arterial oxygen tension typically exceeds 1,500 mm Hg and achieves tissue oxygen tensions of 200 to 400 mm Hg—more than fivefold higher than when breathing air. The primary effect of HBO is to increase the dissolved oxygen content of plasma. In addition, HBO affects neutrophil adhesion to blood vessels and restores mitochondrial, neutrophil, and immunologic disturbances caused by CO poisoning.

### Pharmacokinetics

Oxygen inhaled at hyperbaric pressure is rapidly absorbed. Application of each additional atmosphere of pressure while breathing 100% oxygen increases the dissolved oxygen concentration in the plasma by 2.2 mL $O_2$/dL (vol%). Animal models of ischemia suggest that HBO rapidly distributes $O_2$ to target organs to improve penumbral oxygenation.

### Pharmacodynamics

There are transient benefits from HBO for reducing bubble volume in disorders such as air embolism and oxygenating tissues in conditions in which hemoglobin-based $O_2$ delivery is impaired. These rather straightforward mechanisms form the basis for using HBO for patients with massive ingestions of $H_2O_2$ associated with intravascular gas embolism and for life-threatening poisonings from cyanide (CN), $H_2S$, and exposure to oxidizers causing methemoglobin. Hyperbaric oxygen is also used for $CCl_4$ poisoning, in which acute application of oxygen and pressure inhibit the cytochrome P450 oxidase system responsible for producing hepatotoxic free radicals. Hyperbaric oxygen also has well-described vasoconstriction effects compared with dynamic CO-associated effects on cerebral vasodilation.

There are several mechanisms supporting the use of $O_2$ when treating CO poisoning. Elevated COHb results in tissue hypoxia, and exogenous $O_2$ both hastens dissociation of CO from hemoglobin and provides enhanced tissue oxygenation directly through the increased $PaO_2$. Hyperbaric oxygen causes COHb dissociation to occur at a rate greater than that achievable by breathing 100% $O_2$ at sea level pressure. Additionally, HBO accelerates restoration of mitochondrial oxidative processes. Among the earliest events observed in both an animal model and in humans with CO poisoning is platelet–neutrophil interactions that mediate intravascular neutrophil activation. These changes precipitate neutrophil adherence to blood vessel walls that initiate vascular changes, leading to a cascade of localized changes in brain that cause neurologic dysfunction (Fig. A40–1). Rapid intervention with HBO in animal models causes improvement in cardiovascular status, leads to lower mortality rates, reduces platelet–neutrophil activation, and preserves synthesis of nerve growth factors. Exposure to 2.8 to 3.0 ATA $O_2$ for 45 minutes temporarily inhibits neutrophil adherence to endothelium mediated by the activation-dependent $\beta_2$-integrins on the neutrophil membrane in both rodents and humans. The ability of HBO to inhibit function of neutrophil $\beta_2$-integrin adhesion molecules in animal models forms the basis for amelioration of encephalopathy resulting from CO poisoning. It is important to comment that use of HBO at less than 2.8 ATA, as used in several clinical HBO studies, does not inhibit neutrophil adherence functions.

## ROLE IN CARBON MONOXIDE POISONING

Survivors of CO poisoning are faced with potential impairments to cardiac and neurologic functions. Events that follow an initial period of symptomatic CO poisoning that occur after a clear or "lucid" interval are termed "subacute" or "delayed" neurologic sequelae. The efficacy of HBO for acute CO poisoning is supported in animal trials, and studies provide a mechanistic basis for treatment. Unfortunately, only one clinical trial of significantly poisoned patients satisfies all items deemed to be necessary for the highest quality of randomized controlled trials. This double-blinded, placebo-controlled clinical trial involved 152 patients who received treatment (initiated within 24 hours of the end of exposure) with either three sessions of HBO therapy or normobaric $O_2$

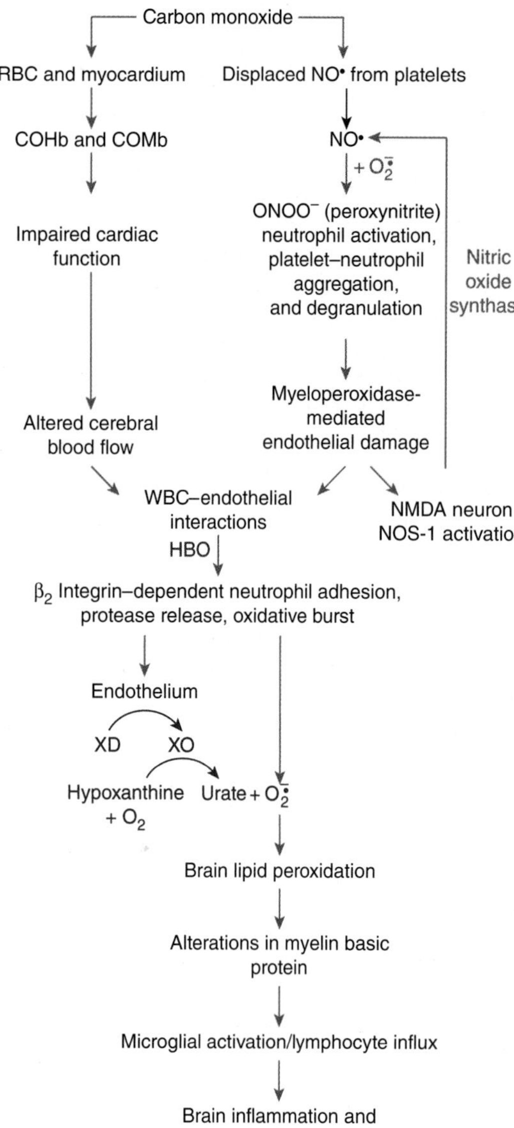


**FIGURE A40–1.** The pathway demonstrating concurrent events leading to vascular injury with carbon monoxide poisoning and the sequence of events leading to neurologic injuries. COHb = carboxyhemoglobin; COMb = carboxymyoglobin; NMDA = *N*-methyl-D-aspartate neurons; NO• = nitric oxide; $NO_2$ = nitrite (major oxidation product of NO•); NOS-1 = neuronal nitric oxide synthase; $O_2^{\bullet -}$ = superoxide radical; $ONOO^-$ = peroxynitrite; RBC = erythrocyte; WBC = leukocyte; XD = xanthine dehydrogenase; XO = xanthine oxidase.

with sham pressurization to maintain blinding. The group treated with HBO had a lower incidence of cognitive sequelae than the group treated with NBO. Other clinical trials suffered from a significant loss of patients to follow-up, a lack of blinding, or the use of subtherapeutic pressures. In a trial involving mildly to moderately poisoned patients, 23% of patients (7 of 30) treated with ambient pressure oxygen developed neurologic sequelae, but no patients (0/30; $P < 0.05$) who were treated with HBO (2.8 ATA) developed sequelae.

We recommend that HBO be administered in all cases of serious acute CO poisoning ideally within 6 hours of diagnosis but certainly up to 24 hours after the end of the exposure. Normobaric 100% oxygen should be continued until the onset of HBO administration.

Risk factors for long-term cognitive impairment in patients not treated with HBO include age older than 36 years, exposure longer than 24 hours, loss of consciousness, COHb greater than 25% on arrival to medical care, and an elevated troponin. Pregnancy poses another special situation in that CO readily crosses the placenta and may cause fetal distress and fetal death. Hyperbaric oxygen has been administered safely to pregnant women, but there are no prospective studies of efficacy. In CO-poisoned pregnant women, HBO is recommended for all of the indications listed above with the exception that a lower COHb threshold (15%) is reasonable as an extra safety measure for the fetus.

## ROLE IN METHYLENE CHLORIDE POISONING

Methylene chloride ($CH_2Cl_2$) is an organic solvent used commercially in aerosol sprays, as a solvent in plastics manufacturing, in photographic film production, in food processing as a degreaser, and as a paint stripper. It is readily absorbed through the skin or by inhalation. Immediate effects of methylene chloride are attributable to the direct depressant actions of this solvent on the central nervous system (CNS) and resulting hypoxia. However, metabolism of methylene chloride produces CO. Production of CO is slow, and peak COHb levels of 10% to 50% are reportedly delayed for 8 hours or more. Hyperbaric oxygen treatment recommendations follow those in patients meeting the aforementioned considerations in CO poisoning. The occurrence of ongoing CO production and persistent or recurring symptoms will likely necessitate additional treatments as the methylene chloride is mobilized from peripheral stores and undergoes metabolism. In patients with contraindications to HBO, prolonged normobaric 100% oxygen therapy is reasonable until COHb levels remain withing normal limits.

## ROLE IN COMBINED CARBON MONOXIDE AND CYANIDE POISONING

Carbon monoxide and CN poisonings can occur concomitantly from smoke inhalation, and experimental evidence suggests that they can produce synergistic toxicity. Hyperbaric oxygen appears to either have direct effects on reducing CN toxicity or augments the effects of other antidotes, including hydroxycobalamin. However, animal studies have not uniformly found that HBO improves outcome, and clinical experience regarding CN treatment with HBO is sparse.

Methemoglobin formation with the standard antidote treatment involving nitrite is not thought to generate high enough methemoglobin concentrations to be of concern, but in the setting of concomitant COHb, the additional reduction of oxygen-carrying capacity poses a potential risk. Hence, there is a special advantage for hydroxycobalamin use in combined poisonings. Hyperbaric oxygen is reasonable in any case of dual (CO and CN) poisoning and in CN poisoning when vital signs and mental status do not improve with antidote treatment, especially in locations that only have the nitrite/thiosulfate antidotes.

## ROLE IN HYDROGEN SULFIDE POISONING

Hydrogen sulfide binds to cytochrome a-$a^3$. This is similar to CN, although it is more readily dissociated by $O_2$. Clinical manifestations of toxicity are also similar to those of CO and CN. Hyperbaric oxygen is more effective than sodium nitrite in preventing death in animals. Several clinical reports indicate that HBO, sometimes in conjunction with supplemental oxygen and blood pressure support, appears to be beneficial. No definitive data regarding use of HBO for $H_2S$ poisoning are available, but HBO is reasonable when altered mental status or unstable vital signs persist after standard resuscitation measures.

## ROLE IN OXIDANT-INDUCED METHEMOGLOBINEMIA

Oxidation of ferrous ($2^+$) heme to the ferric ($3^+$) form renders hemoglobin nonfunctional, and the presence of oxidized hemoglobin varieties causes a left shift of the oxyhemoglobin dissociation curve. Hence, the manifestations of toxicity from acquired methemoglobinemia are usually more severe than those produced by a corresponding degree of anemia. There are numerous anecdotal accounts of clinical improvement with HBO in patients with life-threatening methemoglobinemia. Ongoing exposure to any oxidants and the potential need for methylene blue to treat methemoglobinemia (Antidotes in Brief: A43) should also be addressed.

## ROLE IN CARBON TETRACHLORIDE POISONING

Experimentally induced $CCl_4$ hepatotoxicity is diminished by HBO. There are also several case reports of patients surviving potentially lethal ingestions with HBO therapy. Because there are no proven antidotes for $CCl_4$ poisoning, we only recommend HBO for patients with confirmed $CCl_4$ exposures. However, because of a delicate balance between oxidative processes that are therapeutic and those that mediate hepatotoxicity, HBO should ideally be instituted before the onset of liver function abnormalities.

## ROLE IN HYDROGEN PEROXIDE INGESTION

Ingestion of concentrated $H_2O_2$ solutions (eg, 35%) can result in venous and arterial gas embolism because of liberation of large volumes of $O_2$. At standard temperature and pressure, ingestion of 1 mL of household 3% $H_2O_2$ liberates approximately 10 mL of oxygen gas; by comparison, each milliliter of 35% $H_2O_2$ yields 115 mL of oxygen gas. Hyperbaric oxygen is a successful intervention for portal venous gas, and in some cases of impaired consciousness and/or with focal neurologic findings. Hyperbaric oxygen reduces the volume of offending gas and improves solubility of gas into tissues and plasma. We recommend HBO in patients with neurologic symptoms, and it is reasonable in patients with severe abdominal discomfort despite conservative care.

## ADVERSE EFFECTS AND SAFETY ISSUES

Many HBO facilities have equipment and treatment protocols and abilities analogous to those found in an intensive care unit. The inherent toxicity of $O_2$ and potential for injury resulting from elevations of ambient pressure must be addressed whenever HBO is used therapeutically. Preexisting conditions that require evaluation for possible management before initiation of HBO include claustrophobia, sinus congestion, and patients with scarred or noncompliant structures in the middle ear, such as otosclerosis. Middle ear barotrauma is the most common adverse effect of HBO treatment, and it occurs in 1.2% to 7% of patients. Unconscious patients should be evaluated for prophylactic myringotomy prior to HBO. Toxicity resulting from $O_2$ is manifested by injuries to the CNS, lungs, and eyes. Central nervous system $O_2$ toxicity manifests as a generalized seizure and occurs at an incidence of approximately 1 to 4 per 10,000 patient treatments.

## PREGNANCY AND LACTATION

Hyperbaric oxygen in pregnant patients presents the additional risks of fetal CNS, ocular, pulmonary, and cardiac toxicity. In CO poisoning, these must be weighed against the potentially devastating fetal outcomes such as spontaneous abortion, intrauterine fetal demise, anatomic malformations, CNS injury, respiratory distress, and neonatal jaundice, which occur even in only mildly symptomatic CO-poisoned mothers. For these reasons, COHb thresholds (eg, 15%–20%) for HBO therapy are often set lower for pregnant patients than for other adults in HBO treatment algorithms. The authors of this text recommend treating a pregnant woman with HBO when COHb levels are greater than or equal to 15%. Treatment decisions will ultimately be made on an individual case basis after weighing potential risks and benefits. There are no data regarding the effects of HBO on lactation.

## DOSING AND ADMINISTRATION

Hyperbaric oxygen efficacy is a time- and pressure-dependent phenomenon. Rodent and human studies demonstrate that exposure to 2.8 to 3.0 ATA $O_2$ for 45 minutes is required to temporarily inhibit neutrophil adherence to endothelium mediated by the activation-dependent $\beta_2$-integrins on the neutrophil membrane and to ameliorate metabolic insults leading to loss of neuronal growth factors. Clinical trials using HBO at only 2 ATAs have been unable to demonstrate a benefit of HBO, likely because it is an inadequate dose to achieve biochemical effects on cellular responses as discussed earlier. Multiple trials using HBO (2.5 ATA or above) have demonstrated efficacy. One trial using HBO (2.8 ATA) was unable to demonstrate benefit, because of incomplete followup and poor randomization. If undertaken, HBO therapy (2.5–3.0 ATA, weighted toward the latter) should be provided as early as possible because a mortality benefit is demonstrated if HBO is administered within 6 hours of the CO exposure. Clinical trials that have initiated therapy within 24 hours of the end of CO exposure show improvement of neurologic toxicity. The use of more than one treatment is supported by retrospective and prospective analysis, although clinical practice is highly variable in this regard.

## FORMULATION AND ACQUISITION

Hyperbaric oxygen therapy is provided in monoplace or multiplace chambers, which are considered class II medical devices. For sites not possessing HBO capacity, various online organizational and professional directories may assist in locating hyperbaric facilities in the absence of preexisting HBO transfer protocols.

# 96 CYANIDE AND HYDROGEN SULFIDE

| | |
|---|---|
| **Cyanide** | |
| Normal | < 1 µg/mL |
| Whole blood | < 38.43 µmol/L |
| Concentrations | |
| Airborne | |
| Immediately fatal | = 270 ppm |
| Life threatening | = 110 ppm > 30 minutes |
| **Hydrogen Sulfide** | |
| Airborne | |
| Odor threshold | = 0.01–0.3 ppm |
| Olfactory paralysis | = 100–150 ppm |
| Immediately fatal | = 1,000 ppm |

## CYANIDE POISONING

### History and Epidemiology

Cyanide (CN) exposure is associated with smoke inhalation, laboratory mishaps, industrial incidents, suicide attempts, and criminal activity. Inorganic CNs (also known as CN salts) contain CN in the anion form ($CN^-$) and are used in industries, such as metallurgy, photographic developing, plastic manufacturing, fumigation, and mining. Ingestion of cyanogenic chemicals (ie, acetonitrile, acrylonitrile, and propionitrile) is another source of CN poisoning. Acetonitrile ($C_2H_3N$) and acrylonitrile ($C_3H_3N$) are themselves nontoxic, but biotransformation via CYP2E1 liberates CN (Fig. 96–1). Many plants, such as the *Manihot* spp and *Prunus* spp, contain cyanogenic glycosides such as amygdalin. When ingested, amygdalin is biotransformed to CN (Fig. 96–1). Iatrogenic CN poisoning occurs during prolonged or high-dose nitroprusside therapy for the management of hypertension. Each nitroprusside molecule contains five CN molecules, which are slowly released in vivo.

Napoleon III was the first to use hydrogen cyanide (HCN) in chemical warfare, and it was subsequently used on World War I battlefields. During World War II, hydrocyanic acid pellets caused more than one million deaths in Nazi gas chambers. In 1978, KCN was used in a mass suicide led by Jim Jones of the People's Temple in Guyana, resulting in more than 900 deaths.

### Pharmacology

Cyanide is an extremely potent toxin, with even small exposures leading to life-threatening symptoms. The adult oral lethal dose of KCN is approximately 200 mg. Acute toxicity occurs through a variety of routes, including inhalation, ingestion, dermal, and parenteral.

### Toxicokinetics

Cyanide is eliminated from the body by multiple pathways. The major route for detoxification of CN is the enzymatic conversion to thiocyanate. Two sulfurtransferase enzymes, rhodanese (thiosulfate–CN sulfurtransferase) and β-mercaptopyruvate–CN sulfurtransferase, catalyze this reaction. In acute poisoning, the limiting factor in CN detoxification by rhodanese is the availability of adequate quantities of sulfur donors. The endogenous stores of sulfur are rapidly depleted, and CN metabolism slows. Thiocyanate is eliminated in urine. Elimination follows first-order kinetics, although it varies widely in reports (range, 1.2–66 hours). The volume of distribution of the CN anion varies according to species and investigator, with 0.075 L/kg reported in humans.

### Pathophysiology

Cyanide is an inhibitor of multiple enzymes, including succinic acid dehydrogenase, superoxide dismutase, carbonic anhydrase, and cytochrome oxidase. Cytochrome oxidase is an iron-containing metalloenzyme essential for oxidative phosphorylation and hence aerobic energy production. Cyanide induces cellular hypoxia by inhibiting cytochrome oxidase by binding to the ferric ion on the cytochrome $a_3$ portion of the electron transport chain (Fig. 96–2). Hydrogen ions that normally would have combined with oxygen at the terminal end of the chain are no longer incorporated. Thus,

A: Acetonitrile —CYP2E1→ Hydrogen cyanide + Formaldehyde

B: Amygdalin —β-d-glucosidase→ Glucose (2) + Hydrogen cyanide + Benzaldehyde

**FIGURE 96-1.** Biotransformation of cyanogens acetonitrile (**A**) and amygdalin (**B**) to cyanide.

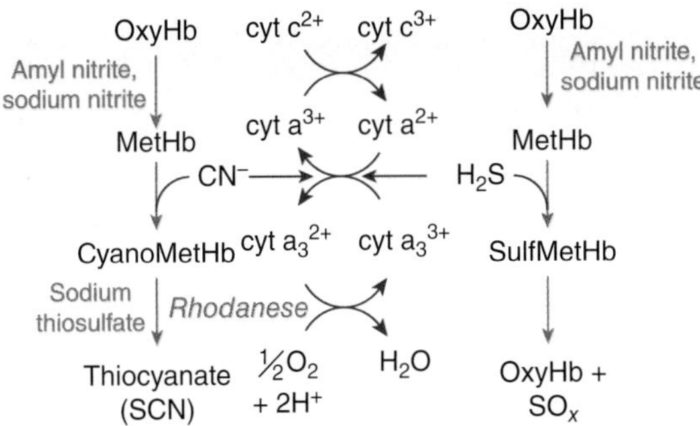


**FIGURE 96-2.** Pathway of cyanide and hydrogen sulfide toxicity and detoxification. MetHb = methemoglobin; OxyHb = oxyhemoglobin; SulfMetHb = sulfmethemoglobin.

despite sufficient oxygen supply, oxygen cannot be used, and ATP molecules are no longer formed. Unincorporated hydrogen ions accumulate, contributing to acidemia.

The lactate concentration increases rapidly following CN poisoning because of failure of aerobic energy metabolism. During aerobic conditions, when the electron transport chain is functional, lactate is converted to pyruvate by mitochondrial lactate dehydrogenase. In this process, lactate donates hydrogen moieties that reduce nicotinamide adenine dinucleotide ($NAD^+$) to nicotinamide adenine dinucleotide (NADH). Pyruvate then enters the citric acid cycle, with resulting ATP formation. When cytochrome $a_3$ within the electron transport chain is inhibited by CN, there is a relative paucity of $NAD^+$ and predominance of NADH, favoring the reverse reaction, in which pyruvate is converted to lactate.

Cyanide is also a potent neurotoxin. It enhances *N*-methyl-D-aspartate (NMDA) receptor activity and directly activates the NMDA receptor, which results in $Ca^{2+}$ entry into the cytosol of neurons.

## Clinical Manifestations

***Acute Exposure to Cyanide.*** The initial clinical effects of acute CN poisoning are nonspecific, generalized, and nondiagnostic, thereby making the correct diagnosis difficult to obtain. Clinical manifestations reflect rapid dysfunction of oxygen-sensitive organs, with central nervous system (CNS) and cardiovascular findings predominating. The time to onset of symptoms typically is seconds with inhalation of gaseous HCN or IV injection of a water-soluble CN salt and several minutes after ingestion of inorganic CN. The clinical effects of cyanogenic chemicals often are delayed, and the time course varies among individuals (range, 3–24 hours), depending on their rate of biotransformation.

Central nervous system signs and symptoms are typical of progressive hypoxia and include headache, anxiety, agitation, confusion, lethargy, nonreactive dilated pupils, seizures, and coma. A centrally mediated tachypnea occurs initially followed by bradypnea and apnea. Cardiovascular responses to CN are complex. An initial period of tachycardia and hypertension usually occurs followed by hypotension with reflex tachycardia, but the terminal event is consistently bradycardia and hypotension. Gastrointestinal toxicity occurs after ingestion of inorganic CN and cyanogens and includes abdominal pain, nausea, and vomiting. These symptoms are caused by hemorrhagic gastritis, which is secondary to the caustic nature of CN salts. Cutaneous manifestations vary. A cherry red skin color is described as a potential finding as a result of increased venous hemoglobin oxygen saturation, which results from decreased utilization of oxygen at the tissue level.

***Delayed Clinical Manifestations of Acute Exposure.*** Survivors of serious, acute poisoning develop delayed neurologic sequelae. Parkinsonian symptoms, including dystonia, dysarthria, rigidity, and bradykinesia, are most common. Response to pharmacotherapy with antiparkinsonian drugs is generally disappointing.

***Chronic Exposure to Cyanide.*** Chronic exposure to CN results in insidious syndromes, including tobacco amblyopia, Konzo, and Leber hereditary optic neuropathy. Chronic exposure to CN is also associated with thyroid disorders. Thiocyanate is a competitive inhibitor of iodide entry into the thyroid, thereby causing the formation of goiters and the development of hypothyroidism (Chap. 26).

## Diagnostic Testing

Because of nonspecific symptoms and delay in laboratory CN confirmation, the clinician must rely on historical circumstances and some initial findings to raise suspicion of CN poisoning and institute therapy (Table 96–1). Laboratory findings suggestive of CN poisoning reflect an increased anion gap metabolic acidosis and elevated lactate concentration. Elevated venous oxygen saturation results from reduced tissue extraction. The finding of a small arterial–venous oxygen difference is also suggestive of CN toxicity. Hyperlactatemia is found in numerous critical illnesses and typically is a nonspecific finding. However, a significant association exists between blood CN and serum lactate concentrations. A lactate greater than 8 mmol/L following ingestion or greater than 10 mmol/L following smoke inhalation is highly suggested of cyanide toxicity. A determination of the blood CN concentration will confirm toxicity, but this determination is not available in a sufficiently rapid manner to affect initial treatment.

## Management

First responders should exercise extreme caution when entering potentially hazardous areas such as chemical plants and laboratories where a previously healthy person is "found down." Because CN poisoning is rare, it is easy to overlook the diagnosis unless there is an obvious history of exposure. Thus, the most critical steps in treatment are considering the diagnosis in high-risk situations (Table 96–1) and initiating empiric therapy with 100% oxygen and either hydroxycobalamin (preferably) or the sodium nitrite and sodium thiosulfate combination. The initial care (Table 96–1) of a CN-poisoned patient begins by directing attention to airway patency, ventilatory support, and oxygenation.

Instillation of activated charcoal often is considered by other authors to be ineffective because of low binding of CN (1 g of activated charcoal only adsorbs 35 mg of CN). However, a potentially lethal oral dose of CN (ie, a few hundred

**TABLE 96–1 Cyanide Poisoning: Emergency Management Guidelines**

***When to Suspect Cyanide***

Sudden collapse of laboratory or industrial worker

Fire victim with coma or acidemia

Suicide with unexplained rapid coma or acidemia

Ingestion of artificial nail remover

Ingestion of seeds or pits from *Prunus* spp

Patient with altered mental status, hyperlactatemia, acidemia, and tachyphylaxis to nitroprusside

***Supportive Care***

Control airway, ventilate, and give 100% oxygen

Crystalloids and vasopressors for hypotension

Administer sodium bicarbonate; titrate according to pH and serum [$HCO_3^-$]

***Antidotes***

1) Hydroxocobalamin (preferred)

Initial adult dose: 5 g IV over 15 min; pediatric dose 70 mg/kg up to 5 g; to be repeated if necessary

or

2) Cyanide Antidote Kit

Amyl nitrite pearls are included in the kit for prehospital use only. For hospital management, sodium nitrite is the preferred methemoglobin inducer and is given in lieu of the pearls.

Give sodium nitrite ($NaNO_2$) as a 3% solution over 2–4 min IV: Adult dose: 10 mL (300 mg) (see Table 96–2 for pediatric dosing)

*Caution:* Monitor blood pressure frequently and treat hypotension by slowing infusion rate and giving crystalloids and vasopressors. Obtain methemoglobin level 30 min after dose; excess methemoglobin formation will cause deterioration during therapy. Withhold nitrites if COHb is suspected to be present (eg, fires).

Give sodium thiosulfate ($NaS_2O_3$) as a 25% solution IV:

Adult dose: 50 mL (12.5 g)

Pediatric dose: 1.65 mL/kg up to 50 mL

***Decontamination***

Protect healthcare provider from contamination

Cutaneous: Carefully remove all clothing and flush the skin

Ingestion: Oro- or nasogastric lavage and instill 1 g/kg activated charcoal

***Laboratory***

ABG or VBG

Electrolytes and glucose

Blood lactate

Whole-blood cyanide concentration (for later confirmation only)

ABG = arterial blood gas; COHb = carboxyhemoglobin; IV = intravenous; VBG = venous blood gas.

**TABLE 96–2 Sodium Nitrite Guidelines for Managing Cyanide Poisoning in Children**

| *Hemoglobin (g/100 mL)* | *Sodium Nitrite 3% Solution (mL/kg)* |
|---|---|
| 7 | 0.19 |
| 8 | 0.22 |
| 9 | 0.25 |
| 10 | 0.27 |
| 11 | 0.30 |
| 12 | 0.33 |
| 13 | 0.36 |
| 14 | 0.39 |

Sodium thiosulfate 25% solution: 1.65 mL/kg IV.

Repeat sodium thiosulfate once at half dose (0.825 mL/kg) if symptoms persist.

(Reproduced with permission from Tintinalli JE et al. *Tintinalli's Emergency Medicine: A Comprehensive Study Guide*, 9e. New York, NY: McGraw Hill; 2020.)

milligrams) is within the adsorptive capacity of a typical 1-g/kg dose of activated charcoal. Although either hydroxocobalamin or sodium nitrite and sodium thiosulfate combination should be administered as soon as CN poisoning is suspected, hydroxocobalamin is preferred. Hydroxocobalamin has few adverse effects, which include rashes and a transient reddish discoloration of the skin, mucous membranes, and urine. No hemodynamic adverse effects other than a potential mild transient rise of blood pressure are observed in those who are not poisoned. Adverse effects of nitrites include excessive methemoglobin formation and, because of potent vasodilation, hypotension and tachycardia. Avoiding rapid infusion, monitoring blood pressure, and adhering to dosing guidelines limit adverse effects. Because of the potential for excessive methemoglobinemia during nitrite treatment, pediatric dosing guidelines are available (Table 96–2). More detailed discussions of cyanide antidotes can be found in the Antidotes in Brief: A41 and A42.

## HYDROGEN SULFIDE POISONING

### History and Epidemiology

Hydrogen sulfide ($H_2S$) exposures are often dramatic and fatal. Most of $H_2S$ exposures occur through workplace exposures, but they also occur in environmental disasters and suicides. Bacterial decomposition of proteins generates $H_2S$. Thus, decay of sulfur-containing products such as fish, sewage, and manure produces $H_2S$. Industrial sources include pulp paper mills, heavy-water production, the leather industry, roofing asphalt tanks, vulcanizing of rubber, viscose rayon production, and coke manufacturing from coal. It is a major industrial hazard in oil and gas production, particularly in sour gas fields (natural gas containing sulfur). Natural sources of $H_2S$ are volcanoes, caves, sulfur springs, and underground deposits of natural gas. More recently, a large number of suicides called "chemical suicides" or "detergent suicides" were attributed to mixing common household chemicals such as pesticides or fungicides and toilet bowl cleaners to create $H_2S$ gas.

Up to 25% of fatalities involve rescuers. For example, a leaking food waste pipeline in the propeller room of a cruise ship released $H_2S$, killing three workers attempting to repair the pipe. The emergency response resulted in injury to 18 crew members, including a physician and a nurse rushing into the dangerous environment without personal protective equipment.

### Pharmacology and Toxicokinetics

Hydrogen sulfide is a colorless gas, more dense than air, with an irritating odor of "rotten eggs." It is highly lipid soluble, a property that allows easy penetration of biologic membranes. Systemic absorption usually occurs through inhalation, and it is rapidly distributed to tissues.

Hydrogen sulfide binds to the ferric ($Fe^{3+}$) moiety of cytochrome $a_3$ oxidase complex with a higher affinity than does CN. The resulting inhibition of oxidative phosphorylation produces cellular hypoxia and anaerobic metabolism. Besides producing cellular hypoxia, $H_2S$ alters brain neurotransmitter release and neuronal transmission through potassium channel–mediated hyperpolarization of neurons, NMDA receptor potentiation, and other neuronal inhibitory mechanisms. The olfactory nerve is a specific target of great interest. Not only does the toxic gas cause olfactory nerve paralysis, but it also provides a portal of entry into the CNS because of its direct contact with the brain. In addition to systemic effects, $H_2S$ reacts with the moisture on the surface of mucous membranes to produce intense irritation and corrosive injury. The eyes and nasal and respiratory mucous membranes are the tissues most susceptible to direct injury. Despite skin irritation, it has little dermal absorption.

Inhaled $H_2S$ enters the systemic circulation where, at physiologic pH, it dissociates into hydrosulfide ions ($HS^-$). After dissociation, hydrosulfide ions interact with metalloproteins, disulfide-containing enzymes, and thio dimethyl S transferase. Hydrogen sulfide and dissociation products are then metabolized by multiple enzymes, including mitochondrial sulfide quinone oxireductase, sulfur dioxygenase to form sulfate ($SO_2^{4+}$), and thiosulfate-CN sulfurtransferase (rhodanese) to form thiosulfate ($SSO_3^{2-}$). The most specific marker of $H_2S$ metabolism is thiosulfate. Sulfhemoglobin is not found in significant concentrations in the blood of animals or fatally poisoned humans.

## CLINICAL MANIFESTATIONS

***Acute Manifestations.*** Hydrogen sulfide poisoning should be suspected whenever a person is found unconscious in an enclosed space, especially if the odor of rotten eggs is noted. The primary target organs of hydrogen sulfide poisoning are those of the CNS, cardiac system, and respiratory system. The clinical findings reported in two large series are listed in Table 96–3. Hydrogen sulfide poisoning has a distinct dose response, and the intensity of exposure likely accounts for the diverse clinical findings in the reports. The odor threshold is between 0.01 and 0.3 ppm, and a strong intense odor is noted at 20 to 30 ppm. Mucous membrane and eye irritation occurs at 20 to 100 ppm. Olfactory nerve paralysis occurs at 100 to 150 ppm, rapidly extinguishing the ability to perceive the gas odor at higher concentrations. Prolonged exposure occurs when the extinction of odor recognition is misinterpreted as dissipation of the gas. Strong irritation of the upper respiratory tract and eyes and acute respiratory distress syndrome (ARDS) occur at 150 to 300 ppm. At greater than 500 ppm, $H_2S$ produces systemic effects, including rapid unconsciousness ("knockdown") and cardiopulmonary arrest. At 1,000 ppm, breathing ceases after one to two breaths. The rapid and deadly onset of clinical effects of $H_2S$ are termed the "slaughterhouse sledgehammer" effect.

**TABLE 96–3 Hydrogen Sulfide Poisoning**

| *When to Suspect Hydrogen Sulfide Poisoning* | |
|---|---|
| Rapid loss of consciousness ("knocked down") and abrupt awakening | |
| Rapid loss of consciousness ("knocked down") and apnea | |
| Rotten egg odor | |
| Rescue from enclosed space, such as sewer or manure pit | |
| Multiple victims with sudden death | |
| Collapse of a previously healthy worker at work site | |
| *Clinical Manifestations* | |
| *System* | *Signs and Symptoms* |
| Cardiovascular | Chest pain, bradycardia, sudden cardiac arrest |
| Central nervous | Headache, weakness, syncope, convulsions, rapid onset of coma ("knockdown") |
| Gastrointestinal | Nausea, vomiting |
| Ophthalmic | Conjunctivitis |
| Pulmonary | Dyspnea, cyanosis, crackles, apnea |
| Metabolic | Metabolic acidosis, elevated serum lactate |

***Chronic Manifestations.*** Most data about chronic low-level exposures to $H_2S$ come from oil and gas industry workers and sewer workers. Mucous membrane irritation seems to be the most prominent problem in patients with low-concentration exposures. The chronic irritating effects of $H_2S$ are proposed to be the cause of reduced lung volumes observed in sewer workers. Rapid loss of consciousness from $H_2S$ exposure was a well-known and, amazingly, accepted part of the workplace in the gas and oil industry for many years. Single or repeated high-concentration exposures resulting in unconsciousness cause serious cognitive dysfunction. Case series suggest that low-concentration exposures cause subtle changes that are only measured by the most sensitive neuropsychiatric tests.

### Diagnostic Testing

Diagnostic testing is of limited value for clinical decision making after acute exposures, but can be used for confirmation of acute exposures, occupational monitoring, and forensic analysis after fatal events. Clinicians must base management decisions on history, clinical presentation, and diagnostic tests that infer the presence of $H_2S$ because no method is available to rapidly and directly measure the gas or its metabolites (Table 96–3). Specific tests for confirming $H_2S$ exposure are not readily available in clinical laboratories.

In acute poisoning, readily available diagnostic tests that are biomarkers of $H_2S$ poisoning are useful but are nonspecific. Arterial or venous blood gas analysis demonstrating acidemia with an associated elevated serum lactate concentration is expected, and oxygen saturation should be normal unless ARDS is present. Hydrogen sulfide, like CN, decreases oxygen consumption and is reflected as an elevated mixed venous oxygen measurement. Because sulfhemoglobin (Chap. 97) typically is not generated in patients with $H_2S$ poisoning, an oxygen saturation gap is not expected.

### Management

The initial treatment (Table 96–4) is immediate removal of the victim from the contaminated area into a fresh air environment. High-flow oxygen should be administered as soon as possible. Optimal supportive care has the greatest influence on the patient's outcome. Because death from inhalation of

| TABLE 96–4 Hydrogen Sulfide Poisoning: Emergency Management |
|---|
| **Supportive care** |
| Prehospital |
| Attempt rescue only if using appropriate respiratory protection |
| Move victim to fresh air |
| Administer 100% oxygen |
| During extrication, evaluate for traumatic injuries from falls |
| Apply ACLS protocols as indicated |
| Emergency department |
| Maximize ventilation and oxygenation |
| Utilize PEEP or BiPAP for ARDS |
| Administer sodium bicarbonate; titrate according to ABG or VBG, and serum [$HCO_3^-$] |
| Administer crystalloid and vasopressors for hypotension |
| **Antidote** |
| 1) It is reasonable to administer sodium nitrite (3% $NaNO_2$) IV over 2–4 min |
| Adult dose: 10 mL (300 mg) |
| Pediatric dose: **Table 96–2**; if hemoglobin unknown, presume 7 g/dL for dosing |
| Caution: |
| Monitor blood pressure frequently |
| Obtain methemoglobin level 30 min after dose |

ABG = arterial blood gas; ACLS = advanced cardiac life support; ARDS = acute respiratory distress syndrome; Hb = hemoglobin; IV = intravenous; PEEP = positive end-expiratory pressure; VBG = venous blood gas.

$H_2S$ is rapid, a limited number of patients reaching the hospital for treatment are reported in the literature. Most patients experience significant delays before receiving treatment. Therefore, specific treatments and antidotal therapies do not show definitive improvement in patient outcome.

The affinity of $H_2S$ for methemoglobin is greater than that for cytochrome oxidase. Nitrite-induced methemoglobin protects animals from toxicity of $H_2S$ poisoning in both pre- and postexposure treatment models. Because $H_2S$ poisoning is rare, no studies have evaluated the clinical outcomes of patients treated with sodium nitrite. However, several human case reports showed rapid return of normal sensorium when nitrites were administered soon after exposure. Sodium nitrite treatment is reasonable to administer to patients with suspected $H_2S$ poisoning who have altered mental status, coma, hypotension, or dysrhythmias but should be given cautiously because of the potential for nitrite-induced hypotension during the infusion.

Treatment of patients with $H_2S$ poisoning requires optimal supportive care. Beyond supportive care, no definitive evidence of significant clinical benefit exists in humans, and additional research is needed to determine efficacy of specific treatments for $H_2S$ poisoning.

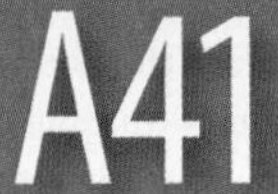

Antidotes in Brief

A41

# HYDROXOCOBALAMIN

## INTRODUCTION

Cyanocobalamin, vitamin $B_{12}$, is formed when hydroxocobalamin combines with cyanide (CN), quickly diminishing CN concentrations and improving hemodynamics. Hydroxocobalamin is now the antidote of choice in fire victims and most other cases of CN toxicity as the previous antidotes based on nitrites therapy have the disadvantage of purposefully inducing methemoglobin.

## HISTORY

The antidotal actions of cobalt as a chelator of CN were recognized as early as 1894. Development of cobalt-containing cyanide antidotes such as cobalt-EDTA were hampered by poor side effect profiles. Hydroxocobalamin was studied in France as a safer cobalt-containing antidote and became the drug of choice there, first as a sole agent and then in combination with sodium thiosulfate. Hydroxocobalamin was approved for use in the United States (US) by the Food and Drug Administration (FDA) in December 2006 and is available under the trade name Cyanokit.

## PHARMACOLOGY

### Chemistry

The hydroxocobalamin molecule shares structural similarity with porphyrin, with a cobalt ion at its core. The difference between cyanocobalamin (vitamin $B_{12}$) and hydroxocobalamin (vitamin $B_{12a}$) is the replacement of the CN group with an OH group at the active site in the latter.

### MECHANISM OF ACTION

The cobalt ion in hydroxocobalamin combines with CN in an equimolar fashion to form nontoxic cyanocobalamin—one mole of hydroxocobalamin binds one mole of CN. Thus, given the molecular weights of each, 52 g of hydroxocobalamin is needed to bind 1 g of CN. So, a standard 5 g of hydroxocobalamin would be expected to bind 96 mg of CN, which is on the order of a typical lethal inhaled dose.

Hydroxocobalamin also binds the vasodilator nitric oxide (NO), which is structurally similar to CN, causing vasoconstriction both in the presence and in the absence of CN. This property contributes to its beneficial effects by increasing systolic and diastolic blood pressure and improving the hemodynamic status of CN-poisoned patients.

## PHARMACOKINETICS AND PHARMACODYNAMICS

In human volunteers given a 5-g IV dose, the peak hydroxocobalamin concentrations averaged 813 μg/mL (604 μmol/L), with an average volume of distribution (Vd) of 0.38 L/kg. A mean of 62% of the hydroxocobalamin dose was recovered in the urine in 24 hours. In a pharmacokinetic study of adult victims of smoke inhalation, the elimination half-life of hydroxocobalamin was 26.2 hours and the Vd was 0.45 L/kg. In the one patient who was subsequently determined not to be exposed to CN, the hydroxocobalamin elimination half-life was 13.6 hours, and the Vd was 0.23 L/kg. Renal clearance of hydroxocobalamin was 37% in the CN-exposed patients compared with 62% in the unexposed patient.

## ROLE IN CYANIDE TOXICITY

### Animals

The ability of hydroxocobalamin to bind CN and produce beneficial effects on mortality and hemodynamics is demonstrated in many animal species, including rabbits, swine, dogs, and baboons.

### Humans

Many case reports and studies document the efficacy of hydroxocobalamin combined with sodium thiosulfate for treatment of CN toxicity. An observational case series reviewed 69 adult smoke inhalation victims suspected of CN poisoning who were treated with a median dose of 5 g of hydroxocobalamin. Of 42 patients with confirmed CN concentrations greater than 39 μmol/L (1 μg/mL, a potentially fatal concentration), 28 (67%) survived. An 8-year retrospective analysis of the use of hydroxocobalamin in the prehospital setting concluded that the risk-to-benefit ratio favors its use in smoke inhalation victims with suspected CN poisoning.

There are currently no studies comparing the nitrite plus sodium thiosulfate regimen with hydroxocobalamin in patients with CN poisoning. There are no studies comparing hydroxocobalamin with or without sodium thiosulfate to sodium thiosulfate alone in smoke inhalation victims presumed to be CN toxic.

## ADVERSE EFFECTS AND SAFETY ISSUES

Hydroxocobalamin has a wide therapeutic index. Large doses were administered to animals with no adverse effects. The $LD_{50}$ (median lethal dose in 50% of test subjects) in mice is 2 g/kg. Red discoloration of mucous membranes, serum, and urine is expected and lasts from 12 hours to many days after therapy. Colorimetric assays are adversely affected because both hydroxocobalamin and cyanocobalamin have an intensely red color. Many clinical chemistry laboratory analyses are artificially increased, decreased, or unpredictable. Hematology analyses including hemoglobin, mean corpuscular hemoglobin (MCH), mean corpuscular hemoglobin concentration (MCHC), and basophils are artificially increased. Coagulation tests are unpredictable. Urinalysis analyses are usually artificially increased, but pH can also be artificially low with low doses of hydroxocobalamin. An in vitro study found statistically significant alterations in serum concentrations of aspartate aminotransferase (AST), total bilirubin, creatinine, magnesium, and iron after hydroxocobalamin administration. Although an in vitro study demonstrated a considerable false increase in carboxyhemoglobin (COHb) levels after hydroxocobalamin administration when measured by cooximetry, other authors suggest that the interference is minimal and results in slight overestimations depending on the instrument and the concentration of hydroxocobalamin. However, more worrisome is the report of two instances in which the COHb levels were falsely low by a factor of 4 to 14 times. An in vitro experiment using human blood confirmed a substantial false decrease in the COHb levels depending on the specific cooximeter tested. Because of the inaccuracies in laboratory determinations, blood should be drawn before hydroxocobalamin administration whenever possible. Because of the deep red color of hydroxocobalamin, hemodialysis machines often sound a false "blood leak" alarm depending on the wavelength of light that the optical emitter detects. Nephrologists should be aware of this possibility.

## PREGNANCY AND LACTATION

Hydroxocobalamin is US FDA Pregnancy Category C.

## DOSING AND ADMINISTRATION

### Cyanide Toxicity

The initial dose of hydroxocobalamin in adults is 5 g IV. A second dose of 5 g should be repeated as clinically necessary. Based on case reports and animal studies, intraosseous administration is anticipated to be of comparable efficacy to IV administration. In children, a dose of 70 mg/kg of hydroxocobalamin up to the adult dose is recommended. Sodium thiosulfate is often administered in addition to hydroxocobalamin, but the administration of hydroxocobalamin should always take precedence. However, the two drugs should not be administered simultaneously through the same IV line because the sodium thiosulfate will inactivate the hydroxocobalamin. The adult dose of sodium thiosulfate is 12.5 g (50 mL of 25% solution) and should be administered intravenously as either a bolus injection or infused over 10 to 30 minutes, depending on the severity of the situation. The dose of sodium thiosulfate in children is 1 mL/kg using a 25% solution (250 mg/kg or approximately 30–40 mL/$m^2$ of body surface area) not to exceed 50 mL (12.5 g) total dose.

### Nitroprusside-Induced Cyanide Toxicity

Nitroprusside-induced CN toxicity should be treated like CN toxicity from any other cause: stop the nitroprusside dosage and administer hydroxocobalamin according to the doses and precautions listed. A dose of hydroxocobalamin of 25 mg/h concurrent with nitroprusside administration (~0.6 mg/kg total dose) was sufficient in one study to decrease the red blood cell and serum CN concentrations and to prevent the development of a metabolic acidosis. We recommend continuing the hydroxocobalamin for 10 hours after the discontinuation of the nitroprusside based on the normal elimination rate of cyanide. However sodium thiosulfate works well for prevention of CN toxicity without producing issues associated with the color changes introduced by hydroxocobalamin.

## FORMULATION AND ACQUISITION

Cyanokit contains 5 g of lyophilized dark red hydroxocobalamin crystalline powder for injection.

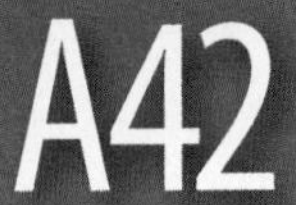



# A42 NITRITES (AMYL AND SODIUM) AND SODIUM THIOSULFATE

## INTRODUCTION

Sodium nitrite is an effective cyanide (CN) antidote that acts best when administered in a timely fashion and is followed by sodium thiosulfate. Although there has never been a head-to-head study in humans comparing hydroxocobalamin with the combination for the treatment of CN toxicity, the two main advantages of hydroxocobalamin are that it works quickly and inactivates CN directly by forming non-toxic cyanocobalamin without impairing oxygen-carrying capacity.

## HISTORY

In 1895, Lang reported the efficacy of sodium thiosulfate in detoxifying hydrocyanic acid. Later, inhaled amyl nitrite was demonstrated to protect canines from up to four minimum lethal doses of sodium CN. Subsequent animal experiments demonstrated improved efficacy of combined nitrite and thiosulfate therapy.

## PHARMACOLOGY OF THE NITRITES

### Mechanism of Action

Cyanide quickly and reversibly binds to the ferric iron ($Fe^{3+}$) in cytochrome oxidase, inhibiting effective energy production throughout the body. Nitrites oxidize the iron in hemoglobin to produce methemoglobin ($Fe^{3+}$). Methemoglobin preferentially combines with CN, producing cyanomethemoglobin. Because nitrites were accepted antidotes for CN poisoning, for many years, methemoglobin formation was assumed to be their sole mechanism of antidotal action. However, when methylene blue is administered to prevent methemoglobin formation, nitrite remains an effective antidote. This led to the hypothesis that nitrite-induced vasodilation might be part of the mechanism of action. Experimental evidence in hypoxia- or hypotension-induced organ damage suggests that the benefits of nitrites are related to their conversion to nitric oxide (NO), a potent vasodilator. Pretreatment with an NO scavenger negated the effects of the nitrite.

## PHARMACOLOGY OF SODIUM THIOSULFATE

### Mechanism of Action

The sulfur atom provided by sodium thiosulfate binds to CN with the help of rhodanese (CN sulfurtransferase) and mercaptopyruvate sulfurtransferase. This produces thiocyanate, which is minimally toxic and renally eliminated. Because sodium thiosulfate does not compromise hemoglobin oxygen saturation, it should be used without nitrites in circumstances when the formation of methemoglobin would be detrimental, as in patients who have elevated levels of carboxyhemoglobin (COHb) from smoke inhalation or preexistent methemoglobinemia congenital dyshemoglobinemias, and when hydroxocobalamin is unavailable.

Sodium thiosulfate is used prophylactically with nitroprusside to prevent CN toxicity. Sodium thiosulfate is also used to treat calcific uremic arteriolopathy (calciphylaxis), by increasing the solubility of calcium deposits, inducing vasodilation, and acting as a free radical scavenger.

## PHARMACOKINETICS AND PHARMACODYNAMICS OF NITRITES

Inhalation of crushed amyl nitrite ampules in human volunteers produced insignificant amounts of methemoglobin and caused headache, fatigue, dizziness, and hypotension. In one study, 300 mg of IV sodium nitrite produced peak methemoglobin levels of 10% to 18% in healthy adults and values of 7% when 4 mg/kg was administered.

## PHARMACOKINETICS AND PHARMACODYNAMICS OF SODIUM THIOSULFATE

### Animal Studies

In canine studies, sodium thiosulfate rapidly distributes into the extracellular space and then slowly into the cell. When administered before CN, thiosulfate converted more than 50% of the CN to thiocyanate within 3 minutes and increased the endogenous conversion rate more than 30 times. Thiosulfate is filtered and secreted in the kidneys.

### Human Studies

After injection of 150 mg/kg in volunteers, the volume of distribution (Vd) was 0.15 L/kg, the distribution half-life was 23 minutes, and the elimination half-life was 3 hours. Approximately 50% of the drug was eliminated in 18 hours unchanged in the urine, most of that was within the first 3 hours. Oral bioavailability is about 8% and was calculated after 5 g of the IV solution was diluted in 100 mL of water and ingested rapidly. In another study using a population pharmacokinetic model, the Vd was 0.226 L/kg. Total-body clearance in the hemodialysis (HD) patients undergoing HD was double that of the same patients not receiving HD.

## ROLE OF NITRITES AND SODIUM THIOSULFATE IN CYANIDE TOXICITY

In the few reported cases of CN ingestion treated solely with sodium thiosulfate, the patients had favorable outcomes. However, we recommend administration of sodium nitrite before sodium thiosulfate. As early as 1952, the literature reported 16 CN-poisoned patients who survived after administration of nitrites and sodium thiosulfate. Case reports attest to the ability of amyl nitrite, sodium nitrite, and sodium thiosulfate to jointly reverse the effects of CN if they are administered sequentially in a timely fashion.

## ROLE OF SODIUM THIOSULFATE IN NITROPRUSSIDE-INDUCED CYANIDE TOXICITY

When nitroprusside (which contains five CN ions) infusion rates are less 0.5 mg/kg/h, there is a minimal rise in CN concentrations. Prolonged infusion or doses in excess of the detoxifying capability of the body lead to thiocyanate or CN toxicity. Coadministration of sodium thiosulfate with sodium nitroprusside in a 5:1 molar ratio prevents the rise in CN concentration. Adding 0.5 g of sodium thiosulfate to each 50 mg of nitroprusside is effective in most cases. Although this dose of sodium thiosulfate usually is sufficient to prevent CN toxicity from nitroprusside, thiocyanate can accumulate, especially in critically ill patients and in those with kidney insufficiency. Although thiocyanate is relatively nontoxic compared with CN, it produces dose-dependent tinnitus, miosis, hyperreflexia, and hypothyroidism, especially at serum concentrations greater than 60 μg/mL. Thiocyanate is hemodialyzable. Nitroprusside-induced CN toxicity should be treated by stopping the nitroprusside and administering standard doses of hydroxocobalamin with or without sodium thiosulfate.

## ROLE OF SODIUM THIOSULFATE IN CALCIFIC UREMIC ARTERIOLOPATHY (CALCIPHYLAXIS)

Calciphylaxis is a rare vascular disease associated with chronic kidney failure that is defined as calcification of the medial layer of arteries, leading to subcutaneous nodules that typically progress to necrotic skin ulcers. Sodium thiosulfate in a typical dose of 5 to 25 g IV in adults during or after HD is used to treat this disease. Thiosulfate likely increases the water solubility of calcium, leading to enhanced excretion of calcium thiosulfate, which induces vasodilation and acts as a free radical scavenger.

## ADVERSE EFFECTS AND SAFETY ISSUES: SODIUM THIOSULFATE

The toxicity of sodium thiosulfate is low. The $LD_{50}$ (median lethal dose in 50% of test subjects) for animals is approximately 3 to 4 g/kg, with death attributed to metabolic acidosis, elevated serum sodium concentration, and decreased blood pressure and oxygenation. Sodium thiosulfate is hyperosmolar, delivering a significant sodium load, resulting in an osmotic diuretic effect. Administering the infusion over 10 to 30 minutes limits some of these adverse effects. Adverse effects associated with therapeutic doses include hypotension, nausea, vomiting, and prolonged bleeding time (1–3 days after a single dose) without changes in other hematologic parameters.

## ADVERSE EFFECTS AND SAFETY ISSUES: NITRITES

Amyl nitrite and sodium nitrite work in part by inducing methemoglobinemia, but excessive methemoglobinemia is potentially lethal. Therefore, nitrite dosages must be carefully calculated to avoid excessive methemoglobinemia, especially in cases in which other coexisting conditions, such as COHb, sulfhemoglobin, and anemia, might compromise hemoglobin oxygen saturation. Children are particularly at risk for medication errors because of dosage miscalculations. Nitrites are potent vasodilators, resulting in transient hypotension. Other common adverse effects include headache, tachycardia, palpitations, dysrhythmias, blurred vision, nausea, and vomiting.

## PREGNANCY AND LACTATION: NITRITES

The nitrites are United States (US) Food and Drug Administration (FDA) Pregnancy Category C. Fetuses are particularly sensitive to methemoglobinemia with the potential for prenatal hypoxia. Hydroxocobalamin is also US FDA Pregnancy Category C; however, even with the limited data available, it likely has a lesser risk than nitrite use for a pregnant woman. It is not known whether nitrites are excreted in breast milk.

## PREGNANCY AND LACTATION: SODIUM THIOSULFATE

Sodium thiosulfate is US FDA Pregnancy Category C. It is not known whether sodium thiosulfate is excreted in breast milk.

## DOSING AND ADMINISTRATION OF NITRITES AND SODIUM THIOSULFATE

### Adults

Amyl nitrite is no longer recommended in medical settings but may have a role as a prehospital antidote in industrial settings. Sodium nitrite 300 mg (10 mL of 3% solution) should be administered intravenously at a rate of 2.5 to 5 mL/min. We recommend repeating sodium nitrite at half the initial dose if manifestations of CN toxicity persist or reappear. Immediately after the completion of the sodium nitrite infusion, 50 mL of 25% solution (12.5 g) sodium thiosulfate should be infused intravenously. The dose of the thiosulfate should be repeated at half the initial dose if manifestations of CN toxicity persist or reappear. In situations in which additional methemoglobin formation would be harmful, as in patients with carbon monoxide poisoning, it is recommended to withhold the nitrite and only administer the IV hydroxocobalamin with or without sodium thiosulfate.

### Children

Intravenously infuse 0.2 mL/kg (6–8 $mL/m^2$ body surface area {BSA}) or 6 mg/kg of 3% sodium nitrite solution at a rate of 2.5 to 5 mL/min, not to exceed 10 mL or 300 mg. We recommend repeating sodium nitrite at half the initial dose if manifestations of CN toxicity persist or reappear. The dose of sodium thiosulfate in children is 1 mL/kg using a 25% solution (250 mg/kg or ~30–40 $mL/m^2$ of BSA) not to exceed 50 mL (12.5 g) total dose immediately after administration of sodium nitrite. We recommend repeating sodium thiosulfate at half the initial dose if manifestations of CN toxicity persist or reappear. In situations in which additional formation of methemoglobin would be harmful, as in patients with smoke inhalation from a fire in which unknown toxic gases exist, we recommend withholding the nitrite and administering hydroxocobalamin with or without sodium thiosulfate.

## FORMULATION AND ACQUISITION

Sodium nitrite is available in vials containing 300 mg in 10 mL of water for injection (USP). Sodium thiosulfate is available in 50-mL vials containing 12.5 g in water for injection (USP). In 2011, the FDA approved Nithiodote, a copackaged vial of sodium nitrite (300 mg in 10 mL water for injection) with one vial of sodium thiosulfate (12.5 g in 50 mL of water) for injection.

# 97 METHEMOGLOBIN INDUCERS

## HISTORY AND EPIDEMIOLOGY

Methemoglobinemia is a disorder of the red blood cells (RBCs). Although methemoglobin is always present at low concentrations in the body, methemoglobinemia is defined herein as an abnormal elevation of the methemoglobin level above 1%. The ubiquity of oxidants, both in the environment and xenobiotics prescribed in the hospital, has increased the number of cases of reported methemoglobinemia.

Methemoglobin was first described by Felix Hoppe-Seyler in 1864. In the late 1930s, methemoglobinemia was recognized as a predictable adverse effect of sulfanilamide use, and methylene blue was recommended for treatment of the ensuing cyanosis. Methemoglobinemia is either hereditary or acquired, is relatively common, and often produces no clinical findings when present at less than 5%. In hospitalized patients, benzocaine spray accounted for the most seriously poisoned patients, whereas dapsone accounted for the largest number of cases. Of the patients who had elevated methemoglobin levels, 8% had symptomatic methemoglobinemia, and approximately one-third received methylene blue. In a large study of children between the ages of 2 and 5 years old admitted to the hospital for fever, elevated methemoglobin levels were detected in 43% of patients. Vomiting, poor capillary refill, metabolic acidosis with an elevated lactate concentration, severe anemia, and malaria were reported in this population. Acute pesticide poisoning leading to methemoglobinemia is common in many parts of the world. In Sri Lanka, a large, multicenter study followed patients with intentional propanil (a herbicide) ingestions and found a 10.7% mortality rate in those with methemoglobinemia.

## HEMOGLOBIN PHYSIOLOGY

Hemoglobin consists of four polypeptide chains noncovalently attracted to each other. Each of these subunits carries one heme molecule deeply within the structure. The polypeptide chain protects the iron moiety of the heme molecule from inappropriate oxidation. The iron is held in position by six coordination bonds. Four of these bonds are between iron and the nitrogen atoms of the protoporphyrin ring with the fifth and sixth bond sites lying above and below the protoporphyrin plane. The fifth site is occupied by histidine of the polypeptide chain. The sixth coordination site is where most of the activity within hemoglobin occurs. Oxygen transport occurs here, and this site is involved with the formation of methemoglobin or carboxyhemoglobin (Fig. 97–1). It is at this site that an electron is lost to oxidant xenobiotics, transforming iron from its ferrous ($Fe^{2+}$) to its ferric ($Fe^{3+}$) state, which defines methemoglobin.

## METHEMOGLOBIN PHYSIOLOGY AND KINETICS

Because of the spontaneous and xenobiotic-induced oxidation of iron, the erythrocyte has multiple mechanisms to maintain its normal low concentration of methemoglobin.

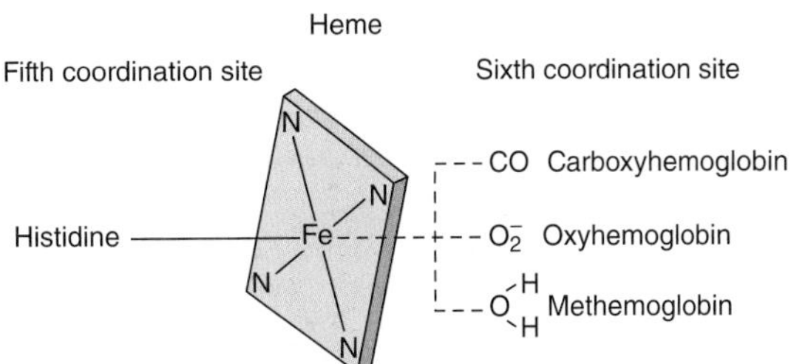


**FIGURE 97–1.** Heme molecule depicted with its bonding sites. Oxyhemoglobin, carboxyhemoglobin, and methemoglobin all involve the sixth coordination bonding site of iron.

All these systems donate an electron to the oxidized iron atom. Because of these effective reducing mechanisms, the half-life of methemoglobin acutely formed as a result of exposure to oxidants is between 1 and 3 hours. With continuous exposure to the oxidant, the apparent half-life of methemoglobin is prolonged. Quantitatively, the most important reductive system requires nicotinamide adenine dinucleotide (NADH), which is generated in the Embden-Meyerhof glycolytic pathway (Fig. 97–2).

Nicotinamide adenine dinucleotide (NADH) serves as an electron donor, and along with the enzyme NADH methemoglobin reductase, reduces $Fe^{3+}$ to $Fe^{2+}$. There are numerous cases of hereditary deficiencies of the enzyme NADH methemoglobin reductase (cytochrome $b_5$ reductase). Individuals who are homozygotes for this enzyme deficiency usually have methemoglobin levels of 10% to 50% under normal conditions without any clinical or xenobiotic stressors. Individuals who are heterozygotes do not ordinarily demonstrate methemoglobinemia except when they are subject to oxidant stress. Additionally, because this enzyme system lacks full activity until approximately 4 months of age, even genetically normal infants are more susceptible than adults to oxidant stress.

Within the RBC is another enzyme system for reducing oxidized iron that is dependent on the nicotinamide adenine dinucleotide phosphate (NADPH) generated in the hexose monophosphate shunt pathway. Although this system reduces only a small percentage of methemoglobin under normal circumstances, it plays a more prominent role in maintaining oxidant balance in the cell and is involved in the mechanism of modulating vascular tone during low oxygen delivery to the capillary beds. However, when the NADPH methemoglobin reductase system is provided with an exogenous electron carrier, such as methylene blue, this system is accelerated and greatly assists in the reduction of oxidized hemoglobin (Antidotes in Brief: A43).

## XENOBIOTIC-INDUCED METHEMOGLOBINEMIA

Nitrates and nitrites are powerful oxidizers that are two of the most common methemoglobin-forming compounds. Sources of nitrates and nitrites include well water, food, industrial compounds, and pharmaceuticals. Nitrogen-based

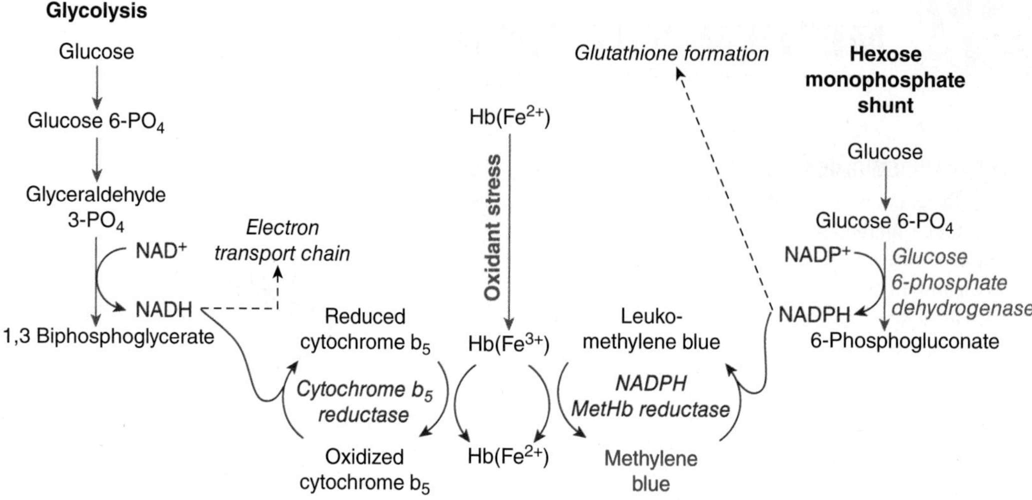


**FIGURE 97–2.** Role of glycolysis (the Embden-Meyerhof pathway) and the role of methylene blue in the reduction of methemoglobin using nicotinamide adenine dinucleotide phosphate (NADPH) generated by the hexose monophosphate shunt. Hb ($Fe^{3+}$) is methemoglobin.

fertilizers and nitrogenous waste from animal and human sources may contaminate shallow rural wells. In the past, nitrate-contaminated well water was associated with infant fatalities because of methemoglobinemia. Topical anesthetics continue to be a problem despite numerous case studies and recommendations by authors and manufacturers about safe use standards. Cetacaine spray (14% benzocaine, 2% tetracaine, 2% butylaminobenzoate) and 20% benzocaine sprays commonly produce methemoglobinemia. Dapsone is implicated as a common cause of methemoglobinemia. Cases of prolonged methemoglobinemia from dapsone ingestion are related to the long half-life of dapsone and the slow conversion to its methemoglobin-forming hydroxylamine metabolites. Predispositions for methemoglobinemia are listed in Tables 97–1 and 97–2.

## METHEMOGLOBINEMIA AND HEMOLYSIS

The enzyme defect responsible for most instances of oxidant-induced hemolysis is glucose-6-phosphate dehydrogenase (G6PD) deficiency. Reviews of hemolysis addressed the confusion regarding the relationship between hemolysis and methemoglobinemia. Both hemolysis and methemoglobinemia are caused by oxidant stress, and hemolysis sometimes occurs after episodes of methemoglobinemia. Another source of confusion concerning hemolysis and methemoglobinemia is that reduced glutathione is required

**TABLE 97–1** Some Physiologic and Epidemiologic Factors That Predispose Individuals to Methemoglobinemia

| | |
|---|---|
| Acidosis | Diarrhea |
| Advanced age | Hospitalization |
| Age < 36 mo | Kidney failure |
| Anemia | Malnutrition |
| Concomitant oxidant use | Sepsis |
| | Xenobiotics |

**TABLE 97–2** Common Causes of Methemoglobinemia

***Hereditary***
Hemoglobin M
NADH methemoglobin reductase deficiency (homozygote and heterozygote)
***Acquired***
Medications
- Amyl nitrite
- Local anesthetics (benzocaine, lidocaine, prilocaine)
- Dapsone
- Nitric oxide
- Nitroglycerin
- Nitroprusside
- Phenazopyridine
- Quinones (chloroquine, primaquine)
- Sulfonamides (sulfanilamide, sulfathiazide, sulfapyridine, sulfamethoxazole)

Other Xenobiotics
- Aniline dye derivatives (shoe dyes, marking inks)
- Chlorobenzene
- Copper sulfate
- Fires (heat-induced denaturation)
- Organic nitrites (eg, amyl, isobutyl nitrite, butyl nitrite)
- Naphthalene
- Nitrates (eg, well water)
- Nitrites (eg, foods)
- Nitrophenol
- Nitrogen oxide gases (occupational exposure in arc welders)
- Propanil
- Silver nitrate
- Trinitrotoluene
- Zopiclone

***Pediatric***
Reduced NADH methemoglobin reductase activity in infants (< 4 mo)
Associated with low birth weight, prematurity, dehydration, acidosis, diarrhea, and hyperchloremia

NADH = nicotinamide adenine dinucleotide.

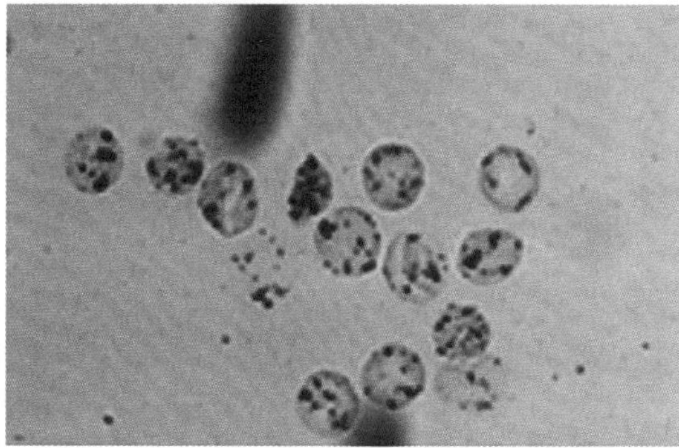

**FIGURE 97–3.** Heinz bodies are particles of denatured hemoglobin, usually attached to the inner surface of the red blood cell membrane. Xenobiotics that result in the oxidative denaturation of hemoglobin in normal (eg, phenylhydrazine) or glucose-6-phosphate dehydrogenase (G6PD)-deficient (primaquine) individuals and unstable hemoglobin mutants are prone to develop these bodies. The Heinz bodies are identified when blood is mixed with a supravital stain, notably crystal violet. The Heinz bodies appear as purple inclusions. *(Reproduced with permission from Lichtman MA. Lichtman's Atlas of Hematology, 1st ed. New York, NY: McGraw-Hill, Inc; 2007.)*

to protect against both toxic manifestations. This codependence on the reducing power of NADPH links these two disorders. Although it is easier to consider hemolysis and methemoglobin formation as subclasses of disorders of oxidant stress, they are separate clinical entities sharing limited characteristics.

Oxidative damage to erythrocytes occurs at different locations in the two disorders. Hemolysis occurs when oxidants damage the hemoglobin chain acting directly as electron acceptors or through the formation of hydrogen peroxide or other oxidizing free radicals. This results in oxidants forming irreversible bonds with the sulfhydryl group of hemoglobin, causing denaturation and precipitation of the globin protein to form Heinz bodies within the erythrocyte (Fig. 97–3). Cells with large numbers of Heinz bodies are removed by the reticuloendothelial system, producing hemolysis. Methemoglobinemia does not necessarily progress to hemolysis even if untreated.

Numerous cases describe the occurrence of hemolysis after methemoglobinemia. The combined occurrence is reported with dapsone, phenazopyridine, amyl nitrite, copper sulfate, and aniline. Currently, it is not possible to predict when hemolysis will occur after methemoglobinemia with any degree of certainty, and markers of hemolysis should be followed for several days.

## CLINICAL MANIFESTATIONS

The clinical manifestations of methemoglobinemia are related to impaired oxygen-carrying capacity and delivery to the tissue (Table 97–3). The clinical manifestations of acquired methemoglobinemia are usually more severe than those produced by a corresponding degree of anemia. This discordance occurs because methemoglobin not only decreases the available oxygen-carrying capacity but also increases the affinity of the unaltered hemoglobin for oxygen. This shifts the oxygen–hemoglobin dissociation curve to the left. Cyanosis typically occurs when just 1.5 g/dL of methemoglobin is present. This represents only 10% conversion of hemoglobin to methemoglobin if the baseline hemoglobin is 15 g/dL. By contrast, 5 g/dL of deoxyhemoglobin (which represents 33% of the total hemoglobin concentration) is needed to produce the same degree of cyanosis from hypoxia.

**TABLE 97–3** Signs and Symptoms Typically Associated with Methemoglobin Levels in Healthy Patients with Normal Hemoglobin Concentrations[a]

| *Methemoglobin Level (%)* | *Signs and Symptoms* |
|---|---|
| 1–3 (normal) | None |
| 3–15 | Possibly none<br>Pulse oximeter reads low $SaO_2$<br>Slate gray cutaneous coloration |
| 15–20 | Chocolate brown blood<br>Cyanosis |
| 20–50 | Dizziness, syncope<br>Dyspnea<br>Exercise intolerance<br>Fatigue<br>Headache<br>Weakness |
| 50–70 | Central nervous system depression<br>Coma<br>Dysrhythmias<br>Metabolic acidosis<br>Seizures<br>Tachypnea |
| >70 | Death<br>Grave hypoxic symptoms |

[a]Associated illness and comorbid diseases produce more severe symptoms at lower levels of methemoglobin.

Because the symptoms associated with methemoglobinemia are related to impaired oxygen delivery to the tissues, concurrent diseases such as anemia, congestive heart failure, chronic obstructive pulmonary disease, and pneumonia increase the clinical effects of methemoglobinemia (Fig. 97–4). Predictions of symptoms and recommendations for therapy are based on methemoglobin level in previously healthy individuals with normal total hemoglobin concentrations.

## DIAGNOSTIC TESTING

Arterial blood gas sampling usually reveals blood with a characteristic chocolate brown color. However, in patients who are clinically stable and not in need of an arterial puncture, a venous blood gas will be accurate in demonstrating the methemoglobin level. The arterial $PO_2$ should be normal, reflecting the adequacy of pulmonary function to deliver dissolved oxygen to the blood. However, arterial $PO_2$ does not directly measure the hemoglobin oxygen saturation ($SaO_2$) or oxygen content of the blood. When the partial pressure of oxygen is known and oxyhemoglobin and deoxyhemoglobin are the only species of hemoglobin, oxygen saturation can be calculated accurately from the arterial blood gas. If, however,

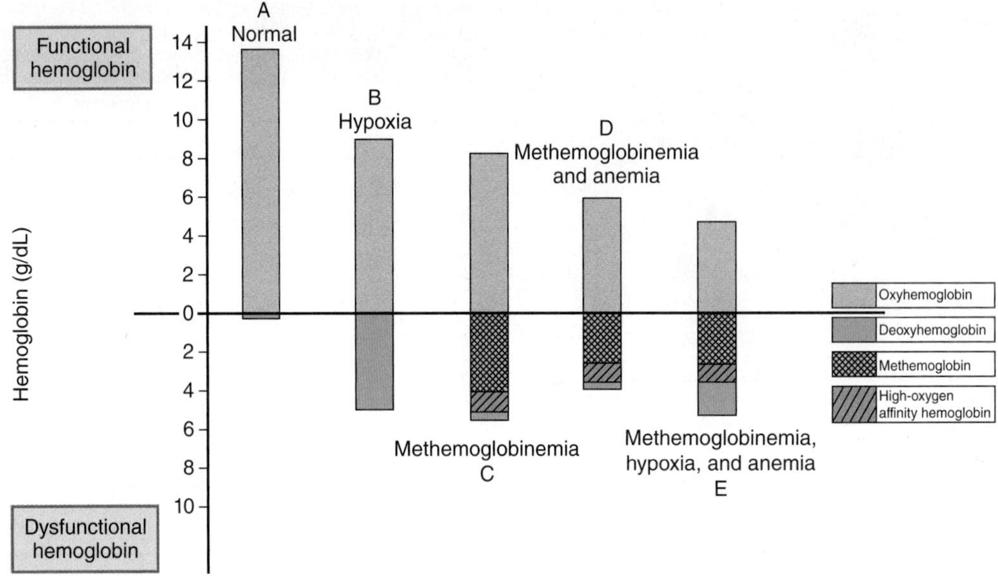


**FIGURE 97–4.** Clinical manifestations of methemoglobinemia depend on the level of methemoglobin and on host factors such as preexisting disease, anemia, and hypoxemia. Five examples of arterial blood gases and cooximeter analyses are presented. (**A**) Blood gas from a normal individual with 14 g/dL of hemoglobin. Almost all hemoglobin is saturated with oxygen. (**B**) Blood gas from a patient with cardiopulmonary disease producing cyanosis in which only 9 g/dL of hemoglobin is capable of oxygen transport. (**C**) Methemoglobin level of 28% in an otherwise normal individual will reduce hemoglobin available for oxygen transport to less than 9 g/dL (~4 g/dL of methemoglobin and 1.3 g/dL of high oxygen affinity hemoglobin because of the left shift of the oxyhemoglobin dissociation curve). (**D**) Same degree of methemoglobin as in ***C*** but in a patient with a hemoglobin of 10 g/dL. Only 6 g/dL of hemoglobin would be capable of oxygen transport. (**E**) Methemoglobinemia and anemia to the same degree as ***D*** but in a patient with hypoxia.

other dyshemoglobins are present, such as methemoglobin, sulfhemoglobin, or carboxyhemoglobin, then the fractional saturation of the different hemoglobin species must be determined by cooximetry.

The pulse oximeter applied to a patient's finger at the bedside was developed to estimate oxygen saturation trends in critically ill patients. Most pulse oximeters in use today use two different wavelengths to determine $O_2$ saturation, and the manufacturers do not provide validation data for situations in which any dyshemoglobin is present. All manufacturers disclaim accuracy under such circumstances. In the dog model, the pulse oximeter oxygen saturation ($SpO_2$) values decrease with increasing methemoglobin levels. This decrease in $SpO_2$ is not exactly proportional to the percentage of methemoglobin. However, the pulse oximeter overestimated the level of actual oxygen saturation at low methemoglobin levels. As the methemoglobin level approached 30%, the pulse oximeter saturation values decreased to about 85% and then leveled off, regardless of how much higher the methemoglobin level became. From our experience and that of others, in humans, much lower levels of oxygen saturation ($SpO_2$) than 85% can be displayed by pulse oximetry when methemoglobin levels increase above 30%.

Although the pulse oximeter reading in patients with methemoglobinemia is not as accurate as desired, it remains helpful when it is compared with that of the arterial blood gas: if there is a difference between the *measured* oxyhemoglobin saturation of the pulse oximeter ($SaO_2$) and the *calculated* oxyhemoglobin saturation of the arterial blood gas ($SpO_2$), then a "saturation gap" exists. The calculated $SaO_2$ of the blood gas will be greater than the measured $SpO_2$ if methemoglobin is present (Table 97–4).

Several manufacturers developed pulse oximeters that read multiple wavelengths to identify other hemoglobin species such as methemoglobin, carboxyhemoglobin, and total hemoglobin concentration. Validation studies using human volunteers with these new pulse oximeters suggest that the accuracy for detecting methemoglobin is acceptable. While imperfect, these devices can be used for screening in high-risk patients or circumstances.

Methemoglobin produces a color change that can be observed when a drop of blood is placed on absorbant white paper. In one study, when various levels of methemoglobin from 10% to 100% were produced in vitro and a drop of each concentration was placed on a white background, a color chart was developed that could reliably be used to predict methemoglobin levels (Fig. 97–5). In situations in which laboratory evaluation is limited, such a bedside test is useful because a determination of the exact methemoglobin level is rarely needed.

## MANAGEMENT

For most patients with mild methemoglobinemia of approximately 10%, no therapy is necessary other than withdrawal of the offending xenobiotic because reduction of the methemoglobin will occur by normal reconversion mechanisms (NADH methemoglobin reductase). However, in some patients, even small elevations of methemoglobin are problematic because they suggest the individual is at a point at which further oxidant stress will cause methemoglobin levels to increase. Patients should be examined carefully for signs of

**TABLE 97–4 Hemoglobin Oxygenation Analysis**

| *Measuring Device* | *Source* | *What Is Measured* | *How Data Are Expressed* | *Benefits* | *Pitfalls* | *Insight* |
|---|---|---|---|---|---|---|
| Blood gas analyzer | Blood | Partial pressure of dissolved oxygen in whole blood | $PO_2$ | Also gives information about pH and $PCO_2$ | Calculates $SaO_2$ from the partial pressure of oxygen in blood; inaccurate if forms of Hb other than OxyHb and DeoxyHb are present | An abnormal Hb form may exist if a gap exists between ABG and pulse oximeter |
| Cooximeter | Blood | Directly measures absorptive characteristics of oxyhemoglobin, deoxyhemoglobin, methemoglobin, and carboxyhemoglobin and in some cases other hemoglobins (fetal hemoglobin, sulfhemoglobin) at different wavelength bands in whole blood | $SaO_2$, %MethHb, %COHb, %OxyHb, %DeoxyHb | Directly measures hemoglobin species | Provides data on hemoglobin only; most instruments will not measure sulfhemoglobin, HbM, and some other forms of Hb | Most accurate method of determining the oxygen content of blood |
| Pulse oximeter | Monitor sensor on patient | Absorptive characteristics of oxyhemoglobin in pulsatile blood assuming the presence of only OxyHb and DeoxyHb in vivo<br>Newer pulse oximeters measure methemoglobin | $SpO_2$ | Moment-to-moment bedside data | Inaccurate data if interfering substances are present (methemoglobin, sulfhemoglobin, carboxyhemoglobin, methylene blue) | Maximum depression, 75%–85% regardless of how much methemoglobin is present |

ABG = arterial blood gas; COHB, carboxyhemoglobin; DeoxyHb = deoxygenated hemoglobin; Hb = hemoglobin; HbM = hemoglobin M; MethHb = methemoglobin; OxyHb = oxygenated hemoglobin; $SaO_2$ = hemoglobin oxygen saturation; $SpO_2$ = pulse oximeter oxygen saturation.

physiologic stress related to decreased oxygen delivery to the tissue. Obviously, changes in mental status or ischemic chest pain necessitate immediate treatment, but subtle changes in behavior and inattentiveness are also signs of global hypoxia and should be treated. Patients with abnormal vital signs such as tachycardia and tachypnea or an elevated lactate concentration thought to be caused by tissue hypoxia or the functional anemia of methemoglobinemia should be treated more aggressively. A mildly elevated methemoglobin level alone generally is not an adequate indication of need for therapy, but when levels exceed 30%, treatment is almost always indicated (Fig. 97–4).

The most widely accepted treatment of methemoglobinemia is administration of 1 to 2 mg/kg body weight of methylene blue infused intravenously over 5 minutes. The use of a slow 5-minute infusion and flushing the line after administration help prevent painful local responses from rapid infusion. Clinical improvement should be noted within minutes of methylene blue administration. If cyanosis has not disappeared within 15 to 30 minutes of the infusion, then a second dose is recommended (Fig. 97–6). Methylene blue causes a transient decrease in the pulse oximetry reading because of its blue color.

The use of methylene blue in patients with G6PD deficiency is controversial. Glucose-6-phosphate dehydrogenase (G6PD)-deficient patients were once excluded from most treatment protocols because methylene blue is a mild oxidant and case reports suggested the toxicity of methylene blue. However, because of the lack of immediate availability of G6PD testing, most patients who need treatment receive methylene blue therapy before their G6PD status is known. Although many patients with G6PD deficiency undoubtedly have been treated unknowingly, few case reports of toxicity are described. Therefore, we believe that the judicious use of methylene blue is recommended in most patients with G6PD deficiency and symptomatic methemoglobinemia.

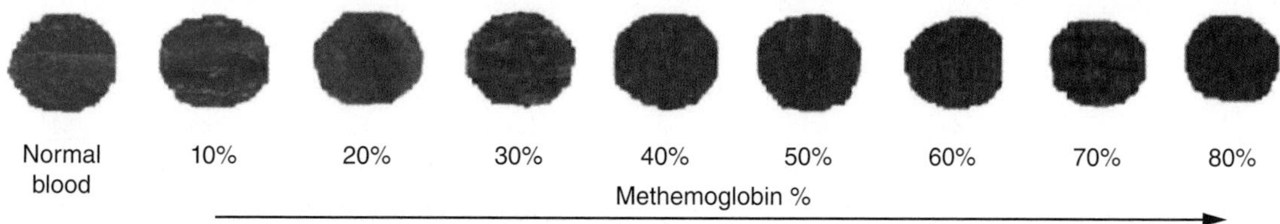


**FIGURE 97–5.** The relationship between methemoglobin level and blood color. This figure demonstrates the relationship between methemoglobin level and the color of blood. If blood from an anticoagulated tube is placed on a white background, the methemoglobin level can be estimated accurately by comparison with the scale. It is important to note that although normal anticoagulated venous blood oxygenates spontaneously (ie, becomes redder over time), if exposed to room air, methemoglobin is incapable of extracting oxygen from air and will remain dark over time. *(Reproduced with permission from Shihana F, Dissanayake DM, Buckley NA, et al. A simple quantitative bedside test to determine methemoglobin. Ann Emerg Med. 2010;55(2):184-189.)*

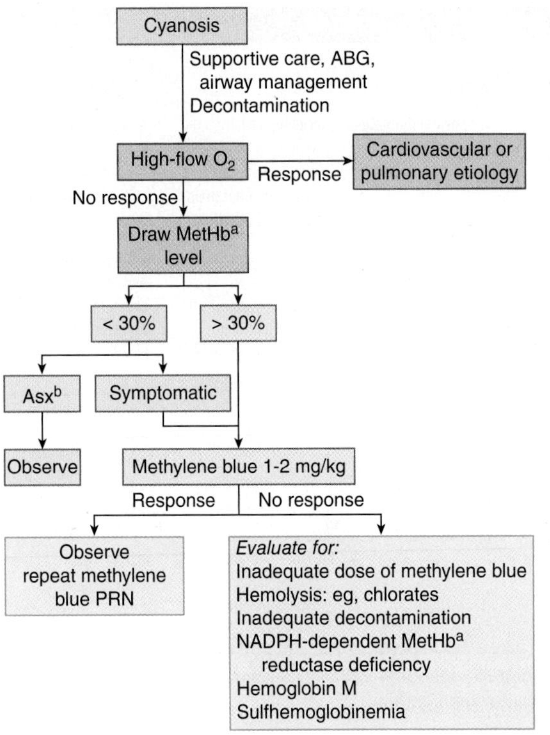


**FIGURE 97–6.** Toxicologic assessment of a cyanotic patient. [a] = MetHb = methemoglobin; [b] = Asx = asymptomatic.

If methylene blue treatment fails to significantly reverse methemoglobinemia, other possibilities should be evaluated. Theoretically, exchange transfusion or hyperbaric oxygen (HBO) would be expected to be beneficial when methylene blue is ineffective. Both interventions are time consuming and costly, but HBO allows the dissolved oxygen time to protect the patient while endogenous methemoglobin reduction occurs. Ascorbic acid is not recommended in the management of acquired methemoglobinemia if methylene blue is available because the rate at which ascorbic acid reduces methemoglobin is considerably slower than the rate of normal intrinsic mechanisms.

Treatment with dapsone deserves special consideration because of its tendency to produce prolonged methemoglobinemia. *N*-Hydroxylation of dapsone to its hydroxylamine metabolite by CYP2C9 and CYP3A4 is mainly responsible for methemoglobin formation in both therapeutic and overdose situations. Both the parent compound and its metabolites are oxidants with long half-lives. Cimetidine is a competitive inhibitor in the cytochrome P450 metabolic pathway and reduces methemoglobin concentrations during therapeutic dosing because less dapsone will be metabolized by the route. In situations of overdose, cimetidine in therapeutic doses will likely exert some protective effects and is reasonable to use with methylene blue. When dapsone is therapeutically indicated but low levels of methemoglobin are found, cimetidine is a reasonable method for reducing oxidant stress. Additionally, cimetidine is responsible for many drug interactions so dosing of other medications often needs adjustment.

## SULFHEMOGLOBIN

Sulfhemoglobin is a variant of hemoglobin in which a sulfur atom is incorporated into the heme molecule but is not attached to iron. Sulfhemoglobin is a darker pigment than methemoglobin, producing cyanosis when only 0.5 g/dL of blood is affected. Sulfhemoglobin also reduces the oxygen saturation determined by the pulse oximeter. The diagnosis is often established based on the patient's failure to improve with methylene blue.

Sulfhemoglobin is an extremely stable compound that is eliminated only when RBCs are removed naturally from circulation. Although the oxygen-carrying capacity of hemoglobin is reduced by sulfhemoglobinemia, unlike in methemoglobinemia, the oxyhemoglobin dissociation curve is shifted to the right. This makes oxygen more available to the tissues. This phenomenon reduces the clinical effect of sulfhemoglobin in the tissues.

A number of xenobiotics induce sulfhemoglobin in humans, including acetanilid, phenacetin, nitrates, trinitrotoluene, and sulfur compounds. Most of the xenobiotics that produce methemoglobinemia are reported in various degrees to produce sulfhemoglobinemia.

Sulfhemoglobinemia usually requires no therapy other than withdrawal of the offending xenobiotic. There is no antidote for sulfhemoglobinemia because it results from an irreversible chemical bond that occurs within the hemoglobin molecule. Exchange transfusion would lower the sulfhemoglobin concentration, but this approach usually is unnecessary.

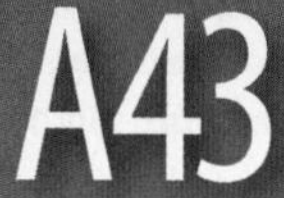



# A43 METHYLENE BLUE

## INTRODUCTION

Methylene blue is an extremely effective antidote for acquired methemoglobinemia. Methylene blue has other actions, including the inhibition of nitric oxide synthase and guanylyl cyclase and the inhibition of the generation of oxygen free radicals.

## HISTORY

Methylene blue was initially recommended as an intestinal and urinary antiseptic and subsequently recognized as a weak antimalarial. In 1933, Williams and Challis successfully used methylene blue for the treatment of aniline-induced methemoglobinemia.

## PHARMACOLOGY

### Chemistry

Methylene blue is a basic thiazine dye that is a deep blue color in the oxidized state but is colorless when reduced to leukomethylene blue.

### Mechanisms of Action

Methylene blue is an oxidizing agent, which, in the presence of nicotinamide adenine dinucleotide phosphate (NADPH) and NADPH methemoglobin reductase, is reduced to leukomethylene blue (**Fig. 97–2**). Leukomethylene blue effectively reduces methemoglobin to hemoglobin. More recent attention has focused on the ability of methylene blue to reverse refractory hypotension from many causes, including drug overdose, vasoplegia, and sepsis. Methylene blue inhibits nitric oxide synthase and guanylyl cyclase in vascular smooth muscle to reduce the amount and effect of vasodilatory nitric oxide.

### Pharmacokinetics

Methylene blue exhibits complex pharmacokinetics, consistent with extensive distribution into deep compartments, followed by a slower terminal elimination, with a half-life of 5.25 hours. Interindividual variability is significant. Total urinary excretion at 24 hours accounts for 28.6% of the drug after IV administration.

### Pharmacodynamics

The onset of action of methylene blue for the reversal of methemoglobin is often within minutes. Maximum effects usually occur by 30 minutes.

## ROLE IN XENOBIOTIC-INDUCED METHEMOGLOBINEMIA

Methylene blue is indicated in patients with symptomatic methemoglobinemia. This usually occurs at methemoglobin levels greater than 20%, but symptoms often occur at lower levels in anemic patients or those with cardiovascular, pulmonary, or central nervous system compromise. The risk-to-benefit ratio of using methylene blue in a patient for methemoglobinemia must always be weighed as with any other xenobiotic. In almost all cases, the benefit of use for a patient with significant methemoglobinemia will almost always outweigh the risks.

## ROLE IN HYPOTENSION

Methylene blue has successfully reversed a low systemic vascular resistance in a few case studies and case reports. A recent review of human data suggests that although blood pressure responds to methylene blue in patients with distributive shock, a prospective study is needed to establish whether better oxygen delivery and improved survival occur.

## ADVERSE EFFECTS AND SAFETY ISSUES

The most common adverse effects reported in healthy volunteers who were administered 2 mg/kg methylene blue were extremity pain at the site of IV administration, chromaturia, dysgeusia, dizziness, feeling hot, diaphoresis, nausea, skin discoloration, headache, and back pain.

Reports of the paradoxical induction of methemoglobinemia by methylene blue suggest an equilibrium between the direct oxidization of hemoglobin to methemoglobin by methylene blue and its ability (through the NADPH and NADPH methemoglobin reductase pathway and leukomethylene blue production) to reduce methemoglobin to hemoglobin.

Methylene blue does not produce methemoglobin at doses of 1 to 2 mg/kg. Limited studies support the avoidance of doses higher than 7 mg/kg. In these high doses, methylene blue induces acute hemolytic anemia independent of the presence of methemoglobinemia. Because methylene blue is a dye, it will transiently alter pulse oximeter readings. Large doses often interfere with the ability to detect a clinical decrease in cyanosis; therefore, repeat cooximeter measurements and arterial or venous blood gas analysis should be used in conjunction with clinical findings to evaluate for improvement. Methylene blue leads to a bluish-green discoloration of the urine and often causes dysuria. Intravenous methylene blue is often painful, but can be given in any sized catheter. It rarely causes local tissue damage even in the absence of extravasation.

Recent reviews reveal an association between an encephalopathy and the use of methylene blue for the staining and localization of parathyroid tumors in women receiving serotonin reuptake inhibitors. Doses of 3 to 7.5 mg/kg were commonly used for this indication. An in vitro study documented the ability of methylene blue to competitively bind to monoamine oxidase A, raising the possibility that methylene blue might interact with serotonergic xenobiotics by acting as a monamine oxidase inhibitor. The United States Food and Drug Administration added a black box warning regarding potential serious or fatal serotonin toxicity when methylene blue is given to patients receiving selective serotonin reuptake inhibitors, serotonin-norepinephrine reuptake inhibitors, or monoamine oxidase inhibitors.

### Use in Patients with Glucose-6-Phosphate Dehydrogenase Deficiency

Methylene blue is frequently hypothesized to be ineffective in reversing methemoglobinemia in patients with glucose-6-phosphate dehydrogenase (G6PD) deficiency because G6PD is essential for generation of NADPH. Without NADPH, methylene blue cannot reduce methemoglobin. However, G6PD deficiency is an X-linked hereditary deficiency with more than 400 variants. The red blood cells containing the more common G6PD $A^-$ variant that are found in 11% of African Americans retain 10% residual activity, mostly in young erythrocytes and reticulocytes. By contrast, the enzyme is barely detectable in those of Mediterranean descent who have inherited the defect. Therefore, it is impossible to predict before the use of methylene blue which persons will or will not respond and to what extent. It appears that most individuals have adequate G6PD, and a variable expression of their deficiency allows an effective response to most oxidant stresses. In addition, in theory, normal cells might convert methylene blue to leukomethylene blue, which might diffuse into G6PD-deficient cells and effectively reduce methemoglobin to hemoglobin. However, when therapeutic doses of methylene blue fail to have an impact on the methemoglobin levels, the possibility of G6PD deficiency should be evaluated, and further doses of methylene blue should not be administered because of the risk of methylene blue–induced hemolysis. In these cases, exchange transfusion, vitamin C, and hyperbaric oxygen are potential alternatives for treating methemoglobinemia (Chap. 97).

## PREGNANCY AND LACTATION

Methylene blue is listed as a Category X drug in pregnancy. Intraamniotic injection has led to fetal abnormalities, including atresia of the ileum and jejunum, ileal occlusions, hemolytic anemia, hyperbilirubinemia, and methemoglobinemia, and should be avoided. Intravenous methylene blue should only be used to treat pregnant women with methemoglobinemia when the benefit outweighs the potential risk to the fetus.

There are no data available with regard to use during lactation. However, it is currently recommended to discontinue breastfeeding when methylene blue has been used and not to resume breastfeeding for 8 days after use.

## DOSING AND ADMINISTRATION

### Methemoglobinemia

The dose of methylene blue is 1-2 mg/kg given IV over 5 minutes followed immediately by a fluid flush of 15 to 30 mL to minimize local pain. This dose can be repeated in 15 to 30 minutes if necessary, based on clinical signs and symptoms and a consequential methemoglobin level. (A total doses greater than 7 mg/kg is not advised). If there is no effect after two sequential doses of 1 mg/kg, then subsequent dosing should be halted, and the diagnosis reexamined or the possibility of severe G6PD deficiency considered. However, repeated dosing of methylene blue is often required in conjunction with efforts to decontaminate the gastrointestinal tract when there is continued absorption or slow elimination of the xenobiotic producing the methemoglobinemia, such as with dapsone. Intraosseous administration is acceptable if IV access is unavailable.

### Vasodilatory Shock

The dose of methylene blue for refractory hypotension is not established. Doses of 1 to 3 mg/kg increase systemic vascular resistance and mean arterial pressure and improve tissue oxygenation.

## FORMULATION AND ACQUISITION

Methylene blue is available in 10-mL vials of a 1% solution for injection, containing 10 mg/mL (100 mg total in 10 mL), and in a 0.5% solution containing 5 mg/mL (50 mg total in 10 mL).

# 98 CHEMICAL WEAPONS

## HISTORY AND EPIDEMIOLOGY

The first well-documented intentional use of chemicals as weapons occurred in 423 B.C. when Spartans besieging Athenian cities burned pitch-soaked wood and brimstone to produce sulfurous clouds. Large-scale chemical warfare began in World War I when the Germans released chlorine near Ypres, Belgium, killing hundreds of people and forcing 15,000 troops to retreat. Both sides rapidly escalated the use of toxic gases released from cylinders or by artillery shells, including various pulmonary irritants, lacrimators, arsenicals, and cyanides.

The Germans first used sulfur mustard in 1917, again near Ypres, and caused more than 20,000 deaths or injuries. The Allies soon responded in kind. By the end of the war, chemical weapons caused more than 1.3 million casualties and approximately 90,000 deaths. Germany began producing nerve agents just before World War II.

Terrorist groups have also used chemical weapons. Sarin was released twice by the Aum Shinrikyo cult in Japan. Chemical weapons are particularly appealing to terrorist groups because the technology and financial outlay required to produce them is much less than for nuclear weapons, and the potential morbidity, mortality, and societal impact remain high (Table 98–1). Biological weapons share some characteristics with chemical weapons (Table 98–2) and are covered in Chap. 99.

## GENERAL CONSIDERATIONS

### Physical Properties

The term *war gas* is generally a misnomer. Sulfur mustard and nerve agents are liquids at normal temperatures and pressures, and many riot-control agents are solids. These weapons are most efficiently dispersed as aerosols, which probably leads to the confusion with gases. Some chemical weapons such as chlorine, phosgene, and hydrogen cyanide are true gases, and although they are generally considered obsolete for battlefield use, they might still be used as improvisational chemical weapons, especially in terrorist attacks. Liquid chemical weapons have a certain degree of volatility and evaporate into poisonous vapors. Aerosols, gases, and vapors are highly subject to local atmospheric conditions. Except for hydrogen cyanide, chemical weapon (CW) gases and vapors are all denser than air and collect in low-lying areas.

### Preparation for Chemical and Biological Weapons (CBW) Incidents

A rational medical response to CBW events differs from the common response to isolated toxicologic incidents. Healthcare professionals must learn about these unconventional weapons and the expected "toxidromes" that they produce. In addition, healthcare professionals must protect themselves and their facilities first, or ultimately no one will receive care.

Recommendations for sustained healthcare facility domestic preparedness include improved training to promptly recognize CBW mass casualty events, efforts to protect healthcare professionals, and establishment of decontamination and triage protocols. Table 98–3 lists some specific recommendations. Individual clinicians and hospitals caring for victims of known or suspected CBW incidents should contact their local department of health, which will likely report the incident to outside agencies such as the United States (US) Federal Bureau of Investigation and the Centers for Disease Control and Prevention (Table 98–4).

### Decontamination

Decontamination serves two functions: (1) to prevent further absorption and spread of a noxious substance on a given casualty and (2) to prevent spread to other persons. Chemical weapons that are exclusively gases at normal temperatures and pressures only require removing the victim from the area of exposure. Isolated aerosol or vapor exposures, as from volatilized nerve agents or sulfur mustard, are also terminated by leaving the area and may require no skin decontamination of the victims. Chemical weapons dispersed as liquids present the greatest need for decontamination. Liquid-contaminated clothing must be removed, and, if able, victims should remove their own clothing to prevent cross-contamination.

Decontamination should be done as soon as practicable to prevent progression of disease and should occur outside of healthcare facilities to prevent contamination of the working environment and secondary casualties. Decontamination near the incident scene would be ideal in terms of timeliness, although logistically, this will not be possible in many situations. Field decontamination before transport will also help to avoid loss of vehicles from being contaminated and taken

| TABLE 98–1 | Unconventional Weapons: Definitions and Acronyms |
|---|---|
| Chemical warfare | Intentional use of weapons designed to kill, injure, or incapacitate on the basis of toxic or noxious chemical properties |
| Biologic warfare | Intentional use of weapons designed to kill, injure, or incapacitate on the basis of microorganisms or xenobiotics derived from living organisms |
| Terrorism | The unlawful use of force against persons or property to intimidate or coerce a government, the civilian population, or any segment thereof, in furtherance of political or social objectives |
| CW | Chemical warfare, or chemical weapon |
| BW | Biological warfare, or biological weapon |
| CBW | Chemical and/or biological warfare or weapons |
| NBC | Nuclear, biological, and/or chemical; usually in reference to weapons |
| CBRNE | Chemical, biological, radiologic, nuclear, and explosive; usually in reference to weapons |
| WMD | Weapon of mass destruction; nuclear, radiologic, chemical, or biological weapon intended to produce mass casualties |

**TABLE 98–2 Chemical Versus Biological Weapons: Comparison and Contrast**

| ***Similarities*** | | |
|---|---|---|
| Xenobiotics most effectively dispersed in aerosol or vapor forms | | |
| Delivery systems frequently similar | | |
| Movement of xenobiotics highly subject to wind and weather conditions | | |
| Appropriate personal protective equipment prevents illness | | |
| ***Differences*** | ***Chemical Weapons (CWs)*** | ***Biological Weapons (BWs)*** |
| Rate at which attack results in illness | Rapid, usually minutes to hours | Delayed, usually days to weeks |
| Identifying release | *Relatively easy:*<br>Rapid clinical effects<br>Possible chemical odor<br>Commercially available chemical detectors | *More difficult:*<br>Delayed clinical effects<br>Lack of color, odor, or taste<br>Limited development of real-time detectors |
| Xenobiotic persistence | Variable<br>Liquids semipersistent to persistent<br>Gases nonpersistent | Generally nonpersistent; most BW xenobiotics are degraded by sunlight, heat, or desiccation (exception: anthrax spores) |
| Victim distribution | Near and downwind from release point | Victims may be widely dispersed by the time disease is apparent |
| First responders | EMTs, hazard materials teams, firefighters, law enforcement officers | Emergency physicians and nurses, primary care practitioners, infectious disease physicians, epidemiologists, public health officials (but will likely be same as CW if release is identified immediately) |
| Decontamination | Critically important in most cases | Not needed in delayed presentations; less important for acute exposures |
| Medical treatment | Antidotes, supportive care | Vaccines, antibiotics, supportive care |
| Patient isolation | Unnecessary after adequate decontamination | Crucial for easily communicable diseases (eg, smallpox, pneumonic plague); however, many BW agents are not easily transmissible |

EMT = emergency medical technician.

out of service. Evidence supports the likelihood that contaminated victims will present to healthcare facilities on their own or be transported for care without decontamination.

The degree of protective gear required by the decontamination personnel cannot be predicted in advance and may be difficult to objectively determine at the time of the incident. Level C personal protective equipment may be sufficient for most hospital settings when the source is defined (eg, receiving and decontamination areas); however, if healthcare professionals begin to develop clinical effects, level B gear with supplied air would become necessary (Chap. 101). When the source of the contamination is not yet known, level B gear should be used.

Chemically contaminated victims presenting to a healthcare facility should, if possible, be denied entrance until decontaminated. Patients who have already entered a healthcare facility and are only later determined to be a contamination hazard present a more difficult problem. If the situation allows, such patients should be taken outside for decontamination before returning and the previous care area cordoned off until any remaining safety hazard is assessed and eliminated. Although special decontamination solutions are preferable if available, rapid washing is more important than the choice of cleaning solution. Care should be taken to clean the hair, intertriginous areas, axillae, and groin. With small numbers of victims, ocular decontamination after lacrimator exposure is ideally performed with topical anesthesia and

**TABLE 98–3 Recommendations for Healthcare Facility Response to Chemical and/or Biological Warfare or Weapons Incidents**

- Immediate access to personal protective equipment for healthcare professionals
- Decontamination facilities that can be made operational with minimal delay
- Triage of victims into those able to decontaminate themselves (decreasing the workload for healthcare providers) and those requiring assistance
- Decontamination facilities permitting simultaneous use by multiple persons and providing some measure of visual privacy
- A brief registration process when patients are assigned numbers and given identically numbered plastic bags to contain and identify their clothing and valuables
- Provision of food, water, and psychological support for staff, who will likely be required to perform for extended periods
- Secondary triage to separate persons requiring immediate medical treatment from those with minor or no apparent injuries who are sent to a holding area for observation
- Providing victims with written information regarding the agent involved, potential short- and long-term effects, recommended treatment, stress reactions, and possible avenues for further assistance
- Careful handling of information released to the media to prevent conflicting or erroneous reports
- Instituting postexposure surveillance

**TABLE 98–4 Chemical and/or Biological Warfare or Weapons Phone Numbers/Contacts**

***Centers for Disease Control and Prevention (CDC)***

800-CDC-INFO (800-232-4636); https://www.cdc.gov

CDC Emergency Operations Center: 770-488–7100

CDC Division of Preparedness and Emerging Infections: 404-639–0385

***US Army Medical Research Institute of Chemical Defense***

410-436-3276 (duty hours), 410-436-3277 (Off Duty Hours)

***Federal Bureau of Investigation (FBI)***

Find your local FBI field office at http://www.fbi.gov/contact-us/field/field-offices

a specially designed contact lens that facilitates irrigation. Decontamination wastewater should ideally be contained and treated, but few facilities have the capability or funds to do this. However, wastewater is a minor issue because with large-scale CWs events, the wastewater represents only a small percentage of the total environmental impact.

### Risk of Exposure

The actual release of chemical or biologic weapons can be characterized as a low-probability, high-consequence event. Potential sources for civilian exposure include terrorist attacks, inadvertent releases from domestic stockpiles, direct military attacks, and industrial events. The chemicals most likely to be used militarily appear to be sulfur mustard and the nerve agents. A "low-tech" terrorist attack could involve the release of toxic industrial chemicals, such as chlorine, phosgene, or ammonia gas, as chemical "agents of opportunity."

### Psychological Effects

Either the threat or the actual use of CBW agents presents unique psychological stressors. Even among trained persons, a CBW-contaminated environment will produce high stress through the necessity of wearing protective gear, potential exposure to weapons, high workload intensity, defensive posture, and interactions with dead and dying patients. The psychological casualties will probably outnumber victims requiring medical treatment. Psychiatrists and other disaster mental health personnel should be enlisted in plans to manage CBW incidents for their expertise in treating anxiety, fear, panic, somatization, and grief. Uncontrolled release of information will compound terror and increase psychological casualties. Examples the influx of patients resulting from a news report suggesting that anyone with dizziness or nausea be checked for cholinesterase inhibitor toxicity or that fever and cough indicate infection with anthrax.

### Israeli Experience during the 1990 to 1991 Gulf War

Israel is probably one of the best prepared countries for CBW disasters. In late 1990, the civilian population was supplied with rubber gas masks, atropine syringes, and Fuller's earth decontamination powder. Thirty-nine ballistic missiles with conventional warheads were launched against Israel from Iraq in early 1991, with only six missiles causing direct casualties. Many more injuries resulted from CBW defensive measures and psychological stress than from physical trauma. Of 1,060 injuries reported from emergency departments (EDs) during this time period, 234 persons were directly wounded in explosions, and there were only two fatalities from trauma. More than 200 people presented for medical evaluation after self-injection of atropine, a few requiring admission to the hospital. About 540 people sought care for acute anxiety reactions. Some suffocated from improperly used gas masks, fell and injured themselves when rushing to rooms sealed against CBW agents, or were poisoned by carbon monoxide in these airtight rooms.

### Special Populations

Pregnancy does not appear to be a significant factor in the treatment of women victims of CWs. Children differ substantially from adults with regard to the effects of CWs and decontamination efforts. Children breathe at a lower ground elevation above the ground and at a higher rate than adults. Because nearly all CW gases and vapors are heavier than air, children are exposed to higher concentrations than adults in the same exposure setting and generally exhibit symptoms earlier. Children are also more susceptible to vesicants and nerve agents than adults with equivalent exposures. Children have thinner and more delicate skin, allowing for more systemic absorption and more rapid onset of injury with sulfur mustard. Decontamination of children is another feature that requires an age-adjusted approach. Most children will need assistance and supervision during decontamination procedures; keeping a mother or other adult guardian with a child should help with both decontamination and thermoregulation.

## NERVE AGENTS

### Physical Characteristics and Toxicity

Nerve agents are extremely potent organic phosphorus compound cholinesterase inhibitors and are the most toxic of the known CWs. Pure nerve agents are clear and colorless. Tabun has a faint fruity odor, and soman is variably described as smelling sweet, musty, fruity, spicy, nutty, or like camphor. Most subjects exposed to sarin and VX were unable to describe the odor. The G agents tabun (GA), sarin (GB), and soman (GD) are volatile and present a significant vapor hazard. Sarin is the most volatile, only slightly less so than water. VX is an oily liquid with low volatility and higher environmental persistence.

### Pathophysiology

The pathophysiology of nerve agents is essentially identical to that from organic phosphorus compound insecticides (Chap. 83), differing only in terms of potency, kinetics, and physical characteristics of the xenobiotics.

### Clinical Effects

Nerve agent vapor exposures produce rapid effects, within seconds to minutes, but the effects from liquid exposure are delayed as the xenobiotic is absorbed through the skin. Aerosol or vapor exposure initially affects the eyes, nose, and respiratory tract. Miosis is common, resulting from direct contact of the xenobiotic with the eye and may persist for several weeks. Ciliary spasm produces ocular pain, headache, nausea, and vomiting, often exacerbated by near-vision accommodation. Rhinorrhea, airway secretions, bronchoconstriction, and dyspnea occur with increasing exposures. With a large vapor exposure, one or two breaths may produce loss of consciousness within seconds followed by seizures, paralysis, and apnea within minutes.

Liquid nerve agents permeate ordinary clothing, allowing for percutaneous absorption and rendering the clothing of patients potential hazards to healthcare personnel before proper decontamination. Mild dermal exposure produces localized sweating and muscle fasciculations after an asymptomatic period lasting up to 18 hours. Moderate skin exposure produces systemic effects with nausea, vomiting, diarrhea, and generalized weakness. Substantial dermal contamination will produce earlier and more severe effects, often with an abrupt onset. Severe toxicity from any route of exposure causes loss of consciousness, seizures, generalized fasciculations, flaccid paralysis, apnea, and/or incontinence. Cardiovascular effects are less predictable because either bradycardia (muscarinic) or tachycardia (nicotinic) may occur. Long-term effects from nerve agent exposure are mostly limited to psychological sequelae.

### Treatment of Nerve Agent Exposure

***Decontamination.*** In some critically ill patients, antidotal treatment will be necessary before or during the decontamination process; but generally, decontamination should occur before other treatment is instituted.

***Atropine.*** Atropine (Antidotes in Brief: A35) is the standard antidote for the muscarinic effects of nerve agents. Atropine does not reverse nicotinic effects but does have some central effects and will thus assist in halting seizure activity. We recommend an initial minimum dose of 2 mg atropine in adults; dosing in children begins at 0.05 mg/kg for mild to moderate symptoms and 0.1 mg/kg for severe symptoms, up to the adult dose. An initial dose of 5 to 6 mg is given for severely poisoned adult patients. Repeat doses are given every 2 to 5 minutes until resolution of muscarinic signs of toxicity. Neither reversal of miosis nor development of tachycardia is a reliable marker to guide atropine therapy. An autoinjector provides atropine (2.1 mg) plus pralidoxime chloride (600 mg) (Antidotes in Brief: A36).

In a mass casualty incident, IV atropine supplies will likely be rapidly depleted from hospital stocks. Alternative sources include atropine from ambulances, ophthalmic and veterinary preparations, or substituting an antimuscarinic such as glycopyrrolate. Facilities expecting large numbers of casualties should store atropine as a bulk powder formulation and rapidly reconstitute it for injection when needed.

***Oximes.*** Oximes are nucleophilic compounds that reactivate organic phosphorus compound–inhibited cholinesterase enzymes by removing the dialkylphosphoryl moiety. The only oxime approved in the US is pralidoxime (2-PAM). Other oximes include trimedoxime (TMB4) and obidoxime (toxogonin) used in some European countries. The Hagedorn (H-series) oximes, particularly HI-6 and HLö-7, are also studied in the context of nerve agent toxicity. Oximes should be given in conjunction with atropine because they are not particularly effective in reversing muscarinic effects when given alone. Oximes are the only antidotes that can reverse the neuromuscular nicotinic effects of fasciculations, weakness, and flaccid paralysis (Antidotes in Brief: A36).

***Antiepileptics.*** Severe human nerve agent toxicity rapidly induces convulsions, which persist for a few minutes until the onset of flaccid paralysis. The US military doctrine is to administer 10 mg of diazepam intramuscularly by autoinjector at the onset of severe toxicity whether seizures are present or not. We recommend midazolam for IM use and any available parenteral benzodiazepine for IV use (Antidotes in Brief: A26). Although diazepam is the most well-studied benzodiazepine in the treatment of nerve agent toxicity, lorazepam and midazolam have similar or improved beneficial effects in animal studies.

***Pyridostigmine Pretreatment.*** The first large-scale use of pyridostigmine as a pretreatment for nerve agent toxicity occurred during Operation Desert Storm in 1991. Whereas pyridostigmine is a carbamate acetylcholinesterase inhibitor that is freely and spontaneously reversible, organic phosphorus compound inhibition is permanent after "aging" occurs. Toxicity from rapidly aging weapons such as soman (GD) can probably not be reversed by standard oxime therapy in realistic clinical situations. Almost paradoxically, then, a carbamate can occupy cholinesterase, blocking access of nerve weapons to the active site, and thereby protect the enzyme from permanent inhibition. After nerve agent exposure, pyridostigmine is allowed to rapidly hydrolyze from acetylcholinesterase and can also be easily displaced by oximes, regenerating functional enzyme. Some US troops in the 1990 to 1991 Gulf War took 30 mg pyridostigmine bromide orally every 8 hours when under threat of nerve agent attack because of concern for potential exposure specifically to soman, which has a short aging half-life. Pyridostigmine pretreatment is not recommended in the civilian sector.

## VESICANTS

Vesicants are historically designated as "blister agents" because they manifest with blistering of skin and mucous membranes.

### Sulfur Mustard

Sulfur mustard is a vesicant alkylating compound similar to nitrogen mustards used in chemotherapy. Sulfur mustard caused over 1 million casualties in World War I and was later used by the Italians and Japanese in the 1930s, by Egypt in the 1960s, and by Iraq in the 1980s. Nonbattlefield exposures also occurred among Baltic Sea fishermen while recovering corroding shells dumped after World War II and to persons unearthing or handling old chemical warfare ordinance.

***Physical Characteristics.*** Sulfur mustard is a yellow to brown oily liquid with an odor resembling mustard, garlic, or horseradish. Mustard has relatively low volatility and high environmental persistence. Mustard vapor is 5.4 times denser than air. Mustard freezes at 57°F (13.9°C), so it is sometimes mixed with other substances, such as chloropicrin or Lewisite, to lower the freezing point and permit dispersion as a liquid.

***Pathophysiology.*** Sulfur mustard is an alkylating agent, forming bonds with sulfhydryl (–SH) and amino ($-NH_2$) groups. This mechanism is the same as occurs with the nitrogen mustards, first developed as cancer chemotherapy agents in the 1940s. The most important acute manifestation is indirect inhibition of glycolysis. Sulfur mustard rapidly alkylates and crosslinks purine bases in nucleic acids. This activates DNA repair mechanisms, including the activation of the enzyme poly(ADP-ribose) polymerase, depleting nicotinamide adenine dinucleotide ($NAD^+$), which in turn inhibits glycolysis and ultimately leads to cellular necrosis from adenosine triphosphate depletion.

***Clinical Effects.*** The organs most commonly affected by mustard are the eyes, skin, and respiratory tract. Incapacitation is severe in terms of number of lost person-days, time for lesions to heal, and increased risk of infection. In contrast, the mortality rate is rather low. Most deaths occur several days after exposure from respiratory failure, secondary bacterial pneumonia, or bone marrow suppression.

Dermal exposure produces dose-related injury. After a latent period of 4 to 12 hours, victims develop erythema that progresses to vesicles or bullae formation and skin necrosis. If decontamination is not performed immediately after exposure, injury cannot be prevented. However, later decontamination limits the severity of lesions and further spread of the chemical weapon to develop new lesions. Skin exposure to vapor typically results in first- or second-degree burns, although liquid exposure more commonly results in full-thickness burns.

Signs and symptoms of ocular and respiratory tract exposures also occur after a latent period of several hours. Ocular effects include pain, miosis, photophobia, lacrimation, blurred vision, blepharospasm, and corneal damage. Permanent blindness is rare, with recovery generally occurring within a few weeks. Inhalation of mustard results in a chemical tracheobronchitis. Hoarseness, cough, sore throat, and chest pressure are common initial complaints. Bronchospasm and obstruction from sloughed membranes occur in more serious cases, but lung parenchymal damage occurs only in the most severe inhalational exposures. Productive cough associated with fever and leukocytosis is common 12 to 24 hours after exposure and represents a sterile bronchitis or pneumonitis. Nausea and vomiting are common within the first few hours. High-dose exposures also cause bone marrow suppression.

Factory workers chronically exposed to mustard have increased risk of respiratory tract carcinomas. Respiratory sequelae include chronic bronchitis, emphysema, tracheobronchomalacia, and bronchiolitis obliterans. Some mustard victims also develop a delayed and often recurrent keratitis. Chronic dermatologic complications include scarring, pigmentation changes, chronic neuropathic pain, and pruritus.

***Treatment.*** Decontamination is essential in treating the sulfur mustard exposures, even among asymptomatic victims. Further treatment is largely supportive and symptomatic.

***Lewisite.*** Lewisite was developed as a less persistent alternative to avoid some shortcomings in the use of sulfur mustard in World War I. Lewisite was never used in combat because the first shipment was en route to Europe when the war ended, and it was intentionally destroyed at sea. British anti-Lewisite (BAL, dimercaprol) was developed as a specific antidote and remains in use for chelation of arsenic and other metals.

Pure Lewisite is an oily, colorless liquid. Impure preparations are colored from amber to blue-black to black and have the odor of geraniums. Lewisite is more volatile than mustard and is easily hydrolyzed by water and by alkaline aqueous solutions such as sodium hypochlorite.

Lewisite toxicity is similar to that of sulfur mustard, resulting in dermal and mucous membrane damage, with conjunctivitis, airway injury, and vesiculation. An important clinical distinction is that Lewisite is immediately painful, while initial contact with mustard is not.

Treatment consists of decontamination with copious water or dilute hypochlorite solution, supportive care, and dimercaprol. Dimercaprol is given parenterally for systemic toxicity and is also used topically for dermal or ophthalmic injuries (Antidotes in Brief: A28).

### Phosgene Oxime

Although classified as a vesicant, phosgene oxime (CX) does not cause vesiculation of the skin. Phosgene oxime is more properly an urticant or "nettle" weapon, in that it produces erythema, wheals, and urticaria likened to stinging nettles. It produces immediate irritation of the skin and mucous membranes. This vesicant has never been used in battle, and little is known about its mechanism or effects on humans.

## CYANIDES (CHEMICAL ASPHYXIANTS)

Several cyanides have been used as CWs. The clinical effects and treatment of cyanide toxicity are covered elsewhere (Chap. 96) and do not differ significantly if used as a weapon. Hydrocyanic acid gas persists for only a few minutes in the atmosphere because it is lighter than air and rapidly disperses. Cyanogen chloride additionally causes ophthalmic and respiratory tract irritation and with sufficiently high exposures is reported to produce delayed acute respiratory distress syndrome (ARDS) in victims who are not rapidly killed.

## PULMONARY IRRITANTS

Chlorine, phosgene, and diphosgene were used as war gases in World War I. Chlorine, phosgene, diphosgene, various organohalides, and nitrogen oxides belong to a group of toxic chemicals designated "pulmonary irritants" because they can all induce delayed ARDS from increased alveolar-capillary membrane permeability. Chapter 94 provides clinical details for this class of xenobiotics.

When released on the battlefield, chlorine forms a yellow-green cloud with a distinct pungent odor detectable at concentrations that are not immediately dangerous. Phosgene is either colorless or seen as a white cloud as a result of atmospheric hydrolysis. Phosgene, which is reported to smell like grass, sweet newly mown hay, corn, or moldy hay, accounted for about 85% of all World War I deaths attributed to CWs. Phosgene produces injury by hydrolysis in the lungs to hydrochloric acid and by forming diamides that cross-link cell components. Battlefield exposure triggers cough, chest discomfort, dyspnea, lacrimation, and the peculiar complaint that smoking tobacco produces an objectionable taste. Prolonged observation after phosgene exposure is the rule because some casualties initially appeared well and were discharged, only to return in severe respiratory distress a few hours later.

## RIOT CONTROL AGENTS

Riot control agents are intentionally nonlethal chemicals that temporarily disable exposed individuals through intense irritation of exposed mucous membranes and skin. These weapons are also known as lacrimators, irritants, harassing agents, human repellents, and tear gas. They are solids at normal temperatures and pressures but are typically dispersed as aerosols or as small solid particles in liquid sprays.

Chloroacetophenone (military designation CN) and *o*-Chlorobenzylidene malononitrile (CS) are the two common riot control agents. When used for crowd control, both CN and CS are disseminated as aerosols or as smoke from incendiary devices. Dibenzoxazepine (CR) is a similar weapon with prominent skin irritation. Exposed persons develop burning irritation of the eyes, progressing to conjunctival injection, lacrimation, photophobia, and blepharospasm. Inhalation causes chest tightness, cough, sneezing, and increased secretions. Dermal exposure causes a burning sensation, erythema, or vesiculation, depending on the dose. Victims generally remove themselves from the offensive environment and recover within 15 to 30 minutes. Deaths are rare and typically occur from respiratory tract complications in closed-space exposures where exiting the area is impossible.

Law enforcement agencies and private citizens have access to oleoresin capsicum (OC), also known as pepper spray. Oleoresin capsicum is the essential oil derived from pepper plants (*Capsicum anuum*), which contains capsaicin, a naturally occurring lacrimator. Capsaicin activates the TRPV1 receptor, a heat-dependent nociceptor, explaining why exposures are experienced as "hot." Severe skin injuries, respiratory tract injuries, and fatalities are occasionally reported from exposures, typically only with prolonged or highly concentrated exposures.

Chloropicrin (PS) is another lacrimator that occasionally causes human toxicity through its use as a broad-spectrum fumigant and soil insecticide, as well as a warning agent associated with structural fumigants such as sulfuryl fluoride. 10-Chloro-5,10-dihydrodiphenarsazine (DM) induces vomiting in addition to irritant effects. Because symptoms are delayed, victims remain in the area, and the likelihood of significant absorption is increased. In addition to upper respiratory and ocular irritation, DM causes more prolonged systemic effects with headache, malaise, nausea, and vomiting.

The primary treatment for all riot control agents is removal from exposure. Contaminated clothing should be removed and placed in airtight bags to prevent secondary exposures. Skin irrigation with copious cold water should be used for significant dermal exposures. Symptomatic treatments, such as with topical ophthalmic anesthetics, nebulized bronchodilators, or oral antihistamines and corticosteroids, are indicated for directed therapy in more severely affected victims.

## INCAPACITATING AGENTS

3-Quinuclidinyl benzilate (BZ QNB) is an antimuscarinic compound that was developed as an incapacitating CW agent. It is 25-fold more potent centrally than atropine, with an $ID_{50}$ (dose that incapacitates 50% of those exposed) of about 0.5 mg. Clinical effects are characteristic for anticholinergics, with drowsiness, poor coordination, and slowing of thought processes progressing to delirium. Following exposure there is a delay of at least 1 hour for initial manifestations, which peak at 8 hours, continue to incapacitate for 24 hours, and takes 2 to 3 days to fully resolve.

Ultrapotent opioids can be used as incapacitating CWs. In 2002, Russian security forces used a fentanyl derivative (carfentanil and/or remifentanil) to end a 3-day standoff with terrorists in a Moscow theater in which Chechen rebels held more than 800 hostages.

Lysergic acid diethylamide (LSD) has also been investigated as an incapacitating weapon. Although effective at very low doses, battlefield use of LSD is impractical because poisoning will not reliably prevent a soldier from participation in combat.

Table 98–5 summarizes the various toxic syndromes associated with use of CWs.

**TABLE 98–5** Chemical Weapons Toxic Syndromes

| | | Organ System | | | | | | |
|---|---|---|---|---|---|---|---|---|
| *Chemical Weapon* | *Onset* | *Eyes* | *Upper Airways and Mucous Membranes* | *Lungs* | *Skin* | *CNS* | *GI Tract* | *Other* |
| ***Nerve Agents*** | | | | | | | | |
| Tabun (GA), Sarin (GB) | | | | | | | | |
| Soman (GD), VX | | | | | | | | |
| Aerosol/vapor (mild/moderate exposure) | Rapid (seconds–minutes) | Miosis, eye pain, dim or blurred vision | Rhinorrhea, ↑secretions | Dyspnea, cough, wheezing, bronchorrhea | — | Headache | Nausea, vomiting, abdominal cramps | — |
| Dermal exposure (mild to moderate exposure) | Delayed (minutes–hours) | — | — | — | Localized sweating | — | — | — |
| Severe exposure (any route) | As above (by route) | Miosis | ↑Secretions | Apnea | — | Sudden collapse, seizures | Nausea, vomiting, diarrhea, cramping, incontinence | Subjective weakness, local muscle fasciculations, generalized fasciculations, weakness, flaccid paralysis |

(*Continued*)

**TABLE 98–5 Chemical Weapons Toxic Syndromes (*Continued*)**

| | | Organ System | | | | | | |
|---|---|---|---|---|---|---|---|---|
| ***Chemical Weapon*** | ***Onset*** | ***Eyes*** | ***Upper Airways and Mucous Membranes*** | ***Lungs*** | ***Skin*** | ***CNS*** | ***GI Tract*** | ***Other*** |
| ***Vesicants*** | | | | | | | | |
| Sulfur mustard (H, HD) | Delayed (hours) | Conjunctivitis, eye pain, blurred vision, blindness (temporary) | Irritation, hoarseness, barky cough, sinus tenderness tracheobronchitis | (More severe exposures) Productive cough, pseudomembrane formation, airway obstruction | Erythema, vesicles, bullae, necrosis | — | Nausea, vomiting | Bone marrow suppression (in severe exposures) |
| Lewisite (L) | Immediate irritation<br>Delayed vesication | Pain, blepharospasm conjunctivitis, eyelid edema | (Same as sulfur mustard) | (Same as sulfur mustard) | Erythema, vesicles | — | — | Shock (in severe exposures) |
| Phosgene oxime (CX) | Immediate irritation<br>Delayed urticaria | Pain, corneal damage | Irritation | ARDS | Pain, blanching, erythema, urticaria, necrosis | — | — | — |
| ***Toxic Inhalants*** | | | | | | | | |
| Phosgene (CG) | Immediate Irritation | Irritation | Irritation | Dyspnea, cough, ARDS | — | — | — | Chlorine effects more rapid than phosgene |
| Chlorine (CL) | Delayed ARDS | — | Stridor | Dyspnea, cough, ARDS | — | — | — | |
| ***Cyanides*** | | | | | | | | |
| Hydrogen cyanide (AC) | Rapid (seconds–minutes) | — | — | Hyperpnea and then apnea | — | Anxiety, agitation, sudden collapse, seizures | — | — |
| Cyanogen chloride (CK) | Rapid (seconds–minutes) | Irritation | Irritation | Hyperpnea and then apnea | — | Anxiety, agitation, sudden collapse, seizures | — | — |
| ***Riot Control Agents*** | | | | | | | | |
| Lacrimators (CN, CS)<br>Capsaicin (OC) | Immediate | Pain, lacrimation, blepharospasm, conjunctivitis | Irritation | Cough, chest pain | Burning pain, erythema<br>Vesiculation (severe exposures) | — | Nausea, retching (may occur with CN or CS) | — |
| Adamsite (DM) | Rapid (minutes) | Irritation | Irritation, sneezing | Cough, chest pain | — | Headache | Nausea, vomiting, abdominal cramps | — |
| ***Incapacitating Agents*** | | | | | | | | |
| 3-Quinuclidinyl benzilate (BZ) | Delayed (hours) | Mydriasis | Dry mouth | — | — | Anticholinergic delirium | — | — |
| Ultrapotent opioids | Rapid (seconds–minutes) | Miosis | — | Hypoventilation | — | CNS depression | — | — |

— = not an expected major finding; ARDS = acute respiratory distress syndrome; CN = chloroacetophenone; CNS = central nervous system; CS = *o*-chlorobenzylidene malononitrile; GI = gastrointestinal.

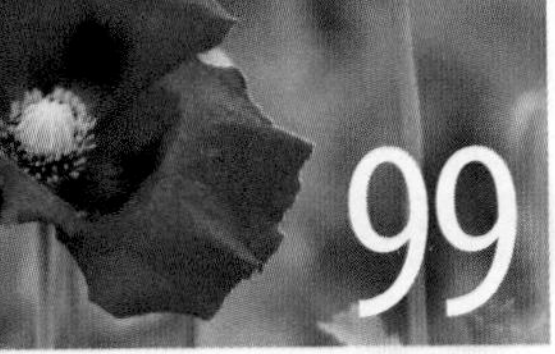

# 99 BIOLOGICAL WEAPONS

Expertise in dealing with biological weapons (BWs) requires specific knowledge from the fields of infectious disease, epidemiology, toxicology, and public health. Biological and chemical weapons share many characteristics in common, including intent of use, some dispersion methods, and initial defense based on adequate personal protective equipment and decontamination (**Tables 98–2** and **98–3**). However, key differences between biological and chemical weapons involve a greater delay in onset of clinical symptoms after exposure to BWs. Additionally, a few BWs can reproduce in the human host and cause secondary casualties, and disease after exposure to certain BWs can be prevented by the timely administration of prophylactic medications.

Biological weapons may be bacteria, fungi, viruses, or toxins derived from microorganisms. Some fungi are listed as potential BWs; however, none are known to have been developed into weapons to date. Because toxin weapons are not living organisms, some authorities classify them as chemical weapons rather than BWs. For the purpose of discussion in this chapter, toxin weapons derived from microorganisms will be considered BWs.

## HISTORY

Biological warfare has ancient roots. Missile weapons poisoned with natural toxins were used as early as 18,000 years ago. Other uses of biological warfare before the modern era relied mainly on poisoning water supplies with natural toxins or spreading naturally occurring epidemic infections to the enemy by hurling infected corpses over battlements or through the intentional transfer of disease-contaminated goods (eg, smallpox-contaminated blankets).

During World War I, Germany was the only combatant nation with an active BW program; however, by World War II, many nations had BW research programs, including Japan, the Soviet Union, Germany, France, Britain, Canada, and the United States (US).

In 1979, an outbreak of human anthrax caused at least 66 fatalities in the Russian city of Sverdlovsk. Autopsies revealed that the deaths were from inhalational anthrax, and epidemiologic investigation demonstrated that almost all the cases occurred downwind from a military facility. These data were consistent only with a release of aerosolized anthrax, which has since been confirmed by Russian authorities. In 2001, closely following the September 11, 2001, attack, a bioterrorist attack occurred in the US resulting in several cases of inhalational and cutaneous anthrax, with five fatalities.

## GENERAL CONSIDERATIONS

### Differences Between Biological Weapons Incidents and Naturally Occurring Outbreaks

Because the clinical effects of BWs are often delayed for several days after exposure, it may be difficult to differentiate an occult BW release from a naturally occurring disease outbreak. Several epidemiologic criteria are proposed to aid in such determinations, many of which should be identifiable in a BW incident (Table 99–1).

### Preparedness

Many BWs initially produce nonspecific symptoms, and diseases that rarely, if ever, occur in clinical practice. Inhalational anthrax and pneumonic plague, for example, could easily be misdiagnosed as influenza or acute bronchitis. Providers in emergency departments and primary care medicine should be educated to recognize the signs, symptoms, and clinical progression of diseases caused by BW. Clear identification, isolation, and aggressive treatment early after exposure within the first 24 to 48 hours are the best and only means of reducing mortality rates and, in the case of smallpox or plague, preventing secondary or tertiary cases.

### Decontamination

Biological weapons are most effective when dispersed by aerosol and, as such, produce little surface contamination. Simple removal of clothing will eliminate a high proportion of deposited particles, and subsequent showering with soap and water will probably remove 99.99% of any remaining organisms on the skin. Contaminated clothing should be removed and placed in airtight bags or containers to prevent resuspension in the air. After an occult BW release, victims are identified late after exposure; decontamination will obviously not be helpful and may only serve to delay care.

## BIOLOGICAL WARFARE AGENTS

### Bacteria

***Anthrax.*** Anthrax is caused by *Bacillus anthracis*, a gram-positive spore-forming bacillus found in soil worldwide. *B. anthracis* causes disease primarily in herbivorous animals.

**TABLE 99–1 Epidemiologic Clues Suggesting Biological Weapon Release**

- Large epidemic with unusually high morbidity, mortality, or both
- Epidemic curve (number of cases vs time) showing an "explosion" of cases, reflecting a point source in time rather than insidious onset
- Tight geographic localization of cases, especially downwind of potential release site
- Predominance of respiratory tract symptoms because most BWs are transmitted by aerosol inhalation
- Simultaneous outbreaks of multiple unusual diseases
- Immunosuppressed and elderly persons more susceptible
- Nonendemic infection ("impossible epidemiology")
- Nonseasonal time for endemic infection
- Organisms with unusual antimicrobial resistance patterns, reflecting BW genetic engineering
- Animal casualties concurrent with disease outbreak
- Absence of normal zoonotic disease host
- Low attack rates among persons incidentally working in areas with filtered air supplies or closed ventilation systems, using HEPA masks, or remaining indoors during outdoor exposures
- Delivery vehicle or munitions discovered
- Law enforcement or military intelligence information
- Claim of BW release by a belligerent force

BW = bioweapon; HEPA = high-efficiency particle absorbing.

Human anthrax cases generally occur in farmers, ranchers, and among workers handling contaminated animal carcasses, hides, wool, hair, and bones.

**Clinical Manifestations.** A few clinically distinct forms of anthrax occur, depending on the route of exposure. Cutaneous anthrax results from direct inoculation of spores into the skin via abrasions or other wounds and accounts for about 95% of endemic (naturally occurring) human cases. Patients develop a painless red macule that vesiculates, ulcerates, and forms a 1- to 5-cm brown-black dermatonecrotic eschar surrounded by edema. Most skin lesions heal spontaneously, although 10% to 20% of untreated patients progress to septicemia and death. When treated with antibiotics, cutaneous anthrax rarely results in fatalities. Anthrax is not transmissible among humans.

Gastrointestinal (GI) anthrax results from ingesting insufficiently cooked meat from infected animals. Patients develop nausea, vomiting, fever, abdominal pain, and mucosal ulcers, which can cause GI hemorrhage, perforation, and sepsis. The mortality rate from GI anthrax is at least 50%, even with antibiotic treatment.

Inhalational anthrax results from exposure to aerosolized *B. anthracis* spores. Although this form of anthrax is very rare, it is so closely associated with occupational exposures that it is called "wool-sorter's disease." Inhalational anthrax is also likely to be the form that occurs in a BW attack because the anthrax spores would be most effectively disseminated by aerosol. After an incubation period of 1 to 6 days, the patient develops fever, malaise, fatigue, nonproductive cough, and mild chest discomfort. The initial symptoms may briefly improve for 2 to 3 days, or the patient may abruptly progress to severe respiratory distress with dyspnea, diaphoresis, stridor, and cyanosis. Bacteremia; shock; metastatic infection such as meningitis, which occurs in about 50% of cases; and death may follow within 24 to 36 hours. Before the 2001 bioterrorist outbreak, the mortality rate from inhalational anthrax was expected to be nearly 100%, even with antibiotics, after symptoms develop. With appropriate antibiotic therapy and supportive care, 5 of 11 patients with inhalational anthrax in 2001 died.

**Pathophysiology.** Inhaled spores are taken up into the lymphatic system, where they germinate and the bacteria reproduce. *B. anthracis* produces three toxins: protective antigen (PA), edema factor, and lethal factor. Protective antigen is so named because antibodies against it protect the individual from the effects of the other two toxins. Protective antigen forms a heptamer that inserts into plasma membranes, facilitating endocytosis of the other two toxins into target cells (Fig. 99–1). Edema factor increases intracellular cyclic adenosine monophosphate (AMP), upsetting water homeostasis, which leads to massive edema and impaired neutrophil function. Lethal factor is a zinc metalloprotease that stimulates macrophages to release tumor necrosis factor α and interleukin-1β, contributing to death in systemic anthrax infections.

**Treatment.** The primary antibiotics used to treat anthrax are ciprofloxacin and doxycycline. Although other fluoroquinolones would be expected to have similar activity

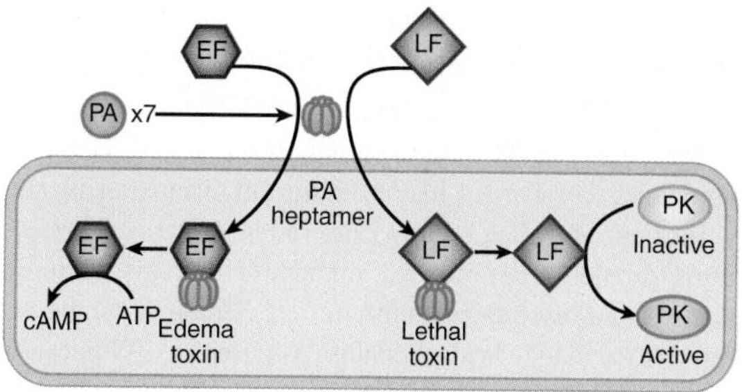


**FIGURE 99–1.** Model of action of anthrax toxins. Edema factor (EF) and lethal factor (LF) are unable to enter cells until they complex with a protective antigen (PA) heptamer, forming edema toxin and lethal toxin, respectively. When intracellular, release from PA allows EF and LF to exert their intracellular effects. Antibodies against PA confer resistance to the toxic effects of anthrax. ATP = adenosine triphosphate; cAMP = cyclic adenosine monophosphate; PK = protein kinase.

against anthrax, ciprofloxacin, levofloxacin, and doxycycline are US Food and Drug Administration (FDA)–approved for use in this infection. In a mass casualty setting or for postexposure prophylaxis, adults should receive ciprofloxacin 500 mg orally (PO) every 12 hours. Alternate therapies are doxycycline 100 mg PO every 12 hours or amoxicillin 500 mg PO every 8 hours if the anthrax strain is proven susceptible. The recommended duration of therapy is 60 days. Children should also be treated with ciprofloxacin (15 mg/kg; maximum, 500 mg/dose) or amoxicillin (80 mg/kg/day divided every 8 hours; maximum, 500 mg/dose). Cutaneous anthrax is treated similarly.

Inhalational anthrax should be treated initially with intravenous antibiotics. Adults receive ciprofloxacin 400 mg intravenously (IV) or doxycycline 100 mg IV every 12 hours, along with one or two additional antibiotics with in vitro activity against anthrax (eg, rifampin, vancomycin, penicillin, ampicillin, chloramphenicol, imipenem, clindamycin, clarithromycin). Children are given ciprofloxacin 10 mg/kg IV (maximum, 400 mg/dose) or doxycycline 2.2 mg/kg IV (maximum, 100 mg/dose) and additional antibiotics, as indicated earlier. Raxibacumab and obiltoxaximab monoclonal antibodies that blocks binding of the anthrax PA to its host cell receptor and are US FDA approved for inhalational anthrax in combination with appropriate antibiotics.

**Anthrax Vaccine.** An effective vaccine against anthrax is available. In human and animal experiments, the vaccine is highly effective in preventing all forms of anthrax, and the vaccine is recommended for workers in high-risk occupations. Anthrax Immune Globulin Intravenous (Human) is also approved for use.

**Lessons from the 2001 Anthrax Bioterrorism Event.** Although the overall number of individuals infected was relatively low, the psychosocioeconomic impact was exceptionally high. Several hundred postal and other facilities were tested for *B. anthracis* spore contamination, and public health authorities recommended antibiotic prophylaxis be initiated for approximately 32,000 persons. As predicted, the psychological impact far exceeded the actual medical consequences, and events with a modest number of medical patients are probably more likely than true mass casualty BW incidents.

Published estimates of tens of thousands of deaths from a military-style anthrax attack depend on efficient BW dispersion.

***Plague.*** *Yersinia pestis* is a gram-negative bacillus responsible for more than 200 million human deaths and three major pandemics in recorded history. Naturally occurring plague is transmitted by flea vectors from rodent hosts or by respiratory droplets from infected animals or humans. Bubonic plague could result from an intentional release of plague-infested fleas. Plague is a particularly frightening BW because it can be released as an aerosol to cause a fulminant communicable form of the disease for which no effective vaccine exists. Antibiotics must be initiated early after exposure because when symptoms develop, mortality rates are reportedly extremely high.

**Clinical Presentation.** Plague occurs in three clinical forms: bubonic, septicemic, and pneumonic. Bubonic plague has an incubation period of 2 to 10 days, followed by fever, malaise, and painful, enlarged regional lymph nodes called buboes. Secondary septicemia occurs in 23% of patients presenting with bubonic plague. Distal gangrene occurs from small artery thromboses, explaining why plague pandemics are sometimes called the Black Death. If left untreated, bubonic plague carries a 60% mortality rate. Pneumonic plague is an infection of the lungs that occurs through septicemic spread of the organism or from inhalation of either infected respiratory droplets or an intentionally disseminated BW aerosol. The incubation period of pneumonic plague is 2 to 3 days after inhalation. Patients develop fever, malaise, and cough productive of bloody sputum, rapidly progressing to dyspnea, stridor, cyanosis, and cardiorespiratory collapse. Plague pneumonia is almost always fatal unless treatment is begun with 24 hours of symptom onset.

**Diagnosis and Treatment.** Plague can be diagnosed by various staining techniques, immunologic studies, or culturing the organism from blood, sputum, or lymph node aspirates. In a mass casualty setting or for postexposure prophylaxis, treatment should be with doxycycline 100 mg or ciprofloxacin 500 mg PO twice daily for adults. Children should be given doxycycline 2.2 mg/kg or ciprofloxacin 20 mg/kg, up to a maximum of the adult doses. Chloramphenicol 25 mg/kg PO four times daily is an alternative. The durations of treatment are 7 days for postexposure prophylaxis and 10 days for mass casualty incidents. Patients with pneumonic plague need to be isolated to prevent secondary cases. In a contained-casualty setting, patients with pneumonic plague should be treated with parenteral streptomycin or gentamicin; alternative antibiotics include doxycycline, ciprofloxacin, and chloramphenicol.

***Tularemia.*** *Francisella tularensis* is a small, aerobic, gram-negative coccobacillus weaponized by the US and probably other countries as well. Tularemia occurs naturally as a zoonotic disease spread by blood-sucking arthropods or by direct contact with infected animal material. Tularemia in humans may occur in ulceroglandular or typhoidal forms, depending on the route of exposure. Ulceroglandular tularemia is more common, occurring after skin or mucous membrane exposure to infected animal blood or tissues. Patients develop a local ulcer with associated lymphadenopathy, fever, chills, headache, and malaise. Typhoidal tularemia presents with fever, prostration, and weight loss without adenopathy. Diagnosing tularemia is often difficult because the organism is hard to isolate by culture and the symptoms are nonspecific. In mass casualty settings or for postexposure prophylaxis, treatment should be doxycycline 100 mg twice daily or ciprofloxacin 500 mg PO twice daily for 14 days for adults. Pediatric dosing for doxycycline is 2.2 mg/kg or ciprofloxacin 15 mg/kg (maximum, adult dose) twice daily. When dealing with a limited number of casualties, the preferred antibiotics are streptomycin 1 g intramuscularly (IM) twice daily or gentamicin 5 mg/kg IM or IV once daily. Alternatives include parenteral doxycycline, chloramphenicol, and ciprofloxacin.

***Brucellosis.*** Brucellosis could potentially be used as an incapacitating BW because it causes disease with low mortality but significant morbidity. Brucellae (*Brucella melitensis, abortus, suis,* and *canis*) are small, aerobic, gram-negative coccobacilli that generally cause disease in ruminant livestock. Humans develop brucellosis by ingesting contaminated meat and dairy products or by aerosol transmission from infected animals. Brucellosis presents with nonspecific symptoms such as fever, chills, and malaise, with either an acute or insidious onset. The diagnosis is established by serologic methods or culture. Patients should be given doxycycline 200 mg/day PO, plus rifampin 600 to 900 mg/day PO for 6 weeks, or doxycycline 200 mg/day PO for 6 weeks, with either streptomycin 15 mg/kg twice daily IM or gentamicin 1.5 mg/kg IM every 8 hours for the first 10 days.

***Rickettsiae.*** Features of rickettsiae favoring their use as BW include environmental stability, aerosol transmission, persistence in infected hosts, low infectious dose, and high associated morbidity and mortality. Rickettsiae that have been weaponized include *Coxiella burnetii*, the causative organism of Q fever, and *Rickettsia prowazekii*, the causative organism of louseborne typhus.

***Q Fever.*** Q fever occurs naturally as a self-limited, febrile, zoonotic disease contracted from domestic livestock. Q fever is caused by *C. burnetii*, a unique rickettsialike organism that can persist on inanimate objects for weeks to months and can cause clinical disease with the inhalation of only a single organism. After a 10- to 40-day incubation period, Q fever manifests as an undifferentiated febrile illness, with headache, fatigue, and myalgias. Patchy pulmonary infiltrates on chest radiography that resemble viral or atypical bacterial pneumonia occur in 50% of cases, although only half of patients have cough, and even fewer have pleuritic chest pain. Uncommon complications include hepatitis, endocarditis, meningitis, encephalitis, and osteomyelitis. Patients are generally not critically ill, and the disease can last as long as 2 weeks. Treatment with antibiotics will shorten the course of acute Q fever and can prevent clinically evident disease when given during the incubation period. Tetracyclines are the mainstay of therapy, and either tetracycline 500 mg PO every 6 hours or doxycycline 100 mg PO every 12 hours should be given for 5 to 7 days.

## Viruses

***Smallpox.*** Smallpox is caused by the variola virus, a large DNA orthopoxvirus with a host range limited to humans. Before global World Health Organization (WHO) efforts to eradicate naturally occurring smallpox by immunization, recurrent epidemics were common, and the disease carried roughly a 30% fatality rate in unvaccinated populations. Smallpox is highly contagious, with 10 to 20 secondary cases per index case. The Soviet Union is known to have weaponized smallpox, and other countries are believed to maintain stocks of variola virus.

**Pathophysiology.** Transmission of smallpox typically occurs through inhalation of droplets or aerosols but may also occur through contaminated fomites. After a 12- to 14-day incubation period, the patient develops fever, malaise, and prostration with headache and backache. Oropharyngeal lesions appear, shedding virus into the saliva. Two to 3 days after the onset of fever, a papular rash develops on the face and spreads to the extremities (Fig. 99–2). The fever continues while the rash becomes vesicular and then pustular. Scabs form from the pustules and eventually separate, leaving pitted and hypopigmented scars. Death usually occurs during the second week of the illness. The diseases most likely to be confused with smallpox are chickenpox (varicella) and monkeypox. The lesions of smallpox should all appear at the same stage of development (synchronous), but chickenpox lesions occur at varying stages (asynchronous). Smallpox lesions tend to be found in a centrifugal distribution (face and distal extremities), but chickenpox lesions are more centripetal, tend to appear first on the trunk, and are pruritic. Until 2022 outbreaks of monkeypox were uncommon. This self-limited disease resembles smallpox except for the prognosis, which is excellent in immunocompromised individuals.

Three antivirals commercially available in the US, cidofovir, tecovirimat, and ribavirin, are effective in vitro against variola. Even a single case of smallpox should be considered a potential international health emergency and immediately reported to the appropriate public health authorities.

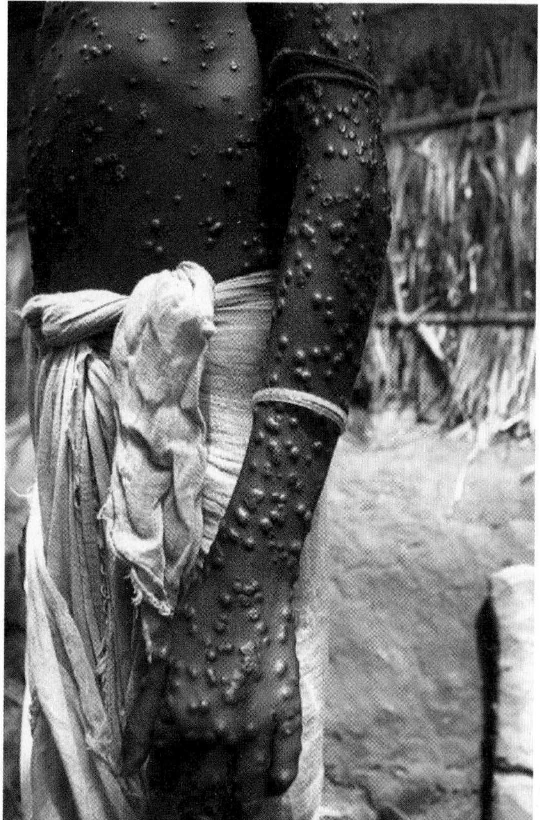

**FIGURE 99–2.** Smallpox rash demonstrating nonpruritic, synchronous tense vesicles.

**Smallpox Vaccination.** Rapid postexposure vaccination confers excellent protection against smallpox. The older smallpox vaccine uses a live vaccinia virus (derived from cowpox vaccine) rather than the actual variola virus that causes smallpox. The two most serious reactions are postvaccinal encephalitis and progressive vaccinia. Progressive vaccinia (Fig. 99–3) can occur in immunosuppressed individuals and is treated with vaccinia immune globulin (VIG). The current vaccine contains a live, but replication-incompetent vaccinia virus, that was US FDA-approved in 2019. It is not associated with vaccinia infection.

***Viral Hemorrhagic Fevers.*** Viral hemorrhagic fevers (VHFs) are all highly infectious by the aerosol route, making them candidates for use as BW. These include the viruses causing Lassa fever, dengue, yellow fever, Crimean-Congo hemorrhagic fever, and the Marburg, Ebola, and Hanta viruses. Clinical features, such as the extent of renal, hepatic, and hematologic involvement, vary according to the specific virus, but they all carry the risk of secondary infection through droplet aerosols. Ribavirin is reasonable for some VHFs, but supportive care is the mainstay of therapy. A vaccine for Ebola is now available.

***Viral Encephalitides.*** Three antigenically related $\alpha$ viruses of the Togaviridae family pose risks as BWs: western equine encephalitis (WEE), eastern equine encephalitis (EEE), and Venezuelan equine encephalitis (VEE). Birds are the natural reservoir of these viruses, and natural outbreaks occur among equines and humans by mosquito transmission. Adults infected with VEE usually develop an acute, febrile, incapacitating disease with prolonged recovery.

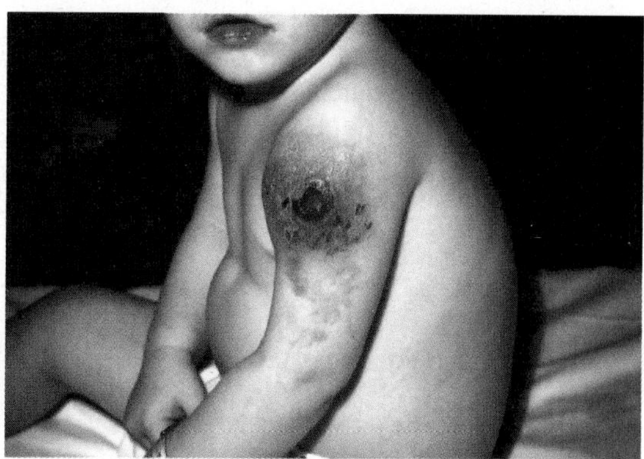

**FIGURE 99–3.** Progressive vaccinia.

Venezuelan equine encephalitis is considered the most likely BW threat among the viral encephalitides. After a 1- to 5-day incubation period, victims experience the sudden onset of malaise, myalgias, prostration, spiking fevers, rigors, severe headache, and photophobia. Nausea, vomiting, cough, sore throat, and diarrhea may follow. This acute phase lasts 24 to 72 hours. Between 0.5% and 4% of patients develop encephalitis, with meningismus, seizures, coma, and paralysis, which carries up to a 20% fatality rate. The diagnosis is usually established clinically, although the virus can sometimes be isolated from serum or from throat swabs, and serologic tests are available. The white blood cell count often shows a striking leukopenia and lymphopenia. Treatment is supportive. Person-to-person transmission can theoretically occur from droplet nuclei. Recovery takes 1 to 2 weeks.

### Toxins

Several toxins derived from bacteria, plants, fungi, and algae could theoretically be used as BWs if produced in sufficient quantities. Because of their high potency, only small amounts would be needed to kill or incapacitate exposed victims. Fortunately, obstacles in manufacturing weaponizable amounts limit the number of toxins that are practical for use as BWs. Discussion here is limited to those toxins known or highly suspected to have been weaponized.

***Botulinum Toxin.*** The US and some other countries developed botulinum toxin as a potential BW. The two most likely means of using botulinum toxin are by food contamination or by aerosol. Either method would result in the clinical syndrome of botulism (Chap. 11).

***Ricin.*** Ricin is derived from the castor bean plant (*Ricinus communis*) (Chap. 91) and is the only biological toxin to exist naturally in more than microscopic quantities. Its easy accessibility, relative ease of preparation, and low cost may make ricin an attractive BW for terrorists or poor countries. Although ricin has never been used in battle, it has attracted the attention of domestic extremists and terrorists and was used in some politically motivated assassinations. Ricin is a glycoprotein lectin (or toxalbumin) composed of two protein chains linked by a disulfide bond. The B chain facilitates cell binding and entry of the A chain into cells. The A chain inhibits protein synthesis, inactivating eukaryotic ribosomes by removing an adenine residue from ribosomal RNA. Inhalation of aerosolized ricin results in increased alveolar–capillary permeability and airway necrosis after a latent phase of 4 to 8 hours. Ingestion causes GI hemorrhage with necrosis of the liver, spleen, and kidney. Intramuscular administration produces severe local necrosis with extension into the lymphatics.

***Staphylococcal Enterotoxin B.*** Staphylococcal enterotoxin B (SEB) is an enterotoxin produced by *Staphylococcus aureus* that is recognized as a "superantigen" because of its profound activation of the immune system. As a BW, SEB could be ingested through contaminated food or water, resulting in acute gastroenteritis identical to classic staphylococcal food poisoning. If inhaled as an aerosol, SEB produces fever, myalgias, and a pneumonitis after a 3- to 12-hour latent period.

### Fungi and Other Fungal Toxins

Fungi may at first appear to be ideal BW, given their relative ease of handling, dissemination, and resistance of spores to physical stressors. The only fungi to be included on lists of microbes with potential use as BWs are *Coccidioides* spp, probably based on the high incidence of symptomatic infection in endemic areas. Nevertheless, the risk of serious disease is low, limiting the utility of *Coccidioides* spp as an effective weapon. Among the fungal toxins, trichothecene mycotoxins, aflatoxins, and amanita toxins, only trichothecene mycotoxins are noteworthy.

***Trichothecene Mycotoxins.*** The trichothecene mycotoxins are produced by filamentous fungi (molds) of various genera, including *Fusarium, Myrothecium, Phomopsis, Trichoderma, Tricothecium*, and *Stachybotrys*. Tricothecene mycotoxins are unusual among potential BWs in that toxicity can occur with exposure to intact skin. Naturally occurring trichothecene toxicity results from ingesting contaminated grains or by inhaling toxin aerosolized from contaminated hay or cotton. Outbreaks of ingested trichothecene toxins result in a clinical syndrome called alimentary toxic aleukia, characterized by gastroenteritis, fevers, chills, bone marrow suppression with granulocytopenia, and secondary sepsis—a syndrome clinically similar to acute radiation poisoning. Survival beyond this stage is characterized by the development of GI and upper airway ulceration and intradermal and mucosal hemorrhage. Trichothecene toxins are potent inhibitors of protein synthesis in eukaryotic cells, producing widespread cytotoxicity, particularly in rapidly proliferating tissues.

Several reports from the 1970s and 1980s suggested that Soviet-supported forces were using trichothecene mycotoxins as a BW. Aerosol and droplet clouds called Yellow Rain were associated with mass casualty incidents in Southeast Asia. Such incidents would involve multiple routes of exposure, with skin deposition likely being the major site. Early symptoms included nausea, vomiting, weakness, dizziness, and ataxia. Diarrhea would then ensue, at first watery and then becoming bloody. Within 3 to 12 hours, victims would develop dyspnea, cough, chest pain, sore mouths, bleeding gums, epistaxis, and hematemesis. Exposed skin areas would become intensely inflamed, with the appearance of vesicles, bullae, petechiae, ecchymoses, and necrosis. The use of trichothecene mycotoxins was never confirmed.

# 100 RADIATION

We use radiation and radionuclides for a vast array of purposes, ranging from mundane household uses such as detecting smoke to powering satellites, treating cancer, and examining the physical properties of individual molecules. Unfortunately, as our knowledge of how to use radiation has expanded, so too has our awareness of radiation as a toxin. The particles of radiation, their sources, and the mechanisms by which they pose a health risk are the subjects of the following discussion.

## HISTORICAL EXPOSURES

Soon after x-rays were discovered in 1895, a deepening understanding of radiation and radionuclides led to their wider use and resulting injuries. Clarence Dally was the first known radiation-induced death in 1904 after repeated exposures to Thomas Edison's early fluoroscopes. By 1927, nearly 100 women employed to create illuminated instrument dials became ill or died after exposure to radium-containing paint. After the use of the two atomic bombs in Japan at the end of World War II, estimates of dead and injured for both cities were well over 200,000. Most of the deaths were from the bomb blast, but many thousands died from acute radiation syndrome (ARS) and others subsequently from radiation-induced cancers. In the radioactive cobalt incident beginning in Juarez, Mexico, thousands of tiny metal pellets were spilled in a scrapyard and melted with other metals into table legs later shipped throughout Mexico and the United States (US). In the radioactive cesium incident in Goiânia, Brazil, scavengers were fascinated by the bluish glow of the material. Ultimately, 250 individuals were contaminated, 46 were treated with a chelator, and 4 died. More recently in the post–nuclear testing era, large radiation incidents occurred at the sites of nuclear reactors, such as Chernobyl in 1986 and Fukushima in 2011. Perhaps one of the most notorious deaths from radiation was that of Alexander Litvinenko, a former Soviet KGB operative who was living in London. It was only after a protracted illness and his death that radioactive polonium was discovered to be the cause.

## PRINCIPLES OF RADIOACTIVITY

*Radiation* is energy sent out in the form of waves or particles. Despite the *strong nuclear force* that holds atoms together, many isotopes are unstable. Various influences such as quantum fluctuations and the *weak nuclear force* can tip the balance toward instability to transform an isotope. This process can be intentional, as with the criticality events in a nuclear reactor or nuclear bomb, but mainly occurs spontaneously in nature as the process called radioactive decay.

### Radioactive Decay

In 1900, Marie Curie discovered that unstable nuclei decay or transform into more stable nuclei (daughters) via the emission of various particles or energy. Radioactive decay occurs mainly through five nuclear mechanisms: emission of gamma rays, alpha particles, beta particles, or positrons or by capture of an electron. The emission of these various particles makes radioactive decay dangerous because these particles *are* ionizing radiation. The half-life ($t_{1/2}$) is the period of time it takes for a radioisotope to lose half of its radioactivity. In every case, the activities of radioactive isotopes diminish exponentially with time (Table 100–1).

*Photons* are elementary particles that mediate electromagnetic radiation. Depending on their energy, the radiation has different names ranging from extremely long radio waves to high-energy gamma rays. X-rays and gamma rays are high-energy photons and are only distinguishable by their source. Gamma radiation is emitted by unstable atomic nuclei via radioactive decay and has a fixed wavelength depending on the energy that formed it. X-rays come from atomic processes outside the nucleus. Because of their nature, high-energy gamma and x-rays can penetrate several feet of insulating concrete. *Beta particles* are electrons. Electrons have less penetrating ability than gamma radiation but can still pass several centimeters into human skin. *Alpha particles* are helium nuclei (two protons and two neutrons) stripped of their electrons. These particles are the most easily shielded of the emitted particles mentioned and can be stopped by a piece of paper, skin, or clothing. *Neutrons* are primarily released from nuclear processes. The natural decay of radionuclides does not include emission of neutrons, which is mainly a health hazard for workers in a nuclear power facility or victims of a nuclear explosion. Unique among the particles of radioactivity, when neutrons are stopped or captured,

**TABLE 100–1 Physical Properties of Radioisotopes**

| *Isotope* | *Half-Life* | *Mode of Decay* | *Decay Energy (MeV)* |
|---|---|---|---|
| ***Medicine and Research Radioisotopes*** | | | |
| $^{2}H$ | Stable | | |
| $^{131}I$ | 8 days | $\beta^-$ | 0.97 |
| $^{201}Tl$ | 73 hours | EC | 0.41 |
| $^{99m}Tc$ | 6 hours | IT | 0.14 |
| $^{133}Xe$ | 5.27 days | $\beta^-$ | 0.43 |
| $^{67}Ga$ | 78 hours | EC | 1.00 |
| $^{137}Cs$ | 30.17 years | $\beta^-$ | 1.17 |
| $^{18}F$ | 109 months | $\beta^-$, EC | 1.65 |
| ***Military Radioisotopes*** | | | |
| $^{3}H$ | 12.26 years | $\beta^-$ | 0.02 |
| $^{90}Sr$ | 28.79 years | $\beta^-$ | 0.55 |
| $^{235}U$ | $7.1 \times 10^8$ years | $\alpha$, SF | 4.68 |
| $^{238}U$ | $4.51 \times 10^9$ years | $\alpha$, SF | 4.27 |
| $^{210}Po$ | 138 days | $\alpha$ | 5.307 |
| $^{239}Pu$ | 24,400 years | $\alpha$, SF | 5.24 |
| $^{241}Am$ | 470 years | $\alpha$, $\gamma$ | 5.14/0.02 |

EC = electron capture; IT = isomeric transition from upper to lower isomeric state; MeV = megaelectron volts; SF = spontaneous fission.

they can cause a previously stable atom to become radioactive in a process known as neutron activation. *Cosmic rays* are streams of electrons, protons, and alpha particles thought to emanate from stars and supernovas.

Isotopes and nuclides are very closely related terms, and most experts in the field use them interchangeably. Isotopes are two or more species or variants of a particular chemical element (same number of protons) that have different amounts of neutrons (eg, $^{123}I$, $^{125}I$, $^{127}I$, $^{131}I$). *Nuclide* is a more general term that may or may not be isotopes of a given element, such as *fissile nuclides* or *primordial nuclides.* Radioisotopes are isotopes that are radioactive, that is, they spontaneously decay and emit energy. Finally, radionuclides are simply nuclides that are radioactive.

## Ionizing Radiation Versus Nonionizing Radiation

*Ionizing radiation* refers to any radiation with sufficient energy to disrupt an atom or molecule with which it impacts. Hydroxyl free radicals, formed by ionizing water, are responsible for biochemical lesions that are the foundation of radiation toxicity.

The space between collisions of ionizing radiation and their target molecules varies with the particle type and its energy. A charged particle, such as an alpha particle, loses kinetic energy through a series of small energy transfers to other atomic electrons in the target medium, such as tissues. Because of its large size, collisions along the path of an alpha particle are clustered together, impeding its ability to penetrate tissue. By comparison, collisions along the path of gamma rays are spread out, increasing their ability to penetrate tissue. This ability to penetrate tissue and transfer energy accounts for the relative dangers of the forms of radiation and tissue susceptibility.

For a source of radiation to pose a threat to tissue, the ionizing particle must be placed in close proximity to vital components of tissue to inflict damage. High-energy photons penetrate deeply, so they pose a similar risk whether they come from an external source or from an incorporated source. Because alpha particles have much more limited tissue penetration, alpha emitters, radionuclides that radiate these particles, must first be incorporated to pose a threat to tissue.

Generally, nonionizing radiation consists of relatively low-energy photons and is used safely in cell phone and television signal transmission, radar, microwaves, and magnetic fields that emanate from high-voltage electricity and metal detectors. These photons lack the necessary energy required to cause ionization and cellular damage.

## Radiation Units of Measure

The units used to measure radiation are shown in Figure 100–1.

## Protection from Radiation

*Shielding* refers to the process by which one limits the amount of unwanted ionizing radiation in a given setting. Placing a specific material between a radiation source and a target will limit the amount of ionizing radiation that will interact with the target. *Distance* is an important safety factor in limiting radiation exposure. Because of their mass and electric charge, alpha and beta particles have a high probability of interacting with matter, such as the atmosphere. The result is that these particles do not travel more than a few centimeters through air and, in general, moving a few feet from the source of this

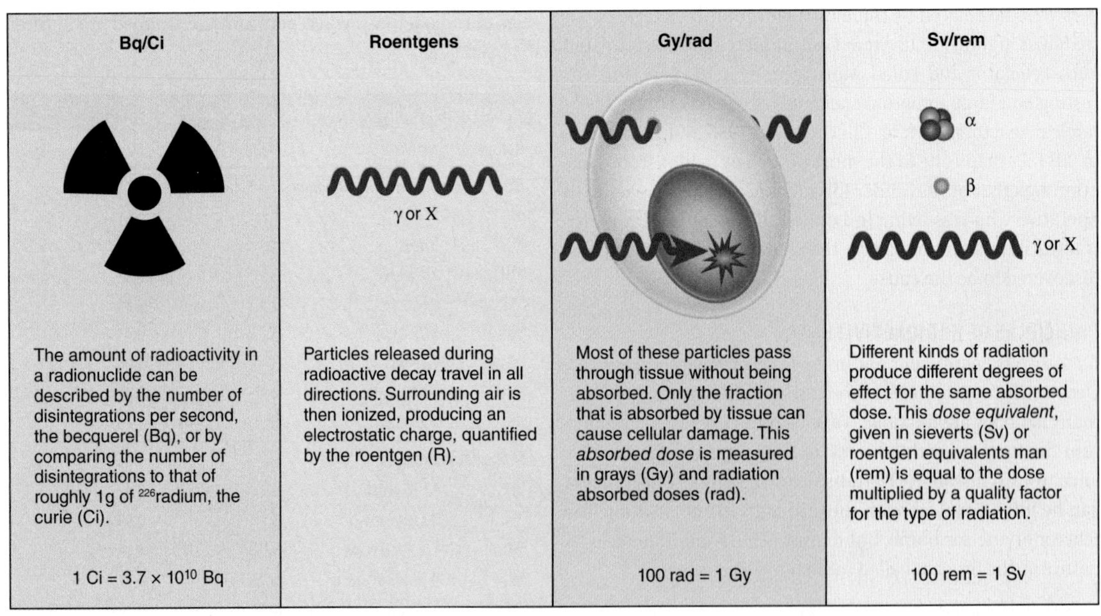


**FIGURE 100–1.** The definitions associated with radiation. Both curies and becquerels describe a quantity of radionuclide in terms of the number of disintegrations rather than mass. Roentgens describes the amount of charge per volume of air ionized by either γ- or x-rays, which indirectly quantifies the amount of radiation in the air around a source. Rads and grays (Gy) describe the fraction of radiation that actually interacts with cellular material and potentially causes injury. Roentgen equivalents man (rem) and sieverts (Sv) calculate the effective dose, taking into account the different particles. For example, a 100-keV alpha particle causes more damage to cellular material than a 100-keV beta particle.

kind of radiation is enough protection by distance. However, x-rays and gamma rays are uncharged and have no rest mass, greatly reducing their probability of interacting with matter, resulting in an unlimited range in space. Photon radiation that is emitted from a point source diverges from that source to cover an increasingly wider area. For example, if the intensity of radiation 1 m from a source is 1 Gy, its intensity would be 0.11 Gy at 3 m from the source. *Time of exposure* is another important safety factor in limiting radiation exposure. Obviously, the longer a person is exposed to radiation, the greater the exposure.

### Irradiation, Contamination, and Incorporation

An object is *irradiated* when it is exposed to ionizing radiation. The risk of tissue damage depends on the total amount of radiation and the tissue type because each tissue type has its own intrinsic resistance to radiation damage. An irradiated object does not become radioactive itself unless exposed to neutrons, and therefore, irradiated individuals pose no risk to others. *Contamination* occurs when a radioactive substance covers an object completely or in part. In these similar cases, the source of radiation is the nuclide undergoing its normal decay process, and the individual is exposed to particles such as those mentioned in Table 100–1. The risk of tissue damage from the radiation particles is usually quite low, assuming that the contamination is detected and appropriate measures for decontamination are instituted. *Incorporation* occurs when a radionuclide is taken up by tissue via some route that permits the radionuclide to enter the body. This principle is used in many diagnostic and therapeutic procedures such as a thallium stress test, gallium scan, or thyroid ablation therapy. Depending on the dose and type of radionuclide, incorporation may lead to tissue damage.

**TABLE 100–2 Annual Estimated Average Effective Dose Equivalent in the United States**

| Source | Dose[a] mSv/year | mrem/year | % of Total Dose |
|---|---|---|---|
| ***Natural*** | | | |
| Cosmic | 0.27 | 27 | 5 |
| Internal | 0.31 | 31 | 5 |
| Radon[b] | 2.29 | 233 | 37 |
| Terrestrial | 0.19 | 19 | 3 |
| ***Subtotal*** | 3.10 | 310 | 50 |
| ***Human-Made*** | | | |
| Consumer products | 0.12 | 12.4 | 2 |
| Nuclear medicine | 0.74 | 74.4 | 12 |
| Occupational | < 0.01 | 0.62 | 0.1 |
| Medical procedures | 2.23 | 223.2 | 36 |
| ***Subtotal*** | 3.10 | 310 | 50 |
| **Total** | 6.20 | 620 | 100 |

[a]All doses are averages and contain some variability within the measurement.

[b]Average effective dose to bronchial epithelium.

mSv = millisieverts; mrem = millirem.

Data from Mettler FA, Bhargavan M, Faulkner K, et al. Radiologic and nuclear medicine studies in the United States and worldwide: frequency, radiation dose, and comparison with other radiation sources—1950-2007. *Radiology.* 2009;253(2):520-531.

## EPIDEMIOLOGY

Everyone is exposed to radiation in one form or another each day (Table 100–2). In the US, the estimated annual dose equivalent of radiation is now considered to be 6.2 mSv, a number revised sharply upward by the National Council on Radiation Protection and Measurement (NCRP) in 2009.

### Natural Sources of Radiation

A wide variety of natural sources expose humans on a daily basis to ionizing radiation. Terrestrial sources of radiation originate from radionuclides in the Earth's crust that move into the air and water. Radon, a radioactive noble gas, accounts for most of the human exposure to radiation from natural sources. This gas, a natural decay product of uranium and thorium, enters homes and other buildings from the building materials themselves or through microscopic cracks in the building's structures. With a relatively short half-life of 3.82 days, $^{222}$Rn poses a health risk if decay occurs while in the respiratory space and one of its solid daughter isotopes deposits on respiratory tissue. These radon daughters emit alpha particles as they decay and are the principal causes in the associated increased incidence of lung cancer in those exposed to radon.

The second largest natural source of radiation originates from ingested radionuclides, of which $^{40}$K, a naturally occurring isotope, is the most abundant. The lifetime cancer mortality risk calculated for $^{40}$K is 4 in 100,000 from external exposure.

### Human-Made Sources

The estimated annual dose of radiation exposure from human-made sources of radiation is increasing, largely from the steeply rising use of computed tomography (CT) (Table 100–3). One retrospective study found an increased relative risk of these cancers resulting from accumulated doses of just a few CT scans. Perhaps influenced by data like these, accompanied by increased availability of other alternative imaging modalities, such as magnetic resonance imaging, several studies report trends of decreasing use of CT for children.

***Nuclear Occupational Exposure.*** Estimates of the annual number of workers occupationally exposed to radiation worldwide are several million. On average, the occupations with the highest exposures (about 4 mSv/year) are uranium miners and millers. Despite the many factors that play a role in occupational exposure at more than 1,200 nuclear reactors worldwide, the estimated effective dose to measurably exposed workers fell to 2.7 mSv/year. *Medical occupational exposure* principally includes physicians, nurses, radiology technologists, and laboratory workers who receive an additional effective dose of about 0.5 mSv/year. Fluoroscopy constitutes less than 10% of all examinations in the US but remains the largest source of occupational exposure in medicine. Worldwide, nearly 500,000 workers are monitored for exposures during dental radiography, but the annual effective dose averaged over 5 years has declined to 0.05 mSv.

*Depleted uranium* (DU) is used by the US military and by several other governments. Uranium ore mined from the earth is about 99% $^{238}$U and 1% $^{235}$U. Enrichment involves separating the isotopes so that $^{235}$U can be used as nuclear fuel

**TABLE 100–3 Diagnostic Imaging Procedures: Type and Amount of Radionuclide or Radiation**

| | | Amount | | Effective Dose | |
|---|---|---|---|---|---|
| *Test* | *Radionuclide* | *MBq* | *mCi* | *mSv* | *mrem* |
| Thyroid scan | $^{123}$I | 25 | 0.68 | 1.9 | 191 |
| Cardiac stress-rest test | $^{201}$Tl | 185 | 5 | 40.7 | 4,070 |
| Lung perfusion | $^{99m}$Tc | 185 | 5 | 2.0 | 200 |
| Lung ventilation | $^{133}$Xe | 740 | 20 | 0.5 | 50 |
| Bone scan | $^{99m}$Tc | 1,110 | 30 | 6.3 | 630 |
| Gallium scan | $^{67}$Ga | 150 | 4.05 | 15 | 1,500 |
| Tumor (PET) | $^{18}$F | 740 | 20 | 14.1 | 1,410 |
| ***Radiographs*** | | | | | |
| Posteroanterior and lateral study of the chest | | | | 0.1 | 10 |
| Abdomen | | | | 0.7 | 70 |
| Pelvis | | | | 0.6 | 60 |
| Lumbar spine | | | | 1.5 | 150 |
| ERCP | | | | 4.0 | 400 |
| ***Computed Tomography*** | | | | | |
| Head | | | | 2 | 200 |
| Cervical spine | | | | 3 | 300 |
| Chest | | | | 7 | 700 |
| Chest for pulmonary embolism | | | | 15 | 1,500 |
| Abdomen | | | | 8 | 800 |
| Pelvis | | | | 6 | 600 |
| Coronary angiography | | | | 16 | 1,600 |

ERCP = endoscopic retrograde cholangiopancreatography; MBq = megabequerel; mCi = millicuries; mSv = millisievert; mrem = millirem; PET = positron emission tomography.

and the leftover $^{238}$U can be used in munitions. Consequently, although DU is radioactive, it is 40% less so than naturally occurring uranium. The Depleted Uranium Follow-Up Program that has surveyed exposed veterans since 1994 has not discovered any consistent, clinically significant illness.

## EXPOSURE LIMITS

The Nuclear Regulatory Commission (NRC) established the "Standards for Protection against Radiation," which regulates radiation exposures using a twofold system of dose limitation: doses to individuals shall not exceed limits established by the NRC, and all exposures shall be kept *as low as reasonably achievable* (ALARA). The total effective dose equivalent may not exceed 50 mSv/year to reduce the risk of stochastic effects (see Stochastic Versus Deterministic Effects of Radiation). The dose to the fetus of a pregnant radiation worker may not exceed 5 mSv over 9 months and should not substantially exceed 0.5 mSv in any 1 month.

## REGULATION AND REPORTING

The use of ionizing radiation, radiation sources, and the by-products of nuclear energy are among the most heavily regulated processes worldwide. Among the international groups are the United Nations Scientific Committee on the Effects of Atomic Radiation (UNSCEAR), the International Commission on Radiological Protection (ICRP), the Biological Effects of Ionizing Radiation (BEIR) Committee, the International Commission on Radiological Units and Measurements (ICRU), the Radiation Effects Research Foundation (RERF), and the International Radiation Protection Association (IRPA). National regulatory agencies include the NRC, Environmental Protection Agency (EPA), Occupational Safety and Health Administration (OSHA), and Food and Drug Administration (FDA).

The Oak Ridge Institute for Science and Education (ORISE) supports the NRC by maintaining the NRC website for Radiation Exposure Information and Reporting System (REIRS) and the database of radiation exposure from NRC licensees (http://www.reirs.com). The Oak Ridge Institute for Science and Education's Radiation Emergency Assistance Center/Training Site (REAC/TS) and the International Atomic Energy Agency (IAEA) both maintain radiation incident registries that track US and foreign radiation incidents.

## PATHOPHYSIOLOGY

Ionizing radiation causes damage to tissue by several mechanisms called direct or indirect effects. *Direct effects* are when particles physically damage the DNA in a cell. When this kind of damage occurs, a mutation can arise, which may then result in alteration of a germline, development of a neoplasm, or cell death. The risk of these consequences overall, however, is low because of the relative paucity of DNA within a cell, the even smaller percentage of active DNA within a given cell, and the ability of DNA to repair itself.

Although DNA represents a low-probability target for radiation, the rest of the cell media represents a higher probability target. *Indirect effects* are when radiation impacts a molecule and creates a reactive species, which then chemically reacts with organic molecules in cells altering their structure or function. Water, which is in great abundance within cells, can transform into a hydroxyl radical (OH·) after interaction with incident radiation.

*The bystander effect* refers to cellular damage in unirradiated cells proximate to irradiated cells. Studies demonstrate the bystander effect for proton beams, x-rays, and low energy transfer radiation. *Genomic instability* is a single mutation followed by a cascade of further mutations altering the fidelity of genomic replication. Although any molecule can be damaged in a variety of ways that may lead to cell injury of varying severity, double-stranded breaks in DNA are the type of damage most likely to cause chromosomal aberrations or cell death.

Dose–response relationships for mutation are approximately linear down to about 25 mGy, the statistical limit of these studies. Although repair mechanisms reduce substantially the radiation risk of mutation, there is no evidence yet that these mechanisms eliminate those risks at low doses, although some question this conclusion.

## STOCHASTIC VERSUS DETERMINISTIC EFFECTS OF RADIATION

The radiation damage just described has two consequential results: it kills cells, or it alters cells and causes cancer. Injuries that do not require a threshold limit to be exceeded include mutagenic and carcinogenic changes to individual cells in which DNA is the critical and ultimate target. This is the *stochastic effect* of radiation. Theoretically, there is no dose of radiation too small to have the potential of causing cancer in an exposed individual. Whereas the stochastic effects of radiation can follow less severe exposures, the *deterministic effects* of radiation usually follow a large whole-body exposure. In terms of cell death, a relatively large number of cells of an organ system must be killed before an effect becomes clinically evident. This number of killed cells constitutes a threshold limit that must be exceeded, and this is what is known as the deterministic or nonstochastic effects of radiation.

## ACUTE RADIATION SYNDROME

Acute radiation syndrome (ARS) involves a sequence of events that varies with the severity of the exposure. Generally, more extensive exposures lead to more rapid onset of symptoms and more severe clinical features. Four classic clinical stages are described, which begin with the early prodromal stage of nausea and vomiting. Although the time to onset postexposure is inversely proportional to the dose received, the duration of the prodromal phase is directly proportional to the dose. That is, the greater the dose received, the more rapid the onset of symptoms, and the longer their duration, except in cases in which death follows rapidly. The latent period follows next as an apparent improvement of symptoms, during which time the patient appears to have recovered and has no clinically apparent difficulties. The duration of this stage is inversely related to dose and can last from several days to several weeks. The third stage usually begins in the third to fifth week after exposure and consists of manifest illness described in subsequent paragraphs. If the patient survives this stage, recovery, the fourth stage, is likely but can take weeks to months before it is completed. Those exposed to supralethal amounts of radiation can experience all the phases in a few hours before a rapid death.

The cerebrovascular syndrome describes the manifestations of injury to the central nervous system after massive irradiation. This syndrome, after exposure to doses of about 15 to 20 Gy or greater, is characterized by rapid or immediate onset of hyperthermia, ataxia, loss of motor control, apathy, lethargy, cardiovascular shock, and seizures. The mechanism of this injury may be a combination of radiation-induced vascular lesions and free radical–induced neuronal death and cerebral edema.

The pulmonary system is not spared injury from irradiation. Pneumonitis can occur within 1 to 3 months after a dose of 6 to 10 Gy. This can lead to respiratory failure, pulmonary fibrosis, or cor pulmonale months to years later.

The gastrointestinal (GI) syndrome begins after an exposure to about 6 Gy or more when GI mucosal cell injury and death occur. Findings and effects include anorexia, nausea, vomiting, and diarrhea. As the mucosal lining is sloughed, there is persistent bloody diarrhea, hypersecretion of cellular fluids into the lumen, and a loss of peristalsis, which can progress to abdominal distension and dehydration. Destruction of the mucosal lining allows for colonization by enteric organisms with ensuing sepsis.

The hematologic changes that occur after an exposure to about 1 Gy or greater are called the hematopoietic syndrome. Hematopoietic stem cells are highly radiosensitive, in contrast to the more mature erythrocytes and platelets. Lymphocytes are also radiosensitive and can die quickly from cell lysis after an exposure. The main effect of radiation-induced hematopoietic syndrome is pancytopenia, leading to death from sepsis complicated by hemorrhage. The lymphocyte nadir typically occurs 8 to 30 days postexposure, with higher doses achieving earlier nadir.

The cutaneous syndrome, a local radiation injury, can develop shortly after exposure or can take years to manifest fully. Target cells include all layers, including the epidermis, hair follicle canals, and subcutaneous tissue. Signs and symptoms include bullae, blisters, hair loss, pruritus, ulceration, and onycholysis. Skin injury ranges from epilation beginning at doses of 3 Gy to moist desquamation at about 15 Gy, to necrosis at greater than 50 Gy.

## DOSE ESTIMATION

Determining an accurate dose of radiation exposure is critical to providing the best care for the irradiated patient because increasing radiation exposure will affect different organ systems, call for different therapies, require different levels of monitoring, and assign different prognoses.

*Biodosimetry* is the use of physiological, chemical, or biological markers to reconstruct radiation doses to individuals or populations and assess the probability of developing ARS. Key elements of dose estimation include time to onset of vomiting, lymphocyte depletion kinetics, and chromosomal assays. Today, there are numerous tools available on the Internet to assist with dosimetry, including the Biological Assessment Tool available at the Armed Forces Radio-biology Research Institute's website (https://www.usuhs.edu/afrri/biodosimetrytools), guidelines from the International Atomic Energy Agency, the Radiation Emergency Medical Management website (https://www.remm.nlm.gov), and the CDC guidance (https://www.cdc.gov/nceh/radiation/emergencies/clinicians.htm).

## CARCINOGENESIS

Radiation was recognized as a carcinogen soon after it was initially discovered in 1895. After decades of research, including animal models, epidemiologic studies, and the lifespan studies of Japanese nuclear bomb survivors, radiation was shown to be a "universal carcinogen" able to induce tumors in nearly every tissue type in nearly every species at all ages.

## COMMONLY ENCOUNTERED RADIONUCLIDES

Americium (symbol Am, atomic number 95, and atomic weight 243) was discovered in 1944 in Chicago during the Manhattan Project. Its most stable nuclide, $^{243}$Am, has a half-life of more than 7,500 years, although $^{241}$Am, with a half-life of 470 years, decays by alpha and gamma emission and will accumulate in bone if incorporated. It is used to test machinery integrity, glass thickness, and in smoke detectors (about 0.26 μg per detector).

Cesium (symbol Cs, atomic number 55, and atomic weight 132) was discovered by Bunsen in 1860. It decays by beta and gamma emissions and is used as a radiation source in radiation therapy and as a radionuclide source for atomic clocks.

Iodine (symbol I, atomic number 53, and atomic weight 126.9) was discovered by Courtois in 1811. Of the 23 isotopes of iodine, $^{127}$I is the only one that is stable. $^{129}$I and $^{131}$I are fission products that are released into the environment during an event. These isotopes will accumulate in thyroid tissue if incorporated and can cause local damage to thyroid tissue.

Polonium (symbol Po, atomic number 84, and atomic weights range from 192 to 218) was discovered by Marie Curie. Polonium has 27 isotopes, the most isotopes of all the elements, and all are radioactive. The short half-life of $^{210}$Po, 138 days, and high specific activity of 4,490 Ci/g means it emits a great deal of high-energy alpha particles (5.3 MeV) that produce 140 W/g. For example, a capsule containing 500 mg of $^{210}$Po reaches a temperature of 932°F (500°C).

Radon (symbol Rn, atomic number 86, and atomic weights range from 204 to 224) was discovered in 1900 by Dorn and is the heaviest noble gas. $^{222}$Radon decays by alpha and gamma emissions. Exposure of radon gas to the pulmonary epithelium is associated with an increased incidence of lung cancer in both uranium miners and in those who dwell in residences with increased concentrations of radon. Damage to bronchial epithelium results from the alpha emissions of radon and radiation from radon daughters that precipitate as solids and remain in the lungs.

Technetium (symbol Tc, atomic number 43, and atomic weight 98.9) was discovered in 1937 and was the first element to be produced artificially. Unusual among the lighter elements, Tc has no stable isotopes and is therefore found on earth as a product of spontaneous uranium fission. Most human contact with Tc is in medical scans in which Tc has a biological half-life of about 1 day.

Thallium (symbol Tl, atomic number 81, and atomic weight 204) was discovered by Crookes in 1861. $^{201}$Tl is used for cardiac imaging, has a half-life of 73 hours, and decays by electron capture and gamma emission.

Tritium is an isotope of hydrogen whose nucleus contains one proton and two neutrons, and its symbol is $^{3}$H. Tritium decays by beta activity and is used in basic science research as a radioactive label, for luminous dials, and for self-powered exit signs, which can contain as much as $9.3 \times 10^{11}$ Bq (25 Ci). Tritium has a half-life of 12.3 years. Tritium emits very weak radiation in the form of 18.6 KeV beta particles, which are easily stopped by thin layers of material, and is safe for glow-in-the-dark watches. When absorbed as tritiated water, tritium tends to follow the water cycle in humans, providing a whole-body dose if incorporated.

## MANAGEMENT

### Initial Assessment and Early Triage

The initial management of patients exposed to radiation will depend on a number of factors, including the amount of radiation in the exposure and the number of casualties in the event. Small-scale exposures to radiation still require at least a brief evaluation for burns and trauma, depending on the circumstances surrounding the nature of the exposure. Calls to the poison center from a residence require referral to emergency services for an expert evaluation of the extent of the contamination of the site and appropriate decontamination measures. Exposures in the laboratory or nuclear medicine suites require referral to the radiation safety officer (RSO) in the building for a similar evaluation.

When considering a local incident involving nuclear material, first responders will likely include a hazardous materials team (HAZMAT) and local police and fire departments. Hospitals should involve their RSO, and public officials will involve a state agency such as the State Department of Environmental Protection. As part of its primary mission for the US Department of Energy, REAC/TS offers consultation with anyone on a 24/7 basis on questions regarding radiation exposure. Its emergency phone number is 865-576-1005 (ask for REAC/TS). For large incidents, other federal agencies will be involved led by the Federal Emergency Management Agency. Additional radiation expertise can be provided via the Department of Energy, and if applicable, the Federal Bureau of Investigation will be called to protect against further threats.

In a mass casualty event, established prehospital plans should be followed to provide the best management for the large numbers of variably injured given that an explosion of potentially catastrophic size also accompanies the radiation exposure. First responders must use universal precautions and should assume that all victims are contaminated; most events will only require C- or D-level protection (Chap. 101). Field triage protocols tailored to the kind of event in question will designate patients as minor, delayed, immediate, or deceased and should not be altered because of radiation exposure.

Preliminary decontamination, including removal of clothing and washing the victim, should be performed before transportation to a medical facility, taking care not to contaminate prehospital providers or equipment. Uninjured patients who are contaminated should be relocated upwind of the incident site for further care.

### Initial Emergency Department Management

It is not considered a medical emergency to have been irradiated or contaminated; even highly irradiated patients take days to die, which is why standard protocols regarding trauma and other medical complaints continue to be followed even in mass casualty events. In the event of a radiation incident, there will likely be little warning of these patients arriving, and information will be incomplete. Ideally, the emergency department (ED) is divided into clean and dirty areas where the floor of the dirty area is covered by plastic or butcher's paper. Staff should don surgical scrubs, gowns, surgical caps, masks, booties, and face shields. Two sets of gloves should be worn, with the inner set taped to the gown. Dosimeters should be worn at the neck for easy access by the RSO, and staff should be reminded that medical personnel have never received a medically significant acute radiation dose when caring for an exposed patient.

When patients arrive to the ED, it is essential to follow an algorithm that takes into account issues of irradiation or contamination and includes data collection specific to biodosimetry. One such algorithm is the REAC/TS patient treatment algorithm at https://orise.orau.gov/reacts/infographics/radiation-patient-treatment-algorithm.pdf. Physical examination, in addition to airway, breathing, and circulation, should focus on vital signs, skin (erythema, blisters, desquamation), GI symptoms (abdominal pain and cramping), neurologic findings (ataxia, headache, motor or sensory deficits), and hematologic signs (ecchymoses or petechiae). Vomiting very early after exposure is considered a sign of the central nervous system subsyndrome and is a poor prognostic indicator.

Recommended initial laboratory testing includes baseline complete blood count (CBC) with differential (including an extra sample in a heparinized tube for cytogenetics), serum amylase (increased from specific salivary gland inflammation and degeneration), urinalysis, baseline radiologic assessment of urine, and starting a 24-hour urine collection. Nasal swabs, emesis, and stool should be collected for radiologic monitoring. For patients with persistent vomiting, erythema, or fever, a repeat CBC with differential is recommended every 4 to 6 hours. If a patient requires surgery, we recommendation that surgery proceed immediately because of the delayed and impaired wound healing expected as a result of decreases in leukocytes and platelets.

## Decontamination

When a patient is medically stable, decontamination should proceed. Patients who were not decontaminated in the prehospital setting but who are grossly contaminated should be fairly easily detected as such by a quick evaluation with an appropriate instrument. As a first step, all clothing should be removed gently by cutting and not tearing as is typically done for trauma patients. Rolling supine patients allows contaminated clothes to be carefully gathered and bagged and marked. Bagged clothes and other contaminated articles should be removed from the ED to a site designated by the RSO so as not to present another source of radiation. A portable dosimeter should assist in external decontamination. After clothing removal, remonitor the patient for contamination, paying attention to exposed areas such as hair. Contaminated hair should be washed with soap and water before washing the body to avoid trickle-down contamination. For patients with contaminated wounds, decontamination should prioritize the wound first, then body orifices around the face, and then intact skin. Always wipe gently away from the wound. Irrigate gently to reduce splashing. Care must be taken not to abrade skin by excessively vigorous scrubbing or shaving of hair.

For patients with smaller exposures to radionuclides, such as laboratory workers, decontamination is often the only management technique required to limit injury. Portable dosimeters will identify contaminated areas, which should be sealed off to limit spread of exposure, especially if the radionuclide is in gaseous form. As with larger exposures, contaminated clothing must be removed and collected. Contaminated skin must be washed with lukewarm soap and water, repeatedly if needed.

## Medical Decision Making

Exposure to radiation can lead to a complex spectrum of organ damage that can be difficult and confusing for physicians when creating a treatment plan. Establishment of guidance in the form of a *response category* (RC) helps clarify a medical plan and disposition (Table 100–4). (For specific suggestions, refer to the interactive version of this assessment tool at the REMM's website at http://www.remm.nlm.gov.)

## Medical Management

*Supportive care* quality will determine the extent of the morbidity and mortality. The majority of patients with ARS who succumb usually do so from fluid loss, infection, or bleeding. Irradiated patients require treatment for nausea and vomiting, diarrhea, pain, and fluid and electrolyte losses. Vomiting is thought to occur as a result of serotonin release from damaged gut tissue. The 5-$HT_3$ antagonists are the most effective medications to control vomiting. Loperamide, anticholinergics, and aluminum hydroxide are reasonable to treat diarrhea. Mild pain should be managed with acetaminophen, but we recommend against the use of aspirin and nonsteroidal drugs because they exacerbate gastric bleeding. An opioid is recommended for the management of more severe pain.

*Probiotic* use introduces selective nonpathogenic strains of *Lactobacillus* and *Bifidobacteria* into the GI tract to suppress the number of pathogens. Based on the existing data, it would be reasonable to treat patients who develop diarrhea with probiotics. Intravenous access should be established and maintained with care because these patients are prone to infection. Fluid replacement begins with crystalloid solution with the goal of replacing GI losses. Cutaneous injuries are cared for depending on the nature, location, and extent of the wounds. Surgical consultation or referral to a burn center should be offered early in the clinical course.

Prevention of infection includes attention to several aspects of care. Maintain the patient in a clean environment and institute reverse isolation for patients with at least moderate exposure or when neutrophil counts decline below 1,000/μL. Prophylactic antibiotics and antifungals are recommended for neutropenic patients, as well as acyclovir or a similar antiviral for herpes simplex virus–positive patients. If neutropenic patients become febrile, we recommend following the Infectious Diseases Society of America guidelines for antibiotic choices. It is reasonable to administer broad-spectrum prophylactic antibiotic coverage, including anaerobic coverage, for patients with burns.

*Cytokine therapy* (colony-stimulating factor {CSF}) use in radiation-exposed patients is based on demonstrated enhancement of neutrophil recovery in patients with cancer, a perceived benefit in a small number of radiation-incident victims, and several prospective trials using different animal models involving radiation exposure. Colon stimulating factors such as filgrastim should be started as soon as possible for patients exposed to a survivable dose of radiation who are at risk for hematopoietic syndrome, that is, more than 3 Gy.

*Use of blood products* is required for patients with significant blood loss or for those experiencing radiation-induced aplasia. Use of leukoreduced and (ironically) irradiated blood products should be the rule to prevent transfusion-associated graft-versus-host disease. *Stem cell transplantation* (SCT) can be used to treat patients with severe bone marrow injury, but the decision to use this therapy is very complicated. If conditions are favorable and resources are available, it would be reasonable to attempt SCT in patients with a severe radiation exposure who have an otherwise grave prognosis.

**TABLE 100–4 Grading System for Organ System Dysfunction and Response Category for Disposition**

| *Symptom* | *Degree 1* | *Degree 2* | *Degree 3* | *Degree 4* |
|---|---|---|---|---|
| ***Neurovascular System*** | | | | |
| Anorexia | Able to eat | Decreased | Minimal | Parenteral |
| Nausea | Mild | Moderate | Severe | Excruciating |
| Vomiting | 1/day | 2–5/day | 6–10/day | > 10/day |
| Fatigue | Able to work | Impaired | Assisted ADLs | No ADL |
| Fever | (< 38°C) | (38°–40°C) | (> 40°C) < 24 hours | (> 40°C) > 24 hours |
| Headache | Minimal | Moderate | Severe | Excruciating |
| Hypotension (BP, mm Hg) (Adult) | > 100/70 | < 100/70 | < 90/60 | < 80 systolic |
| Cognitive deficits | Minor | Moderate | Major | Complete |
| Neurological deficits | Barely detectable | Easily detectable | Prominent | Life threatening |
| ***Hematopoietic System (all counts × $10^9$/L)*** | | | | |
| Lymphocytes | 1.5–3.5 | 0.5–1.5 | 0.25–1 | 0.1–0.25 |
| Granulocytes | 4–9 | < 1[a] | < 0.5[a] | 0–0.5 |
| Platelets | 150–350 | 50–100 | 0–50 | Very low[b] |
| ***Gastrointestinal System*** | | | | |
| Diarrhea | | | | |
| Frequency (/day) | 2–3 | 4–6 | 7–9 | ≥ 10 |
| Consistency | Bulky | Loose | Loose | Watery |
| Bleeding | Occult | Intermittent | Persistent | Large, persistent |
| Abdominal cramps/pain | Minimal | Moderate | Severe | Excruciating |
| ***Cutaneous System*** | | | | |
| Erythema | Minimal | < 10% BSA | 10%–40% BSA | > 40% BSA |
| Edema | Asymptomatic | Symptomatic | Secondary dysfunction | Total dysfunction |
| Blistering | Rare, sterile | Rare, bloody | Bullae, sterile | Bullae, bloody |
| Desquamation | Absent | Patchy, dry | Patchy, moist | Confluent, moist |
| Ulceration or necrosis | Epidermal | Dermal | Subcutaneous | Muscle or bone |
| Hair loss | Absent | Partial | Partial | Complete |
| ***Response Category*** | 1 | 2 | 3 | 4 |
| ***Triage and Monitoring*** | Ambulatory | Ambulatory vs. hospitalized | Hospitalized<br>ICU | Hospitalized<br>Specialized hospitals[c] |
| | | Supportive care<br>Blood products | Blood products<br>CSFs | Blood products<br>CSFs or SCT |

[a]An abortive rise in cell counts begins between days 5 and 10, which lasts about 8 to 12 days. Afterward, cell counts decline slowly, reaching a nadir around day 20. [b]Cell counts decline faster, reaching lower nadir for more severe exposures at about days 22, 16, and 10 for grades 2 to 4. [c]"Specialized hospitals" refers to those with experience in all areas of intensive care medicine, particularly allogenic stem cell transplantation (SCT).

ADL = activity of daily living; BP = blood pressure; BSA = body surface area; CSF = colony-stimulating factor; ICU = intensive care unit.

### Management of Internal Contamination

Internal contamination cases are assessed differently from external doses in that they are not measured but rather are calculated. These calculations are performed by a health physicist on samples such as nasal swabs, urine, or stool to estimate how much activity entered the body. Doses are termed *committed doses*, defined as the doses received that last more than 50 years because of the internal deposit of the radionuclide. That is, the radionuclide dose is protracted and remains until it decays or is eliminated via normal kinetic processes. These doses are compared with the annual limits on intake (ALIs) provided by the EPA as a benchmark for medical decision making. Interpretation of committed doses from contaminated wounds requires special conversion factors provided by the NCRP. Management of internal contamination is isotope dependent (Antidotes in Brief: A44 and A45).

## PROGNOSIS

Survival is inversely proportional to the radiation dose absorbed. Historically, the mean lethal dose required to kill 50% of humans at 60 days was about 3.5 Gy without supportive care. The addition of antibiotics and blood products increases that mean to 6 to 7 Gy. This dose is likely to be even higher for those treated early with CSFs in a specialized hospital. An acute dose of 20 Gy or more is considered supralethal.

During a catastrophic radiation incident, resources will likely become depleted to the extent that not all patients who require certain medical treatments to survive will be able to receive them. The REMM Scarce Resources Triage Tool is available online for assistance in evaluating a patient's prognosis, in which a patient's injury extent may indicate an expectant prognosis, assisting clinicians to help those who may survive instead.

## CONSIDERATION OF THE DECEASED

Contaminated bodies should be placed in a temporary morgue that is refrigerated. Use of the hospital morgue will lead to contamination there. These bodies *should not* be cremated because this will only redistribute the nuclear material, which is not destroyed by fire.

## PREGNANCY AND RADIATION

In general, radiation effects to an embryo or fetus are dependent on its stage of development and the dose received. The medical decision to perform imaging or a diagnostic procedure that exposes any patient to radiation is always based on a risk-to-benefit analysis with a given patient's situation. Very early in a pregnancy before implantation, the embryo is in an "all-or-none" period of development in which the greatest risk from radiation is miscarriage but not greater than baseline risk. Older than this, the fetus is next at greatest risk between 8 and 15 weeks of gestation, during which major neuronal migration takes place.

The NCRP considers risk to fetuses to be negligible compared with other risks of pregnancy when the dose to a fetus is less than 50 mGy (5 rad), which corresponds to 50 mSv from x-ray examination, compared with about 6 mSv effective dose from a CT examination of the pelvis. The risk of malformation is increased only at doses above 150 mSv. The vast majority of routine diagnostic imaging procedures impart less than 5 mSv to a fetus, increasing baseline risk by about 0.17%. Shared decision making should always balance the potential maternal benefit of the radiologic procedure and the potential risk to the fetus.

## PEDIATRICS AND RADIATION

The use of CT scanning in children has markedly increased over the past 30 years. Estimates calculate an increased risk of lifetime mortality rate in the range of 0.04% for a head CT for a young female patient (1 in 2,500) compared with a normal lifetime cancer mortality risk of 20% (1 in 5). This excess relative risk was supported by a large retrospective study of a pediatric population that found increased incidence of certain leukemias and certain brain tumors attributed to CT scans over a 23-year period. Radiographic studies should continue to be ordered in the best interest of the patient, although it is likely that the number of scans performed could safely be diminished without compromising care. Reports on this topic commonly include problems with ordering unnecessary multiple CTs, follow-up CT scans, and CT scans that occur simply because of a lack of communication among the patient, healthcare professional, and technician. These problems, compounded by inappropriate CT protocol for pediatric patients, suggest that the medical community must be more proactive in reducing the health risk of those in our charge.

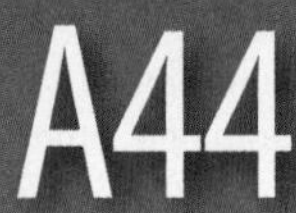

Antidotes in Brief

# POTASSIUM IODIDE

## INTRODUCTION

Potassium iodide (KI) is the antidote to radioactive iodine that is released into the atmosphere after a nuclear incident. It functions as a competitive inhibitor of thyroid uptake of radioiodine to reduce the risk of thyroid cancer.

## HISTORY

Following the study of thyroid cancers in Pacific Islanders who were subjected to fallout from nuclear testing, scientists concluded in 1957 that KI could effectively protect the thyroid from radioactive iodine. The National Council on Radiation Protection and Measurements reported in 1977 that the sudden release of radionuclides, including radioiodine, could affect large numbers of people after a nuclear incident (Fig. A44–1). The following year, the United States (US) Food and Drug Administration (FDA) requested the production and storage of KI for the purpose of blocking the effects of radioiodine on the thyroid gland when needed.

## PHARMACOLOGY

### Chemistry

Iodine (I), atomic number 53, derives from the Greek *iodes* meaning violet, owing to the violet color of elemental iodine vapor. Similar to other halogens, iodine occurs mainly as a diatomic molecule $I_2$. The term *iodide* refers to the ion $I^-$, which forms inorganic compounds with iodine that is in the oxidation state −1, such as KI. Only $^{127}I$ is stable.

### Mechanism of Action

Neonates, children, and adolescents are particularly susceptible to developing thyroid cancer following radioactive iodine exposure because during rapid developmental periods, the thyroid gland grows and accumulates a larger percentage of exogenously ingested iodide as it increases thyroglobulin and iodothyronine stores. Similarly, during pregnancy, the maternal thyroid gland is stimulated and takes up more iodide compared with other adults.

Exposure to radioactive iodine occurs via inhalation or via ingestion of contaminated food. After being incorporated into the thyroid gland, radioiodine exposes thyroid tissue to β and γ emissions, potentially leading to cancer. Because the chemical properties of radioactive iodine are unchanged from stable iodine, prophylaxis with KI is effective through isotopic dilution. That is, KI competes with radioactive iodine for the active iodide transport system to reduce the concentration of radioiodine in the serum, making the uptake of radioiodine much less likely.

### Pharmacokinetics

Dietary iodide distributes selectively into the thyroid gland but also to a lesser extent into salivary glands, choroid plexus, and gastric mucosa with a volume of distribution of 0.3 L/kg. During pregnancy and lactation, iodide distribution to the mammary glands and ovaries increases. Iodide that is not concentrated in the thyroid is excreted 80% in urine and 20% in feces.

### Pharmacodynamics

Iodide ($I^-$), an essential nutrient present in minute total-body amounts of 15 to 25 mg, is required for the synthesis of the thyroid hormones L-thyroxine ($T_4$) and L-triiodothyronine ($T_3$). Iodide is actively transported into thyroid follicular cells and concentrated 20- to 40-fold compared with the serum. It is then transported into the follicular lumen, where it iodinates thyroglobulin to form $T_4$ and $T_3$ (Chap. 26).

## ROLE IN RADIOACTIVE IODINE EXPOSURE

Radioactive iodine uptake is effectively blocked by KI supplementation. The 1986 Chernobyl incident remains the largest experience of KI distribution following a nuclear incident from which data and recommendations are derived. After Chernobyl, the Polish government distributed nearly 18 million doses of KI in its most affected provinces, but none was distributed in Ukraine and Belarus. Studies demonstrated not only a dose–response relationship between radiation dose and the relative risk of thyroid cancer, but also a threefold reduction of this risk through use of KI supplementation.

## ADVERSE EFFECTS AND SAFETY ISSUES

### Thyroidal Effects

Extensive experience with treating goiter and the use of iodized salt demonstrates that both hyper- and hypothyroidism result from supplementation with KI. Both the prevalence of goiter and subclinical hypothyroidism increase when iodine intake is chronically high. A large study in Poland after the Chernobyl incident investigated the risks and benefits of KI prophylaxis. Of the thousands of men, women, and children who were studied, the vast majority of whom received a single dose of KI, no statistical differences were found between treated and untreated groups when thyroid-stimulating hormone (TSH) concentrations were measured among all populations.

### Extrathyroidal Effects

"Iodide mumps," is an inflammation of the salivary glands and appears to be unpredictable. Iododerma is a rare and

$$^{235}U + {}^{1}n \longrightarrow {}^{131}In \xrightarrow{0.28\ s} {}^{131}Sn \xrightarrow{56\ s} {}^{131}Sb \xrightarrow{23\ m} {}^{131}Te \xrightarrow{25\ m} \boxed{^{131}I} \xrightarrow{8.02\ d} {}^{131}Xe$$

**FIGURE A44–1.** The decay pathway that describes how $^{131}I$ is derived from nuclear fuel (whether in a bomb or a reactor) and ultimately decays to stable xenon. s = seconds; m = months; d = days. U = uranium; In = indium; Sn = tin; Sb = antimony; Te = tellurium; Xe = xenon; N = neutron.

**TABLE A44–1 Threshold Radiation Exposure Doses and Recommended KI Doses for Different Risk Groups**

| | *Predicted Thyroid Exposure (Gy, rad)* | | | | |
|---|---|---|---|---|---|
| | *Gy* | *rad* | *KI Dose (mg)* | *No. of 130-mg Tablets* | *Milliliters of Oral Solution, 65 mg/mL* |
| Adults > 40 yr | ≥ 5 | ≥ 500 | 130 | 1 | 2 |
| Adults 18–40 yr | ≥ 0.1 | ≥ 10 | 130 | 1 | 2 |
| Pregnant or lactating women | ≥ 0.05 | ≥ 5 | 130 | 1 | 2 |
| Children and adolescents 3–18 yr | ≥ 0.05 | ≥ 5 | 65 | 1/2[a] | 1 |
| Children 1 mo to 3 yr | ≥ 0.05 | ≥ 5 | 32 | Use KI oral solution[b] | 0.5 |
| Birth to 1 mo | ≥ 0.05 | ≥ 5 | 16 | Use KI oral solution[b] | 0.25 |

[a]Adolescents approaching adult size (70 kg) should receive a full dose of 130 mg. [b]For smaller, more precise dosing, a potassium iodide (KI) oral solution is available with a dropper marked for 1-mL, 0.5-mL, and 0.25-mL dosing. Gy = Gray = 100 rads.

Modified from Food and Drug Administration. Guidance. Potassium Iodide as a Thyroid Blocking Agent in Radiation Emergencies. http://www.fda.gov/downloads/Drugs/GuidanceComplianceRegulatoryInformation/Guidances/ucm080542.pdf.

reversible acneiform eruption related to iodine ingestion that may result from nonspecific immune stimulation, which is similar to bromoderma. Other reactions reported in association with KI use include gastrointestinal disturbances, fever, and shortness of breath.

"Allergy" to radiocontrast media is actually an anaphylactoid (nonimmune hypersensitivity) response to the high osmolarity of these xenobiotics. Although seafood contains iodide, allergy to fish or shellfish is caused by specific marine proteins and not sensitivity to iodide. Patients manifesting allergic contact dermatitis resulting from iodine-containing cleaning preparations such as povidone–iodine do not react to patch testing with KI. Therefore, the decision to administer KI dosing in the event of radioactive iodine exposure should not be based on a history of reactions to radiocontrast media, seafood, and povidone–iodine.

## PREGNANCY AND LACTATION

Potassium iodide is listed as Pregnancy Category D and readily crosses the placenta and distributes into milk. Both the US FDA and World Health Organization (WHO) support the use of KI for pregnant women when the risk is declared substantial by public health authorities.

## DOSING AND ADMINISTRATION

Based on data from Chernobyl regarding estimated doses and cancer risks in exposed children, the WHO in 1999 and the US FDA in 2001 provided recommendations for KI supplementation for various populations, depending on their relative risks (Table A44–1).

### Timing of Administration

For full blocking effect, KI should be administered shortly before exposure or immediatly afterward. Some models describe the blockade of only 50% of iodide uptake when there is a delay of several hours after an exposure. Depending on the duration and type of risk, administration of KI months after an exposure may also partially reduce thyroid cancer risk.

### Daily Versus Single Dosing

The protective effect of KI lasts for about 24 hours, so it should be dosed daily depending on the dosing estimates for exposure in children aged 1 month to 18 years in whom an ongoing risk is perceived. Groups in whom only a single dose is recommended include pregnant women and neonates, in whom there is a significant risk of iodine causing harm to the fetus related to impaired cognitive development. For lactating women, stable iodide will be delivered to the nursing newborn and may cause functional blocking of iodide uptake by an overload of iodine. Therefore, the US FDA recommends that lactating mothers not receive repeated doses except during continuing, severe contamination, which would generally be defined by health officials.

### Monitoring

All neonates who are treated with KI should be monitored for changes in TSH and total $T_3$ and free $T_4$. Likewise, when a lactating mother requires repeat doses of KI, the nursing infant should be monitored for the development of hypothyroidism.

## FORMULATION AND ACQUISITION

Several manufacturers formulate KI and market them as nonprescription, US FDA-approved products with a shelf life of 7 years. Tablets are available in both 130-mg and 65-mg doses, as well as an oral solution in a concentration of 65 mg/mL. Iodide-containing products ***not*** considered useful as radioiodine protective treatments include iodized salt, seaweed, and tincture of iodine.

# A45 PENTETIC ACID OR PENTETATE (ZINC OR CALCIUM) TRISODIUM (DTPA)

## INTRODUCTION

Pentetate zinc trisodium and pentetate calcium trisodium (zinc or calcium diethylenetriaminepentaacetate; Zn-DTPA and Ca-DTPA, respectively) are chelators recommended for the treatment of internal contamination with plutonium (Pu), americium (Am), and curium (Cm).

## HISTORY

First synthesized in 1954, these chelators were used as investigational therapies to enhance elimination of transuranic elements. Over the past decades, hundreds of human exposures to radionuclides as well as numerous animal studies helped to define the best practices for the use of these chelators, culminating in their approval by the United States (US) Food and Drug Administration (FDA) in 2004.

## PHARMACOLOGY

### Chemistry

Pentetic acid is a synthetic polyaminopolycarboxylic acid that bonds stoichiometrically with a central metal ion through the formal donation of one or more of its electrons. The calcium trisodium salt and the zinc trisodium pentetic acid are used therapeutically.

### Related Xenobiotics

Several metal chelators in clinical practice include deferoxamine, dimercaprol, dimercaptopropane sulfonate, edetate calcium disodium, penicillamine, Prussian blue, succimer, and trientine hydrochloride. However, none of these are effective for transuranic metals (elements with atomic numbers greater than 92).

### Mechanism of Action

Pentetic acid wraps itself around the metal, forming up to eight bonds, exchanging its calcium or zinc ions for a metal with greater binding capacity (Fig. A45–1). The chelated complex is then excreted by glomerular filtration into the urine.

### Pharmacokinetics

DTPA is rapidly absorbed via intramuscular, intraperitoneal, and intravenous (IV) routes, but animal studies indicate that DTPA is poorly (< 5%) absorbed by the gastrointestinal (GI) tract. Absorption via the lungs approximates 20% to 30%. Its volume of distribution is small (0.14 L/kg in humans), and it is distributed mainly throughout the extracellular space. The plasma half-life is 20 to 60 minutes, although a small fraction is bound to plasma proteins with a half-life of more than 20 hours. DTPA undergoes minimal, if any, metabolism. Elimination is via glomerular filtration, with more than 95% excreted within 12 hours and 99% by 24 hours. There are no specific data regarding dosing or clearance changes when chelating patients with kidney disease. However, hemodialysis increases elimination. Fecal excretion is less than 3%.

### Pharmacodynamics

DTPA increases the urinary elimination rate of chelated metals. In animals, treatment with Ca-DTPA within 1 hour of internal contamination resulted in 10-fold greater rate of urinary elimination of plutonium compared with Zn-DTPA. The greatest chelating capacity occurred immediately and for the first 24 hours after contamination while the metal was still circulating and available for chelation. Similarly, inhalation of Ca-DTPA followed by a month-long regimen of Zn-DTPA reduced lung deposits of aerosolized plutonium to 2% of control animals.

## ROLE IN RADIONUCLIDE CONTAMINATION

DTPA is recommended and US FDA approved for contamination from plutonium, americium, and curium. For inhaled metals, such as might be experienced after an explosion, treatment with nebulized DTPA is recommended. While chelation is reasonable to increase elimination of the radionuclide and decrease cancer risk, this risk reduction has only been demonstrated in animals. Increased urinary excretion of transuranic elements is a clinically meaningful endpoint for efficacy of DTPA. We recommend against chelation after ingestion of americium, curium, or plutonium, because increased GI absorption will result.

Although data are limited, we agree with the Radiation Emergency Assistance Center/Training Site (REAC/TS) recommendation of DTPA for chelating berkelium, californium, cobalt, einsteinium, europium, indium, iridium, manganese, niobium, promethium, ruthenium, scandium, thorium, and yttrium. Pentetic acid salts are not effective in removing antimony, beryllium, bismuth, gallium, lead, mercury, neptunium, platinum, or uranium.

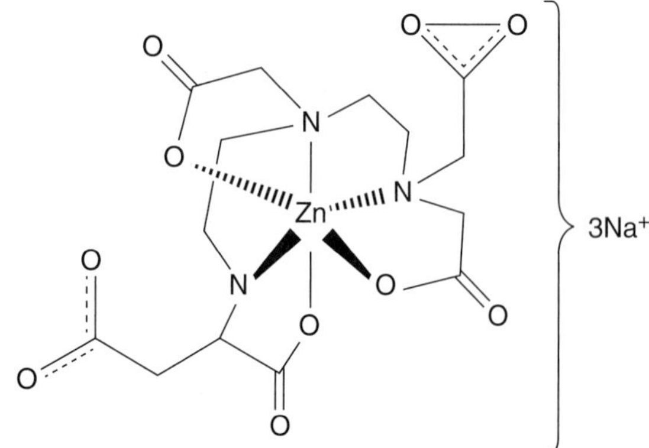


**FIGURE A45–1.** Trisodium zinc diethylenetriaminepentaacetate, in which a transuranic element (Am, Pu, Cm) is substituted for Zn, forming a stable chelate.

DTPA is neither recommended nor approved for treating patients contaminated with uranium or neptunium for several reasons. DTPA mobilizes uranium from tissue stores but does not increase urinary elimination. Chelating incorporated neptunium is problematic because it forms extremely stable complexes with transferrin, making it very difficult to decorporate.

## ADVERSE EFFECTS AND SAFETY ISSUES

No serious toxicity is reported among humans after more than 4,500 Ca-DTPA administrations at recommended doses. Common adverse reactions include nausea, vomiting, diarrhea, chills, cramps, fever, pruritus, and muscle. Doses of 4 g of Ca-DTPA per day in hemochromatosis patients are associated with lethargy, obtundation, oral mucosal ulceration, stomatitis, dermatitis, loss of lower extremity sensation, and three deaths. The nonfatal reactions resolved upon cessation of Ca-DTPA. Injury was attributed to zinc depletion. In animals, Zn-DTPA is approximately 30-fold less toxic than Ca-DTPA.

### Safety

Because of the renal excretion of the radioactive chelate, the kidneys are exposed to potentially higher doses of radiation than other organs, which theoretically increases the risk of malignancy. Additionally, because urine is radioactive during chelation, there are recommendations to use toilets instead of urinals and to flush several times. Any spilled urine or feces should be cleaned promptly and completely, accompanied by thorough hand washing. Patients being chelated should take special care to dispose of any expectorant or breast milk carefully. After nebulization treatments, patients should be cautioned not to swallow any expectorant.

Radiologically contaminated patients do not generally pose a danger to healthcare personnel. Universal precautions, including a gown, a mask, gloves, a head cover, and booties, effectively protect workers from contaminated material. Ambulances, operating rooms, and dialysis machines may become contaminated after providing care to contaminated patients and should be evaluated for decontamination before providing care for the next patient.

## DOSING AND ADMINISTRATION

If the contamination route is mixed (defined as anything in addition to inhalation) or unknown, then intravenous Ca-DTPA is recommended at a dose of 1 g in adults and 14 mg/kg up to the adult dose as a maximum in children younger than 12 years. This dose is administered either undiluted over 3 to 4 minutes or diluted in 100 to 250 mL D5W, lactated Ringer, or 0.9% sodium chloride administered over 30 minutes daily up to 5 days per week for the first week. If subsequent chelation is indicated, a twice-a-week regimen is recommended until the excretion rate of the contaminant does not increase with Zn-DTPA administration. If contamination was solely by inhalation, then we recommend diluting Zn-DTPA 1:1 with sterile water or 0.9% sodium chloride and administering via nebulization. Although Ca-DTPA is recommended as the initial chelator, Zn-DTPA should be used after the first 24 hours, given daily at the same dose because it has less adverse effects on essential metals.

### Timing of Administration and Duration of Therapy

Administration of DTPA should be initiated as soon as possible but remains effective as long as radiocontaminants persist prior to their sequestration in bone and liver. Historically, about 55% of all patients treated with DTPA received only one dose. The decision to continue therapy should be based on radioassay data. This assessment should include collection of 24-hour urine samples, whole-body or chest counting, and close consultation with the hospital radiation safety officer or REAC/TS (865-576–1005). Current recommendations are to continue chelation until the deposition of contaminant is less than 5% of the maximum permissible body burden for each specific contaminant.

### Monitoring

A complete blood count with differential, blood urea nitrogen, serum electrolytes, and urinalysis, as well as blood and urine radioassays should be obtained before initiating treatment. Daily zinc, manganese, and magnesium monitoring should be performed. During treatment, repeated blood, urine, and fecal radioassays should be used to monitor elimination. Zinc supplementation is recommended during therapy. A standard oral multivitamin that contains zinc is considered sufficient.

### Patients with Chronic Kidney Disease

No dose adjustment is needed for patients with chronic kidney disease.

## PREGNANCY AND LACTATION

Calcium-DTPA is listed as US FDA Pregnancy Category C based on animal data. Zinc-DTPA is listed as US FDA Pregnancy Category B, also based on animal data. There are no human pregnancy outcome data from which to draw conclusions regarding the risk of DTPA. Contaminated pregnant women should begin any treatment with Zn-DTPA as opposed to Ca-DTPA because of perceived risks of the latter chelator for adverse reproductive outcome. However, in pregnant women with severe internal contamination in which the risk to the mother and fetus is considered to be high, that is, greater than an expected dose of 200 mSv, it would be reasonable to give Ca-DTPA for a first dose in conjunction with mineral supplements that contain zinc. These chelators do not cross the placental barrier.

There are no studies regarding DTPA excretion in breast milk. However, radiocontaminants are excreted in breast milk. Thus, women with known or suspected contamination should not breastfeed until contamination risk is reduced. Likewise, there are no data regarding safety in lactating women, and data regarding the use in children are extrapolated.

## FORMULATION AND ACQUISITION

DTPA is available as Ca-DTPA or Zn-DTPA as a sterile solution in 5-mL ampules containing 200 mg/mL (1 g per ampule) for IV use. It should be stored in a cool, dry place with an ambient temperature of between 59°F (15°C) and 86°F (30°C) away from sunlight. Several manufacturers formulate DTPA for IV administration. Both chelators are maintained in the US Strategic National Stockpile.

# 101 HAZARDOUS MATERIALS INCIDENT RESPONSE

This chapter focuses on the identification, management, and response to hazardous materials incidents. According to the United States (US) Department of Transportation, a hazardous material is any item or agent that has the potential to cause harm to humans, animals, or the environment, either by itself or through interaction with other agents. These can be chemical, radiologic, or biological. A hazmat incident is the result of an unplanned or uncontrolled release of or exposure to a hazardous material. Although there are no specific requirements for an event to be considered a hazardous materials incident, typically, there must be the potential for many people or a large area to be affected.

Each incident and the associated response are unique. Emergency managers and healthcare professionals must consider all possibilities and adjust the incident response based on the specific xenobiotics involved, the route of the exposure, and other variables (eg, time, location, and weather conditions). This chapter discusses the basic principles used for a confined and quickly identifiable hazardous materials incident.

In general, a hazardous materials incident response focuses on the care of patients exposed to xenobiotics in the prehospital setting, prepares for multiple casualties, and emphasizes patient decontamination while at the same time trying to prevent exposure and contamination of first responders and healthcare professionals.

## DISASTER MANAGEMENT AND RESPONSE

Local resources and agencies such as police, fire, and emergency medical services (EMS) provide initial disaster management preparedness and response. If necessary, local agencies can escalate response to the county, state, or federal level. The US Federal Emergency Management Agency (FEMA) within the US Department of Homeland Security is the lead federal agency for emergency management in the US.

According to FEMA, disaster management contains four phases: (1) mitigation, (2) preparedness, (3) response, and (4) recovery. Mitigation measures are plans and efforts that attempt to prevent and reduce or eliminate the effects of a potential hazard from becoming a disaster. Preparedness involves creating action plans to be initiated when a disaster occurs, as well as testing plans with mock exercises and run-throughs. The response phase includes the mobilization of appropriate resources and the coordinated management of the incident. A hazardous materials incident response must include the containment of the xenobiotic followed by neutralization, removal, or both. The recovery phase occurs after the immediate needs and threats to human life are addressed in the response phase and entails the restoration of property, infrastructure, and the environment.

Limiting the loss of life is dependent on all responding agencies and personnel working efficiently and effectively together. The coordination of federal, state, and local governments is mandated by the National Incident Management System (NIMS), which uses a systematic approach designed to allow agencies to work together and manage incident response. The National Incident Management System provides for an incident command system (ICS) to be used during a disaster response. The ICS is a standardized, on-scene, all-hazards approach to incident management. The goal of the ICS is to enable a coordinated response among agencies and jurisdictions. It provides a common organizational structure and integrates equipment personnel, facilities, procedures, and communication. During a response, an incident commander (IC) is responsible for managing the incident, establishing objectives, and implementing tactics. Four subsections report to the IC: operations, planning, logistics, and finance and administration. The planning section supports the incident action planning process, collects and analyzes information, and tracks resources. The logistics section arranges for resources and services, and the finance and administration section monitors costs related to the incident.

Medical professionals are a necessary part of all hazardous materials incident responses because patient assessment and treatment are typically the highest priority. Unsolicited medical personnel at the scene of a hazardous materials incident, although well intentioned, may actually harm the coordinated response and interfere with operational efforts. The plan for mobilization, management, and use of volunteer medical personnel at the scene of a disaster should be created in advance, especially for events that might reasonably be expected to require resources. Disaster plans incorporate the use of local medical assets such as hospitals and clinics. Therefore, communities are best served if medical providers respond to their respective institutions during an incident.

## RESPONSE COMPONENTS

After the identification of a release of a hazardous material, there must be a notification to emergency response personnel. Typically, an individual activates the emergency response system by calling 9-1-1. Initially, first responders are often not aware that an incident involves hazardous materials. For instance, a responder to an unconscious patient may be unaware that the cause of the medical emergency was a chemical exposure. First responders must consider that every incident may have a hazardous materials etiology.

Extensive knowledge, training, and judgment are requirements for all emergency personnel, especially those responding to a hazardous material incident. They must follow basic response paradigms. Personnel should approach the scene from uphill and upwind if possible. Personnel should not immediately rush to the scene because the rescuer may become an additional victim. Establishment of a perimeter is essential to scene security to prevent uncontaminated individuals from becoming exposed. First responders and prehospital personnel must also consider other aspects of incident response, including the need for escalation to other emergency response agencies, weather and wind conditions, terrain, confinement of the release, intentionality, and the need for rapid rescue and evacuation of casualties.

## Identification of Hazardous Materials

Identification of the specific xenobiotic(s) involved is of the highest priority because many of the response components depend on the properties and potential health effects of the xenobiotic itself. This information can be gleaned from placards, container labels, shipping documents, material safety data sheets (MSDSs), detector devices, personnel at the scene, patients' signs and symptoms, and odors at the scene (eg, the rotten egg smell of hydrogen sulfide). In the US, first responders are required to be familiar with the use of the *Emergency Response Guidebook*, which is an aid for quickly identifying the hazards of the material(s) involved in a transportation incident.

Hazardous materials may be classified as radioactive, flammable, explosive, asphyxiating, pathogenic, and biohazardous. Although most hazardous materials incidents involve only one hazardous material, more than one xenobiotic may be encountered at an incident. For consequential hazardous materials, the vast majority are caused by gases, vapors, or aerosols. Inhalation is the most common route of exposure at hazardous materials incidents.

Because the number of hazardous materials is large, it is efficient to group hazardous materials according to their toxicologic characteristics. The International Hazard Classification System (IHCS) is the most commonly used system (Table 101–1).

**TABLE 101–1 International Hazard Classification System**

| |
|---|
| ***Class 1: Explosives*** |
| Division 1.1: Mass explosion hazard |
| Division 1.2: Projection hazard |
| Division 1.3: Predominantly a fire hazard |
| Division 1.4: No significant blast hazard |
| Division 1.5: Very insensitive explosives |
| Division 1.6: Extremely insensitive detonating articles |
| ***Class 2: Gases*** |
| Division 2.1: Flammable gases |
| Division 2.2: Nonflammable compressed gases |
| Division 2.3: Poisonous gases |
| Division 2.4: Corrosive gases (Canada) |
| ***Class 3: Flammable or Combustible Liquids*** |
| ***Class 4: Flammable Solids*** |
| Division 4.1: Flammable solid |
| Division 4.2: Spontaneously combustible materials |
| Division 4.3: Dangerous when wet materials |
| ***Class 5: Oxidizers and Organic Peroxides*** |
| Division 5.1: Oxidizers |
| Division 5.2: Organic peroxides |
| ***Class 6: Poisonous Materials and Infectious Substances*** |
| Division 6.1: Poison materials |
| Division 6.2: Infectious substances |
| ***Class 7: Radioactive Substances*** |
| ***Class 8: Corrosive Materials*** |
| ***Class 9: Miscellaneous Hazardous Materials*** |

***Chemical Names and Numbers.*** Chemical compounds may be known by several names, including the chemical, common, generic, or brand (proprietary) name. The Chemical Abstracts Service (CAS) of the American Chemical Society assigns a unique CAS registry number (CAS#) to chemicals in order to overcome the confusion regarding multiple names for a single chemical. Identifying a chemical by name and CAS# is critical because one must be as specific as possible about the hazardous material in question.

CHEMTREC provides essential chemical information and is available at 800-424-9300 or at http://www.chemtrec.org. A regional poison center is also a valuable source of medically relevant information. Other information sources include local and state health departments, the American Conference of Governmental and Industrial Hygienists, the Occupational Safety and Health Administration (OSHA), the National Institutes of Occupational Safety and Health (NIOSH), the Agency for Toxic Substances and Disease Registry, and the Centers for Disease Control and Prevention.

***Vehicular Placarding: United Nations Numbers, North American Numbers, and Product Identification Numbers.*** Xenobiotics in each hazard class of the IHCS (Table 101–1) are assigned four-digit identification numbers, which are known as United Nations, North American, or Product Identification Numbers, and are displayed on characteristic vehicular placards. This system is used by the US Department of Transportation in the *Emergency Response Guidebook*. Unfortunately, this system provides very little guidance in treating poisonings caused by hazardous materials.

***National Fire Protection Association 704 System for Fixed Facility Placarding.*** Fixed facilities, such as hospitals and laboratories, use a placarding system that is different from the vehicular placarding system. The National Fire Protection Association (NFPA) 704 system is used at most fixed facilities. The NFPA system uses a diamond-shaped sign that is divided into four color-coded quadrants: red, yellow, white, and blue. The red quadrant on top indicates flammability; the blue quadrant on the left indicates health hazard; the yellow quadrant on the right indicates reactivity; and the white quadrant on the bottom is for other information, such as OXY for an oxidizing product, W for a xenobiotic that has unusual reactivity with water, and the standard radioactive symbol for radioactive substances. Numbers in the red, blue, and yellow quadrants indicate the degree of hazard: numbers range from 0, which is minimal, to 4, which is severe, and indicate specific levels of hazard. Similar to all placarding systems, this one also has limitations. It does not name the specific hazardous substances in the facility and gives no information about the quantities or locations of the materials.

***United Nations.*** Recognizing that the transport of chemicals often occurs across international boundaries, the United Nations developed a chemical classification system in an attempt to harmonize an approach to classification and labeling. The Globally Harmonized System of Classification and Labelling of Chemicals classifies substances and mixtures by their health, environmental, and physical hazards.

## Exposure and Contamination

*Primary contamination* is contamination of people or equipment caused by direct contact with the initial release of a hazardous material by direct contact at its source of release. Primary contamination occurs whether the hazardous material is a solid, a liquid, or a gas. *Secondary contamination* is contamination of healthcare personnel or equipment caused by direct contact with a patient or equipment covered with adherent solids or liquids removed from the source of the hazardous material spill. For instance, if a patient arrives at a healthcare facility and is not decontaminated, the hospital and healthcare providers are at risk for secondary contamination.

Secondary contamination generally occurs only with solids or liquids, but as noted later, some "gaseous" xenobiotics are actually suspended liquids or solids. Aerosols are airborne xenobiotics, not gases. Aerosols are suspensions of solids or liquids in air, such as solid dusts or liquid mists, that can cover victims with these adherent solids or liquids, which cause secondary contamination.

## Hazardous Materials Site Operations

Limiting dispersion of the hazardous material is critical to prevent further consequences. The physical state of a material determines how it will spread through the environment and gives clues to the potential route(s) of exposure. Unless moved by physical means such as wind, ventilation systems, or people, solids usually stay in one area. Solids can cause exposures by inhalation of dusts, by ingestion, or rarely by absorption through skin and mucous membranes. A vapor is defined as a gaseous dispersion of the molecules of a substance that is normally a liquid or a solid at standard temperature and pressure. Uncontained liquids will spread over surfaces and flow downhill. Liquids that evaporate create a vapor hazard.

**TABLE 101–2 Nomenclatures of the Hazardous Materials Control Zones**

| *Temperature Terminology System*[a] | *Color Terminology System* | *Explanatory Terminology System* |
|---|---|---|
| Hot zone | Red zone | Exclusion or restricted zone |
| Warm zone | Yellow zone | Decontamination or contamination reduction zone |
| Cold zone | Green zone | Support zone |

[a]Data from the National Institutes of Occupational Safety and Health and the Environmental Protection Agency.

The vapor pressure (VP) is useful to estimate whether enough of a solid or liquid will be released in the gaseous state to pose an inhalation risk. The lower the VP, the less likely the xenobiotics will volatilize and generate a respirable gas. Standard references (eg, *NIOSH Pocket Guide to Chemical Hazards and the Merck Index*) list VPs for commonly encountered chemicals.

## Hazardous Materials Scene Control Zones

Scene management is a fundamental feature of hazardous materials incident response. Three control zones are established around a scene and are described by "temperature," "color," or "explanatory terminology" (Table 101–2 and Fig. 101–1).

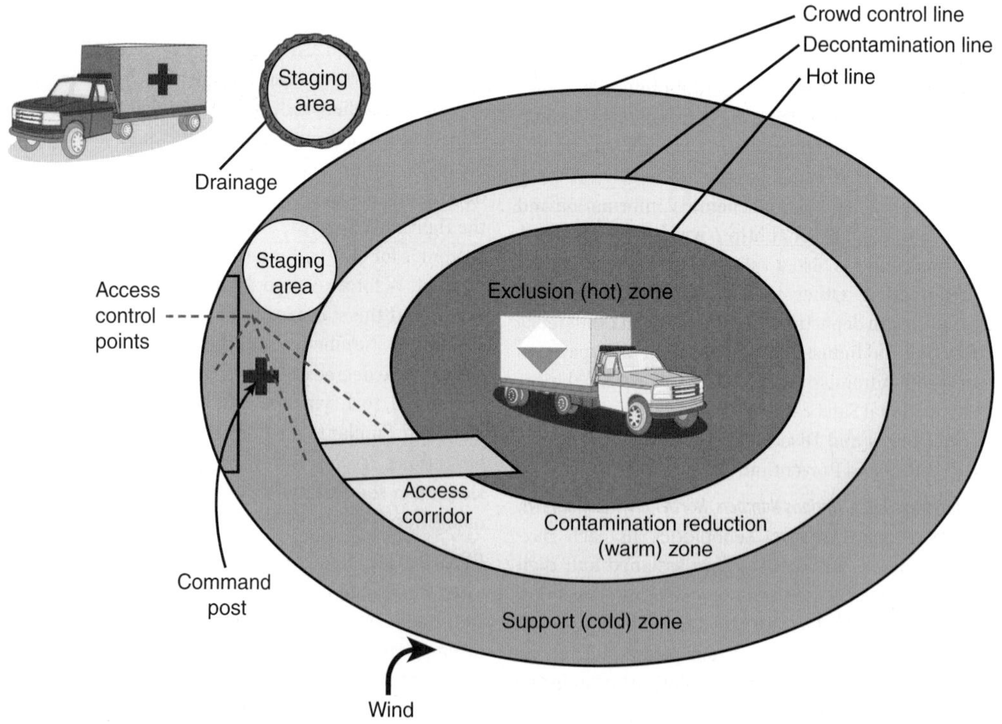


**FIGURE 101–1.** National Institutes of Occupational Safety and Health/Occupational Safety and Health Administration recommended hazardous materials control zones.

**TABLE 101–3 Personal Protective Equipment**

| | Protects Skin and Eyes From | | | Protects Respiratory System From | |
|---|---|---|---|---|---|
| Level[a] | Select Vapors and Aerosols | Gases, Vapors, and Aerosols | Oxygen-Deficient Atmospheres | Liquids and Solids | Gases and Vapors |
| D | | | | | |
| C | + | | | + | |
| B | + | | + | + | + |
| A | + | + | + | + | + |

[a]Level A is a self-contained breathing apparatus (SCBA) worn under a vapor-protective, fully encapsulated, airtight, chemical-resistant suit. Level B is a positive-pressure supplied-air respirator with an escape SCBA worn under a hooded, splash-protective, chemical-resistant suit. Level C is an air-purifying respirator worn with a hooded, splash-protective, chemical-resistant suit. Level D is regular work clothing (offers no protection).

## Personal Protective Equipment

A critical goal of hazardous materials emergency responders is protecting themselves and the public. Safeguarding hazardous materials responders includes wearing appropriate PPE to prevent exposure to the hazard and prevent injury to the wearer from incorrect use of or malfunction of the PPE equipment. Donning PPE poses significant health hazards for the provider, including loss of cooling by evaporation, heat stress, physical stress, psychological stress, impaired vision, impaired mobility, and impaired communication. Because of these risks, individuals involved in hazardous materials emergency response must be properly trained regarding the appropriate use, decontamination, maintenance, and storage of PPE.

***Levels of Protection.*** The US EPA defines four levels of protection for PPE: levels A (greatest protection) through D (least protection) (Table 101–3). *Level A* provides the highest level of protection and is airtight and fully encapsulating. A breathing apparatus must be worn under the suit. *Level B* uses chemical-resistant clothing. *Level C* protection should be used when the type of airborne xenobiotic is known, its concentration can be measured, the criteria for using air-purifying respirators (APRs) are met, and skin and eye exposures are unlikely. *Level D* is basically a regular work uniform.

***Personal Protective Equipment Respiratory Protection.*** Level A PPE mandates the use of a self-contained breathing apparatus (SCBA) composed of a face piece connected by a hose to a compressed air source. Disadvantages of the SCBA include its bulkiness and heaviness and a limited time period of respiratory protection because of the limited amount of air in the tank. A supplied-air respirator (SAR) may be used in level B PPE and differs from SCBA in that air is supplied through a line that is connected to a source located away from the contaminated area (Fig. 101–2). One major advantage of SARs over SCBA is that they allow an individual to work for a longer period. However, a hazardous materials worker must stay connected to the SAR and cannot leave the contaminated area by a different exit. An APR may be used in level C PPE

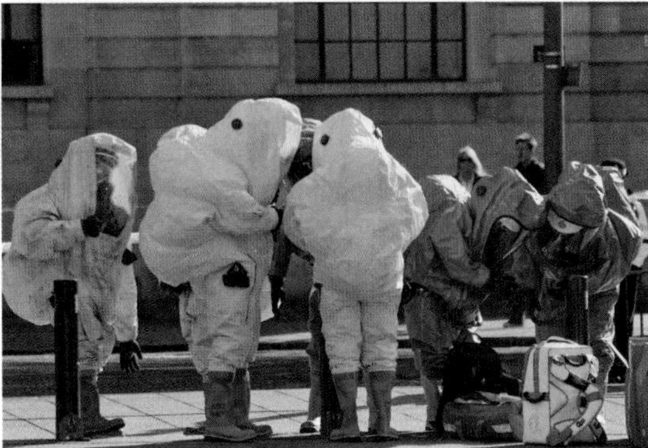

**FIGURE 101–2.** Individuals wearing level A PPE. *(Used with permission from Chris McLoughlin/Alamy Stock Photo.)*

and allows breathing of ambient air after inhalation through a specific purifying canister or filter. Powered devices reduce the work of breathing, which can significantly limit an individual's performance while wearing PPE.

### Decontamination

One of the most important and essential aspects of hazardous materials response is decontamination of patients. Not only does decontamination reduce the health consequences for the patient (by reducing absorption or exposure time), but it also prevents secondary contamination. Decontamination of equipment, the environment, and the entire area (ie, hot zone) is necessary but is secondary in priority to the decontamination of victims.

An estimated 75% to 90% of contaminants can be removed simply by removing clothing and garments. Subsequent decontamination is most commonly accomplished by using water to copiously irrigate the skin of a patient, thereby physically washing off, diluting, or hydrolyzing the xenobiotic. All exposed skin, including the skin folds, axillae, genital area, and feet, should be decontaminated. Lukewarm water should be used with gentle water pressure to reduce the risk of hypothermia. Water should be applied systematically from head to toe while the airway is protected if necessary. Exposed, symptomatic eyes should be continuously irrigated with water throughout the patient contact, including transport, if possible. Remember to check for and remove contact lenses.

Providers should use care with chemical contaminants because some solid contaminants react with water and create an increased hazard. Some xenobiotics are better removed mechanically by physically wiping them from the skin while avoiding smearing the xenobiotic or abrading the skin. Some contaminants may be chemically "inactivated" by applying another chemical, such as a 0.5% hypochlorite solution (see extensive discussion in Special Considerations: SC1).

***Scene Triage.*** Victim decontamination and movement from a scene require an organized methodology for categorization of medical severity. The most common triage method used is the Simple Triage and Rapid Treatment (START) system, although many others exist. This system follows a simple algorithm that allows for a color categorization based upon respiration, perfusion, and mental status: immediate (red), delayed (yellow), walking wounded or minor (green), and deceased or expectant (black). Victims may be initially triaged in the contaminated zone and then retriaged after decontamination.

## HAZARDOUS MATERIALS INCIDENT RESPONSE RULES AND STANDARDS

Occupational Safety and Health Administration and the NFPA have developed rules and guidelines, respectively, regarding hazardous materials incident response. Occupational Safety and Health Administration rules are mandated as law and must be followed. Meeting NFPA guidelines will ensure OSHA compliance. The Superfund Amendments and Reauthorization Act of 1986 (SARA) required OSHA to develop and implement standards to protect employees responding to hazardous materials emergencies. This resulted in the *Hazardous Waste Operations and Emergency Response* standard, 29 CFR 1910.120, or HAZWOPER. NFPA 471, *Recommended Practice for Responding to Hazardous Materials Incidents*, outlines the following tactical objectives: incident response planning, communication procedures, response levels, site safety, control zones, PPE, incident mitigation, decontamination, and medical monitoring. NFPA 472, *Standard on Professional Competence of Responders to Hazardous Materials Incidents*, helps define the minimum skills, knowledge, and standards for training outlined in HAZWOPER for three types of responders.

### Prehospital Hazardous Materials Emergency Response Team Composition, Organization, and Responsibilities

***First Responder at the Awareness Level.*** First responders at the awareness level are expected to recognize the presence of hazardous materials, protect themselves, secure the area, and call for better-trained personnel. They must take a safe position and keep other people from entering the area.

***First Responder at the Operational Level.*** These individuals are additionally trained to protect nearby persons, the environment, and exposed property from the effects of hazardous materials releases. They are expected to assume a defensive posture, control the release from a safe distance, and keep the hazardous material from spreading. Operational level individuals are trained on the following aspects of material containment: absorption of liquids, containment of the spill, vapor suppression, and vapor dispersion. They do not operate within the hot zone.

***Hazardous Materials Technician.*** Hazardous materials technicians are trained in the use of chemical-resistant suits, air-monitoring equipment, mitigation techniques, and the interpretation of physical properties of hazardous materials. Technicians are capable of containing an incident, making safe entry into a hazardous environment, determining the appropriate course of action, victim rescue, and cleaning up or neutralizing the incident to return property to a safe and usable status, if possible. These individuals are trained to operate within the hot zone to mitigate the incident.

### Advanced Hazardous Materials Components

***Advanced Hazardous Materials Providers.*** Paramedics are trained in the recognition of signs and symptoms caused by exposure to hazardous materials and the delivery of antidotal therapy to victims of hazardous materials poisonings. Ideally, entry into hazardous atmospheres should not be performed until appropriately trained paramedics are on the scene with resuscitative equipment in place, including a drug box containing essential antidotes for specific hazardous materials.

***Patient Care Responsibilities of the Prehospital Decontamination Team and the Hazardous Materials Entry Team.*** Hazardous material incident responders should identify the entry and exit areas by controlling points for the access corridor (decontamination corridor) from the hot zone, through the warm zone, to the cold zone (Fig. 101–1). This corridor should be upwind, uphill, and upstream from the hot zone, if possible. Hazardous materials technician entry team members should remove victims from the contaminated hot zone and deliver patients to the inner control point of the access (decontamination) corridor. Hazardous materials decontamination team members decontaminate patients in the decontamination (access) corridor of the contamination reduction (warm zone).

The primary responsibility of the prehospital hazardous materials sector is the protection of the hazardous materials entry team personnel. In some systems, the hazardous materials entry team may include specialized providers who have the ability to provide lifesaving patient care within the hot zone. The ability to perform triage or cardiopulmonary resuscitation or to provide any medical care is greatly limited by the PPE being worn. Therefore, only immediately lifesaving procedures should be considered, such as intubation or antidote administration.

***Patient Care Responsibilities of Emergency Medical Services Providers at Hazardous Materials Incidents.*** Emergency medical services providers who are not part of the hazardous materials team should report to the incident staging area and await direction from the IC. They should approach the site from upwind, uphill, and upstream, if possible. Emergency medical services providers should remain in the cold zone until properly protected hazardous materials incident responders arrive, decontaminate, and deliver patients to them for further triage and treatment. Ideally, EMS response for an event will involve direct communication with the EMS medical director or medical control; this physician will assist with coordination of appropriate care with the hospital, regional poison centers, and toxicologists.

Patients with skin contamination should not be transported from the hazardous materials site without being properly decontaminated. Before transportation, EMS should notify the receiving hospital of the number of victims being transported and their toxicologic history, patient assessments, and treatment rendered.

***Hospital Responsibilities for Hazardous Materials Victims.*** Ideally, local or regional emergency department (ED) physicians and personnel will receive prompt advanced notification about a hazardous materials incident before any victims arrive at the hospital. The notification should include, if known, information regarding the event, hazardous materials involved, number and condition of casualties to be transported to the hospital, and estimated time of arrival, as well as information regarding the decontamination completed. The mnemonic ETHANE (exact location; type of incident; hazards, access route; numbers of casualties; emergency services on site) is one way to remember these required elements. Assistance of a poison control center and a medical toxicologist is generally recommended.

Victims may leave an incident scene and subsequently present to a hospital. The hospital must have a preestablished protocol by which hospital response teams will decontaminate patients who arrive at the hospital if not previously decontaminated or if field decontamination is believed to be insufficient. Patients who require skin decontamination should be denied entry to the ED until they are decontaminated by an appropriately trained and equipped hazardous materials response team. Treatment should not be initiated until the patient is in the cold zone.

Special Considerations

# SC10 ASSESSMENT OF ETHANOL-INDUCED IMPAIRMENT

## INTRODUCTION

This discussion describes the history and use of assessments of ethanol-induced impairment, primarily in a legal context. Throughout this chapter, the terms *ethanol* and *alcohol* are used interchangeably and words such as *drunk* and *punishable* are used to preserve the specific language from early studies and legal writings.

## HISTORY

Although the intoxicating effects of ethanol have been known for centuries, the advent of mechanized transportation spawned increased public and legal scrutiny. Although railroads had regulations against the operation of equipment while intoxicated dating back to at least the 1850s, the first arrest for drunk driving in an automobile was a London taxicab driver in 1897. In 1910, New York was the first state in the United States (US) to enact a "drunken driving" law.

Prior to the landmark work by Widmark in Sweden and by Heise in the US, evaluations of driver impairment were predominantly based on the "expert" testimony of an evaluating physician and the arresting police officer, as well as behaviors reported by witnesses. The development of analytical technology capable of measuring the concentration of alcohol in blood gave rise to the idea that diagnosis of intoxication might be assisted by an objective chemical test result. The greater the blood alcohol concentration (BAC), the more drinks the individual must have consumed and, therefore, the greater the degree of impairment. Although the assignment of a specific clinical effect to a given BAC is not rigorously applicable to evaluation of an individual case, the general trends when examined across a population formed the foundation of many modern driving while intoxicated (DWI) laws. Despite centuries' worth of knowledge of the effects of alcohol and decades of efforts to articulate drunk driving standards, a single universal definition of "alcohol intoxication" does not exist.

## *PER SE* LIMITS

The first US states to incorporate BAC into drunk-driving statutes were Indiana and Maine, which did so in 1939. The approach taken by the Indiana legislature resulted in a three-tiered statute, which stated that a BAC of less than 50 mg/dL (10.9 mmol/L) was considered presumptive evidence of no intoxication, a BAC between 50 and 100 mg/dL was considered supportive evidence of intoxicated driving, and a BAC of greater than 150 mg/dL (32.6 mmol/L) was considered *prima facie* (ie, obvious and evident without proof) evidence of guilt. From a legal perspective, *prima facie* evidence shifts the burden of proof from the accuser having to substantiate the charge to the defense to rebut the allegation. It is this legal perspective from which the so-called *per se* standards are derived—that is, an individual whose BAC exceeds a predetermined concentration is deemed guilty of driving while impaired by alcohol, even without any other evidence of intoxication or impairment.

However, by 1960, as data regarding alcohol-related motor vehicle crashes became available, most states adopted a more rigorous *per se* BAC driving standard of 100 mg/dL (21.7 mmol/L). Epidemiologic assessments demonstrate that the probability of causing an alcohol-related motor vehicle crash increases slightly at a breath alcohol concentration (BrAC) of 50 mg/dL. The risk of causing a crash is increased by roughly 4-fold at a BrAC of 80 mg/dL, 7-fold at a BrAC of 100 mg/dL, and 25-fold at a BrAC of 150 mg/dL. In 1994, all states in the US lowered the BAC used to define *per se* intoxicated driving to 80 mg/dL (17.4 mmol/L). Lower *per se* BACs are applied to interstate commercial drivers (40 mg/dL) (8.7 mmol/L) and pilots of aircraft (40 mg/dL, with no alcohol consumed within 8 hours prior to acting as pilot in command), as well as minors (10–20 mg/dL, depending on the state, and 20–50 mg/dL (5.4-10.9 mmol/L) in some European countries).

Laws addressing *per se* driving under the influence (DUI) limits are based on ethanol concentrations measured in whole blood. BrAC limits (which are arithmetically linked to BAC) are also frequently specified in *per se* statutes. It is, however, imperative to understand that *per se* BACs do *not* define drunkenness or alcohol intoxication in nondriving situations, and their use in circumstances not involving motor vehicle operation is generally inappropriate.

The legal significance of a *per se* limit is that there is no requirement for behavioral evidence of intoxication, as long as the measured BAC exceeds that established by the legislature.

## ANALYTICAL CONSIDERATIONS

Accurate measurement of ethanol concentration in various biological matrices can be done using a number of analytical techniques. Enzymatic ethanol assays based on alcohol dehydrogenase (ADH) are commonly used, especially in high-throughput laboratories. The greater selectivity for ethanol of gas chromatographic (GC) methods makes these techniques the mainstay for quantitative analysis in most forensic laboratories. As ethanol distributes based on total body water, the water content of the matrix will affect the amount of ethanol present in a given volume or mass of biological sample. A common circumstance in which this is observed is in the difference between a whole blood ethanol determination and a plasma or serum ethanol determination. The water content of serum and plasma is 10% to 12% higher than whole blood, meaning that serum or plasma ethanol concentrations will be correspondingly higher than whole blood concentrations. Clinical laboratories most often use serum and plasma for analysis, whereas *per se* driving under the influence (DUI) statutes are written in terms of whole blood. Therefore, if a comparison is to be made between a serum or plasma analytical result and a legal standard, the result must be converted to an approximated whole blood ethanol concentration. Typically, a ratio of 1.16 is used for this conversion, and no significant difference appears to exist between the serum-to-whole blood and plasma-to-whole blood ratios.

Breath testing is commonly performed to assess BAC because of its relative simplicity and less invasive collection compared to urine or blood. The analytical basis for sampling exhaled breath is that, at equilibrium, alcohol in expired air is present at a predictable ratio with blood. In the US, a blood-to-breath alcohol ratio of 2,100:1 is commonly used in the calibration of breath alcohol testing devices, although experimental evidence suggests that the actual ratio is closer to 2,300:1. As such, a systematic underestimation of BAC is expected when breath alcohol results are converted to whole blood alcohol results. Several studies document this underestimation with data from suspected impaired drivers and evidential breath alcohol testing instruments. In 1983, Britain adopted a legal limit in breath of 35 μg/100 mL, which corresponds to a blood alcohol of 80 mg/dL, using a 2,300:1 blood-to-breath ratio. Legal statutes that include in their offense definition breath alcohol results expressed in units of grams/210 L of exhaled air eliminate the need to convert breath alcohol to blood alcohol, largely mitigating arguments based on the breath-to-blood ratio.

## BREATH-TESTING DEVICES

Breath-testing instruments are generally divided into four broad categories: passive alcohol sensors (PASs), screening devices (preliminary breath testers {PBTs}), breath alcohol ignition interlock devices (BAIIDs), and evidential breath testers (EBTs).

A PAS device may be concealed in a device such as a modified police flashlight and is used to detect alcohol on or in the immediate vicinity of a subject through passive means (ie, with no requirement for subject cooperation). Breath alcohol ignition interlock devices are used to prevent drinking and driving by requiring the driver to blow into a sensor in order to start the ignition of the vehicle. The PBT and EBT devices are the most common breath alcohol–testing devices encountered in cases of DUI arrest. In this setting, PBT results are used in conjunction with observation and field sobriety tests to establish probable cause for DUI arrest. In contrast to PBT results, measurements from an EBT device are admissible in court and administrative proceedings and can be used as the basis for establishment of *per se* DUI cases without the necessity of blood collection and analysis. Although mobile EBT devices are available, most often the EBT is maintained in a fixed location such as a police station. Required procedures for the use of EBT devices exist for the subject as well as the instrument. The subject must have a period of alcohol deprivation of at least 15 to 20 minutes during which trained personnel observe him or her to ensure not only that no additional ethanol is consumed but also that no regurgitation, emesis, or eructation occurs, which could result in residual ethanol in the mouth prior to breath alcohol analysis.

## STANDARDIZED FIELD SOBRIETY TESTS

A driver whose BAC exceeds the established legal standard is considered *per se* intoxicated and often convicted without behavioral evidence of intoxication. However, some objective findings of impairment assist in establishing probable cause to demand chemical testing, initiate a DUI arrest, or prosecute a charge of impairment, without invoking *per se* limits. In these settings, results of a specific group of behavioral tests are of value in discriminating and prosecuting or refuting an impaired driving charge, although submitting to these behavioral tests is typically voluntary. The three tests comprising the standardized field sobriety tests are the one-leg stand (OLS), walk-and-turn (WAT), and horizontal gaze nystagmus (HGN). Descriptions of these tests are provided in Table SC10–1.

## ESTIMATING THE AMOUNT OF ALCOHOL INGESTED

The kinetic profile of ethanol in the blood has been extensively studied. In general, it is known that when blood ethanol concentration is greater than 20 mg/dL (4.3 mmol/L), it follows a zero-order elimination profile and then converts to first-order elimination when the concentration drops below this threshold. In the zero-order portion of the curve, typical elimination rates range from 10 to 20 mg/dL/h in social drinkers, whereas in chronic users, the rate is higher. The estimation of the

**TABLE SC10–1 Standardized Field Sobriety Tests**

| *Test* | *Test Description* | *Test Scoring ("clues")* |
|---|---|---|
| One-leg stand (OLS) | With the arms at sides, raise one foot at least 6 inches off the ground and stand on the other foot for at least 30 seconds. | 4-point scale<br>1. Putting foot down<br>2. Hopping<br>3. Swaying<br>4. Raising arms<br>Any 2 "clues" is failure. |
| Walk-and-turn (WAT) | Balance with feet heel-to-toe and listen to test instructions.<br>Walk 9 steps heel-to-toe in a straight line, turn 180 degrees, and walk 9 more steps heel-to-toe, while counting steps, watching feet, and keeping hands at sides. | 8-point scale<br>1. Inability to maintain balance in the starting position<br>2. Starting too soon (eg, prior to completion of instructions)<br>3. Stepping off the line<br>4. Not touching toe to heel<br>5. Raising arms<br>6. Improper turn<br>7. Stopping<br>8. Wrong number of steps<br>Any 2 "clues" is failure. |
| Horizontal gaze nystagmus (HGN) | Angle of onset of nystagmus is determined for each eye. | 6-point scale (3 points for each eye)<br>1. Lack of smooth pursuit<br>2. Distinct nystagmus at maximum deviation<br>3. Onset of nystagmus before 45 degrees<br>Cutoff is 4 "clues." |

Reproduced with permission from Rubenzer SJ. The standardized field sobriety tests: a review of scientific and legal issues. *Law Hum Behav.* 2008;32(4):293-313.

number of drinks ingested to achieve a given BAC or back calculation from a current concentration to a previous moment in time has been extensively studied, but the results are too imprecise for and individual legal argument.

Some legal arguments have quite incorrectly suggested that ethanol is odorless. Ethanol has a characteristic pleasant smell, with an odor threshold of approximately 50 ppm. The presence or absence of breath alcohol odor is often used by police officers in the decision to proceed further with sobriety testing. In one study, 20 experienced police officers assessed alcohol odor on 14 subjects with BACs ranging from 0 to 130 mg/dL (28.2 mmol/L) after drinking beer, wine, bourbon, or vodka. Assessments were initiated 30 minutes after cessation of drinking. The strength of breath alcohol odor was determined to be an unreliable indicator of BAC. Correct detection of the presence of alcohol was 85% for BACs at or above 80 mg/dL but declined with decreasing BAC or the presence of food.

## DRAM SHOP

Liquor liability or "dram shop" laws hold the server of alcoholic beverages liable for damages or injuries caused by an individual who was provided alcohol when such service should have been refused. In the 19th century, laws were enacted to punish tavern owners who contributed to the downfall of patrons. By contrast, current application of the laws is typically as a means to compensate innocent victims injured by an intoxicated patron. This action on behalf of the innocent victim is why liquor liability law is sometimes referred to as "third party" liability.

Direct comparison of the efficacy of dram shop liability laws between states is difficult as liability laws and insurance vary widely. One study concluded that dram shop liability and responsible beverage service (RBS) laws were associated with significant reduction in *per capita* beer consumption and fatal crash ratios in drivers under age 21.

## INTOXICATION AND ESTIMATION OF BLOOD ALCOHOL CONCENTRATION

The ability of an individual to accurately estimate his or her own BAC is poor. Drivers who underestimate their own BAC are more impulsive and riskier drivers than those who overestimate their BAC. A lack of accuracy in estimating BAC is also observed in trained medical providers and police officers. A large confounding factor in these observations is tolerance. Greater tolerance, as occurs in people with alcohol use disorder, imparts greater difficulty in detecting the clinical effects associated with a given alcohol concentration. However, tolerance has no bearing on the potential prosecution of a DUI case on a *per se* BAC or BrAC basis.

The central nervous system effects of alcohol intoxication are typically more pronounced on the ascending portion of the blood alcohol kinetic curve than on the descending side due to the development of acute tolerance. In other words, the clinical effect of intoxication is greater during the absorptive arm of the kinetic curve than on the elimination arm, even though the same blood alcohol concentration is measured in both kinetic phases. This principle is known as acute tolerance, or the Mellanby effect.

Multiple studies have examined the likelihood of alcohol sales to obviously intoxicated individuals (typically, paid professional actors pretending to be drunk) by various commercial entities for consumption on-premise (bars, restaurants, outdoor events like festivals) and off-premise (liquor stores, grocery stores, and convenience stores). The results are fairly uniform in that the majority of the time the alcohol was sold or served to the "intoxicated" individual. Additionally, it was noted that male servers/clerks who appeared younger than age 31 were reportedly more likely to make such sales and the sales were more likely to occur in off-premise establishments.

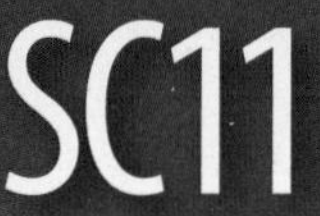

Special Considerations

# SC11 ORGAN PROCUREMENT FROM POISONED PATIENTS

Xenobiotic poisonings can cause brain death. However, with supportive care, poisoned patients may be suitable candidates for organ donation depending on the xenobiotic and the target organ involved. Early identification of donors is critical as the viability of transplantable tissue diminishes as duration of brain death progresses and may be further complicated by the presence of xenobiotics that mimic brain death (Table SC11–1).

Published brain death protocols require exclusion of poisoning, but obtaining and interpreting xenobiotic concentrations is complex and, in many circumstances, not feasible in a clinically meaningful timeframe. Although other methods of establishing brain death such as cerebral blood flow are utilized, the effects of xenobiotics on these studies are not well described. Once brain death is established, organ procurement personnel assist in obtaining familial consent, deciding which organs are most suitable for transplant, and maximizing physiological support and perfusion until organ procurement occurs. Successful transplantation of organs is reported from poisoned donors associated with a variety of xenobiotics (Tables SC11–2 and SC11–3).

The 1-year survival in recipients from poisoned donors approximates that from nonpoisoned donors and was reported as 75% in one series. Additionally, in most transplant failures from poisoned donors, the causes are rejection, sepsis, or technical reasons, not the initial xenobiotic.

Waitlists for organs are far greater than the number of available organs. Finding consensus on the ethics of procuring organs from poisoning fatalities is challenging. Patients who suffer brain death from poisoning are potentially suitable donors, and exclusion of this population for organ procurement should not be defined or limited by the xenobiotic.

**TABLE SC11–2 Organs Transplanted After Donor Poisonings**

| *Organ* | *Xenobiotics Identified in Donors* |
|---|---|
| [a]Cornea | Brodifacoum, cyanide |
| Heart | Acetaminophen, β-adrenergic antagonists, alkylphosphate, benzodiazepines, brodifacoum, carbamazepine, carbon monoxide, chlormethiazole, cyanide, digitalis, digoxin, ethanol, glibenclamide, insulin, meprobamate, methanol, propoxyphene, thiocyanate |
| [a]Kidney | Acetaminophen, brodifacoum, carbon monoxide, *Conium maculatum*, cyanide, ethylene glycol, insulin, malathion, methanol, cyclic antidepressants |
| Liver | Brodifacoum, carbon monoxide, *Conium maculatum*, cyanide, ethylene glycol, insulin, malathion, methanol, methaqualone, cyclic antidepressants |
| Lung | Brodifacoum, carbon monoxide, methanol |
| Pancreas | Acetaminophen, brodifacoum, carbon monoxide, *Conium maculatum*, cyanide, ethylene glycol, methanol, cyclic antidepressants |
| Skin | Cyanide, methanol |

[a]Can be cadaveric procurement.

**TABLE SC11–1 Xenobiotic Mimics[a] of Clinical Brain Death**

| |
|---|
| Amitriptyline |
| Baclofen |
| Barbiturates |
| Bupropion |
| Lidocaine |
| Phorate |
| Snake envenomation[b] |
| Valproic acid |
| Vecuronium |

[a]Based on reported cases. [b]Case from India, species not identified.

**TABLE SC11–3 Xenobiotic-Related Deaths With Successful Organ Donation**

| | |
|---|---|
| β-Adrenergic antagonists | Ethanol |
| Alkylphosphate | Ethylene glycol |
| Barbiturates | Glibenclamide |
| Benzodiazepines | Ibuprofen |
| Brodifacoum | Insulin |
| Carbamazepine | Malathion |
| Carbon monoxide | Methaqualone |
| Cardioactive steroids | Meprobamate |
| Chlormethiazole | Methanol |
| *Conium maculatum* | Nicotine |
| Cyanide | Opioids |
| Cyclic antidepressants | Propoxyphene |

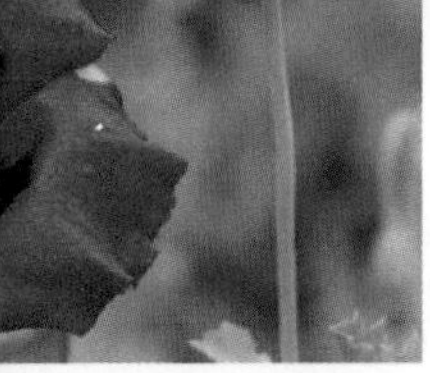

# INDEX

*Note:* Page numbers followed by *f* indicate figures; and page numbers followed by *t* indicate tables.

**M**